NEUROLOGIC REHABILITATION
Neuroscience and Neuroplasticity in Physical Therapy Practice

Second Edition

Edited and Authored by

Deborah S. Nichols-Larsen, PT, PhD, FAPTA
Director and Professor Emeritus
School of Health & Rehabilitation Sciences
The Ohio State University
Columbus, Ohio

Authored by

D. Michele Basso, PT, EdD
Professor
School of Health and Rehabilitation Sciences
The Ohio State University
Columbus, Ohio

John A. Buford, PT, PhD, FAPTA
Professor and Director
Division of Physical Therapy
School of Health & Rehabilitation Sciences
The Ohio State University
Columbus, Ohio

Jill C. Heathcock, MPT, PhD
Professor
Division of Physical Therapy
School of Health & Rehabilitation Sciences
The Ohio State University
Columbus, Ohio

Deborah A. Kegelmeyer, PT, MS, DPT
Board-Certified Clinical Specialist in Geriatric
Physical Therapy
Professor, Clinical Physical Therapy Division
School of Health & Rehabilitation Sciences
The Ohio State University
Columbus, Ohio

Anne D. Kloos, PT, PhD
Board-Certified Clinical Specialist in Neurologic
Physical Therapy
Professor, Clinical Physical Therapy Division
School of Health & Rehabilitation Sciences
The Ohio State University
Columbus, Ohio

New York Chicago San Francisco Athens London Madrid Mexico City
New Delhi Milan Singapore Sydney Toronto

1 2 3 4 5 6 7 8 9   DSS   28 27 26 25 24 23

ISBN 978-1-260-46139-8
MHID 1-260-46139-4

Notice

Medicine is an ever-changing science. As new research and clinical experience broaden our knowledge, changes in treatment and drug therapy are required. The authors and the publisher of this work have checked with sources believed to be reliable in their efforts to provide information that is complete and generally in accord with the standards accepted at the time of publication. However, in view of the possibility of human error or changes in medical sciences, neither the authors nor the publisher nor any other party who has been involved in the preparation or publication of this work warrants that the information contained herein is in every respect accurate or complete, and they disclaim all responsibility for any errors or omissions or for the results obtained from use of the information contained in this work. Readers are encouraged to confirm the information contained herein with other sources. For example and in particular, readers are advised to check the product information sheet included in the package of each drug they plan to administer to be certain that the information contained in this work is accurate and that changes have not been made in the recommended dose or in the contraindications for administration. This recommendation is of particular importance in connection with new or infrequently used drugs.

This book was set in Minion Pro by MPS Limited.
The editors were Michael Weitz and Peter J. Boyle.
The production supervisor was Catherine Saggese.
Project management was provided by Monika Chaudhari, MPS Limited.

Library of Congress Control Number: 2023945576

This book is dedicated to the physical therapy students over the years,
who have challenged us to keep it relevant;
the MS and PhD students, who have challenged us to keep it fresh;
our colleagues, who have helped us think more clearly;
our friends and families, who have allowed us the time and space to write;
and most especially, our patients
who have allowed us to see the miracle of the nervous system in action
as we helped guide their recovery.

Contents

Preface vii

SECTION I
Introduction to the Neuroscience
of Physical Therapy 1

1   **Introduction to Neuroanatomy 3**
    John A. Buford

2   **Neuronal Structure and Function 25**
    John A. Buford and D. Michele Basso

3   **Somatosensory Pathways and Perception 43**
    Deborah S. Nichols-Larsen

4   **Sensorimotor Systems of the Spinal Cord 63**
    D. Michele Basso

5   **Motor Control and the Descending Systems 75**
    John A. Buford

6   **The Special Senses 93**
    Deborah S. Nichols-Larsen and Anne D. Kloos

7   **Cognition, Emotion, and Language 119**
    Deborah S. Nichols-Larsen

8   **Child Development 133**
    Deborah S. Nichols-Larsen

9   **Neuroplasticity 159**
    Deborah S. Nichols-Larsen and D. Michele Basso

SECTION II
Neurologic Conditions – Neuropathology and
Physical Therapy Management 177

10   **Neurologic Exam 179**
     *Deborah A. Kegelmeyer, Jill C. Heathcock, and
     Deborah S. Nichols-Larsen*

11   **Stroke 211**
     *Deborah S. Nichols-Larsen and
     Deborah A. Kegelmeyer*

12   **Brain Injury: Trauma, Anoxia, and Neoplasm 265**
     *Deborah A. Kegelmeyer and
     Deborah S. Nichols-Larsen*

13   **Spinal Cord Injury 303**
     D. Michele Basso

14   **Multiple Sclerosis 361**
     Anne D. Kloos and Deborah A. Kegelmeyer

15   **Basal Ganglia Disorders: Parkinson and
     Huntington's Diseases 393**
     Anne D. Kloos and Deborah A. Kegelmeyer

16   **Motor Neuron Disease and Neuropathies 445**
     *Anne D. Kloos, Deborah A. Kegelmeyer,
     John A. Buford, and Jill C. Heathcock*

17   **Vestibular/Cerebellar Disorders 513**
     Anne D. Kloos

18   **Age-Related Neurologic Changes 557**
     *Deborah A. Kegelmeyer and
     Deborah S. Nichols-Larsen*

19   **Neural Tube Disorders and Hydrocephalus 579**
     Jill C. Heathcock and Deborah S. Nichols-Larsen

20   **Cerebral Palsy 611**
     Jill C. Heathcock and Deborah S. Nichols-Larsen

21   **Developmental Disabilities 641**
     Deborah S. Nichols-Larsen and Jill C. Heathcock

Appendix 667
Adult Outcome Measures by ICF Category and
Diagnostic Group

Index 671

Preface

The practice of neurologic physical therapy relies on the growing body of evidence from the field of neuroscience. This text uniquely brings the fields of neuroscience and neurologic physical therapy practice together in a single volume that explores neurologic pathologies and their management across the lifespan. This field is crucial to our understanding of neurologic function, the effects of neurologic damage, and the plasticity of the nervous system as it responds to growth, development, aging, damage, and activity. Therapists need a strong foundation in neuroscience to maximize their treatment methods and efficacy, so this text includes seven introductory chapters that provide a neuroscience foundation along with an overview of neonatal and child development in Chapter 8, and an introduction to the concepts of neuroplasticity in Chapter 9. Chapter 10 is an overview of the neurologic physical therapy evaluation that affords the foundation for disease-specific assessment, which are incorporated into the remaining eleven chapters. These eleven chapters delineate common neurologic disease and injury processes, the current medical management, and the targeted physical therapy evaluation and treatment for each, examining the emerging evidence of how physical therapy can influence neuroplasticity. Each chapter is anchored by clinical cases, following a patient through the diagnostic process, physical therapy assessment, and potential treatment options across stages of the condition. Cases progress from acute care through inpatient and outpatient rehabilitation for conditions such as stroke or spinal cord injury, from infancy through adolescence for developmental disorders, and from early diagnosis through disease progression for degenerative conditions such as Parkinson disease or multiple sclerosis. In addition, this text includes a lifespan approach, encompassing changes associated with aging (Chapter 18) and three chapters on common pediatric conditions that affect the nervous system (Chapters 19-21), including myelomeningocele, cerebral palsy, intellectual developmental disability, autism spectrum disorder, and others. There are also videos to illustrate many of the conditions discussed, including cerebral palsy, myelomeningocele, spinal cord injury, stroke, and Parkinson Disease, and an accompanying lab manual to facilitate active learning in the laboratory. To view the videos, click on the *Multimedia* tab at the top of the Access Physiotherapy page and then select *Neurologic Rehabilitation Videos*. Ultimately, this text unites the fields of neuroscience, neurologic rehabilitation, and neuroplasticity to guide the physical therapy student into their career as evidence-based practitioners.

INTRODUCTION TO THE NEUROSCIENCE OF PHYSICAL THERAPY

SECTION 1

INTRODUCTION TO THE NEUROSCIENCE OF PHYSICAL THERAPY

Introduction to Neuroanatomy

John A. Buford

1

OBJECTIVES

1) Identify and name the major parts of the central and autonomic nervous systems

2) Use terms for direction in the nervous system, such as rostral, caudal, dorsal, ventral, along with the cardinal plane directions appropriately when referring to the structures in the CNS

3) Identify the lobes of the cerebral hemispheres, including the landmarks that form their boundaries, and list the main functions for each lobe

4) Identify and relate functional areas of the brain to support future discussions of neural activities and pathologic conditions

5) Identify and describe the general functions of selected subcortical nuclei and white matter structures

6) Identify the main parts of the ventricular system

7) Identify the lobes and functional divisions of the cerebellum and provide a general description of their functions

8) Identify the main parts of the brainstem along with selected nuclei and white matter structures for sensorimotor systems

9) Identify the main gray matter and white matter structures in the spinal cord, including the organization of a typical spinal segment

10) Identify and describe the basic structures and functions of the peripheral and autonomic nervous system

● INTRODUCTION TO NEUROANATOMY

The brain is an amazing structure. With levels of organization ranging from the brain to the spinal cord, white matter to gray, axons to synapses, and at countless other levels, understanding neuroanatomy is a prerequisite to understanding brain function. In this chapter, the reader is introduced to the major parts of the nervous system with relevance for the rehabilitation professional. For this purpose, the focus will be on sensory and motor systems. Structures associated with the special senses, learning, memory and cognition, language, and other systems with strong relevance to physical rehabilitation will be addressed in some detail, with additional coverage in later chapters. However, details of systems in neuroscience such as vision, hormonal regulation, and others are not covered in detail here. For a broader coverage of neuroscience across all systems, the reader is referred to *Principles of Neural Science*.

Directions and Planes in the Nervous System

In musculoskeletal anatomy, the cardinal plane directions are anterior–posterior, superior–inferior, and medial–lateral. In the nervous system, we can use these same directions. However, because of the way the nervous system curves around from the front of the skull to the back and then turns to descend into the spinal canal, a directional system relative to the nervous system itself, independent of the **cardinal planes**, is often more useful. Rather than anterior–posterior, it is often more useful to refer to ventral–dorsal directions (Figure 1-1). For the spinal cord in a person standing up, anterior and ventral are equivalent, as are dorsal and posterior. However, in the brain, the top surface of the brain would still be the **dorsal** side, but this would be **superior** in the anatomical planes. Likewise, the lower, undersurface of the brain is **ventral** but also **inferior**. Dorsal and ventral allow for more consistent localization of relevant structures across regions of the nervous system, so this directional system is typically used rather than the cardinal planes. Likewise, the front of the brain right behind the forehead is **anterior**, and the back of the brain, **posterior**. However, the brainstem and spinal cord curve downward as they form and emerge from the foramen magnum, so anterior–posterior no longer describes the direction we would move in going from the brain to the spinal cord. Instead, we use the terms rostral and caudal. **Rostral** means toward the nose, whereas **caudal** means toward the tail (or in the human, toward the coccygeal segments). In this frame of reference, the brain is always rostral to the spinal cord, no matter what posture the person adopts. The relative directional terms dorsal–ventral and rostral–caudal are useful at any stage of embryologic development, and in any vertebrate species, when studying the nervous system.

Gray Matter and White Matter

The first distinction we make in examining tissues in the nervous system is whether we are looking at **gray matter** or **white matter** (Figure 1-2). Gray matter is composed of a variety of structures including: (1) neurons – the active, information-processing cells of the nervous system with both the cell bodies of large projecting neurons and entire smaller interneurons; (2) glial cells – cells that provide immune, metabolic, and structural

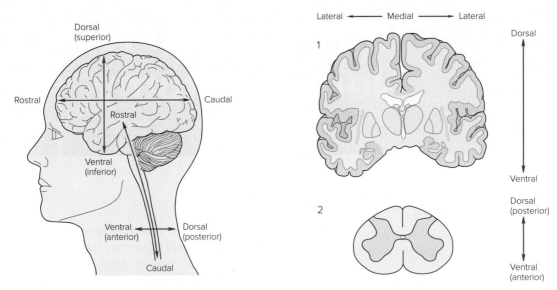

FIGURE 1-1 The directions used in the nervous system. The rostral direction is toward the nose and caudal is toward the tail. Within the head of a person standing, in the cerebrum, rostral and anterior are roughly the same direction, and caudal and posterior are also the same. However, as the brainstem forms and descends toward the spinal cord, the meaning of rostral and caudal shifts. In the brainstem, rostral would be closer to the cerebrum and caudal would be closer to the spinal cord. Within the spinal cord, rostral would be toward the brainstem and caudal would be toward the coccygeal segments. In the person standing, for the spinal cord, rostral and superior are the same, and caudal and inferior are the same. The other directions used in the nervous system are dorsal, toward the back, and ventral, toward the front. The ventral side of the nervous system is the anterior part of the brainstem and spinal cord and the inferior part of the cerebrum. The dorsal part is the superior part of the cerebrum and the posterior part of the brainstem and spinal cord. Medial and lateral directions in the nervous system have the same meaning as in the regular cardinal planes. (Reproduced with permission from Kandel ER, Schwartz JH, Jessell TM, et al. *Principles of Neural Science*, 5th ed. New York, NY: McGraw-Hill; 2013.)

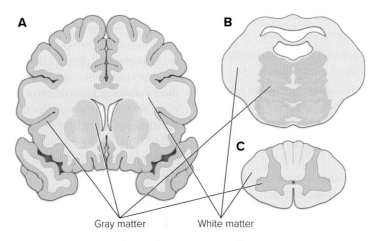

FIGURE 1-2 Brain, brainstem, and spinal cord sections showing gray and white matter. All levels of the central nervous system have a combination of gray matter and white matter. Gray matter is composed of the neurons and the supporting cells, along with the connections between neurons. The gray matter is where the information processing of the brain occurs. White matter is composed of axons carrying information between parts of the nervous system. In the cerebral hemispheres, there is white matter inside forming connections, and gray matter at the surface and in nuclei within the brain. In the brainstem and spinal cord, there is white matter on the outside, and gray matter within. (**B:** Used, with permission, of John A. Buford, PT, PhD. **C:** Reproduced with permission, from Kandel ER, Schwartz JH, Jessell TM, Siegelbaum SA, Hudspeth AJ. *Principles of Neural Science*, 5th ed. New York, NY: McGraw-Hill; 2013.)

support to neurons; (3) axons and their synapses (connections) coming into the gray matter; and (4) the axons leaving the gray matter. White matter, in contrast, is composed of axons and the fatty substance called **myelin** that insulates them, along with the glial cells that produce and sustain the myelin. On the first examination, white matter is relatively uniform in its appearance throughout the nervous system. On closer examination, the physical structure of large groups of axons that might take a straight path versus a curved or crossing path does provide some variation in the gross appearance of certain sections of white matter. Gray matter, in contrast, is quite variable in appearance, just as the sizes and shapes of neurons and the patterns of incoming and outgoing axons are quite variable in the various regions of the nervous system.

Key Terms

Understanding how structures relate to each other and work together for function is the essence of neuroscience, the fascinating field dedicated to understanding the brain. As is often the case in science; however, there is a large amount of nomenclature to be learned before we can develop our understanding. Fortunately, there are some key terms that are used repeatedly in neuroscience, and these are provided in Table 1-1.

TABLE 1-1	Major Structures and Landmarks in the Nervous System, with Emphasis on Function in Sensory and Motor Systems	
STRUCTURE	**FUNCTIONS**	
Meninges	Protect the brain and spinal cord	
Lobes of the Cerebrum		
Frontal	Motor planning and initiation and production of movement, language output, personality, problem-solving, insight, and foresight	
Parietal	Sensory perception and integration, visual location, auditory location, music appreciation	
Occipital	Vision (primary visual cortex and visual association cortex)	
Temporal	Auditory processing, especially language, identification of objects, learning, and memory	
Regions of the Cerebrum		
Insular	Gustatory (taste) perception	
Limbic	Emotional responses, drive-related behavior, and emotional memory	
Major Cortical Landmarks		
Central sulcus	Divides frontal and parietal lobes	
Parieto–occipital sulcus	Divides parietal and occipital lobes	
Lateral sulcus	Superior border of temporal lobe	
Cingulate sulcus	Superior border of limbic lobe	
Precentral gyrus	Primary motor cortex	
Postcentral gyrus	Primary sensory cortex	
Posterior parietal association area	Integration of body awareness with visual perception	
Subcortical Structures		
Lateral ventricle	C-shaped chambers in each cerebral hemisphere where most of the cerebrospinal fluid (CSF) is made; there is one on the left and another on the right; each one communicates with the third ventricle (a midline structure) via an interventricular foramen	
Third ventricle	Midline cavity in diencephalon that connects with the fourth ventricle via the cerebral aqueduct	
Fourth ventricle	Tent-like cavity between the cerebellum posteriorly and the pons and rostral medulla anteriorly that communicates with subarachnoid space via the median and lateral apertures	
Choroid plexus	Vascularized tissue that secretes CSF; found within the lateral ventricles and the fourth ventricle	
Cerebral aqueduct	Narrow channel through the midbrain that connects the third and fourth ventricles	
Foramen of Magendie	Median aperture (opening) of fourth ventricle through which CSF flows into the subarachnoid space dorsal to the lower medulla	
Foramina of Luschka	Two lateral apertures of fourth ventricle through which CSF flows into the subarachnoid spaces ventrolateral to the upper medulla	
Basal Ganglia	Reward-based motor learning, initiation and selection of thoughts and especially actions, switching from one thing to another, esp. sequencing	

(Continued)

TABLE 1-1	Major Structures and Landmarks in the Nervous System, with Emphasis on Function in Sensory and Motor Systems *(Continued)*
STRUCTURE	**FUNCTIONS**
Caudate nucleus	Receives information primarily from association areas of the cerebral cortex; important for cognitive functions of the basal ganglia
Head	Rostral – main target for prefrontal cortex
Body	Superior – parietal areas
Tail	Wraps around into the temporal lobe – temporal areas
Putamen	Functionally and cellularly just like the Caudate, but anatomically separated from Caudate by fibers of the internal capsule. Receives information primarily from motor and somatosensory areas of the cerebral cortex; important for motor functions of the basal ganglia
Striatum	A name used to refer to the caudate and putamen in combination
Globus pallidus – external segment (GPe)	One target of output from striatum. Involved in intermediate stage of basal ganglia processing
Globus pallidus – internal segment (GPi)	Final output nucleus targeted by GPe and STN – has neurons with axons leaving basal ganglia to go to the thalamus and thereby influence cortex and the control of movement
Subthalamic nucleus	Works with GPe for intermediate steps in basal ganglia processing
Substantia nigra	The largest nucleus in the midbrain
Pars compacta (SNpc)	Location of dopamine-producing cells that project into the striatum (caudate and putamen) to control movement
Pars reticulata (SNpr)	Just like cells in GPi but SNpr cells control eye movements, while GPi cells are for the rest of the body
Internal Capsule	Funnel-shaped region separating the thalamus from the basal ganglia; contains fiber tracts that relay almost all of the information going to and from the cerebral cortex and other (non-cortical) parts of the brain
Hippocampus	Memory formation (declarative)
Amygdala	Emotions, learning whether something is "good" or "bad," aggression
Thalamus	Receives, filters, and distributes information bound for the cerebral cortex
Hypothalamus	Autonomic functions, drives, hormones
Cerebellum	Receives information from sensory systems, the cerebral cortex and other sites, and participates in the planning and coordination of movement
Cerebellar Cortex	Three-layered structure that receives cerebellar inputs and projects them to the deep cerebellar nuclei
Folia	Repeated horizontal folds of the cerebellum
Vermis	Midline lobe of the cerebellum important for cerebellar control of body and posture
Flocculonodular lobe	Cerebellar control for vestibular responses and eye movements
Spinocerebellum	Consists of the vermis and medial parts of the lateral cerebellar hemispheres that receive spinal inputs; involved with regulation of posture and coordination of limb movements
Lateral cerebellar hemispheres	Main lobes of the cerebellum on each side of the vermis; medial part is part of spinocerebellum as stated above; lateral parts are part of the cerebrocerebellum, a functional division that communicates with the cerebral cortex for the coordination of motor planning and to some extent the coordination of higher-order thought processes
Deep cerebellar nuclei	Location for cells sends axons projecting out of the cerebellum to affect other parts of the nervous systems, especially the brainstem and (via the thalamus) the cortex
Brainstem	Consists of the midbrain, pons, and medulla

(Continued)

TABLE 1-1	Major Structures and Landmarks in the Nervous System, with Emphasis on Function in Sensory and Motor Systems *(Continued)*
STRUCTURE	**FUNCTIONS**
Midbrain	The most rostral of the three subdivisions of the brainstem
Cerebral peduncles	Two large fiber bundles on ventral surface of midbrain containing descending motor fibers from the cortex
Red nucleus	Involved in cerebellar circuitry and in control of limb movements, especially rapid error correction and shaping the hand during reaching
Cerebral aqueduct – PAG	Site of origin of a descending pain-control pathway
Superior colliculi	Involved in directing visual attention and controlling eye movements
Inferior colliculi	Major link in the auditory system
Pons	The second of the three parts of the brainstem, continuous rostrally with the midbrain and caudally with the medulla
Pontine nuclei	Nuclei in the basal pons that receive inputs from the cerebral cortex and project to contralateral cerebellum
Cerebellar peduncles	Three paired fiber bundles connecting the cerebellum and brainstem via cerebellar afferents and efferents
Vestibular nuclei	Involved in regulating posture and coordinating eye and head movements
Reticular formation	Complex network of nuclei involved in integrative functions such as control of complex movements, transmission of pain information, vital functions, and arousal and consciousness
Medulla	The most caudal of the three subdivisions of the brainstem
Pyramids	Two rounded masses on the ventral surface of the medulla containing motor fibers projecting from the cerebral cortex to the spinal cord via the corticospinal tracts
Inferior olivary complex	Origin of "climbing fibers" to the cerebellum that are involved in motor learning
Dorsal column nuclei	Nuclei for relay of proprioceptive and discriminative touch for dorsal column-medial lemniscus system
Vestibular nuclei	Involved in regulating posture and coordinating eye and head movements
Reticular formation	Complex network of nuclei involved in motor functions such as posture and postural set and control of whole limb or whole body movements, including locomotion. Also contains nuclei important for transmission and regulation of pain, vital functions, and arousal and consciousness
Spinal Cord	Conducts sensory/motor information to/from the brain; contains central pattern generators for control of walking
White matter	Fiber tracts (i.e., myelinated axons) that carry information up and down
Grey matter (aka gray matter)	Contains neuronal cell bodies and reflex circuits
Cervical enlargement (C5–T1)	Expanded gray matter to control the arms, and expanded white matter for incoming and outgoing information
Lumbar enlargement (L2–S3)	Expanded gray area to control the legs, and expanded white matter for incoming and outgoing information
Dorsal roots	Incoming (sensory) information
Ventral roots	Outgoing (motor) commands
Spinal nerves	Where dorsal and ventral roots fuse before exiting the intervertebral foramina
Cauda equina	Spinal nerves in lower vertebral column on their way to their original foramina (vertebral column longer than spinal cord in adults)
Sympathetic chain	Series of interconnected ganglia that lie ventral and lateral to the vertebral column that contains cell bodies of postganglionic neurons in the sympathetic nervous system
Corpus callosum	White matter fiber tracts connecting left and right cerebral hemispheres

● PARTS OF THE BRAIN

Cerebral Hemispheres

The **cerebral hemispheres** are the large structures at the most rostral end of the nervous system (Figure 1-3). They are bilateral, with a **left** and a **right** hemisphere. The cerebral hemispheres contain the structures that provide for consciousness, voluntary actions, intelligence, memory, movement, sensation, feelings and emotions, and more. When we think of things we need our "brain" to accomplish, we are usually thinking of something that happens in the cerebral hemispheres. Another term used for both hemispheres together is the **cerebrum**. In general, the structure of the hemispheres is characterized by an external layer of gray matter called the **cerebral cortex**. In shorthand parlance, rather than saying "the cerebral cortex," people often simply say, "the cortex." While the outer layer of the cerebral hemispheres is the cell-rich cortex, they also contain many **nuclei**, including the basal ganglia. Inside the cerebral hemispheres, there is a great deal of **white matter** connecting the various components of the hemispheres and other brain regions. The cerebral hemisphere also contains parts of the **ventricular system**, fluid-filled cavities that can be found within certain parts of the brain (described in a later section of this chapter).

Cerebellum

The cerebellum is found within the cranial cavity, posterior and inferior to the cerebrum (Figure 1-3). Literally, cerebellum means little brain. The cerebellum is primarily associated with motor function and motor learning. Evidence from functional imaging studies shows it may also play a role in the imagination of movements.[1] The cerebellum connects to the rest of the nervous system through the brainstem and has pathways connecting it with the spinal cord, brainstem, and cerebrum. Like the cerebrum, the cerebellum has an outer layer of gray matter called the **cortex**, inner nuclei called the **deep cerebellar nuclei**, and of course **white matter** for connections. Even though the cerebellum also has a cortex, it is generally understood that when people say, "the cortex," they mean "the cerebral cortex." To refer to the cortical tissue of the cerebellum, one should always say, "the cerebellar cortex."

Brainstem

The brainstem includes nuclei and white matter structures and forms the physical connection between the cerebral hemispheres, the spinal cord, and the cerebellum (Figure 1-3). It is home to a wide variety of complex nuclei and circuits for functions such as hearing, respiration, arousal, posture and locomotion, chewing, and many others. In addition, there are 12 cranial nerves that together make connections with the face, mouth, and throat, the nose, eyes, ears, and balance organs as well as the internal organs. Most of these cranial nerves have nuclei in the brainstem, and nerves that exit or enter the brainstem.

Spinal Cord

The spinal cord is the final source of direct connections between the brain and the body (Figure 1-3A). A large portion of the

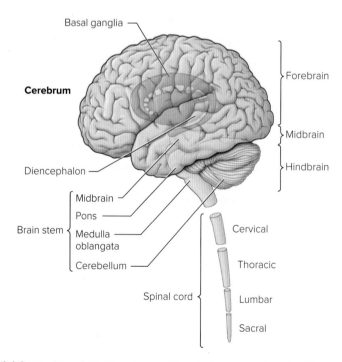

FIGURE 1-3 Gross anatomical divisions of the CNS. The cerebral hemispheres are found at the rostral end of the nervous system. The basal ganglia are contained within the cerebrum. The midbrain, pons, and medulla oblongata together are called the brainstem, and caudal to that is the spinal cord. Rostral to the midbrain is the diencephalon, the thalamus, and hypothalamus, which together with the cerebrum is called the forebrain. In this nomeclature (forebrain, midbrain, and hindbrain), the midbrain is itself, and the hindbrain is the pons, medulla, and cerebellum. (Reproduced with permission, from Kandel ER, Schwartz JH, Jessell TM, Siegelbaum SA, Hudspeth AJ. *Principles of Neural Science*, 5th ed. New York, NY: McGraw-Hill; 2013.)

physical structure of the spinal cord is dedicated to these connections. Spinal nerves projecting from the left and right sides of each vertebral segment allow connection with peripheral muscles and sensory receptors; long fiber tracts within the cord convey information between the brain and the spinal cord. Functionally, however, the spinal cord is much more than this set of physical connections. The spinal cord contains complex neural circuits within its central gray matter that can coordinate complex behaviors like withdrawing a limb from a painful stimulus, reflexive control of bowel and bladder function, and even the rudimental elements for the neural control of walking (discussed in detail in Chapter 2).

● THE MENINGES

The central nervous system is encased in bone, so the outermost protective structure is bone, either the skull or the vertebral column. The meninges are a multilayered set of membranes that enclose the nervous system and separate it from the protective bony structures. If a window in the bone is opened to reveal the central nervous system, the outermost structure seen will be the **dura mater** (Figure 1-4A). The dura mater is a tough, relatively inelastic tissue that is several layers thick. In addition to surrounding the brain, there are some large infoldings of the dura mater to further protect and stabilize certain brain structures. For example, in between the two cerebral hemispheres is the **falx cerebri** (Figure 1-4B, C). Lying over the top of the cerebellum is the **cerebellar tentorium** (Figure 1-4C). The dura mater also surrounds and protects several large venous sinuses that collect blood from the brain to return it to the venous circulation. The dura mater forms a seal around the outside of the brain through which fluid will not pass, except through blood vessels.

The innermost layer of the meninges is the **pia mater**. The pia is very thin and adheres directly to the underlying nervous tissue, even in its deeper enfolding on the cerebral cortex. It takes a microscope to view the pia. In a gross dissection, the pia matter would appear to be the surface of the brain. The pia also seals the brain as a part of the blood–brain barrier.

In between the dura mater and the pia mater is the **arachnoid mater** (Figure 1-4B). The arachnoid is a loose layer of tissue immediately below the dura. It does not extend to all brain surfaces like the pia mater does and more closely follows the dura mater. Underneath the arachnoid and above the pia is where the cerebrospinal fluid (CSF) is found. Arteries along the surface of the nervous system travel through the space between the arachnoid and the pia. The arachnoid forms into small tubes called **villi** that conduct CSF out of the subarachnoid space and into the dural sinuses, where the CSF eventually mixes with the venous blood to return to the circulation (see discussion in Chapter 18).

When the meninges become infected, the result is called meningitis. This can be life-threatening because the inflammation within the enclosed cranial cavity puts pressure on the brain, and if pressure is high enough, brain damage and even death can occur. There are both viral and bacterial forms of meningitis. If the pathogen gets through the pia mater and infects the brain tissue directly, this is called encephalitis.[2]

● LOBES OF THE BRAIN

The cerebral hemispheres are divided into lobes. Modern nomenclature indicates four lobes, the frontal, parietal, occipital, and temporal. There are two other regions which were once considered lobes, the insular region and the limbic region. These are indicated in Figure 1-5.

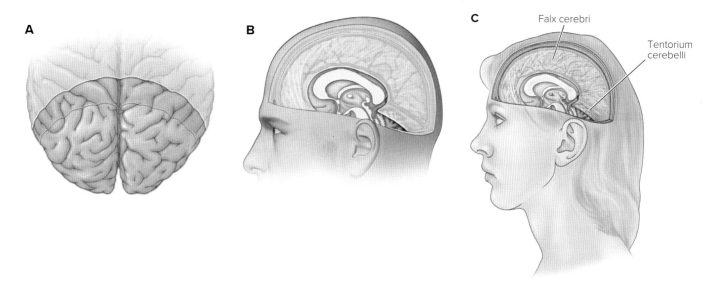

FIGURE 1-4 The meninges. A and **B**. This image of a brain shows layers of meninges removed, revealing the tough dura matter and the thinner arachnoid. The pia is continuous with the brain surface and cannot be distinguished without a microscope. **C**. The falx cerebri is a dura mater structure that separates the two cerebral hemispheres. (**C:** Reproduced, with permission, from Martin JH. *Neuroanatomy Text and Atlas*, 4th ed. New York: McGraw-Hill; 2012, Fig. 1-15.)

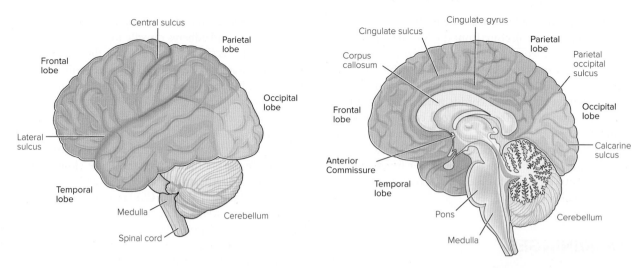

FIGURE 1-5 **Lobes of the cerebral cortex and the landmarks structures that form their boundaries.** On the left, a lateral view of the brain shows the four major lobes. The central sulcus and the lateral sulcus are visible here. On the right, the medial view of the brain is shown, with the brain split in the sagittal plane, along the midline. The parietal–occipital sulcus is visible here, along with the cingulate gyrus. (Reproduced with permission from Martin JH. *Neuroanatomy Text and Atlas*, 3rd ed. New York, NY: McGraw-Hill; 2003.)

Frontal

The frontal lobe is associated with thoughts, planning, decisions, and actions, including movement. It is also considered the home to what we think of as the personality. The frontal lobe is relatively large in humans and other animals we would consider intelligent. Most of what we would consider the cortical motor systems, the cortical structures involved in the control of movement, are found in the frontal lobe. The frontal lobe begins at the **central sulcus**, such that everything rostral to the central sulcus is frontal lobe.

Parietal

The parietal lobe is associated with sensation and perception. Because of the critical role that sensation plays in control of movement, the parietal lobe is also critical for control of movement. Reflecting the integration between sensation and motor control, a common term used to categorize research and knowledge in this area is "sensorimotor systems." The parietal lobe is the primary location for the initial sensations coming in from the somatosensory system (skin, muscles, joints, etc.)[3] but not the special senses (vision, hearing, etc.). The parietal lobe does integrate somatosensory sensation with information from the special senses to form an overall perception. Hence, although initial hearing and seeing occurs in other lobes, the parietal lobe is where we would perceive where a sound came from, or where an object was seen, in relation to the position of our body.[3] Higher-order sensory experiences like music appreciation also occur in the parietal lobe.[4] The rostral boundary of the parietal lobe is the central sulcus, and the caudal boundary is the parietal–occipital sulcus, which is most prominent on the mesial surface of the brain. An imaginary line separates parietal and occipital lobes on the lateral aspect of the brain.

Occipital

The occipital lobe is dedicated to vision. There are a variety of stations in the processing of visual information, including the initial perception, the elucidation of color, the recognition of motion, distinguishing objects from the background, and so on. Coming from the occipital lobe, visual information takes two major routes. The dorsal visual stream provides information for the parietal lobe to use in locating objects and integrating vision into perception for action. The ventral visual stream leads to the temporal lobe for the recognition and naming of objects, such as faces, food, predators and prey, tools, etc. The occipital lobe is bounded by the temporal lobe laterally and the parietal lobe medially.[5]

Temporal

The temporal lobe is associated with auditory processing, especially language, as well as memory and the identification of objects. The temporal lobe is separated from the parietal and frontal lobes by the lateral sulcus. There is no clear demarcation between the temporal and occipital lobes; an imaginary line is used to divide these lobes based on local landmarks on the brain.

Special Regions of the Cortex

Insular Cortex

The insular cortex is no longer considered a lobe, but rather, a region (Figure 1-6A, B). It is found deep in the lateral sulcus, in between the temporal and parietal lobes. Cortical tissue here is associated with eating and digestive functions, autonomic function, and feelings such as pain or pleasure, especially when associated with sensory experiences (see Chapter 7 for more information on the insular cortex).

Cingulate Cortex

The cingulate cortex (Figure 1-5, right) is associated with basic drives and motivations such as hunger, emotions, and initiation as well as memory and learning (see chapter 7 for more detail).[6] Once thought of as a part of a lobe called the limbic lobe, the cingulate cortex, like insular cortex, is now considered a region.

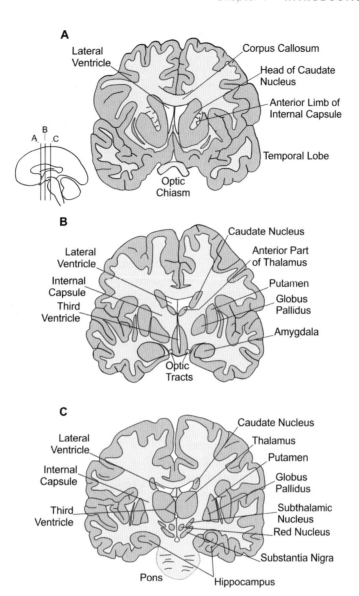

FIGURE 1-6 **Frontal-plane sections through the cerebrum showing selected subcortical structures.** The outline of a lateral view of the brain that is inset at the top left shows where each section was made (A, B, and C). Structures may only be labeled on one side, but most are bilateral.

The cingulate can be found superior to the corpus callosum. The rostral portion of the cingulate cortex is part of the frontal lobe; the caudal portion is part of the parietal lobe.

● SUBCORTICAL STRUCTURES

Within the cerebral hemispheres are a variety of important white and gray matter structures. Those most relevant to this text are listed below.

Thalamus

The thalamus is a major nucleus that receives and processes information that will be sent to the cerebral cortex (Figure 1-6C). Almost all information that comes into the brain must eventually reach the thalamus and synapse on a neuron there. The thalamic neuron will then bring the information to the cortex. The thalamus is comprised of a number of nuclei that serve as relay stations for specific motor and sensory projections.

Basal Ganglia

The basal ganglia are a set of nuclei within the cerebral hemispheres that process cortical information and send it back to the cortex by way of the thalamus (Figures 1-3A, 1-6A–C). There are also some direct outputs from the basal ganglia to the oculomotor and postural control system, but most basal ganglia output goes back to the cortex via the thalamus. The specific nuclei included in the basal ganglia are the **caudate** and **putamen** (together called the **striatum**), the **globus pallidus** (which has external and internal segments), the **subthalamic nucleus**, and the **substantia nigra** (which has a *pars compacta* and a *pars reticulata*). The substantia nigra is located in the dorsal midbrain rather than within the cerebral hemispheres, and the subthalamic nucleus sits just below the thalamus within the portion of the brain, known as the **diencephalon** (e.g., thalamus, hypothalamus, epithalamus, and subthalamus). The caudate borders and follows the lateral ventricles and can be divided into the **head** (anterior portion within the frontal lobes), the **body** (extending back through the parietal lobe), and the **tail** (extending down into the temporal lobe). The globus pallidus and putamen can appear grossly to be a single nucleus, referred to as the **lenticular nucleus**, just medial to the insular region; despite that appearance, the globus pallidus and putamen are distinct nuclei with different functions.

Hypothalamus

The hypothalamus is the region inferior to the thalamus (Figure 1-6B). This is where hormones are regulated by the brain, thirst and hunger are detected based on physiologic signals, sleep–wake cycles are determined, and many other basic physiological functions for homeostasis are regulated. This region has connections to and from many other parts of the brain allowing it to cross-reference many sources of information.

Hippocampal Formation

This region of cortex is in the medial part of the temporal lobe, on the inferior surface of the brain (Figure 1-6C). It is specifically associated with the formation of declarative memory, the ability to memorize information and experiences (see Chapter 7).

Amygdala

The amygdala is a nucleus in the temporal lobe that can be found at the rostral end of the hippocampal formation. The amygdala works with the hippocampal formation in the generation of memories, especially those associated with intense emotional states such as fear and anger (see Chapter 7).

Corpus Callosum

The corpus callosum is the major structure connecting the left and right cerebral hemispheres (Figures 1-5, 1-6A–C). It is comprised entirely of axons passing between the left and right cerebral hemispheres, principally the frontal and parietal lobes.

Anterior Commissure

The anterior commissure is like the corpus callosum but is mainly comprised of axons crossing between the left and right temporal lobes. Because of its regular appearance and location (Figure 1-5), it is often used as a point of reference in brain imaging studies to allow for alignment of the images from an individual at various points in time as well as to align an individual brain with standard images from brain atlases.

Internal Capsule

The internal capsule is a white matter pathway with axons going up to and coming down from the cerebral cortex (Figure 1-6).

Its **anterior limb** becomes evident at the beginning of the separation of the caudate and putamen in the frontal lobe (Figure 1-6A, B). Its **posterior limb** separates the thalamus from the basal ganglia (Figure 1-6C). Axons from neurons of the cerebral cortex pass through the internal capsule on their way to the brainstem and spinal cord. Axons of the sensory systems coming into the brain pass through the internal capsule on the way to thalamus, and thalamic fibers projecting to the cortex are also found in the internal capsule. Lesions in the internal capsule can have severe sensory and motor consequences (see Chapter 11, Stroke).

Corona Radiata

There is a great deal of white matter underneath the cerebral cortex that is not part of the internal capsule. This is not labeled specifically in the diagrams above because that would be impracticable: it comprises the bulk of the subcortical white matter. Most of this is formed by axons from cortical neurons that are projecting from one part of the cortex to another. These cortico-cortical connections do not need to pass through the thalamus, they project straight to the cortex. Projections from cortical tissue to subcortical structures such as the caudate and putamen are also found in this white matter. Compared to these cortico-cortical connections, only a subset of the axons in the white matter of the cerebrum project outside of the cerebral hemispheres to influence other parts of the nervous system.

● VENTRICULAR SYSTEM

As noted above, the brain is surrounded by meninges, and within the meninges, there is CSF. Just as CSF surrounds the brain, it can also be found inside the brain in cavities called the ventricles. The ventricular system includes the ventricles, passageways between the ventricles, the tissue that secretes the CSF, and the system for collecting the fluid to return it to the circulation. In Chapter 19, there are illustrations of the ventricular system, additional discussion of the flow of CSF, and examples of disorders of this flow that result in hydrocephalus. The names of these structures are provided here.

Within the cerebral hemispheres are two large ventricles called the lateral ventricles, one on the left and one on the right. Neither is formally labeled the first or second, but since there are two, the next one is called the third ventricle, and after that comes the fourth. The third ventricle is a midline structure located around the level of the midbrain, and the fourth ventricle is also a midline structure located in between the brainstem and the cerebellum. CSF is secreted within the ventricular system by a type of tissue called the **choroid plexus**. Choroid plexus is found within the lateral ventricles and the fourth ventricle, but usually not in the third. The passage of fluid between the lateral ventricle and the third ventricle on each side occurs through an opening called the **interventricular foramen**. The third and fourth ventricles are connected by the **cerebral aqueduct**.

CSF exits the ventricular system through one of three openings. The largest is the median aperture, also called the **foramen of Magendie**. This is a midline opening from the fourth ventricle to the posterior aspect of the medulla in the brainstem. The space here where CSF collects under the cerebellum and behind the brainstem is called the **cisterna magna**. There are also two lateral apertures, a left and right, coming out from each side of the fourth ventricle in the space between the cerebellum and pons. The lateral apertures are also called the **foramina of Luschka**. The place where CSF collects here, anterior and lateral to the cerebellum, is called the **cerebellopontine angle cistern**. The central canal of the spinal cord, forming in the caudal medulla, is also a place for CSF to leave the fourth ventricle, but it is very small and carries very little fluid compared to the other pathways for CSF to flow within the ventricular system.

Once the CSF has passed outside the ventricular system, through the median or lateral apertures to get outside of the cerebrum and brainstem, the CSF is contained within the meninges. Thus, the brain has a cushion of fluid on the inside and the outside, keeping it essentially floating within the CSF. The subarachnoid space holds the CSF in between the arachnoid mater and the pia mater. Because CSF is constantly being produced, there needs to be a way to return this fluid to the circulation. Much of the venous blood leaving the brain is collected in structures called venous sinuses that form within the dura mater. Small protrusions from the arachnoid, called **arachnoid villi**, reach into these venous sinuses so that the CSF in the subarachnoid space can leak slowly into the venous blood, maintaining the right level of fluid pressure with the ventricular system but allowing for the return of the fluid to the circulation.

● THE CEREBELLUM

The cerebellum, like the cerebrum, has an external layer of gray matter called the cortex, nuclei of gray matter deep within, and white matter structures providing the connections (Figure 1-6D). The best single word to describe cerebellar function is coordination. Literally, this word means to coordinate, to control two or more things at once. The connections and circuitry of the cerebellum serve this purpose in many ways. When a pitcher throws a baseball, (s)he must coordinate anticipatory postural adjustments with the leg and trunk motions of the windup, and the visual scene in the batter's box with the throwing motion of the arm. Speech requires coordination of the muscles of the throat and vocal cords with the movements of the tongue and lips and respiratory muscles for controlled exhalation. Motor learning requires coordination of the experience from past trials with plans for the next attempt. Further details of cerebellar function are provided in Chapter 5. Here, we focus on the anatomy.

Cortex

Cerebellar cortex is simpler and more uniform in structure than cerebral cortex. There are three layers: a parallel fiber layer, a Purkinje layer, and a granular layer, each named for the predominant structural feature. **Granule cells** in that layer, the innermost level, receive the information coming into the cerebellum. The axons of granule cells project to the cerebellar cortex and split in two, running along the surface of the cortex in parallel with the folia, the small enfolding of tissues evident on the surface of the cerebellar cortex. These **parallel fibers** dominate the appearance of the parallel fiber layer, the outmost level. Parallel fibers synapse in the synaptic tree of the **Purkinje cells**. The Purkinje cell bodies are the dominant feature of the Purkinje layer, the middle level. Purkinje cells make axons that project to the nuclei within the cerebellum, often referred to as the deep cerebellar nuclei.

Deep Cerebellar Nuclei (DCN)

The DCN are a group of gray matter structures located inside the cerebellum. In a general sense, all neurons in the DCN are the same kind of cell. The fact that we can observe apparently distinct cerebellar nuclei is simply a consequence of the way the white matter structures pass among these neurons, dividing them into anatomically distinct entities. From a functional standpoint, each of the DCN tends to connect consistently with a certain part of the cerebellar cortex, and to the extent that there is differentiation of the function in parts of the cerebellar cortex, there is also differentiation in function among the DCN. However, this differentiation is a consequence of the connections, not any difference in the neurons themselves. In the human, we can observe four distinct DCN: the **fastigial** nucleus, the **globose** and **emboliform** nuclei, and the **dentate** nucleus. In other animals, these nuclei may be combined in different ways with different names, but the essential function of the deep cerebellar nucleus neurons is the same.

Lobes/Regions of Cerebellum

The cerebellum can be divided according to two schemes, lobes and functional divisions. There are three lobes. The **anterior lobe** is the part underneath the occipital lobe, rostral to a cerebellar cortex structure called the **primary fissure**. The **posterior cerebellum** is everything else, with the exception of a small structure called the **flocculonodular lobe**, which is at the opposite end of the cerebellum from the anterior lobe and can be found on the anterior surface, apposed to the fourth ventricle (Figure 1-7A, B).

For the rehabilitation professional, the functional divisions of the cerebellum are often a more useful way to think about cerebellar anatomy than the anatomical divisions. The functional divisions of the cerebellum are the vestibulocerebellum, the spinocerebellum, and the cerebrocerebellum (Figure 1-7C). The flocculonodular lobe is identical to the **vestibulocerebellum**. The other two include both anterior and posterior cerebellum, but the functional divisions are divided along a mediolateral axis. The **spinocerebellum** includes the midline cerebellar tissue called the vermis, as well as the medial parts of each cerebellar hemisphere, called the paravermis. The **cerebrocerebellum** is the remainder of the cerebellar hemispheres.

Each of the DCN is connected mainly with a certain function division of the cerebellum. The **vestibulocerebellum** is connected to the fastigial nucleus (and also has some direct connections to the vestibular nuclei); thus, its function relates to vestibular control of eye movement, posture, and balance. The spinocerebellum is connected to the fastigial, globose, and emboliform nuclei, receiving postural sensory information via the spinocerebellar tracts and projecting to the medial

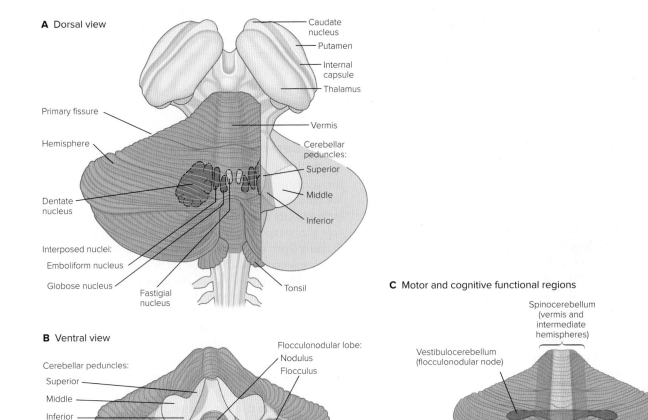

FIGURE 1-7 The cerebellum. A. The deep cerebellar nuclei within the cerebellum are illustrated. On the right, the cerebellum has been removed to show how the cerebellar peduncles come from the brainstem. **B.** This is the view of the cerebellum that would be seen from the front if it was removed from the brainstem. **C.** The functional regions of the cerebellum are shown. (Reproduced, with permission, from Nieuwenhuys R. *Chemoarchitecture of the Brain.* New York: Springer-Verlag; 1985.)

descending system (rubrospinal, vestibulospinal, and reticulospinal tracts) to control postural stability. The cerebrocerebellum is connected to the dentate nucleus, sending efferents via the thalamus to the motor cortex and other cortical areas to participate in motor planning and motor control (see Chapter 5).

Cerebellar Peduncles

On each side, there are three cerebellar peduncles, the white matter connections between the cerebellum and the brainstem; these are the inferior, middle, and superior cerebellar peduncles (Figure 1-7B). The **inferior cerebellar peduncle** contains axons carrying information from the spinal cord with highly detailed sensory information about the body and its position and movements. It also carries information in from a nucleus in the brainstem called the **inferior olivary complex** to convey indications of errors that require improved coordination. The **middle cerebellar peduncle** carries information from nuclei in the pons to the cerebellum. These pontine nuclei are the targets of axons from the cerebral cortex, so the middle cerebellar peduncle is the second leg of the pathway from cortex to cerebellum, which is called the **cortico-ponto-cerebellar pathway**. The **superior**

cerebellar peduncle is mainly comprised of axons exiting the cerebellum from the DCN to project to brainstem and cortical structures for motor control. There are also certain kinds of information from the spinal cord entering through the superior cerebellar peduncle. More information about the cerebellum is provided in Chapter 5.

● THE BRAINSTEM

The brainstem (Figure 1-8) has a wide variety of important structures involved in all types of neural function, including sensory, motor, autonomic, and integrative. Basic functions for taste and eating, hearing, balance, and vision are found here, as are systems for the control of posture and locomotion, perception and modulation of pain, regulation of cardiorespiratory function, and arousal. In addition, all white matter connections between the brain and spinal cord must pass through the brainstem. Any serious injury to the brainstem is usually fatal.

Certain structures span much of the rostro–caudal length of the brainstem and are not confined to any particular region.

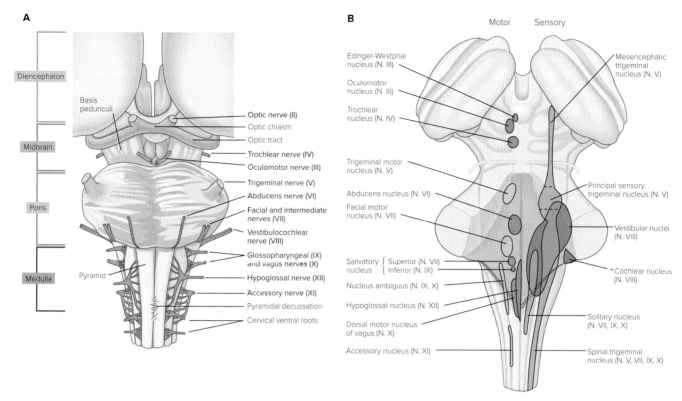

FIGURE 1-8 The cranial nerves. On the left (**A**), a ventral view of the brainstem and diencephalon shows where each of the cranial nerves exits the brainstem. On the right (**B**), a dorsal view shows where the cranial nerve nuclei are located for motor outputs and sensory inputs. (Reproduced with permission from Kandel ER, Schwartz JH, Jessell TM, Siegelbaum SA, Hudspeth AJ. *Principles of Neural Science*, 5th ed. New York: McGraw-Hill, NY; 2013.)

One is the **trigeminal nucleus**, which spans from the midbrain to the medulla. Different regions have different specializations in the trigeminal complex, but overall, this is a very long structure serving all sensory and motor functions of the trigeminal nerve. Another is called the **reticular formation**. This is a long column of gray matter found ventrolateral to the cerebral aqueduct and fourth ventricle extending from the midbrain to the medulla. The reticular formation has a variety of functions. Those of most importance in rehabilitation are the pathways from the brainstem to spinal cord, the **reticulospinal tracts**, which are key sources for the regulation of posture, locomotion, and gross limb movements. Medial and somewhat ventral to the reticular formation in the caudal pons and rostral medulla are the **raphe nuclei**. These have a variety of functions that regulate the state of other parts of the nervous system, including arousal, the spinal cord circuits for control of walking, and the transmission and modulation of pain.

Midbrain

The midbrain is the most rostral level of the brainstem. The most prominent white matter features at this level are the **cerebral peduncles**, containing all axons coming from the cerebrum and projecting to brainstem and spinal cord structures below. Within the midbrain, we find several key nuclei. The **substantia nigra**, part of the basal ganglia, is located at the midbrain level. The **periaqueductal gray**, a central structure involved in pain regulation, is also a midbrain structure. A key motor nucleus

involved in coordination between the cerebrum and cerebellum is called the **red nucleus**, which is a prominent spherical nucleus in the midbrain; the red nucleus is the origin of the rubrospinal tract. On the posterior aspect of the midbrain, we find two dome-like protrusions on each side, the superior colliculus and the inferior colliculus. The **superior colliculus** is for visual function, and the **inferior colliculus** is for auditory function. In addition, two cranial nerve nuclei are found at this level, the oculomotor nucleus (CN III) and the trochlear nucleus (CN IV). The **pedunculopontine nucleus** is a specialized structure in the brainstem that plays a critical role in the initiation of locomotion and the release of acetylcholine in selected brain areas. The **locus coeruleus** projects widely throughout the CNS, releasing a neuromodulator called norepinephrine that regulates overall excitability. Finally, the **ventral tegmental area** is associated with dopamine projections for regulating reward and pleasure and projects through the basal ganglia to the frontal lobe.

Pons and Medulla

The pons and medulla are mainly distinguished from each other by the middle cerebellar peduncle, which is the prominent white matter feature on the anterior aspect of the pons formed by axons exiting the pons to wrap around caudally toward the cerebellum. Within the pons, the ventral region contains the **pontine nuclei**, where corticopontine projections synapse en route to the cerebellum. In the dorsal pons, we find the **trigeminal nucleus** for the fifth cranial nerve (CN V), the nucleus for the sixth cranial nerve, abducens (CN VI), and the nucleus for the seventh cranial nerve, the facial nerve (CN VII). The **vestibular nuclei** are in the pons slightly lateral to midline and just ventral to the fourth ventricle. They receive afferents from the vestibular system and interconnect the vestibulocerebellum with the control of head, neck, and eye movements, as well as postural responses to head movements and position. The **cochlear nucleus** receives incoming auditory information from the cochlea, and the superior olivary complex contains neural circuits used for the initial localization of sound. Special senses, including hearing and the vestibular system, are discussed in Chapter 6.

The **medulla** emerges as the most caudal part of the brainstem, beneath the pons. The most prominent surface features of the medulla anteriorly are the **medullary pyramids** and the **inferior olives**. The pyramids are formed by the axons of the corticospinal tract, fibers for motor control running from the cerebral cortex to the spinal cord. The olives surround an internal structure called the **inferior olivary complex**, a processing center for information about errors to be sent up into the cerebellum. On the dorsal aspect of the brainstem, we see at the most caudal part of the medulla the continuation of two ascending fiber bundles rising from the spinal cord on each side. Below the brainstem, along the midline of the cervical spinal cord, is the **fasciculus gracilis** carrying ascending sensory information from the legs and lower trunk, and lateral to that is the **fasciculus cuneatus** carrying ascending sensory information from the upper trunk and arms. These tracts together are called the dorsal columns in the spinal cord. At the top of the dorsal columns as they reach the caudal medulla, we find the dorsal column nuclei (cuneatus and gracilis). These are evident on the surface of the medulla as small bumps, swellings from the dorsal column nuclei in the tissues underneath. The dorsal column nuclei contain the second sensory neuron in the pathways from the spinal cord to the brain (see Chapter 3).

Within the medulla there are many important nuclei, including the cranial nerve nuclei for nerves IX–XII (glossopharyngeal, vagus, spinal accessory, and hypoglossal). In addition, the cardiorespiratory regulation centers are in the medulla. Details about nuclei and fiber tracts that can be found within the midbrain, pons, and medulla are provided throughout the text as needed.

Cranial Nerves

The first cranial nerve is the **olfactory nerve**. This is somewhat unique among the cranial nerves in that the sensory neurons project to the olfactory bulb, and from there second-order sensory neurons project directly to cerebral cortex. The second cranial nerve is the **optic nerve** from the eyes. This nerve carries the visual information into the brain, and the axons synapse in a structure called the lateral geniculate nucleus, which can be thought of as a part of the thalamus. Some visual fibers also project to midbrain structures, such as the superior colliculus and third cranial nerve nucleus, for subconscious reactions to light such as orienting to a bright light, controlling pupillary constriction, photoregulation of the sleep–wake cycle, etc.

The third cranial nerve is the **oculomotor nerve**. This carries motor axons to four of the six extra-ocular muscles (all except lateral rectus and trochlear muscles.). The third cranial nerve also carries the autonomic nervous system fibers for control of the pupil and lens of the eye, which originate in the nucleus of **Edinger–Westphal**, located in the midbrain near the oculomotor nucleus (N. III) (Figure 1-8). The fourth cranial nerve is the **trochlear nerve**, carrying the motor axons to the trochlear muscle of the eye and originating from the trochlear nucleus in the midbrain (N. IV).

The fifth cranial nerve is the **trigeminal nerve**, which serves sensory and motor functions for much of the face and head. The motor fibers innervate key muscle of mastication, including temporalis, the pterygoids, and the masseter. These come from the trigeminal motor nucleus in the lower mesencephalon. The sensory fibers divide into ophthalmic branches innervating skin and structures of the forehead as well as the nose, maxillary branch for the cheek and upper lip, and the mandibular branch for the jaw and chin. The discriminative touch conveyed by the trigeminal nerve comes into the principal sensory nucleus, whereas information on pain and temperature comes into the spinal nucleus of the fifth cranial nerve.

The sixth cranial nerve is **abducens**, and this carries the motor axons to the lateral rectus muscle of the eye, originating in the abducens nucleus (N. VI) in the pons. The seventh is the **facial nerve**, which projects to all facial muscles not controlled by the trigeminal, focused on facial expressions, and also receives taste from the anterior part of the tongue. The seventh cranial nerve also innervates the lacrimal and salivary glands for tears and saliva. The seventh cranial nerve's motor fibers for the facial muscles originate in the facial nucleus in the pons (N. VII); efferents to the salivary glands projecting through VII come from the **salivatory nucleus**. Afferents for taste project through CN VII to the **solitary nucleus**, and some pain afferents project through CN VII to the spinal trigeminal nucleus in the medulla. The eighth cranial nerve is the **vestibulocochlear** nerve. This carries all the information for the cochlea and from the vestibular apparatus in the inner ear to the corresponding nuclei in the brainstem. The ninth cranial nerve is the **glossopharyngeal nerve**, which receives taste from the posterior tongue and sensation from the soft palate and the pharynx. The motor fibers come from nucleus ambiguous and innervate pharyngeal muscles and the parotid salivary gland. The taste fibers project to the solitary nucleus. Some pain fibers traveling in CN IX reach the spinal trigeminal nucleus in the medulla. The 10th cranial nerve is the **vagus**, which projects from the brainstem to the pharynx and into the thoracic and abdominal cavities. In the pharynx, the vagus controls many of the muscles involved in swallowing, as well as the gag reflex (in response to glossopharyngeal afferents). The motor fibers come from the nucleus ambiguous and the dorsal motor nucleus of the vagus, both in the medulla. Some taste and pain fibers come in through the vagus to reach the solitary nucleus and the spinal trigeminal nucleus, respectively. The vagus reaches the thoracic and upper abdominal cavities for **parasympathetic nervous system** control of the cardiorespiratory and upper digestive systems. The 11th cranial nerve is the **spinal accessory nerve**, which carries motor axons to the upper trapezius muscle and to the sternoclei-domastoid muscle. Its origin is the accessory nucleus, located in the upper few cervical segments. The 12th cranial nerve is the **hypoglossal**, which provides efferent motor control to the tongue. Its motor fibers come from the hypoglossal nucleus in the medulla.

Major Fiber Tracts

As noted above, major fiber tracts evident on the surface of the brainstem include the cerebral and cerebellar peduncles, the medullary pyramids, and the dorsal columns. There are also certain internal white matter tracts of importance in reha-bilitation (Figure 1-9). The **medial lemniscus** is the bundle of axons ascending from the dorsal column nuclei to carry sen-sory information to the thalamus (see Chapter 3). A bundle of fibers along the midline on each side is called the **medial longitudinal fasciculus**. The ascending fibers of the MLF

connect the vestibular nuclei with cranial nerve nuclei and other structures for control of eye movement (see Chapter 6). The descending fibers of the MLF project to the upper parts of the spinal cord to control head and neck movements, and this part of the system is commonly called the medial vestibulo-spinal tract.

● THE SPINAL CORD

Gross Anatomical Features

The spinal cord (Figure 1-10) is surrounded by meninges, including dura, arachnoid, and pia mater layers just like the rest of the CNS. Unique to the spinal cord, small extensions of pia mater extend laterally at each level of spinal cord to form **den-ticulate ligaments** to attach the spinal cord to the dura mater, keeping the cord stable and preventing it from twisting within the spinal column. There is also an extension of pia surrounded by dura at the caudal end of the spinal cord, called the **filum terminale**, which tethers the caudal end of the spinal cord to the lower end of the vertebral canal.

Viewing the spinal cord as a whole, the dorsal aspect reveals the dorsal columns, containing sensory fibers ascending toward the medulla. There is a median fissure evident throughout the rostro–caudal length of the spinal cord. In the upper thoracic and cervical portions of the spinal cord, both gracile (medial) and cuneate (lateral) fasciculi can be appreciated in the dorsal columns. In lower thoracic and lumbosacral spinal cord, there is only a gracile fasciculus.

The dorsal roots are formed by sensory fibers entering the spinal cord, and the dorsal root entry zone forms the lateral bor-der of the dorsal columns. The white matter on the lateral aspect of the spinal cord is called the lateral funiculus. The ventral roots are formed by the efferent axons of motor and autonomic effects projecting from the spinal cord to the body. The white matter on the surface of spinal cord, ventral and medial to the ventral roots, is called the ventral (or anterior) funiculus.

Segmental Organization

The spinal cord is organized into segments named for the verte-bral bone that formed alongside that segment during embryo-logical development. At each segment of the spinal cord, a spinal nerve is formed by the combination of the dorsal and ventral roots. The first spinal nerve exits through the intervertebral foramen above the first cervical vertebra, and the eighth spi-nal nerve exits below the seventh cervical vertebra (above T1). These first eight segments are called the cervical segments, so although there are only seven cervical vertebrae, there are eight cervical spinal segments. From there on, the spinal segment is named by the vertebra above the exit of its spinal nerve. Hence, the first thoracic segment has a spinal nerve that exits below the first thoracic vertebra. The third lumbar segment has a nerve that exits below the third lumbar vertebra, and so on. With this convention, there are 8 cervical, 12 thoracic, 5 lumbar, 5 sacral, and 1 coccygeal segmental levels in the human spinal cord, and an equal number of spinal nerves on each side.

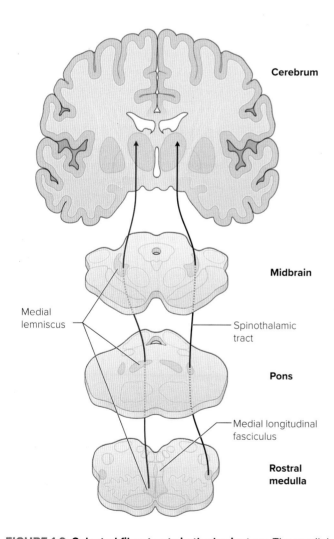

FIGURE 1-9 Selected fiber tracts in the brainstem. The medial lemniscus and spinothalamic tracts carry sensory information upward toward the brain. The medial longitudinal fasciculus carries oculomotor control signals as well as commands for head and neck movements.

Labels in figure: Cerebrum, Midbrain, Pons, Rostral medulla, Medial lemniscus, Spinothalamic tract, Medial longitudinal fasciculus

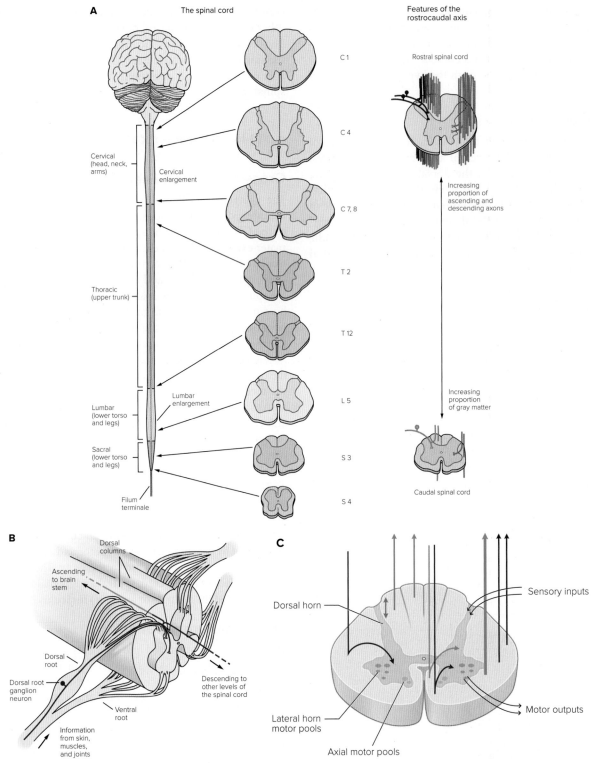

FIGURE 1-10 The spinal cord. A. The spinal cord carries all information between the brain and the body except that carried by the cranial nerves. There are enlargements at the cervical and lumbosacral levels to contain the extra gray and white matter for the arms and legs. Cross-sections representative of each segmental level are illustrated. Note how the relative proportion of white matter decreases at lower levels; few sensory axons have accumulated from below, and most motor axons have already terminated at levels above. **B.** The organization of a typical spinal segment is shown, including the dorsal roots, ventral roots, dorsal root ganglion, and spinal nerve. **C.** The general organization of information moving up and down the spinal cord is shown. Descending fibers (red) can travel in the lateral or ventral funiculus. Ascending fibers travel in the lateral and dorsal funiculus, some bound for the brain (green) and some for the cerebellum (purple). Special systems also descend to release neuromodulators that regulate spinal cord circuits (orange). (**A:** Reproduced permission from Kandel ER, Schwartz JH, Jessell TM, Siegelbaum SA, Hudspeth AJ, eds. *Principles of Neural Science*, 5th ed. New York: McGraw-Hill; 2013, Fig. 16-2, p. 359.) (**B:** Reproduced permission from Kandel ER, Schwartz JH, Jessell TM, Siegelbaum SA, Hudspeth AJ, eds. *Principles of Neural Science*, 5th ed. New York: McGraw-Hill; 2013, Fig. 16-3 p. 360.)

In each segment, the organization is consistent. As noted above, sensory fibers ascend in the dorsal columns. There are also some ascending fibers in the lateral funiculus, some destined for the cerebellum and others for the brainstem and thalamus. Descending fibers from the cortex and brainstem are found in the lateral and ventral funiculus. Some of these descending fibers are for direct motor control, and others are for modulation of spinal cord neurons and circuits. The gray matter is located in the center of the spinal cord. The dorsal horn is dedicated to sensory processing, and the ventral horn is dedicated to motor outputs. In the cervical and lumbosacral regions, the lateral expansion of the ventral horns is where limb muscle motoneurons are located. Throughout the spinal cord, muscles of the vertebral column and trunk have their motoneurons located medially. The organization and function of the spinal cord are discussed in detail in Chapter 2.

THE PERIPHERAL NERVOUS SYSTEM

The peripheral nervous system is formed by the motor and sensory axons coming out of and heading into the central nervous system. An important difference in these two parts of the nervous system is the type of cell that makes myelin. In the central nervous system, myelin is made by **oligodendrocytes**. Each oligodendrocyte will form a part of the myelin sheath around several axons. In the peripheral nervous system, there are **Schwann cells**, instead. Each Schwann cell wraps around a segment of only one axon. In the upper cervical, thoracic, lower sacral, and the coccygeal segments, the spinal nerves are individual, each innervating a defined segment of the body. However, in the lower cervical segments, including T1, and in the lumbosacral segments, the spinal nerves blend and merge into nerve plexuses on the way to the arms and legs. Specific peripheral nerves emerge from these plexuses to innervate the muscles, skin, and other structures.

THE AUTONOMIC NERVOUS SYSTEM

The autonomic nervous system consists of sympathetic and parasympathetic divisions that regulate the visceral organs, vasculature, and glands. In general, the **sympathetic nervous system** is associated with arousal, often referred to as our fight or flight system, and the **parasympathetic** division is associated with relaxation. Arousal would occur, for example, during exercise or in response to fear. Relaxation would be associated with increased digestive function, voiding of excretions, and rest. The parasympathetic parts of the autonomic nervous system are in the cranial nerves and their associated nuclei, along with specialized structures in the sacral spinal cord. Preganglionic neurons exit these areas and project to target ganglia in the periphery; then, postganglionic neurons project to the target organs. The sympathetic nervous system includes the **sympathetic chain ganglia** that run along the spinal cord from the cervical to the

coccygeal segments, some outlying ganglia near the viscera, and specific regions in gray matter of the thoracic and upper lumbar spinal cord that govern these structures. Efferents from the thoracolumbar regions exit the cord with other motor efferents but synapse in a sympathetic ganglion, traveling up or down within the chain to a specific level where they synapse on second-order fibers. Then, the second-order neurons project to target organs. These two systems function in harmony such that an increase in sympathetic activity is associated with a concomitant decrease in parasympathetic activity. For example, when we exercise, our digestive system's activity is diminished while our heart and respiration rates increase, thus targeting blood flow to our heart and muscles rather than our stomach.

SUMMARY

Understanding of the nervous system requires a combined understanding of the anatomical structures along with their functions. This includes understanding how the structures are connected with each other, what kinds of neurons and neural circuits exist within the structure, and how neurotransmitters and neuromodulators function in the structure. From this knowledge, we can understand the alterations in brain structure and function associated with pathologies, and we can see how and why certain approaches to treatment with physical therapy will be beneficial. Overall, the goal of this text is to help the reader see these connections and apply them to practice to help the patient.

REFERENCES

1. Buckner RL. The cerebellum and cognitive function: 25 years of insight from anatomy and neuroimaging. *Neuron*. 2013;80(3):807-815.
2. Richie MB, Josephson SA. A practical approach to meningitis and encephalitis. *Semin Neurol*. 2015;35:611-620.
3. Delhaye BP, Long KH, Bensmaia SJ. Neural basis of touch and proprioception in primate cortex. *Compr Physiol*. 2019;8(4):1575-1602.
4. Tsai CG, Chou TL, Li CW. Roles of posterior parietal and dorsal premotor cortices in relative pitch processing: comparing musical intervals to lexical tones. *Neuropsychol*. 2018;119:118-127.
5. Prasad S, Galetta SL. Anatomy and physiology of the afferent visual system. *Handbook Clin Neurol*. 2011;102:3-19.
6. Rolls ET. The cingulate cortex and limbic systems for emotion, action and memory. *Brain Structure Function*. 2019;224:3001-3018.

SUGGESTED READINGS

Kandel S, Schwartz JH, Jessell TM, Siegelbaum SA, Hudspeth AJ. *Principles of Neural Science*. 5th ed. New York: McGraw-Hill; 2013.

Vanderah T, Gould D. *Nolte's The Human Brain*. 7th ed. Philadelphia, PA: Elsevier; 2015. ISBN-10: 1455728594.

Parent A, Carpenter MB. *Carpenter's Human Neuroanatomy*. Baltimore, MD: Williams and Wilkins; 1996. ISBN 0683067524.

Haines D. *Neuroanatomy in Clinical Context: An Atlas of Structures, Sections, and Systems*. 9th ed. Baltimore: Lippincott Williams and Wilkins; 2015. ISBN 1451186258.

Martin JH. *Neuroanatomy Text and Atlas*. 4th ed. New York, NY: McGraw-Hill; 2012.

Review Questions

1. **In a person standing, what two directions are roughly equivalent in the cerebral hemispheres?**
   A. Anterior–ventral
   B. Inferior–dorsal
   C. Anterior–rostral
   D. Posterior–dorsal

2. **What kind of neural structure can be found in gray matter and in white matter?**
   A. Neuronal cell bodies
   B. Axons
   C. Dendrites of neurons
   D. Synapses

3. **How is a ganglion different from a nucleus?**
   A. A ganglion has neuronal cell bodies.
   B. A ganglion is usually outside the CNS.
   C. A ganglion has incoming and outgoing connections.
   D. A ganglion is for sensory neurons.

4. **The cerebellum is physically connected to the rest of the nervous system at the level of the**
   A. Cerebrum.
   B. Brainstem.
   C. Spinal cord.
   D. All of the above are correct.

5. **Which part of the meninges is toughest and thickest?**
   A. The dura mater
   B. The arachnoid mater
   C. The subarachnoid space
   D. The pia mater

6. **Match the lobe of the cerebral hemisphere with the functions listed.**
   A. Frontal Sensations and perception B
   B. Parietal Forming memories D
   C. Occipital Making decisions A
   D. Temporal Vision C

7. **Which of the following structures is most clearly visible on the mesial surface of the cerebral cortex?**
   A. Lateral sulcus
   B. Central sulcus
   C. Parietal occipital sulcus
   D. Insular cortex

8. **Which part of the basal ganglia is found immediately lateral to the lateral ventricle?**
   A. Caudate nucleus
   B. Putamen
   C. Globus pallidus
   D. Substantia nigra

9. **What structure would not contain any corticospinal fibers passing from the cortex to the spinal cord?**
   A. The internal capsule
   B. The corpus callosum
   C. The cerebral peduncle
   D. The medullary pyramid

10. **What structure is associated with the brain's regulation of hormones in the bloodstream?**
    A. The amygdala
    B. The hypothalamus
    C. The subthalamic nucleus
    D. The nucleus of Edinger–Westphal

11. **What is the name of the tissue that secretes cerebrospinal fluid?**
    A. Ventricular tissue
    B. Choroid plexus
    C. Pia mater
    D. Dural sinus

12. **What is the name of the passageway between the third and fourth ventricles?**
    A. The foramen of Magendie
    B. The interventricular foramen
    C. The cerebral aqueduct
    D. The central canal

13. **Which of the deep cerebellar nuclei is principally connected through the thalamus to the cerebral cortex?**
    A. Fastigial
    B. Globose
    C. Emboliform
    D. Dentate

14. **The vermis is considered part of which functional division of the cerebellum?**
    A. Cerebrocerebellum
    B. Vestibulocerebellum
    C. Spinocerebellum
    D. Paleocerebellum

15. **Which part of the basal ganglia is in the midbrain?**
    A. Caudate
    B. Putamen
    C. Globus pallidus
    D. Substantia nigra

16. **Where are the dorsal column nuclei found?**
    A. Midbrain
    B. Pons
    C. Medulla
    D. Spinal cord

17. **Which cranial nerve carries motor efferents to extraocular muscles and autonomic efferents to the muscles of the pupil and lens?**
    A. Optic nerve (II)
    B. Oculomotor nerve (III)
    C. Trochlear nerve (IV)
    D. Abducens nerve (VI)

18. **Which cranial nerve has a long series of nuclei reaching from the midbrain to the medulla?**
    A. Trigeminal (V)
    B. Facial (VII)
    C. Vestibulocochlear (VIII)
    D. Glossopharyngeal (IX)

19. **Which part of the spinal cord has more spinal cord segments than there are actual vertebral bones for that region?**
    A. Cervical
    B. Thoracic
    C. Lumbar
    D. Sacral

20. **Which structure in the thoracic and abdominal cavities is the initial target for neurons of the part of the autonomic nervous system associated with fight or flight responses in dangerous situations?**
    A. The cephalic ganglion
    B. The dorsal root ganglion
    C. The sympathetic chain ganglion
    D. The epigastric ganglion

Answers

1. C	**2.** B	**3.** B	**4.** B	**5.** A
6. A	**7.** C	**8.** A	**9.** B	**10.** B
11. B	**12.** C	**13.** D	**14.** C	**15.** D
16. C	**17.** B	**18.** A	**19.** A	**20.** C

GLOSSARY

Amygdala. Temporal lobe nucleus associated with memory and emotion

Anterior commissure. White matter projection between the temporal lobes

Arachnoid mater. The middle layer of the meninges

Arachnoid villi. Small tubules that conduct CSF from subarachnoid space to dural sinus

Basal ganglia. Caudate, globus pallidus, putamen, subthalamic nucleus, substantia nigra

Cardinal planes. Anterior–posterior, superior–inferior, medial–lateral

Caudal. Toward the tail (coccygeal segments of spinal cord)

Cerebellar cortex. Gray matter external layer of cerebellar hemispheres

Cerebellar tentorium. Dural extension that lies between cerebellum and the occipital lobe

Cerebellopontine angle cistern. Site of CSF collection anterior and lateral to the cerebellum

Cerebral aqueduct. Passageway between the third and fourth ventricles

Cerebral cortex. Gray matter external layer of cerebral hemispheres

Cerebral peduncles. Bridge containing white matter projecting between the cerebrum and brainstem/spinal cord

Cerebrocerebellum. Lateral portion of cerebellum, connected to the dentate nuclei, associated with higher-order functions

Choroid plexus. Source of cerebrospinal fluid

Cisterna magna. Space between the brainstem and cerebellum where CSF collects

Corona radiate. White matter projections between parts of the cerebral hemispheres

Corpus callosum. Major white matter connection between the cerebral hemispheres

Cortico-ponto-cerebellar pathway. Pathway from cortex, synapsing in the pons, and projecting to the cerebellum

Deep cerebellar nuclei. Dentate, fastigial, globose and emboliform nuclei

Diencephalon. Portion of brain housing the thalamus, hypothalamus, epithalamus, and subthalamus

Dorsal. Superior aspect of brain, posterior aspect of spinal cord

Dura mater. Tough outermost layer of the meninges

Falx cerebri. Dura projection that separates the two cerebral hemispheres

Foramen of Magendie. Opening between the fourth ventricle to the cisterna magna

Foramina of Luschka. Openings from the 4th ventricle to the cerebellopontine angle cistern

Granule cells. Cerebellar cells that receive incoming information

Gray matter. Location of neuron cell bodies

Hippocampus (hippocampal formation). Gray matter in temporal lobe associated with memory

Hypothalamus. Hormone regulation center

Inferior cerebellar peduncle. Contains afferent axons originating in the inferior olivary complex and some coming in from the spinal cord

Inferior colliculus. Midbrain nucleus, associated with hearing

Inferior olivary complex. Medullary structure associated with the cerebellum and movement error detection

Internal capsule. White matter pathway between the brainstem and cerebral hemispheres or thalamus

Interventricular foramen. Passage between the lateral and third ventricle

Locus coeruleus. Midbrain nucleus, associated with norepinephrine release

Medial lemniscus. Fiber bundle conveying sensory information from brainstem to thalamus

Medial longitudinal fasciculus. Fiber bundle carrying control signals for eye movements up from vestibular nuclei up to eye movement centers

Middle cerebellar peduncle. Site of axons from the pons to the cerebellum

Myelin. Covering of neurons that facilitates neural propagation, made by Schwann cells in periphery and oligodendrocytes in CNS

Parallel fibers. Axons of granule cells that synapse on the Purkinje cells

Parasympathetic nervous system. Portion of autonomic nervous system located in cranial nerves and sacral cord, associated with relation

Pedunculopontine nucleus. One of the pontine nuclei in the midbrain, associated with acetylcholine release and locomotor function

Periaqueductal gray. Gray matter surrounding cerebral aqueduct

Pia mater. Innermost layer of meninges that adheres to the brain surface

Purkinje cells. The output cells of the cerebellum that project to the deep cerebellar nuclei

Raphe nuclei. Located in the caudal pons and rostral medulla, associated with arousal and pain transmission/modulation

Red nucleus. Large midbrain nucleus, origin of rubrospinal tract

Reticular formation. A column of nuclei throughout the brainstem associated with many functions; origin of reticulospinal tracts

Rostral. Toward the nose

Spinocerebellum. Midline cerebellar tissue, including the vermis, connects to the fastigial, globose and emboliform nuclei, associated with postural function

Striatum. The caudate and putamen nuclei

Superior colliculus. Midbrain nucleus, associated with vision

Superior cerebellar peduncle. Axons exiting the cerebellum and some coming in from the spinal cord

Sympathetic nervous system. Portion of autonomic nervous system in sympathetic chain ganglia, associated with arousal

Trigeminal nucleus. Sensory and motor nucleus of the trigeminal nerve

Ventral. Inferior aspect of brain, anterior of spinal cord

Ventral tegmental area. Midbrain gray matter, associated with dopamine projections that regulate reward and pleasure

Vestibulocerebellum. The flocculonodular lobe, associated with vestibular function, connected to the fastigial nucleus

White matter. Neuron axons covered with myelin

ABBREVIATIONS

CSF   cerebrospinal fluid
PAG   peri-aqueductal gray

Neuronal Structure and Function

2

John A. Buford and D. Michele Basso

OBJECTIVES

1) Delineate general principles underlying neuronal function and cellular signaling, including passive and active propagation of electrical potentials, communication between neurons, and how information is encoded for transmission through the nervous system

2) Describe the sequence of events for a neuron to receive, integrate, and transmit information, including EPSPs, IPSPs, action potentials, and synaptic transmission

3) Describe the role of glia (aka glial cells) in establishing and maintaining homeostasis in the CNS

4) Synthesize the role of microglia, astrocytes, and oligodendrocytes in motor learning and activity-dependent plasticity

5) Describe the factors that allow glia to communicate with each other and with neurons

● INTRODUCTION

In a multicellular organism, cells communicate with each other. This is true of all cells, and the broad name used in biology to describe this phenomenon is **cellular signaling**. Neurons are cells specialized for cellular signaling so that information can be received, processed, transmitted, stored, and retrieved.

As described in Chapter 3, neurons receive information from receptors in the body. These can be sensitive to internal signals (interoceptors) or external signals (exteroceptors). As described in Chapter 4, sensory neurons that receive certain kinds of input will transmit that information to the spinal cord where it can be processed to produce an outgoing neural command for a reflexive response. And for the reader of this chapter, it is hoped that some of the information coming into the brain through reading this chapter can be stored and later retrieved!

How do neurons do this? This chapter will explain basic mechanisms of neural structure and function. In addition, the structure and function of the glial cells, cells in the nervous system that support the functions of neurons, will also be described.

A Typical Neuron

A typical neuron has five main parts. We will begin our example focusing on cell type A (Figure 2-1A), the **projection interneuron**, and then discuss a few differences in cell types B and C. First, there is the **dendritic tree**. This is a structure of processes resembling the arbor of a tree that emanates from the cell body of the neuron. The dendritic tree is typically where information from other neurons is received (Figure 2-1A, C; blue). Next is the **soma**, the main part of the neuron's cell body (Figure 2-1, black). As with any cell in the body, a neuron will have a cell nucleus and the usual complement of intracellular organelles. These are contained in the soma, so from a biological perspective, the soma is the metabolic center of the cell. In terms of information processing, the soma is thought of as an **integrator** for most neurons (Figure 2-1A, C, green). From a certain point of view, all the information coming into a projection interneuron, at any point in time, is ultimately represented as one number: the voltage level of the cell membrane at the soma. So, the soma integrates all that input to form one result. The next part of the neuron is called the **axon hillock** (Figure 2-1A, gold), which is where the axon comes out of the soma, and ultimately, it can be thought of as the place where the action potential, the electrical event representing excitation of the neuron, is initiated. The next structure is the **axon**, a tubular process coming out of the soma (Figure 2-1, orange). It is the axon that allows for information to be transmitted from one place to another. Finally, there is the **axon terminal**, where packets of neurotransmitters are stored in vesicles that are ready to be released (Figure 2-1, pink). This neurotransmitter release is the typical means by which information from one neuron can be transmitted to another.

Sensory neurons have a slight variation in these parts (Figure 2-1B). The sensory receptor is where information comes in, not the dendritic tree. In fact, a sensory neuron in the somatosensory system does not even have a dendritic tree. The sensory receptor is connected to the axon, where we find a **trigger zone**. If the neuron is myelinated, the trigger zone is the 1st **Node of Ranvier** (Fig 2B, *), as illustrated here, and this is where the action potential is initiated. If the axon is not myelinated, the trigger zone where the action potential is initiated is a segment of axon near the receptor. Therefore, in a sensory neuron found in your body, e.g., coming from your foot, reception, integration, and encoding all occur within this distal region of the axon. The soma of a sensory neuron provides metabolic support but does not serve as an integrator of electrical information. The axon of the sensory neuron transmits information to axon terminals for output.

The parts of a local **interneuron** (Figure 2-1C) have functions like those of the projection interneuron. However, the projection interneuron will typically have a myelinated axon to allow for rapid transmission over long distances, whereas the axons of local interneurons are very short and are not myelinated.

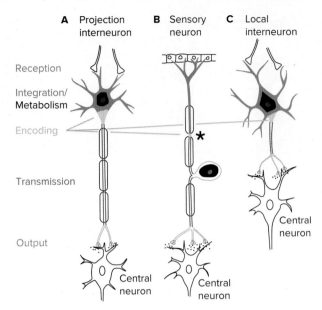

FIGURE 2-1 Picture of typical neuron with parts labeled by function. (A) Projection interneuron. This is the kind of cell that sends information to a relatively long distance in the nervous system. For example, there are projection neurons with their cell bodies in the cerebral cortex that reach the spinal cord with their axons. There are projection neurons in the deep cerebellar nuclei that reach the brainstem, etc. A projection neuron receives information through its dendrites and also on its cell body, the soma. The soma of this type of cell integrates the electrical information and also provides metabolic support for the cell as a whole. The place where the axon comes out of the soma is called the axon hillock, and this is where the information is encoded into action potentials, as explained later in this chapter. A projection neuron sends its output to other neurons. A sensory neuron **(B)** has a different structure. There is a distal projection of the axon to a peripheral receptor (or a free nerve ending), and a central projection into the spinal cord or brainstem (except for special senses, which are covered in later chapters). The cell body of a sensory neuron is located in a ganglion outside the central nervous system, and provides metabolic support, but typically does not serve as a point of connection among neurons. The distal part of the sensory axon is where information is integrated and encoded into action potentials, which travel into the nervous system to affect other cells. Local interneurons **(C)** are like projection interneurons, but much smaller. Their axons travel short distances and do not leave their local structure. The axons of these local cells are not myelinated. For each type of cell, the function served by each part is color coded. (Reproduced with permission from Kandel ER, Schwartz JH, Jessell TM, Siegelbaum SA, Hudspeth AJ. *Principles of Neural Science*. New York: McGraw-Hill; 2013.)

Overview of Neural Function

The Action Potential

Referring back to the parts of the neuron, we can begin to understand its functions. Let us start with the dendrites. For this example, some other neuron in the nervous system will release a neurotransmitter upon the dendrites. The place where this information exchange occurs is called a **synapse**. At the synapse, the neurotransmitter binds to receptor proteins in the cell membrane of the **dendrite**. These receptor proteins respond to the neurotransmitter, and thereby, have an effect on the cell. In

the typical example, this effect would be to open a pore in the cell membrane that allows increased permeability to a certain species of ion, such as sodium, at an active synapse.

At rest, due to metabolic processes and intracellular contents specific to neurons, there will be an **electrical potential** present between the inside and outside of the neuron. Typically, the inside of the cell is resting with a voltage level of about −65 mV compared to the outside. The voltage level across the cell membrane of the neuron is determined by the **electrochemical gradient**, which represents the combined influence of the **concentration gradient** and the **electrical (voltage) gradient**. The concentration gradient is the force that tends to make the concentration of any given ion equal on both sides of the membrane. The voltage gradient is the force that tends to make the voltage the same on both sides of the membrane. Because some ions have a greater affinity for electrons than others, when the influences of the concentration gradient and the voltage gradient are combined, the resulting equilibrium often means that neither the voltage nor the concentrations are both equal across the membrane. There is a compromise resulting in a slight difference in concentrations and a slight difference in voltage. The result is that there will be a voltage present across the cell membrane, and this voltage is what neurons use to represent information. As we will see, neurons can increase or decrease this voltage by increasing or decreasing their permeability to certain kinds of ions. Increased permeability to one kind of ion can cause the voltage to increase, whereas increased permeability to another kind of ion can make the voltage decrease. If sodium is allowed to flow into the cell at an active synapse, this will reduce the relatively negative potential inside the cell. Because the cell was negatively polarized before this event and becomes less negative once sodium starts coming in, this positive deflection of the cell's internal voltage potential is called **depolarization** of the cell.

A single synapse in reality would have an almost imperceptible effect on membrane voltage. Real neurons have thousands, even millions, of incoming synapses. But for the sake of this example, we will think of this one synapse as representing the concerted effort of many.

The depolarization of the dendrites causes a voltage change in the soma and, in turn, at the axon hillock as the electrical potential spreads passively along the membrane of the cell (**passive voltage**). At the axon hillock, there is a strong concentration of special kinds of proteins in the cell membrane. These are called voltage-gated sodium channels. This is a type of **voltage gated ion channel**, a protein that changes its shape, depending on the voltage potential of the cell membrane where it is located. At the relatively negative **resting membrane potential**, the voltage-gated sodium channel is closed, but when the membrane potential **depolarizes** past a certain level, called the **threshold**, the voltage-gated sodium channel snaps open and allows sodium to rush into the cell. This of course makes the cell depolarize even more, and sets off a brief period where there is a positive feedback loop: the rising voltage potential opens more voltage-gated sodium channels, causing an even further rise in potential. During this phase of the action potential, the neuron's membrane potential rises rapidly. At this point, we would say that the **action potential** has been initiated.

As this voltage begins to rise, after it goes above zero, a second type of voltage-gated ion channel opens, the voltage-gated potassium channel. Unlike sodium, which is at a relatively low concentration inside the cell, potassium is at a relatively high concentration inside the cell (an active cellular process called the **sodium potassium pump** maintains this **concentration gradient**). Potassium, therefore, rushes out of the cell, and as this positive charge is lost, the cell's membrane potential is pulled back down toward the resting membrane potential. At the same time, the voltage-gated sodium channels enter a special state called **inactive**. In the inactive state, caused by the very high membrane potential at the peak of the action potential, the sodium channels close and are temporarily stuck that way. In typical neurons like those involved in sensation and movement, the closed and inactive state lasts for about a millisecond. During this time, the potassium rushing out of the cell is able to return the membrane potential to a level at or below its resting potential. When membrane potential falls to a level that is lower than the resting the membrane potential, the cell is said to be **hyperpolarized**. Because the voltage-gated sodium channels are inactive while

this is happening, it is impossible for the cell to make another action potential during this time. We call this the **absolute refractory period.** Then, the voltage-gated potassium channels begin closing, the voltage-gated sodium channels come out of their inactive state, and the sodium potassium pump works to restore the preexisting concentration gradients. At this point, the action potential is over, and the cell is ready to respond again. For a brief time, after the voltage-gated sodium channels are back in their resting state (closed, active) but before the concentration gradients are fully restored, it is still relatively difficult to make a new action potential while the cell reestablishes equilibrium, and this period is called the **relative refractory period** (Figure 2-2).

One thing to bear in mind is that very little actual flow of sodium and potassium ions is required to make the action potential. Remembering from basic physics, voltage (V) is the product of current (I) and resistance (R): $V = I \times R$. The resistance of a cell membrane is very, very high. Therefore, because membrane resistance is very high, it doesn't require very much

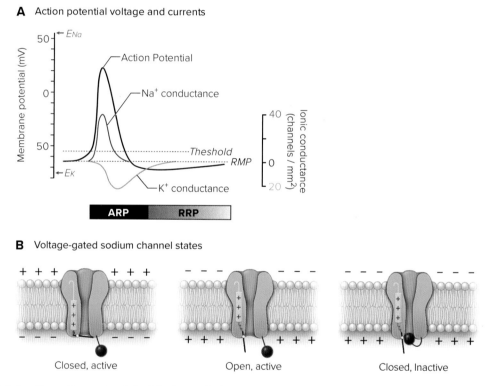

A Action potential voltage and currents

B Voltage-gated sodium channel states

Closed, active   Open, active   Closed, Inactive

FIGURE 2-2 Explaining the action potential with channels, ions, and voltages. In **A**, the voltage that would be recorded between the inside and outside of a single neuron during an action potential is illustrated in black. The red curve indicates how easily Na+ can flow through the cell membrane (i.e., Na+ conductance) during the action potential, and the blue curve shows K+ conductance. Threshold is the voltage level required for an action potential to be initiated. Once the membrane potential exceeds the threshold, and action potential will definitely occur. RMP stands for resting membrane potential. E_K is the voltage the membrane would reach if potassium channels were open and stayed open (called the **equilibrium potential**), and E_{NA} is the equilibrium potential for sodium. ARP stands for absolute refractory period, the time when a new action potential cannot begin. RRP stands for relative refractory period, the time when it is relatively difficult to make a new action potential. In **B**, the three possible states for one type of ion channel, voltage-gated sodium channels, are illustrated. In the resting state, the channel is closed but responsive and can be moved into the open state if the voltage across the cell membrane exceeds threshold. Sodium can only flow during the open, active state, but when the voltage across the membrane gets even more positive and stays that way for a certain amount of time, the channel will enter the inactivated state. Once it becomes inactivated, the channel is closed, and it stays that way for a long enough time to allow the action potential to be completed. (**A.** Reproduced with permission from Kandel ER, Schwartz JH, Jessell TM, Siegelbaum SA, Hudspeth AJ, eds. *Principles of Neural Science.* McGraw Hill; 2013, and Reproduced with permission from Hodgkin AL, Huxley AF. A quantitative description of membrane current and its application to conduction and excitation in nerve. *J Physiol.* 1952;117(4):500-544. **B.** Reproduced with permission from Kandel ER, Schwartz JH, Jessell TM, Siegelbaum SA, Hudspeth AJ. *Principles of Neural Science.* New York: McGraw-Hill; 2013.)

current (I) to get voltage (V) to change. This means that the actual concentrations of sodium and potassium inside and outside of the cell have not changed dramatically during the action potential. There is not much work for the sodium potassium pump to do to restore the resting state.

Propagation of Action Potentials

Once an action potential is initiated, it will spread like a wave along the length of the axon. In some neurons, part of the cell body and even the most proximal parts of the dendrites (**proximal dendrite**) also have the appropriate complement of **ion channels** to create and propagate action potentials. For the purpose of this explanation, we will only consider propagation along an axon.

As explained above, when enough current enters the cell at a synapse to bring the membrane potential above threshold, an action potential is initiated. We can think of the current flowing into the cell through the voltage-gated sodium channels at the initiation of the action potential in the same way. Once membrane potential rises in the part of the membrane where threshold has been reached, the voltage is also felt in the surrounding membrane. However, the farther away we are along the membrane, the more the voltage has decayed. In a healthy axon, the voltage-gated sodium channels are close enough together that, as long as one segment of membrane has reached threshold, there definitely will be enough voltage present at the location of the next voltage-gated sodium channel to bring it above threshold, as well. Hence, if the axon is healthy, once an action potential is initiated, it will propagate all the way to the end of the axon.

In a myelinated axon, special glial cells (explained later) provide an insulating layer around the axon. This helps prevent the passive decay of the potential so that the voltage-gated sodium channels can be spaced farther apart. While it is true that the voltage-gated sodium channels open very quickly once threshold is reached, there is definitely time required for the protein shape to change and the pore to open. The illustration in Figure 2-3 explains how myelin allows for faster propagation of the action potential. The second major factor determining conduction velocity of a nerve is its diameter. Increased diameter of a nerve also allows greater spacing between ion channels, and therefore, also increases conduction velocity. Myelin is much more effective at increasing conduction velocity than size, so myelination allows axons to be both small and fast.

Synaptic Function

When the action potential reaches the end of the axon, its electrical potential arrives at the synaptic terminals. Here, instead of voltage-gated sodium channels, there are **voltage-gated calcium channels**. When these open, the influx of calcium activates a system that transports **synaptic vesicles** full of neurotransmitter to the edge of the synaptic membrane. The vesicles release the neurotransmitter into the gap, called the **synaptic cleft**, between the synaptic terminal and the next neuron. In describing the function of a synapse, we call the cell releasing the neurotransmitter the **presynaptic neuron**, and the cell being affected the **postsynaptic neuron**. The neurotransmitter diffuses to bind with receptors on the postsynaptic neuron in a region called the **postsynaptic terminal**, and this allows the postsynaptic cell to receive the information.

As shown in Figure 2-4A, illustrating the **postsynaptic terminal** the receptor in the membrane of the postsynaptic neuron will have a part outside the membrane, which is the part where the chemical binding occurs with the neurotransmitter, and a part that spans the cell membrane and reaches inside the cell. These are called the **extracellular domain** (outside) and the **intracellular domain** (inside). Some receptors serve as ion channels, such that when the neurotransmitter binds to the receptor, the ion channel opens and current flows to change the membrane potential of the postsynaptic neuron. These are called **ionotropic receptors**. Another name for this is a **ligand-gated ion channel**. In Figure 2-4B, the illustration shows that when a neurotransmitter binds to an ionotropic receptor, there is a change in the physical shape and properties of that molecule so that the ion channel opens and ionic current can flow through the channel. Other kinds of receptors, called **metabotropic receptors**, have extracellular sites that a neuromodulator will bind to and an intracellular domain that influences the postsynaptic neuron. Metabotropic receptors can act on ion channels from the inside of the cell to influence their permeability. Sometimes, this is through a series of proteins that are physically connected to the ion channel on the inside of the cell. In other cases, the intracellular domain acts like an enzyme to influence cellular processes through biochemical pathways. In most cases, the effects of metabotropic receptors are longer lasting than those of ionotropic receptors. When we think of the rapid transmission of information from one neuron to the next, we are usually thinking of functions dominated by ionotropic receptors. When we are thinking of longer-term processes like sleep–wake cycles or learning, these are typically dominated by metabotropic receptor functions.

To this point, we have focused on the ability of the postsynaptic neuron to respond to the presynaptic neuron. It is just as necessary for this response to come to an end. Otherwise, a synapse could be activated only once, and no new information could ever be received. There are two basic processes that lead to the end of the synaptic response. The first is simple **diffusion**. Like any chemical reaction, the binding between the neurotransmitter and the receptor depends on a concentration gradient. The neurotransmitter will not stay bound forever. As time passes, the neurotransmitter molecules diffuse out of the synaptic cleft and can no longer bind with the receptors. The second is **enzymatic degradation**. Enzymes, produced either by neurons or glia, are present in the extracellular space around neurons, and these cleave neurotransmitter molecules into constituent parts, which also lowers the concentration of neurotransmitter. Not every neurotransmitter is subjected to enzymatic degradation. For very small neurotransmitter molecules, diffusion may be sufficient.

In addition to diffusion and enzymatic degradation, the presynaptic neuron will often have a **reuptake** process. Whole or broken-down neurotransmitter will be actively resorbed into the **presynaptic terminal** and repackaged into vesicles. This saves the cell energy compared to reassembling the molecule from scratch. Some neurotransmitters can be reassembled quickly at the terminal of the presynaptic neuron, whereas others must be transported back to the soma by a process called **retrograde axonal transport**. There is also a system that carries proteins from the soma to the terminals, and this is called **anterograde axonal transport**. In this way, the metabolic machinery required for the synapse to function is kept in

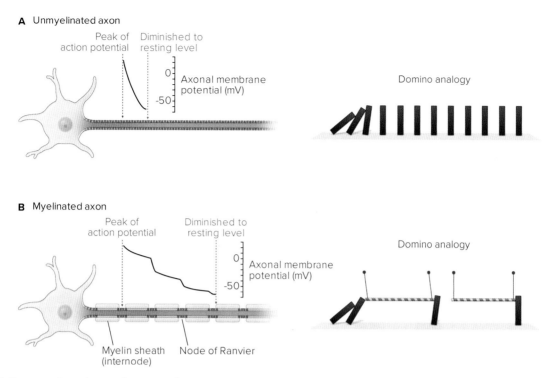

A Unmyelinated axon

Peak of action potential

Diminished to resting level

Axonal membrane potential (mV)

Domino analogy

B Myelinated axon

Peak of action potential

Diminished to resting level

Axonal membrane potential (mV)

Myelin sheath (internode)

Node of Ranvier

Domino analogy

FIGURE 2-3 Propagation of an action potential along an axon, including the function of myelin. In **A**, the function of an unmyelinated axon in propagating an action potential is shown. Blue indicates resting membrane potential (negative), and red indicates depolarization, which is excitatory and relatively positive. If the cell is excited enough to exceed threshold at the axon hillock, an action potential occurs there. At the point of the red arrow, we can imagine this is a place on the axon where this part of the membrane is at the peak voltage of the action potential. If we were to measure the voltage at this precise instant in time at other places on the axon farther away, we would measure lower voltages due to passive decay, such that, at the purple arrow, membrane voltage would appear to be at rest. At that distance, the effect of the action potential occurring at the red arrow would produce no measurable voltage at the purple arrow. However, the voltage-gated sodium channels are spaced closely enough so that the voltage is still above threshold and the next voltage-gated sodium channel will be excited enough to open, allowing the action potential to propagate. In **B**, the effect of myelin is shown. Because myelin reduces passive decay due to leakage, the voltage present at the red arrow doesn't get much smaller even though we are relatively far away. The purple arrow is much farther away in the myelinated axon. This means the voltage-gated sodium channels can be farther away from each other in the myelinated axon. At each node of Ranvier (the gaps between myelin), there is a concentration of the voltage-gated sodium and voltage-gated potassium channels responsible for re-creation of the action potential. Due to the current flow at the node, where there is no myelin, there is more leakage at the node and more voltage is lost at the nodes. But in a healthy neuron, there is enough preservation of voltage to still surpass threshold 2 or 3 nodes away from the peak of the action potential. Thus, we move farther down the axon more quickly. The domino analogy to the right provides a physical phenomenon that does something similar. With voltage-gated sodium channels close together in the unmyelinated axon, the voltage is sufficient to open the next channel, but opening a channel and having enough current flow through to reach a peak at that location takes time. This time is analogous to the time required for one domino to tip far enough to hit the next. With myelin, the distance between channels can be farther. Like the straw transmitting force between the dominos in the lower figure, the myelin allows the voltage to travel farther, so fewer voltage-gated sodium channels are needed. Hence, the last domino will tip over sooner in the lower example, just as the action potential will reach the end of the axon sooner in the myelinated axon. Just like the lower example means fewer dominoes have to go through the time-consuming process of being tipped over, in a myelinated axon, fewer ion channels have to go through the time-consuming process of changing their shape to allow current flow. Therefore, a myelinated axon transmits an action potential faster than an unmyelinated one. (Original figure by John Buford.)

good working order, and a ready supply of neurotransmitter is maintained (see Box 2-1 for more details).

Non-synaptic Communication between Neurons

At some locations in the nervous system, there are connections between dendrites of neurons called gap junctions where the electrical potential of one cell directly affects the other without the need for a chemical synapse. There are also receptors on neurons that are not at synapses. These would be sensitive to hormones and neuromodulators. Neuromodulators are like neurotransmitters, but their action is indirect. A neuromodulator can bind to metabotropic receptors to affect membrane potential indirectly by modifying the effectiveness of a neurotransmitter, or by affecting ion channels that do not have extracellular receptors. Neuromodulators can also have influences on neurons other than changes in membrane potential. There are neurons in the CNS that release neuromodulators in a relatively nonspecific manner into the space around a group of neurons, providing a concentration of the neuromodulator through the local tissue, affecting many neurons in the region simultaneously. In a sense, this allows for a local concentration of a hormone-like substance to regulate a group of cells.

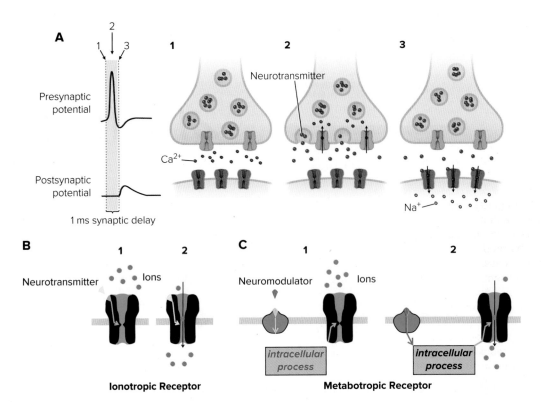

FIGURE 2-4 A. Synaptic function. In 1, the synapse is shown just before an action potential arrives. The voltage is just about to rise in the presynaptic terminal. Synaptic vesicles have neurotransmitter (blue dots) ready to release, and Ca^{2+} is present in the extracellular space. At the time point labeled 2, the action potential has arrived, voltage-gated calcium channels are open, and Ca^{2+} is entering the presynaptic terminal. This causes exocytosis of the neurotransmitter into the synaptic cleft. There is a time delay for diffusion and the binding of the neurotransmitter to the postsynaptic cell's receptors at the **postsynaptic terminal**, before any sodium can enter the postsynaptic cell at time 3 to produce a voltage change in the postsynaptic cell. This time lag is called the synaptic delay. **B. Ionotropic receptors.** For an ionotropic receptor, the ion channel configuration, open or closed, is directly affected by the binding of the neurotransmitter. In the resting state (1), the channel is closed. When the neurotransmitter binds to the receptor (2), it causes the receptor to open so that ions can flow through the channel. **C. Metabotropic receptors.** For metabotropic receptors, the receptor is not an ion channel, but it has the potential to affect ion channels. In (1), the neuromodulator is not bound to the receptor, so there is no link between the receptor and the ion channel; the intracellular process is not activated. In (2), with the neuromodulator bound to the receptor, the intracellular domain of the receptor initiates an intracellular process that opens the ion channel. (**A.** Reproduced with permission from Kandel ER, Schwartz JH, Jessell TM, Siegelbaum SA, Hudspeth AJ. *Principles of Neural Science*, McGraw-Hill; 2013. **B** and **C** originals by John Buford.)

The Integrative Functions of Neurons

As described earlier, in typical synaptic transmission involving ionotropic receptors, the postsynaptic neuron responds because it has a receptor. The action of the receptor on the postsynaptic cell is what determines the response. If the receptor allows positive current to flow into the cell, then it depolarizes the postsynaptic neuron, which is called **excitation**. However, if activating the receptor allows current flow to make the inside of the cell even more negative (hyperpolarized), we call this **inhibition**. Inhibition can occur due to positive ions flowing out of the cell or negative ions flowing into the cell; technically, any ionotropic receptor that produces current flow tending to hold membrane potential at an equilibrium that is below threshold is inhibitory. The potential recorded in the postsynaptic neuron is, therefore, given one of two names, either an **excitatory postsynaptic potential** (EPSP) or an **inhibitory postsynaptic potential** (IPSP).

As we look at the organization of synaptic inputs on a typical neuron, we notice a consistent pattern. Synapses that produce EPSPs tend to be on the dendritic tree but can also be on the soma. However, the synapses that produce IPSPs consistently tend to be on or near the soma. This leads to what is referred to as the **integrative property of neurons**. It takes a concerted effort to generate enough EPSPs to depolarize a neuron above threshold and cause it to generate an action potential. However, inhibition of a neuron can be effective quickly and can efficiently override incoming excitation. Philosophically, this makes sense. Once we take an action in the outside world, there are consequences, and if the action was a mistake, it can be hard to undo. However, if we choose not to take action, there will often be a second chance. Synaptic inputs to neurons are organized in such a manner that there must be strong influence to take action; "no votes" due to inhibition seem to take priority.

Transduction and Encoding of Information by Neurons

Membrane Potential

The ultimate result of the integration of EPSPs and IPSPs by a neuron is the generation of a membrane potential at the axon

Box 2-1   Understanding Pharmacology and Tract Tracing Based on Synaptic Function

As explained in this section, there are receptors in post-synaptic neurons, and neurotransmitters are chemicals that bind to these receptors. For synaptic function to succeed, there is either an active reuptake process or an enzymatic degradation process so that the action of a neurotransmitter can be short lived. Many of the medicines that act on the nervous system do so by affecting synaptic function. Some medicines bind to the receptors in a more durable way than the natural neurotransmitter and are harder for the enzymatic degradation systems to break down. They act like super potent neurotransmitters. Neurotoxins would be the extreme case where potency is so high, the synapse is irreversibly blocked. Another type of medicine will affect the reuptake process, allowing longer lasting effects from the naturally present neurotransmitters. These **reuptake inhibitors** have the advantage that the presence of the neurotransmitter at any given synapse is natural, having been initiated by the nervous system. Ideally, the reuptake inhibitor makes the natural process stronger but does not introduce actions that wouldn't have naturally occurred.

The ability of neuroscientists to trace tracts in the nervous system also stems from what we just learned. Through experimentation, compounds have been discovered that have a part of their molecular structure shaped just right to make the presynaptic neuron absorb and transport the compound back to the soma as if it was needed by the cell. Typically, these compounds are inert and have no effect on neural function, but because they are not natural, histological processing of the tissue, followed by microscopic analysis, can show which neurons have the compound. This is called **retrograde tracing**. In animal models, retrograde tracing has identified the spatial distribution of neurons which make up nuclei in the brain and project to other brain regions and throughout the spinal cord.[1] Likewise, there are compounds that are absorbed by the soma and will be carried through the anterograde axonal transport system, allowing **anterograde tracing**.[2] Through these experimental approaches, scientists have traced many of the pathways in the brain, and this monumental effort continues.

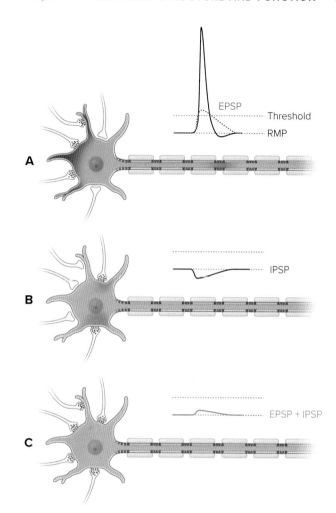

FIGURE 2-5 A cell integrating various inputs. In the upper panel, a cell being excited by multiple excitatory synapses is shown. The EPSP is large and triggers an action potential. In the middle panel, the cell is affected by a pair of inhibitory synapses, and it makes an IPSP. In C, both sets of synapses are active. Because the inhibitory synapses are closer to the axon hillock and because they increase the conductance of the cell, the EPSP is substantially reduced in amplitude and does not produce an action potential. With the ion channels on the soma opened by the inhibitory synapses, membrane resistance is reduced so that passive potentials from the dendrites decay quickly and are not transmitted very effectively to the axon hillock. Hence, inhibition tends to override excitation.

Rate Coding

Rate coding is the principal means by which the excitement level of one neuron is transferred to the next. At a synapse, when action potentials arrive in rapid succession, the concentration of neurotransmitter in the synaptic cleft rises and a higher proportion of the receptors are activated for a greater proportion of the time. This translates into larger EPSPs and a greater depolarization of the postsynaptic cell. In this way, the higher level of excitement is transferred from one cell to the next. Likewise, in sensory receptors, when the stimulus is stronger, more receptor channels are open for a longer time, and the **generator potential** is stronger (Figure 2-6).

How, then, does this higher level of excitement transfer again to the next cell? The greater the level of depolarization at the

---

hillock (Figure 2-5). For a typical neuron within the central nervous system, synaptic inputs are the influences that determine fluctuations in membrane potential. However, there are other means by which the membrane potential can change. Indeed, in some neurons, synaptically driven EPSPs and IPSPs do not even occur. One example is in sensory receptors. For these cells, the adequate stimulus is what creates a change in membrane potential. For a sensory receptor in the skin, mechanical deformation of the receptor channels is what opens the ion channel, allowing sodium to flow in. In this case, the initiation of the action potential actually starts at the end of the axon and proceeds toward the cell body, as explained in Chapter 3. In the vestibular system, hair cells create membrane potential changes in a different manner. Despite these variations, one common principle applies: the more depolarized the cell membrane is, the more excited the cell is, and the nervous system must have a way to transfer that level of excitement from one neuron to the next.

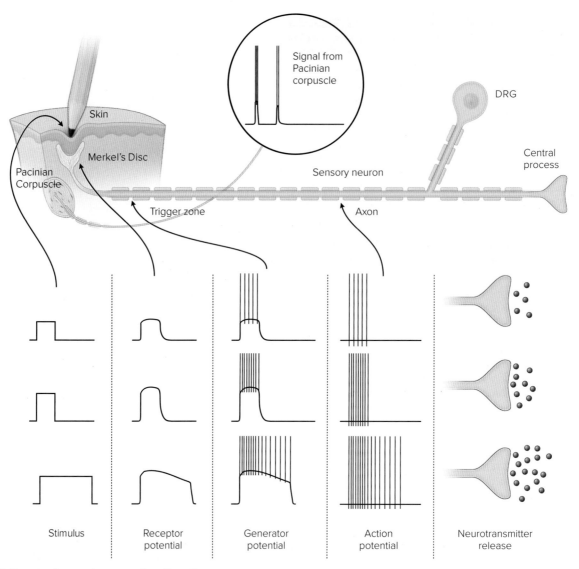

FIGURE 2-6 Rate coding and temporal coding. The encoding of information by a sensory receptor is illustrated. Imagine a pencil touches the skin for a fixed duration, gently in the upper panel, moderately in the middle, and moderately and for a longer duration on the bottom. The receptor potential in the sensory receptor (e.g., Merkel's disc) is proportional in size and duration to the actual stimulus. At the trigger zone, this is translated into a burst of action potentials with a rate that is proportional to the size of the receptor potential. By the time the burst of action potentials is propagated along the axon, the voltage from the receptor potential has passively decayed, but the information about the stimulus is preserved in the rate of action potentials. When this reaches the axon terminal, higher rate and longer burst durations result in higher amounts of neurotransmitter release. This in turn affects EPSP size in the postsynaptic membrane as information is transferred to the next cell. The relationship between stimulus amplitude and the rate of action potentials is called rate coding. The relationship between the onset and offset of the stimulus and the beginning and end of the burst of action potentials is called temporal coding. There is a second aspect to temporal coding, shown by the Pacinian corpuscle. These receptors fire rapidly at the beginning and end of the stimulus, providing increased accuracy in detecting the onset and offset of the stimulus. (Reproduced with permission from Kandel ER, Schwartz JH, Jessell TM, Siegelbaum SA, Hudspeth AJ, eds. *Principles of Neural Science*, McGraw-Hill 2013.)

axon hillock (or for a sensory neuron, at the initial segment), the more rapidly action potentials are created. If the membrane potential is just barely above threshold, then, after the action potential occurs, there will be a relatively weak electrical current flowing to push the membrane potential back over threshold, and the next action potential will not occur right away. However, if the membrane potential is substantially above threshold due to strong excitation, then, there will be a strong electrical current, and the cell will rapidly exceed threshold and fire again. Of course, the relative refractory period will tend to limit the firing

rate once very high rates are reached, and the absolute refractory period places an upper limit on firing rate.

Temporal Coding

Temporal coding, in the simplest sense, means that when the stimulus or neural drive begins, this is signaled by an increase (or decrease) in the firing rate, and the change occurs back to the baseline condition, when the stimulus or period of central drive is finished. In addition, the nervous system frequently uses a secondary means of temporal coding. Some neurons have a rapid burst (or sudden dropout) of activity at the beginning or end of an event. This helps accentuate the beginning and end of a command from one part of the nervous system to the other. In sensory systems, we call these rapidly adapting cells. Within the nervous system, cells that respond like this are often called **phasic neurons**. Other kinds of neurons have more steady responses, continue to make action potentials at a consistent rate as long as the stimulus is present or the command is ongoing. In sensory systems, these are called **slowly adapting cells**. Within the CNS, we call these **tonic neurons**.

Adaptation

Adaptation is a key feature of neural responses that affects rate coding and temporal coding. Turning back to Figure 2-6, examine the **receptor potential** for the lower panel, the moderate and long duration stimulus. Notice how the receptor potential gets smaller over time even though the stimulus strength is constant. Is this a mistake? Is there something wrong with the receptor? No, this is adaptation, and it is a normal and useful feature of sensory receptors. As detailed further in Chapter 3, some sensory receptors are rapidly adapting and some are slowly adapting. As shown in Figure 2-6, the combination of both kinds of receptors for certain kinds of sensory information helps provide more information about the sensory experience.

Temporal Summation

As described above for rate coding, when multiple EPSPs arrive in rapid succession, the response of the postsynaptic cell is stronger. In part, this is because the synapse is fully activated. But another factor is that the membrane potential caused by the first EPSP may still be present when the second EPSP occurs. The voltage from the second rides upon the first, achieving a greater depolarization than either alone could have achieved. This is called temporal summation and will be discussed further in Chapter 4. It can occur for IPSPs as well as for EPSPs. For most central nervous system pathways, arrival of one EPSP on the postsynaptic cell will not be sufficient to generate an action potential. Temporal summation is usually required. The presynaptic neuron might need to send a dozen action potentials in rapid succession to get the postsynaptic cell to make just a few action potentials.

Spatial Summation

Spatial summation occurs when multiple different incoming sources are all trying to excite the cell. For example, your balance control system, your reflexes, and your voluntary effort might all be trying to produce the same response at the same time. In this case, the motoneurons for the relevant muscle will be receiving EPSPs from three separate pathways all at the same time. These synaptic contacts would all be landing on slightly different parts of the motoneuron, so the voltage from these different spatial locations on the cell would all combine to produce a substantial depolarization. This is spatial summation.

Storage of Information: Neural Plasticity

Changes in Synaptic Strengths and Connections between Neurons

Synapses can change over time to become stronger or weaker.[3] The presence of an action potential in a neuron is not only an electrical event, but it is also a metabolic event. Through receptors and biochemical pathways that are sensitive to the intracellular consequences of the action potential, long-term changes in the cell can occur. This can occur through the growth of dendritic spines, such that the postsynaptic cell develops a small outgrowth to make closer contact with the presynaptic terminal. It can also involve expansion of the postsynaptic membrane's receptor zone under the synapse. The postsynaptic cell can make a larger number of receptors so that the response at its synapses is stronger. The presynaptic cell can increase the size of the presynaptic terminal, release higher quantities of neurotransmitter, and sprout new axon terminals to increase the number of contacts with the postsynaptic cell. The postsynaptic cell can increase the number and size of synaptic receptor zones. For each of these instances, there can be a decrease, instead, and these kinds of changes can occur for synapses that make EPSPs or IPSPs. As noted in the section on non-synaptic communication between neurons, neuromodulators can regulate the effectiveness of neurotransmitters. In addition to this short-term effect, they can also stimulate the long-term changes in synaptic function described here (Figure 2-7).

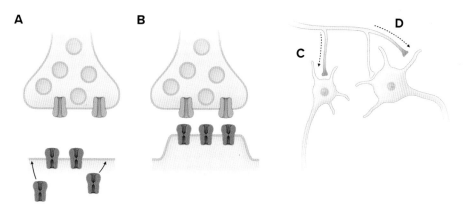

FIGURE 2-7 Changes in synapses and sprouting. In **A**, increased effectiveness of a synapse is illustrated by an increased number of postsynaptic receptors. In **B**, the development of a synaptic spine is shown, such that the size of the synaptic cleft is reduced, making the synapse more efficient. In **C**, an axon collateral sprouts to connect to a nearby cell that was previously not connected. In **D**, the axon sprouts a new branch increasing the number of connections to the postsynaptic cell. (Original figure by John Buford.)

There is also a phenomenon known as a **silent synapse.**[4,5] There are potential connections between neurons in the nervous system that are not functioning because the postsynaptic cell does not have the proper complement of receptors. If a new behavioral pattern develops (e.g., lots of practice of a new skill) such that the activity of the two cells is correlated and they are firing together, the silent synapses can become active. For this to occur, the postsynaptic cell activates metabolic pathways to make receptors and insert them in the postsynaptic membrane to make that synapse active and able to respond to the presynaptic cell.

In sum, connections between neurons change with experience and practice. As an analogy, if you find that every time you take advice from a certain friend, you succeed, you will pay more and more attention to that friend. If activity between a presynaptic and postsynaptic neuron is correlated with success, the connection will become stronger. Synapses that do not become stronger through this process will become weaker in comparison. A common saying that comes from this phenomenon is, "Neurons that fire together wire together," based on the work published by Hebb in 1949 and since confirmed through more basic studies.[6]

GLIAL CELLS

Glia of the Nervous System

The most predominant cells in the central nervous system are not neurons but rather glia – small cells having multiple processes but no axons or dendrites. Their prevalence and size suggested to early scientists that they functioned as "glue" to hold the nervous system together and were given the name for glue in Greek – glia. While there is little evidence that glia work as glue, recent findings are showing that they play important roles in maintaining normal homeostasis within the CNS. In fact, some scientists are beginning to explore whether dysfunction of glia alone can create clinical impairments. There are three types of glia or neuroglia, as they are also called – astrocytes, microglia, and oligodendrocytes.

Astrocytes

Astrocytes are named because of their star-like shape and radial projections. They can be divided into two types, based on differences in shape and location. Protoplasmic astrocytes occupy gray matter regions in the brain and spinal cord and have many main projections with uniform small branches, forming a dense globoid structure (Figure 2-8). Fibrous astrocytes are found in white matter regions and have long, thin fibers. Both of these types of astrocytes place end feet onto blood vessels which allows them to monitor changes in the vasculature. This tight relationship means that astrocytes detect and respond to blood vessel dilation, movement of cells across the vessel wall, and CNS edema. Astrocytes also make contact with neural synapses, in the gray matter, and with nodes of Ranvier, in the white matter. Thus, each astrocyte extends end feet to both vessels and neural structures, comprising the neurovascular unit. In some regions of the brain, a single astrocyte covers more than 100,000 synapses from many different neurons.[7] Astrocytes also extend processes to neighboring astrocytes. In this way, they form a tile-like pattern with astrocytic processes touching, but not overlapping each other, and covering the entire nervous system.

Historically, neuroglia were considered only as structural support for neurons and axons. However, with scientific and technological advances, it is now clear that the structural

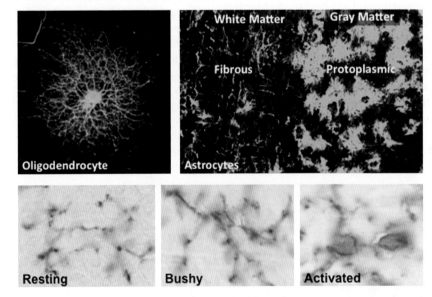

FIGURE 2-8 Microscopic images of oligodendrocytes, astrocytes, and microglia. The oligodendrocyte cell body is centrally located and surrounded by numerous delicate protrusions. Note the different morphology of the fibrous and protoplasmic astrocytes which are located in the white and gray matter, respectively. The tile-like relationship of the protoplasmic astrocytes is clear, with only the end feet in close proximity. Microglia are shown in three states – resting, bushy profile and activated. The activation of microglia includes thickening of the ramifications which presents as a bushy morphology. When they are fully activated, the cell body greatly enlarges and the arms are retracted. Oligodendrocytes and astrocytes were labeled with a green fluorescent protein while the microglia were labeled with a brown chromagen. (Used with permission of D. McTigue and DM Basso, The Ohio State University.)

organization of astrocytes allows them to influence or control a wide number of functions in the CNS. The large number of contacts on both blood vessels and synapses enables them to control blood flow in the brain and spinal cord to match the needs of neural regions with high activity.[8] Greater synaptic activity produces higher calcium levels in the astrocyte that translate into the release of compounds that increase blood vessel dilation to produce greater blood flow in an activity-dependent manner. Astrocytes also release compounds that induce vasoconstriction and appear to finely regulate regional blood flow in the CNS.

Astrocytes play a fundamental role in metabolic and trophic support to neurons. Glycogen storage occurs primarily in astrocytes, and the highest concentrations are found in brain regions with the highest neural activity, and therefore, the greatest metabolic need.[9] Neurotransmitters like glutamate, released during neural firing, modulate glycogen. Astrocytes break down glycogen, producing the metabolite lactate, which is critical for maintaining synapses and promoting new synaptic growth. The **synaptic strength** needed for learning and memory depends on astrocytic metabolic support. The metabolites are transferred to both neurons and axons, where they are used for aerobic metabolism when other sources of energy are low.[10]

One of the most important roles of astrocytes is to maintain normal, nontoxic ionic, fluid, and neurotransmitter levels. Astrocytes shuttle ions like potassium from the extracellular space through transporters on their surface.[9] To control interstitial fluids, water channels, called aquaporin 4, are highly concentrated on astrocytic end feet on blood vessels and reduce fluids. Astrocytes buffer the neurotoxic effects of high levels of neurotransmitters, especially glutamate. Excessive glutamate, as occurs after brain or spinal cord injury, induces pronounced cell death in the CNS and must be quickly and carefully buffered. Astrocytes play a primary role in removing excess glutamate from the extracellular space via transporters that move glutamate into the astrocyte, where it is converted into its precursor, and then, released back into the synaptic space for future use. These homeostatic mechanisms are often overwhelmed in acute CNS trauma and lead to lesion expansion beyond the initial insult. Extensive research is directed toward improving these homeostatic mechanisms in an effort to enhance ion, fluid, and glutamate clearance.[9]

Astrocytes respond to a variety of molecules, including growth factors, inflammatory substances, degeneration substrates, like A beta, and cell death factors, like free radicals. Two important responses emerge in reaction to these events: (1) calcium signaling to neurons and other astrocytes and (2) astrogliosis which means a large increase in astrocytes. By regulating internal calcium concentrations, oscillations develop within the astrocyte that trigger neurotransmitter release that likely changes synaptic activity directly.[9] The internal calcium influx also moves in waves to the neighboring astrocytes through gap junctions and can convey cellular changes over great distances from one part of the nervous system to another. The calcium waves enable signaling in both astrocytes and neurons under normal conditions and during disease or trauma. In times of disease or damage, the astrocytes change their shape, function, and number. The astrocytes closest to the site of injury or

disease have the greatest response, and it gradually decreases the farther away from the site. Here, the astrocytes adopt a reactive phenotype with enlarged cell bodies and processes and increase in number by migrating to the site or through proliferation. Unlike in the normal state, reactive astrocytes overlap extensively, which has important implication for neuropathology of spinal cord injury which will be discussed in Chapter 12. Taken together, these complex changes are called **astrogliosis**. High levels of astrogliosis produce glial scarring, which can be neuroprotective by limiting the spread of toxins, inflammation, and infection. Glial scarring can also be disruptive by preventing axonal growth or synaptic plasticity, producing inflammation, releasing toxic substances, like glutamate, and causing edema.[9]

Microglia

Microglia, under normal conditions, are tiny cells with many, finely ramified processes. Like astrocytes, they are widely distributed, without overlapping, throughout the gray and white matter in the brain and spinal cord. Microglia are the resident immune cells in the CNS and protect the nervous system from infection, disease, and the consequences of injury. In their finely ramified state, they are considered to be "resting microglia" (see Figure 2-8) but routinely perform surprisingly fast movements. The fine microglial endings repeatedly extend to the nearby cells, interstitial fluid, and neuropil to survey for unusual changes. Scientists have been able to label brain microglia, allowing them to capture microglial surveillance movements under normal conditions. These movies are fascinating in how active and expansive the resting microglia movements are.[11]

As resident immune cells, a variety of microbes and substances can activate microglia, and in response, they adopt different shapes and functions along a continuum. From the resting, finely ramified state (Figure 2-8), microglia partially retract their processes becoming thicker and bushy while the cell body enlarges (Figure 2-8). With greater exposure to the signals, microglia become fully activated with fewer protrusions and even larger cell bodies (Figure 2-8). In the final stage, the microglia assume a round, amoeboid shape without any protrusion. In this form, they are called macrophages that phagocytose debris and damaged cells. Interestingly, monocytes from the blood also cross the vasculature into the parenchyma and become macrophages. Resident and blood-borne macrophages are indistinguishable from each other.[12,13]

Activated microglia and macrophages restore homeostasis not only by engulfing damaged cells but also by modulating excitotoxicity and promoting neuroplasticity. Injured neurons emit toxic factors such as excessive glutamate and free radicals, which recruit activated microglia to surround the toxic neuron.[14] This synaptic stripping reduces the toxic cascade and may support neural regeneration. Synaptic stripping also plays a role in plasticity (Chapter 9). Additionally, at least one important signal comes from the neuron and binds to a receptor on the activated microglia/macrophage which is thought to protect the neuron from phagocytosis. Activated microglia also participate in neuroplasticity by pruning synapses or secreting enzymes that open space in the neuropil for new growth. The microglia also appear to preferentially encircle synapses that are highly active, suggesting a role in experience-dependent plasticity.[14]

Microglia defend the CNS against frank disruption from trauma, disease, or infection while also putting mechanisms in place to restore homeostasis. They mediate the immune response in the CNS by presenting antigen-initiating microglial activation and recruiting other cells to the threatened region.[15] Microglia express many substances or receptors in response to changes in homeostasis. These factors are called cytokines and chemokines. **Cytokines** determine the state of activation of microglia and function by activating not only the cell that expresses them but also neighboring microglial. This means they exert autocrine and paracrine effects. Cytokines fall into two broad categories and define microglial function as anti-inflammatory or pro-inflammatory. Microglia also produce **chemokines**, which microglia use to move to areas where the neural tissue is threatened by infection, disease, or injury. Microglia also use chemokines to recruit lymphocytes, monocytes, and neutrophils into the brain and spinal cord to help restore homeostasis. Once these peripheral, blood-borne cells enter the CNS, microglia signal them through cytokines and antigen presentation to determine their role and use chemokines to distribute them anywhere in the nervous system. Once the threat to the CNS has been contained or cleared away, activated microglia return to a resting state and most phagocytic macrophages undergo cell death, thereby, restoring homeostasis.[15]

Oligodendrocytes

Oligodendrocytes (oligos) are the only cells in the CNS that myelinate axons (Figure 2-9A). Their equivalent partners in the periphery are **Schwann cells** (Figure 2-9B). Myelination of peripheral motor and sensory axons is carried out by individual Schwann cells so that a single cell wraps one portion of the axon. The cell body of the Schwann cell is visible at each **internode** so the loss of a single Schwann cell will only demyelinate a small region of the peripheral axon. Oligos are primarily located within the white matter of the CNS and have a small, centralized cell body with multitudes of radial extensions (Figure 2-8). Each extension wraps a different axon, thus, allowing a single oligo to myelinate many neural axons and a single axon to be myelinated by multiple oligos (Figure 2-9A) The loss of a single oligo will mean that large portions of several axons will be demyelinated. Oligos myelinate axons of specific sizes. As in the periphery, small diameter axons are typically unmyelinated. Oligos myelinate axons that are 0.2 μm or larger.[16] While it is unclear what signals the oligos to identify axons of specific sizes, it is clear that axonal activity is an important but indirect regulator. The action potential, traveling down the axon, releases molecules that target astrocytes. In response, the astrocytes express a factor that induces myelin formation around the axon. This close relationship indicates that changes in astrocytes, especially during development or after injury, can cause problems in myelination.

Myelination is very important to the structure and function of the neuron–axon unit. Myelin is mostly comprised of lipid, which serves as an insulator of the axon, enabling the action potential to continue to the terminal. The oligo ensheaths segments of the axon, leaving gaps between myelinated areas.[17] As described previously, within these gaps, called **Nodes of Ranvier**, voltage-gated sodium channels and voltage-gated potassium channels are concentrated. As shown in Figure 2-9, these myelinated segments, separated by nodes of Ranvier, allow the action potential to move down the axon by jumping from one node to the next. This type of progression is called **saltatory conduction** and facilitates much faster axonal conduction. In addition to conduction, myelin also supports anterograde and retrograde axonal transport, which is important for moving proteins, transmitters, and growth factors from the neuronal cell body to the axon terminal (Box 2-1). The **myelin sheath** also provides trophic support to the underlying axon and the neuron by secreting several different types of growth factors.

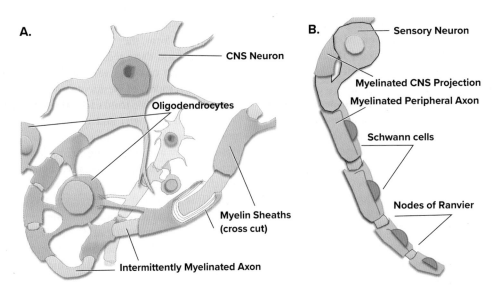

A.

CNS Neuron

Oligodendrocytes

Myelin Sheaths
(cross cut)

Intermittently Myelinated Axon

B.

Sensory Neuron

Myelinated CNS Projection

Myelinated Peripheral Axon

Schwann cells

Nodes of Ranvier

FIGURE 2-9 Cells that produce myelin in the nervous system. (A) An oligodendrocyte in the central nervous system provides the myelin sheath for multiple axons in the central nervous system. Several oligodendrocytes myelinate a single axon. **(B)** In the peripheral nervous system, each Schwann cell provides one segment of myelin wrap for one axon. In sensory neurons, the peripheral branch is myelinated by Schwann cells and the branch projecting in the CNS is myelinated by oligodendrocytes. A segment of myelin wrap is called an internode, while the gaps between internodes where the axon is not wrapped in myelin is called the node of Ranvier.

There is a large demand placed on oligos as they wrap axons in myelin. At least 50 axons are myelinated by a single oligo, which represents a membrane load that is 100 times its cell body weight.[17] This means the oligos have a high metabolic rate and consume high levels of oxygen and ATP for energy, which can create toxic byproducts, called reactive oxygen species. Unfortunately, oligos have very low levels of antioxidants that buffer this toxicity. Thus, oligos are quite vulnerable to shifts in homeostasis, and toxic damage can result in oligo cell death. This type of damage and oligo cell death occurs in multiple sclerosis, injury, and ischemia. Additionally, exposure to inflammation, inflammatory cytokines, or cytotoxic T lymphocytes put oligos at risk for demyelination or cell death.[17]

The central nervous system retains the ability to remyelinate, or restore, myelin to axons that have been demyelinated. Oligodendrocyte precursor cells (OPCs), immature cells found in different regions of the adult brain and spinal cord, receive signals from microglia and astrocytes that cause the OPCs to migrate to affected areas and to increase in number.[17] Once they arrive in the demyelinated zone, the OPCs develop into mature oligos and begin the remyelination process. One consequence of remyelination is that fewer wraps are made around the axons, so they are only thinly myelinated. This difference in thickness slows axonal conduction and may allow the action potential to dwindle away. Over time, the CNS is unable to mount a remyelination response, but it is unclear what factors are responsible.

Oligodendrocytes are the only glial cell to receive neural input. There is mounting evidence that increased neural activity, as occurs during skill learning or adaptation after CNS injury, induces greater myelination.[18] The greater neural drive appears to add internodal segments of myelin to the axon. Not all axons in the adult nervous system are fully myelinated from the neuronal cell body to the axon terminal. In fact, the length of cortical neurons is only intermittently myelinated.[19] One method to enhance learning and neuroplasticity is to add myelin internodes to axons that are only partially myelinated.[18] By adding internodes, the conduction of the action potential increases and the risk of it decaying before it reaches the terminal is reduced. By ensuring synaptic activity and increasing postsynaptic firing, stronger relationships between the cells (neuron-to-neuron or neuron-to-OPC) can occur, in an activity-dependent manner. This synaptic strengthening has important implications for motor learning and recovery after CNS impairment. A pivotal study shows, for the first time, that learning a complex wheel running task increases the number of OPCs in the brain, in mice. To prove that these OPCs were necessary to learn the complex task, the scientists blocked specific genes that allowed maturation. When OPCs were retained in their precursor form and could not mature into myelinating oligos, the mice could not learn the task. This is strong evidence that learning a new skill or relearning functions, during rehabilitation, will be dependent on generating OPCs and converting them into myelinating cells.[20]

In summary, all glia of the nervous system play a crucial role in maintaining a healthy microenvironment so that the neurons can function properly. Under challenging conditions, astrocytes and microglia become activated while OPCs increase in number. These different forms of glia help buffer toxicity, bolster repair processes, and facilitate learning and plasticity.

REFERENCES

1. Basso DM, Beattie MS, Bresnahan JC. Descending systems contributing to locomotor recovery after mild and moderate spinal cord injury in rats: experimental evidence and a review of literature. *Restor Neurol Neurosci.* 2002;20:189-218.

2. Vercelli A, Repici M, Garbossa D, Grimaldi A. Recent techniques for tracing pathways in the central nervous system of developing and adult mammals. *Brain Res Bull.* 2002;51(1):11-28.

3. Merzenich MM, Van Vleet TM, Nahum M. Brain plasticity-based therapeutics. *Front Hum Neurosci.* 2014;8:385.

4. Buno W, Cabezas C, Fernandez de SD. Presynaptic muscarinic control of glutamatergic synaptic transmission. *J Mol Neurosci.* 2006;30(1-2):161-164.

5. Kasten MR, Fan Y, Schulz PE. Activation of silent synapses with sustained but not decremental long-term potentiation. *Neurosci Lett.* 2007;417(1):84-89.

6. Hebb DO. *The Organization of Behavior.* New York, NY: Wiley; 1949.

7. Bushong EA, Martone MA, Jones YZ, Ellisman MH. Protoplasmic astrocytes in CA1 stratum radiatum occupy separate anatomical domains. *J Neurosci.* 2002;22:183-192.

8. Howarth C. The contribution of astrocytes to the regulation of cerebral blood flow. *Front Neurosci.* 2014;8(103):1-9.

9. Sofroniew MV, Vinters HV. Astrocytes: biology and pathology. *Acta Neuropathol.* 2010;119:7-35.

10. Suzuki A, Stern SA, Bozdagi O, Aberini CM. Astrocyte-neuron lactate transport is required for long-term memory formation. *Cell.* 2011;144:810-823.

11. Davalos D, Grutzendler J, Yang G, et al. ATP mediate rapid microglial response to local brain injury in vivo. *Nat Neurosci.* 2005;8(6):752-758.

12. Hansen CN, Norden DM, Faw TD, et al. Lumbar myeloid cell trafficking into locomotor networks after thoracic spinal cord injury. *Exp Neurol.* 2016;282:86-98.

13. Norden DM, Faw TD, McKim DB, et al. Bone marrow-derived monocytes drive the inflammatory microenvironment in local and remote regions after thoracic spinal cord injury. *J Neurotrauma.* 2019;36:937-949.

14. Ziebell JM, Adelson PD, Lifshitz J. Microglia: dismantling and rebuilding circuits after acute neurological injury. *Metab Brain Dis.* 2014. doi:10.1007/s11011-014-9539-y.

15. Rock RB, Gekker G, Hu S, et al. Role of microglia in central nervous system infections. *Clin Microbiol Rev.* 2004;17(4):942-964.

16. Simons M, Trajkovic K. Neuron-glia communication in the control of oligodendrocyte function and myelin biogenesis. *J Cell Biochem.* 2006;119:4381-4389.

17. Bradl M, Lassmann H. Oligodendrocytes: biology and pathology. *Acta Neuropathol.* 2010;119(1):37-53.

18. O'Rourke M, Gasperini R, Young K. Adult myelination: wrapping up neuronal plasticity. *Neural Regen Res.* 2014;9:1261.

19. Tomassy GS, Berger DR, Chen HH, et al. Distinct profiles of myelin distribution along single axons of pyramidal neurons in the neocortex. *Science.* 2014;344:319-324.

20. McKenzie IA, Ohayon D, Li H, et al. Motor skill learning requires active central myelination. *Science.* 2014;346(6207):318-322.

SUGGESTED READINGS

Batool S, Raza H, Zaidi J, Riaz S, Hasan S, Syed NI. Synapse formation: from cellular and molecular mechanisms to neurodevelopmental and neurodegenerative disorders. *J Neurophysiol.* 2019;121:1381-1397.

Bean BP. The action potential in mammalian central neurons. *Nature Rev Neurosci.* 2007;8:451-465.

Jamjoom AAB, Rhodes J, Andrews PJD, Grant SGN. The synapse in traumatic brain injury. *Brain.* 2021;144:18-31.

Raghavan M, Fee D, Barkhaus PE. Generation and propagation of the action potential. *Handb Clin Neurol.* 2019;160:3-22.

Tavee J. Nerve conduction studies: basic concepts. *Handb Clinical Neurol.* 2019;160:217-224.

Review Questions

1. What is the name of the fatty substance the covers axons to improve their ability to conduct action potentials?
   A. Adipose tissue
   B. Extracellular matrix
   C. Myelin
   D. Neurolemma

2. For the type of axon noted above, what is the name of the gap not covered by fatty substance?
   A. Internode
   B. Voltage-gated sodium channel
   C. Axon hillock
   D. Node of Ranvier

3. What is the name of the force that determines which way ions will flow across the neural cell membrane when a certain ion pore opens?
   A. Electrical gradient
   B. Electromechanical gradient
   C. Electrochemical gradient
   D. Concentration gradient

4. What kind of ion channel must be opened to initiate an action potential at the axon hillock of a projection interneuron?
   A. Voltage-gated potassium channel
   B. Voltage-gated sodium channel
   C. Voltage-gated calcium channel
   D. Metabotropic receptors

5. Assuming other characteristics are equal, the neuron with the fastest conduction velocity would be the one with the …
   A. Largest diameter axon.
   B. Longest axon.
   C. Highest number of voltage-gated sodium channels.
   D. Smallest number of inhibitory synapses.

6. What is different about the axon membrane at the nodes of Ranvier than in the axon where it is wrapped with the substance produced by Schwann cells?
   A. There is a high degree of membrane resistance.
   B. There is a high concentration of voltage-gated sodium channels.
   C. There is no passive decay of the membrane potential.
   D. Ligand-gated receptors are present to respond to neurotransmitters.

7. Which one of these processes can NOT contribute to the removal of the neurotransmitter so the synapses can recover to normal?
   A. Diffusion
   B. Enzyme degradation
   C. Reuptake into the presynaptic terminal
   D. Glial cells scavenging up the breakdown products
   E. Absorption of the neurotransmitter into the postsynaptic cell

8. When a neuron is active, the number of action potentials it makes per second should be proportional to the membrane potential at the trigger zone of the cell. What is the name for this relationship?
   A. Temporal coding
   B. Population coding
   C. Rate coding
   D. Amplitude coding

9. Which of these cells would not be found inside the cerebral cortex?
   A. Astrocytes
   B. Schwann cells
   C. Oligodendrocytes
   D. Microglia

10. In learning a new motor skill, what oligodendrocyte changes would be expected?
    A. Increased myelination and a decreased number of internodal segments
    B. Decreased myelination and an increased number of internodal segments
    C. Increased myelination and an increased number of internodal segments
    D. Decreased myelination and a decreased number of internodal segments

11. How do astrocytes react in the presence of injury?
    A. They adsorb glutamate to prevent neuronal death.
    B. They induce excitotoxicity.
    C. They become enlarged and more widely spaced.
    D. They enhance axonal regeneration through the formation of a glial scar.

12. **Which of the following correctly describes the activity of astrocytes during normal conditions?**
    A. Fibrous astrocytes detect fluctuations in blood vessel dilation.
    B. Protoplasmic astrocytes play a primary role in structural support.
    C. Astrocytes recruit lymphocytes and monocytes into the brain.
    D. Both types of astrocytes stimulate free radical release.

13. **Microglia are the resident immune cells in the CNS. What functions do they perform to earn this name?**
    A. Fight infection
    B. Perform surveillance under normal conditions
    C. Perform surveillance under disease conditions
    D. All of the above
    E. None of the above

14. **What does it mean when it says that cytokines have a paracrine effect?**
    A. They activate the microglia that produced and expressed them.
    B. They create an inflammatory environment.
    C. They cause chemotaxis of cells.
    D. They produce glial scarring.

15. **Which glial cell provides the primary metabolic support to CNS neurons?**
    A. Schwann cells
    B. Microglia
    C. Astrocytes
    D. Oligodendrocytes

Answers

1. C	2. D	3. C	4. B	5. A
6. B	7. E	8. C	9. B	10. C
11. A	12. A	13. D	14. A	15. C

GLOSSARY

1st node of Ranvier. The node of Ranvier nearest to the end of a sensory axon, where action potentials are generated.

Action potential. A defined sequence of voltage changes where the cell membrane rises rapidly and then falls rapidly to return to rest. Considered an all-or-none phenomenon, meaning that in general, the size of the action potential is very consistent and does not convey information. Only the frequency of action potential generation is used to carry information.

Anterograde axonal transport. A process by which molecules within an axon move away from the cell body, in the same direction that action potentials would normally be moving.

Astrocytes. Star-shaped glial cells (fibrous and protoplasmic) that provide metabolic and trophic support to neurons.

Axon hillock. The very beginning of the axon as it emerges from the soma; the site where action potentials are initiated in a typical neuron.

Axon terminal. Also called the synaptic bouton (boo – tawn) or the synaptic knob. Emerges from the axon as a swelling where synaptic vesicles filled with neurotransmitter can be found. The place where neurotransmitter is released into the synaptic cleft to affect another neuron.

Axon. The part of the neuron carrying information away from the neuron in the form of action potentials to influence other neurons or external structures like muscles.

Chemokines. Substances produced by microglia to recruit immune cells to the CNS.

Concentration gradient. The force tending to drive the flow of a particular type of ion across the cell membrane because of differences in concentration of that ion inside and outside the cell.

Cytokines. Substances expressed by microglia that are either anti-inflammatory or pro-inflammatory.

Dendrite. A projection from a neuron where information is received – not the axon.

Dendritic tree. All the dendrites coming out of a neuron.

Depolarize. The inside of the neuron becomes less negative (and more positive) than resting membrane potential.

Electrical (voltage) gradient. The force tending to drive the flow of a particular type of ion across the cell membrane because of voltage across the cell membrane. Anions (−) will tend to flow toward the positive side of the cell membrane and cations (+) will tend to flow toward the negative side of the membrane.

Electrical potential. The same as an electrical voltage.

Electrochemical gradient. The combined effect of the electrical and concentration gradient calculated by a special equation (called the Nernst equation) that ultimately determines whether a particular ion species will tend to flow into or out of the cells when its ion channels are open.

Enzymatic degradation. With respect the neurotransmitters and neuromodulators, enzymatic degradation is a deliberate process where an enzyme is present that will break down the neurotransmitter or neuromodulator into components that can no longer bind the receptor so that the effect goes away.

EPSP (Excitatory postsynaptic potential). A voltage change in the postsynaptic cell resulting from a synapse that tends to drive postsynaptic membrane potential more positive to a value that would be above threshold.

Equilibrium potential. For a specific ion species (e.g., sodium, potassium, chloride, calcium, etc.), the voltage that would exist in the membrane if only that ion species was free to flow across the cell membrane and a state of equilibrium was reached in the electrochemical gradient for that type of ion.

Excitation. In a neuron, a change in membrane potential that tends to drive the voltage above the threshold for making an action potential.

Extracellular domain. When a protein has part of its structure inside the cell and part of its structure outside the cell, the part outside is called the extracellular domain.

Generator potential. A passive voltage measured across the neural membrane at the first node of Ranvier, or in an unmyelinated axon, at the trigger zone.

Glia. Small cells within the nervous system with multiple functions (astrocytes, oligodendor cytes, microglia).

Hyperpolarize. The inside of the neuron becomes more negative than resting membrane potential.

Inhibition. In a neuron, a change in membrane potential that tends to drive the membrane potential to a level below the threshold for making an action potential.

Integrator. Something that adds things up (summing). In the nervous system, neuronal cell bodies act as the integrator of positive and negative voltages coming in from the synapses. Typically, in electrical circuits, an integrator can be "reset" back to zero. In neurons, the tendency for inhibitory synapses to be located on the soma plays a comparable role to the electrical reset.

Interneuron. Technically, any neuron in the nervous system that is neither a motoneuron nor a primary sensory neuron is an interneuron. Typically, this word is used to refer especially to local interneurons, cells with an axon that does not go beyond the local structure where the cell body is located. In general, the axons of interneurons are not myelinated.

Internode. A section of axon that is wrapped by a myelin sheath. In the peripheral nervous system, each internode is made by one cell, called a Schwann cell. In the central nervous system, cells called Oligodendrocytes make multiple internodes for axons nearby, and may make multiple internodes per axon. A single oligodendrocyte typically produces 20 to 60 internodes.

Intracellular domain. When a protein has part of its structure inside the cell and part of its structure outside the cell, the part inside is called the intracellular domain.

Ion channel. A special type of protein in a neuron membrane that has a potential hole, in the middle, called a pore, through which certain kinds of ions can flow relatively easily, but other ions will not flow easily (or may not flow at all).

Ionotropic receptor. A type of ligand-gated ion channel that opens or closes to allow ions to flow through the pore based on whether or not something is bound to the receptor on the extracellular domain.

IPSP (Inhibitory postsynaptic potential). A voltage change in the postsynaptic cell that tends to drive postsynaptic membrane potential to a value that would be below threshold.

Ligand-gated ion channels. Ion channels that open or close depending on whether a chemical is bound to them; that chemical could be a neurotransmitter or some type of medicine or drug.

Membrane potential. The voltage measured between on the inside of a neuron relatively to the voltage outside the cell.

Metabotropic receptor. A type of receptor that is not itself an ion channel (not an ionotropic receptor). The effect on the neuron is caused by changes in the intracellular domain of the metabotropic receptor in response to binding of a chemical to the receptor on the extracellular domain.

Microglia. Tiny glial cells that are resident immune cells within the CNS.

Myelin sheath. A wrapping of multiple layers of myelin around an axon. The number of wrappings varies with the size and level of maturation of the axon, and might be just a few wraps to a few dozen or more.

Node of Ranvier. A gap between myelin sheaths along the length of a myelinated axon where the axonal membrane is directly exposed to the extracellular fluid. Ion channels sufficient for the generation of action potentials are concentrated in this part of the axon.

Oligodendrocytes. Glial cells that produce myelin in the CNS.

Passive voltage. A voltage present across a neural membrane that either isn't capable of making an action potential (e.g., the dendritic tree) or is not in the midst of making an action potential. Passive voltage decays exponentially as the distance from the source of the voltage increases.

Phasic neurons. Neurons that tend to fire in brief rapid bursts of activity when changes occur or when activity is needed, but that are silent (not making action potentials) at rest.

Postsynaptic terminal. The part of the postsynaptic neuron's membrane that forms the down-stream side of the synaptic cleft, where receptor molecules are found that the neurotransmitter binds to.

Presynaptic terminal. The part of the synaptic bouton that forms one side of the synaptic cleft.

Projection interneuron (or projection neuron). A type of neuron with an axon long enough to transmits information to some other neuron located in a different part of the nervous system. Some projection neurons may travel a relatively short distance, from one side of the cerebral cortex to the other. Others may travel long distances, from a nucleus in the brainstem all the way to the lumbar spinal cord.

Proximal dendrite. A relatively large dendrite coming from the soma of the neuron itself, before branching begins to form the dendritic tree.

Rate coding. A way of representing the level of excitement of a neuron by how many action potentials per second it is making.

Receptor potential. A passive voltage measured across the neural membrane at or near the receptor, distal from the first node of Ranvier.

Resting membrane potential. The membrane potential of a neuron when it is not in the process of the making an action potential and is not being excited or inhibited, typically about -65 mV.

Retrograde axonal transport. A process by which molecules within an axon move toward the cell body, opposite to the direction the action potentials would normally be moving.

Reuptake. A process by which neurotransmitters or neuromodulators, or their components after enzymatic degradation, are actively transported from the extracellular fluid near the synapse back into the presynaptic neuron for eventual reassembly and repackaging into synaptic vesicles.

Saltatory conduction. Nerve conduction from one node of Ranvier to the next.

Schwann cells. Cells that produce myelin in the peripheral nervous system.

Silent synapse. Non-functioning synapses.

Sodium potassium pump. An active, process-utilizing ATP to move potassium ions into the neuron while at the same time pumping sodium ions out of the neuron to maintain resting membrane potential.

Soma. The cell body of the neuron, where the cell nucleus is located.

Spatial summation. When multiple synapses at multiple locations on the postsynaptic neuron are all receiving action potentials, there is a larger voltage change in the postsynaptic cell than if only one synapse was active.

Synaptic cleft. The space between neurons where the neurotransmitter is released by one neuron (the presynaptic neuron) so that the neurotransmitter can diffuse across the space in the cleft and bind to a receptor on the next neuron (the postsynaptic neuron).

Synaptic strength. For a single synapse, the size of the EPSP (or IPSP) resulting in the postsynaptic cell when an action potential arrives at the presynaptic terminal. Influenced by the size of the presynaptic and postsynaptic terminals, the concentration of receptors in the postsynaptic terminal, the distance of the synaptic cleft, the number of synaptic vesicles released by the presynaptic bouton.

Synaptic vesicle. A small spherical body like a balloon, made of a phospholipid bilayer, with neurotransmitter (or neuromodulator) molecules on the inside, with special proteins on the surface, allowing the vesicle to be transported from the inside of the synaptic bouton to the surface of the presynaptic terminal, where exocytosis puts the neurotransmitter into the synaptic cleft.

Temporal summation. When action potentials occur at a high rate in the presynaptic neuron, the voltage change in the postsynaptic cell is larger than when action potentials arrive at a lower rate or one at a time.

Threshold. A membrane potential above which an action potential will be generated, and below which an action potential will not be generated.

Tonic neurons. Neurons that tend to make action potentials on a steady basis, with their rate going up or down from a steady state to represent changes. Tonic neurons have internal processes that keep them depolarized above threshold and making action potentials even in the absence of incoming EPSPs.

Trigger zone. In an unmyelinated axon, a portion of the neural membrane near the distal end of the axon where there are enough voltage-gated sodium and voltage-gated potassium channels to permit the initial creation of an action potential based on the generator potential.

Voltage-gated ion channels. Ion channels that open or close to ion flow based on the membrane potential.

Somatosensory Pathways and Perception

Deborah S. Nichols-Larsen

3

OBJECTIVES

1) Differentiate the concepts of perception, discrimination, and haptics

2) Differentiate the neuroanatomical structures that support sensory perception, discrimination, and higher-order sensory function

3) Introduce methods of testing sensation

4) Discuss how sensory information contributes to reflexes and function

● INTRODUCTION

Human somatosensation is supported by complex networks, allowing the perception of touch, joint pressure and motion, muscle stretch and tension, pain, pressure, temperature, vibration, and itch. From these simple modalities, the human sensory system can characterize the location of touch, the magnitude of the stimulus, the orientation of the body or limb in space, and the identification of object properties such as texture, roughness, weight, shape, and identity. This chapter will focus on the neural processing of somatosensory sensations and how that processed information is used. We will also address how common tests of sensation can be used to elucidate different sensory abilities.

● SENSATION

To say that sensation is complex is at best an incredible understatement. Think of some of the sensations that you have experienced such as the tickle of hair as the hairdresser cuts your bangs or the feel of an ice cube melting in your hand. Imagine the feel of cool crisp sheets as you climb into bed at night or the rumpled warmth of those same sheets the next morning. Feel the golf club in your hand as you take a long back swing and then swing forward to hit the ball from the tee, immediately sensing whether it is a good or a bad shot. There are an endless number of sensations that can be described, but basically, they fall into two general categories: cutaneous sensation and proprioception.

Cutaneous Sensation

Cutaneous sensation allows the perception of touch (pressure, vibration, tickle, texture), temperature (hot/cold), pain (extreme temperatures, tissue damage, mechanical force), and itch via the activation of specific sensory receptors that respond to unique stimulus characteristics. **Cutaneous receptors** can collectively be referred to as ***mechanoreceptors***, encompassing **Pacinian corpuscles**, **Meissner corpuscles**, **Merkel disks**, and **Ruffini endings** (Table 3-1, Figure 3-1); these receptors, as their name implies, convert mechanical forces to the skin, muscles, and other tissues into neural signals. Mechanoreceptors are also designated by their mode of adaptation (rapid or slow) and their location in the skin (superficial = 1, deep = 2). Slow-adapting receptors are activated by a maintained stimulus and continue firing for the duration of the stimulus; conversely, **rapidly adapting receptors** respond quickly to stimulus change, including the initiation or cessation of a stimulus, but cease activation during a maintained stimulation. Mechanoreceptors project centrally via large diameter, moderately myelinated, **A beta (Aβ) neurons**, which conduct slightly slower than the **A alpha neurons** that are discussed later in relation to muscle spindles and Golgi tendon organs.[1,2] Mechanoreceptors collectively allow humans to discriminate a vast array of sensations, including but not limited to touch perception and localization; two-point, texture, weight, and shape discrimination; and object identification. *Texture discrimination* basically involves distinguishing two dimensions along a continuum of rough to smooth and soft to hard and is derived from activation of Pacinian corpuscles and RA2 afferents.[2] ***Stereognosis*** refers to the ability to identify an object by touch alone; we all do this when we reach into our pocket and distinguish a quarter from the other coins without looking. ***Graphesthesia*** is the ability to identify letters or words drawn on the skin, a common game among school-aged children, and *haptic perception* is the ability to distinguish object or surface characteristics, including shape, texture, and weight, through manipulation. This, of course, is an interaction between the motor system and the sensory system, and therefore, can be interrupted by a disturbance of either system. These higher-order sensory abilities likely result from convergence of information from different classes of mechanoreceptors and their respective afferents within the sensory cortex.[1]

Temperature, pain, and itch activate free nerve endings, located superficially in the skin with small receptive areas that project centrally via **A delta (Aδ)** and **C fibers** that are minimally or nonmyelinated respectively, and therefore, are slow conducting. Nerve endings that react to temperature (**thermoreceptors**) are distinct, responding to either hot or cold; they increase from a steady state of

TABLE 3-1	Receptors and Afferents[1,2]					
RECEPTOR	**ADAPTATION**	**SURFACE LOCATION**	**INNERVATION**	**AFFERENT**	**CUTANEOUS FUNCTION**	**PROPRIOCEPTIVE FUNCTION**
Meissner corpuscles (RA1)	Rapid	Superficial	RA1s innervate corpuscle clusters; corpuscles innervated by > 1 RA1	A beta	Skin motion	
Pacinian corpuscles (RA2)	Rapid	Deep	RA2s innervate 1 corpuscle	A beta	Vibration, texture	Joint perturbations (motion)
Merkel disks (SA1)	Slow	Superficial	SA1 fibers innervate clusters of disks	A beta	Pressure, spatial features, rate and degree of skin displacement	
Ruffini endings (SA2)	Slow	Deep	Innervated by 1 SA2	A beta	Skin stretch	Joint position and rotation
Golgi tendon organ	Rapid	Musculoskeletal junctions		Ib (A alpha)		Muscle tension
Nuclear bags	Rapid or slow	Within spindle in striated muscle		Ia (A alpha)		Muscle length and rate of change
Nuclear chains	Slow	Within spindle in striated muscle		II		Maintained stretch
Free nerve endings	Slow	Superficial	Small receptive areas	A delta	Pain	
				C	Temperature, itch	

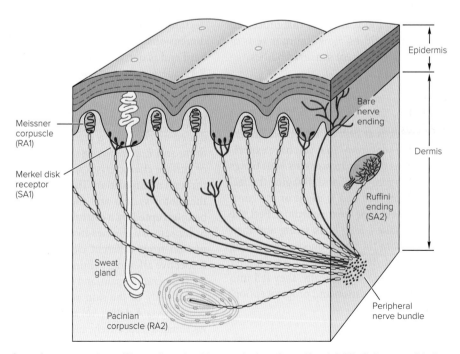

FIGURE 3-1 Illustration of mechanoreceptors. (Reproduced, with permission, from Kandel ER, Schwartz JH, Jessell TM, Siegelbaum SA, Hudspeth AJ. *Principles of Neural Science*, 5th ed. New York: McGraw-Hill; 2013, Fig. 23-1, p. 500.)

activity to a dynamic state, when exposed to hot or cold. Similarly, separate fibers function as thermal **nociceptors** (pain receptors), activated by extremes of temperature that are perceived as painful (either burning or freezing). While other nociceptors (pain receptors) respond to different types of tissue damage from mechanical or chemical sources. It should be noted that nociceptors are also located in tendons, joint capsules, muscles as well as the walls of internal organs and blood vessels.[3] Many nociceptors respond to only one type of noxious stimulation while others respond to several and are referred to as **polymodal nociceptors**.[2]

Aδ fibers are associated with higher threshold and single modality nociceptors; conversely, C fibers attach to polymodal nociceptors.[2,3] Several types of free nerve endings exist that initiate the perception of itch and also project via C fibers. Aδ fibers convey the sharp, acute pain sensation while C fibers are active with slow, aching pain sensations over the chronic phase of pain. Initially, it was thought that the sensation of itch was created only by a histamine reaction, but it has subsequently been noted in the absence of histamine, albeit the precipitating mediator(s) is(are) unclear.[2]

Damage to the somatosensory system can result in peripheral neuropathic pain syndromes that can present with either one condition or a combination of two conditions: **hyperalgesia** and/or **allodynia**. *Hyperalgesia* is an exaggerated response to a painful stimulus likely resulting from changes in the sensory afferents (e.g., ion channel disruption) and/or activation of free nerve endings by inflammatory mediators, such as histamine and substance P; it can be localized to the damaged area (primary hyperalgesia) or in adjacent tissues (secondary hyperalgesia).[2] While hyperalgesia is an exaggerated response to a painful stimulus; *allodynia* is an exaggerated sensitivity, experienced as pain, to stimuli that are typically non-pain–producing, like light touch or clothing covering a region of skin. There is some suggestion that allodynia may involve abnormal function of Aβ afferents, yet its origin is likely multifaceted.[4]

Receptive Fields

A receptive field is the surface area to which a single receptor and its sensory nerve fiber are responsive (Figure 3-2), or in terms of free nerve endings, the area of innervation for a single nerve ending. Each type of mechanoreceptor has a different receptive field with Merkel's disks and Meissner corpuscles having smaller receptive fields than Ruffini endings or Pacinian corpuscles. In turn, receptors are more closely organized in distill body areas (i.e., the hand) than in proximal areas (i.e., the shoulder), and the density of receptors is associated with the tactile sensitivity of the body part. Thus, the hand with its high density of mechanoreceptors is much better at detecting object characteristics than most other areas of the body.[1]

Interestingly, receptors have areas of stronger and lesser sensitivity. For example, Meissner corpuscles have multiple areas of high sensitivity (hot spots), surrounded by areas of lesser sensitivity, while Pacinian corpuscles are most sensitive in their center with decreasing sensitivity toward their periphery. A given stimulus may activate multiple receptors, especially when applied to the fingertip, and their activation will allow localization of the touch and interpretation of the stimulus characteristics, based on the number and type of receptors that are

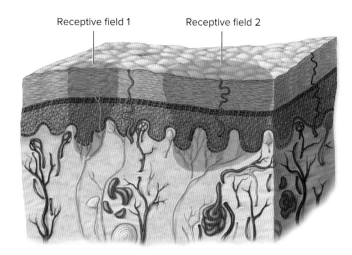

FIGURE 3-2 Illustration of receptive fields. (Reproduced, with permission, from McKinley M, O'Loughlin VD. *Human Anatomy*, 3rd ed. New York: McGraw-Hill; 2012, Fig. 19-1, p. 562.)

activated; more intense stimulation may activate a given receptor multiple times, which contributes to the perception of stimulus intensity and duration.[1,2,5]

Proprioception

Proprioception has had many definitions, and there has been considerable confusion in how this term and that of kinesthesia have been used. Most recently proprioception has been used to embody a comprehensive ability to sense: (1) muscle tension, (2) limb or body position and movement, including the velocity and direction of the movement (**kinesthesia**), (3) muscle or movement effort, and (4) balance.[6,7] This chapter will use this comprehensive definition of proprioception and limit the use of kinesthesia to the perception of limb/body position and movement.

Mechanoreceptors, located within joint capsules and ligaments, contribute to proprioception related to joint compression and movement; however, muscle spindles and Ruffini endings are uniquely activated during limb and trunk movement. Muscle spindles within the striated muscle respond to changes in muscle length; similarly, Ruffini endings are activated by skin stretch. In concert, these two receptor types provide a more complete indication of kinesthesia than either alone.[6–8]

Muscle spindles are unique receptors, located within striated *skeletomotor* **muscle** (those that move the limbs and trunk). They are oriented in parallel to the large striated muscle fibers and attached at each end to the adjacent striated muscle fibers; muscle spindles are encapsulated sensory receptors that house two types of tiny striated muscle fibers (Figure 3-3). To distinguish these tiny spindle muscle fibers from the larger skeletomotor muscle fibers, the spindle fibers are referred to as **intrafusal fibers** (within the spindle) and the skeletomotor muscle fibers as **extrafusal fibers** (outside of the spindle). Intrafusal fibers have two distinct shapes – one is round in the center like a bag with a handle on each end; the other is long and thin like a chain. Therefore, they are referred to as nuclear bags and nuclear chains. Nuclear bags are larger and the central enlargement, or bag, contains the nuclei of the fiber; the nuclear chains are smaller and narrow with nuclei in a central row in the middle section of the fiber. Each muscle spindle contains one

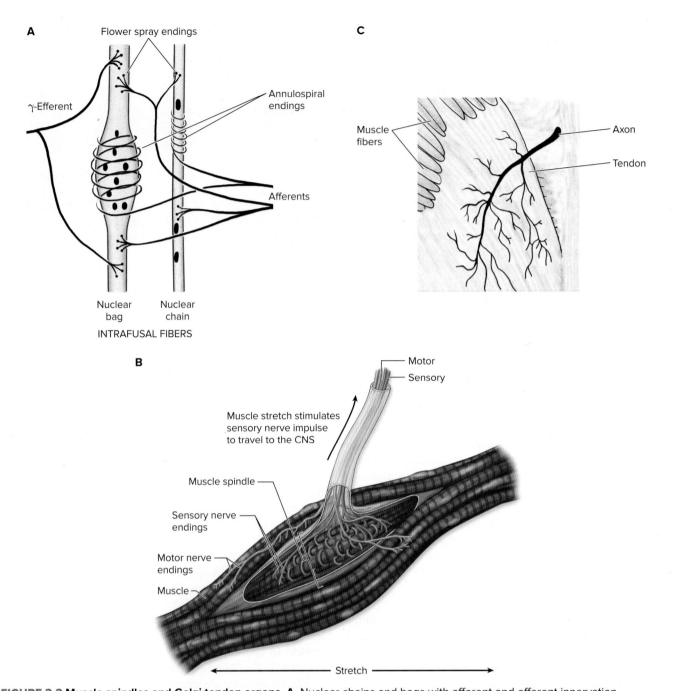

FIGURE 3-3 Muscle spindles and Golgi tendon organs. A. Nuclear chains and bags with afferent and efferent innervation.
B. Muscle spindle illustration within a muscle. (Reproduced, with permission, from Afifi AK, Bergman RA. *Functional Neuroanatomy*.
2nd edition. New York: McGraw-Hill; 2005, Fig. 1-13, p. 17.) **C.** Golgi tendon organ. (Reproduced, with permission, from McKinley M,
O'Loughlin VD. *Human Anatomy*, 3rd ed. New York: McGraw-Hill; 2012, Fig. 16-14, p. 512.)

to two nuclear bags and up to 11 nuclear chains. There are two types of nuclear bags (dynamic – bag 1 and static – bag 2), and it appears that most muscle spindles include one of each.[9]

Muscle spindles project to the spinal cord via two types of afferent fibers (primary and secondary). Each spindle gives rise to a single primary afferent but 0-5 secondary afferents. **Primary afferents (Ia)** spiral around the central portion of each intrafusal fiber (dynamic and static nuclear bags and nuclear chains), and their endings that attach to the intrafusal fibers are often referred to as *annulospiral or spiral endings.* **Secondary afferents** (II) coil primarily around nuclear chains but also some

static nuclear bags, typically on only one fiber, at each side of the central area with endings referred to as *flower spray endings.* The two types of afferents react differently to muscle length, stretch, and maintained tension on the extrafusal fibers. First, stretch of the extrafusal fibers simultaneously stretches the intrafusal fibers, resulting in activation of Ia afferents at a rate comparable to the rate and magnitude of stretch. More specifically, Ia fibers are most responsive at the beginning of a dynamic stretch and decrease their firing rate as the stretch progresses, providing key input toward the perception of movement. They have a brief silent period when the stretch is released and are silent during rapid contractions of their parent muscle. It should be noted that for any joint motion, there are muscles that are being elongated (stretched) with heightened spindle activity and those that are shortened with diminished spindle activity; in fact, during muscle shortening, muscles spindles are unloaded and would cease firing unless otherwise activated (see gamma motor innervation). Conversely, group II fibers respond increasingly over the course of a stretch and maximally when the muscle reaches its final tension or length, and thereby, contribute more to the perception of posture than movement.[6,8,9]

In the simplest form, the muscle spindle serves a reflex function to prevent excessive stretch to the ***homonymous muscle*** (muscle in which the Ia fibers originate). Ia afferents project through the dorsal horn of the spinal cord to synapse directly on **alpha motor neurons** that innervate the homonymous muscle fibers. Once the muscle spindle is activated by stretch, the Ia fiber's conduction induces alpha motor activation to produce a muscle contraction of the muscle, resulting in shortening of the muscle to prevent excessive stretch. This monosynaptic reflex is easily elicited by tapping a striated muscle tendon (i.e., the patellar tendon of the knee) with subsequent muscle contraction (i.e., quadriceps muscle) and is known as a stretch (tendon, monosynaptic or h) reflex. Simultaneously, a collateral projection of the Ia fiber also innervates inhibitory interneurons to the antagonistic (**heteronymous**) muscle's alpha motor neuron to induce relaxation of that muscle to allow the agonist to contract and that heteronymous muscle to elongate. In the case of the patellar tendon reflex, the heteronymous muscle would be the hamstrings.

Secondary afferent (II) fibers synapse within the spinal cord on interneurons that, in turn, project both to the homonymous muscle and heteronymous muscle(s); there is also some evidence that these afferents may project to interneurons at multiple spinal levels. II fibers are smaller and slower conducting than their Ia counterparts. Interestingly, II fibers synapse on both alpha and gamma motor neurons, but, similar to Ia fibers, are primarily excitatory, both to alpha motor neurons and to gamma motor neurons (see subsequent section).[9]

Like extrafusal fibers, nuclear bags and chains are innervated by efferent motor neurons, both **beta** and **gamma**, that project from the ventral horn of the spinal cord along with the alpha motor neurons that innervate extrafusal fibers. Beta motoneurons innervate both intrafusal and extrafusal fibers while gamma motoneurons innervate only intrafusal fibers. Intrafusal innervation allows for the responsiveness of the muscle spindle to be up or downregulated under the control of higher motor centers but independent of the muscle length of the homonymous muscle. The structure of intrafusal fibers is unique to their function as stretch receptors; for both bags and chains, the contractile components of the fibers are located at the ends of the fiber. Thus, gamma activation results in contraction of these distill contractile elements with subsequent stretching of the central region where the afferent endings are located. Thus, intrafusal fiber contraction is perceived as extrafusal fiber stretch or lengthening.[9]

Each intrafusal fiber type shortens in response to gamma or beta activation; however, the impact of that shortening creates a slightly different effect. Notably, gamma motor neurons can be divided into two types: dynamic and static. Dynamic gamma motor neurons innervate dynamic nuclear bags; static gamma motor neurons innervate static nuclear bags and/or nuclear chains. Dynamic gamma activation of type 1 bags enhances Ia firing at the beginning and ending of extrafusal muscle stretch. Conversely, static gamma activation to type 2 bags and nuclear chains is relatively absent during the active stage of stretch but demonstrates heightened activity when a muscle is held at a constant length. Thus, it is hypothesized that dynamic gamma activation assists to support awareness during movement while static gamma activation primarily supports postural awareness.[9]

However, this may be a simplistic view. More specifically, contraction of dynamic nuclear bags in response to gamma activation occurs slowly but increases their overall stiffness such that subsequent extrafusal muscle lengthening rapidly increases the firing of the Ia afferent, and thus, enhances length awareness during motion. When activated by gamma excitation, static nuclear bags rapidly increase the Ia firing rate, facilitating awareness of muscle length, as a muscle shortens, and enhancing force generation within the muscle. Nuclear chain activation, via gamma innervation, is the most rapid of the three intrafusal fiber types and enhances its sensitivity to maintained stretch.[10] Ultimately, the functioning of the muscle spindle components allows for a determination of muscle length at all times during movement and stability. See Box 3-1 for a description of the functional application of gamma motor control.

There is another receptor associated with the proprioceptive system called the **Golgi tendon organ (GTO)**; as its name suggests, it is located in the tendon near the junction with

---

Box 3-1 | **Gamma Motor Control of Muscle Spindles: Why?**

One key question often asked by the student, struggling to understand muscle spindles and their innervation and function, is why change the sensitivity of the muscle spindle? The following example gives an illustration of how this system may be used within complex movement. Visualize, for a moment, a diver on a 10-m platform, preparing to complete a backward 2½ flip. He walks to the end of the platform, turns, and very carefully arranges his feet on the end of the platform, coming to stand precariously on his toes. As he maintains this position, it is critical that he be aware of even the slightest sway of his body so as not to lose his balance. Activation of static nuclear bags will increase his awareness of even minimal muscle length change to assist in balance maintenance as he prepares to dive and enhanced force production as he pushes off of the platform. As he pushes off and leaps up into a pike position (hands on ankles, knees straight), the responsiveness of the spindles needs to be downregulated in the back and hamstring muscles to avoid a stretch response that would pull him out of this position. Yet, toward the end of his second rotation, gamma activation of nuclear chains can enhance his positional awareness in preparation for kicking out of the pike position; similarly, dynamic bags in the hamstrings and back extensors can be activated via dynamic gamma efferents to facilitate his movement into a fully extended position prior to hitting the water. This integration of gamma and alpha motor activity will be further explored in the chapter 5 on motor control.

the muscle, and each is innervated by a single Ib afferent. As described for other afferents, the Ib has its cell body in the dorsal root ganglion with a peripheral projection to the GTO and a central projection into the spinal cord. Unlike the Ia afferent of the muscle spindle, the Ib projects only onto interneurons in the spinal gray rather than directly to alpha motor neurons, creating a polysynaptic reflex loop. Initially, the GTO was thought to serve only as a protective mechanism to prevent excessive tension generation in the homonymous muscle that could lead to muscle or tendon tearing. When activated, it would inhibit the contraction of the homonymous muscle and facilitate the contraction of the heteronymous muscle, known as the **autogenic inhibition reflex**, to protect the homonymous muscle from generating a damaging level of force. This function was largely inferred by the experimental setup used in the original studies that examined whole muscle force as well as the early identification of the Ib's projection onto an inhibitory Ib interneuron (Ib-IN) for the homonymous muscle and an excitatory interneuron to the heteronymous muscle. However, as techniques advanced, researchers were able to examine the activity of GTOs during partial activation of single motor units and found that GTOs were active throughout the contraction, providing constant monitoring of muscle tension with feedback to higher motor centers, both from contracting and at-rest muscles. Thus, the GTO works through a spinal network to produce ongoing force monitoring and a negative feedback loop as force increases, creating homeostasis for force.[11]

The location of each GTO within the tendon may provide differential feedback with activation of those closer to the muscle belly conveying active force generation in motor units and those more distill responding to total force generation from the entire muscle. There is also some evidence that GTOs help to signal tendon length or stretch, since there are no muscle spindles in tendons. To accurately know the end-to-end muscle length, the nervous system must account for, not only the length of the contractile elements of muscle, as sensed by the muscle spindles, but also the length of the tendon. Measuring the force imposed on the tendon may provide an indication of the degree of stretch on the tendon, allowing more complete awareness of total muscle-tendon length.[11,12]

There is also direct evidence that **Ib fibers** connect to another set of interneurons, referred to as Ib excitatory interneurons (Ib-EN), which excite the homonymous muscle to create a positive feedback loop for force; however, this loop is not normally active.[13] Activity in this circuit has been identified during the stance phase of gait in extensor muscles, and is associated with depression of the input from Ib fibers to their Ib-IN and Ib excitation of Ib-EN, thereby, facilitating the homonymous muscle. This is referred to as state-dependent reflex reversal.[11,12] In addition, descending projections from motor centers, including corticospinal collaterals, are able to modify the reflexive activity of the GTO at the Ib–interneuronal synapse, contributing to this reflex reversal or modulating the inhibitory or excitatory activity of the Ib interneurons, see Figure 3-4.

Thus, muscle spindles and GTOs work in concert, providing detailed feedback on muscle length and force generation, using the same excitatory and inhibitory interneurons to integrate muscle responsiveness to length and force changes (see Box 3-2).[11]

Box 3-2 | **Golgi Tendon Organ's Influence on Movement**

If we go back to the diver in Box 3-1 and imagine the contribution of the GTOs to this complex movement, you can expect that they are active throughout the series of muscle contractions. Feedback from GTOs would be necessary to assure appropriate contraction of muscles and that over-contraction that might pull the legs, trunk, or arms out of line with the intended position does not occur. Similarly, muscle spindle activation allows for constant monitoring of each joint's position. Thus, the integration of information from muscle spindles and GTOs along with information from joint and skin receptors allows for ongoing awareness of body position, limb position in relation to the body, muscle length, and force generation from muscle contraction throughout the dive (or any other movement). Of course, when an error starts to occur, this feedback system can allow some degree of correction, during the movement. Obviously, mid-movement correction is not always successful, and divers often miss components of the dive; in that case, feedback from these proprioceptors (GTOs and muscle spindles) allows the motor control system to adapt the motor plan for the next attempt.

In combination, this system of mechanoreceptors can assist the motor control system to plan for appropriate force generation and lengthening within each muscle as well as to allow for minor corrections during the course of the movement. Some level of integration of afferent information from spindles and GTOs occurs within the spinal cord, allowing not just the coordination of muscles at a given joint but actually throughout a limb.[11] See Chapters 2 and 4 for more discussion of how the nervous system incorporates these reflexes into function.

Receptors in the joint also contribute to our sense of proprioception but to a minimal extent. These receptors are Ruffini-like endings (Type I), Pacinian-like corpuscles (Type II), Golgi endings (Type III), and free nerve endings (Type IV).[12] The majority are Ruffini receptors that are slow adapting, located in the capsule, cartilage, and ligaments, and signal both static and dynamic joint position. The Pacinian-like receptors are rapidly adapting and respond to motion in any direction with a short burst of activity. Golgi endings are located in the joint ligaments and, at least at the knee, in the meniscus; they are also slow-adapting receptors with high thresholds and are thought to measure extremes of motion and intra-articular pressure. Free nerve endings, like those in the periphery, are responsive to pain and located throughout the joint components. Interestingly, stretch of the skin, during joint motion, also contributes to the perception of joint movement[8] as does pressure on the joint such as that on the bottom of the foot, during stance.[12-14] It is likely that all inputs enhance our ability to sense the position and movement of our joints.

DERMATOMES AND SPINAL NERVE ORGANIZATION

The afferents from peripheral sensory receptors aggregate and enter the spinal cord as spinal nerves with one spinal nerve per segment of the cord (cervical, thoracic, lumbar,

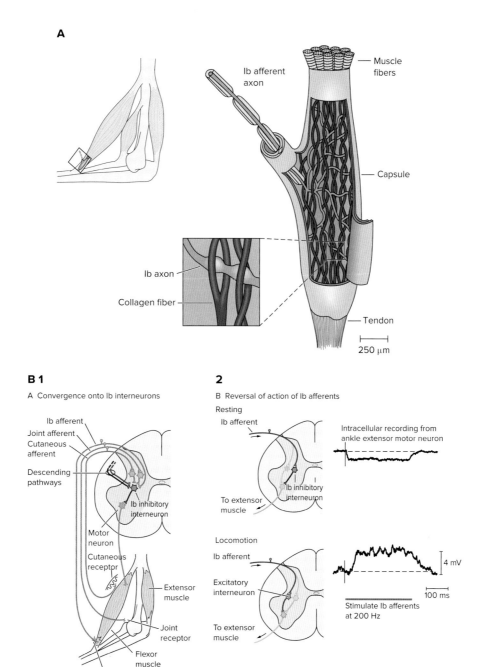

FIGURE 3-4 Golgi tendon organ function. A. Stretching of the Golgi tendon organ, typically from muscle contraction, results in compression of the Ib axon by collagen fibers, increasing its firing rate. **B.** During ambulation Golgi tendon organs modulate Ib activity: (1) Left image – illustrates Ib inhibitory input from GTOs, joint and cutaneous receptors, and descending pathways; (2) Right images – during ambulation, the action of Ib fibers switches from inhibition to excitation on extensor muscles at the ankle. At rest, Ib activation from the ankle extensor muscles inhibits those same muscles through the Ib inhibitory interneuron (hyperpolarization on recording); during ambulation, Ib activity to the excitatory interneuron increases and Ib activity to the inhibitory interneuron decreases so that extensor muscle activity is facilitated (EMG recording). (Reproduced with permission from Kendel ER, Koester JD, Mack SH, Siegelbaum SA. *Principles of Neural Science*. 6ed. New York, NY: McGraw Hill; 2021.)

sacral) except for the first cervical segment (C1), which does not receive sensory projections. Spinal nerves are organized into the many peripheral nerves, learned in gross anatomy and beyond the scope of this text. A dermatome is the area of the skin innervated by a single spinal nerve (Figure 3-5). Surprisingly, multiple dermatome maps exist with varying degrees of commonality. However, recent evidence suggests that the differences in these dermatome maps result from the inherent variability of individual dermatome maps and the significant overlap between adjacent dermatomes, which is greater in the limbs and minimal in the midline of the body.[15]

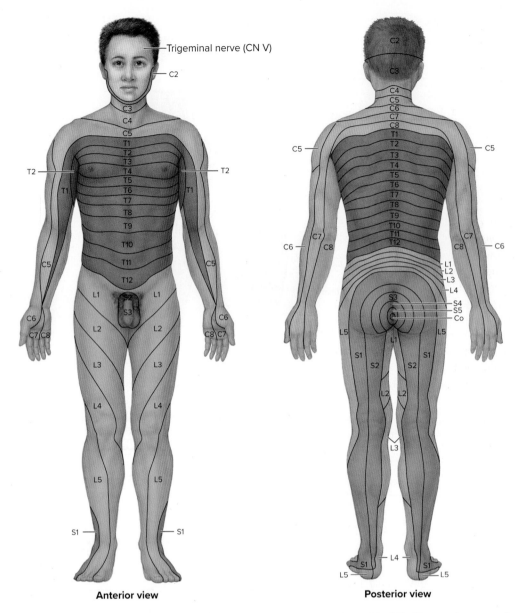

FIGURE 3-5 Dermatome map. (Reproduced, with permission, from McKinley M, O'Loughlin VD. *Human Anatomy*, 3rd ed. New York: McGraw-Hill; 2012, Fig. 16-6, p. 495.)

• DORSAL GRAY MATTER

Sensory fibers from spinal nerves, conveying information from all types of receptors, project either entirely or partially into the gray matter of the spinal cord. The information from more distill receptors projects into more medial areas of the gray matter and that from proximal receptors projects into more lateral areas.[5] Dorsal column fibers send collaterals that contribute to monosynaptic and polysynaptic reflexes. Others synapse on second-order neurons that project to higher centers (i.e., anterolateral pathway). Thus, the dorsal gray is a complexly organized area of cellular activity. It is divided into laminae (I-VI) with smaller diameter pain fibers ending in laminae I and II while A beta fibers end in deeper laminae.[5]

• CENTRAL PROJECTION SYSTEMS

Receptor activation of a magnitude to initiate transduction (the conversion of a stimulus to an action potential within the sensory neuron) is necessary to begin the central conduction of the sensation. Sensory neurons have their cell bodies in the dorsal root ganglia with a long dendritic projection to the periphery, attaching to a mechanoreceptor or ending as a free nerve ending, and an axon or central projection that enters the spinal column through the dorsal root. Within the spinal cord, there are two primary pathways that convey cutaneous sensation from the periphery to the brain: the dorsal-column-medial lemniscal system and the anterolateral system.

Dorsal-Column-Medial Lemniscal Pathway (DCML)

As sensory neurons, conveying tactile sensation, enter the spinal cord, they can project into the cord to synapse directly on alpha motor neurons or interneurons; those from muscle spindles, as previously described, contribute to monosynaptic and polysynaptic reflexes.[12] Additionally, they traverse the dorsal horn and enter the dorsal column in a sequential order from the sacral cord to the cervical cord, beginning medially with the sacral neurons and then filling in toward the lateral margins with fibers from the lumbar, thoracic, and finally cervical regions (Figure 3-6).

From the exterior or cross section, the dorsal column is clearly divided into two columns: the fasciculi **gracilis** (medially located, conveying lower body neurons) and cuneatus (laterally located, conveying upper body neurons). The primary afferents in this system project all of the way to their second-order neurons within three medullary nuclei: **gracilis**, **cuneatus**, and **external cuneatus**, located in the dorsal aspect of the caudal medulla. The second-order neurons exit these dorsal column nuclei and cross over (decussate) to the opposite side, ascending to the thalamus, as the medial lemniscal pathway, where they synapse on third-order neurons in the **ventroposteriolateral (VPL) nucleus**. Notably, the cuneatus receives primarily cutaneous sensation while the external cuneatus receives proprioception from the UE with some second-order neurons that project to the cerebellum (cuneocerebellar tract) and others projecting to the cortex via VPL. The third-order neurons within VPL project through the posterior limb of the internal capsule, as the thalamic radiations, to the primary sensory cortex (SI), located within the postcentral gyrus. The postcentral gyri mirror the primary motor cortices with an inverse body orientation such that the foot is at the top of SI, extending over onto the medial surface of the hemisphere, and the face is located at the bottom of SI (Figure 3-7).[1]

In addition to SI, many other areas assist in determining the characteristics of sensation: (1) **secondary somatosensory cortex (SII)** – located above and within the lateral sulcus; (2) adjacent areas within the lateral sulcus (e.g., ventral parietal area [PV]) and components of the insular cortex; (3) supramarginal gyrus of the temporal lobe; and (4) posterior parietal cortex (Brodmann's areas 5 and 7) – located posterior to SI.[1] There has been much discussion about the projection of sensory information to these higher-level processing areas, specifically whether projections are serial, passing through SI to get to other areas, or parallel with third-order sensory neurons projecting directly to SII and the posterior parietal cortex.[9] Of course, some parallel projections could also emanate from the spinothalamic system (see subsequent section). Notably, SI is known to project to each of these sensory areas and interestingly has strong bilateral projections to SI in each hemisphere. We will pick up this discussion in a subsequent section of this chapter.

Anterolateral System (AL)

As described in the preceding section for the dorsal column system, nociceptive neurons enter the spinal cord via the dorsal root but differentially enter the posterior aspect of the dorsal horn, forming the ***Tract of Lissauer***, which allows them to ascend or descend up to two spinal segments before terminating within the ***posterior marginalis*** (Aδ fibers) or ***nucleus proprious*** (C fibers) of the dorsal horn where they synapse on neurons with cell bodies in multiple laminae (I, II, IV-VI, X). These second-order neurons then cross to the opposite side of the cord via the anterior commissure and ascend within the anterolateral cord (AL) as two

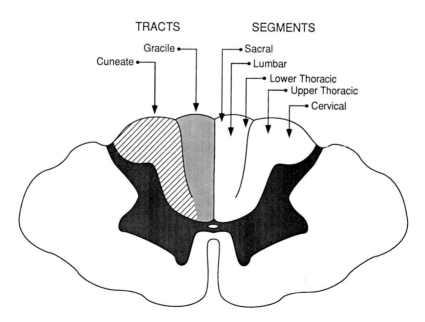

TRACTS   SEGMENTS

Gracile • • Sacral
Cuneate • • Lumbar
           • Lower Thoracic
           • Upper Thoracic
           • Cervical

FIGURE 3-6 Organization of the dorsal column. (Reproduced, with permission, from Afifi AK, Bergman RA. *Functional Neuroanatomy.* 2nd ed. New York: McGraw-Hill; 2005, Fig. 3-8, p. 53.)

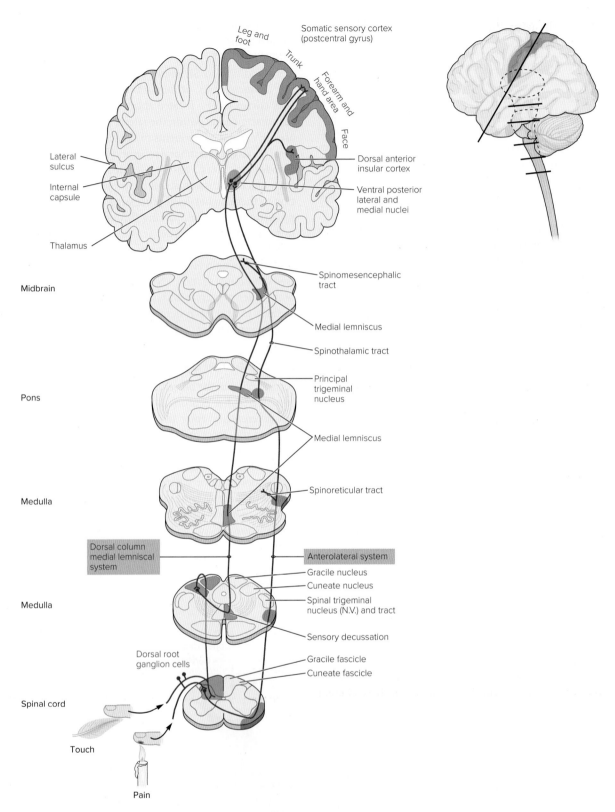

FIGURE 3-7 Ascending somatosensory pathways. (Reproduced, with permission, from Kandel ER, Schwartz JH, Jessell TM, Siegelbaum SA, Hudspeth AJ. *Principles of Neural Science*, 5th ed. New York: McGraw-Hill; 2013, Fig. 22-11, p. 493.)

spinothalamic pathways: anterior and lateral. The anterior spinothalamic tract, located in the most anterior portion of the AL, conveys crude touch information, emanating from second-order neurons in the deeper dorsal horn laminae. The lateral spinothalamic tract conveys pain and temperature and is comprised of neurons originating in the more superficial laminae (I, IV, and V). There are actually three respective components within the lateral AL: the lateral spinothalamic tract, the spinoreticular tract, and the spinomesencephalic tract, descriptive of their terminations – the thalamus, reticular formation, and midbrain (Figure 3-7).[2,16]

The lateral **spinothalamic tract** (LST) also has three segments, based on the termination of the respective fibers within the thalamus: (1) ventral posterolateral nucleus – ventral LST fibers that merge with the medial lemniscal pathway in the brainstem and terminate in the VPL are associated with discrimination of locus and type of painful stimuli ; (2) posterior medial and intralaminar nuclei – dorsal LST fibers project to these nuclei, which are linked to the limbic system and therefore thought to contribute to the motivational and affective responses to painful stimuli; and (3) central medial nucleus (CM) – remaining LST fibers terminate on areas that also projects to the insula and amygdala (limbic centers) and thereby also contribute to the affective response to pain.[17]

While the LST conveys pain and temperature information centrally, the larger **spinoreticular portion** of the AL terminates within the lateral and medial reticular nuclei. The medial nuclei have strong connections to components of the limbic system, and therefore, contribute to the intense emotional responses to persisting pain signals, including depression in chronic pain conditions. The lateral nuclei receive input from multiple areas of the motor system, and therefore, may be more involved in the motor response to pain stimuli (i.e., the change in gait pattern to accommodate a painful joint). Interestingly, spinoreticular neurons send collaterals to multiple parts of the brainstem that are associated with pain inhibition (**anti-nociception**). The **spinomesencephalic** tract also projects to the brainstem, but rather than terminating in the reticular formation, ends in the midbrain, more specifically in the periaqueductal gray (PAG), which surrounds the cerebral aqueduct, and the superior colliculus, in the dorsum of the midbrain. Notably, the PAG is an area of antinociceptive systems; thus, the spinomesencephalic system along with the collaterals of the spinoreticular pathway work together to activate systems that function to decrease the pain experience. Projections to the superior colliculus are responsible for the reflexive visual orientation to a painful stimulus.[17] See Box 3-3 for a description of pain perception and Box 3-4 for pain modulation.

Spinocerebellar Systems

Ia, Ib, and II fibers from muscle spindles and GTOs are not just involved in reflexive mechanisms within the spinal cord; they also contribute to our sense of proprioception through projections to the cerebellum and cortex. Collaterals of these afferent fibers as well as those from mechanoreceptors from the skin and joint receptors convey proprioceptive information to the cortex through the DCML system. Similarly, additional collaterals of the Ia, Ib, and II fibers enter the dorsal spinal gray matter and synapse on second-order neurons that project rostrally. These second-order neurons convey information to the cerebellum within the spinocerebellar system.

For the lower extremities and trunk, some proprioceptive afferents terminate in Clarke's nucleus or column within the lumbar and thoracic dorsal gray matter. Projections from Clarke's nucleus make up both the ventral and dorsal spinocerebellar tracts, conveying information from the lower extremities and trunk to the cerebellum. The ***dorsal spinocerebellar tract*** is located in the dorsolateral aspect of the spinal cord, enters the cerebellum primarily via the inferior peduncle, and terminates

| Box 3-3 | What Happens When We Experience Pain? |

A simple example of the complexity of the pain experience is a paper cut to your finger. The first thing perceived is a tactile sensation, conveyed by the large A fibers from mechanoreceptors in the fingertip, that your fingertip was "touched" by the paper. This is quickly followed by a perception of acute pain, initiated by Aδ fiber projections from nociceptors (free nerve endings); however, even before your primary sensory cortex has processed where and what has happened, your eyes move to look in the direction of your hand, and you have probably sworn or mumbled a verbal response to the pain that you're now experiencing. The reflexive motions of your hand away from the paper, your eye orientation to look at your hand, and the verbal expletive result from the projections of the spinoreticular and spinomesencephalic tracts as well as reflex units in the spinal cord (look for a detailed explanation in Chapter 4, on the sensorimotor systems of the spinal cord.

However, your pain experience has just begun. Once a painful stimulus occurs, your body responds in two ways. One, there is a rush of endogenous molecules to the traumatized tissue, including histamine, bradykinin, substance P, and prostaglandins.[18] These molecules repetitively depolarize nociceptors, activating pain afferent fibers (typically C fibers), and resulting in the ongoing chronic pain perception that will last for several days.

Yet, a second series of events is also in process as collaterals from second-order pain afferents in the brainstem target the sites of powerful endogenous anti-nociceptive (anti-pain) systems, originating in the PAG, reticular formation, and other brainstem nuclei (locus coeruleus, raphe nuclei) (Figure 3-8). These descending pain-modulating systems release serotonin, norepinephrine, and endogenous opiates (opiate-like substances within the body) to decrease the perception of pain. One site of their activity is the synapses in the spinal cord between first- and second-order pain neurons in the anterolateral pathway, where they can act as either presynaptic or postsynaptic inhibitors through multiple mechanisms (e.g., neurotransmitter deregulation, postsynaptic hyperpolarization). Similarly, circulating endogenous opiates, such as beta-endorphin, function at the periphery to impede the action of histamine and other nociceptive molecules' depolarization of nociceptors. Thus, this tiny paper cut induces a battle between nociception and anti-nociception that will continue for several days as the tissue of the cut heals. Without these powerful anti-nociceptive systems, our pain experiences would be much more intense and most likely intolerable; anti-nociceptive activity is noted at every level of the pain projecting pathways to modify our pain experiences. Obviously, a paper cut is a minor pain experience; however, this same process occurs in the presence of larger pain situations, and many current treatments for pain are designed to augment the natural endogenous anti-nociception process.

mainly in the ipsilateral vermis and paravermal cortex but also projects to the deep cerebellar nuclei.[12,20] Both cutaneous and proprioceptive afferents project through the ***ventral spinocerebellar tract*** (VSCT); the second-order neurons that make up this tract are located in laminae V-VII of the dorsal horn. They leave the dorsal gray and cross to the opposite side of the cord

Box 3-4	Pain Modulation: The Gating of the Pain Experience

In 1965, Melzack and Wall proposed the "Gate Theory of Pain," which asserted that large A sensory fibers could decrease the pain experience by "closing the gate" between first- and second-order pain neurons in the spinal cord[19] (see Figure 3-9). This proposal opened the gate, so to speak, to a large amount of research aimed at identifying how this occurred and invited the development of treatment modalities aimed at "closing the gate" (i.e., TENS – transcutaneous electrical nerve stimulation). Since that initial proposal, many inhibitory networks have been identified that modify the pain experience by blocking pain transmission, not only in the spinal cord, but at every level of the pain projecting system to prevent the transmission of pain signals from the spinal cord to higher centers. Descending systems, originating in the brainstem, also contribute to pain modulation by directly synapsing on first-order or second-order pain neurons, inducing presynaptic (disruption of neurotransmitter release) or postsynaptic (disrupting depolarization of the second-order neuron) inhibition or indirectly achieving these changes through the activation of interneurons within the dorsal horn of the spinal cord. Many pharmaceutical and therapy modalities have been derived to augment this natural pain modulation.

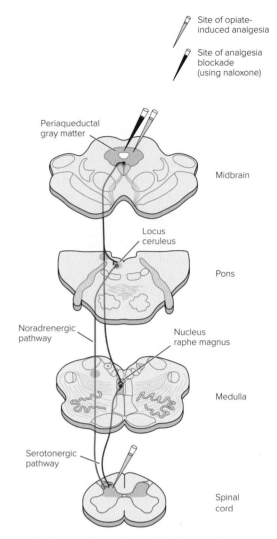

FIGURE 3-8 Descending pain-modulating pathways.
(Reproduced, with permission, from Kandel ER, Schwartz JH, Jessell TM, Siegelbaum SA, Hudspeth AJ. Principles of Neural Science, 5th ed. New York: McGraw-Hill; 2013, Fig. 24-15, p. 548.)

within the anterior commissure, ascending within the anterior funiculus and re-crossing in the brainstem to enter the cerebellum, primarily through the superior cerebellar peduncle,[19] terminating in the anterior portion of the vermis.[12] Notably, the ventral spinocerebellar tract is modulated by collateral projections from both the corticospinal and vestibular systems. In theory, this is thought to convey the motor plan to neural circuits in the cord, during active movement, with neurons in the VSC providing feedback to the cerebellum relative to movement progression, supporting preparation prior to movement and adaptation of the movement as it is occurring.[12,21]

Upper extremity proprioception from Ia, Ib, and II fibers is also conveyed centrally, but the systems conveying this information have received little study in humans, in part, because we do not locomote on all fours, and therefore, unconscious proprioception plays a less significant role in arm control. As mentioned in an earlier section, proprioception from the arms and upper trunk ascends within the dorsal column and synapses within the external, also called the accessory, **cuneate nucleus** (ACN) within the medulla adjacent to the cuneate nucleus. From the ACN, it projects as the **cuneocerebellar tract** to the cerebellum within the inferior cerebellar peduncle, specifically to the interposed nuclei of the cerebellum. A parallel system, also conveying UE proprioception, projects in the ventral funiculus, alongside the VSCT, and is called the **rostral spinocerebellar tract** (RSCT), which terminates in the ipsilateral anterior cerebellum. Like its VSCT counterpart, the RSCT receives modulation from higher centers and is considered to play a role in movement preparation and correction.[22]

Spinoreticular Pathway

Proprioceptive information is also conveyed to the reticular formation of the pons and medulla through another pathway within

the anterolateral portion of the spinal cord. The axons of this pathway originate in dorsal horn neurons that receive incoming afferent collaterals from Ia, Ib, and II fibers. The widespread terminations of these fibers within the reticular formation allow them to contribute to postural reactions (anticipatory and reactive) as well as motor control for posture and movement.[12]

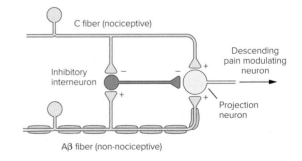

FIGURE 3-9 Schematic of the Gate Theory of Pain.
(Reproduced, with permission, from Kandel ER, Schwartz JH, Jessell TM, Siegelbaum SA, Hudspeth AJ. *Principles of Neural Science*, 5th ed. New York: McGraw-Hill; 2013, Fig. 24-14, p. 548.)

SENSORY PROJECTIONS FROM THE FACE

The preceding discussion of sensory systems has focused on sensation emanating from the extremities and trunk; however, the structures of the face, including the eyes, nose, ears, and oral cavity also have well-organized sensory projections. Tactile sensitivity from the face and many oral structures (2/3 of the tongue as well as the teeth, cheeks, and gums) is conveyed within the trigeminal nerve (cranial nerve V); the remainder of the tongue is conveyed via the glossopharyngeal nerve (IX). The vagus nerve (X) transmits tactile sensation from the external and internal ear as well as the internal organs[21] (Table 3-2).

Similar to what has been described for sensation from the body, sensation from the face and oral structures involves mechanoreceptors, proprioceptors, and free nerve endings to allow detection of cutaneous sensations and proprioception. In fact, it should be evident that the face, and more specifically the mouth, is capable of the highest level of sensory discrimination.

First-order sensory neurons within the trigeminal nerve have their cell bodies in what is known as the **trigeminal ganglion**, located within the temporal skull just above the cheekbone (maxilla), with a central projection that terminates in the trigeminal sensory nuclear complex of cranial nerve V in the pons, medulla, and upper spinal cord. Sensory fibers from both CN IX and X have their cell bodies in the superior and inferior ganglia, located caudal to the trigeminal ganglion, just inside the jugular foramina.[23]

This trigeminal sensory complex is divided into the principal nucleus in the pons and the elongated spinal nucleus in the medulla. Trigeminal sensory fibers enter the brainstem and course upward or downward to these two nuclei within the trigeminal sensory tract, which caudally aligns with the dorsal horn of the spinal cord and is evident in the upper cervical segments (C1–C3). The trigeminal tract also includes fibers from CN VII, IX, and X, which terminate in the solitary tract and reticular formation. The two trigeminal nuclei (principal and spinal) have a somatotropic organization related to the fiber origination from the face; most caudal are the fibers innervating the mandibular area, followed by the maxillary representation and finally the ophthalmic portion most rostral; however, the most ventral segments of the face (e.g., the nose) are more dorsal and the more dorsal aspects (e.g., the ears) are more ventral within the tract.[16,23,24] There is also a separation within the sensory complex of V between large and small diameter neuron projections. The principal nucleus primarily receives information from large-diameter fibers, conveying cutaneous sensation from the face. The most caudal portion of the nucleus (the **spinal trigeminal nucleus** caudalis) receives the smaller diameter fiber projections from the facial structures, associated with nociceptive information. There, they synapse on second-order neurons, which cross and join the lateral spinothalamic tract, terminating in the ventroposteriomedial (VPM) of the thalamus. Proprioceptive information from the muscles of mastication project to the trigeminal mesencephalic nucleus and form a monosynaptic reflex with neurons in the motor trigeminal nucleus.[23]

Second-order cutaneous fibers merge in the rostral or principal portion of the trigeminal complex, decussate upon exiting within the pons, and join the DCML system on their way to the thalamus where they synapse primarily in the VPM; thereafter, their third-order projections travel with those of the DCML to the sensory cortex within the thalamic radiations (Figure 3-10).[23] Within the primary sensory cortex, there is a large somatotopic representation of the face and oral structures, allowing for the high level of sensory processing of sensation from these areas.

Fibers from cranial nerves IX (glossopharyngeal) and X (Vegas) that are conveying pain from the mouth, ear, and internal organs join with those from the face (CN V) within the spinal portion of the trigeminal sensory nucleus. Ultimately these fibers cross to the opposite side within the anterior commissure of the upper cervical segments of the spinal cord and then ascend through the spinal cord and brainstem along with the anterolateral pathway, terminating and sending collaterals to the same areas already discussed for that pathway; however, those aligning with the lateral spinothalamic pathway terminate in VPM along with the facial tactile fibers.[23,24]

HIGHER-LEVEL SENSORY PROCESSING

A growing area of research is aimed at determining how the brain interprets sensation. Our ability to distinguish tactile stimulus characteristics is complex, ranging from the most simple identification of stimulation detection that allows the determination of location, duration, and intensity of the stimulus to the complex determination of multiple object characteristics such as shape, weight, size, texture, and temperature, and the more complex abilities of stereognosis and graphesthesia. Research, using multiple imaging modalities, has allowed us to identify the many areas of the brain involved in these simple and complex sensory perception and discrimination abilities.

S1: Primary Sensory Cortex

As mentioned earlier in the chapter, sensory projecting systems, DCML and AL, have third-order projections that terminate in the primary sensory cortex (SI). Direct thalamic projections

TABLE 3-2	Somatosensory Function from the Head and Internal Organs
CRANIAL NERVE	**AREAS OF SOMATOSENSORY FUNCTION**
V	Ophthalmic branch: Cornea, nose, upper eyelid, forehead, anterior scalpMaxillary branch: Lower eyelid, nasal mucosa, upper lip, palate, gums, cheekMandibular branch: Anterior 2/3 tongue, chin, lower jaw and teeth, 1/3 auricle of ear
IX	Posterior 1/3 of tongue
X	Pharynx, larynx, chest and abdominal organs, external ear

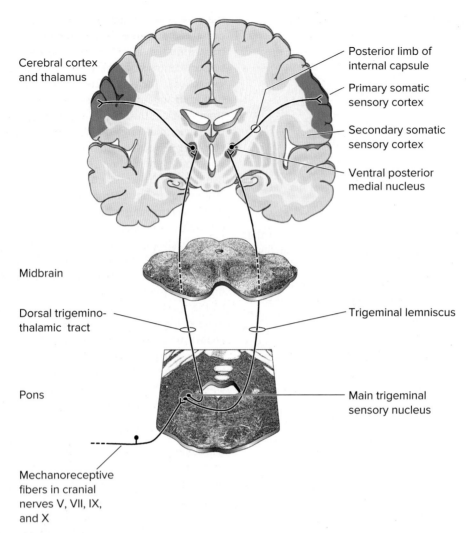

FIGURE 3-10 Trigeminal pathways for somatosensory function. (Reproduced, with permission, from Martin JH. *Neuroanatomy Text and Atlas*, 4th ed. New York: McGraw-Hill; 2012, Fig. 6-8, p. 139.)

have also been found in the secondary sensory cortex (SII), so there is some level of both parallel (at the same time) and sequential (SI first, then SII) sensory processing within these two areas. For the most part, parallel processing is most associated with temperature, pain and vibration perception, and serial processing with most other tactile stimuli.[9] SI is uniquely organized into four distinct sensory areas (3a, 3b, 1, and 2), associated with the originating stimulus, but not necessarily each individual type of receptor, resulting in four somatotopic representations of each area of the body.[17] Proprioceptive projections primarily terminated in 3a, while cutaneous projections primarily terminated in 3b.[12] Damage to area 3b can almost completely eliminate cutaneous perception as well as higher-order abilities such as object discrimination and **haptics**. Area 1, similarly, receives cutaneous information; however, damage to this area results in impaired tactile discrimination while shape discrimination remains intact. Area 2 uniquely receives both cutaneous and proprioceptive information; damage here disrupts coordination, especially of the fingers, and haptics, specifically for size and shape. In addition, SI has strong reciprocal connections back to the thalamus, suggesting that modulation

of sensation can occur through a feedback mechanism activated by the initial sensory stimulation.[1]

Lateral Somatosensory Cortex

SI is also known to project to the ipsilateral posterior parietal cortex (areas 5 and 7), supramarginal gyrus, intraparietal sulcus, and insular cortex; these latter areas are also known as the lateral somatosensory area. Neurons in SI also project to the contralateral SII and posterior parietal cortex. The insular cortex may also receive some direct sensory projections from dorsal column neurons. Notably, there are multiple sensory areas within the lateral sulcus that once were considered to be part of SII and appear to support different aspects of sensory processing. SII and the adjoining ventral area, known as the **parietal ventral (PV) area**, demonstrate mirror images of the body, respectively; their combined central region receives primarily cutaneous information while their outer areas receive proprioceptive information. Interestingly, both areas receive input from all areas of SI, but even more interesting, they receive input from both visual and auditory regions, potentially contributing to higher-level sensory integration.[1] SII appears to contribute to knowing the "what" of an object, facilitating object exploration through its connections to the motor cortex as well as the interpretation of object shape and texture; this is apparent as damage to SII results in impaired texture and shape discrimination. Alternatively, PV has connections with the posterior parietal cortex as well as the premotor cortex and is proposed to play more of a role in the knowing of the "where" of an object (orientation of the object to the body), contributing to the information needed for reaching and grasping.[25]

Posterior Parietal Cortex (PPC)

As the name implies, this area is posterior to SI and includes two regions: Brodmann's area 5, which is more rostral and extends over onto the medial portion of the hemisphere, and area 7, which extends caudally to the lateral sulcus and posteriorly to the visual cortex. Projections from area 2 of SI reach PPC through 2 separate streams: one inferior and one superior. Serial processing exists between the 2 PPC areas with area 5 receiving information from and projecting to area 7. PPC not only receives cutaneous and proprioceptive information but also receives projections from the visual, vestibular, and auditory systems. Thus, PPC is a site of sensory integration; in addition, PPC is reciprocally connected to the premotor and primary motor cortices, linking it to motor planning, especially reaching. Specifically, it seems to encode target location in relation to body position and contributes to object identification through manual exploration (e.g., haptics and stereognosis); it is also a site of integration with visual information to coordinate visually guided motion.[1]

The intricacies in the organization of SI and the connections radiating from its four subareas to SII, the posterior parietal cortex, the lateral sensory area, and the contralateral hemisphere induce activation in an even broader neural network for the determination of object characteristics (Figure 3-11). This network includes dorsal aspects of the prefrontal cortex bilaterally with a dominant level of activity in the right hemisphere.[26,27]

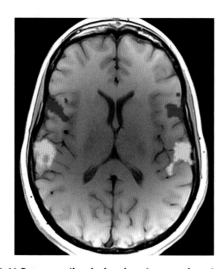

FIGURE 3-11 Sensory discrimination: Is associated with functional magnetic resonance activation in a network of SI and lateral somatosensory area, bilateral SII, and dorsal prefrontal cortex bilaterally. (Used with permission of Deborah S. Nichols Larsen, PT, PhD. The Ohio State University.)

There are also connections with speech centers to allow object identification (naming) and memory areas within the temporal lobe to maintain tactile memories. Tactile memories are also thought to involve SII. Since active touch to identify object characteristics (haptics) involves active manipulation of the object, activity within the primary motor area (M1) is typically reported with this active exploration. Simple touch perception is associated with localized activity in SI contralateral to the stimulation, but any type of tactile discrimination, whether for texture, weight, or size, initiates activation in this broader network of SII, the lateral sensory area, and the dorsal prefrontal cortex. Stereognosis, as one of the most complex sensory discrimination abilities, requires activation in memory and speech centers as well.

There is some support for a dual system for object identification. The "what" system is proposed to involve a circuit of S1 to SII with subsequent projections to areas of the insular cortex and limbic system for object identification. Conversely, projections from primary sensory cortex areas 3a and 2 to the posterior parietal cortex are thought to contribute to the "where" system. So, the first identifies what an object is and the latter provides the relationship between the object's location and the body. While this is likely an oversimplification of the complexities of this system, it allows for the understanding of brain injuries that affect components of these two circuits.[25]

Sensory Testing

Common sensory screening techniques are described in Chapter 10 (Evaluation). Logically, sensory screening focuses on touch localization, the discrimination of sharp versus dull stimuli, hot/cold discrimination, and simple proprioception and kinesthesia, and sometimes stereognosis. Proprioception and kinesthesia are often assessed superficially by having patients identify where a limb or body part is in space, after it has been moved by the therapist, or by mirroring passive movement of a limb or body part by the examiner with movement of the opposite limb or body part. This method of screening provides insight into potential sensory deficits; however, further testing is warranted, if any of these simple screening methods identify deficits. Notably, some sensory deficits are missed when only these screening tests are completed, since there are conditions that disrupt higher-level sensory discrimination ability but have little impact on touch localization or proprioception. Table 3-3 highlights a few tests that can be used in the clinic to evaluate sensory skills; these are especially focused on hand and upper extremity function, since most higher-level sensory discrimination involves use of the hands. For many of these tests, there are commercial items available for purchase; a few that should be used in the clinic are described. However, adequate testing can often be completed with constructed materials or items easily available to the practitioner. Some of these methods are also described in Table 10-4. It is important for the clinician to incorporate these methods into their assessment and progressive evaluation during treatment to determine improvement in dysfunction and improvement in many neurologic conditions. Recently, training paradigms that focus on improving sensation and movement have been described; these paradigms are included in the latter chapters on specific disorders of this text.

TABLE 3-3	Somatosensory Testing Methods	
DOMAIN	**TEST**	**DESCRIPTION**
Touch Perception	Semmes Weinstein Monofilaments™	Monofilaments applied in a descending order until the subject is unable to detect a stimulus; identifies the lightest filament detected.[28]
	WEST (Weinstein enhanced Sensory Test)™	Five monofilaments have been selected from the Semmes Weinstein battery to provide an abbreviated testing procedure; sensitivity is identified as the smallest filament detected.[29]
	Locognosia	The fingertip is divided into specific areas and the individual detects the area of the touch. Stimulus is a monofilament determined to be detectible by the individual.[31]
Two-Point Discrimination	Static	Testing is done with a Disk-Criminator™ (or other device) to allow the smallest distance that two points of contact on the skin can be differentiated from a single point. Norms are available.[30]
	Moving	Similar to static testing, a device is used with two points separated by different distances versus a single point. The smallest two-point separation that can be distinguished as they are drawn across the hand or other body part is recorded.
Sensory Discrimination	Sharp/dull	Frequently uses random application of a pencil eraser and a pin for discrimination of the two sensations. Used frequently with spinal cord injuries to screen the integrity of the two ascending systems.
	Hot/Cold	Multiple testing methods are available for purchase, but testing can include hot/cold water tubs or test tubes, plastic "ice" cubes frozen versus room temperature, or another method.
	Tactile Grating Orientation	Typically uses a set of plastic domes. Each dome has groves/ridges of equal width. The widths vary in decreasing distances. The domes are oriented either parallel or perpendicular to the finger alignment. Response as to orientation is recorded.[19]
	Roughness	There are a variety of commercially available devices to test roughness discrimination, including the domes used for tactile grating orientation. Some involve a continuous progressive grating device engraved with wide to small ridges; testing involves swiping the fingertip across the device and stopping when the ridges can no longer be detected.
	Weight	Can be done with different weights in each hand or comparing weights with the same hand. The heavier the weights, the larger the difference necessary for a detectable difference (e.g., at <10 g, a 1-g difference can be detected; at 100 g, a 7–10 g difference can be detected).
	Stereognosis	A variety of familiar objects can be used that should fit into the hand (e.g., paperclip, coin, marble); verbal influences can be eliminated by providing a picture array of included objects (some non-included objects in the picture array will make the task more challenging). Also, familiar/unfamiliar shapes can be used (circle, oval, square, octagon, or irregular shapes such as a puzzle piece) as well as letters (e.g., plastic or wood children's toys). Commercially available tests can be used.
	Graphesthesia	Letters or numbers can be drawn with the tester's fingertip or utensil (i.e., eraser end of a pencil) on hand or other body part. Verbal response or matching to a visual array can be used.

REFERENCES

1. Delhaye BP. Long KH, Bensmaia SJ. Neural basis of touch and proprioception in primate cortex. *Compr Phyiol.* 2018;8(4):1575-1602.

2. McGlone F, Reilly D. The cutaneous system. *Neurosci Behav Rev.* 2010; 34:148-159.

3. Godfrey H. Understanding pain, part 1: physiology of pain. *Brit J Nursing.* 2003;14(16):846-852.

4. Jensen TS, Finnerup NB. Allodynia and hyperalgesia in neuropathic pain: clinical manifestations and mechanisms. *Lancet Neurol.* 2014;13:924-935.

5. Abraira VE, Ginty DD. The sensory neurons of touch. *Neuron.* 2013; 78(4):618-639.

6. Fortier S, Basset FA. The effects of exercise on limb proprioceptive signals. *J Electromyogr Kinesiol.* 2012;22:795-802.

7. Gilman S. Joint position sense and vibration sense: anatomical organization and assessment. *J Neurol Neurosurg Psychiatry.* 2002;73:473-477.

8. Proske U, Ganegia SC. The kinaesthetic senses. *J Physiol*. 2009;17:4139-4146.

9. Macefield VG, Knellwolf TP. Functional properties of human muscle spindles. *J Neurophysiol*. 2018;120:452-467.

10. Banks RW. The innervation of the muscle spindle: a personal history. *J Anat*. 2015;227:115-135.

11. Nichols TR. Distributed force feedback in the spinal cord and the regulation of limb mechanics. *J Neurophysiol*. 2018;119:1186-1200.

12. Mackinnon CD. Sensorimotor anatomy of gait, balance, and falls. *Handb Clin Neurol*. 2018;159:3-26.

13. Gossard JP, Brownstone RM, Barajon I, Hultborn H. Transmission in a locomotor-related group Ib pathway from hindlimb extensor muscles in the cat. *Experimental Brain Res*. 1994;98:213-228.

14. Johannsson H. Role of knee ligaments in proprioception and regulation of muscle stiffness. *J Electromyogr Kinesiol*. 1991;1(3):158-179.

15. Lee MWL, McPhee RW, Stringer MD. An evidence-based approach to human dermatomes. *Clin Anat*. 2008;21:363-373.

16. Al-Chalabi M, Reddy V, Gupta S. *Neuroanatomy, Spinothalamic Tract*. StatPearls. Treasure Island FL: StatPearls. https://www.ncbi.nlm.nih.gov/books/NBK507824. Accessed May 4, 2023.

17. Almeida TF, Roizenblatt S, Tufik S. Afferent pain pathways: a neuroanatomical review. *Brain Res*. 2004;1000:40-56.

18. Pergolizzi J, Ahlbeck K, Aldington D, et al. The development of chronic pain: physiological CHANGE necessitates a multidisciplinary approach to treatment. *Curr Med Res Opin*. 2013;1-9.

19. Melzack R, Wall PD. Pain mechanisms: a new theory. *Science*. 1965;150:971-979.

20. Bosco G, Poppele RE. Proprioception from a spinocerebellar perspective. *Physiol Rev*. 2001;81(2):539-568.

21. Stecina K, Fedirchuk B, Hultborn H. Information to cerebellum on spinal motor networks mediated by the dorsal spinocerebellar tract. *J Physiol*. 2013;591(22):5433-5443.

22. Cohen O, Harel R, Aumann TD, Israel Z, Prut Y. Parallel processing of internal and external feedback in the spinocerebellar system of primates. *J Neurophysiol*. 2017;118:254-266.

23. Bičanič I, Hladnik A, Domagoj D, Petanjek Z. The anatomy of orofacial innervation. *Acta Clin Croat*. 2019;58(Suppl. 1):35-42.

24. DaSilva AFM, Becerra L, Makris N, et al. Somatotopic activation in the human trigeminal pain pathway. *J Neurosci*. 2002;22(18):8183-8192.

25. Disbrow E, Litinas E, Recanzone GH, Padberg J, Krubitzer L. Cortical connections of the second somatosensory area and the parietal ventral area in Macaque monkeys. *J Comp Neurol*. 2003;462:382-399.

26. Harada T, Saito DN, Kashikura K, et al. Asymmetrical neural substrates of tactile discrimination in humans: a functional magnetic resonance imaging study. *J Neurosci*. 2004;24(34):7524-7530.

27. Borstad A, Schmalbrock P, Choi S, Nichols-Larsen DS. Neural correlates supporting sensory discrimination after left hemispheric stroke. *Brain Res*. 2012;1460:78-87.

28. Baseline® Tactile™ Semmes-Weinstein Monofilaments. Available at https://www.performancehealth.com/baseline-tactile-semmes-weinstein-monofilaments. Accessed May 28, 2020.

29. Weinstein Enhanced Sensory test (WEST) Monofilament D Evaluator™. Available at https://www.rehabmart.com/product/west-d-monofilaments-22194.html. Accessed on May 28, 2020.

30. Disk-Criminator™. Available at https://www.medexsupply.com/diagnostic-tools-neurological-diagnostic-instruments-dellon-2-point-disk-criminator-set-of-2-x_pid-44822.html. Accessed on May 28, 2020.

31. Jerosch-Herold C, Rosén B, Shepstone L. The reliability and validity of the locognosia test after injuries to peripheral nerves in the hand. *J Bone Joint Surg*. 2006;88-B:1048-1052.

Review Questions

1. **Your patient is experiencing contralateral loss of pain and ipsilateral loss of touch on their right leg; where would a lesion be to produce these symptoms?**
   A. Spinal cord
   B. Upper medulla
   C. Ventroposterior nucleus of the thalamus
   D. Sensory cortex

2. **Similarly, at what level in the projections of sensation, would you expect a lesion to create contralateral loss of both pain/temperature and touch?**
   A. Above the lower medulla
   B. Below the lower medulla

3. **If there were a condition that resulted in the absence of Ruffini receptors, what types of sensation would be disrupted?**
   A. Tension and touch
   B. Touch and stretch
   C. Pain and touch
   D. Tension and pain

4. **Which is a monosynaptic reflex?**
   A. Ib activation of the heteronymous muscle
   B. Ib activation of the homonymous muscle
   C. Ia activation of the heteronymous muscle
   D. Ia activation of the homonymous muscle

5. **Which commonly used sensory test requires no additional equipment to perform?**
   A. Sharp/dull
   B. Graphesthesia
   C. Stereognosis
   D. Two-point discrimination

6. **A stroke disrupting the medial posterior thalamic nucleus would disrupt sensation from which part of the body?**
   A. Arms
   B. Legs
   C. Face
   D. Trunk

7. Your patient is experiencing hyperalgesia on the left side of her face, occurring when her hair touches it. Damage to what cranial nerve, associated with facial sensation, would it most likely be associated with?

A. Cranial nerve V

B. Cranial nerve VII

C. Cranial nerve IX

D. Cranial nerve X

8. Damage to the most medial part of the dorsal column in the cervical spinal cord would disrupt sensation from which spinal nerve roots?

A. Cervical

B. Thoracic

C. Lumbar

D. Sacral

9. Damage to Clarke's nucleus would disrupt what sensory function emanating from the legs?

A. Pain

B. Proprioception

C. Touch perception

D. Stereognosis

10. Of the components of the anterolateral pathway, which is most associated with the emotional aspects of our pain experience?

A. Lateral Spinothalamic tract

B. Spinomesencephalic tract

C. Spinoreticular tract

D. Ventral spinothalamic tract

11. The Golgi tendon organ is known to respond to what aspect of muscle activity?

A. Length change during a muscle contraction

B. Velocity of the muscle contraction

C. Force of a muscle contraction

D. Joint position during a muscle contraction

12. The posterior parietal cortex receives what kind of sensory information?

A. Cutaneous

B. Cutaneous and proprioceptive

C. Cutaneous, proprioceptive, and auditory

D. Cutaneous, proprioceptive, auditory, and visual

13. Cutaneous information is processed in which areas of SI?

A. Area 1

B. Areas 1 and 2

C. Areas 1, 2, and 3b

D. Areas, 1, 2, 3a, and 3b

14. Which of the following correctly describes the Ruffini endings?

A. Slowly adapting mechanoreceptor that responds to skin stretch

B. Rapidly adapting mechanoreceptor that responds to vibration

C. Slowly adapting mechanoreceptor that responds to pressure

D. Rapidly adapting mechanoreceptor that responds to skin motion

15. Your patient is demonstrating incoordination of the left arm; damage to which of the following might be implicated?

A. Cuneocerebellar and ventral spinocerebellar tracts

B. Cuneocerebellar and rostral spinocerebellar tracts

C. Rostral spinocerebellar and ventral spinocerebellar tracts

D. Dorsal spinocerebellar and ventral spinocerebellar tracts

Answers

1. A	2. A	3. B	4. D	5. B
6. C	7. A	8. D	9. B	10. B
11. C	12. D	13. C	14. A	15. B

GLOSSARY

A alpha neurons. Heavily myelinated large sensory (afferent) neurons.

A beta neurons. Moderately myelinated mid-sized neurons from cutaneous mechanoreceptors.

A delta neurons. Small, diameter, minimally myelinated neurons.

Allodynia (hyperalgesia). Exaggerated pain sensitivity.

Alpha motor neurons. Large A fibers to striated muscle.

Anterolateral system. System conveying pain and temperature information from the spinal cord to brain centers, includes lateral spinothalamic tract, spinoreticular tract, and spino-mesencephalic tract.

Anti-nociception. Pain modulation, arising from multiple systems.

Autogenic Inhibition. Protective reflex induced by excessive stretch, leading to contraction of the homonymous muscle and inhibition of the heteronymous muscle.

Beta motor neurons. Mid-sized motor neurons that innervate both extrafusal and intrafusal fibers.

C Neurons fibers. Small diameter, unmyelinated.

Cuneatus. Dorsal column funiculus, conveying upper body somatosensory information.

Cuneate nucleus (nucleus cuneatus). Medullary nucleus, site of synapse between first- and second-order neurons conveying cutaneous sensation.

Cuniocerebellar tract. Projection of upper limb fibers, conveying proprioceptive information from external cuneate nucleus to cerebellum.

Cutaneous sensation. Touch, temperature, pain, and itch.

Cutaneous/touch receptors (mechanoreceptors). Meissner corpuscles, Merkel disks, and Ruffini endings.

Dermatomes. Area of skin innervated by one spinal nerve.

Dorsal-column-medial lemniscal pathway. Conveys cutaneous and proprioceptive information to the cortex.

Dorsal spinocerebellar tract. Conveys lower extremity proprioception to ipsilateral vermis and paravermal cortex.

External cuneate nucleus (external cuneatus). Medullary nucleus, site of synapsing for upper limb proprioceptive first- and second-order neurons from dorsal column.

Extrafusal fibers. Skeletomotor muscle fibers.

Gamma motor neurons (γ). Motor neurons to muscle spindles.

Gracilis. Dorsal column funiculus, conveying lower extremity sensation.

Gracilis nucleus. Medullary nucleus, site of synapse between first- and second-order somatosensory neurons of the dorsal column-medial lemniscal pathway.

Golgi tendon organ (GTO). Receptor for muscle force.

Graphesthesia. Identification of drawing of letters or words on the skin.

Haptics. Detection of object characteristics (shape, texture, roughness, weight) through touch.

Heteronymous muscle. Antagonistic muscle.

Homonymous muscle. Muscle of origin for a Ia fiber.

Hyperalgesia. Exaggerated response to a painful stimulus.

Ib fibers. Large alpha afferent that innervates Golgi tendon organ.

Intrafusal fibers. Tiny muscle fibers within muscle spindles.

Kinesthesia. A component of proprioception, involving posture and movement awareness.

Lateral spinothalamic tract. Conveys pain and temperature information; comprised of three components that terminate in either the ventral posterolateral nucleus of thalamus, posterior medial, and intralaminar nuclei of thalamus, or central medial nucleus of thalamus.

Mechanoreceptors. Cutaneous receptors, convert mechanical force applied to the skin, muscle, tendons, or joint capsule to neural signals.

Meissner corpuscles (RA1). Rapidly adapting superficial mechanoreceptors, activated by skin motion.

Merkel disks (SA1). Slowly adapting superficial mechanoreceptors, activated by pressure.

Muscle spindles. Encapsulated receptors in skeletomotor muscles that respond to muscle length.

Nociceptors. Pain receptors.

Nucleus proprious. Site of termination for C fibers within dorsal gray matter of spinal cord.

Pacinian corpuscles (RA2). Rapidly adapting deep mechanoreceptors, responsive to vibration and texture.

Parietal ventral area. Located in the lateral sulcus; a component of the "where" system.

Polymodal nociceptors. Nociceptors responding to multiple types of pain sensations.

Posterior marginalis. Site of termination for Aδ fibers within dorsal gray matter of spinal cord.

Posterior parietal cortex. Posterior to SI, site of sensory integration and linked to motor planning.

Primary afferent (Ia). Large-diameter fiber innervating central portion of intrafusal fibers.

Primary sensory cortex (S1). Postcentral gyrus, Brodmann's areas 3a, 3b, 2, and 1.

Principal nucleus of CN V. Locus of second-order neurons for cutaneous sensation.

Proprioception. Ability to sense muscle tension, limb/body position and motion, muscle movement and effort, and balance.

Rapidly adapting mechanoreceptors. Respond quickly to stimulus change (Pacinian and Meissner Corpuscles).

Receptive field. Surface area for which a single receptor or a single free nerve ending responds.

Rostral spinocerebellar tract. Conveys upper extremity proprioception to the ipsilateral anterior cerebellum.

Ruffini endings (SA2). Slowly adapting mechanoreceptors, located deep in skin, activated by skin stretch.

Secondary afferents (II). Large-diameter fiber innervating nuclear chains and static bags of muscle spindle.

Secondary somatosensory cortex (SII). Involved in knowing the "what" about objects due to its ties with language and memory areas

Skeletomotor muscle. Striated muscle that moves limbs or trunk.

Slow-adapting mechanoreceptors. Activated by a maintained stimulus and continue firing for the duration of the stimulus (Ruffini endings, Merkel disks).

Spinal Trigeminal Nucleus. Locus of second-order neurons for nociception for the face.

Stereognosis. Object identification and object characteristic identification through touch.

Thermoreceptors. Temperature receptors.

Tract of Lissauer. Most dorsal aspect of dorsal gray matter, pathway for primary pain afferents to ascend 1-2 segments within spinal cord.

Trigeminal ganglion. Locus for the cell bodies of the first-order sensory neurons of the trigeminal nerve.

Ventral spinocerebellar tract. Project cutaneous and proprioceptive information from lower extremities to the anterior vermis of cerebellum.

Ventroposteriolateral nucleus. Thalamic nucleus; site of synapsing between second and third-order sensory neurons from the extremities and trunk.

Ventroposteriomedial nucleus. Thalamic nucleus; site of synapsing between second- and third-order sensory neurons from the face.

Sensorimotor Systems of the Spinal Cord

4

D. Michele Basso

OBJECTIVES

1) Describe cellular structures that support movement

2) Characterize the neural firing properties that modulate contraction force

3) Differentiate between spinal interneurons and their role in movement

4) Evaluate how the spinal cord produces simple and complex movements

INTRODUCTION

This chapter will explore how the spinal cord is organized to produce complex movements. There is an orchestrated, precise balance between the type of afferent information entering the cord and how it is integrated by neurons in the gray matter of the spinal cord to activate muscles. The difference between a simple movement like the patellar tendon reflex and running on a treadmill can be as little as adding a set of interneurons to the monosynaptic circuit. We will consider how the spinal cord is designed to support multi-joint movements that adapt to the changing environment and unexpected perturbations within milliseconds. This chapter will show you that the spinal cord is organized in remarkable ways so that even a few neurons can mediate and sustain intricate, complex movements without input from the brain. Probably the most exciting feature we will consider is that the spinal cord can learn tasks independent of the brain. With this functional capacity existing in the cord, the brain can provide descending input and create even more complex, skilled movements.

Structure and Organization of the Spinal Cord

The human spinal cord extends from the base of the skull to the vertebral level between L1 and L2. It is made up of cervical, thoracic, lumbar, and sacral regions, which receive afferent information and send motor signals to nearby muscles – **cervical** supplies the arms and hands; **thoracic** supplies the trunk; **lumbar** supplies the legs and feet; and **sacral** supplies the bowel, bladder, and genitalia. The spinal cord has unique features in each region based on the shape and size of **gray matter** and the amount of surrounding **white matter, comprised** of myelinated axons that ascend to the brain, descend from the brain, and propriospinal axons connecting different regions of the cord (Figure 4-1).

In regions that supply many muscles as in the upper and lower extremities, the gray matter will be larger in the cervical and lumbar cord. Specifically, greater motor neurons reside in the ventral horn of the gray matter in these regions. Smaller gray matter and thin ventral horns appear in the thoracic cord, which primarily supplies intercostal muscles. The white matter is also larger in cervical and lumbar enlargements than in the thoracic cord due to increased myelinated axons to innervate motor neurons and sensory axons ascending to the brain, associated with the enlargements. Therefore, the cervical cord is larger in diameter than all other segments and has a greater risk of compression injury due to whiplash or spinal stenosis (canal narrowing).

The **dorsal horn** consists of several layers of neurons that receive afferent input, described in detail in Chapter 3, Somatosensory Pathways and Perception. The **ventral horn** contains alpha and gamma motor neuron pools for each of the muscles in the body (Figure 4-2). These pools are generally divided into **medial groups** that supply axial muscles and **lateral groups** that innervate distal muscle groups. The **spinal interneurons** in the **intermediate zone** make up networks for organization of multi-joint muscle synergies within a limb and other typical movement patterns. They connect both sides of the cord and coordinate the action of the axial motor pools to allow for alternating movements of the legs and arms, while walking, as well as other actions. In contrast, the lateral motor pools have few interneuronal connections with the opposite side of the cord. This allows us to move each hand or foot independent of the other. In the thoracic and upper lumbar regions of the cord, the intermediate gray matter has a prominent lateral horn where neurons of the autonomic nervous system are located. These neurons make up the sympathetic nervous system that controls body responses in emergency situations like dilating the pupils and increasing the heart rate as introduced in Chapter 1.[1]

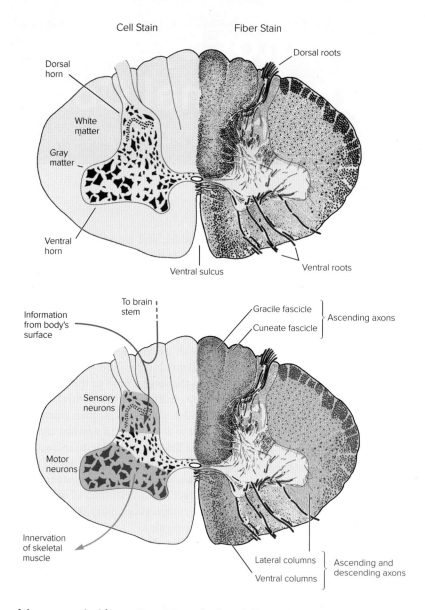

FIGURE 4-1 Organization of the gray and white matter of the spinal cord. (Reproduced with permission from Kandel ER, Schwartz JH, et al., *Principles of Neural Science*, 5th ed. New York, NY: McGraw-Hill; 2013.)

● BUILDING BLOCKS OF MOVEMENT: MUSCLES AND MOTOR NEURONS

In normal movement, we do not recruit one muscle cell at a time; we recruit an entire **motor unit**, which is defined as one alpha motoneuron and the muscle cells it innervates. In the normal, healthy condition, each time that an alpha motoneuron generates an action potential at the neuromuscular junctions of the innervated muscle, a muscle twitch occurs in every one of its muscle cells. This is the most basic level of movement that can occur. The job of the nervous system is to organize the multitude of twitches into simple movements like finger tapping as well as the precise movements of ballet or the strength and agility of a running back.

Not all motor units are identical. Several factors differ between motor units, including the number and type of muscle fibers that make up the unit. Some have a relatively small number of muscle

fibers in the motor unit, and some have many. Some are comprised of small, **slow twitch** muscle fibers with good endurance that produce low force while some are composed of large, **fast twitch** muscle fibers with high force production capacity but fatigue quickly. And, some are intermediate in these properties.[2] As illustrated in Table 4-1, these properties all go together in certain combinations that provide the nervous system with a menu of choices for the control of movement. For example, whether standing in front of a class or sitting on a stool, we control posture using relatively low force and lasting endurance, recruiting primarily muscle tissue that is highly resistant to fatigue. Smaller motor units with slow twitch muscle fibers are ideally suited to this task. If the person who is standing or sitting reaches for a pen, a greater force impulse will be needed to launch the hand on its trajectory while maintaining a stable posture, but full-blown effort won't be used. Here, a combination of small and intermediate motor units would be recruited to perform these postural

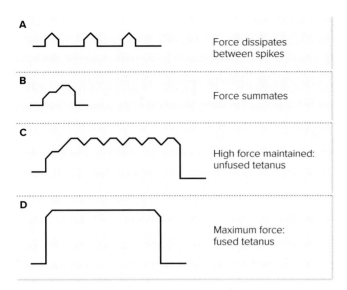

FIGURE 4-2 Muscle activation and force production relationship. A. Slow firing rate with muscle relaxation between next action potential. **B.** Intermediate firing rate with summation of muscle contraction and greater force. **C.** Fast firing rate with only minimal relaxation and greater force production. **D.** Maximal firing rate and maximal force.

and reaching tasks. This reaching task would not require much, if any, recruitment of the largest motor units. However, if we were to throw a ball across the room from our standing or sitting posture, we would need to recruit additional motor units that produce high force for brief periods. Thus, layered with small, slow motor units for postural control, we would add intermediate motor units to initiate arm trajectory and lastly, our largest, fast twitch-high force motor units would be needed to produce enough arm velocity to propel the ball a long distance.

One of the more convenient tricks of biology for the control of muscle recruitment is described in a phenomenon called the **size principle**, which was extensively studied by E. Henneman.[3] As described above, we would like the first motor units brought into use for the control of low-level effort, where subtle modulation of force is required, to be the smaller motor units with slow twitch muscle fibers. We would not want the largest motor units to be active in this situation because they would make us overshoot the mark. Conversely, if we are in a circumstance where we need maximum muscle force, the slow twitch, smaller motor units are welcome to join in the effort, but we will ultimately need the largest, fast twitch units to get the job done. With few exceptions, the nervous system follows this principle of size in recruitment order.

This occurs somewhat automatically because the alpha motoneurons for the smaller, slow twitch motor units are smaller neurons. With a given amount of synaptic drive for excitation, a smaller motoneuron experiences a more substantial voltage change and is, therefore, easier to bring above threshold for an action potential. A larger motoneuron requires a greater amount of synaptic input to become excited. Hence, if the nervous system simply targets small and large motoneurons equally and drives them all without distinction, the natural result is that with low levels of drive to the motoneurons, only the smaller ones will be activated. With a full-blown effort, the small and the large will be activated. Hence, the proper recruitment order comes about naturally, simply based on the sizes of the alpha motoneurons.[2,3]

Putting the Building Blocks Together

The nervous system activates the different motor units in a selective, organized way to produce finely graded force. For small precise movements like those of the eye and eardrum, small motor units are recruited that have very few muscle fibers. A motor unit in an extraocular muscle has about 10 fibers. When intermediate control is needed, such as hoisting a hammer, units with more muscle fibers will be recruited. The intrinsic muscles of the hand have a few hundred fibers in each motor unit. When general motor function with a high level of force is required like jumping up to catch a rebound, motor units with a high number of muscle fibers will be activated. In the gastrocnemius, a single motor unit contains about 2000 muscle fibers.[2,4] We can now see that the muscular system is capable of contracting in a graded fashion to produce forces that match the needs of the task. These gradations are determined by the firing rate of the alpha motor neuron.

The force, speed, and duration of muscle contraction are determined in the spinal cord. The firing rate of the alpha motor neuron modulates muscle force. A slow firing rate of the motor neuron means that the time between one action potential and the next is long enough to allow the motor unit (all muscle cells innervated by a single alpha motor neuron) to fully relax before the next action potential arrives. The long intervals and slow firing rate produce low levels of muscle force that quickly dissipate (Figure 4-2). This type of activity would be a muscle twitch. When the firing rate is increased to an intermediate level, the interval between action potentials shortens and the muscle doesn't fully relax before the second action potential causes a contraction. The contractile force from the second impulse piggybacks on the first, which is known as **summation**, and causes greater force production. In this way, even a slightly faster firing rate can produce

TABLE 4-1	Classification of Motor Units[2]		
	SLOW	**FAST FATIGABLE**	**FAST FATIGUE RESISTANT**
Fiber type	Type 1; red	Type IIb, IIx; white	Type IIa; red
Motor unit size	Small	Intermediate	Large
Oxidative capacity	High, aerobic	Low, anaerobic	Mix, anaerobic
Force production	Low	High	Intermediate
Contraction time	Long	Rapid	Rapid

substantially higher contraction forces. This type of activity would occur when standing upright to overcome gravity. With a fast firing rate of the motor neuron, the interval between action potentials is very short, so muscle force increases quickly and very little relaxation occurs. Therefore, force levels remain high and each successive action potential produces small fluctuations in force. This is called **unfused tetanus** and occurs during high force activities like weightlifting or a maximal voluntary contraction. There is also an experimental condition that can produce even greater contractile forces; the motor axon is stimulated at a very fast rate, which is higher than the motor neuron can produce on its own. In this condition, there is almost no interval between action potentials and maximum force is immediately generated. Because there is no relaxation, the force is sustained without fluctuation and is called **fused tetanus**.[5]

How much does the firing have to change to produce gradations in muscle force? Even very small changes to the firing rate can modulate muscle force and produce different patterns of movement. Adding an extra action potential or eliminating one from a train of impulses will reset the contractile force. In studies by Burke, adding a single extra impulse to a high firing rate caused the force to summate. This higher level of force was maintained throughout the train of impulses (Figure 4-3A). Likewise, removing a single impulse from a train of action potentials immediately reduces muscle force that is sustained with each subsequent impulse (Figure 4-3B).[6] This means that if the alpha motor neuron simply adds or omits a single action potential from a group of impulses, then a substantial and sustained change in muscle force occurs. The next chapter will consider how features of the muscle and motor neuron recruitment contribute to contractile force determination.

We know that muscle activity is dictated by the firing rate and pattern of the alpha motor neuron, so the next factor to consider is how alpha motor neuron firing is controlled. There are three sources of input that drive motor neuron activity – descending axons from nuclei in the brain, sensory afferents from the periphery, and interneurons within the spinal cord. Descending brain systems will be discussed in the next chapter.

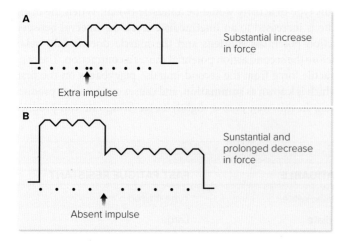

FIGURE 4-3 Gradations in force. Changes in force generation accompany changes in action potential train generation. **A.** An additional impulse creates an increase in force. **B.** An omitted impulse will decrease force.

Afferent Drive

Organization of complex movements begins at the level of the spinal cord and builds upon the simplest movement – the muscle spindle stretch reflex. As we have seen in Chapter 3, the stretch reflex is monosynaptic, meaning that the primary sensory afferents from the muscle spindle synapse directly on the motor neuron. A quick stretch of the muscle stimulates the Ia afferent, which elicits firing of the alpha motor neurons that innervate the stretched muscle. The resulting muscle contraction relieves the stretch. This monosynaptic relationship allows for rapid changes in motor neuron firing based on proprioceptive feedback from the periphery. Small stretches of the muscle will change the firing rate, which in turn will produce gradations in force and movement. In this way, proprioceptive input to the cord influences motor neuron activation. It is upon this background that all volitional, purposeful movement is orchestrated.

To engage in purposeful movement, the activation and coordination of many motor neurons and the muscles they innervate must occur. One process, called **divergence**, creates widely distributed motor neuron ensembles. In divergence, axon collaterals from a single neuron synapse on specific, distributed groups of neurons and, when activated, produce coordinated responses. Divergence occurs in the monosynaptic reflex where the afferent axon sends collateral branches to motor neurons of synergist muscles and to interneurons in the gray matter.[7] The input to the synergistic motor neurons enables a more effective movement. Divergence of afferent drive also occurs within a single muscle that has several divisions like the extensor digitorum (ED) of the hand. By ordering synaptic input to subsets of motor neurons for the ED, extension of one finger is synchronized with the other fingers.[8] Thus, we can begin to see that sending common proprioceptive input to distributed neurons will produce coordinated, synchronized muscle action across multiple joints. Divergence of synaptic input occurs in all neurons in the nervous system.

Spinal Interneurons

Interneurons are located in the gray matter of the spinal cord and receive inputs from peripheral afferents and descending axons from brain nuclei. Interneurons consolidate these multiple signals, compare them, and determine whether the signal is passed onto the motor neuron. Interneurons can be defined by their relationship to the motor neuron, the type of afferent input they receive, and whether they are excitatory or inhibitory. The last interneuron to synapse onto the motor neuron is called the **last order interneuron**, and these have been the most studied type of interneurons in the spinal cord. While many last order interneurons have been identified in mammals (Figure 4-4), three have been characterized in terms of their role in modulating muscle contraction: the 1a inhibitory interneuron, the Renshaw cell, and the 1b inhibitory interneuron.

Ia Inhibitory Interneuron

The Ia inhibitory interneuron plays an important role in the stretch reflex (see Chapter 3). If we consider a stretch reflex of the biceps tendon, the Ia afferent from the muscle spindle sends axon collaterals not only to the motor neurons of the biceps and the synergistic brachioradialis muscle but also sends a branch to the Ia inhibitory interneuron (Figure 4-4). The Ia

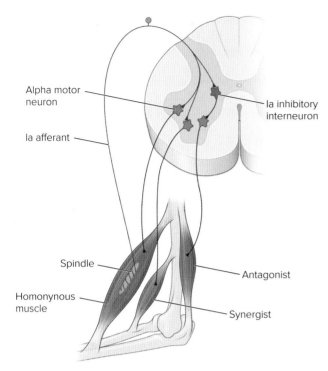

FIGURE 4-4 Diagram of the Ia inhibitory interneuron. The Ia inhibitory interneuron is activated by a collateral of the Ia afferent and serves to inhibit the antagonistic muscle to allow the reflexive contraction of the homonymous muscle and its agonists.

inhibitory interneuron synapses on the motor neurons of the antagonist triceps muscle and stops its activity. This is another example of the process of divergence used by the nervous system to produce coordinated, distributed control because at the same time the elbow flexors are contracting, the extensor is relaxed. In this way, there is little opposing force to overcome as the elbow flexes.

The spinal cord interneurons play an important role in goal-directed movements. The Ia inhibitory interneuron receives a convergence of synapses from the primary afferents, corticospinal axons, other descending axons from the brain and brainstem as well as other interneurons (Figure 4-5A). The output of the Ia interneuron is the sum of these excitatory and inhibitory inputs. The higher brain centers control the activity of the opposing muscle at a joint through a single command. A descending signal that stimulates muscle contraction at a joint will also simultaneously relax the opposing muscle.

Renshaw Cells

Renshaw cells are inhibitory and synapse back on alpha and gamma motor neurons of the agonist and synergists, which is called **recurrent inhibition**; they receive input from descending brainstem nuclei and are also stimulated by motor neurons (Figure 4-5B). The Renshaw cell also inhibits Ia inhibitory interneurons to the antagonist, thereby facilitating their activation. Thus, activation of the Renshaw cell controls the excitability of the agonist and antagonist around the joint.[9]

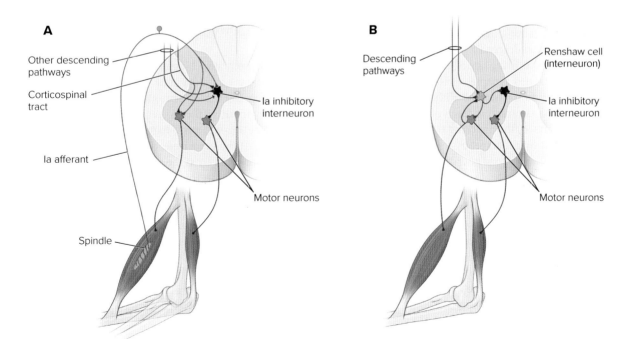

FIGURE 4-5 Illustration of Ia inhibitory neuron and Renshaw cell control. A. Convergence of input from descending pathways and primary afferents converge on the Ia inhibitory interneuron as part of coordinated movement; the sum of these inputs will excite or inhibit the Ia inhibitory interneuron. **B.** Renshaw cells serve to inhibit their agonist and synergists and inhibit the antagonist, which serves to protect the homonymous muscle(s) from excessive exertion or to refine movement; they are activated by motor neurons and descending brainstem pathways.

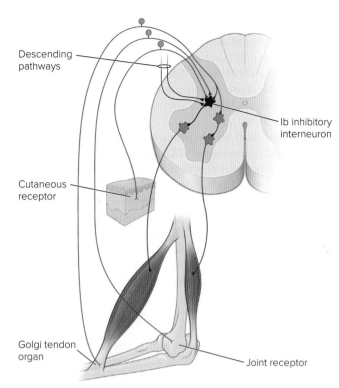

FIGURE 4-6 Ib inhibitory interneurons. The Ib inhibitory interneuron is part of the Golgi tendon organ's homonymous inhibitory circuit, decreasing activation to the homonymous muscle and its synergists while facilitating the antagonist; descending motor systems also can activate the Ib inhibitory interneuron to achieve coordinated muscle activity.

Group Ib Inhibitory Interneurons

Group Ib inhibitory interneurons are innervated by afferent axons from the Golgi tendon organ as well as ipsilateral corticospinal and rubrospinal descending axons (Figure 4-6). These interneurons decrease the firing rate of the homonymous motor neuron. The Ib axons also synapse on Ib excitatory interneurons to stimulate the motor neuron of the antagonist muscle. In this way, while the contracting force of the agonist muscle is controlled or decreased, the opposing resistance is increased. Convergence of input from cutaneous afferents and joint afferents also occurs on Ib inhibitory interneurons to reinforce and integrate multiple inputs.

Importance of Interneurons

Remarkably intricate and orchestrated multi-joint movements emerge by combining excitatory and inhibitory interneurons into circuits within the spinal cord. The spinal cord controls bilateral limb movements without descending brain input by using interneurons to take a single input and convey it throughout a limb and to the opposite limb. This is called divergence.

The flexor withdrawal reflex is a good example of how the spinal cord integrates afferent input through the interneuronal networks to produce coordinated movement across both legs. Figure 4-7 shows the interneuronal pathways activated by a painful stimulus. By stepping on a tack, action potentials in

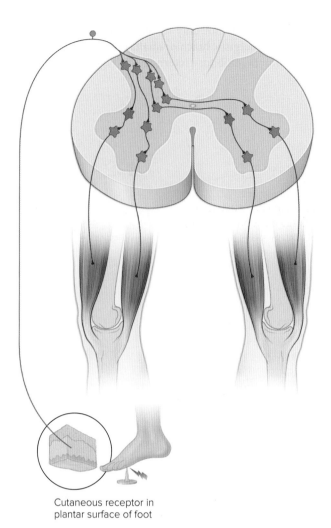

Cutaneous receptor in plantar surface of foot

FIGURE 4-7 Interneuronal network for the spinal flexor withdrawal reflex.

small unmyelinated A-delta fibers from the skin are transmitted to many excitatory and inhibitory interneurons. On the painful leg, the motor neurons that control the flexors receive excitatory input so the leg can be lifted off the tack. However, raising the leg will only happen if the extensor muscles are inhibited. At the same time, the painful input diverges through interneurons that cross the gray matter to the motor neurons of the opposite leg. In this limb, the extensor motor neurons are activated and the flexor motor neurons are inhibited. In this way, the spinal cord ensures that while the painful leg is lifted off the tack, the opposite leg is stiffened to support the weight of the person. Otherwise, the person literally wouldn't have a leg to stand on.

These interneuronal networks are not only used to control reflexes but also to coordinate, complex voluntary movements. Depending on the convergence and divergence in the circuit, a single input signal can create a response that outlasts the stimulus (Figure 4-8). This type of processing is called a **reverberating circuit** and is made up of at least three excitatory interneurons. Excitation of the first interneuron diverges and causes excitation of other interneurons that converge back on the original interneuron.

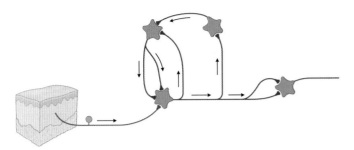

FIGURE 4-8 Illustration of a reverberating excitatory circuit. Initial sensory neuron activation can induce activity in a reverberating circuit that produces ongoing excitation as the circuit feeds back onto the original second-order neuron; this type of activity plays a role in ongoing pain experiences that continue long after the pain stimulus is removed.

Adding inhibitory interneurons to a reverberating circuit converts afferent activity or tonic, continuous neural drive into alternating activation of flexor and extensor muscle groups (Figure 4-9). This type of organization is thought to be part of the **central pattern generator** (CPG). A CPG produces rhythmic motor patterns without input from the brain or sensory input. Once they receive a "go signal," they become self-stimulating and produce repetitive synchronized activity that continues until a "stop signal" occurs. While there are examples of CPGs in various parts of the nervous system, the CPGs in the spinal cord produce locomotion (Figure 4-10; Box 4-1).

The influence of a small portion of descending motor axons from the brain on spinal cord plasticity and learning was recently shown, using a sensitive indicator of learning. In rats with a spinal cord injury in the thoracic region, some descending axons are spared and reach the lumbar enlargement where they change lumbar cord functions. In one group, the lumbar cord had recovered for several weeks in the presence of spared axons. In the other group, recovery occurred in the absence of spared axons. Next, the lumbar cord was isolated from the brain by complete transection and a learning test was applied to show the capacity of the lumbar cord in these groups (Figure 4-11). In the learning test, the hindlimb is suspended over a saline solution and a contact rod was taped to the paw. When the limb dangles in an extended position, the rod contacts the solution, which completes an electrical circuit and delivers a small electrical stimulation to the leg. If the lumbar cord learns, the leg will

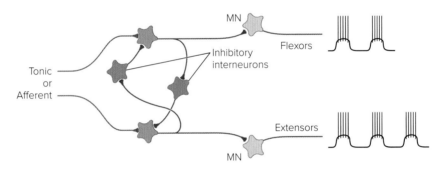

FIGURE 4-9 Inhibitory interneurons within a reverberating circuit. When inhibitory interneurons exist within a reverberating circuit, they induce alternating inhibition within the existing excitation of the circuit, consistent with the repetitive excitation–inhibition of the gait cycle.

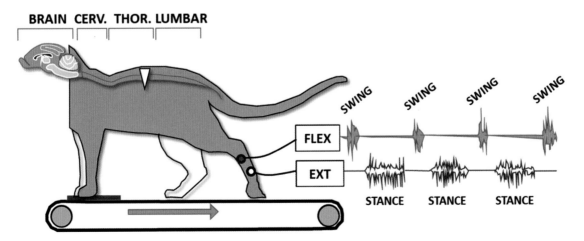

FIGURE 4-10 Evidence of Central Pattern Generator (CPG) in the spinal cord that produces locomotion. Complete transection of the thoracic cord (THOR.) at the white point isolates the lumbar cord that innervates hindlimb muscles from brain and cervical (CERV.) cord motor systems. The CPGs in the isolated cord activate hindlimb flexor muscles (Flex; blue EMG bursts in swing) and extensor muscles (Ext; white EMG bursts instance). EMG = Electromyography

---

Box 4-1   Evidence of CPGs for Locomotion

The first and best evidence of CPGs for locomotion within the spinal cord were identified in animals. In these experiments, the spinal cord was cut to prevent any input moving from and to the brain; this is called **spinal cord transection**. In this way, the lumbar spinal cord is isolated and only receives input from the peripheral muscle, cutaneous, and joint receptors. To understand the motor control of the spinal cord, the animal was placed on a moving treadmill. If brain input is required to produce locomotion, then the hindlegs with only isolated lumbar cord control would not step. Scientists were surprised to find that the animals were able to step with both hindlimbs in a coordinated, alternating pattern.[10] Using this transection paradigm, scientists also showed that isolated spinal cord circuits can adapt to changing environments.

For example, hindlimb locomotion increases when the treadmill speeds up and stepping movements change to overcome obstacles placed on the belt.[11] These findings mean that information from the peripheral receptors can modulate spinal cord neurons on a step-by-step basis to produce purposeful movements. Next, scientists set out to determine whether the isolated spinal cord could be trained to generate specific tasks.[12] After spinal cord transection, animals underwent daily training for several

weeks. One group was trained to step with the hindlegs on a moving treadmill while another group was trained to stand and support the hindquarters on a stationary treadmill. With intensive training, the stepping group showed steady increase in the number of consecutive alternating steps of the hindlegs, and the stand-trained group had regular increases in time of independent weight support. Thus, the spinal cord can respond to task-specific sensory input from peripheral receptors to learn coordinated, multi-joint movements without any input from the brain. This task-specific learning was maintained for several weeks after training ended; then, the groups were tested and trained on the opposite task. Interestingly, both groups learned the new task but were unable to retain the previously learned task. This finding indicates that the isolated spinal cord continues to be able to learn new tasks but has a limited capacity. Learning of a new task extinguishes the old task. These experiments lay the foundation for an activity-based rehabilitation after CNS injury or disease. They demonstrate that the spinal cord retains a remarkable ability to learn motor tasks even in the most severe condition of complete loss of input from the brain. In conditions where partial input from the brain is spared, even greater capacity for motor relearning at the spinal level is likely to exist.

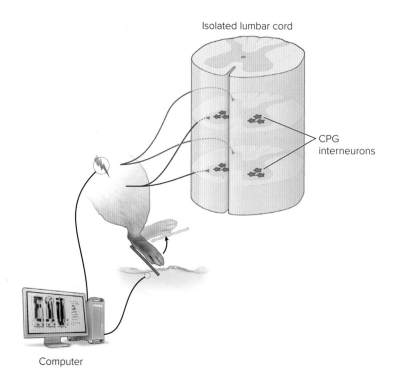

FIGURE 4-11 Experimental test of learning and plasticity in the lumbar cord. A mild stimulus over the front of leg activates lumbar interneurons. With good learning and plasticity, the motor neurons are activated and the paw is held out of the water to avoid the stimulus.

be held out of the solution to avoid the stimulation, but if there is no learning, stimulation time will be greater. In this study, the lumbar cord that recovered in the presence of some sparing was able to keep the limb elevated out of the solution longer and make fewer mistakes than when no sparing occurred. This study is important because it shows that even small amounts of sparing can greatly change the functional plasticity of neural systems that are likely part of CPGs for walking. It is this plasticity that rehabilitation may be able to capitalize on to improve function.[13]

What Are the Clinical Implications of CPGs and Spinal Learning?

Central pattern generators for locomotion have been well-described in a variety of animals but cannot be definitively proven in the human spinal cord because all input from the brain must be eliminated. To assure complete transection of the cord after injury and isolation from brain input, microscopic examination of the injury is required that cannot be performed in people living with spinal cord injury. The best evidence of CPG in the human cord is provided by Blaire Calancie's report from 1994.[14] This study is of a man who experienced a spinal cord injury 17 years earlier that resulted in incomplete paralysis below the injury. He started intensive gait training, and shortly thereafter, found that when he laid supine with his hips fully extended, his legs began moving. The movements were involuntary and moved in an alternating, stepping-like manner. He could not voluntarily suppress these rhythmic movements, and they would continue until he moved out of supine or hip extension. These stepping-like movements emerged during sleeping and awakened him several times a night. Several characteristics of these movements match those produced by CPGs in animal studies, including the fact that rhythmicity occurred without brain input, the stepping movements responded to hip angle, and muscle activation occurred in a strict timing pattern. Availability of human CPGs for locomotion holds promise for improving recovery after CNS injury, since they would remain largely intact after brain or spinal cord injury and be capable of producing coordinated, functional leg movements that respond to changes in the environment.

SKILL LEARNING AND SENSORIMOTOR INTEGRATION

The organization of sensory and motor systems in the spinal cord can produce complex functions, tasks and actions with remarkable efficiency. Afferent input from the periphery plays a pivotal role when learning new tasks and consolidating the learning into skilled, error-free performance. In fact, recent research shows that adding electrical stimulation to somatosensory nerves in the forearm of healthy adults, improved motor skill learning by increasing sensorimotor integration in the cortex.[15] New research has also focused on learning in natural/actual settings. The influence of the environment on motor learning is a foundational part of motor control[16] and is more recently being examined through ecological dynamics research.[17] Given the importance of the environment on movement, it seems that afferent input to the cord is an important neurophysiology mechanism for motor learning and relearning. Exposure to natural/realistic conditions during training in healthy or CNS impairment will improve motor unit recruitment, appropriate force modulation, and transference between upper limb, trunk, and lumbosacral muscles. This ecological approach is one rationale for task-specific training during rehabilitation (e.g., to better entrain the CNS for skill acquisition rather than simply neural and muscle activation). Likewise, training with virtual reality (VR) may not faithfully engage the CNS due to simulated rather than real world conditions. It is clear that benefits of VR include greater motivation to practice, capturing skill learning as play, improvement in acuity (rate of accurate performance).[18]

However, translation to real world performance is especially difficult when haptics are a major part of the task. Haptics include the perception of vibration, temperature, texture, and heft of objects.[19] Technical advances to improve haptics in the virtual environment are critically needed and are under development.[20,21]

REFERENCES

1. Cho TA. Spinal cord functional anatomy. *Continuum (Minneap Minn)*. 2015;21(1):13-15.
2. Monti RJ, Roy RR, Edgerton VR. Role of motor unit structure in defining function. *Muscle Nerve*. 2001;24:848-866.
3. Henneman E, Somjen G, Carpenter DO. Functional significance of cell size in spinal motoneurons. *J Neurophysiol*. 1965;28:560-580.
4. Enoka RM. Morphological features and activation patterns of motor units. *J Clin Neurophys*. 1995;12(6):538-559.
5. Celichowski J. Mechanisms underlying the regulation of motor unit contraction in the skeletal muscle. *J Physiol Pharmacol*. 2000;51:17-33.
6. Burke RE. Composite nature of the monosynaptic postsynaptic potential. *J Neurophysiol*. 1967;30(5):1114-1137.
7. Mendell LM, Henneman E. Terminals of single Ia fibers: location, density, and distribution within a pool of 300 homonymous motoneurons. *J Neurophysiol*. 1971;34:171-187.
8. Keen DA, Fuglevand AJ. Role of intertendinous connections in distribution of force in the human extensor digitorum muscle. *Muscle Nerve*. 2003;28:614-622.
9. Alvarez FJ, Fyffe REW. The continuing case for the Renshaw cell. *J Physiol*. 2007;584(1):31-45.
10. Stuart DG, Hultborn H. Thomas Graham Brown (1882-1965), Anders Lundberg (1920-), and the neural control of stepping. *Brain Res Rev*. 2008;59:74-95.
11. Zhong H, Roy RR, Nakada KK, et al. Accommodation of the spinal cat to a tripping perturbation. *Front Physiol*. 2012;3:112.
12. Hodgson JA, Roy RR, Dobkin B, Edgerton VR. Can the mammalian lumbar spinal cord learn a motor task? *Med Sci Sports Exerc*. 1994;26:1491-1497.
13. Hansen CN, Faw TD, White S, Buford JA, Grau JW, Basso DM. Sparing of descending axons rescues interneuron plasticity in lumbar cord to allow adaptive learning after thoracic spinal cord injury. *Frontiers Neural Circuits*. 2016;10:11.
14. Calancie B, Needham-Shropshire B, Jacobs P, Willer K, Zych G, Green BA. Involuntary stepping after chronic spinal cord injury. Evidence for a central rhythm generator for locomotion in man. *Brain*. 1994;117:1143-1159.
15. Veldman MP, Maurits NM, Zijdewind I, et al. Somatosensory electrical stimulation improves skill acquisition, consolidation, and transfer by increasing sensorimotor activity and connectivity. *J Neurophysiol*. 2018;120:281-290.
16. Gentile AM. Skill acquisition: action, movement, and the neuromotor processes. In: Carr JH, Shepherd RB, Gordon J, Gentile AM. Held JM, eds. *Movement Science: Foundations for Physical Therapy in Rehabilitation*. Rockville: Aspen; 1987.
17. Renshaw I, Keith D, O'Sullivan M, Maloney MA, Crowther R, McCosker. An ecological dynamics approach to motor learning in practice: reframing the learning and performing relationship in high performance sport. *Asian J Sport Exerc Psychol*. 2022;2:18-26.
18. Listman JB, Tsay JS, Kim HE, Mackey WE, Heeger DJ. Long-term motor learning in the "Wild" with high volume video game data. *Front Hum Neurosci*. 2021;15:777779.
19. Michalski SC, Szpak A, Loetscher T. Using virtual environments to improve real-world motor skills in sports: a systematic review. *Front Psychol*. 2019;10:2159.
20. Haar S, Sundar G, Faisal AA. Embodied virtual reality for the study of real-world motor learning. *PLoS One*. 2021;16:e0245717.
21. Wang, D, Schostak M, Steiner U, et al. Haptic display for virtual reality: progress and challenges. *VRIH*. 2019;1:136-162.

Review Questions

1. **In an elite weight lifter, name a mechanism to increase force when most or all motor units have been activated.**
   A. Modulate the firing rate through summation
   B. Recruit primarily slow twitch motor units
   C. Use short muscle length
   D. Activate small motor neurons only

2. **Part of any purposeful movement is to adapt to the demands of the environment. How does afferent input from the muscle spindle help to produce purposeful movement?**
   A. Alpha-gamma co-activation helps detect the rate of change in limb position.
   B. Afferents converge to activate agonist motor neurons.
   C. Afferents diverge to activate inhibitory interneurons to agonist motor neurons.
   D. All of the above are correct.

3. **In a patient that has sustained a partial spinal cord injury, how would inhibitory interneurons be affected?**
   A. Descending drive to the inhibitory interneurons will increase.
   B. Inhibitory interneurons will increase in number.
   C. Excitatory interneurons will increase in number.
   D. Descending drive to the inhibitory interneurons will decrease.

4. **What organizational structures within the spinal cord can produce complex limb movements?**
   A. Central pattern generators
   B. Muscle spindles
   C. Gamma motor neurons
   D. All of the above

5. **How will treadmill training change neural systems in the lumbar cord after spinal cord injury?**
   A. Alternating contraction patterns between muscles of the legs will increase.
   B. Neural activation will adapt to afferent input according to the environmental context.
   C. Learning and plasticity will occur.
   D. All of the above are correct.

6. **Increased muscle tone and spasticity typically occurs after spinal cord injury. What spinal cord structures are affected and how?**
   A. Direct damage and loss of alpha motor neurons occur which innervate the spastic muscle.
   B. Muscle atrophy results in loss of motor neurons and their neural input shifts to nearby neurons causing higher firing frequencies.
   C. Inhibitory interneurons receive less descending input which lowers their firing rate and allows increased motor neuron firing.
   D. None of the above are correct.

7. **Which area of the spinal cord is most likely to be impinged by stenosis?**
   A. Medulla at the foramen magnum
   B. Cervical cord
   C. Thoracic cord
   D. Sacral cord

8. **In motor learning, being in a realistic or "ecological" environment improves skill acquisition by which of the following:**
   A. Simplifying the task by removing haptics
   B. Relying on practicing the skill in parts
   C. Using sensory afferents to recruit motor units according to the size principle
   D. All of the above
   E. None of the above

9. **Decreasing the alpha motor neuron firing rate by a single impulse will greatly reduce muscle force production.**
   A. True
   B. False

10. **Divergence organizes movement by:**
    A. Summation.
    B. Unfused Tetanus.
    C. Reciprocal Inhibition.
    D. Coordinated activation of multiple muscles.

Answers

1. A	**2.** B	**3.** D	**4.** A	**5.** D
6. C	**7.** B	**8.** C	**9.** A	**10.** D

GLOSSARY

Central pattern generator. A reverberating circuit that includes inhibitory interneurons, creating alternating rhythmic motor patterns (e.g., gait).

Divergence. Coordinated response, generated by a single neuron synapsing on a distributed group of neurons to synergistic muscles.

Fast twitch muscle fiber. High force production, easily fatigued.

Fused tetanus. Sustained force generated by a sustained muscle contraction without any relaxation due to a high frequency of action potentials.

Ia inhibitory interneuron. An interneuron, located in the spinal gray matter, that is activated by a Ia afferent to relax the antagonist muscle, during a stretch reflex, and is inhibited by the Renshaw cell to facilitate its muscle activation.

Ib inhibitory interneuron. An interneuron within the spinal gray matter that receives input from muscle sensory afferents and inhibits the alpha motor neuron innervating the same muscle.

Last order interneuron. The interneuron that synapses on a motor neuron.

Motor unit. Alpha motoneuron and the muscle cells it innervates.

Recurrent inhibition. Inhibition of the homonymous muscle (agonists and synergists).

Reverberating circuit. Activity in a neural network that outlasts the initial signal.

Size principle. Activation of motor units, based on their size.

Slow twitch muscle fiber. Produce low force and have good endurance.

Summation. The production of greater force when the firing rate of motor units occurs close together such that the fiber doesn't fully relax between contractions.

Unfused tetanus. A summation of action potentials that generates small incremental increases in muscle force.

ABBREVIATIONS

CPG   central pattern generator

Motor Control and the Descending Systems

5

John A. Buford

OBJECTIVES

1) Understand general principles underlying control of movement, including motor planning, motor performance, anticipatory postural adjustments, feedback, and reflexes

2) Describe the neuroanatomy and general functional roles of the descending systems for motor control

3) Describe the roles of the basal ganglia and cerebellum in motor control

4) Explain control of the movement based on the shared interactive control from the motor systems described

OVERVIEW OF MOTOR CONTROL

The primary difference between animals and plants is the ability to move, and the organ most responsible for this difference is the brain. Some have argued, in fact, that the entire purpose of the nervous system is the control of movement. Perhaps it is no coincidence, then, that the earliest studies of neuroscience began with studies of the control of movement.

To understand the control of movement, one must first have an appreciation for the musculoskeletal system. While that is beyond the scope of this text, a few important principles are worth emphasizing before we explore in any detail what the nervous system does to control movement.

Motor Control Inherent in the Musculoskeletal System

- Many of the characteristics of movements observed are dictated by the biomechanical constraints of the musculoskeletal system, which simplifies the problem of neural control.

- Muscle is the source of power for movement. The nervous system must control the muscles, and therefore, some understanding of muscle physiology is required to understand neural control of movement. In particular, the recruitment of alpha motoneurons for the production of force is described in Chapter 4.

- The nervous system devotes considerable resources to proprioception, the conscious and subconscious sensation of the state of the muscles, and the musculoskeletal system, in order to provide accurate feedback for motor control. Details of these systems were covered in Chapter 3.

The student of motor control should already possess a basic understanding of the musculoskeletal system and of muscle physiology, sensory systems, especially proprioception, and motor systems in the spinal cord including alpha motoneurons, reflexes, and central pattern generators. As we consider the systems for control of movement, we will refer to and expand upon these concepts from previous chapters in this text.

AN EXAMPLE OF A COMMON MOVEMENT TASK

What is required to sit in a chair and press a specific key on a computer keyboard, and then reach for the computer mouse (Figure 5-1)? First, we need to have the postural control system sufficient to hold our trunk and lower limbs stable in the sitting position. Details of the postural control system are provided in Chapter 11 on the vestibular system, but some things are self-evident. A stable postural base for accurate reaching will require steady, low-level activation of trunk and lower limb muscles and the ability to modulate muscle activity as our body sways about in space. We will need the ability to sense body position and a sense of balance to keep upright against gravity. We would also like to be able to do this efficiently, with very little mental or physical effort.

We will simultaneously need to be able to see the keyboard, or perhaps having memorized it, recall the layout from memory as we look at the screen. Either way, we will need to know where the key is that we would like to press. We will need a stable position of our head, from which to direct the gaze of our eyes, as well as a stable position of our shoulders and arms, from which to direct our hand and finger movements. Most likely, in order to simplify the task, we will have our forearms and wrists resting in front of the keyboard so that only a combination of wrist and finger movements is needed to reach the key. Nonetheless, there is subtle modulation of shoulder and arm muscle activity to provide that stability.

As we go to strike the key, we will need to recruit a very specific subset of wrist and finger muscles in a controlled, delicate manner to position the finger over the key and depress it with sufficient but not excessive force. We will pay close attention to the sensory feedback from our fingers, and perhaps use auditory feedback from the key if it clicks, and vision of the character appearing on the screen for confirmation that the key was really pressed.

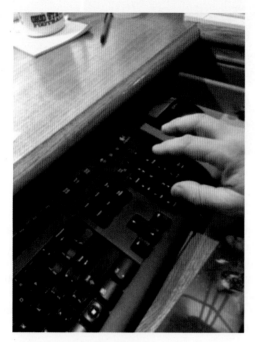

FIGURE 5-1 As a person performs even a seemingly simple task, typing and then reaching for a computer mouse, a complex series of sensory and motor actions is required throughout the central nervous system to control the musculoskeletal system for successful performance. (Used, with permission, of John A. Buford, PT, PhD.)

Having accomplished that task and seeing the feedback on the screen, we are now ready to reach for the mouse. We will need to pick up our hand and begin to move it in space toward the mouse. Again, we would like to do this efficiently. Our peripheral vision has already located the mouse, and we do not need to look directly at it to know where to put our hand. Before we finish pressing the key, the brain has already plotted a trajectory for the hand to reach the mouse, probably in our subconscious, so we have this movement planned and prepared before we make it.

A problem to be solved here is that the inertial mass of our arm, being accelerated toward the mouse, will tend to drive our body in the opposite direction. This introduces a more dynamic trajectory control problem. Over time, our brain has become familiar enough with the mass properties of our arm that it can predict quite accurately what those inertial consequences will be. Rather than initiating the movement and waiting for the consequences to occur, the brain will actually employ a predictive strategy called **feedforward control**. We will initiate a slight trunk and shoulder lean toward the mouse immediately prior to reaching. If we execute this feed-forward strategy perfectly, this preparatory movement will be just enough to counteract the inertial consequences of the reach so that, to the outside observer, there will appear to be no disturbance of trunk position caused by the reach. This amazing process occurs without our conscious effort and occupies perhaps a tenth of a second, playing out before we even realize that we have begun to reach.

As our hand begins to move toward the mouse, two things are happening at once. First, the hand is being transported along an efficient trajectory, avoiding obstacles on the way to the mouse. For a short movement like this to an object in a known location, we are probably not expecting to make corrections along the way. If it was a living mouse and we were trying to catch it, then that would be a different problem! But with a computer mouse, our plan is likely to succeed without the need to watch the movement and initiate corrections along the way. The reaching movement occurs with a smooth acceleration profile such that there is very little jerkiness evident in the movement, and the hand comes to rest over the mouse without knocking the mouse out of position in the process. A second aspect of this control process occurs in parallel with the reach. The shape of the hand is being morphed from the shape appropriate for typing into a shape intended to hold the mouse in a gentle grasp, with the index and long fingers free to use the buttons. Having worked with the mouse extensively, we have that shape memorized, and our hand is shaped for the mouse before it gets there. As our hand grasps the mouse, we need sensation to tell us that we have completed the task and to help finish the completion of the grasp with the appropriate positioning and force.

If we break this task down, we will see that we need a number of capabilities to succeed. We need a system for posture and balance that helps us stay upright in a stable position, and we would prefer not to have to give this very much thought or energy. We need the ability to use spatial memory to plan and guide movements in space, or as a novice, the ability to locate a thing in space, usually based on vision, and guide our movement to that spot. We need some knowledge of the way our musculoskeletal system works, how much force our muscles can produce, and what the inertial properties of our limbs are, in order to plan and control movements. We need the capacity to do more than one thing at a time to both transport the hand and shape it. And we need sensory feedback to guide movement and to give us knowledge of the outcome of our effort.

As we work through this chapter, we will see how the motor control system is organized in a manner to help us accomplish all of these aspects of the neural control of movement. Before we can integrate our knowledge at that level, however, we will need a foundation. There are certain facts to be learned about the nervous system and its pathways for control of movement. The reader must first understand the muscles and the motoneurons, the means by which the nervous system produces the forces to control movement. This is covered in Chapter 4. From there, we can consider the **descending systems for motor control**, the pathways from the brain that control the recruitment of motoneurons. Finally, we will consider systems within the brain that organize the control of movement.

MAJOR DESCENDING SYSTEMS FOR MOTOR CONTROL

There are four major descending systems for motor control: the corticospinal system, the rubrospinal tract, the reticulospinal system, and the vestibulospinal system. Each of these systems has distinct functions.

There are certain tools we have available to us in neuroscience to reveal the functions of a particular descending system for motor control. One key set of facts we use to understand the functions of each descending system comes from the field of neuroanatomy, specifically, tract tracing. In early studies, before modern tract-tracing techniques were developed, the only way to trace a particular tract was to find places in the nervous system where there was evidence of the degeneration of axons resulting from lesions deliberately made in experimental animal models or revealed from human beings in autopsy after death (*c.f.* Kuypers 1981,[1]). While the data collected from these early approaches remains invaluable, often the only direct anatomical evidence from human tissues, much more detail is available with current tract-tracing approaches in comparable animal models.[2,3] In these studies, the axonal transport system described in Chapter 2, Box 2-1 is harnessed to reveal the axons in greater detail, including not only their pathways, but their origins and **terminations**.

Understanding the organization of the spinal gray helps to understand the functions of the descending systems. For example, the vestibulospinal system is important in postural reactions for standing balance.[1,4] As such, it sends axons to control recruitment of both axial and limb muscles, including the muscles of the ankle joint. It should be no surprise, based on the organization shown in Figure 1-10, to find that vestibulospinal projections can be found in the medial and lateral parts of the ventral horn, as well as in the intermediate zone.[1] Hence, one of the basic anatomical facts we must know about a descending system is where its axons terminate. We will want to know this both in terms of the regions of the gray matter, as described in Chapter 4 and above, and in terms of the segmental levels of the spinal cord contacted. For example, a system that terminates only in cervical levels could not be expected to control the legs.

Another fact about descending systems that we will need to know is where the cells originate. In some cases, this will be a particular nucleus in the brain, and in others, it will be a specific type of neuron. Sometimes, we will know both. In order to appreciate the literature, where these terms may be used interchangeably, we will need to be well-versed in the most common ways of speaking about the origins of the descending systems. If a certain part of the brain is lesioned that we know is the location for neurons with axons of a certain descending system, then we will understand why there would be certain deficits in motor control.

We will also want to know the pathways through the nervous system by which the axons of the descending system travel to reach the spinal cord. This will include the names of the major structures through which the axons travel, their general location in that structure, and the location of the axons in the white matter of the spinal cord. Again, this will make it possible to make sense out of the deficits that result from lesions in certain places in the nervous system.

Finally, where possible, we would like to know something about how the axon terminals of any particular descending system ultimately influence the **motor neurons** (aka motoneurons). Are there direct connections to the motoneurons themselves, or does a particular descending system only work through the interneuronal networks? Or, is there some combination of both kinds of projection? Does the descending system have a tendency to

contact interneurons in the medial gray matter that cross over to the other side, thereby exerting bilateral control, or does the descending system only influence movement on one side at a time? Where possible, integrating an understanding of how a particular descending system ultimately connects to the motoneurons will help explain why that descending system has certain functions.

In addition to this type of neuroanatomical information derived from noting the consequences of lesions and from tract tracing, we can add information from electrophysiology, pharmacology, clinical studies, and neural imaging. **Electrophysiology** can involve recording the electrical activity of neurons during activity to see what kinds of movements engage those structures, or electrically activating one or more neurons to see what happens. For example, if we discover that neurons in a certain region are most electrically active when skilled hand movements are being made, and that stimulating neurons in that region results in finger movements, we would infer that this region, and the tracts that originate from it, is important for skilled hand movements. Pharmacology can involve measuring the kinds of neurotransmitters or receptors present in a certain part of the nervous system, or applying pharmacologic agents systemically or locally to reveal the effects on movement. Clinical studies examine disease states or the consequences of injury, comparing the part(s) of the nervous system involved to the symptoms. Neural imaging approaches capitalize on local changes in cerebral blood flow that is regulated to supply more blood to more active areas of the brain to reveal local regions of the brain that are more or less active for certain kinds of activities (see Chapter 9 for discussion on imaging methods). Our current understanding of the descending motor systems is derived from a synthesis of the results of all of these kinds of studies.

On the following pages, there are diagrams of the cortical motor areas (Figure 5-2) and the four major descending systems

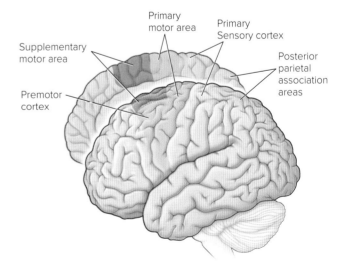

FIGURE 5-2 Cortical motor areas. The lower part of the image represents a lateral view of the left brain. The upper part shows the mesial surface as a reflection. (Reproduced with permission from Kandel ER, Schwartz JH, et al., *Principles of Neural Science*, 5th ed. New York, NY: McGraw-Hill; 2013.)

(Figure 5-3), and there are also tables, detailing the origins and destinations of these pathways, along with details of how the system travels through the nervous system. In the text, we will describe one system at a time, integrating this information to paint a functional picture at the end.

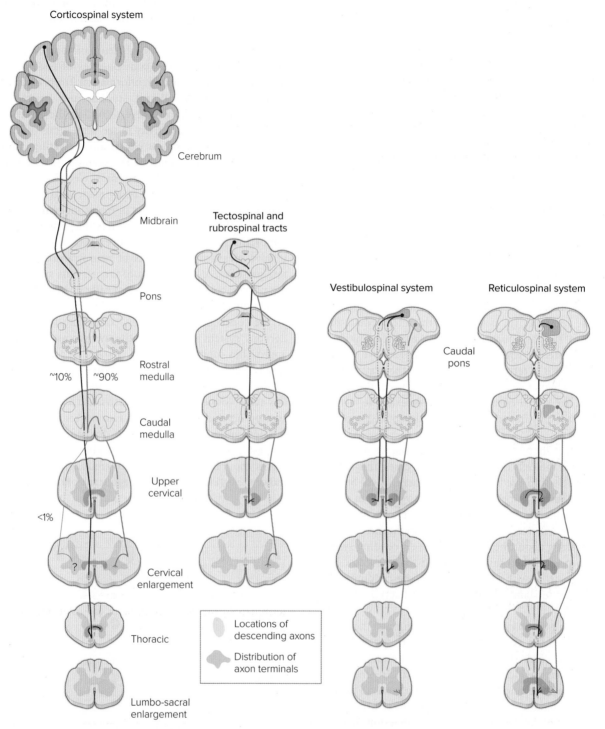

FIGURE 5-3 Descending systems for motor control. For each system, the path of an axon for a typical neuron is illustrated, along with the pattern of terminations. For the corticospinal system, the lateral corticospinal tract is illustrated in blue, and the anterior corticospinal tract is magenta. From the midbrain, the tectospinal tract is magenta, and the rubrospinal tract is blue. For both the vestibulospinal and reticulospinal systems, the lateral tract is blue, and the medial tract is magenta. In addition to the paths of a typical axon for each system, the locations of all fibers in the tract are shown by shading in the white matter of the spinal cord sections, and the overall sphere of influence of axon terminals from each tract is shown by shading in the gray matter.

DESCENDING SYSTEMS FOR MOTOR CONTROL

Corticospinal Tract

Origins and Inputs

A single neuron in the corticospinal system will have its cell body in the gray matter of the cerebral cortex, and by definition, will produce an axon that ultimately reaches the gray matter of the spinal cord.[1,4] The type of cell that makes a corticospinal axon is a **pyramidal cell**. The cell body of a pyramidal neuron will be in layer 5 of the cortical gray matter (cortical tissue in this part of the brain has six layers).

About 30% to 40% of corticospinal neurons have their cell body in the **precentral gyrus**, also known as the **primary motor cortex** (Brodmann's Area [BA] 4).[4–6] This may be called M1 ("M-one") or simply "the **motor cortex**." The precentral gyrus is the strip of brain tissue just rostral to the central sulcus. A subset of corticospinal cells synapses directly on **motoneurons**, and these are called **corticomotoneuronal cells**.[5,7] As described below, not all corticospinal cells make these direct contacts; most synapse on interneurons in the spinal cord, and in many cases, those interneurons in turn then connect to motoneurons.[8] Therefore, a corticomotoneuronal cell is a special type of corticospinal cell. The vast majority of corticomotoneuronal cells in the corticospinal system will emanate from M1, principally from areas devoted to control of the hand and face, and predominately from the part of M1 found buried within the rostral wall of the central sulcus.[5]

M1 contains neurons projecting to **motor pools** for control of virtually any muscle in the body. These are organized in a **somatotopic** map of the body that is arranged, at the macroscopic level, in a consistent manner among individuals. The foot and leg are most medial, on the mesial surface. The trunk is around the top of the cortex, and then come arm, hand, face, and mouth. A disproportionately large area of cortex in the human and other dexterous primates is devoted to the hand, largely in the part that is enfolded into the central sulcus. Functionally, when MI is activated and these corticospinal cells are creating action potentials, the synaptic strength of connection to the motor pools is such that movement will invariably occur. Electrical stimulation with a microelectrode placed with its tip in layer 5 of M1 will elicit visible muscle twitches with very low currents, ranging from a few microamperes up to about 30 microamps.[7,9–12] With this method of intracortical microstimulation, a very fine-grained map of the motor cortex outputs can be revealed. Comparable maps on a much grosser scale can also be obtained with noninvasive methods such as transcranial magnetic stimulation.

But with only 30% to 40% of the corticospinal tract originating from the primary motor cortex, where does the rest of it come from? About 30% of the corticospinal cells originate from areas rostral to M1. In Brodmann's numbering system, most of this broad region is called area 6. In general, this region is active for motor planning in advance of movement, and many of the neurons in area 6 project to MI to govern movement.[9–12] There are also many corticospinal neurons in area 6. Modern neuroscientists have found several subdivisions of area 6, but for this chapter we will consider two.

On the mesial surface of the superior frontal gyrus, there is a region of area 6 called the **supplementary motor area**, abbreviated SMA.[11–14] This is also called M2 (M-"two"). This area is sensitive to electrical stimulation, but more current (40-80 microamps) is typically required to evoke movement. The SMA is the second largest contributor to the corticospinal tract and also contains a somatotopic map. This map is less detailed, however, and it is typical to elicit multi-joint or even bilateral movements from SMA. SMA is most concerned with motor planning and performance for complex, memorized movements such as sequences, and is also critical for bimanual tasks where both hands must be used in conjunction (e.g., buttoning a shirt).[1,14]

The remainder of area 6 is typically called the **premotor cortex** (PM), which is located on the lateral surface of the cortex rostral to M1.[4,9,11,14–16] This area is concerned with planning for movements like reaching to an object or kicking a ball, where the limb movement must be directed at an external object, especially if the object must be moved in certain directions with respect to the outside world. PM is especially interested in learning arbitrary links between external stimuli and responses, such as learning to respond to traffic lights, turn signals, horns, and brake lights to drive a car in city traffic.[16] In the area for hand control, there is a concentration of the ability to imagine moving, based on observation and imitation.[17] As with SMA, much of the output from PM is directed toward MI to coordinate motor outputs there, but some corticospinal neurons emanate directly from PM itself.[4]

With about 70% of the corticospinal tract emanating from these and other frontal lobe areas that have clear relationships to motor control, where does the rest of the corticospinal tract come from? Surprisingly, much of the corticospinal tract comes from the parietal lobe,[1,4] which is typically associated with sensory function, not motor function. Some of these corticospinal projections from sensory areas are thought to help the nervous system focus on aspects of sensory information critical to movement.[18] Further, in order to have control over movement, one must control reflexes. In this regard, it makes sense that the sensory areas of the cerebral cortex contribute to the corticospinal tract. Indeed, in lower animals, the corticospinal tract has no projections directly to motoneurons and has as many terminals in the dorsal horn as in the intermediate zone.[19] In this sense, regulation of reflexes as a prerequisite to voluntary motor control may be the original purpose of the corticospinal tract. Direct voluntary control of motor pools seems to be a more recent development.

In sum, the corticospinal tract originates from a wide region of the parietal and frontal lobes. Most of the projections come from MI and SMA, but the premotor cortex and sensory cortical areas also make substantial contributions. The various cortical areas contributing to the corticospinal tract operate in parallel to govern this one descending system just as the four major descending systems work together on a larger scale.

Each of these cortical motor areas that contributes to the corticospinal system receives inputs that are specific to its functions. All receive input to a greater or lesser extent from the basal ganglia and cerebellum via relays in the thalamus. A detailed description of these brain areas is covered later, but a simple characterization is that the basal ganglia are important for selection of movement components and switching from one movement to the next, whereas the cerebellum coordinates movement as it occurs and learns to anticipate coordination required for upcoming movements. Through interactions at the level of shared structures like the motor cortex, basal ganglia, and cerebellar function are ultimately integrated for overall control of movement.[20]

Among the cortical motor areas, M1 is principally concerned with real-time performance of movement.[21] In other words, if M1 is activated, then there is movement being produced. The major sources of input to M1 are SMA and PM, which relay the movement plans to M1. M1 also receives detailed sensory perceptions from the primary sensory cortex (S1). The premotor cortical areas receive higher-order perceptual information that combines things such as whole-body image for SMA to govern memorized movements and the perception of the body's position with respect to the outside world for PM to govern targeted limb movements. These integrated perceptions come from the posterior parietal area (PPA; BA 5, 7; Figure 5-2).[17] The prefrontal cortex (PF) is also a strong source of input to SMA and PM. PF is the source of executive functions such as decision making to choose the appropriate action from among many possibilities. In essence, PF chooses what we should do, SMA and PM figure out how, and MI does it.[22-24] These areas can be subdivided further into parts that parcel out certain aspects of the function, but that level of detail is beyond the scope of this chapter.

Destinations

From the primary motor cortex, corticospinal cells often make strong synaptic connections directly to alpha motoneurons for the limb muscles, especially muscles of the hands and feet.[5,12,25-27] As noted above, these corticospinal cells with direct connections to motoneurons are called corticomotoneuronal cells. This type of direct connection means increased corticospinal activity can reliably and specifically recruit muscles in these body parts, potentially overwhelming competing influences from other descending systems. However, even for the hands, 50% or more of the corticospinal cells will not contact the motoneurons directly.[8] Instead, they will work through interneuronal networks, described in Chapter 4, to have their influence. In other words, the corticospinal cells will synapse on a set of local neurons in the spinal cord and those cells will, in turn, connect to the motoneurons. Corticomotoneuronal cells themselves will also send collateral branches of their axons to interneuronal networks to recruit these in parallel with the motor pool. The primary motor cortex (M1) is where most corticomotoneuronal cells are found, but these can also originate from the supplementary motor area (SMA) and the premotor cortex (PM). When the corticospinal projections from areas other than M1 are considered (SMA, PM, etc.), it becomes even more uncommon for corticospinal cells to synapse directly on alpha motoneurons, and even more likely that this will only occur for control of the hands and feet.[12,13] The point here is that to a great extent, the corticospinal system relies upon well-established networks of neural connections in the spinal cord to produce most movements. Only for the details of the hand and finger movements, and to a lesser extent for limb movements, does

the corticospinal system take it upon itself to choose relatively specifically which muscles to recruit for a particular movement.

For control of proximal limb girdle muscles and muscles of the trunk and spinal column, there is very little potential for corticospinal cells to directly control motoneurons. Rather, the corticospinal system works through spinal networks that are responsible for coordination of responses among these axial muscles. Indeed, other descending systems are probably more influential on these girdle and core muscles than the corticospinal tract. Finally, a substantial portion of the corticospinal tract is targeted for the intermediate zone and dorsal horn of the gray matter in the spinal cord. In other words, a large responsibility of the corticospinal tract is to govern the neurons that are involved in reflexes and sensory inputs.

There are actually two main divisions of the corticospinal tract. The **lateral corticospinal tract** is almost completely a contralateral system, with the left brain projecting to the right half of the spinal cord, and the right projecting to the left.[1,4,6,27] In total, about 85% to 90% of the corticospinal tract decussates and comprises the lateral corticospinal tract, which is located in the white matter of the lateral funiculus in the spinal cord.[1,4,6] There are a very small number of corticospinal axons that travel in the ipsilateral lateral funiculus, perhaps 1% to 2%.[1,6,27] We have no direct data about what these do; we can only say that anatomical studies reveal their presence. The remainder of the corticospinal tract, approximately 10% to 15%, stays ipsilateral and descends in the ventral funiculus; this is called the **ventral** (or anterior) **corticospinal tract**.[1,4,6,8] There appears to be some individual variation in how much of the corticospinal tract is ipsilateral, and in recovery from injury, the effect of rehabilitation may be in part to increase the influence of the ipsilateral, uninjured fibers on motor control.[6,8] The ventral corticospinal tract is mainly concerned with control of axial muscles and terminates medially in the gray matter of the spinal cord, in Rexed's lamina number VIII, which is where motoneurons and interneurons concerned with trunk and proximal limb girdle muscles are located.[1,4] The lateral corticospinal tract, in contrast, terminates in the motor pools of the ventral horn, as well as in the intermediate zone and in the dorsal horn.[1,4] The lateral portions of the ventral horn are where the motoneurons for limb, and especially distal muscles, are located.[1]

Single corticospinal cells in the lateral corticospinal tract will terminate in just a few motor pools spanning just a few spinal segments. This provides a substrate for single corticospinal neurons of the lateral corticospinal tract to recruit just a few muscles at a time. For the ventral corticospinal tract, the terminations in the medial part of the spinal cord often contact interneurons that cross to influence movements on the other side. In other words, the ventral corticospinal tract can influence both sides of the body, but typically only for the trunk and proximal muscles to which it connects.[13] However, in recovery from cortical injury, the ipsilateral components of the corticospinal tract may take on increased importance.[6,27,28]

Functions

From the preceding discussion of the sources and inputs to the corticospinal tracts and their destinations in the spinal cord, we can already glean a good idea of the function of the corticospinal tract. Not surprisingly, the corticospinal tract is critical for

skilled, voluntary movement throughout the body. This is not to say that voluntary movement cannot occur if the corticospinal tract is damaged, but the movement will not be as well controlled. Movements made in the absence of corticospinal function occur in gross, stereotyped synergies reflective of patterns of connections in the brainstem and spinal cord.[4,30,32] These **gross movements** are useful in functional tasks such as weight-bearing but are not specific enough to allow the kinds of arbitrary, learned movements that humans rely upon for things like skilled use of tools or competitive sports. Control of the hand and finger movement is dramatically impaired by damage to the corticospinal tract. Reaching in a variety of directions with reasonably equal accuracy is also impaired when the corticospinal tract is damaged.[29]

In addition to problems with motor control, there are problems in the regulation of reflexes when the corticospinal tract is damaged,[33] and this should not be surprising given the large number of corticospinal projections to the intermediate zone and dorsal horn of the spinal cord. The most common symptom is spasticity, an inability to govern the stretch reflex.[34–36] Interestingly, the size of the stretch reflex can be learned with practice, and the corticospinal tract is critical for this learning to occur and for its preservation.[35,36] In other words, part of learning a new skill is not just learning how to turn on the proper muscles in the proper sequence, it is also learning how to set up the strengths of the reflexes that will be occurring in parallel with the movement. When the corticospinal tract is damaged, this aspect of motor control is impaired, and patients will have difficulty regulating muscle tone in concert with movement. When we see this, we call it **spasticity**. This emphasizes that regulation of reflexes, and more generally, attention to and regulation of incoming proprioceptive and cutaneous information in concert with movement, is also a part of the motor control problem for the nervous system.

Rubrospinal Tract

The rubrospinal tract is greatly overshadowed by the corticospinal tract in the human and does not appear to be as large, in relative terms, as it is in the cat.[1] However, this is a poor standard by which to judge importance. There is a tract called the raphe spinal system that descends from the brainstem to the dorsal horn of the spinal cord. This system is critical for modulation of pain and is much smaller than the rubrospinal tract, but does this make it unimportant? A better question would be, "what is the function of the rubrospinal tract, and is that type of thing critical to human function?"

Origins and Inputs

The rubrospinal tract originates from the **red nucleus**, which is in the midbrain. Like the lateral corticospinal tract, the rubrospinal tract is a crossed system. The neurons that contribute to the rubrospinal tract are called **magnocellular neurons** because they are large; parvocellular neurons in the red nucleus are part of a circuit with the cerebellum. There are two principal sources of input to the rubrospinal system. One is the cortical motor areas in the frontal lobe. The other main source of input to the red nucleus is the cerebellum. The cerebellum uses the rubrospinal tract as one of its outputs for the coordination of movement. Hence, the red nucleus is a center for integrating the motor commands from the motor cortex with coordination from the cerebellum.

Destinations

The rubrospinal tract projects to the lateral motor pools in the anterior horn of the spinal cord, as well as to interneurons projecting to the motor pools. Many of the rubrospinal projections are monosynaptic.[26] In higher primates, including humans, the rubrospinal tract has little to no influence below the cervical spinal cord.[1] Unlike the corticospinal system, rubrospinal connections are not typically sent to motoneurons for distal muscles intrinsic to the hands. Rather, rubrospinal connections are to the **extrinsic muscles** of the hand, wrist, and upper limb (shoulder/elbow).[26] Like corticospinal cells, rubrospinal projections are to selected groups of muscles, but single rubrospinal tract cells are more likely to affect muscles at multiple joints (e.g., shoulder, elbow, and wrist), whereas corticospinal projections are more likely to allow for control of one joint at a time.

Functions

There have been many ideas in the literature about the potential function of the rubrospinal tract. Current evidence is that it is important for rapid, coordinated movement of the entire limb, especially when the reach must be set so the hand can be adapted to the shape of an object.[37,38] Also, early findings noted that the rubrospinal tract was highly active during the swing phase of walking in the cat. The conclusion was erroneously drawn that rubrospinal tract cells might be important for control of flexors. There seems to have been a desire in the field, in the early studies of motor control, to say that one tract controls flexors and another controls extensors, etc. These simple ideas have been largely discarded. In the cat, as in the human, the end of swing phase is a time of rapid, accurate limb movement where limb positioning must be precisely controlled.[39,40] For the forelimb in particular (the upper limb in the cat), this is like a reaching movement, and there is as much or more extensor activity as flexor activity at this point in the gait cycle. From detailed studies in nonhuman primates, it is clear that rubrospinal tract neurons are quite effective at recruiting extensor muscles around the wrist, not just flexors.[26] Hence, by integrating commands from the cerebellum and MI to affect muscles throughout the limb, it seems likely that the rubrospinal tract is used for rapid correction of limb movements, especially when there is a requirement for both speed and distal accuracy in the movement. In particular, the parallel coordination for shaping of the hand, during a reaching movement, seems to make rubrospinal cells more active than either task, reaching or hand shaping, alone.[37,38] Increased cortical projections to the red nucleus and an increased role for the rubrospinal system in the control of distal movements may also be a part of the substrate for motor recovery.[28] With a function in shaping the hand for rapid, skilled reaching and a potential role in recovery of distal control after injury, even though the rubrospinal tract is small in the human, it still may be quite important.

Vestibulospinal Tracts

The **vestibular nuclei** in the pons and medulla are centers of integration for inputs from the vestibular system (utricle, saccule, semicircular canals) with the control of eye movements, head and neck movements, and postural reactions for balance. Cortical projections to the vestibular nuclei are sparse and thought to subconsciously inhibit vestibular reflexes that would interfere with voluntary movement; the vestibulospinal tracts are not traditionally thought to be under direct conscious control,[41,42] but there do appear to be a small number of projections to the vestibular nuclei from the motor contex.[43] Vestibulospinal systems may serve mainly in an automatic, regulatory fashion based on inputs from the vestibular system and other sources, but that does not mean the vestibulospinal systems are not important for motor learning. Rather, for these systems to make their respective contributions to learning and adaptation, practice is required.

Origins and Inputs

Much of the vestibular system is devoted to internal processing of vestibular information and control and coordination of eye movements, but there are two components that descend to the spinal cord for control of the trunk and limbs. The **medial vestibulospinal tract** is an extension of the head and eye control and coordination system. It originates from the **medial vestibular nucleus**.[43] Inputs to the medial vestibular nucleus arise from all components of the vestibular apparatus, including the semicircular canals, sensing head rotation, as well as the utricle and saccule, sensing linear acceleration of the head in up/down and anterior/posterior directions (see Chapter 6 for details). The **lateral vestibulospinal tract** originates in the **lateral vestibular nucleus** and receives mainly utricle and saccule inputs, so it senses mainly the linear acceleration components of head movement.[43] The other strong source of input to the vestibular nuclei, in addition to the vestibular apparatus, is the cerebellum. Hence, to the extent the cerebellum is involved in coordination of limb and body movements for postural reactions and adjustments in support of movement, some of that cerebellar influence is exerted through the descending control afforded by the vestibulospinal systems.[43]

Destinations

The medial vestibulospinal system is bilateral. Cells in the medial vestibular nucleus project to the left and right sides of the spinal cord. These projections are limited to the cervical and upper thoracic segments where motor pools to be recruited in support of head movements are located.[44] Medial vestibulospinal projections are concentrated in the medial part of the spinal gray, lamina VIII, where axial muscles are controlled.[44,45] The lateral vestibulospinal tract projects through the length of the spinal cord and can influence muscles throughout the body.[44] It provides ipsilateral projections, so the left lateral vestibular nucleus projects to the left side of the body. These projections are targeted to facilitate extensor muscles used for postural reactions.[44] Many synapse directly on the motoneurons of the extensor muscles for rapid and secure control of these muscles. Another output of the lateral vestibular nucleus is the reticulospinal system, which, as we will see below, also contributes to postural reactions.

Functions

The medial vestibulospinal tracts govern head and neck movements used to maintain a stable position of gaze, despite fluctuations imposed from the outside. Functionally, this is called the **vestibulo-ocular reflex** (VOR). If something turns your body to the right, your eyes and head will counter-rotate to the left to keep your vision on the same object.

The lateral vestibulospinal tracts are used for the control of antigravity muscles necessary for posture and balance. For example, when something perturbs the body and pitches you forward, you will need to recruit the plantarflexors to restrain that movement. Much of this may be accomplished by the stretch reflex to the extent the ankles themselves sense the change in body position.[46,47] However, when the perturbation is felt by the head, then the lateral vestibulospinal tracts will be driven to recruit extensor muscles in an effort to resist falling.

Reticulospinal Tracts

The reticulospinal tracts are the last of the descending systems we will consider in detail. As with the vestibulospinal tracts, they are divided into two parts, but unlike the vestibulospinal tracts, the reticulospinal tracts receive extensive projections from motor and especially premotor cortical areas (SMA and PM) and are thought to be under some degree of conscious control.[48] In lower animals, the reticulospinal system is the principal descending system for motor control. It has access to a variety of information from the cortex, cerebellum, vestibular systems, and somatosensory systems. And, it has outputs directed toward the limbs and the trunk throughout the body. Hence, the reticulospinal system plays a supporting role, and sometimes a leading role, in control of virtually every functional movement.

Origins and Inputs

The **reticular formation** is a network of neurons located in the core of the brainstem, especially in the pons and medulla. In the caudal part of the pons and rostral medulla, in the vicinity of the vestibular nuclei around the dorsal aspect of the reticular formation, there is an area called **Nucleus Reticularis Pontis Caudalis**. In this region, there are large neurons that produce reticulospinal axons that form one part of the reticulospinal-system, the **medial reticulospinal tract**. Moving slightly caudally into the medulla and somewhat ventrally toward the medullary pyramids, we find a nucleus called **Nucleus Reticularis Gigantocellularis**. This is also a source of reticulospinal neurons. Some of these contribute to the medial reticulospinal tracts, whereas others descend through the **lateral reticulospinal tracts**.

Destinations

Many texts seem to tell a compellingly simple story about the differences between the functions of the lateral and medial reticulospinal tracts. A careful reading of the original literature, however, reveals no such simple story. It appears to be more based on legend than fact. Modern studies have yet to provide a means to reliably test the differences in function between these two parts of the reticulospinal system; in fact, some argue that the lateral vestibulospinal system and the reticulospinal system may be inter-related.[43] A few findings about the reticulospinal systems, however, seem reliable and may reveal some insight, and these are described below.

Neurons of the lateral reticulospinal system tend to have relatively small axons with slower conduction velocities, whereas the medial reticulospinal system is comprised of large axons, often larger and faster than those of the corticospinal system.[1,48] Medial reticulospinal tract axons often travel the length of the spinal cord and deliver collateral branches at multiple levels.[49,50]

These single cells may have axons that influence cervical, thoracic, lumbar, and sacral segments of the spinal cord. In many cases, there may be branches on the ipsilateral and contralateral sides of the spinal cord. Lateral reticulospinal tract cells do not seem to have this pattern. Rather, they tend to terminate at only a few levels on the ipsilateral side, and therefore, have a more limited sphere of influence.[44,48]

For the medial reticulospinal tract, the typical destination is motoneurons and interneurons for motor control in lamina VIII of the spinal gray, where proximal limb muscles and axial muscles are controlled. There are also interneurons called commissural interneurons that coordinate responses between the left and right sides of the spinal cord. For example, in the flexor withdrawal and crossed extension response (described in Chapter 4), stepping on a nail with your right foot causes right leg flexion and left leg extension. The left leg response is mediated through these commissural interneurons. The reticulospinal tract uses commissural interneurons as well to produce bilateral influences.[51] For the medial reticulospinal tract, there are also some fibers that produce terminals in both sides of the spinal cord, so responses are promoted on both sides simultaneously in response to the activity of single neurons. The medial reticulospinal neurons are rapidly conducting, so that responses may occur almost simultaneously in the arms and legs.

The lateral reticulospinal tract tends to have more limited influences at a smaller number of spinal segments. Lesioning of the spinal cord laterally, where this tract descends, is particularly detrimental to the brain's ability to activate the spinal central pattern generator for locomotion.[52]

Based on physiological data and anatomical connections, a reasonable hypothesis is that the **lateral reticulospinal tracts** may be the route for activation of **central pattern generation circuits** (defined in Chapter 4) in control of locomotion, and the **medial reticulospinal tracts** are more for **rapid postural reactions** and cortico-reticular pathways for **gross limb movements**.

Functions

As those involved in neurological rehabilitation well know, a critical part of distal mobility is proximal stability. Hence, while the person who is making a reaching movement is thinking about what to do with the hand, there are postural responses and coordination of shoulder girdle and arm movements that must occur for the reach to succeed. The person may be subtly aware that these components of movement are occurring but does not usually think about them overtly. But when a clinician sees a person moving, we often pay more attention to these proximal bases of the movement than to exactly what is going on with the hand because we know that problems with proximal stability are going to lead to problems with distal control. These proximal adjustments that occur in conjunction with skilled movement are largely the domain of the reticulospinal system.

There are projections from the cortical motor areas to reticulospinal neurons in the brainstem, especially from PM and SMA.[48] There are also projections from the cerebellum to the reticulospinal neurons.[44] Thus, as we begin to plan movement and make the early parts of movement, we are typically making postural adjustments that we have learned through practice must precede

and accompany our limb movement. Otherwise, the limb movement will destabilize the trunk, and our limb will not go where we expect. Reticulospinal neurons are activated in the early stages of movement, even when the movement is just being planned,[48] presumably to help set up the right state in the postural control system and the proximal limb to support the distal movement that is about to occur. Reticulospinal outputs can coordinate trunk and limb movements bilaterally. The typical output of the reticulospinal system to the upper limb is a reciprocal action that resembles the asymmetric tonic neck reflex: ipsilateral limb flexion and contralateral limb extension.[53] This typical reticulospinal output pattern is an obvious component of the basic alternating limb movements that have their roots in locomotion. In fact, the neural systems that initiate and regulate locomotion depend heavily on the reticulospinal tracts to do so.[52]

⬤ FUNCTIONAL SCHEME FOR UNDERSTANDING THE TRACTS

One useful way for dividing the descending systems is into the **lateral systems**, including the lateral corticospinal and rubrospinal systems, and the **ventromedial systems**, including the ventral corticospinal, vestibulospinal, and reticulospinal systems.[1] The following sections integrate the details for the descending systems into this functional scheme for understanding.

Lateral Systems: Corticospinal and Rubrospinal

Lateral Systems Govern Voluntary Movements and Fine Motor Control

Working together, the lateral systems are most responsible for controlling the distal components of limb movements, especially the parts we think about and try to control voluntarily. The extreme example of this is using the hands with **fine movements** to manipulate small objects. Whenever we make a **discrete movement** such as reaching out for an object or placing our foot in a particular spot such as a rung on a ladder, we are depending on the corticospinal system.

Lateral Systems Are Especially Important for Limb Movement

As indicated by the location of projections to the spinal cord in the lateral parts of the spinal gray, the lateral systems are especially important for limb movement. For the corticospinal system, this is evident in the homunculus by the amount of cortex devoted to the limbs, especially the hands and feet, and also the face. For the rubrospinal tract, it is mainly concerned with reaching movements, especially rapid movements to position the limb.

Lateral Systems Are Focused on Distal Muscles and Parametric Motor Control at the Interface with the Environment

The corticospinal system, in particular, controls our ability to produce finely graded amounts of force in specific directions for specific periods of time. To accomplish this, the lateral systems employ the immense sensory systems devoted to conscious perception of the hands and feet. Consider this: take a small sewing needle and try to thread it with poor lighting. You probably will not succeed. Now, add bright light, stick the needle in a pin cushion, and use a magnifying glass. You will find yourself able to thread the needle straight through the middle of the hole. Why should it be possible for us to visually control our fingers with many times the accuracy than we could ever expect to have in a natural environment? Normally, we use the immensely accurate sensory perceptions from our fingers to control precision grip of small objects. When the nervous system is provided visual input at a level of accuracy to match, it has more than enough precision in motor control and proprioceptive acuity to capitalize on the augmented visual feedback. All of this interaction is occurring in the cerebral cortex. Without the corticospinal tract, a magnifying glass would mainly make it easier to see how badly you were missing the hole with the thread.

Ventromedial Systems: Vestibulospinal and Reticulospinal

The ventromedial system includes the reticulospinal and vestibulospinal tracts, as well as the ventral corticospinal tract. The ventromedial systems operate in parallel with the lateral systems, and to a great extent are governed by different subsystems in the brain. While lateral systems are mainly driven by the cortex with modulation by subcortical systems, the ventromedial systems are in some cases completely dependent on subcortical centers such as the cerebellum and vestibular system. Even for the reticulospinal tract, which does receive cortical control via **corticobulbar tracts**, the cerebellar inputs are highly influential.[1,44] Hence, a large proportion of control over neural activity levels in the ventromedial system is not directly accessible to our consciousness. We will tend to do things in the way we have practiced, not always the way we intend, for movements where the ventromedial systems are a strong component of control.

Ventromedial Systems Govern Whole Body Postural Reactions, Trunk Control

When the surface under your body moves, such as an elevator or a moving walkway, you need a whole-body reaction to maintain your balance as you reach for the elevator button or struggle to control your luggage. Likewise, when your body is perturbed from above, like having a patient slip while you hold her gait belt, you also need a whole-body reaction to remain stable. These kinds of movements are the domain of the ventromedial systems. Of course, to do this, these systems connect preferentially to trunk and proximal limb muscles and have relatively weak influence in the hands or feet. Further, it makes little sense to move one side of your trunk at a time, and it may rarely be useful to react with only one limb. Hence, single neurons from the ventromedial systems tend to have bilateral influences and may even affect the upper and lower limbs simultaneously.

Ventromedial Systems Produce Gross Limb Movements in Synergy

The ventromedial systems can move the limbs, to some extent under voluntary control through cortical projections to the reticulospinal system. However, the limb movements produced are stereotyped into **synergies**, organized through the interneuronal networks in the spinal cord. During walking, there are also basic limb synergies that dominate the motor pattern. These gross limb movements show the prevalent outputs of the ventromedial systems. The lateral systems depend on these basic limb movement synergies as a starting point upon which to superimpose control for specific skills.

Ventromedial Systems May Provide Most of the Power for Functional Tasks, Especially Trunk Stability Required for Limb Movement

When it comes to control of the trunk, one need only look at the homunculus of the cerebral cortex to realize that something else is in charge of trunk movement. Many functional tasks, such as getting in and out of bed or walking, require substantial trunk control. Neurologic rehabilitation is often focused on trunk control for these tasks, and our clients often have trouble controlling their trunk in the ways we ask. When we stop to realize that trunk control is largely subconscious and under the control of the ventromedial systems, not the lateral systems, this should come as no surprise. This means we cannot expect to make much progress in these tasks by talking to the patient. We need to create situations where they can practice the skill in a way that demands and promotes the components they lack, and then, keep them working on it to develop the skill. When a limb movement must be made, the ventromedial systems may be engaged right away by the SMA and PM projections to reticulospinal systems and by cerebellar coordination produced in anticipation of the movement. These components of movement to achieve stability of the trunk will actually precede the movement of the limb.

Elements of Control for Reaching

Control of reaching provides an example that contrasts the roles of the lateral and ventromedial systems. Here, we are considering a movement largely driven by the lateral systems, where support from the ventromedial systems is crucial for success.

Endpoint Accuracy – Lateral Systems

Generally, when reaching, we look at an object and reach out to grasp it in some way. The endpoint accuracy of our movement is the domain of the lateral systems. Without the lateral systems functioning properly, our movement will tend to go the wrong distance and to the wrong location, though we may still grossly extend the limb in an effort to make the reach. Our PM will use perception of the object to recruit the motor cortex to produce the proper limb movements to make the reach and shape the hand as needed to conform to the object to be reached. With coordinated control from the cerebellum and motor cortex, rubrospinal systems will participate and help coordinate the actions and adjust to errors made along the way.

Dynamic Postural Control – Ventromedial Systems

As the premotor cortex is preparing in advance of the reach, part of its responsibility is to engage in preparatory actions in the trunk and proximal limb. Not surprisingly, the premotor cortex is a strong source of control over the reticulospinal system, which has access to these parts of the body. By pre-engaging well-established trunk movement and gross limb movements in synergy, the problem faced by the cerebral cortex to govern movement through the lateral systems is simplified.

In engineering terms, this is called constraining the **degrees of freedom**. With an automated system, such as the ventromedial system, taking care of details such as setting up the posture and recruiting limb extensors in a coordinated synergy, the lateral systems can focus on details of the distal limb, such as putting a key in a lock. Without the ventromedial systems providing their influence, the arm would tend to hang limp at the side, with the hand moving well, but not enough power or proximal stability to support extending the limb in space.

Elements of Control for Gait

For gait, the situation is almost the opposite. Gait is a gross motor behavior relying heavily on trunk control and movement of all four limbs in a stereotyped pattern. The ventromedial systems are really the principal systems governing the behavior, and the lateral systems play a supporting role.

Central Pattern Generation – Ventromedial Systems

At the heart of neural control for locomotion is a set of neural circuits known as a **central pattern generator,** as described in Chapter 4. The existence of a central pattern generator for locomotion has been confirmed for every animal in which it has been studied. In humans with spinal cord injuries that are apparently motor complete, treadmill training with a body-weight supported harness system can lead to reemergence of locomotor **electromyogram** patterns, and in some cases, a return to independent locomotion with assistive devices even in patients who are years out from their injury. When various aspects of the neuromotor control patterns in these patients are probed, certain features of the responses mimic what has been observed in animal models with a complete spinal cord transection. Tonic stimulation of the lumbar spinal cord in a spinal cord–injured adult can lead to alternating left and right kicking movements.[54,55] These findings make it hard to argue that there is not a central pattern generator for locomotion in the human.

Interestingly, in the animal models, the evidence is clear that the locomotion-initiating systems in the brainstem rely upon the reticulospinal tracts as the principal route for initiation and regulation of locomotion.[52] It seems clear that the reticulospinal systems are part of the normal route for activation of the central pattern generators in the spinal cord. If this is true, then, it would be unnatural to ask a person to try to voluntarily use a little more dorsiflexor effort during swing. Their normal means of walking is not to have their corticospinal tract control that muscle in swing. The recruitment of the proper muscles in the proper sequence is built into the brainstem and spinal cord, and the ventromedial systems utilize that for control. To increase a certain element of the locomotor pattern, the client should practice with a task that demands the missing component, such as walking up a ramp.

The Obstacle Course – Lateral Systems

When walking must occur on unusual surfaces, such as an obstacle course, then the lateral systems are required to translate the visual perception of the safe places to step into accurate placement of the foot.[39] In this situation, the central pattern generator continues to operate, but the lateral systems make specific adjustments as required. When running or walking, the adjustments we can make voluntarily, in deviation from the typical pattern, are limited. The ventromedial systems and central pattern generators have largely taken over the circuits in the spinal cord, and the lateral systems can add or subtract from what is already going on but will have a hard time completely changing the motor pattern.

● FUNCTIONS OF THE BASAL GANGLIA AND CEREBELLUM IN MOTOR CONTROL

The basal ganglia and the cerebellum play key roles in motor control. The **basal ganglia** are a set of large nuclei within the cerebral cortex. In general, they provide a set of pathways for information, originating in the cerebral cortex, to be processed and relayed through the thalamus back up to the cerebral cortex. There are many theories of basal ganglia function. Two, which we will consider here, are that this system helps select certain actions, to the exclusion of others, and helps regulate the effort for movement.[56–58] The **cerebellum** is a structure attached to the dorsal aspect of the brainstem. This complex structure receives sensory inputs from the spinal cord and information about the movements, being planned and performed from the cortex, and it is able to influence and adjust planning and performance of movement to provide for better coordination and control.

Basal Ganglia

For the basal ganglia, there are two pathways, the direct and the indirect (Figure 5-4). For the **direct pathway**, cortical neurons

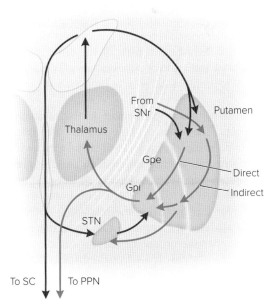

FIGURE 5-4 Basal ganglia loops. In the diagram, pink arrows show excitatory effects, blue arrows inhibitory. GPi, globus pallidus internal segment; GPe, globus pallidus external segment; SNr, substantia nigra pars reticulata; STN, subthalamic nucleus; SC, spinal cord; PPN, pedunculopontine nucleus. (Reproduced with permission from Kandel ER, Schwartz JH, et al., *Principles of Neural Science*, 5th ed. New York, NY: McGraw-Hill; 2013.)

send information through the basal ganglia, and the net result is increased facilitation sent back to the cortex. For the **indirect pathway**, the net result is decreased cortical excitation. At the simplest level, we can understand this as a way to promote activity in certain cortical neurons while suppressing activity in others. Hence, this system can help select certain actions to the exclusion of others.[56,57] At the same time, the relative strength with which one activity is promoted and competing activities are suppressed can result in larger or smaller efforts being required.

Consider our example of typing and using the mouse. The most natural way to use the hand is either to extend all the fingers or to flex them all. Selecting one finger to the exclusion of others requires more control. As we move to strike one key to the exclusion of others, circuits in the direct pathway would be promoting movement of one finger while activation of nearby circuits through the indirect pathway would be suppressing similar movements in other fingers. If we move our example to the difference between typing and reaching for the mouse, then in the motor planning areas, to move the hand, without also reaching, requires a selection, promoting the plan to move the hand while suppressing nearby plans to move the arm. But then to reach, the active area would need to be switched. Hence, not only can the basal ganglia help us choose to move one body part and not another, it can help us choose one action and not another, and then, to switch to the reverse actions.

Dopamine is a neuromodulator that is critical to normal function of the basal ganglia. Dopamine regulates the transmission of information through the direct and indirect loops. Normally, dopamine makes it easier for information to pass through the direct loop but more difficult for it to pass through the indirect loop. In a normal nervous system, the precise location of dopamine release is regulated in concert with the movement such that only certain parts of the direct pathway and certain parts of the indirect pathway are affected, so we can choose what to promote and what to suppress and how strongly to do so.

The cells that make dopamine are in the substantia nigra, pars compacta. The axons of these neurons terminate in the caudate and putamen, the nuclei in the basal ganglia where the cortical information is first delivered. In parkinsonism, these dopamine-producing neurons begin to be lost, and the overall number of these cells is reduced. At first, the nervous system can compensate for this by having the remaining dopamine-producing cells work harder. Eventually, however, there are simply not enough dopamine-producing cells for sufficient dopamine release. The result of this is a relative imbalance between promotion of the direct pathway and suppression of the indirect. As it so happens, the imbalance favors the lack of suppression of the indirect pathway, and the result is a stiff state known as rigidity, with difficulty relaxing and activating the muscles to produce one movement to the exclusion of others. When the patient attempts to move, not only are the agonists recruited, the antagonists are, as well.

Another consequence of basal ganglia dysfunction is slow movement (bradykinesia) and reduced movement amplitude (hypokinesia). In part, this may be a consequence of the excessive co-contraction and rigidity, but another factor seems to be an altered perception of movement velocity and amplitude. The person with parkinsonism thinks he is moving faster and farther than he really is.[58] Basal ganglia circuits are also connected to frontal and parietal lobe areas related to regulation and perception of sensation, so it is not unexpected that there would be some alterations in this system, as well. As described in Chapter 14's discussion of Parkinson Disease, a deliberate and practiced attempt to make big movements can result in some improvement.

Cerebellum

The cerebellum is a structure attached to the back of the brainstem. Its first recognized role was in balance and motor coordination, but it is now accepted that some functions associated with motor planning, which might be considered cognitive, also engage the cerebellum.[20,59] The cerebellum has three main functional divisions. The **vestibulocerebellum** receives information from the vestibular nuclei about balance and eye/head movements and helps regulate these. The **spinocerebellum** receives sensory and proprioceptive inputs from the spinal cord and influences the activity of the descending systems through the reticulospinal system, rubrospinal system, and via the motor cortex, the corticospinal system. The **cerebrocerebellum** receives inputs from the cerebral cortex and projects back up to the cerebral cortex in order to help maintain coordinated neural activity in support of movement and motor planning.

At its core, the cerebellum helps improve motor control in two ways, adjustment and coordination. **Adjustment** is the ability to do slightly more or less. For example, in trying to thread a needle, you will watch the thread as you move it toward the needle's eye. If you are slightly left of the target, you will adjust to move slightly right. **Coordination** is the ability to link together control of two or more actions. If a glass is tipping over and you reach out to grab it, you will not only need to move your arm rapidly to the proper location, you will need your trunk to support the reaching action and your hand to open in preparation. There are two distinct features of the circuits through the cerebellum that support adjustment and coordination. The same circuits are used in each functional division of the cerebellum.

The first circuit is shown in Figure 5-5. The inputs to the cerebellum come in via axons that are called **mossy fibers**. These come from one of the three places mentioned above, the vestibular nuclei, spinal cord, or brainstem. In the case of the vestibular nuclei, the mossy fibers come directly from vestibular nucleus neurons. For the spinal cord and cerebrum, there will be at least one synapse between the origin of the information (a primary sensory neuron or a cortical neuron) and the mossy fiber. For the spinocerebellum, the mossy fiber will come from a cell in **Clarke's column** of the lumbar spinal cord or from the **accessory cuneate nucleus** for upper thoracic and cervical segments. For information coming from the cerebrum, the synapse will be in the pontine nuclei.

Once the mossy fiber carries its information into the cerebellum, it will make excitatory synapses in two places.

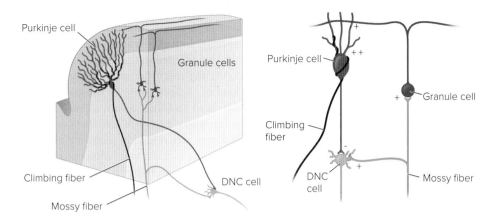

FIGURE 5-5 Cerebellar circuits. On the left, an anatomical cross-section of the cerebellar cortex is illustrated, and on the right, a schematic diagram of the circuit is shown. For simplicity, this diagram shows only a part of the cerebellar circuit.

One branch will go to a neuron in a **deep cerebellar nucleus** (DCN), and the other will synapse in the cerebellar cortex on a type of cell called a **granule cell**. The cell in the DCN will convey the output of the cerebellum, so for this part of the circuit, a higher level of activity coming in on the mossy fiber will tend to lead to a higher level of activity going out. At the same time, however, the activity from the mossy fiber is driving the granule cell. The granule cell will, in turn, synapse on a type of cell in the cerebellar cortex called the **Purkinje cell**. The Purkinje cells make inhibitory synapses on the neurons in the DCN, so through this side of the circuit, increased activity on the mossy fiber coming in will lead to less output from the DCN. The ultimate effect is a contest. Through a process described below, the relative strengths of the excitatory and inhibitory drive to the DCN cells are adjusted with practice so that the proper amount of DCN output is produced. For DCN output cells with influence over the position of the fingers, decreased activity might move the thread slightly left, and increased activity might move it slightly right. Hence, this circuit is well suited for adjustments in motor control.

The feature of cerebellar circuitry that supports coordination of actions across joints is the way in which the granule cells themselves connect to the Purkinje cells. When the granule cell's axon reaches the upper layers of the cerebellar cortex, it splits into two branches, each of which runs parallel to the folia of the cerebellar cortex. These axons are thus aptly named **parallel fibers**. The parallel fibers are what synapse on the Purkinje cells. Each parallel fiber spans relatively far, as much as one-third the width of the cerebellum. Across this large span, there is the possibility that a single parallel fiber in the spinocerebellum could contact various Purkinje cells to influence motor outputs for the legs, trunk, and arms. As such, parallel fibers provide the substrate for coordination of activity across these body parts. In the vestibulocerebellum, the parallel fibers could link balance and postural reactions to movements of the eyes and the head. And in the cerebrocerebellum, they could link past experience with future expectations to provide for anticipatory motor control.

The last aspect of cerebellar function that we will consider is the basis for motor learning provided by the climbing fibers. A **climbing fiber** is a special type of axon that climbs up and around the soma and proximal dendrites of each Purkinje cell. There is only one climbing fiber per Purkinje cell. The **inferior olivary nucleus** in the medulla is the location of the cell bodies of the neurons that produce the climbing fibers. As noted earlier, for adjustments to occur, the relative strengths of the Purkinje cell and mossy fiber influences on the DCN cell must be adjustable. There are two ways in which this occurs. First, there is a principle of operation in the nervous system called **long-term potentiation**. A simple catch phrase used to describe this is that "neurons that fire together wire together." What this means is that if a Purkinje cell tends to make an action potential every time a particular parallel fiber fires to excite it, that synapse will strengthen over time. At first glance, this might seem inevitable, but there are millions of parallel fibers for each Purkinje cell. One parallel fiber firing alone, therefore, is not sufficient to make the Purkinje cell fire. But if the whole set of parallel fibers' influence is such that the Purkinje cell fires, then those parallel fibers that are active, when the Purkinje cell makes an action potential, will tend to see their synaptic influence increase over time. Hence, there is a natural way for synapses between parallel fibers and Purkinje cells that are involved in similar actions to strengthen their connections with each other.

However, what if the action made was a mistake? This is where the climbing fibers come in. Projections to the inferior olivary nucleus will produce action potentials in climbing fibers going to Purkinje cells that were active in association with the mistake. When the climbing fiber makes an action potential, its influence upon the Purkinje cell is profound. The electrical potential created by the climbing fiber is so strong that it creates a special kind of action potential in the Purkinje cell called a **complex spike**. After a complex spike occurs, any parallel fiber synapses that were recently active in that Purkinje cell get weaker, and this is called **long-term depression**. Presumably, these were parallel fiber inputs to the Purkinje cell that were associated with the mistake, so in a way of thinking, they get the blame.

Thus, parallel fiber to Purkinje cell synapses that are not associated with errors will naturally tend to get stronger via long-term potentiation, and those that are associated with errors are made weaker through long-term depression initiated by complex spikes.[60] This allows the adjustment of Purkinje cell influence on the DCN cell. And just as this can occur in any given Purkinje cell to make adjustments in the control of a single aspect of the motor control problem, it can occur in a whole set of parallel fiber to Purkinje cell connections all at once as a means to adjust the coordination of activity among the Purkinje cells, and hence, coordination among multiple aspects of the motor control task.

● PUTTING IT ALL TOGETHER

We now return to the example of the person typing and reaching for the mouse. At this point, we can attach specific tracts and their functions to the example. As the person is typing, there will be tonic activity in the ventromedial systems, including the reticulospinal and vestibulospinal systems, to maintain a stable sitting posture. The primary motor cortex and supplementary motor areas will be active on both sides to select the appropriate sequencing of finger movements to type the text. There will be engagement of the basal ganglia circuits to select the sequence of keystrokes for typing and to select the particular muscles to recruit and relax to perform the actual wrist and finger movements. While the typist will be somewhat unaware of this, there will also be subtle modulation of shoulder and upper trunk activity so that the small shifts in hand and forearm position are made from a stable base. Cerebellar activity will be constantly coordinating these actions, maintaining appropriate forces of the keystrokes and locations of the keys as time passes.

When it is time to reach for the mouse, cortical sensory areas will have a memory of the mouse's location and weight and size and will transfer this memory to the frontal lobe, which will engage motor memory of the action to grasp the mouse through basal ganglia (selection and initiation) and cerebellar (anticipation, coordination, and adjustment) circuits as soon as the desire to use the mouse enters the author's mind. The trajectory to the mouse will be planned, and before the hands are raised from the keyboard, neural activity in the PM and supplementary motor areas will begin to create a subtle postural shift of the shoulders and upper trunk to prepare for the expected inertial consequence of moving the arm. These outputs will be conveyed to some extent through the corticospinal system, which does originate, in part, from these premotor areas. In addition, corticoreticular projections will engage the reticulospinal system to provide the dynamic, anticipatory postural adjustment prior to the reach.

As the reach for the mouse occurs, the author will most likely maintain a visual gaze toward the computer monitor. To the extent that the anticipatory postural adjustment, prior to reaching, along with the arm movement itself, during the reach, results in subtle head movements in reaction, the VOR will operate through the medial vestibulospinal tracts to help keep the eyes pointed to the correct location.

As the reach occurs, the lateral corticospinal tract will be heavily engaged to move the arm in the proper direction and the hand and fingers into a position to grasp the mouse. The rubrospinal tract will also help with this rapid, coordinated reaching action to help shape the hand for grasping the mouse. Cerebellar circuits will help coordinate the forces and torques throughout the upper limb for a smooth movement, making adjustments along the way. As the mouse is grasped, sensory systems will be attuned to the shape and texture of the mouse, helping guide the motor actions required for final placement of the hand around the mouse to use it properly. This seemingly simple action requires cooperation throughout the motor system.

REFERENCES

1. Kuypers HG. Anatomy of descending pathways. In: Brooks V, ed. *Handbook of Physiology. Sect. I. The Nervous System. Vol. II. Motor Control, pt 1.* Bethesda: The American Physiological Society; 1981:597-666.

2. Köbbert C, Apps R, Bechmann I, Lanciego JL, Mey J, Thanos S. Current concepts in neuroanatomical tracing. *Prog Neurobiol.* 2000;62(4):327-251.

3. Saleeba C, Dempsey B, Le S, Goodchild A, McMullan S. A student's guide to neural circuit tracing. *Front Neurosci.* 2019;13:897. https://www.frontiersin.org/articles/10.3389/fnins.2019.00897. Accessed May 5, 2023.

4. Lemon RN. Descending pathways in motor control. *Ann. Rev Neurosci.* 2008;31(1):195-218.

5. Bortoff GA, Strick PL. Corticospinal terminations in two new-world primates: further evidence that corticomotoneuronal connections provide part of the neural substrate for manual dexterity. *J Neurosci.* 1993;13:5105-5118.

6. Jang SH. The corticospinal tract from the viewpoint of brain rehabilitation. *J Rehabil Med.* 2014;193-199.

7. Fetz EE, Cheney PD. Postspike facilitation of forelimb muscle activity by primate corticomotoneuronal cells. *J Neurophysiol.* 1980;44(4):751-772.

8. Martin J. Neuroplasticity of spinal cord injury and repair. *Handb Clin Neurol.* 2022;184:317-330.

9. Dum RP, Strick PL. Motor areas in the frontal lobe of the primate. *Physiol Behav.* 2002;77(4-5):677-682.

10. Strick PL. Stimulating research on motor cortex. *Nat Neurosci.* 2002;5(8):714-715.

11. Freund HJ. Premotor areas in man. In: Evarts EE, Wise SP, Bousfield D, eds. *The Motor System in Neurobiology.* New York: Elsevier; 1985:332-335.

12. Maier MA, Armand J, Kirkwood PA, Yang HW, Davis JN, Lemon RN. Differences in the corticospinal projection from primary motor cortex and supplementary motor area to macaque upper limb motoneurons: an anatomical and electrophysiological study. *Cereb Cortex.* 2002;12(3):281-296.

13. Dum RP, Strick PL. Spinal cord terminations of the medial wall motor areas in macaque monkeys. *J Neurosci.* 1996;16(20):6513-6525.

14. Roland PE, Larsen B, Lassen NA, Skinhoj E. Supplementary motor area and other cortical areas in organization of voluntary movements in man. *J Neurophysiol.* 1980;43(1):118-136.

15. Cheney PD, Hill-Karrer J, Belhaj-Saif A, McKiernan BJ, Park MC, Marcario JK. Cortical motor areas and their properties: implications for neuroprosthetics. *Prog Brain Res.* 2000;128:135-160.

16. Wise SP, di Pellegrino G, Boussaoud D. Primate premotor cortex: dissociation of visuomotor from sensory signals. *J Neurophysiol.* 1992;68(3):969-972.

17. Halsband U, Lange RK. Motor learning in man: a review of functional and clinical studies. *J Physiol Paris*. 2006;99(4-6):414-424.

18. Vaseghi B, Zoghi M, Jaberzadeh S. Does anodal transcranial direct current stimulation modulate sensory perception and pain? A meta-analysis study. *Clin Neurophysiol*. 2014;125(9):1847-1858.

19. Courtine G, Bunge MB, Fawcett JW, et al. Can experiments in nonhuman primates expedite the translation of treatments for spinal cord injury in humans? *Nat Med*. 2007;13(5):561-566.

20. Bostian AC, Strick PL. The basal ganglia and cerebellum: modes in an integrated network. *Nat Rev: Neurosci*. 2018;19(6):338-350.

21. Schwartz AB. Useful signals from motor cortex. *J Physiol*. 2007;579(Pt 3): 581-601.

22. Seidler RD, Bo J, Anguera JA. Neurocognitive contributions to motor skill learning: the role of working memory. *J Mot Behav*. 2012;44(6):445-453.

23. Petrides M. Lateral prefrontal cortex: architectonic and functional organization. *Philos Trans R Soc Lond B Biol Sci*. 2005;360(1456):781-795.

24. Goldman-Rakic PS. Motor control function of the prefrontal cortex. *Ciba Found Symp*. 1987;132:187-200.

25. Buys EJ, Lemon RN, Mantel GW, Muir RB. Selective facilitation of different hand muscles by single corticospinal neurons in the conscious monkey. *J Physiol*. 1986;381:529-549.

26. Fetz EE, Cheney PD, Mewes K, Palmer S. Control of forelimb muscle activity by populations of corticomotoneuronal and rubromotoneuronal cells. *Prog Brain Res*. 1989;80:437-449.

27. Isa T, Mitsuhashi M, Yamaguchi R. Alternative routes for recovery of hand functions after corticospinal tract injury in primates and rodents. *Curr Opin Neurol*. 2019;32(6):836-843.

28. Williams PTJA, Jian Y, Martin JH. Motor system plasticity after unilateral injury in the developing brain. *Dev Med Child Neurol*. 2017;59:1224-1229.

29. Ellis MD, Lan Y, Yao J, DeWald JPA. Robotic quantification of upper extremity loss of independent joint control or flexion synergy in individuals with hemiparetic stroke: a review of paradigms addressing the effects of shoulder abduction loading. *J Neuro Engineering Rehabil*. 2016;13:95.

30. McKiernan BJ, Marcario JK, Karrer JH, Cheney PD. Corticomotoneuronal postspike effects in shoulder, elbow, wrist, digit, and intrinsic hand muscles during a reach and prehension task. *J Neurophysiol*. 1998;80(4):1961-1980.

31. Jankowska E, Edgley SA. How can corticospinal tract neurons contribute to ipsilateral movements? A question with implications for recovery of motor functions. *Neuroscientist*. 2006;12(1):67-79.

32. Denny-Brown D. *The Cerebral Control of Movement*. Springfield: Charles C Thomas; 1966.

33. Bourbonnais D, Vanden Noven S, Pelletier R. Incoordination in patients with hemiparesis. *Can J Public Health*. 1992;83(Suppl 2):S58-S63.

34. Porter B. A review of intrathecal baclofen in the management of spasticity. *Br J Nurs*. 1997;6(5):253-260, 262.

35. Thompson AK, Wolpaw JR. Operant conditioning of spinal reflexes: from basic science to clinical therapy. *Front Integr Neurosci*. 2014;8:25.

36. Chen XY, Chen Y, Wang Y, et al. Reflex conditioning: a new strategy for improving motor function after spinal cord injury. *Ann N Y Acad Sci*. 2010;1198(Suppl 1):E12-E21.

37. Van Kan PL, McCurdy ML. Role of primate magnocellular red nucleus neurons in controlling hand preshaping during reaching to grasp. *J Neurophysiol*. 2001;85(4):1461-1478.

38. Van Kan PL, McCurdy ML. Discharge of primate magnocellular red nucleus neurons during reaching to grasp in different spatial locations. *Exp Brain Res*. 2002;142(1):151-157.

39. Drew T, Andujar JE, Lajoie K, Yakovenko S. Cortical mechanisms involved in visuomotor coordination during precision walking. *Brain Res Rev*. 2008;57(1):199-211.

40. Rho MJ, Lavoie S, Drew T. Effects of red nucleus microstimulation on the locomotor pattern and timing in the intact cat: a comparison with the motor cortex. *J Neurophysiol*. 1999;81(5):2297-2315.

41. Fukushima K. Corticovestibular interactions: anatomy, electrophysiology, and functional considerations. *Exp Brain Res*. 1997;117(1):1-16.

42. Sugiuchi Y, Izawa Y, Ebata S, Shinoda Y. Vestibular cortical area in the periarcuate cortex: its afferent and efferent projections. *Ann N Y Acad Sci*. 2005;1039:111-123.

43. McCall AA, Miller DM, Yates BJ. Descending influences on vestibulospinal and vestibulosympathetic reflexes. *Frontiers in Neurology*. 2107;8:112.

44. Wilson VJ, Peterson BW. Vestibulospinal and reticulospinal systems. In: Brooks V, ed. *Handbook of Physiology. Sect. I. The Nervous System. Vol. II. Motor Control, pt 1*. Bethesda: The American Physiological Society; 1981:667-702.

45. Jang SH, Kwon JW, Yeo SS. Three dimensional identification of medial and lateral vestibulospinal tract in the human brain: a diffusion tensor imaging study. *Front Human Neurosci*. 2018;12:229.

46. Horak FB. Postural compensation for vestibular loss. *Ann N Y Acad Sci*. 2009;1164:76-81.

47. Horak FB, Henry SM, Shumway-Cook A. Postural perturbations: new insights for treatment of balance disorders. *Phys Ther*. 1997;77(5):517-533.

48. Buford JA. Reticulospinal system. In: Squire L, ed. *The New Encyclopedia of Neuroscience*. Elsevier; 2008. Available at http://store.elsevier.com/product.jsp?isbn=9780080446172. Accessed May 5, 2023.

49. Matsuyama K, Takakusaki K, Nakajima K, Mori S. Multi-segmental innervation of single pontine reticulospinal axons in the cervico-thoracic region of the cat: anterograde PHA-L tracing study. *J Comp Neurol*. 1997;377(2):234-250.

50. Matsuyama K, Mori F, Kuze B, Mori S. Morphology of single pontine reticulospinal axons in the lumbar enlargement of the cat: a study using the anterograde tracer PHA-L. *J Comp Neurol*. 1999;410(3):413-430.

51. Jankowska E. Spinal interneuronal networks in the cat: elementary components. *Brain Res Rev*. 2007;57:46-55.

52. Steeves JD, Jordan LM. Localization of a descending pathway in the spinal cord which is necessary for controlled treadmill locomotion. *Neurosci Lett*. 1980;20(3):283-288.

53. Herbert WJ, Davidson AG, Buford JA. Measuring the motor output of the pontomedullary reticular formation in the monkey: do stimulus-triggered averaging and stimulus trains produce comparable results in the upper limbs? *Exp Brain Res*. 2010;203:271-283.

54. Angeli CA, Edgerton VR, Gerasimenko YP, Harkema SJ. Altering spinal cord excitability enables voluntary movements after chronic complete paralysis in humans. *Brain*. 2014;137(Pt 5):1394-1409.

55. Edgerton VR, Roy RR. A new age for rehabilitation. *Eur J Phys Rehabil Med*. 2012;48(1):99-109.

56. Mink JW. The basal ganglia: focused selection and inhibition of competing motor programs. *Prog Neurobiol*. 1996;50(4):381-425.

57. Mink JW. The basal ganglia and involuntary movements: impaired inhibition of competing motor patterns. *Arch Neurol*. 2003;60(10):1365-1368.

58. Konczak J, Corcos DM, Horak F, et al. Proprioception and motor control in Parkinson's disease. *J Mot Behav*. 2009;41(6):543-552.

59. Bostan AC, Dum RP, Strick PL. Cerebellar networks with the cerebral cortex and basal ganglia. *Trends Cogn Sci*. 2013;17(5):241-254.

60. Medina JF, Lisberger SG. Links from complex spikes to local plasticity and motor learning in the cerebellum of awake-behaving monkeys. *Nat Neurosci*. 2008;11(10):1185-1192. doi:10.1038/nn.2197. Epub 2008 Sep 21. Erratum in: *Nat Neurosci*. 2009 Jun;12(6):808.

Review Questions

1. **What is the best example of feed-forward control?**
   A. A stretch reflex resisting forward sway when a person is pushed from behind
   B. Looking at a mouse before reaching for it
   C. Leaning forward before reaching forward
   D. Moving one finger while holding the wrist stable

2. **Which of the cortical motor areas is most likely to produce a corticospinal cell that synapses directly on an alpha motoneuron?**
   A. Primary motor cortex
   B. Supplementary motor area
   C. Premotor cortex
   D. All are equal in this regard

3. **Which body area has a disproportionately small representation in the primary motor cortex?**
   A. Face (mouth)
   B. Arm and hands
   C. Trunk
   D. Legs and feet

4. **In which part of the spinal cord would we expect to find a complete absence of the ventral (anterior) corticospinal tract?**
   A. Upper cervical
   B. Cervical enlargement
   C. Thoracic
   D. Lumbosacral enlargement

5. **Which of the descending systems listed here has bilateral influence?**
   A. Rubrospinal
   B. Lateral reticulospinal
   C. Medial reticulospinal
   D. Lateral vestibulospinal

6. **A patient in a neurologic clinic has trouble moving the right side of her body, reaches with her right arm in a very limited way, and does not seem able to use her right hand. She can sit and can walk with a cane, but there is** also some difficulty in the right leg. She is speaking and her eye movements and facial function seem fairly normal. Where would you most expect the lesion in this person's nervous system to be found?
   A. Left cervical spinal cord
   B. Left motor cortex
   C. Left brainstem
   D. Left cerebellum

7. **What additional motor deficit would you expect to discover upon testing this individual?**
   A. Marked weakness in the left hand
   B. Spasticity (difficulty regulating reflexes) in the right arm and/or leg
   C. Inability to swallow
   D. Ataxia (discoordinated, flailing movements) on the left side

8. **In the basal ganglia, which pathway includes the subthalamic nucleus?**
   A. The direct pathway
   B. The indirect pathway
   C. The thalamocortical pathway
   D. The substantia nigra pathway

9. **What happens when a climbing fiber sets off a complex spike in a Purkinje cell?**
   A. Synapses of mossy fibers on DCN cells get stronger if they were silent.
   B. Synapses of parallel fibers on the Purkinje cell get weaker if they were active.
   C. Synapses of the Purkinje cell on the DCN cell get stronger.
   D. Synapses of the granule cell on the climbing fiber get weaker.

10. **The ventromedial systems for motor control serve what general function?**
    A. Control of the adductor and extensor muscles
    B. Control of the postural and proximal limb muscles
    C. Control of the distal hand and foot muscles
    D. Control of the abdominal and low back muscles

Answers

1. C	**2.** A	**3.** C	**4.** D	**5.** C
6. B	**7.** B	**8.** B	**9.** B	**10.** B

GLOSSARY

Corticobulbar tracts. Groups of neurons with their cell bodies in the cerebral cortex and axon terminals in the brainstem. May terminate in motor pools for cranial nerves or in other brainstem structures such as the reticular formation to influence other system.

Corticomotoneuronal cells. A special type of corticospinal cell that synapses directly onto an alpha motoneuron. These are typically associated with fine control of hand, face, and to some extent foot muscles. They are the minority compared to the typical pattern, which is corticospinal neurons that synapses on interneurons that in turn influence motoneurons. In most regions of the spinal cord, only about 5% of corticospinal cells are corticomotoneuronal neurons, but in the lower cervical enlargement, this may reach 30% to 40%.

Corticospinal system. A group of axons that have neuronal cell bodies in the cerebral cortex and axons terminating in the spinal cord. Some of these axons terminate (synapse) on motoneurons, but most terminate (synapse) on interneurons in the spinal cord that in turn influence motoneurons.

Degrees of freedom. The number of things that can happen or must be controlled. In motor control, the degrees of freedom could be represented by the number of muscles that need to be controlled or the possible combination of joint movements. It could also represent the number of movement patterns possible.

Descending systems (for motor control). Groups of axons referred to as tracts that have neurons in the cerebrum or brainstem with axons projecting to motor pools in the brain stem or spinal cord.

Direct pathway (basal ganglia). A pathway from through the basal ganglia to the thalamus involving two neurons. The first is in the striatum (either in the caudate nucleus or the putamen) and synapses in the internal segment of the globus pallidus. The second is the neuron in the globus pallidus – internal segment, which in turn synapses in the thalamus.

Discrete movement. A movement that has a definite beginning and end, where it would make sense to talk about counting "repetitions" or "trials" of that movement.

Electrophysiology (in neuroscience). An approach to studying the function of the nervous system that involves measuring electrical activity of neurons and/or stimulating neurons with electrical potentials to produce measurable responses. May also involve measuring electrical activity of muscles. More generally, electrophysiology is any study of a physiological system by measuring or applying electrical energy. Also used in cardiology to refer to studies of the conduction system of the heart.

Electromyogram. The electrical pattern of activation measured from a muscle.

Feedforward control. Issuing an early control signal, such as a set of muscle activations, based on prediction from past experience, to counteract the expected consequences of the main command (e.g., shift the trunk forward prior to a forward reaching.

Fine movements. Typically referring to skilled movements of the hands but could include any movement where the intent is a carefully controlled, very accurate movement of a specific body part in a skilled, voluntary manner.

Gross movements. Large movement patterns of a whole limb, or even of the whole body. Things like pushing with the arms, standing up, and rolling over are considered gross movements.

Indirect pathway (basal ganglia). A pathway from the basal ganglia to the thalamus involving four neurons. The first is in the striatum (either in the caudate nucleus or the putamen) and synapses in the external segment of the globus pallidus. The second is the neuron in the globus pallidus – external segment, which in turn synapses in the subthalamic nucleus. The third is the neuron in the subthalamic nucleus, which synapses in the internal segment of the globus pallidus. The fourth is the neuron in the globus pallidus – internal segment, which synapses in the thalamus.

Medial vestibular nucleus. A part of the vestibular system where afferents from all components of the vestibular system (utricle, saccule, semicircular canals) converge to provide complete information about head position and acceleration. Coordinates head and neck movements, including the vestibulo-ocular reflex (VOR). Source of the medial vestibulospinal tracts (and the origin of the medial longitudinal fasciculus).

Lateral vestibular nucleus. A part of the vestibular system where afferents from the otolith organs (utricle and saccule) of the vestibular system converge. Responds to head acceleration by recruiting head, body, and limb movements to maintain upright posture. Source of the lateral vestibulospinal tract.

Motor cortex (general). In a general sense, motor cortex can refer to all of the frontal lobe areas involved in the control of movement, including the primary motor cortex, the supplemental motor area, the premotor cortex, and other cortical areas in that region.

Motoneuron (aka motor neuron). A neuron in the central nervous system producing an axon that projects through the peripheral nervous system to synapse on a muscle. Includes alpha motoneurons, which synapse on skeletal muscle, and gamma motoneurons, which synapse on intrafusal muscle fibers of the muscle spindle.

Motor pool. A local group of motoneurons projecting to a particular muscle.

Precentral gyrus. The strip of brain tissue rostral to the central sulcus but caudal to the pre-central sulcus. Generally, corresponds with primary motor cortex.

Premotor cortex (aka PM). A region of the brain located lateral to the supplementary motor area and rostral to primary motor cortex. A source of motor control for newly learned movements and movements that require real-time adjustments to external information, especially visual information.

Pyramidal cell. A type of neuron found within the cerebral cortex (typically in cortical layer III or V). The cell body of a pyramidal neuron has a shape resembling a pyramid. These are the kinds of neurons that produce the output of the cerebral cortex to project to other part of the brain locally or in distant structures. Corticospinal and corticobulbar cells are pyramidal neurons.

Primary motor cortex. Also called "M1 [M one]" and sometimes called "the motor cortex [specific]." This is the precentral gyrus and the tissue in the rostral bank of the central sulcus from which the most specific cortical control of voluntary movement originates. Corresponds to Brodmann's Area 4.

Somatotopic. A level of organization in the nervous system where neurons (or axons) related to a specific part of the body are grouped together in the same general location. For example, in the cerebral cortex, in primary motor cortex, the leg is represented most medially, the trunk is lateral to the leg, the arm and hand are lateral to that, and the face is represented most laterally.

Spasticity. A hyperactivity of the muscles, especially characterized by stretch reflexes that are too strong, interfering with the ability to move efficiently or as desired. Also described as "increased muscle tone" – indicating the muscles are overly active and the person has difficulty maintaining relaxed muscles, especially during movement. Also used to describe a difficulty regulating the amount of muscle activation, where the movement might require mild muscle activation but the individual produces strong muscle activation.

Supplementary motor area. Also called "SMA," or "M2 [M-two]." A region in the brain located on the dorsal-medial and mesial surface of the superior frontal gyrus, rostral to the primary motor cortex. A source of motor control that helps produce well-learned movements, movements requiring bimanual coordination, and movements in sequences.

Synergies. Patterns of movement in which particular muscle groups are recruited (activated) together, and in some cases, other muscle groups might also be inhibited (relaxed) together; typically refers to coordinated muscle actions across multiple joints in a limb. Often these synergies are a normal part of motor control such that the nervous system can employ circuits that produce synergies for common activities like pushing with the arm or standing on the leg. In neurologic pathology, synergy can have a negative connotation, meaning that even when the person wants to recruit one muscle without the others, they cannot do that very well; the synergy can dominate the movement pattern even when the person wants to move only one joint.

Terminations. When discussing a tract, terminations refer to the general location where axons make synapses in the target structure. A termination is a place where something ends.

Vestibulospinal tract. A descending system for motor control with neuronal cell bodies originating in the medial or the lateral vestibular nucleus with axons terminating in the gray matter of the spinal cord. There is a medial vestibulospinal tract from the medial vestibular nucleus and a lateral vestibulospinal tract from the lateral vestibular nucleus.

Vestibular nuclei. A group of nuclei in the caudal pons and rostral medulla located in the tissues near the fourth ventricle that receive and process afferent information from the vestibular system (semicircular canals, utricle, saccule) of the inner ear. Includes the superior, inferior, medial, and lateral vestibular nuclei.

Voluntary movement. A movement that you can choose to perform or choose not to perform. Not a reflex, not automatic.

The Special Senses

Deborah S. Nichols-Larsen and Anne D. Kloos

6

OBJECTIVES

1) Review the neuroanatomical basis of vision, hearing, smell, taste, and vestibular system function

2) Develop a foundation for the discussion of sensory dysfunction associated with neurologic conditions

3) Examine common testing methods to identify sensory system integrity

In this chapter, we will review the organization and function of the special senses, focusing on vision, vestibular, hearing, taste, and proprioception. These special senses, like somatosensation, each have specific receptors that translate external stimuli to neural coding, neural projections that convey these neural impulses centrally, and brain networks that decode the sensation. This review should help the reader with later chapters when these systems are disrupted by neurologic injury or disease.

● VISION

The Eye

The visual system, of course, starts with the eye. The eye is uniquely shaped to allow perception of our environment; its rounded shape allows the projection of almost 180 degrees of horizontal vision without head or eye movement and nearly 130 degrees of vertical vision. The eye is protected from the environment by a tough external membrane, the **sclera**, which is opaque (white); interestingly, the sclera is continuous with the dura mater (the protective covering of the brain). A clear mucous membrane, the **conjunctiva**, covers the sclera. The **cornea** is transparent and makes up the most central portion of the sclera, covering the iris and refracting light toward the lens as it enters the pupil. The eye and, more specifically, the retina are nourished by the **choroid** underlying the sclera, which is a highly vascular tissue that secretes a thin liquid, called **aqueous humor**, which provides critical nutrients to maintain eye health and helps maintain pressure in the eye. Light is projected by the cornea, through the **pupil** (the central opening of the eye) onto the **lens**, which in turn, focuses it onto the retina (Figure 6-1). The pupil is surrounded by the iris, which is comprised of muscles that control the pupil's size: the **sphincter pupillae muscle** constricts the pupil in bright light, and the dilator pupillae muscle dilates the pupil when light is low. Although the pupil determines the amount of light that enters the eye, it does not play a critical role in focusing the light. This is done by the cornea and the lens. The **lens** sits behind the pupil and is controlled by the ciliary muscles, located within the ciliary body, which surrounds the lens. Both the muscles of the iris and those for the pupil are controlled by the autonomic nervous system: sympathetic activity, originating in the superior ganglion, dilates the pupil; parasympathetic activity via CN III constricts the pupil and contracts the ciliary muscle to thicken the lens to allow focus on near objects (see Box 6-1). Although the greatest amount of light refraction occurs at the cornea, the lens is critical for finely focusing light on the fovea. In the center of the eye, between the lens and retina, there's a gelatinous substance, known as the **vitreous humor or body** that serves to maintain the shape of the eye. The **retina** is a layered structure at the rear of the eye that contains the photosensitive receptors of the eye and the transmission neurons of optic projections.[1,2]

Visual Field(s)

The shape of the eye along with the unique characteristics of the cornea and lens allows for projection of our visual environment with duplication of the central portion of our visual field onto the retinas of both eyes; this explains our enhanced central vision, compared to our peripheral vision, and allows some visual preservation with certain neural injuries. The view of our environment that is visible without eye movement is referred to as our *visual field* (Figure 6-2). Information from the right visual field is conveyed to the nasal retina of the right eye and the temporal retina of the left eye and vice versa for the left visual field; there is a portion of the extreme peripheral visual field that is only projected to the ipsilateral eye because the nose blocks its projection to the opposite eye; this information is projected to the most nasal portion of the ipsilateral eye. For the most part, however, our visual field is binocular. Notably, as light passes through the cornea, it bends such that the upper visual field is projected to the lower retina and the lower visual field is projected to the upper retina; basically, this means that the image projected to the retina is upside down and also reversed (right is left), since the peripheral field is on the nasal retina and the central field is on the temporal retina.[2,4]

Visual Receptors

The eye possesses a unique filtering system and sensory receptors that encode light into neural signals. As light enters the

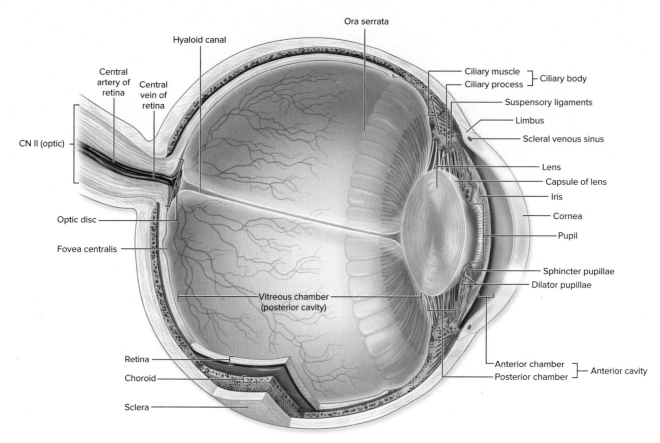

FIGURE 6-1 Anatomy of the eye. (Reproduced with permission from McKinley M, O'Laughlin VD. *Human Anatomy*, 3rd Ed, New York, NY: McGraw-Hill; 2012.)

<table>
<tr><td colspan="2">Box 6-1   Pupil and Lens Control</td></tr>
</table>

Pupillary reflexes:

Constriction: When a strong light hits the retina, it induces constriction of the pupil through a reflexive response. This reflex is mediated by sequential projections from the retina to the midbrain's pretectal olivary nucleus, to a pupillary region dorsal to the Edinger–Westphal nuclei (also in the midbrain), to the ciliary ganglion and ultimately to the ciliary muscles that constrict the pupil via parasympathetic fibers in CN III. Each midbrain pupillary region connects to its counterpart on the opposite side such that pupillary constriction occurs bilaterally and symmetrically.[3]

Dilation: Dilation can be achieved by inhibition of the reflexive loop that produces constriction or by activation of the iris dilator muscle via the sympathetic nervous system component of the ciliary ganglion. This pathway originates in the hypothalamus, synapses in the superior cervical ganglion, and passes through the ciliary ganglion to the dilator muscle.[4]

Accommodation:

Changing the shape of the lens within the eye allows us to orient to objects near to us as well as those far away. To allow us to focus on objects in the distance, the lens becomes elongated, associated with ciliary muscle relaxation, while focus on near objects is achieved by a thickening of the lens via ciliary muscle contraction; both of these changes serve to focus the image on the retina. The ciliary muscles of the lens create this change in lens shape through the same series of projections that control the pupillary reflexes; in fact, accommodation for near vision is also associated with pupil constriction and eye convergence (slight adduction), requiring integration via these brainstem nuclei.[2]

Myopia (nearsightedness): Light is focused short of the retina, making distance vision poor, associated with poor elongation of the lens or an eye that is too long.

Hyperopia (farsightedness): Poor near vision caused by poor accommodation (inability of the lens to achieve a sufficiently round shape) or an eye that is too short.

Presbyopia: Age-induced change in the ability to accommodate, resulting in poorer near vision.

---

eye through the pupil, the lens focuses the incoming image centrally, aiming for the tightest cluster of receptors, located in the central portion of the retina, known as the **fovea**. The fovea is the central area of the **macula; the macula is** a lightly colored area in the central retina that is dense with receptors and **ganglion cells**. The receptors of the eye are **rod and cone cells;** both are photosensitive due to special pigments within them. The fovea contains only cones, which are color receptors that are less sensitive to light but provide better visual acuity. There are three types of cones, responding to different portions of the light spectrum: red – longest rays of the spectrum, L cones; green – middle portion of the spectrum, M cones; blue – shortest rays of the spectrum, S cones. However, since cones are less light-sensitive, they are inactive in dim light, rendering us "color most posterior retinal layer, just behind these photoreceptors, is a dark layer of epithelium, called the **pigment epithelium**, which is a structural support and metabolic hub for the retina but also absorbs light to preserve the projected image and prevent light from "bouncing back" through the eye. The middle cellular layer of the retina houses the interneuronal complex that transmits signals from the receptors to the ganglion cells. This interneuronal complex is comprised of three types of interneurons: bipolar, horizontal, and amacrine cells. **Bipolar cells** are the primary transmission interneurons, connecting the receptors to the ganglion cells that make up the **optic nerve**; the **horizontal** and **amacrine** cellular networks function as modulators of neural transmission by increasing or decreasing the effectiveness of bipolar cell activation of ganglion cells, and thereby, adjusting spatial sensitivity and acuity. Ganglion cells are more superficial in the retina, closest to the incoming light; their axons come together in the optic disc, also known as the **blind spot** of the eye, as they exit the eye to convey visual information centrally as the optic nerve (CN II).[2]

Optic Projections and Visual Processing

As mentioned, the visual environment is projected such that each eye receives information from the right and left environment: ipsilateral peripheral vision to the nasal retina and contralateral central vision to the temporal retina. As the ganglion cell axons merge into the optic nerve, those from the nasal retina are more medial and those from the temporal retina more lateral. Just above the pituitary gland, the two optic nerves come together in the **optic chiasm**; it is here that the central fibers cross and merge with the temporal fibers of the contralateral eye. This crossing brings all of the fibers for a **hemifield** (1/2 of the entire visual field) into the contralateral **optic tract** that projects to the **lateral geniculate** of the thalamus; a small number of fibers bypass the lateral geniculate and project to the **superior colliculus**, which is involved in the assessment of object versus self-movement and visual reflexes. Visual neurons from the lateral geniculate project as the **optic radiations** to the primary visual cortex in the occipital lobe (Brodmann's area 17; striate cortex); the optic radiations split as they leave the lateral geniculate, to accommodate the lateral ventricles, with the upper visual field fibers (lower retinal fibers) traversing laterally within the temporal lobe as **Meyer's loop** and the lower visual field fibers (upper retinal fibers) coursing superiorly through the parietal lobe (**parietal radiations**) to the striate (calcarine) cortex of the occipital lobe (Figure 6-4). It is referred to as the **calcarine cortex** because it straddles the calcarine sulcus on the medial surface of the hemisphere as well as the striate cortex because of its layered or striped appearance. Terminations of the optic radiations place the information from the fovea more posteriorly and that from the periphery more anteriorly with the upper visual field in the lower striate cortex and the lower visual field in the upper striate cortex; thus, the visual image is upside down in the primary visual cortex.[4] Visual processing begins in the striate cortex but relies heavily on the surrounding occipital lobe, or non-striate cortex (areas 18 and 19). The cortical processing of visual stimuli occurs through interconnections within these three occipital areas to separately decode for color, shape, and location/movement. Additional connections between the two hemispheres allow for a complete reproduction of the visual environment to occur. More sophisticated analysis of object

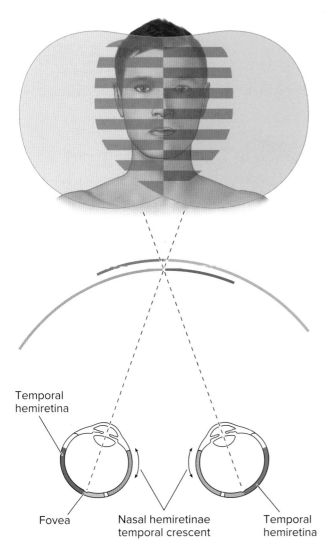

Temporal hemiretina

Fovea   **Nasal hemiretinae temporal crescent**   **Temporal hemiretina**

FIGURE 6-2 Schematic of visual field projections. Projections to the retina: The central striped area illustrates the overlapping binocular visual field, conveyed to the temporal retina of each eye. The solid-colored fields are unique to each eye. The right monocular visual field (green) is transmitted to the right nasal retina while the left (blue) is transmitted to the left nasal retina. This allows the projections from the right field to come together as the nasal fibers cross at the optic chiasm. (Reproduced with permission from Martin JH. *Neuroanatomy Text and Atlas*, Ed 4. New York, NY: McGraw-Hill; 2012.)

blind" in low levels of light. Conversely, rods are highly light sensitive, capable of being activated by a single photon of light, and responsible for our vision at night and in poorly lit environments. However, they quickly become saturated, and therefore inactive, in bright light. Notably, cones are clustered tightly in the fovea and then progressively decrease toward the periphery of the retina; conversely, rods are absent in the fovea, more dense in the area surrounding it, and also become progressively less dense toward the periphery.[2,4]

The Retina

Although rods and cones are the photosensitive receptors for vision, light must travel through multiple cellular layers of the retina before reaching these critical receptors (see Figure 6-3). The

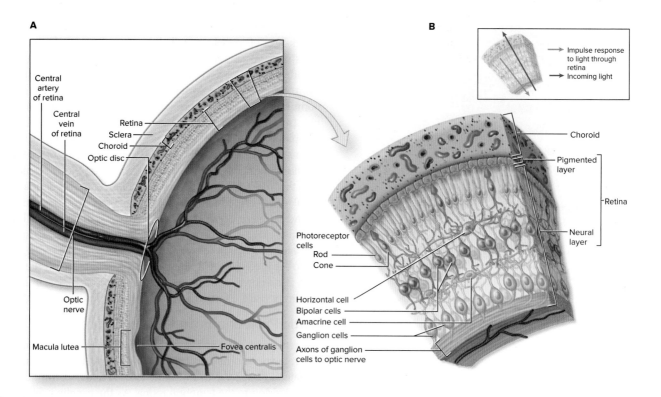

FIGURE 6-3 Diagram of eye and retina. Light enters the front of the eye and passes through the lens, vitreous humor to the retina, where it passes first through the interneural complex of ganglion, bipolar, and horizontal cells before hitting the photosensitive rods and cones. Transduction retraces this pathway with sequential activation of the bipolar cells and then the ganglion cells that form the optic nerve. Horizontal and amacrine cells modulate the cellular activity between the bipolar and ganglion cells. (**A.** Reproduced with permission from McKinley M, O'Laughlin VD. *Human Anatomy*. 3rd ed. Mew York, NY: McGraw Hill,2012. **B.** Reproduced with permission from Saladin KS. *Human Anatomy*, 6ed, New York, NY: McGraw-Hill; 2020.)

recognition and localization relies on two separate networks between the occipital lobe and the temporal and parietal lobes, respectively (Figure 6-5). According to this model, object recognition (what) involves the ventral stream, which ties the occipital lobe to the temporal lobe, while spatial orientation of the object (where) involves the dorsal stream, which involves the occipital and parietal lobes.[4]

One method of testing for visual system integrity is through the **visual evoked potential** (VEP). The VEP measures the time it takes a presented stimulus to move through the visual system to the occipital cortex, using electroencephalographic (EEG) measurement. The typical stimulus is a checkerboard pattern, introduced in an alternating fashion to each eye, or a flashing light, used mostly in children. The P100 wave is a spike that can be seen when the visual signal reaches the occipital cortex, named for the characteristic 100 seconds this transmission takes in most people. A delay in the P100 is indicative of disruption in the visual projections, associated with multiple sclerosis, optic neuritis, or other conditions that impede neuronal transmission.[5]

Eye Movement and Visual Pursuit

The eye has a dynamic group of six muscles, innervated by three cranial nerves (III, IV, and VI) that allow its unique and complex movement abilities: superior rectus, inferior rectus, medial rectus, and inferior oblique, innervated by CN III; superior oblique (CN IV); and lateral rectus (CN VI). The medial and lateral recti produce medial (adduction) and lateral (abduction)

horizontal movements, consistent with their names. Similarly, the superior and inferior recti pull the eye upward (elevation) and downward (depression), respectively, but due to their off-center insertions on the eye, also pull the eyes inward, so with superior rectus contraction the eye moves up and in, and conversely, the inferior rectus contraction pulls the eye down and in to look at the tip of the nose. Both of the oblique muscles attach to the eye on the posterolateral surface and have actions in opposition of their name but consistent with their attachment on the eye. The superior oblique attaches on the superior aspect of the eye and orients the eye downward and laterally (lower corner of the room) by pulling the back of the eye up and in, while the inferior oblique attaches on the inferior aspect and orients the eye upward and laterally (to look at the upper corner of the room) by pulling the back of the eye down and medially.[6]

Although these extraocular muscles can be controlled individually or in combination through upper motor neuron activation of their respective cranial nuclei and nerves, eye control is also maintained through a series of brainstem networks, and as you have likely experienced, moving just one eye is very difficult as they are controlled in tandem through these networks. First, the paramedian pontine reticular formation controls lateral eye coordination, referred to as **horizontal saccades**, through its projections to the abducens nucleus; neurons within this nucleus directly produce lateral rectus contractions of the ipsilateral eye and indirectly produce medial rectus contractions of the contralateral eye via the oculomotor nucleus. A group of

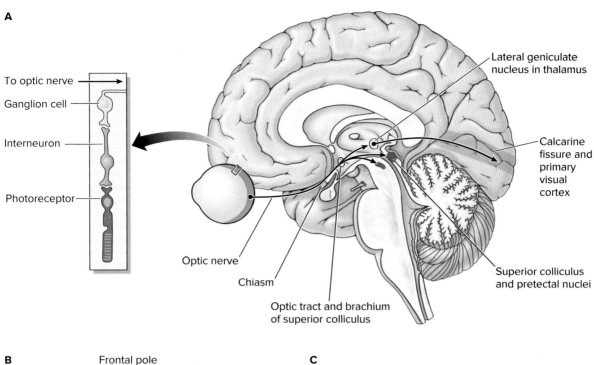

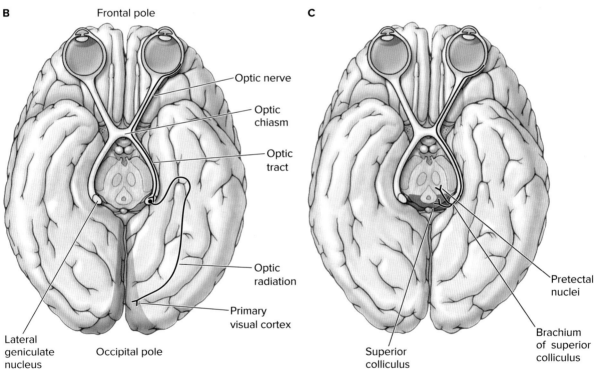

FIGURE 6-4 Visual projections from the retina to the visual cortex. (Reproduced with permission from Martin JH. *Neuroanatomy Text and Atlas*, 4th ed, New York, NY: McGraw-Hill; 2012.)

neurons within the abducens nucleus, known as internuclear neurons, decussate and project to the contralateral oculomotor nucleus, thus activating the medial rectus of the opposite eye. Thus, abduction of the ipsilateral eye and adduction of the contralateral eye can be produced in unison to achieve smooth horizontal motion of the eye. Horizontal saccades can be initiated via projections from the frontal eye fields within the frontal lobe to the superior colliculi in the midbrain but are also controlled by projections from the medial vestibular nuclei in the

adjacent brainstem and ultimately their cerebellar connections to maintain vision when the head is turned[6] (see vestibular section of this chapter).

Similarly, smooth **vertical saccades** (upward–downward motions) of both eyes are achieved by a network that includes the mesencephalic reticular formation (MRF), the medial longitudinal fasciculi, and the oculomotor nuclei bilaterally. The mesencephalic reticular formations of each side of the brainstem interconnect via projections through the posterior

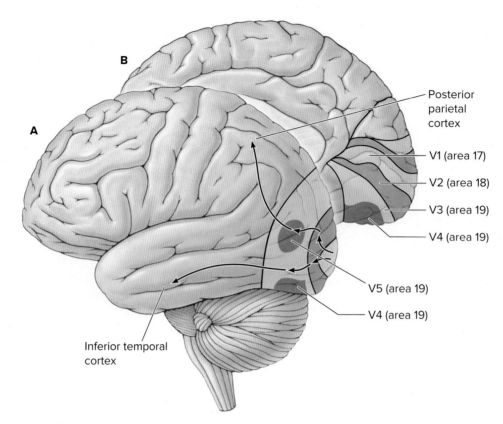

FIGURE 6-5 Areas involved in visual image processing. V1, primary visual cortex (area 17); V2, secondary visual cortex (area 18); V3, V4, V5, distinct regions of area 19. V2-V5 are referred to as the extrastriate cortex as well as visual association cortex. Areas 18 and 19 surround area 17 in a circular fashion. These areas are highly interconnected with many subdivisions, allowing for the complex interpretation of object shape, color, orientation, and movement. Ventral projections to the temporal lobe are associated with object recognition. Dorsal projections to the posterior parietal cortex are associated with object location. (Reproduced with permission from Martin JH. *Neuroanatomy Text and Atlas*, 4th ed, New York, NY: McGraw-Hill; 2012.)

commissure in the midbrain, allowing bilateral control of vertical saccades. The medial longitudinal fasciculus runs between the MRF and the ipsilateral oculomotor nucleus on each side of the brainstem, which innervates both the superior and inferior recti. Thus, simultaneous activation of the respective oculomotor neurons will generate smooth up and down movements. Vertical saccades are also controlled by the frontal eye field via the superior colliculus as well as through inputs from the cerebellum and vestibular nuclei.[6]

This link between eye movement and the vestibular system serves to facilitate eye orientation with head movement via a reflexive response known as the optokinetic reflexes (see vestibular section of this chapter).

Multiple areas of the cerebral hemispheres also contribute to the control of eye movements. First, projection of an image to the striate cortex is necessary for visually guided eye movements; damage to the striate cortex impairs or eliminates these movements, depending on the degree of damage. The **temporo-parietal-occipital junction** serves to interpret the speed of moving objects; damage in this area is associated with impaired ability to track moving objects but maintained ability to focus on a stationary object. In addition, multiple areas of the parietal lobe contribute to eye movement control, including the **posterior parietal cortex** (PPC). Unilateral damage to the PPC impedes visual pursuit to the contralateral environment, especially when damage is in the right hemisphere, contributing to contralateral

visual neglect. Neurons in the **intraparietal sulcus** contribute to object memory, allowing the shifting of attention to a new target and back to a previously viewed object. Similarly, multiple areas of the frontal lobes contribute to smooth eye movements, including the frontal eye field in the middle frontal gyrus and precentral sulcus, the dorsomedial prefrontal cortex, and the supplementary cortex. These frontal lobe areas may modulate reflex activity and inhibit misdirected eye movements.[6]

Visual Testing

Evaluation of visual function and system integrity is highly complex; here we will discuss briefly some of the measures currently used to examine visual acuity, which should look at each eye and both eyes together, color vision, the ophthalmoscopic assessment of the inner eye, visual field analysis, ocular motility, and pupil responsiveness. Almost everyone has experienced a **high-contrast visual acuity** examination, using a Snellen Chart (lines of letters and numbers of progressively diminishing size) with each line marked by an acuity level. Normal vision is 20/20 or the ability to read at 20 ft which is considered "typical." If you have a visual acuity deficit, this is represented by an increase in the denominator of this fraction (e.g., 20/40), indicating that you see at 20 ft what others see clearly at 40 ft; over-correction or enhanced vision is similarly represented by a smaller denominator (e.g., 20/10), indicating that you see at 20 ft what others must be at 10 ft to see. Visual acuity can also be examined at bedside, using a Rosenbaum visual acuity card held 14 inches from the face with a similar acuity outcome measure to a Snellen chart. Visual acuity testing is also the best way to confirm CN II function.[7,8]

Color perception is trichromatic (red, green, blue) and achieved by the sensitivity of different cone subtypes to specific light spectra; color "blindness" results from a change in the prevalence or functioning of a cone subtype. For many of those affected, the deficit is incomplete with three cone subtypes present but one is impaired, resulting in what is known as an **anomalous trichromatic** deficit; in others, there is an absence of one cone subtype, which is referred to as **dichromatic vision**. For these individuals, they perceive the two remaining color spectra but see the missing spectra as gray or black. Although true color blindness is rare, partial deficits are present in up to 10% of the male population; females rarely experience this deficit because red and green deficits are primarily genetically acquired via X-linked inheritance so that females are carriers but males are affected. Blue color blindness is associated with chromosome 7 mutation, so may be found in both men and women but is much rarer than red or green deficits. Testing for color vision is typically done with Ishihara plates, which are spheres with a background of multicolored dots with an embedded number or letter, also constructed of multicolored dots. The plates are designed to distinguish the different color deficits, listed in Table 6-1 so that the background would be shades of one hue (e.g., green) and the embedded figure would be shades of another (e.g., red) to identify those with an anomalous trichromatic deficit or dichromatic deficit (e.g., protanomaly).[8,9]

The **ophthalmoscope assessment** of the inner eye allows magnified scrutiny of the external (cornea) and internal eye (lens, vitreous humor, retina), with close attention paid to the **fundus** of the eye, which includes the fovea, macula, optic disk, retina, and retinal blood vessels, and is a critical part of evaluation of eye integrity. This exam is looking for edema, inflammation, infarcts, and vascular changes within the retina.[8]

To assess **visual fields**, it is best to have the individual look straight ahead; the examiner can then introduce one to three fingers from the left and right above and below eye level (upper and lower visual fields), thus, checking peripheral vision by quadrant. It is important that no eye movement be allowed so that "true" peripheral vision is tested.[8]

Optic muscle function should first be evaluated by assessing the resting position of the eye when the individual is looking straight ahead. Second, having the individual track your finger as it moves in all directions will identify disparities between the two eyes indicative of cranial nerve dysfunction and subsequent muscle dysfunction, since these are typically unilateral. Eye motion should be evaluated with only one eye moving (the other eye is covered) and with both eyes following.[8] Table 6-2 provides details on loss of function with cranial nerve damage.

Pupillary responsiveness should be evaluated in a semi-darkened room with the person looking at an object straight

TABLE 6-1	Color Vision Deficits[9]		
TERM		**CONES/WAVELENGTH DISRUPTED**	**COLOR VISUAL DEFICIT**
Protanomaly		L Cones – long wavelength	Red
Deuteranomaly		M Cones – middle wavelength	Green
Tritanomaly		S Cones – short wavelength	Blue
Achromatopsia (complete loss of color discrimination)	Rod monochromatism	Loss of all cone function	Photophobia Nystagmus Poor acuity No color vision
	Cone monochromatism	Blue cone function without red or green function but very few blue cones so primarily rod vision	

TABLE 6-2	Ocular Cranial Nerve Function and Dysfunction[6]	
CRANIAL NERVE	**FUNCTION**	**DYSFUNCTION**
III	Medial, inferior, and superior recti, and inferior oblique; pupil constriction; eyelid lifting (opening); accommodation	Pupil dilation; at rest, pull of superior oblique and lateral rectus is unopposed, so eye looks down and outward
		Can't look directly downward due to absence of inferior rectus (eye deviates outward due to pull of superior oblique), medially or upward
		Pupil is dilated; eyelid droops; and vision is blurry (lack of accommodation)
IV	Superior oblique	At rest, eye is elevated
		When eye is adducted, elevation increases
		When eye is abducted, elevation decreases
VI	Lateral rectus	Unable to abduct eye

ahead on the wall; this will produce pupil dilation. Then, introduce a penlight from below and watch for the response; both pupils should constrict equally. It is not unusual for people to have a slight difference in the size of their pupils, but the degree of the response should be the same.[7]

OLFACTION: THE SENSE OF SMELL

Our sense of smell, or olfaction, is phylogenetically the oldest sensory system, and in nonhumans plays a critical role in survival, enabling the identification and location of food. Thus, in most animals, the olfactory system is much larger, respectively, than in humans, who rarely rely on their nose to find their food except perhaps when they are awakened by the smell of fresh coffee brewing or bacon frying.

Olfactory Receptors

Olfaction originates in the **bipolar cells** of the nasal epithelium. While the nasal cavity is lined with epithelium, only a small part (olfactory epithelium) on the superior aspect of the nasal cavity contains the bipolar cells, supporting olfaction; much of the remainder is associated with respiration. The olfactory bipolar cells project multiple **cilia** (stiff hair-like projections) into the mucosa that covers the epithelial layer. Only airborne chemicals, known as **odorants**, that are soluble in the mucosa can activate the olfactory neurons, yet the wide degree of odors perceived and the sensitivity of the olfactory system to minor variations of odor is quite impressive. The mucosa, itself, facilitates the transportation of these soluble chemicals toward the

epithelial layer. Odorants enter the nose through breathing or sniffing as well as through the nasopharyngeal corridor during eating. The axons of the olfactory bipolar cells bundle together into axons that pass through the bony cribriform plate at the top of the nasal passage; these bundled axons, though not tightly organized, make up the **olfactory nerve** (CN I), synapsing on second-order neurons, called **mitral cells**, in the olfactory bulb. The connection between the mitral cells and bipolar axons is quite complex with multiple bipolar axons synapsing on each mitral cell, serving to magnify the olfactory signal. The mitral cell axons merge to form the olfactory tract as it exits the olfactory bulb and projects directly to cortical processing centers. See Figure 6-6 for the olfactory projections. Notably, the sense of smell is the only sense that does not project initially to the thalamus before proceeding to the cortex; however, there are projections from the olfactory cortical areas to the thalamus.[10]

Cortical Processing of Olfaction

The areas of the cortex that receive direct olfactory projections are collectively called the olfactory cortex and are located together in the dorsal aspect of the brain: (1) the anterior olfactory nucleus (AON), which sits just above the olfactory bulb; (2) the olfactory tubercle, which is medial to the anterior olfactory nucleus, and (3) the pyriform cortex (primary olfactory cortex), which is lateral to the AON.[11] The AON not only receives projections from the olfactory tract but also projects multiple projections back to the olfactory bulbs bilaterally, and thereby, may serve most to modulate our olfactory experience, either enhancing or diminishing it. Other areas that receive secondary projection are the amygdala, insular cortex, rostral entorhinal cortex

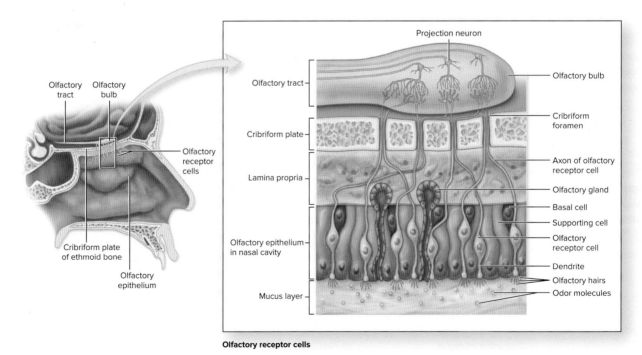

FIGURE 6-6 Olfactory receptors and projections. Bipolar cells within the nasal epithelium project through the cribriform plate to the olfactory tubercle, activating mitral cells that project as the olfactory tract to the olfactory cortex in structures on the dorsum of the brain. (Reproduced with permission from McKinley M, O'Laughlin VD. *Human Anatomy* 3rd Ed, New York, NY: McGraw-Hill; 2012.)

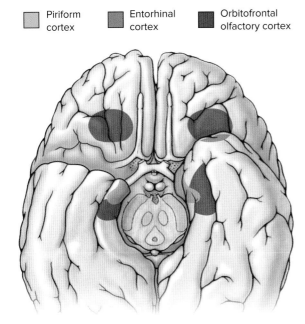

Piriform cortex ▢ Entorhinal cortex ▢ Orbitofrontal olfactory cortex ▢

FIGURE 6-7 Olfactory cortex. (Reproduced with permission from Martin JH. *Neuroanatomy Text and Atlas*, 4th ed, New York, NY: McGraw-Hill; 2012.)

(medial temporal lobe), and the orbitofrontal cortex (Figure 6-7). The connections with the amygdala and olfactory tubercle are likely related to the strong emotional responses generated by many smells, while the piriform cortex is thought to be the source of odor identification and intensity determination, and the entorhinal cortex is the source of memories, associated with specific smells.

The orbitofrontal olfactory cortex receives secondary and tertiary projections from the other olfactory cortices as well as the gustatory (taste) cortex and the thalamus; it is thought that this area is critical in olfactory discrimination and identification. Primarily, it encodes the association between a source and its emitted odor as well as the positive/negative value of an odor. In combination with taste perception, the orbitofrontal cortex seems to encode our definition of "flavor."[12]

Olfactory Testing

Testing olfactory function is relatively simple: choose common liquids with distinct and familiar odors (e.g., vanilla, peppermint extract, or diluted ammonia); wet a cotton swab with the liquid and bring it to a distance of about 1 inch from each nostril. The other nostril should be pushed close with the tester's finger. Using several different odors will yield a more reliable measure.

● GUSTATION: THE SENSE OF TASTE

Similar to olfaction, our perception of taste is based on the transduction of chemicals (**tastants**) within food to neural signals and starts with the taste (gustatory) receptors that are arranged within taste buds. **Taste buds** are located on the tongue, pharynx, soft palate, epiglottis, and larynx; the taste buds on the tongue are located within papillae while those on the other surfaces are

embedded in the epithelium. Each taste bud is made up of 50 to 100 neuroepithelial cell clusters. There are three kinds of taste bud papillae on the tongue: (1) circumvallate – most dense (48% of taste buds) found centrally at the back of the tongue; foliate – located on the lateral aspect of the dorsal tongue bilaterally, second most dense (28%); and fungiform (mushroom-shaped) – found on the anterior 2/3 of the tongue and least dense (24%). The density of receptors on the posterior tongue suggests that it plays a more critical role in taste. The role of taste buds in the epithelium of the oral cavity (soft palate, epiglottis, larynx, pharynx) is less well understood. Notably, taste buds only survive 8 to 22 days, and then, are replaced; there is some suggestion that the ability to replace taste buds diminishes with aging and may contribute to appetite changes in older adults.[13] See Box 6-2 for the relationship between taste and smell.

Taste Receptors

There are five identified taste qualities perceived by specific taste receptors: salty – responding to potassium, sodium, or other ionized metals; sweet – responding to sugars; sour – responding to acid-released hydrogen ions; bitter – responding to toxins or alkaloids; and umami, which is a Japanese word that translates as a pleasant or savory taste, typically associated with meats and cheeses due to their amino acid content. In addition, there is a suggestion that fatty acids and calcium may also elicit a specific taste. Some taste receptors respond to only one quality while others respond to several.[14] The rapid turnover of taste receptors most likely assures ongoing responsiveness to tastants.

Why is taste so important? It allows us to identify potential poisons or impurities in our food.

Central Processing of Taste

Taste is projected centrally via three cranial nerves: VII (anterior 2/3 of the tongue), IX (posterior 1/3 of tongue, pharynx), and X (epiglottis, larynx). Figure 6-8 illustrates these projections. Analogous to the primary sensory receptors, these are pseudounipolar neurons with cell bodies in peripheral ganglia encased within the skull; their central projections all terminate in the solitary nucleus of the medulla. Indeed, these fibers not only convey taste but also somatosensory information from the oral structures. Second-order neurons project from the solitary nucleus to the ventral posterior medial nucleus of the thalamus along with somatosensory information from the face, nose, and mouth. Tertiary projections convey information from the thalamus to the gustatory cortex within the insula and adjacent operculum.[15] This primary gustatory cortex determines taste identity, intensity, and temperature. It is also connected to

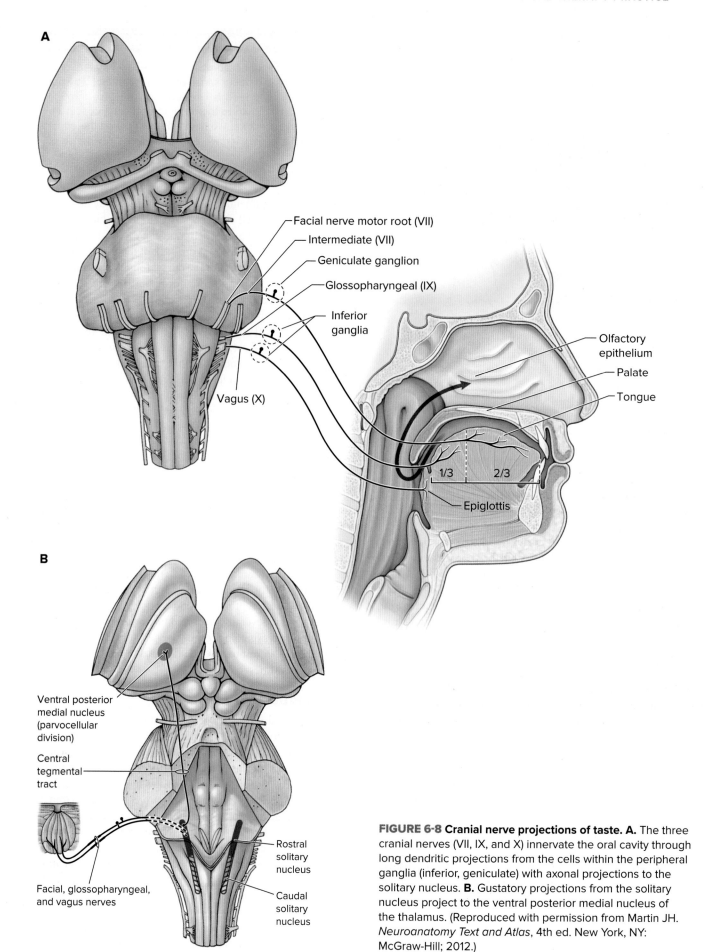

A

Facial nerve motor root (VII)
Intermediate (VII)
Geniculate ganglion
Glossopharyngeal (IX)
Inferior ganglia
Vagus (X)

Olfactory epithelium
Palate
Tongue
1/3   2/3
Epiglottis

B

Ventral posterior medial nucleus (parvocellular division)
Central tegmental tract
Facial, glossopharyngeal, and vagus nerves
Rostral solitary nucleus
Caudal solitary nucleus

FIGURE 6-8 Cranial nerve projections of taste. A. The three cranial nerves (VII, IX, and X) innervate the oral cavity through long dendritic projections from the cells within the peripheral ganglia (inferior, geniculate) with axonal projections to the solitary nucleus. **B.** Gustatory projections from the solitary nucleus project to the ventral posterior medial nucleus of the thalamus. (Reproduced with permission from Martin JH. *Neuroanatomy Text and Atlas*, 4th ed. New York, NY: McGraw-Hill; 2012.)

the orbitofrontal cortex, similar to olfaction, where the reward value of a taste, including that of the texture, is assigned (pleasantness or unpleasantness).[12]

Taste Testing

Similar to the testing of smell, taste can easily be tested by wetting a cotton swab with water flavored with sugar, salt, or lemon juice. Due to the complexity of the innervation for taste, testing should include the anterior 2/3 of the tongue (CN VII) as well as the posterior 1/3 of the tongue (CN IX); although taste also originates from receptors in the epiglottis and throat, testing here is most likely to cause gagging, and therefore, is not done.

● HEARING: THE AUDITORY SYSTEM

The Ear's Organization and Auditory Apparatus

The ear is the location for two sensory functions: hearing and vestibular. This section will address the sense of hearing. The external ear (**auricle**) and the **external acoustic meatus** (ear canal) are uniquely funnel-shaped, directing sound inward and toward the **tympanic membrane** (eardrum). The narrowing of the canal compresses the sound wave to increase the pressure impact on the tympanic membrane. Thus, sound waves press upon the tympanic membrane, and this pressure-release phenomenon creates a chain reaction vibration within the middle ear's three ossicles (tiny bones): **stapes**, **incus**, and **malleus**. The vibrating of these tiny auditory ossicles further amplifies the sound wave and causes the stapes (the third bone in the chain) to push in and out of the **oval window**, which is the membranous covering for the inner ear. The middle ear is also connected to the nasopharynx via the **Eustachian tube**, which allows the relief of pressure that can develop in the ear (e.g., changes in external pressure while flying) as well as a means of clearing mucus from the middle ear.[16]

The inner ear is comprised of the cochlea and vestibular apparatus or labyrinths that are part of what is referred to as the **bony labyrinth**, a part of the temporal bone that is pitted with cavities and tunnels, lined with a **membranous labyrinth, comprised of interconnected sacs and ducts**. The space between the bony and membranous labyrinths is fluid-filled with a substance known as **perilymph** that serves as a protective cushion for the membranous labyrinth. The membranous labyrinth is also filled with fluid, called **endolymph**. The **cochlea** is coiled like a snail with the **cochlear duct** (scalia media) in its center, enclosed by the thin vestibular membrane above and thick basilar membrane below. These two membranes also partition the cochlea into two additional chambers, the **vestibular scala** and **tympanic scala** that are connected by a tiny opening. The cochlear duct has an area of thick epithelium, called the **spiral organ** or **organ of Corti** that is embedded with **hair cells**, which are the sensory receptors for sound. The hair cells lie in a supporting matrix of cells just above the basilar membrane but project tiny extensions (stereocilia) upward into a gelatinous mass, known as the **tectorial membrane**. When the oval window is struck by the stapes, vibrations are transmitted into

the vestibular duct and successively to the tympanic duct via movement of the endolymph, which, in turn, generates movement of the basilar membrane and the hair cells resting above it. However, the stereocilia are more rigid within the tectorial membrane, causing a shearing force between them and their respective hair cell; this shearing activates the hair cell and induces transduction of the vibration to a neural impulse. There are two types of hair cells, identified by their location as inner and outer hair cells. The **inner cells** are fewer but receive extensive innervation from CN VIII fibers; these cells are principally responsible for the transduction of auditory information. **Outer hair cells** outnumber inner cells 3:1 but appear to have more of an efferent function, modulating the activity of inner cells, and thereby, enhancing the amplification of the auditory signal. The vibration dissipates as it passes through the tympanic duct and, then, dissipates through the **round window**, back into the middle ear cavity.[2,17] See Figure 6-9 for the components of the ear and Figure 6-10 for the auditory apparatus.

Central Processing of Hearing

Similar to other cranial nerves, the neurons that make up the cochlear portion of CN VIII have their cell bodies in peripheral ganglia, the **spiral ganglia**, with long central axons that terminate in the ipsilateral ventral and dorsal **cochlear nuclei** of the rostral medulla. CN VIII neurons convey information from specific areas of the cochlea, associated with sound frequencies, with

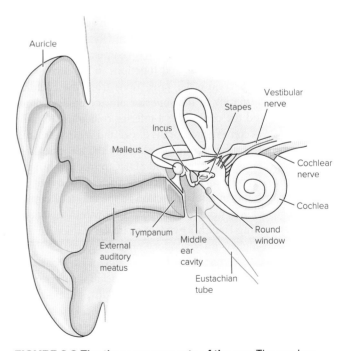

FIGURE 6-9 The three components of the ear. The ear has three functional components: (1) the external ear (auricle, external acoustic meatus, and tympanic membrane) that funnels sound to the interior of the ear; (2) the middle ear (auditory ossicles – malleus, incus, and stapes) that transmits vibration to the eardrum; and (3) the inner ear (cochlea) that allows the transduction of sound to neural signals. (Reproduced with permission from Kandel ER, Schwartz JH, et al, *Principles of neural Science*, 5th Ed.,New York, NY: McGraw-Hill; 2013.)

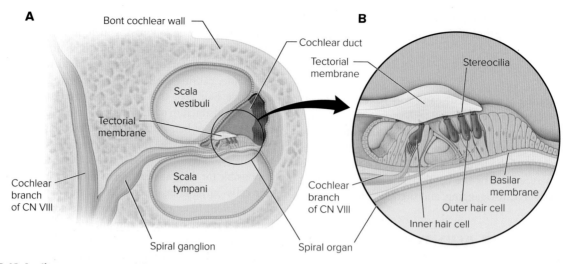

FIGURE 6-10 Auditory apparatus of the cochlea. A. A cross-section and close-up view of the cochlea with the membranous labyrinth dividing it into the cochlear duct, vestibular duct (scala vestibuli), and tympanic duct (scala tympani). **B.** The spiral organ houses the hair cells that transduce sound vibration to a neural signal within cranial nerve VIII. (Reproduced with permission from McKinley M, O'Laughlin VD. *Human Anatomy*. 3rd ed. New York, NY: McGraw-Hill; 2012.)

those transmitting low frequencies originating from the apical portion of the cochlea (narrow tip) and those transmitting higher frequencies originating from the basal cochlea (area closest to the middle ear). Similarly, these projections terminate within the cochlear nuclei such that the ventral portion receives the apical projections and the dorsal portion receives basal projections. This organization is referred to as tonatopic, meaning it is organized by the tone of the sounds. In addition to this tonatopic organization, the anterior division of the cochlear nucleus and the ventral auditory stream function in sound localization, while the dorsal stream synapses in the posteroventral and dorsal divisions of the cochlear nucleus and functions in the analysis of complex sounds. Second-order projections from the cochlear nuclei project bilaterally to the **superior olivary nuclear complex (SONC)** and the contralateral inferior colliculus (IC); the latter is the site of convergence for the dorsal and ventral streams, initiating the integration of sound localization and identification. Tertiary projections from the IC and SONC project within the lateral lemniscus to **the medial geniculate nucleus (body)** of the thalamus with a fourth-level projection to the auditory cortex, located in Herschl's gyrus of the temporal lobe within the lateral sulcus. Surrounding Herschl's gyrus in a circular fashion are the secondary and higher-order auditory processing areas.[16] From these initial auditory processing cortices, auditory information is projected to numerous areas of the brain, including other parts of the temporal lobe involved in language skills, the posterior parietal cortex, prefrontal and cingulate cortex, occipital cortex, amygdala, and striatum. Within the prefrontal and posterior parietal cortices, it is integrated with somatosensory and visual information to support object identification, language, and spatial orientation.[18] See Figure 6-11 for central auditory projections.

Sound Localization

The localization of sound is complex since most sounds are transmitted to both ears. However, sound to the right of the midline will reach the right ear before it hits the left ear, and vice versa, resulting in an interaural time difference. The more lateral

a sound, the greater the interaural difference. For higher frequencies, location is primarily determined by what is referred to as an interaural intensity difference with a stronger signal received by the closest ear. Either way, we can determine the horizontal location of sound, based on the difference in interaural activation.

Auditory Testing

The complexity of the hearing apparatus requires complex testing to assure adequate analysis of the different parts of the system. The first step in an auditory assessment is typically **behavioral audiometry**, also known as air conduction testing or pure tone audiometry; this is the presentation of sounds via earphones or headphones, at a range of frequencies (0.25-8 Hz), to each ear in a random order; patients are instructed to raise their hand on the side that the sound is heard. **Speech audiometry** may be done to further clarify a hearing deficit, identified through behavioral audiometry, and includes two components: (1) **speech recognition** – the ability to repeat word phrases heard through the audiometry headphones at different decibel levels; and (2) **word recognition** – the ability to hear single words in a quiet environment. Also, if behavioral audiometry is abnormal, a second measure, known as **bone conduction**, may be completed. With bone conduction, vibration is introduced to the forehead or mastoid via a tuning fork or audiometer to activate the cochlea while bypassing the external and middle ear. An audiograph is developed that illustrates the perceived frequencies from both tests in comparison to normal levels. A hearing loss characterized by an abnormal pure tone audiometry but normal bone conduction is referred to as a **conductive loss**, associated with abnormalities of the middle ear. When the two tests yield similar results, it is most likely that there is a **sensorineural hearing loss**, involving the cochlea or other neural projections; however, some hearing deficits result from a combined loss (both conductive and sensorineural). Further clarification of a sensorineural hearing loss may be provided by the auditory brainstem evoked potential, also known as the

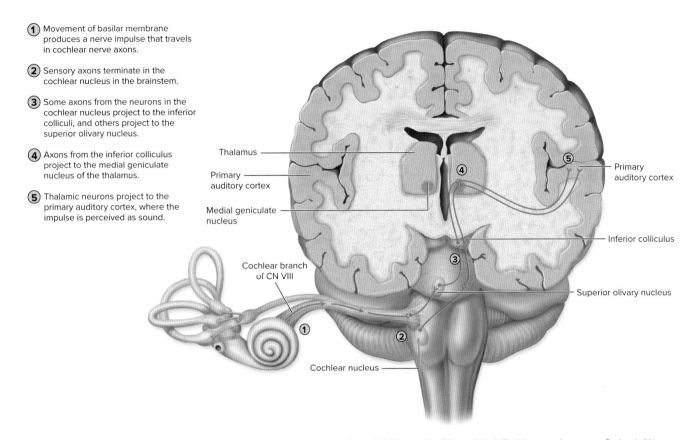

① Movement of basilar membrane produces a nerve impulse that travels in cochlear nerve axons.

② Sensory axons terminate in the cochlear nucleus in the brainstem.

③ Some axons from the neurons in the cochlear nucleus project to the inferior colliculi, and others project to the superior olivary nucleus.

④ Axons from the inferior colliculus project to the medial geniculate nucleus of the thalamus.

⑤ Thalamic neurons project to the primary auditory cortex, where the impulse is perceived as sound.

Thalamus

Primary auditory cortex

Medial geniculate nucleus

Cochlear branch of CN VIII

Cochlear nucleus

Primary auditory cortex

Inferior colliculus

Superior olivary nucleus

FIGURE 6-11 Auditory projections. (Reproduced with permission from McKinley M, O'Laughlin VD. *Human Anatomy* 3rd ed, New York, NY: McGraw-Hill; 2012.)

auditory brainstem response (ABR). Similar to the VEP, the ABR tracks the neural conduction of sound from its presentation to sequential neural structures: CN VIII, cochlear nucleus in the medulla, superior olivary complex, and inferior colliculi in the midbrain; each of these structures is associated with a specific wave change with a predictable time delay.[19]

● HEAD POSITION AND MOVEMENT: THE VESTIBULAR SYSTEM

The purpose of the vestibular system is to detect the position and motion of your head in space. It does this by measuring **linear** and **angular acceleration** of the head through five receptor organs in the portion of the inner ear called the **vestibular labyrinth**. Information conveyed by the vestibular system helps us to maintain balance through its roles in our subjective perceptions of movement and spatial orientation, in postural reflexes that allow us to adjust muscle activity and body position to stay upright, and in control of reflex eye movements that stabilize the eyes in space during head movements.

The Vestibular Labyrinths

The vestibular labyrinths are mirror-symmetric structures on both sides of the head that are composed of three **semicircular canals** (SCCs) and two **otolithic organs**, the **utricle** and **saccule** (Figure 6-12). The vestibular portion of the **bony labyrinth** consists of a central area called the **vestibule** and the three SCCs

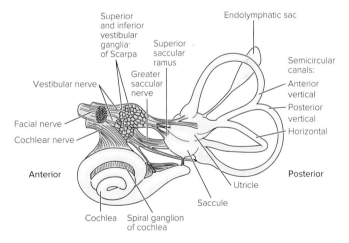

Superior and inferior vestibular ganglia of Scarpa

Superior saccular ramus

Vestibular nerve

Greater saccular nerve

Facial nerve

Cochlear nerve

Anterior

Cochlea   Spiral ganglion of cochlea

Endolymphatic sac

Semicircular canals:
Anterior vertical
Posterior vertical
Horizontal

Posterior

Utricle

Saccule

FIGURE 6-12 Vestibular labyrinths: This schematic illustrates the relationship of the cochlea and the components of the vestibular labyrinth: the vestibule with its saccule and utricle and the three semicircular canals. (Reproduced with permission from Kandel ER, Schwartz JH, et al., *Principles of Neural Science*, 4th Ed., New York, NY: McGraw-Hill; 2000.)

that are attached to the vestibule. Suspended within each SCC is a semicircular duct that corresponds to the **membranous labyrinth discussed earlier in relation to hearing**. The two otolithic organs, the **utricle** and **saccule**, are each a dilation of the membranous labyrinth within the vestibule. As in the cochlea, the space between the bony and membranous labyrinths is

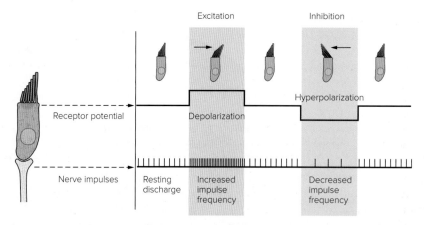

FIGURE 6-13 Hair cells of the vestibular labyrinth. In the resting state, the stereocilia are upright, with depolarization they bend in the direction of the kinocilium, and with hyperpolarization they bend away from the kinocilium. (Adapted, with permission, from Flock A. 1965. Transducing mechanisms in the lateral line canal organ receptors. *Cold Spring Harbor Symp Quant Biol.* 30:133-145.)

fluid-filled with **perilymph** while the membranous labyrinth is filled with **endolymph**.[20]

The sensory cells in each organ are specialized epithelial cells called **hair cells** which transduce mechanical signals into neural signals. Similar to the hair cells in the cochlea for hearing, each hair cell in the vestibular labyrinth has a graduated array of **stereocilia**, protruding into the endolymph-filled space within the membranous labyrinth. At one end of the stereocilia is a particularly long process called the **kinocilium**. When a hair cell is in a resting state (i.e., no deflection of sterocilia) there is generally some amount of tonic firing, recorded from the connecting vestibular nerves. Displacement of the sterocilia toward the kinocilium elicits a depolarization (i.e., excitation) of the hair cell membrane and leads to greater release of an excitatory neurotransmitter onto the vestibular nerve endings, which in turn, increase their firing frequencies. In contrast, deflection of

stereocilia away from the kinocilium causes hyperpolarization (i.e., inhibition) and leads to a reduction in neurotransmitter release, thereby decreasing vestibular nerve firing rate[20] (see Figure 6-13).

Semicircular Canals Detect Angular Acceleration

Angular accelerations caused by rotations of the head, such as when you turn or tilt your head, rotate your body, or make turns during walking, are measured by the SCCs. The three SCCs – horizontal, anterior, and posterior – are oriented almost precisely perpendicular to each other (analogous to the spatial relationship between two walls and the floor of a rectangular room) so that each canal detects motion in a single plane (Figure 6-14). The horizontal canal as its name implies is roughly horizontal (although it's actually tilted backwards about 30 degrees)

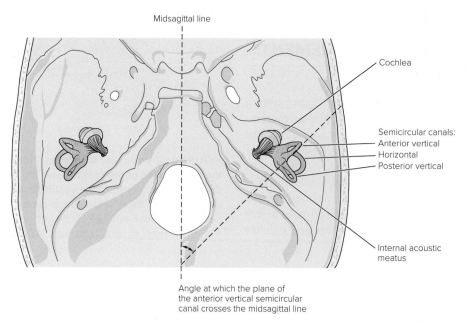

FIGURE 6-14 Alignment of the anterior semicircular canal. With the head upright, the anterior vertical canal is at a 45-degree angle from the sagittal plane as is the posterior vertical canal (angle not drawn). (Reproduced with permission from Kandel ER, Schwartz JH, et al., *Principles of neural Science*, 5th Ed., New York, NY: McGraw-Hill; 2013.)

when the head is in its typical, upright position. This canal is, therefore, sensitive to head rotations about a vertical axis. Each anterior and posterior canal is roughly vertical. However, the anterior and posterior canals are oriented at 45-degree angles from the sagittal plane in opposite directions from each other. The anterior canal of one side is, therefore, parallel to the posterior canal of the other side, so movements that affect one will affect the other. Thus, the two horizontal canals lie in the same plane and function together, while the anterior canal of one side functions as a pair with the contralateral posterior canal.[20]

Each SCC is a continuous endolymph-filled hoop that connects with the utricle. At one end of each semicircular duct is a swelling called the **ampulla**. Within each ampulla is a **crista**, a saddle-shaped ridge of tissue that contains the sensory hair cells. The hair cells are arranged as a single tuft that projects up into the **cupula**, a gelatinous mass that stretches from the crista to the root of the ampulla (Figure 6-15). Rotation of a SCC around an axis perpendicular to it (like a wheel on an axis) is the best way to deflect a cupula. Consider the example of a person sitting in a chair that spins. At the beginning of such a spin, the horizontal SCCs will rotate around their vertical axes. However, movement of the endolymph inside the canals lags behind because of inertia, which causes it to slosh against the cupula and deflect the hair cells to stimulate them. With continued rotations, the endolymph will eventually "catch up" so that the cupula is no longer deflected and stimulation of hair cells ceases. When the rotation stops, the endolymph sloshes up against a suddenly still cupula (again because of inertia), and the cupula bulges in the opposite direction causing a sensation of turning in the other direction. Thus, each SCC responds best to changes in the speed of rotation in a particular plane (i.e., angular acceleration), making them particularly sensitive to higher-frequency motion, such as head movements that occur during walking. The SCCs are normally insensitive to linear accelerations or gravitational forces because the densities of the cupula and endolymph are equal. Since all of the hair cells of a given crista are aligned so that their kinocilia are facing in the same direction, angular acceleration in one direction causes the vestibular afferents that innervate the crista to increase their firing rates, while acceleration in the opposite direction causes them to decrease their firing rates. Because the three SCCs are oriented in roughly orthogonal planes (Figure 6-14), a different canal can be stimulated by head movements in different planes, and multiple canals can be stimulated if movement is off those planes. Horizontal canals detect rotations in a vertical axis (yaw) such as shaking the head left and right, anterior canals detect rotation in a sagittal plane (pitch) such as nodding the head or doing a somersault, and posterior canals detect rotations in the coronal plane (roll) such as moving your head to touch your shoulders or doing a cartwheel. Since most head movements have a rotational component, movements in any direction can be detected.[20] The fact that the SCC cannot detect maintained rotation is not very consequential since most people don't typically experience maintained rotations (except at amusement parks).

Each coplanar pair of canals (i.e., right and left horizontal, left anterior and right posterior, and left posterior and right anterior) on either side of the head will generally be operating

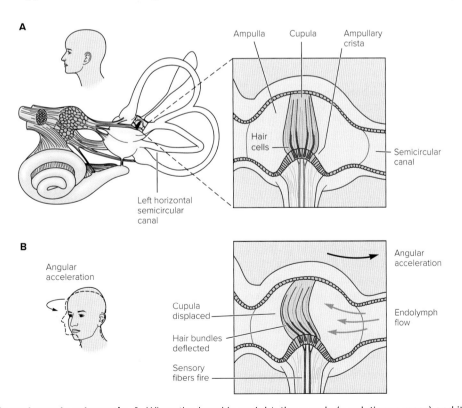

FIGURE 6-15 Ampulla and cupula schematic. A. When the head is upright, the cupula (a gelatinous mass) and its hair cells are stationary within the ampulla (swelling within the canals). **B.** As the head moves, the ampulla and its hair cells are moved by the motion of the endolymph. (Reproduced with permission from Kandel ER, Schwartz JH, et al., *Principles of neural Science*, 5th Ed., New York, NY: McGraw-Hill; 2013.)

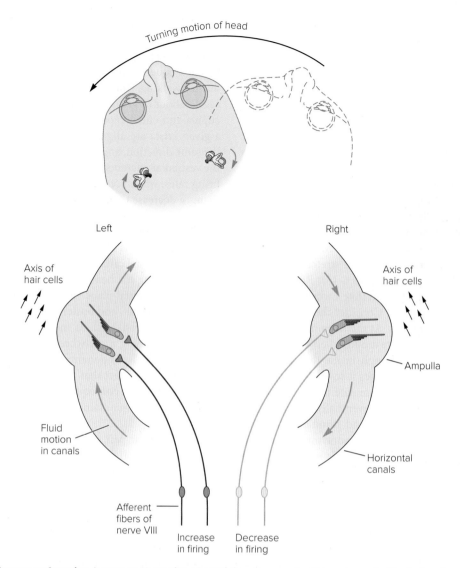

FIGURE 6-16 Complimentary function between the pairs of semicircular canals. This schematic illustrates the push–pull relationship of the complimentary SCC pairings. With a slight head turn to the left, the left hair cells are excited, moving toward the kinocilium while the hair cells in the right canal are inhibited (moving away from the kinocilium) in association with the movement of the endolymph. (Reproduced with permission from Kandel ER, Schwartz JH, et al., *Principles of Neural Science*, 5th ed., New York, NY: McGraw-Hill; 2013.)

in a push–pull rhythm; when one is excited, the other is inhibited. This occurs because head motion within their shared plane causes the endolymph of the pair to be displaced in opposite directions with respect to their ampullae, resulting in increased firing in one vestibular nerve and decreased firing in the other (Figure 6-16). Disruption of this relationship between sides, as in vestibular neuritis, will cause a person to feel debilitating vertigo and nausea.[20]

The Utricle and Saccule Detect Linear Acceleration and Static Head Position

Linear accelerations, such as when a person steps onto a moving sidewalk or when you lean to one side, and static head positions are detected by the utricle and the saccule. Each organ has a sheet of hair cells located in a portion of its wall called the **macula**. Macular hair cells are also embedded in a gelatinous mass similar in composition to the cupula. However, the gelatinous

substance also contains clumps of small crystals of calcium carbonate, called **otoconia** or **otoliths**, and thus, is called an **otolithic membrane**, from which the otolithic organs get their name. The otoconia make the otolithic membrane denser than endolymph, thereby, making the otolithic organs sensitive to gravity and linear accelerations such as experienced in elevators and automobiles. When the head changes position or begins a movement, the weight of the membrane bends the stereocilia of the macular hair cells (Figure 6-17). This stimulates the hair cells, which then signal the new head position. The orientation of the utricular macula is roughly horizontal (near the plane of the horizontal SCCs), while that of the saccular macula is roughly vertical when the head is in its typical upright position. Thus, in the upright position, the utricle is particularly sensitive to any accelerations in the horizontal plane (i.e., side-to-side and anterior–posterior motions) and the saccule particularly senses any accelerations along a sagittal plane (i.e., up and down

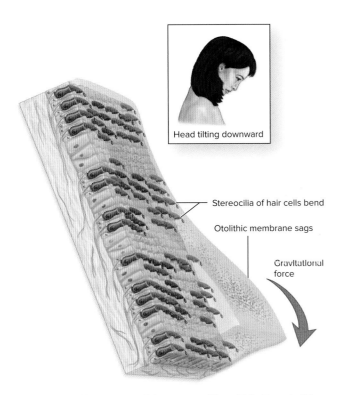

FIGURE 6-17 Movement of the stereocilia within the otolith. (Reproduced with permission from McKinley M & O'Loughlin VD. *Human Anatomy* 3rd ed. New York, NY: McGraw-Hill; 2012.)

In the figure: Head tilting downward; Stereocilia of hair cells bend; Otolithic membrane sags; Gravitational force

Box 6-3	What Would Be the Pattern of Stimulation of the Vestibular Labyrinths When a Person Arises from the Driver's Seat of an Automobile?

As a person begins to swivel toward the door, both horizontal SCCs are strongly stimulated. Simultaneous lateral movement out of the car's door stimulates hair cells in both utricles in a pattern that changes as the head turns with respect to the direction of bodily movement. Vertical acceleration to arise to the standing position stimulates certain hair cells in the saccules, while oppositely oriented saccular hair cells are inhibited. As the movement is completed, linear and angular accelerations in the opposite direction to the initial movement stimulate other hair cells in the utricles and SCCs.

motions) as well as anterior–posterior motions. As in the SCCs, there is push–pull processing of the otolithic organs between the two sides of the head. In addition, the hair cells within each otolithic macula are oriented with their kinocilia in different directions along a curving zone called the **striola**, so that head movement causes excitation of a group of hair cells from one portion of the macula while those in another portion of the same macula are inhibited. This extra redundancy probably explains why the otolithic organs are less impacted by unilateral vestibular lesions than the SCCs. The otoliths are most sensitive to lower-frequency motion, such as motion that occurs while standing in place, and thus, they are particularly important for postural control.[20]

As the head tilts, the otolithic membrane sags, bending the stereocilia of the hair cells and generating activation of these receptors.

Although the actions of the vestibular labyrinths have been discussed separately, most human movements produce complex patterns of excitation and inhibition in several receptor organs on both sides of the body (see Box 6-3 for an example).

Vestibular Pathways

Vestibular primary afferents have cell bodies in the vestibular ganglion (also called Scarpa's ganglion), which lies in a swelling of the nerve within the internal auditory canal (Figure 6-15). Their central processes travel within the eighth cranial nerve and enter the brainstem at the pontomedullary junction.[21]

Most primary vestibular afferents project to the vestibular nuclear complex, a large structure containing four main nuclei (superior, medial, lateral, and inferior) located within the pons and medulla. The vestibular nuclei integrate inputs from the primary vestibular afferents with those from the visual system, spinal cord, and cerebellum and project to several central targets: the oculomotor nuclei (i.e., cranial nerves III, IV, and VI), the spinal cord (via the lateral and medial vestibulospinal tracts), parts of the cerebellum (i.e., same areas as do primary vestibular afferents), the parietal cortex (via the thalamus), and the contralateral vestibular nuclear complex.

The major vestibular nuclei subserve different functions (Figure 6-18A). The superior and medial nuclei receive inputs primarily from the SCCs and send ascending projections via the **medial longitudinal fasciculus** (MLF) to the oculomotor nuclei (i.e., cranial nerves III, IV, VI) that are responsible for mediating the VOR. In addition, the medial nucleus sends descending projections via the **medial vestibulospinal tract** that travel within the MLF to cervical areas of the spinal cord. These projections function to stabilize the head position, during activities like walking, and to coordinate head with eye movements. The lateral nucleus (Deiter's nucleus) receives inputs from the SCCs and the otolithic organs and projects via the **lateral vestibulospinal tract** to the motor neurons for antigravity muscles at all areas of the spinal cord (Table 6-3). This tract, along with the medial vestibulospinal tract, is responsible for mediating the vestibulospinal reflexes that compensate for tilts and movements of the body. The inferior nucleus receives predominantly input from the otolithic organs and projects to the cerebellum, reticular formation, spinal cord, and contralateral vestibular nuclei. This nucleus primarily functions to integrate vestibular and central motor system activity for postural control.[20,21]

Vestibular afferents to the cerebellum enter through the inferior cerebellar peduncle and terminate in the flocculonodular lobe (or vestibulocerebellum) and other parts of the cerebellar vermis (i.e., middle part of the cerebellum). The primary roles of the cerebellum, related to the vestibular system, are to monitor vestibular performance and make adaptive adjustments to central vestibular processing as needed. More specifically, the cerebellar flocculus maintains, and when necessary, tunes the gain (ratio of head to compensatory eye movement) of the vestibulo-ocular reflex (VOR). The anterior–superior portion of the vermis of the cerebellum regulates the vestibulospinal reflex (VSR) to maintain postural and gait stability, and the cerebellar

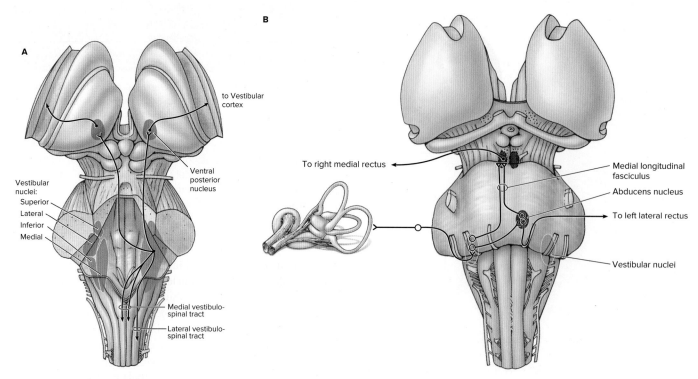

FIGURE 6-18 The vestibular nuclei. A. The four vestibular nuclei can be visualized in this diagram along with their projections to the thalamus and spinal cord. **B**. The superior and medial vestibular nuclei send projections ipsilaterally and contralaterally respectively, via the medial longitudinal fasciculus, to oculomotor nuclei. (Reproduced with permission from Martin JH. *Neuroanatomy Text and Atlas*, 4th Ed. New York, NY: McGraw-Hill; 2012.)

TABLE 6-3	Vestibular Nuclei Efferents and Functions[23–25]	
NUCLEUS	**EFFERENTS**	**FUNCTIONS**
Superior	Axons ascend in ipsilateral MLF to nuclei of extraocular muscles (CN III, IV, VI) and bilateral thalamus	Mediates vestibulo-ocular reflex (VOR)
Lateral	Axons descend in lateral vestibulospinal tract to anterior horns cells throughout cord	Mediates vestibulospinal reflex (VSR)
Medial	Axons ascend in contralateral MLF to nuclei of extraocular muscles and descend in medial vestibulospinal tract to cervical area of cord	Mediates VOR and VSR reflexes, coordinates eye and head movements that occur together
Inferior (Spinal)	Axons project to reticular formation, cerebellum, and contralateral medial, lateral, and inferior vestibular nuclei	Mediates postural adjustments via reticular formation; allows sharing of information between vestibular nuclei bilaterally

nodulus regulates the duration of VOR responses and processing of otolith input.[22]

The vestibular nuclei and vestibular cerebellum send projections to multiple regions of the thalamus, which in turn, send ascending projections to areas of the cortex. Clinical evidence in humans suggests that the posterolateral thalamus (i.e., ventral posterolateral and ventral intermediate nuclei) is a major relay station for vestibular information.[23] Unlike visual and auditory systems, there is no single primary cortical area processing vestibular system information. Cortical areas that receive vestibular information have been found in the temporo–parietal junction,

the insula, the somatosensory cortex, posterior parietal cortex, and lateral and medial frontal cortices.[23]

Vestibulo-ocular Reflex

The vestibulo-ocular reflex (VOR) is the means by which a person's gaze can stay fixed on a target even though his or her head is moving or is being moved. To illustrate how the eyes are kept still by the VOR, shake your head side to side quickly while you read this paragraph. The VOR allows you to continue reading even with head movement. However, if you move this book at the same speed and try to read it, you will have difficulty because

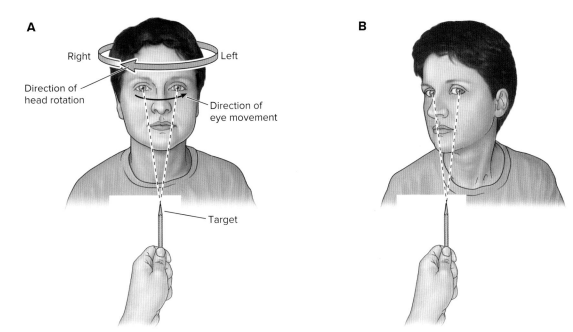

FIGURE 6-19 VOR and its neural connections. A. The person in the picture is asked to keep the eyes focused on the tip of the pencil while turning the head to the right. **B.** Head rotation to the right excites hair cells in the right horizontal SCC and signals are sent via the right vestibular nerve to the right medial and lateral vestibular nuclei. Neurons from these nuclei in turn stimulate neurons in the right oculomotor nucleus to excite the right medial rectus muscle and simultaneously stimulate neurons in the left abducens nucleus to excite the left lateral rectus muscle, thereby, evoking conjugate eye movements to the left. At the same time, neurons that excite the right lateral rectus and left medial rectus muscles are inhibited. This allows the person to keep the eyes focused on the target. (Reproduced with permission from Martin JH: *Neuroanatomy Text and Atlas*, 4th Ed. New York, NY: McGraw-Hill; 2012.)

visual processing takes longer and is less efficient than vestibular processing for image stabilization. The neural pathways of the reflex are shown in Figure 6-1B. The directions of the three planes of the SCCs are matched closely by the directions of motion of the three pairs of muscles that control eye movements (medial/lateral recti; superior/inferior recti; inferior/superior obliques), so that a single canal interacts with a single muscle pair. Each horizontal canal controls motoneurons that innervate the ipsilateral medial rectus (via ipsilateral CN III) and contralateral lateral rectus muscles (via contralateral CN VI). At the same time, they inhibit the antagonist eye muscles (Figure 6-19). Anterior canals control motoneurons to ipsilateral superior rectus and contralateral inferior oblique muscles (via contralateral CN III), while posterior canals control motoneurons to ipsilateral superior oblique (via contralateral CN IV) and contralateral inferior rectus muscles (via contralateral CN III). Thus, downward rotation of the head stimulates the anterior canals and causes compensatory upward eye movement, while upward head rotation stimulates the posterior canals and the eyes move downward. There are also VOR reflexes that involve the otolithic organs to compensate for linear and head tilt away from the vertical movements. The "gain" of the rotational VOR is defined as the change in the eye angle divided by the change in the head angle, during the head turn, and is normally 1.0. There are some situations where a VOR is not a good thing, such as when we want to direct our gaze in the same direction that our head is turning. In that case, the VOR is suppressed by the central nervous system, which is referred to as **VOR cancellation**. Two mechanisms that have been proposed to explain this cancellation are a reduction of the VOR gain by the flocculus of the cerebellum or activation of smooth pursuit eye movements in the opposite direction.[24] Individuals who lose this reflex experience **oscillopsia**, in which the visual world is unstable and objects appear blurry. In comatose individuals, the VOR can be used to test the integrity of brainstem eye movement pathways. The **oculocephalic reflex**, a form of the VOR, is tested by holding the person's eyes open and rotating the head quickly from side to side or up and down. The reflex is present if the eyes move in the opposite direction of the head movements, and it is often referred to as **doll's eyes**. Doll's eyes are typically not present in conscious individuals because they will usually suppress the reflex. Thus, the absence of doll's eyes suggests brainstem dysfunction in the comatose person but can be normal in the conscious individual. The afferent limb of the oculocephalic reflex probably also includes proprioceptors of the neck because some reflex movement can be elicited in individuals with nonfunctioning labyrinths.[25]

Vestibulospinal Reflex

The vestibulospinal reflex (VSR) functions to help us maintain our balance. For example, consider the situation where a person is walking and slips on an icy sidewalk. The person's feet fly to the right and his or her upper body and head fly to the left (left ear down). The head movement to the left will stimulate the vestibular labyrinths on the left side and increase the firing rate of the left vestibular nerve, which in turn will increase activity in the left vestibular nuclei. Activation of neurons in the lateral and medial vestibular nuclei that project to the spinal cord (via the lateral and medial vestibulospinal tracts respectively) will excite motoneurons to extensor muscles and inhibit motoneurons to the flexor muscles in the left arm and leg in order to right the person and prevent the person from falling.[22]

Nystagmus

With sustained head rotations that are too large to be compensated for by the vestibulo-ocular reflex, the VOR is periodically interrupted by rapid eye movements in the opposite direction. The back-and-forth eye movements, with a slow phase in one direction and a fast phase in the other, are called **nystagmus**. The eye movements of nystagmus can be in any direction (i.e., horizontal, vertical, or torsional). Eye movements of nystagmus may be faster in one direction, or the movements in both directions may be the same. Certain types of nystagmus are a normal physiological response to vestibular or visual system stimulation, but other types of nystagmus are due to neuropathology.

There are three main ways to cause nystagmus physiologically, two of which are induced by vestibular system stimulation and one by visual system stimulation. Examples of vestibular-induced physiological nystagmus are sustained head rotation and caloric testing. Consider again the person sitting in a chair that spins. As the person begins to rotate to the left, the VOR, as explained previously, will cause compensatory deviation of the eyes to the right. As rotation to the left continues, one would think that the person's eyes would move to the edge of the orbit and stay there. However, this doesn't happen because the eyes make a very rapid or **saccadic** resetting movement to the left back across the center of the gaze. The nystagmus is named for the direction of rapid movement (i.e., in this case, the eyes move slowly to the right and rapidly back to the left, so it would be called **nystagmus to the left** or **left-beating nystagmus**). During the period of sustained rotation, when the cupula "catches up" and is not deflected, the eye movement response depends on the light condition. In the dark or with the person's eyes closed, nystagmus would cease; with visual input, for reasons explained below, left-beating nystagmus might continue throughout the rotation. When the rotation is suddenly stopped, movement of the cupula in the opposite direction tricks the brainstem into thinking that the direction of head rotation has reversed (to the right), which causes a brief period of right-beating **postrotatory nystagmus**. The person will also tend to fall in the direction of the previous rotation when walking. Thus, if the rotation was to the left, the person will tend to fall to the left when walking. The postrotatory falling is due to an imbalance of the lateral vestibulospinal tracts.

A second way to cause physiological nystagmus through vestibular stimulation is by means of the **caloric test**. For this test, a person's head is tilted backward by about 60 degrees to bring the horizontal SCCs into a vertical position. Cold or warm water or air is then introduced into the person's ear. The temperature difference between the body and the injected water or air creates a convective current in the endolymph of the nearby horizontal SCC. Hot and cold water produce currents in opposite directions, and therefore, a horizontal nystagmus in opposite directions. If the water is warm (44°C or above), endolymph in the ipsilateral horizontal SCC rises, causing an increased rate of firing in the vestibular afferent nerve. This situation mimics a head turn to the ipsilateral side, creating horizontal nystagmus to the ipsilateral ear. For example, irrigation of the left ear

with warm water will cause the endolymph in the left horizontal SCC to move in the direction that causes an increased rate of firing in the left vestibular nerve, mimicking a left head turn. This, in turn, will cause conjugate eye movements to the right via the VOR followed by fast saccadic movements to the left or left-beating nystagmus. If the water is cold (3°C or below), the endolymph falls within the SCC, decreasing the rate of vestibular afferent firing. The eyes then deviate toward the ipsilateral ear, with horizontal nystagmus induced to the contralateral ear.[26] One mnemonic used to remember the fast direction of nystagmus with caloric testing is *COWS*. With **C**old water irrigation, the fast phase of nystagmus is to the **O**pposite side from the filled ear; with **W**arm water irrigation the fast phase of nystagmus is to the **S**ame side as the filled ear.

A third way to cause physiological nystagmus is with a moving visual stimuli. Consider the situation of a person sitting in a rapidly moving bus who is watching regularly spaced telephone poles fly by. The person's eyes will slowly follow a particular pole toward the rear of the bus and then rapidly flick back toward the front of the bus to find a new pole to fixate on. If the individual is seated on the right side of the bus, looking out the window, the movement of the series of telephone poles to the right across the person's visual field would cause slow pursuit tracking eye movements to the right followed by fast saccadic "reset" movements to the left or nystagmus to the left. Because it is induced by moving visual stimuli, it is called **optokinetic nystagmus** (OKN) and the reflex that causes OKN is called the **optokinetic reflex**. In the clinic, a rotating striped drum or moving piece of striped cloth is typically used to test the reflex. OKN is the reason for the continued nystagmus, during sustained rotations in a lighted room.[27]

Nystagmus can be caused by pathology to a variety of nervous system structures including the labyrinths, vestibular nerves, vestibular nuclei, oculomotor nerves, and the cerebellum. Peripheral vestibular disorders involve the vestibular nerve and all distal structures. Patients with a unilateral peripheral disorder typically demonstrate horizontal nystagmus to the contralateral side which suppresses with visual fixation. Unlike peripheral lesions, nystagmus of central pathology usually changes direction with gaze, is unaffected by fixation, and may be purely vertical or torsional.[27]

Balance Control

The ability to balance or maintain vertical orientation of the body requires perception and action. Perception is the integration of sensory information to assess the position and motion of the body in space, involving sensory and higher-level cognitive processes. Action is the ability to generate forces for controlling body position, involving motor systems. The main sensory inputs that the central nervous system uses for determining the body's position and movement in space are visual, somatosensory, and vestibular. The visual system provides information about body movement with respect to surrounding objects and helps us determine what is upright. The vestibular system provides information about head position with respect to gravity and inertial forces and about head movement. The somatosensory system (i.e., proprioception, touch) provides information about the body with reference to supporting surfaces (i.e., weight-bearing) and the relative positions of body parts. Auditory inputs assist with maintenance of upright posture by alerting us to objects in the environment (i.e., cars, buses) that might destabilize us.[28]

REFERENCES

1. Riordan-Eva, P. Anatomy & embryology of the eye. In: Riordan-Eva P, Augsburger JJ, eds. *Vaughan & Asbury's General Ophthalmology*. 19th ed. McGraw Hill; 2017. https://accessmedicine.mhmedical.com/content.aspx?bookid=2186&sectionid=16551577. Accessed September 27, 2021.

2. Saladin KS. *Chapter 17 – Sense organs*. In: *Human Anatomy*. New York, NY: McGraw-Hill; 2020:456-492.

3. Wilhelm H. Disorders of the pupil. *Handb Clin Neurol*. 2011;102(3):427-461.

4. Prasad S, Galetta SL. Anatomy and physiology of the afferent visual system. *Handb Clin Neurol*. 2011;102:3-19.

5. Creel DJ. Visually evoked potentials. *Handb Clin Neurol*. 2019;160:501-522.

6. Horn AKE, Leigh RJ. The anatomy and physiology of the ocular motor system. *Handb Clin Neurol*. 2011;102:22-68.

7. Corbet JJ. The bedside and office neuro-ophthalmology examination. *Semin Neurol*. 2003;22(1):63-76.

8. Rucker JC, Kennard C, Leigh RJ. The neuro-ophthalmological examination. *Handb Clin Neurol*. 2011;102:71-94.

9. Melamud A, Hagstrom S, Traboulsi EI. Color vision testing. *Ophthalmic Genet*. 2004;25(3):159-187.

10. Smith TD, Bhatnagar KP. Anatomy of the olfactory system. *Handb Clin Neurol*. 2019;164:18-28.

11. Brunjes PC, Illig KR, Meyer EA. A field guide to the anterior olfactory nucleus(cortex). *Brain Res Rev*. 2005;50:305-335.

12. Rolls ET. Taste and smell processing in the brain. *Handb Clin Neurol*. 2019;164:97-118.

13. Witt M. Anatomy and development of the human taste system. *Handb Clin Neurol*. 2019;164:147-171.

14. Iwata S, Yoshida R, Ninomiya Y. Taste transductions in taste receptor cells: basic tastes and moreover. *Curr Pharm Des*. 2014;20:2684-2692.

15. Vincis R, Fontanini A. Central taste anatomy and physiology. *Handb Clin Neurol*. 2019;164:187-204.

16. Pickles JO. Auditory pathways: anatomy and physiology. *Handb Clin Neurol*. 2015;129:3-25.

17. Ekdale EG. Form and function of the mammalian inner ear. *J Anat*. 2016;228:324-337.

18. Hackett TA. Anatomic organization of the auditory cortex. *Handb Clin Neurol*. 2015;129:27-53.

19. Baiduc RR, Poling GL, Hong O, Dhar S. Clinical measures of auditory function: the cochlea and beyond. *Dis Mon*. 2013;59(4):147-156.

20. Kingma H, Van de Berg R. Anatomy, physiology and physica of the peripheral vestibular system. *Handb Clin Neurol*. 2016;137:1-16.

21. Hain TC, Helminski JO. Anatomy and physiology of the normal vestibular system. In: Herdman SJ, ed. *Vestibular Rehabilitation*. 3rd ed. Philadelphia, PA: FA Davis Co; 2007.

22. Khan S, Chang R. Anatomy of the vestibular system: a review. *NeuroRehabilitation*. 2013;32:437-443.

23. Lopez C, Blanke O. The thalamocortical vestibular system in animals and humans. *Brain Res Rev*. 2011;67(1-2):119-146.

24. Gordon CR, Caspi A, Levite R, Zivotofsky AZ. Mechanisms of vestibulo-ocular reflex (VOR) cancellation in spinocerebellar ataxia type 3 (SCA-3) and episodic ataxia type 2 (EA-2). *Prog Brain Res*. 2008;171:519-525.

25. Singh HH. The comatose patient (Chapter 13). In: *Clinical Examination: A Practical Guide to Medicine*. New Delhi, India: Jaypee Brothers Medical Publishers; 2011.

26. Goncalves DU, Felipe L, Lima TMA. Intepretation and use of caloric testing. *Rev Bras Otorrinolaringol*. 2008;74(3):440-446.

27. Strupp M, Kremmyda O, Adamczyk C, et al. Central ocular motor disorders, including gaze palsy and nystagmus. *J Neurol*. 2014;261(Suppl 2):S542-S558.

28. Peterka RJ. Sensory integration for human balance control. *Handb Clin Neurol*. 2018;159:27-42.

Review Questions

1. **Which two structures are responsible for focusing light onto the retina of the eye?**

   A. Iris and pupil

   B. Pupil and cornea

   C. Cornea and lens

   D. Lens and vitreous humor

2. **Which of the following correctly describes the projection of the right visual field onto the retina of the eye?**

   A. The right monocular visual field projects to the temporal retina of the left eye.

   B. The right monocular visual field projects to the nasal retina of the left eye.

   C. The right monocular visual field projects to the temporal retina of the right eye.

   D. The right monocular visual field projects to the nasal retina of the right eye.

3. **Meyer's loop contains what aspect of the visual field?**

   A. The ipsilateral upper visual field (lower retinal fibers)

   B. The contralateral upper visual field (lower retinal fibers)

   C. The ipsilateral lower visual field (upper retinal fibers)

   D. The contralateral lower visual field (upper retinal fibers)

4. **The lateral rectus muscle of the eye is innervated by what cranial nerve?**

   A. CN II

   B. CN III

   C. CN IV

   D. CN VI

5. Which sense discussed in this chapter projects directly to the cortex without going through the thalamus?

A. Hearing

B. Olfaction

C. Taste

D. Vestibular

E. Vision

6. The strong emotional response that we have to many smells is most likely associated with what part of the olfactory system?

A. Amygdala

B. Entorhinal cortex

C. Olfactory tubercle

D. Piriform cortex

7. Which of the cells listed below is the receptor cell for the sense that it is paired with?

A. Bipolar cells – vision

B. Hair cells – hearing

C. Mitral cells – olfaction

D. Papillae – taste

8. The gustatory cortex (taste) is located where?

A. Dorsal temporal cortex

B. Insular cortex

C. Anterior frontal lobe

D. Posterior occipital lobe

E. Ventral parietal lobe

9. Taste receptors are more dense on what aspect of the oral structures?

A. Tip of the tongue

B. Anterior 2/3 of tongue

C. Posterior 1/3 of tongue

D. Inner cheeks

E. Inner gums

10. What nucleus in the brainstem receives all gustatory projections?

A. Abducens

B. Cochlear

C. Solitary

D. Superior colliculus

11. The middle ear cavity contains which of the following structures?

A. Bony labyrinth

B. Incus, malleus, and stapes

C. Eustachian tube

D. Tympanum

12. The thick epithelium that holds the auditory receptors is called what?

A. Bony labyrinth

B. Cochlear duct

C. Endolymph

D. Spiral organ

13. The otolithic organs (utricle and saccule):

A. Are part of the central vestibular system.

B. Detect rotational movement and velocity of the head.

C. Detect linear acceleration and static position of the head.

D. Mediate the vestibulo-ocular reflex.

14. In a healthy individual, rotation of the head to the right produces which of the following in the hair cells in the horizontal semicircular canals (SCCs):

A. Hyperpolarization of hair cells in the right SC; depolarization of hair cells in the left SC

B. Depolarization of hair cells in the right SC; hyperpolarization of hair cells in the left SC

C. No change in the activity of the hair cells on either side

D. Depolarization of the hair cells on both sides

15. When the stereocilia on a hair cell are bent toward the kinocilium, the vestibular nerve endings:

A. Depolarize and increase their firing rate.

B. Hyperpolarize and decrease their firing rate.

C. Stay at a tonic level and do not change their firing rate.

D. Either increase or decrease their firing rate depending on the person's head position.

16. The type of gelatinous material that the hair cells of the semicircular canals are embedded in is called the:

A. Otolithic membrane.

B. Tectorial membrane.

C. Cupula.

D. Basilar membrane.

17. The major function of the lateral vestibulospinal tract is to control:

A. Eye movements.

B. Balance and upright posture.

C. Head and neck movements.

D. Central pattern generators for walking.

18. The combination of semicircular canals (SCCs) that have a push-pull relationship is the:

A. Left anterior SCC and right anterior SCC.

B. Left horizontal SCC and right horizontal SCC.

C. Left posterior SCC and right horizontal SCC.

D. Left posterior SCC and right posterior SCC.

19. **The slow phase of the nystagmus induced by looking at a rotating strip drum is due to:**
    A. Smooth pursuit eye movements.
    B. The vestibulo-ocular reflex.
    C. Saccadic eye movements.
    D. The oculocephalic reflex.

20. **The parasympathetic nervous system has what effect on the visual system?**
    A. Constricts the pupil and thickens the lens for near vision
    B. Dilates the pupil and relaxes the lens for night vision
    C. Dilates the pupil and thickens the lens for far vision
    D. Constricts the pupil and relaxes the lens for night vision

21. **Damage to what critical connection would impair one's ability to locate an object in space?**
    A. The dorsal stream connection between the occipital lobe and the parietal lobe
    B. The dorsal stream connection between the occipital lobe and the temporal lobe
    C. The ventral stream connection between the occipital lobe and the parietal lobe
    D. The ventral stream connection between the occipital lobe and the temporal lobe

22. **Which of the higher processing visual areas is correctly paired with its function?**
    A. Frontal eye fields – object speed interpretation
    B. Intraparietal sulcus – object memory
    C. Posterior parietal cortex – modulation of visual reflex activity
    D. Temporo-parietal-occipital junction – contralateral visual neglect

Answers

1. C	2. D	3. B	4. D	5. B
6. A	7. B	8. B	9. C	10. C
11. B	12. D	13. C	14. B	15. A
16. C	17. B	18. B	19. A	20. A
21. C	22. B			

GLOSSARY

Accommodation. Elongation of the lens in the eye to allow near vision due to ciliary muscle relaxation.

Ampulla. The jug-like swellings at the base of the semicircular canals that contain the hair cells and cupula.

Angular acceleration. The change in angular (rotational movement) velocity divided by the time.

Aqueous humor. Thin liquid from the choroid that provides critical nutrients to the eye.

Auditory brainstem response (ABR). Tracking of neural projection to sequential structures.

Auricle. External ear.

Behavioral audiometry (air conduction testing; pure tone audiometry). Sounds presented at a range of frequencies.

Bipolar cells of nasal epithelium. First-order cells for olfaction.

Bipolar cells of retina. Retinal interneurons.

Blind spot (optic disc). Location where optic nerve fibers come together to exit the retina.

Bone conduction. Testing for sound conduction induced by vibration.

Bony labyrinth. A bony cavity within the petrous portion of the temporal bone that contains the membranous labyrinth of the inner ear and is divided into the vestibule, cochlea, and semicircular canals.

Calcarine cortex. Striated primary visual cortex in the occipital lobe (Brodmann's area 17).

Caloric test. A test of the vestibulo-ocular reflex that involves irrigating cold or warm water or air into the external auditory canal to induce a convective current in the endolymph of the adjacent horizontal semicircular canal that produces horizontal nystagmus, in a direction that is dependent on the temperature. Absent or reduced reactive eye movements indicate vestibular hypofunction of the horizontal semicircular canal of the side being stimulated.

Choroid. Vascular tissue under the sclera that secrete aqueous humor.

Cochlea. A portion of the bony labyrinth, shaped like a snail.

Cochlear duct. Center of cochlea.

Conductive hearing loss. Pure tone loss with normal bone conduction.

Cone. Color photoreceptor with less light sensitivity.

Conjunctiva. Clear mucous membrane that covers the sclera of the eye.

Cornea. Transparent central portion of sclera; refracts light into the pupil.

Crista. A ridge within each ampulla of the semicircular canals in the inner ear where hair cells are located.

Cupula. A gelatinous mass that overlies the hair cells in the cristae of the ampullae of the semicircular canals in the inner ear.

Dichromatic vision. An absence of one cone subtype, resulting in inability to perceive one color.

Doll's eyes reflex. See oculocephalic reflex.

Endolymph. The potassium-rich fluid filling the membranous labyrinth of the inner ear; bathes the apical end of the hair cells.

Eustachian tube. Connection between middle ear to nasopharynx.

External acoustic meatus. Funnel-shaped ear canal.

Fovea. Central portion of the macula of the retina.

Ganglion cells. Projection cells from superficial retina that give rise to the optic nerve.

Gustation. Sense of taste.

Hair cells. The sensory cells within the inner ear that transduce mechanical displacement into neural impulses.

Hemifield. Half of the visual field conveyed to the ipsilateral nasal retina and the contralateral temporal retina.

Hyperopia. Farsightedness due to poor accommodation.

Incus. Middle ossicles in middle ear.

Kinocilium. The longest cilium next to the 40 to 70 stereocilia of the hair cells located in the cristae of the ampullae of the semicircular canals and the maculae of the utricle and saccule.

Lateral vestibulospinal tract. A descending motor tract that originates from the lateral vestibular nucleus and projects ipsilaterally to all levels of the spinal cord to facilitate extensor muscles for postural control and balance.

Lens. Located in the center of the eye, focuses light onto the retina.

Linear acceleration. The change in linear (movement in a straight line) velocity divided by time.

Macula (eye). Lightly colored area in the center of the retina with dense photoreceptors.

Macula (inner ear). A neuroepithelial sensory area within the utricle and saccule in the inner ear where hair cells are located.

Malleus. First ossicles in middle ear.

Medial longitudinal fasciculus. A bilateral tract located near the midline within the midbrain and pons that interconnects the oculomotor nuclei (i.e., oculomotor, trochlear, and abducens) for coordination of conjugate eye movements.

Medial vestibulospinal tract. A descending motor tract that originates from the medial vestibular nucleus and projects bilaterally to cervical and upper thoracic levels of the spinal cord to activate motor neurons that control head and neck movements for gaze stabilization.

Membranous labyrinth. A collection of tubes and chambers located within the bony labyrinth of the inner ear that contains the sensory receptors for the auditory and vestibular systems.

Mitral cells. Second-order neurons in the olfactory bulb.

Myopia. Nearsightedness secondary to poor elongation of the lens or an eye that is too long.

Nystagmus. Involuntary, rapid, rhythmic eye movements (horizontal, vertical, rotatory, or combinations) that can be physiological (normal) or pathological.

Oculocephalic reflex (also called dolls' eyes reflex). A form of the vestibulo-ocular reflex performed in comatose individuals by opening the eyes and turning the head to one side. If the brainstem is intact, the eyes will move conjugately away from the direction of turning. A negative oculocephalic reflex is when the eyes stay fixed midorbit, indicating that the brainstem is not intact.

Odorants. Airborne chemicals that stimulate olfactory neurons.

Olfaction. Sense of smell.

Olfactory nerve. CN I, carries olfaction.

Ophthalmoscope. Instrument used to magnify eye features for assessment.

Optic chiasm. Intersection of right and left optic nerves where the nasal fibers cross to the opposite side, bringing all of a hemifield to the contralateral hemisphere.

Optic nerve. CN II. Conveys vision from retina to optic chiasm.

Optic radiations. Projections from the lateral geniculate of the thalamus to the occipital cortex.

Meyer's loop. Optic radiations that traverse the temporal lobe, conveying upper visual field.

Parietal radiation. Optic radiations that traverse the parietal lobe, conveying lower visual field.

Optokinetic nystagmus. Multi-direction (horizontal, vertical, rotatory) nystagmus in response to looking at a succession of objects moving across the visual field (e.g., a moving strip or drum with parallel stripes). The nystagmus consists of a slow phase, with slow pursuit eye movements in the direction of strip movement, followed by a fast phase with rapid saccadic eye movements back to midline.

Optokinetic reflex. See optokinetic nystagmus.

Organ of Corti (spiral organ). Thick epithelium in cochlear duct with hair cell.

Oscillopsia. A subjective report that objects viewed are oscillating back and forth, when in fact they are not.

Otoconia (also called otoliths). The calcium carbonate crystals that rest on the otolithic membrane overlying the hair cells of the utricle and saccule.

Otolithic organs. The utricle and saccule.

Oval window. Membranous covering for the inner ear.

Perilymph. The potassium-poor fluid that fills the space between the bony and membranous labyrinths within the inner ear.

Pigment epithelium. Dark posterior layer of retina that provides structural and metabolic support.

Postrotatory nystagmus. Horizontal nystagmus that occurs with a rapid stop to a unidirectional head rotation, causing the fast phase to be in the opposite direction of the head rotation.

Presbyopia. Poor accommodation due to aging that results in poor near vision.

Pupil. Central opening in the iris that allows light to enter the eye; controls the amount of light that enters the eye.

Pupillary constriction. A reflexive decrease in the size of the pupil in the presence of bright light.

Pupillary dilations. A sympathetic response to widen the pupil in situations of poor light.

Retina. Layered structure at the back of eye; contains photoreceptors.

Rod. Highly light-sensitive photoreceptor responsible for night vision.

Round window. Embedded in cochlea, dissipates vibration back into middle ear.

Saccades. Coordinated eye movements (horizontal or vertical).

Saccule. The otolith organ that detects linear accelerations and head tilts in the vertical plane.

Semicircular canals. The vestibular end organs within the inner ear that sense rotational accelerations of the head.

Sclera. Opaque external membrane of the eye.

Sensorineural hearing loss. Hearing deficit associated with disrupted function of the cochlea and/or neural projections.

Sphincter pupillae muscle. Constricts pupil.

Spiral ganglia. Location of cell bodies for CN VIII.

Stapes. Third ossicle in inner ear; pushes oval window.

Stereocilia. The actin-rich processes that, along with the kinocilium, form the hair bundle extending from the apical surface of the hair cell; site of mechanotransduction.

Striola. A line found in both the utricle and saccule that divides the hair cells into two populations with opposing hair bundle polarities.

Tastants. Chemicals within foods that activate taste buds.

Taste buds. Hold taste receptors; located in papillae of tongue and epithelium of oral structures.

Tympanic membrane. Eardrum.

Utricle. The otolith organ that senses linear accelerations and head tilts in the horizontal plane.

Vestibular labyrinth. The utricle and saccule and semicircular canals.

Vestibule. An oval cavity in the middle of the bony labyrinth of the inner ear that contains the utricle and saccule.

Vestibulo-ocular reflex. A reflex that produces eye movements in the direction opposite to head movements to stabilize images on the retinas of the eye during head movement.

Vestibulo-ocular reflex cancellation. A visually-mediated override of the vestibulo-ocular reflex; it is tested by asking individuals to keep their gaze fixated on an object while their body rotates *en bloc* from side to side.

Visual field. Environment visible without eye movement.

Vitreous humor. Gelatinous substance within eye that maintains the shape of the eye.

ABBREVIATIONS

MLF	medial longitudinal fasciculus
OKN	optokinetic nystagmus
SCC	semicircular canal
VOR	vestibulo-ocular reflex
VSR	vestibulospinal reflex

Cognition, Emotion, and Language

Deborah S. Nichols-Larsen

7

1) Differentiate the abilities that comprise cognition, including executive function and memory, and the neural networks that support them

2) Distinguish the neural networks responsible for language production and language comprehension

3) Discern feelings from emotions and the neural networks that support these concepts

This chapter focuses on the most complex of abilities (cognition, emotion, and language), and in many ways, the areas of functioning that most differentiate humans from other animals, or at least we like to think so. Although these functions are highly interrelated, we will talk about each and the neural networks that support them individually.

COGNITION

Cognition is an expansive term used to describe our ability to perceive the world around us, interact with it, remember our past experiences in it, and imagine potential experiences with it; the concepts of learning, thinking, attention, memory, imagery, problem-solving, and decision-making are all included within the term cognition.[1] Obviously, these skills are extensive and span multiple neural networks. Within this chapter, we will discuss some of the components of cognition and the neural networks that are involved in cognitive processes, specifically executive function, language, emotion, learning, and memory.

Executive Function

Executive function (EF) refers to our ability to respond appropriately to changing circumstances and includes a spectrum of abilities, including attention, working memory, inhibition, **task switching**, abstract thought, and behavioral regulation as well as decision-making, sequence planning and initiation.[2,3] First, we will explore these skills under the EF umbrella, and then we'll look at the complex neural networks that give rise to these abilities.

Attention is the ability to focus your awareness on visual, auditory, tactile, or other sensory stimuli (**sustained attention**) but also involves the ability to prioritize your attention on one among competing stimuli as well as to switch your attention from one stimulus to another[1] (see Box 7-1).

Task or set switching, just as it sounds, is the ability to focus on one task and then respond to different cues or demands for another task. For example, if I asked you to sort playing cards by suit and then by number, you would first pay attention to the suit designation without need to look at the number, and then, you would focus on the number while disregarding the suit. This requires an integration of attention, inhibition, and working memory so that you can adjust your attention to the right cues, inhibit your tendency to respond to the previous cues, and keep the "rules" of the task in memory.[2] **Perseveration** occurs when we fail to switch our attention to the appropriate cue(s) and continue to sort by suit instead of by number. The more similar the task, the more likely we are to make perseverative errors.

Working memory refers to the ability to retain or manipulate information cognitively for immediate use; the most common example used to illustrate this is retaining a phone number for the brief amount of time needed to punch it into your cell phone, after your friend gives it to you. How many times have you been distracted in this process and forgotten the number, requiring you to ask your friend to repeat it? Thus, working memory is of short duration, for small amounts of information, and does not indicate that learning has taken place; also, any disruption will typically impede our ability to retain information within the working memory circuits.[2] **Inhibition** is a complex ability that involves delaying our verbal or physical

Box 7-1	Types of Attention[1]

As you read this paragraph, let's propose that you are also listening to the radio (a cognitive-cognitive dual task); this requires **divided attention** between the two activities, yet, to fully understand the words on the page, you will need to focus more of your attention on the printed word than on the music (**selective attention**). However, if your favorite song comes on the radio, you are able to switch your attention quickly to listen to the song and then switch back to prioritizing reading again, once the song is done (**shifting attention**). This ability to divide, prioritize, and switch your attention from one stimulus to another is critical for functioning in our complex environment and often disrupted in many neurologic conditions. However, as the many instances of accidents when driving or walking while texting or talking on the phone indicate, there are limitations in our ability to divide our attention, and at times, we prioritize the wrong task (e.g., texting when we need to focus on driving).

response to a stimulus, or in many instances, simply waiting; interestingly, we are constantly in a state of cognitive inhibition. How many times do you think of something but know not to say it, or similarly, how many times do you find yourself doing something (e.g., tapping your pencil), when you are really focused on something else? The first is an example of inhibition; the second, an example of failure of inhibition or **disinhibition**. Thus, inhibition is a willful blockade of attention, movement, verbalization, or other behavior, while disinhibition is a failure of inhibition. Disinhibition is also apparent in young children, who are likely to say whatever they are thinking or to reach out and touch things, even after being told "no," because they haven't yet learned to inhibit their behavior.[2] Inhibition is tightly linked to **behavioral or self-regulation**, which refers to our ability to learn the rules of behavior in society and respond accordingly, even in novel situations.[3] For example, we learn to take turns in conversations – listening and then talking; we learn to be quiet in libraries and cheer at sporting events; we learn to sit quietly in school and run freely at recess. And perhaps most importantly, we learn to observe others' behavior in new situations and regulate our own in accordance with their example. Finally, **abstract thought** is the highest of human abilities; it refers to our ability to combine information in novel ways so as to generalize to new situations, to use logic or deductive reasoning to solve problems, or to be adaptable in one's thinking such that new information can be used to form new opinions.[4,5] All of these abilities, along with memory, contribute to the capacity for **decision-making**, based on relevant information, past experience, potential for reward or punishment, environmental factors, and our current emotional state; decision-making requires the comparison of current factors with past experience to make a choice between multiple potential solutions.[4-7] The terms crystallized and fluid intelligence are used to describe certain aspects of cognitive ability that change as we age. **Crystallized intelligence** refers to those things that are well-learned such as our life experiences and general knowledge (e.g., language) and accumulates over our lifetime; **fluid intelligence** refers to our ability to use reasoning to solve problems, so EF is a component of fluid intelligence along with memory and is impacted by processing speed. Crystallized intelligence continues to expand until late in our lives; however, fluid intelligence declines with aging.[1]

The Neural Networks Supporting EF

With the vast capabilities subsumed in the term EF, it should not be surprising that they are supported by a series of complex networks. Notably, the frontal lobe has three areas that play critical roles in these functions: the dorsolateral prefrontal cortex, the orbitofrontal or ventromedial prefrontal cortex, and the medial prefrontal and anterior cingulate cortex[7,8] (Figures 7-1 and 7-2). Each of these areas is linked to multiple other areas that appear to contribute to our EF abilities.

Dorsolateral Prefrontal Cortex (DLPFC)

As indicated by its label, the DLPFC is located just in front of the premotor cortex on the dorsolateral aspect of the frontal lobe and includes the medial frontal gyrus (BA 9 & 46).[7,9] It has projections to and from the temporal and parietal lobes,

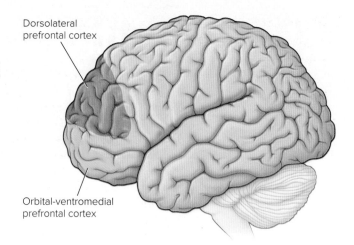

Dorsolateral prefrontal cortex

Orbital-ventromedial prefrontal cortex

FIGURE 7-1 Frontal areas associated with executive function.

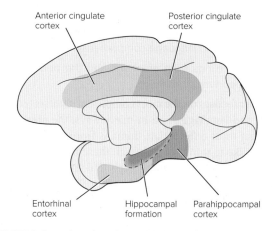

Anterior cingulate cortex

Posterior cingulate cortex

Entorhinal cortex

Hippocampal formation

Parahippocampal cortex

FIGURE 7-2 Anterior cingulate (ACC) and its connections with the limbic system. The ACC, as depicted here, is the anterior portion of the cingulate gyrus within the frontal lobe on the medial surface of the hemisphere. Its interconnections with the medial temporal lobe structures of the limbic system contributes to our awareness of emotion. (Reproduced with permission from Kandel ER, Schwartz JH, et al., *Principles of Neural Science*, 5th Ed. New York, NY: McGraw-Hill; 2013.)

the basal ganglia (globus pallidus and substantia nigra), and the hypothalamus.[3] The temporal lobe is our emotional center, and the DLPFC has connections to temporal structures, including the nucleus accumbens, the **hippocampus**, the amygdala, and the entorhinal cortex, all of which are implicated in emotion.[3,7] The DLPFC is critical in working memory as well as memory retrieval from the temporal and posterior association cortices for use in synthesizing information for problem-solving activities, especially when assessing unfamiliar or ambiguous cues to make a difficult decision or calculation.[4,7,9] The DLPFC has also been linked to cognitive flexibility.[3] Damage to the DLPFC is associated with perseveration, lack of attention, difficulty following instructions or maintaining the goal of a task in mind, poor planning or strategy development, impaired decision-making, especially related to moral dilemmas, and changes in personality. Along with these, there is an obvious loss of inhibition. This myriad of deficits has been referred to as **frontal dysexecutive syndrome**.[7]

Orbitofrontal Cortex (OFC)

The OFC encompasses Brodmann's areas 11–14 and 47 and can be visualized as the most ventral part of the frontal lobes; in association with the anterior cingulate cortex and frontal polar cortex, it is referred to as the **orbitofrontal ventromedial cortex (OFVMC)** or **ventromedial prefrontal cortex (VMPC or VMPFC)**. The OFC is an area of integration for sensory processing of visual, auditory, and somatosensory stimuli, receiving information from the inferior temporal lobe, secondary and tertiary auditory cortex, and the parietal lobe's secondary somatosensory area, each conveying their respective information. The VMPC is also interconnected with the DLPFC; areas of memory in the insular cortex, temporal lobe, and hippocampus; as well as areas associated with emotion and homeostasis in the amygdala and hypothalamus. Ultimately, this area is active in determining the motivational aspects of decision-making, whether for reward or to avoid punishment; it is also involved in the regulation of negative emotions (e.g., fear).[10] The VMPFC and its connection to the bilateral anterior cingulate cortex assists in making familiar or intuitive decisions.[9] Damage to this region impairs social awareness (**acquired sociopathy** Happaney), reflected as the inability to interpret other people's emotions and to demonstrate appropriate behavior in social situations.[8] This also manifests as impulsive behavior and risk-taking due to the inability to see the potential consequences of actions.[7,8]

Anterior Cingulate Cortex (ACC)

Located on the medial surface of the frontal lobe, the ACC is an area of convergence for projections from the other two critical areas, the DLPFC and OFVMC, but also has reciprocal connections to these areas. It appears to contribute to our ability to shift our attention from one task feature to another and also has been associated with our awareness of emotion, resulting from its strong connections to the **limbic system**, including the amygdala, hippocampus, entorhinal cortex, and parahippocampal cortex[3] (see Figure 7-2). It works with the DLPFC and OFVMC for EF but seems particularly essential for decisions where the outcome is ambiguous or incongruent (e.g., reading the word RED when printed in blue as in the Stroop test).[7] Damage to the anterior cingulate exacerbates the poor social awareness, demonstrated with OFVMC damage, and results in a condition, referred to as **alexithymia**, which is the inability to describe one's emotions.[11]

Other Networks Involved in EF

It is too simplistic to think that the three areas discussed in the previous sections act exclusively to mediate EF. First, as mentioned, these three areas of the prefrontal cortex are interconnected with multiple other regions of the cerebral cortex, basal ganglia, and limbic system. In addition, the **posterior parietal cortex**, with its links to the DLPFC, contributes to working memory, and more specifically is thought to be active when we compare, evaluate, or manipulate information held in working memory (e.g., picking out a picture of an object recently held in the hand). An adjacent area within the intraparietal sulcus has been linked to our ability to orient to objects and space, including our ability to mentally realign objects to their appropriate orientation, if they are presented upside down or sideways, as well as contributing to our ability to manipulate or compare memories. The basal ganglia also plays a role in EF through its many corticostriatal connections. First, the ventral caudate and nucleus accumbens form a **limbic loop** with the VLPFC that contributes to memory retrieval, the production of stereotypical behavior, attention, and motivated behavior. Similarly, a second loop, known as the **associative loop**, links the caudate and putamen to the DLPFC, contributing to working memory and our ability to benefit from errors while learning a task as well as shifting from one strategy to another, as in the card sorting task described earlier. Such learning contributes to the development of behavioral habits, primarily controlled by the limbic loop.[3]

Somewhat surprisingly, the cerebellum, known most for its role in balance and coordination, also plays a role in EF. The lateral portions of the posterior lobes, the cognitive cerebellum, contribute to task shifting and working memory, sequence planning, visuospatial orientation, and word finding and speech fluency. It's theorized that the cerebellum contributes to cognition, much as it does to motor planning and execution, by controlling and revising the rate and sequencing of cognitive activities. Damage to the posterior cerebellum results in a return to concrete thinking, problem-solving deficits, and impaired multi-tasking as well as disrupted working memory and long-term memory retrieval. Through its connections to the limbic system, the posterior vermis and fastigial nuclei participate in behavioral regulation and inhibition. Damage to this area results in disinhibition and impulsivity. Extensive damage to the posterior lobes and vermis results in cerebellar cognitive affective syndrome with a combination of the deficits discussed for both the cognitive and limbic areas.[12,13]

Learning and Memory

The concepts of learning and memory are linked; historically, learning has been defined as a permanent change in behavior that results from experience or practice with memory being the method by which learning is stored. Even memory is not a simple concept because we have different types of learning and thereby memory. Do you know how to ride a bicycle? Most of us do, but if asked to describe how it is done, we would all struggle a bit with verbalizing the combination of movements and awareness necessary to successfully ride a bike. Such a skill is typically learned by practice through what is referred to as **procedural learning** and stored as a **nondeclarative** or **implicit** memory. On the other hand, when we learn facts or remember events from our childhood, it is much easier to verbalize them; this type of learning and memory is referred to as **declarative, conscious,** or **explicit**. The neural structures and networks supporting these two types of memory are different. It should be noted that memories are not stored in a single region; rather, memory seems to be a distributed function with many brain regions involved. Memory duration also differentiates memory characteristics, and neural networks that support working (short-term) memory are different from those supporting long-term memory. We have already discussed the network associated with working memory, so in this section we will focus on long-term memory and the networks that support procedural versus declarative memory.[1]

Declarative (Explicit) Memory

Declarative memory includes retention of our personal experiences (**episodic memory**) as well as retention of facts and concepts (**semantic memory**). Further, declarative memory involves at least three separate processes. The initial phase is known as **encoding**, referring to the neural process of translating what is to be remembered to activity in neural circuits that link new experiences/information to prior related memories. Second, permanent changes in synaptic activity occur as the "new memory" is **consolidated** into a more stable memory within widespread neural areas with similar memories aligned in given brain networks.[14] Ultimately, our ability to recall our memories in the future is based on the process of **retrieval**. These sequential stages of memory (encoding, consolidation, and retrieval) help to explain why some events or facts are well remembered and others not. If we lack related memories with which to link new information, we are likely to lay down a weak memory or one that is difficult to retrieve. Further, if the process of consolidation is disrupted, as often happens with a brain injury, a stable memory may fail to form, resulting in the common inability to remember the accident that produced the brain injury as well as events leading up to the accident. Lastly, our ability to retrieve a memory is reliant on appropriate cues that direct our recall; if there aren't appropriate cues, we are unlikely to retrieve the memory.[14] Recalling a memory provides an opportunity for reconsolidation, which allows for strengthening or modification of the memory. Modification can involve adding more details to the stored memory.[15] For example, when you sit with friends and discuss a shared experience, each may add details that can then be stored with your own original memory. Interestingly, perceived or imagined events can disrupt the **consolidation** of memories, leading to a "false" memory; similarly, competing information/events can disrupt the encoding or consolidation of memories. Sleep can facilitate memory consolidation but has also been found to distort memories as perceived attributes may be added to the "true" memory.[16]

Structures in the medial temporal lobe are critical for declarative memory; these include the **hippocampal formation** (hippocampus, dentate gyrus, and subiculum) as well as the lateral entorhinal, perirhinal, medial entorhinal, and parahippocampal cortices (Figure 7-3). These medial temporal lobe structures have reciprocal connections with the association cortices that are areas of convergence for sensory, motor, emotion, and cognitive brain regions. Notably, these temporal lobe areas appear to be differentially responsible for separate aspects of a given experience with the entorhinal and perirhinal cortices active in response to "what" was experienced and the medial entorhinal and parahippocampal cortices active with regard to the spatiotemporal context or the "where/when" of the experience.[14] Each of these areas has reciprocal connections with the hippocampus, which, in turn, is reciprocally connected to the prefrontal cortex via the subiculum. The prefrontal cortex appears instrumental in both memory consolidation and retrieval, likely playing a role in organizing similar memories and their respective/distinctive features and helping us to discern critical cues to achieve memory retrieval. However, the locus of memories seems well distributed throughout many cortical areas, protecting us from losing all of our memories with any focal injury.

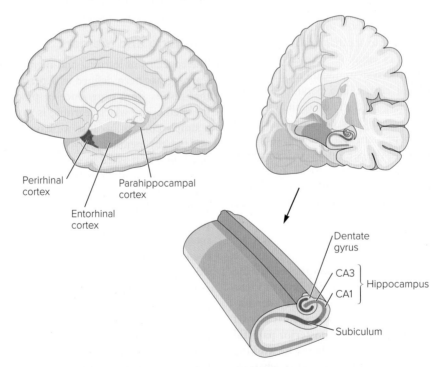

FIGURE 7-3 Medial temporal lobe structures associated with memory. Within the medial temporal lobe, the hippocampal formation, and the surrounding cortex – rhinal (perirhinal, entorhinal) and parahippocampal – are critical for the encoding of memories. The hippocampal formation consists of the dentate gyrus, subiculum, and hippocampus, which has two layers of pyramidal neurons (CA1 and CA3). These pyramidal neurons are activated by projections from the entorhinal cortex and subsequently activate projection fibers that exit through the subiculum to the prefrontal cortex. (Reproduced with permission from Kandel ER, Schwartz JH, et al., *Principles of Neural Science*, 5th Ed. New York, NY: McGraw-Hill; 2013.)

Yet, damage to the medial temporal lobe will disrupt memory encoding (**anterograde amnesia**) and may disrupt access to some recent memories as the hippocampus continues to play a role in memory retrieval for some time after the memory origin. Over time, as memories are consolidated, they become "cortical," losing some of the contextual details of the original experience and becoming less reliant on the hippocampus for retrieval. However, memories that retain a strong emotional context for us may always rely on the hippocampus for retrieval.[17]

Other anatomic regions linked to declarative memory function are the anterior and mediodorsal nuclei of the thalamus and the mammillary bodies. The mammillary bodies are part of the diencephalon and seem to serve a relay function between the hippocampus and the anterior thalamus, which, in turn, projects to the cingulate cortex, another area implicated in memory recall. The mediodorsal nuclei have reciprocal projections to both the prefrontal cortex and the medial temporal lobe structures; this network is active in distinguishing novel from familiar events or objects.[18] One can also make a distinction between recollection of an event and the determination of something as familiar; in recollecting an event, all of the characteristics of the event would be remembered. However, there is a lack of detail associated with the determination of something as familiar versus novel. We have all experienced this phenomenon, while at a party, where we are meeting new people; we often recognize someone later in the evening that we met earlier without remembering the details of the introduction (name, relationship to the host, etc.). Anatomically, the hippocampus is routinely active in recollection but not in determining familiarity, which is associated more with activity in the rhinal cortex.[14,19]

Nondeclarative (Implicit) Memory

Nondeclarative or implicit learning and memory refers to our ability to learn without conscious awareness of that learning. Although much of implicit learning is related to the learning of movements or procedures, and often referred to as **procedural**

Box 7-2	**Implicit Learning Letter Sequence**

When presented with a random series of letters, participants will react similarly to each new letter presentation; however, when a repeating sequence of letters is embedded in the series, participants will demonstrate less cortical activity to the embedded repeating series than the others, demonstrating that the series is familiar and not novel. However, they are typically unable to explicitly describe the repeating series.

altpri**jgft**mniqr**jgft**drjoplwaxdmkytei**jgft**

---

learning, we are also capable of learning other types of information in this manner, including habits, classical conditioning responses, mirror reading, distinguishing familiar from novel stimuli, and many others. For example, when presented with a hidden repeating sequence of letters within a long series of letters, most people will not be able to verbalize the sequence but will react to it as familiar when presented with it later (Box 7-2). While explicit learning and the resultant memories have been well documented to incorporate the two systems described in the preceding section, implicit learning is thought to be independent of a specific system. In fact, it is thought that implicit learning is the result of neural plasticity throughout brain regions, which is why localized lesions don't disrupt implicit or procedural learning or memories[20] (Figure 7-4).

The synaptic changes, responsible for implicit learning, can largely be defined by two mechanisms: long-term potentiation and long-term depression, as initially discussed in Chapter 5. **Long-term potentiation (LTP)** results from an increased level of activity within a synapse in response to a given stimulus. Conversely, **long-term depression (LTD)** is associated with a decreased level of responsiveness within a synapse.[21] Both are long-lasting and occur in response to repeated exposure to specific stimuli. [**It should be noted that explicit memory consolidation also involves these mechanisms.**] Thus, groups of neurons that are activated or inhibited in the presence of a given sensory or motor experience will

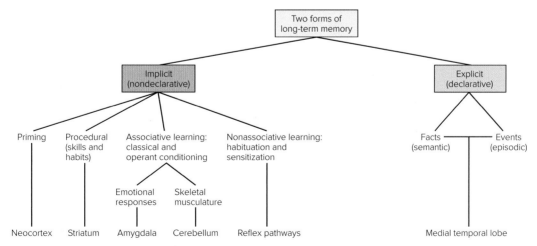

FIGURE 7-4 Schematic of implicit and explicit memory systems. Long-term memory can be divided into explicit (semantic – facts; episodic – events) and implicit (procedural) memories. Explicit memories are encoded by the medial temporal lobe structures and their connections to the anterior cingulate and prefrontal cortices. Implicit memories are generated within an array of networks, including the sensory cortices (priming), striatum of the basal ganglia and cerebellum (motor skills, habits), the cerebellum and amygdala (classical and operant conditioning), and reflex networks of the brainstem. (Reproduced with permission from Kandel ER, Schwartz JH, et al., *Principles of Neural Science*, 5th Ed. New York, NY: McGraw-Hill; 2013.)

begin to fire as a group with subsequent exposure to the same or very similar experiences. Based on this premise, implicit learning can involve almost any area of the brain. For **sensorimotor skills**, the cerebellum, basal ganglia, and the premotor and motor cortices are active during learning and remembering of these skills. The striatum of the basal ganglia is active when **habits** are learned, such as our method of combing our hair or brushing our teeth. Both the visual and auditory sensory cortices have been found to develop specific neuronal responses, known as **priming**, to repeated exposure to a given salient stimulus; priming results in less neural activity to a repetition of the stimulus that is characterized by fewer neurons firing for a shorter length of time, but the onset of the activity is quicker than for novel stimuli. These changes are thought to represent efficiency within the sensory system. Similar priming effects are also thought to mediate other types of implicit learning like the response to the hidden sequence of letters within the implicit learning paradigm, described in Box 7-2.[20] Notably, repeated exposure to sensory stimuli can result in decreased responsiveness (**habituation**) or increased responsiveness (**sensitization**); these terms have been generated from animal experiments where animals are presented with threatening or nonthreatening stimuli. Over time, they ignore the nonthreatening stimuli (habituation) but show heightened responses to the threatening stimuli (sensitivity).[22] An example for humans may be a young child's initial fear response to fireworks on the 4th of July that over time becomes an enjoyable experience with limited response to each "pop" (habituation). Conversely, a bumble bee may be just another pretty insect to a young child, but once stung, sighting a bee may elicit a strong fear response (**sensitivity**). This type of classical or operant conditioning, where a neutral stimulus is associated with a reward or punishment, is linked to activity in both the cerebellum (motor response) and the amygdala (emotional response). As a reminder, classical conditioning involves the presentation of a neutral stimulus followed by the presentation of another stimulus (positive or negative), where the response to the second stimulus becomes tied to the first. Similarly, operant conditioning is behavior that is developed as a result of the consequence of that behavior. So, a young child may initially grab a bee, but after being stung, may cry at the sight of a bee (operant conditioning). The pretty firework, followed by the loud sound, may generate a fear response to the sight of the firework (classical conditioning).[22]

Forgetting

Forgetting is a common occurrence for all of us and is likely an important process that allows us to keep needed memories and eliminate unwanted ones; however, it is also a frustrating thing when we wish to recall something and cannot. Forgetting can be an active or a passive process. **Passive forgetting** is thought to result from one of three processes: (1) failure to identify appropriate cues for retrieval; (2) memory interference from related memories; or (3) decaying of the memory trace over time, if unused. Multiple processes are also thought to support **active forgetting**. First explicit memories are proposed to involve two components: the spatial-contextual component, which relies on the hippocampus, and a content component encoded in the cerebrocortex. One cause of active forgetting is thought to involve suppression of the hippocampal contextual trace such that the cerebrocortical component can't be retrieved.

Much of this appears to happen during sleep so that unneeded memories from our many activities each day are removed to maintain optimal functioning. A second process involves **retroactive interference**, by which a memory trace is suppressed or replaced by newer similar or competing memories.[23] A third process involves deliberate forgetting via inhibitory mechanisms, originating from the dorsolateral prefrontal cortex, to suppress memory encoding or retrieval – likely a method to avoid remembering unpleasant experiences. A fourth process involves retrieval competition, whereby contextual cues connect to multiple memories. With retrieval practice, inhibitory processes eliminate the connection to the weaker or less desirable memories (retrieval-induced forgetting).[24]

Emotion

Emotions are complex learned responses elicited by sensory stimuli that produce physiologic changes (heart and respiration rate, sweating, etc.) and motor responses (muscle tensing, facial expression, movement); they motivate us to action (attraction, avoidance), involving many neurologic systems.[6] The reaction to these physiologic, motor, and attentional changes are interpreted cognitively, whereby each situation is evaluated for its potential impact on the individual and the long-term outcome possibilities. This involves an integration between cognition (situation analysis) and memory (past experiences in similar situations), ultimately culminating in an emotional response,[6] or what humans call feelings, ranging from happiness to sadness, confidence to fear, attraction to disgust, and gratitude to anger.

At the forefront of any discussion on emotional control is the limbic system, which includes the hippocampus, amygdala, striatum, fornix, hypothalamus, mammillary bodies, anterior thalamic nuclei, areas of the cingulate gyrus, and the insular cortex. These structures contribute to three primary networks with distinct functions: (1) **hippocampal-parahippocampal-retrosplenial network**; (2) **temporal-amygdala-orbitofrontal network**; and (3) **dorsomedial default-mode network**. For the first network, fibers from the hippocampus, the surrounding parahippocampal cortex, and the adjacent retrosplenial cortex project through the fornix to the mammillary bodies, thalamus, and hypothalamus and ultimately to the cingulate cortex, which, in turn, connects to the prefrontal cortex. This circuit primarily supports spatial orientation and the ability to use current environmental cues to determine location by comparing them to cues stored in memory (Figure 7-5). Thus, although the limbic system is often solely referred to as our emotional system, it is important to remember its critical role in memory.[25]

The temporal-amygdala-orbitofrontal network links the amygdala to the insular and orbitofrontal cortices via the uncinate fasciculus (a fiber bundle running from the temporal lobe to the orbitofrontal cortex at the base of the frontal lobe). This network integrates our visceral sensations with our cognitive activities, linking the outcome (reward or punishment) and the emotional response (satisfaction, fear) to the behavior/situation and ultimately to the stored memory (Figure 7-5). The dorsomedial default-mode network, which includes the anterior cingulate and medial prefrontal cortex, is active in the absence of goal-directed activity, as the name implies, and seems to be responsible for internalized activities such as daydreaming or

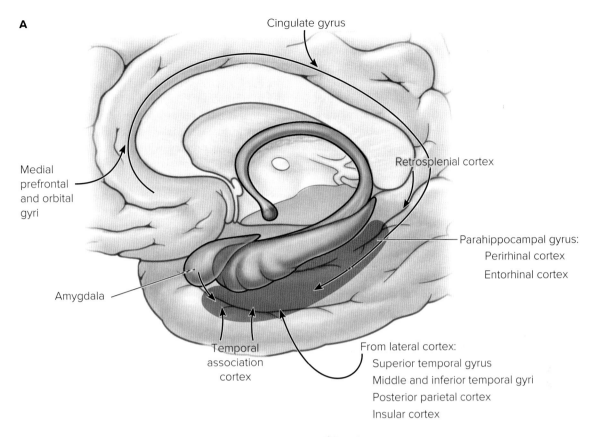

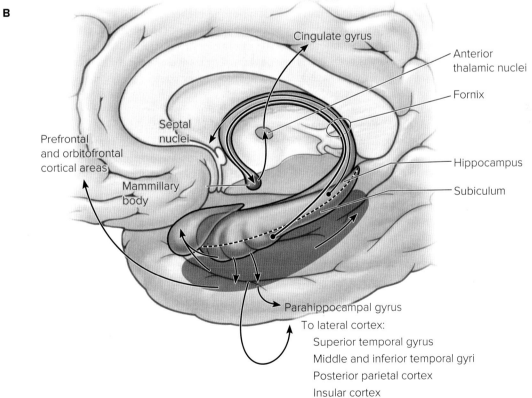

FIGURE 7-5 Circuits of the limbic system. These two figures schematically illustrate the two circuits of the limbic system: **A** illustrates the temporo-amygdala-orbitofrontal network that supports emotions (especially fear) and impacts learning related to reward and punishment. **B** illustrates the hippocampal formation's connections to the mammillary bodies and areas of the cingulate and insular cortex; this network subserves memory and emotion. (Reproduced with permission from Martin JH. *Neuroanatomy Text and Atlas*, 4th Ed. New York, NY: McGraw-Hill; 2012.)

introspection, which likely contributes to the monitoring of our ongoing emotional state (Figure 7-5).[25]

The **amygdala** is adjacent to the hippocampus in the medial temporal lobe and has reciprocal connections to the medial prefrontal and orbitofrontal cortices; it also projects, along with the hippocampus, to the hypothalamus and brainstem nuclei that contribute to the control of respiration, heart rate, postural muscle control, and other autonomic responses (e.g., sweating, chills). The hippocampus is active during stress responses and, through its connections with the hypothalamus, modulates the release of stress hormones; in turn, these stress hormones provide a negative feedback loop to the hippocampus, decreasing its activity. Notably, the ventral hippocampus is specifically associated with emotional regulation; damage to this area results in decreased responsiveness to fear or anxiety-producing situations.[26] The amygdala is core to our fear responses and to the heightened vigilance that we display in fearful situations; for example, when you are walking down a dark alley by yourself, your heart rate increases, you may have goosebumps, and are likely to react in an exaggerated way to any noise. This vigilance and hyper-responsiveness are triggered by activity in the amygdala through its connections to the hypothalamus and critical brainstem nuclei. Notably, the afferent connections from the medial prefrontal cortex to the amygdala are critical for suppression of these natural fear and avoidance responses, suggesting that stimuli are analyzed by the frontal cortex with subsequent inhibition of amygdala activity.[27] The amygdala also appears to contribute to the analysis of social situations as well as encoding the emotional components of memory via its connections with the hippocampus, which may explain why some of our strongest memories are associated with fearful experiences. Increased activity in the amygdala has been found in those diagnosed with anxiety disorders. Similarly, damage to both the hippocampus and amygdala along with decreased prefrontal and ACC activity has been associated with post-traumatic stress disorder (PTSD); in combination, these changes result in a heightened response to stressful or fearful situations with an inability to inhibit this response via the prefrontal cortex – amygdala/hippocampal connections. An increase in default-mode network activity, during rest, is also noted in PTSD.[27]

Similar to the amygdala's connection to fear responsiveness, other areas of the limbic system seem to be linked to specific emotions. The **ACC** is most active when people describe sadness and has been found to be less active in those diagnosed with depression, increasing its level of activity in the presence of antidepressant medications.[28] In addition, the ACC seems to be involved in our conscious awareness of our emotions and their regulation. Damage to the dorsal ACC has been associated with alexithymia, the inability to describe emotions (one's own or others').[29,30] The **basal ganglia** is linked to happiness or positively motivating activities but is also tied to our disgust response.[28] This activity in the basal ganglia may be related to the potential motor response to situations/things that elicit happiness (movement toward) or avoidance of those that elicit disgust (movement away). The basal ganglia exerts its role in emotion through projections from the dorsal caudate to the amygdala, insular cortex, and prefrontal cortex. In addition, this dorsal caudate–limbic connection is active during habit learning, based on reward motivation (praise or punishment). Interestingly, this

connection between the dorsal caudate and the limbic areas has been found to have exaggerated activity in response to pictures of food in morbidly obese individuals, which was associated with greater connectivity between the amygdala and insula. In addition, there was a decreased level of activity within the dorsofrontal and orbitofrontal cortices in obese subjects, which are two areas that inhibit reward-seeking behavior through their connections to the amygdala.[31] Thus, there is substantial evidence that the dorsal caudate with its links to the prefrontal cortex and amygdala plays a significant role in behavioral motivation and learning as well as emotion. Disorders of the basal ganglia, such as Parkinson's disease, are often associated with emotional changes, further illustrating its contributory role in emotion.

Finally, the **medial prefrontal cortex** appears to have a significant role in emotional processing that may comprise the analysis of contextual cues to determine the appropriate emotion, including the comparison of the current situation to our memories of similar situations, as well as self-assessment of our current emotional state. Its interconnections with the hippocampus likely facilitate this comparison. The **insular cortex** is an area of convergence for visceral sensations (e.g., heart and respiration rate, sweating), which contribute to our interpretation of our emotional response. Further, this area of the brain seems to play a critical role in our interpretation of reward and punishment and interestingly appears to also contribute to the development of addiction.[28]

Language

Of all of the higher level skills that differentiate humans from other animals, none is as obvious as language. Our understanding of the neural substrates that support our language abilities continues to evolve as our ability to image and use electrical stimulation to evaluate this system expands. A few common terms, associated with language, will be important for our discussion of the neural systems supporting our language abilities. **Phonology** or **phonetics** refers to the way sounds are put together to form words while **syntax**, also known as grammar, is the way words are organized within a phrase or sentence. **Semantics** refers to the meaning of words or sounds, such as "un" referring to "not."

Our language skills and the systems that support them are typically divided into reception (our ability to recognize and understand language) and production (our ability to produce speech). In the 1800s two centers were identified that seemed to support these two functions, based on the presentation of patients that had damage to one or the other area. **Broca's area**, named for Paul Broca, is located in the frontal lobe, just anterior to the primary motor area on the lateral surface of the hemisphere, and was linked to language production; damage to this area was reported to result in difficulty with word selection and, thereby, limited speech output but good speech understanding (**non-fluent aphasia**). **Wernicke's area**, named for Carl Wernicke, is located in the posterior aspect of the temporal lobe and associated with language reception. Damage to this area resulted in loss of speech understanding with fluid but nonsensical speech production; this was thought to result from limited comprehension of what others say as well as the inability to monitor self-generated speech (fluent aphasia/Wernicke's aphasia/**receptive aphasia**). These two areas were found to interconnect via the **arcuate fasciculus** and damage to these fibers resulted in **conductive aphasia**, associated with disordered verbalizing of syllables (phonology). Further, the left hemisphere was found to be dominant for language in most individuals, but with a small percentage of left-handed individuals showing right dominance. However, several hundred years of research, since these early descriptions, has determined them to be a simplistic view of human language systems, so our complex language abilities are now believed to be supported by a more expansive neural network that spans the temporal, parietal, and frontal lobes as well as some subcortical structures.[32] However, many clinicians still rely on these original definitions of **aphasia** (disrupted speech; see Chapter 11 (Stroke) for more descriptions of speech disorders).

According to Hickok and Poeppel (2007), the neural networks, supporting language perception and production, involve two projection streams and their respective connections. Although speech sounds are processed initially by the same neurologic substrates as any other sounds within the auditory cortex of the temporal lobes, as described in Chapter 6, the superior temporal gyrus (STG) is active bilaterally when speech is heard and appears to be the first processing area of our language system, although with a slight dominant hemisphere bias, likely playing a role in distinguishing verbal from nonverbal stimuli. In fact, damage to the STG bilaterally results in **word deafness**, which literally is the inability to distinguish speech from other sounds. Fortunately, this is an extremely rare disorder.[33]

Subsequent to activity in the STG, verbal processing appears to use two projection streams, one bilateral and one unilateral, within the dominant hemisphere (left for most people). A **dorsal stream**, in the dominant hemisphere, connects structures in the temporal lobe (ventral supramarginal gyrus) to the parietal lobe (sylvian parietal temporal region) and insula as well as portions of the frontal lobe (inferior frontal gyrus [inclusive of Broca's area] and ventral precentral gyrus) via the arcuate fasciculus and posterior components of the **superior longitudinal fasciculus**. This stream is critical for transforming what we want to say into appropriately articulated sentences (syntax), requiring sensorimotor mapping

of speech sounds into articulation.[33,34] In line with the earlier section of this chapter that discussed the role of the prefrontal cortex in working memory, the inferior frontal cortex is associated with verbal working memory as well as the planning of speech vocalizations, including semantics and phonology. Interestingly, it is also active during silent reading, especially in novice readers, which may suggest that they are mapping the pronunciation of the words as they read them; mature readers demonstrate very little activity in this area, when reading silently. In summary, the historic non-fluent (Broca's) aphasia is a disruption of the dorsal stream, resulting in disrupted articulation (disordered syntax).[33-35]

The **ventral stream, present bilaterally, connects the anterior middle temporal gyrus and anterior inferior temporal sulcus to** the posterior middle temporal and inferior temporal gyri. These temporal lobe regions are tightly linked to semantic memory areas and visual areas in the frontal, parietal, and occipital lobes. This ventral stream principally supports the conversion of what is heard and seen to its meaning for both understanding what is said (semantics) and planning what one wants to say, including naming visually presented objects. Thus, the fluent aphasia, previously associated with Wernicke's area, results from disruption of the ventral stream with subsequent disordered semantics. It's important to note that the original site for Wernicke's area was in the posterior aspect of the STG, now known to be the site where speech sounds are identified bilaterally, subsequently initiating activity in both the ventral and dorsal streams; yet, the classic impairment of disrupted understanding of speech primarily accompanied by jargon speech production aligns with damage to the ventral stream. Both streams are bidirectional, allowing for the integration of speech production with speech perception. Obviously, damage to many areas, surrounding the historic Broca's and Wernicke's areas, will result in disruption of language abilities (Figure 7-6). However, this expanded network also explains the preservation of many language skills after brain damage as well as the more variable presentations of some survivors of stroke, brain injury, or other disorders.[33]

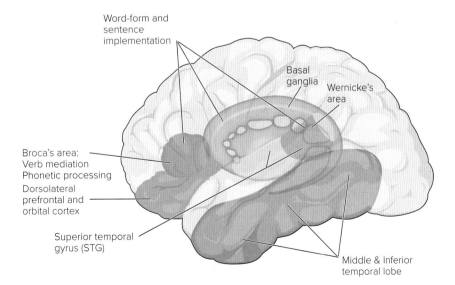

FIGURE 7-6 Language centers. The historic Broca's and Wernicke's areas are depicted in association with the surrounding areas that contribute to language skills (dorsolateral and orbitofrontal cortex, middle and inferior temporal lobes, basal ganglia). (Reproduced with permission from Kandel ER, Schwartz JH, et al., *Principles of Neural Science*, 5th Ed. New York, NY: McGraw-Hill; 2013.)

Extensive damage to the dominant hemisphere, involving both the frontal and temporal lobes, can result in a complex loss of language skills, referred to as **global aphasia**, and presenting with impaired speech production with impaired speech reception; typically, reading and writing are also affected.

Historically, **conduction aphasia** was thought to be caused by damage to the arcuate fasciculus, which, in effect, disrupted the connection between speech perception centers in the temporal lobe and speech production centers in the frontal lobe. This resulted in impaired speech production that included difficulties in repeating what someone else has said, disordered phonology (syllable ordering within a word or word order within a sentence), and problems with naming of objects. More recent evidence suggests that conduction aphasia is more likely the result of damage to the superior temporal sulcus and subsequently the temporal–parietal lobe interconnections rather than the arcuate fasciculus.[36]

Interestingly, multiple other areas contribute to our language abilities, including the basal ganglia and cerebellum, which play a role in the fluidity of our speech. Both contribute to the rate at which we say words as well as word spacing via their connections with the frontal lobe's motor planning centers. Damage to the basal ganglia results in **hypokinetic dysarthria**, characterized by abrupt stoppage of verbalization in the middle of syllables, words, or phrases, and is thought to be a disruption in the motor planning of speech as well as of the execution of the motor plan.[36] Similarly, the cerebellum contributes to phonology and sequence formation through connections between the right superior cerebellum and the frontal lobe. Damage to the superior cerebellum results in an irregular timing of speech, known as **ataxic dysarthria**, also called scanning or staccato speech, with varying emphasis on different syllables and/or words.[36] Other contributions of the cerebellum to speech and language are thought to include motor speech planning, processing of syntax and grammatical rules, reading, and production of writing. Similarly, the thalamus in the dominant hemisphere serves as a relay station in support of language; thalamic nuclei involved include the posterior ventrolateral, and pulvinar and anterior ventrolateral nuclei, among others. Damage to the thalamus can be associated with anomia, word omission in sentences, and verbal memory encoding errors.[37]

Reading is also associated with a complex network, involving the temporal, parietal, occipital, and frontal cortices. Occipital–temporal connections link sounds to printed words or symbols while temporal–parietal areas, including the angular gyrus, map those sounds into verbal words, which activates the inferior frontal cortex. In early readers, there is considerable activity in the frontal cortex even with silent reading, suggesting that readers are "speaking" the words silently; once reading is mature, there is much less inferior frontal lobe activity, indicating a decreased reliance on articulation for word processing. Notably, other areas of the frontal lobe, related to attention, EF, and memory, are necessary for mature reading.[34]

● SUMMARY

The higher level functions discussed in this chapter – EF, memory, emotion, and language – demonstrate the complexity of the human brain. They also illustrate the multiple interconnections between these functions and the neural systems that support them, which is the reason that they were presented in a single chapter. In the presence of neurologic injury or disease, these higher level functions are often disrupted in combination with highly variable presentations, since brain damage is rarely the same between individuals with similar conditions. In the disease-focused chapters of this text, the impact of brain damage on higher level functions will be discussed.

REFERENCES

1. Harada CN, Love MCN, Triebel K. Normal cognitive aging. *Clin Geriatr Med*. 2013;29(4):737-752.

2. Rabinovici GD, Stephens ML, Possin KL. Executive dysfunction. *Continuum*. 2015;21(3)646-659.

3. Leh SE, Petrides M, Strafelia AP. The neural circuitry of executive functions in healthy subjects and Parkinson's disease. *Neuropsychopharmacology*. 2010;35:70-85.

4. Kroger JK, Nystrom LE, Cohen JD, Johnson-Laird PH. Distinct neural substrates for deductive and mathematical processing. *Brain Research*. 2008:1243:86-103.

5. Vendetti MS, Bunge SA. Evolutionary and developmental changes in the lateral frontoparietal network: a little goes a long way for higher-level cognition. *Neuron*.2014;84(5):906-917.

6. Brosch T, Scherer KR, Grandjean D, Sander D. The impact of emotion on perception, attention, memory, and decision-making. *Swiss Med Wkly*. 2013;143:w13786.

7. Rosenbloom MH, Schmahmann JD, Price BH. The functional neuroanatomy of decision-making. *J Neuropscyh Clin Neurosci*. 2012;24(3):266-277.

8. Happaney K, Zelazo PD, Stuss DT. Development of orbitofrontal function: current themes and future directions. *Brain Cognition*. 2004;55:1-10.

9. Erdeniz B, Done J. Common and distinct functional brain networks for intuitive and deliberate decision making. *Brain Sci*. 2019;9 (7):174-184.

10. Hiser J, Koenigs M. The multifaceted role of ventromedial prefrontal cortex in emotion, decision-making, social cognition, and psychopathology. *Biol Psychiatry*. 2018;83(8):638-647.

11. Meriau K, Wartenburger I, Kazzer P, et al. A neural network reflecting individual differences in cognitive processing of emotions during perceptual decision making. *Neuroimage*. 2006;33(3):1016-1027.

12. Bodranghien F, Bastian A, Casali C, et al. Consensus paper: revisiting the symptoms and signs of cerebellar syndrome. *Cerebellu*. 2016;15(3):369-391.

13. Buckner RL. The cerebellum and cognitive function: 25 years of insight from anatomy and neuroimaging. *Neuron*. 2018;80:807-815.

14. Preston AR, Eichenbaum H. Interplay of hippocampus and prefrontal cortex in memory. *Current Biol*. 2013;23:R764-R773.

15. Gavin CF, Theibert AB. Learning and memory. In: *Essentials of Modern Neuroscience*. McGraw Hill; 2021 Downloaded 2021-5-18.

16. Staube B. An overview of the neuro-cognitive processes involved in the encoding, consolidation and retrieval of true and false memories. *Behav Brain Funct*. 2012;8:35-45.

17. Winocur G, Moscovitch M, Bontempi B. Memory formation and long-term retention in humans and animals: convergence towards a transformation account of hippocampal-neocortical interactions. *Neuropsychologia*. 2010;48:2339-2356.

18. Metzger CD, van der Werl YD, Walter M. Functional mapping of thalamic nuclei and their integration into cortico-striatal-thalamo-cortical loops via ultra-high resolution imaging: from animal anatomy to in vivo imaging in humans. *Front Neurosci*. 2013;7:1-14.

19. Ranganath C, Ritchey M. Two cortical systems for memory-guided behavior. *Nature Reviews: Neuroscience*. 2017;13:713-726.

20. Reber PJ. The neural basis of implicit learning and memory: a review of neuropsychological and neuroimaging research. *Neuropsychologia.* 2013;51:2026-2042.

21. Gold MG. A frontier in the understanding of synaptic plasticity: solving the structure of the postsynaptic density. *Bioessays.* 2012;34:599-608.

22. Kandel ER, LeDoux JE. Cellular mechanisms of implicit memory storage and the biological basis of individuality. In: Kandel ER, Koester JD, Mack SH, Siegelbaum SA, eds. *Principles of Neural Science.* 6th ed. McGraw Hill; 2021.

23. Hardt O, Nader K, Nadel L. Decay happens: the role of active forgetting in memory. *Trends Cogn Sci.* 2013;17(3):111-120.

24. Anderson MC, Hulbert JC. Active forgetting: adaptation of memory by prefrontal control. 2021;72:1-36.

25. Catani M, Dell'Acqua F, deSchotten MT. A revised limbic system model for memory, emotion and behavior. *Neurosci Biobehav Rev.* 2013;37:1724-1737.

26. Fanselow MS, Dong HW. Are the dorsal and ventral hippocampus functionally distinct structures? *Neuron.* 2010;65(1):7-19.

27. Kim MJ, Loucks RA, Palmer AL, et al. The structural and functional connectivity of the amygdala: from normal emotion to pathological anxiety. *Behav Brain Res.* 2011;223(2):403-410.

28. Phan KL, Wager T, Taylor SF, Liberzon I. Functional neuroanatomy of emotion: a meta-analysis of emotion activation studies in PET and fMRI. *Neuroimage.* 2002;16:33-348.

29. Dalgleish T. The emotional brain. *Perspectives.* 2004;5:582-589.

30. Meriau K, Wartenburger I, Kazzer P, et al. A neural network reflecting individual differences in cognitive processing of emotions during perceptual decision making. *Neuroimage.* 2006;33:1016-1027.

31. Nummenmaa L, Hirvonen J, Hannukainen JC, et al. Dorsal striatum and its limbic connectivity mediate abnormal anticipatory reward processing in obesity. *PLoS One.* 2012;7(2):e31089.

32. Dick F, Bates E, Wulfeck B, Utman JA, Dronkers N, Gernsbacher MA. Language deficits, localization and grammar: evidence for a distributive model of language breakdown in aphasic patients and neurologically intact individuals. *Psychol Rev.* 2001;108(4):759-788.

33. Hickok G, Poeppel D. Dorsal and ventral streams: a framework for understanding aspects of functional anatomy of language. *Cognition.* 2004;92:67-99.

34. D'Mello AM, Gabriel DE. Cognitive neuroscience of dyslexia. *Lang Speech Hear Serv Sch.* 2018;49:789-809.

35. Tippett DC, Hillis AE. Where are aphasia theory and management "headed"? *F1000Research.* 2017;1038. doi:10.12688/f1000research.11122.1.

36. Reilly KJ, Spencer KA. Speech serial control in healthy speakers and speakers with hypokinetic or ataxic dysarthria: effects of sequence length and practice. *Front Hum Neurosci.* 2013;7(article 665):1-17.

37. Chang EF, Raygor KP, Berger MS. Contemporary model of language organization: an overview for neurosurgeons. *J Neurosurg.* 2015;122:250-261.

Review Questions

1. **Failure to switch attention from one cue to another in a task switching paradigm is known as:**

   A. Disinhibition

   B. Dysregulation

   C. Perseveration

   D. Prioritization

2. **Frontal dysexecutive syndrome is associated with damage to:**

   A. Anterior cingulate cortex

   B. Dorsolateral prefrontal cortex

   C. Orbitofrontal cortex

   D. Premotor cortex

3. **Our memories for general knowledge and our own life experiences are also known as:**

   A. Crystallized intelligence

   B. Fluid intelligence

   C. Implicit knowledge

   D. Procedural knowledge

4. **What brain region is critical to working memory?**

   A. Anterior cingulate

   B. Dorsolateral prefrontal cortex

   C. Orbitofrontal cortex

   D. Ventromedial cortex

5. **Our ability to remember a skill, like how to hit a baseball, is referred to as:**

   A. Declarative memory

   B. Episodic memory

   C. Implicit memory

   D. Semantic memory

6. **Permanent changes in synaptic activity, in association with memory creation, are associated with what process?**

   A. Consolidation

   B. Encoding

   C. Retrieval

   D. Priming

7. **A patient demonstrates poor social awareness but also the inability to describe their own emotions. This is likely due to damage in what area?**

   A. Amygdala

   B. Anterior Cingulate Cortex

   C. Prefrontal Cortex

   D. Striatum

8. **Anterograde amnesia is associated with damage to what anatomical area?**

   A. Amygdala

   B. Hippocampus

   C. Mammillary bodies

   D. Thalamus

9. Increased responsiveness of a synapse to a given stimulus, associated with memory, is known as:
   A. Long-term depression
   B. Long-term excitation
   C. Long-term potentiation
   D. Priming

10. What changes in behavior might be associated with damage to the vermis and fastigial nuclei of the cerebellum?
    A. Concrete thinking
    B. Disrupted working memory
    C. Impulsive behavior
    D. Scanning speech

11. Passive forgetting includes which of the following processes?
    A. Decaying of an unused memory trace
    B. Inhibition from the prefrontal cortex
    C. Retroactive interference
    D. Suppression of the contextual trace

12. The amygdala is most strongly linked to what emotion?
    A. Disgust
    B. Fear
    C. Happiness
    D. Sadness

13. Monitoring of our internal emotional state is likely related to what emotional network?
    A. Caudate-amygdala-prefrontal cortex network
    B. Dorsomedial default-mode network
    C. Hippocampal-mammillary body-hypothalamus-cingulate network
    D. Temporo-amygdala-orbitofrontal network

14. What area of convergence for visceral sensation is active in our interpretation of reward and punishment?
    A. Anterior cingulate
    B. Basal ganglia
    C. Insular cortex
    D. Medial prefrontal cortex

15. In language, the way sounds are organized into words is known as what?
    A. Grammar
    B. Phonetics
    C. Semantics
    D. Syntax

16. Which language network supports syntax?
    A. Dorsal stream
    B. Fronto-occipital stream
    C. Uncinate stream
    D. Ventral stream

17. Fluent aphasia is characterized by disruption of what language skill?
    A. Phonetics
    B. Reception
    C. Semantics
    D. Syntax

18. Someone with basal ganglia damage is likely to present with what speech impairment?
    A. Ataxic dysarthria
    B. Fluent aphasia
    C. Hypokinetic dysarthria
    D. Receptive aphasia

19. Which area of the brain has been found to be associated with learning, emotion, language, and working memory?
    A. Amygdala
    B. Basal ganglia
    C. Hippocampus
    D. Parietal cortex

20. As children become mature readers, what area of the brain decreases its level of activity?
    A. Frontal lobe
    B. Occipital lobe
    C. Parietal lobe
    D. Temporal lobe

Answers

1. C	2. B	3. A	4. B	5. C
6. A	7. B	8. B	9. C	10. C
11. A	12. B	13. B	14. B	15. B
16. A	17. A	18. C	19. B	20. A

GLOSSARY

Abstract thought. To combine information in novel ways

Acquired sociopathy. Loss of social awareness due to damage of the ventromedial prefrontal cortex

Active forgetting. Forgetting that involves intentional neural activity (suppression of contextual cues, retroactive interference, retrieval competition, or inhibition of encoding or retrieval).

Alexithymia. The inability to describe one's emotions.

Amygdala. Temporal lobe limbic structure adjacent to hippocampus; involved in emotions.

Anterior cingulate cortex. On medial surface of frontal lobe; involved in attention shifting and emotional awareness; contributes to decision-making when the outcome is ambiguous.

Anterograde amnesia. Disruption of memory encoding.

Aphasia (dysphasia). Impaired speech.

Arcuate fasciculus. White matter projection system between temporal and frontal lobes; part of dorsal stream.

Ataxic dysarthria. Scanning or staccato speech resulting from damage to the right superior cerebellum.

Attention. Ability to focus on visual, auditory, tactile, or other sensory stimuli.

Behavioral (self) regulation. Adapting behavior to social situations.

Broca's area. Frontal lobe region originally thought to be the site of origin for speech articulation; included in dorsal stream.

Crystallized intelligence. Well-learned general knowledge or life experiences.

Cognition. Expansive term that includes learning, thinking, attention, memory, imagery, problem-solving, and decision-making.

Conductive aphasia. Disrupted speech related to damage of the superior temporal sulcus.

Consolidation. Laying down memories with permanent synaptic changes.

Disinhibition. A failure of inhibition often seen in young children or after brain injury.

Divided attention. Ability to attend to more than one stimulus at a time.

Dorsal stream. Language network linking temporal lobe structures to the parietal and frontal lobes to generate speech in the dominant hemisphere.

Dorsolateral prefrontal cortex (DLPFC). Located anterior to the premotor cortex on the dorsolateral aspect of the frontal lobe; involved in working memory, memory retrieval for problem-solving, and cognitive flexibility.

Dorsomedial default-mode network. Areas of anterior cingulate cortex and medial prefrontal cortex that are active in the absence of any goal-directed behavior; associated with internalized activities (e.g., daydreaming).

Encoding. Neural activity that links a new activity to related memories.

Episodic memory. Memories for personal experiences.

Executive function. The ability to respond appropriately to changing circumstances, including attention, working memory, inhibition, task switching, abstract thought, behavioral regulation, decision-making, sequence planning, and initiation.

Explicit memory (declarative, conscious). Memory for facts and personal experiences.

Expressive aphasia (Broca's, non-fluent). Disrupted speech articulation with intact understanding of speech caused by disruption of the dorsal stream.

Fluid intelligence. Reasoning to solve problems.

Frontal dysexecutive syndrome. Damage to the dorsolateral prefrontal cortex that disrupts executive function.

Global aphasia. Loss of expressive and receptive language as well as reading and writing abilities with extensive damage to the dominant hemisphere.

Habituation. Decreased responsiveness to a repeated sensory stimulus.

Hippocampal formation. Hippocampus, dentate gyrus, and subiculum, associated with memory.

Hippocampal-parahippocampal-restrosplenial network. Active in spatial orientation.

Hippocampus. Medial temporal lobe structure associated with memory.

Hypokinetic dysarthria. Abrupt pauses of speech in the middle of words or sentences, associated with basal ganglia injury.

Implicit memory (nondeclarative, procedural). A memory for movement or a task that is acquired through repetition or practice.

Inhibition. Delaying or blocking a response.

Limbic system. The emotional hub (hippocampus, amygdala, striatum, fornix, hypothalamus, mammillary bodies, anterior thalamic nuclei).

Orbitofrontal cortex (OFC). Brodmann's areas 11-14 and 47; most ventral part of frontal lobes; integrates visual, auditory, and somatosensory stimuli.

Orbitofrontal ventromedial cortex (OFVMC). The OFC plus the anterior cingulate cortex and frontal polar cortex; also referred to as VMPFC or VMPC; involved in motivational decision-making and social awareness.

Passive forgetting. Forgetting that doesn't require inhibitory processes from higher centers (decay, memory interference, cue inadequacy).

Perseveration. Continuing to focus on a prior stimulus when directed to switch to a new characteristic or cue.

Phonology (phonetics). The combination of sounds to form words.

Priming. Decreased neural activity (fewer neurons active) to a repetitive stimulus.

Receptive aphasia (Wernicke's, fluent). Inability to understand verbal language; articulation is intact but produces jargon speech; associated with disruption of the ventral stream.

Retrieval. The ability to recall a memory.

Selective attention. Ability to prioritize attention to one stimulus over another.

Semantics. Meaning of words.

Semantic memory. Memory for facts and concepts.

Sensitization. Increased responsiveness to a repeated sensory stimulus.

Superior longitudinal fasciculus. White matter pathway linking temporal, parietal, occipital, and frontal lobes; supports dorsal stream for language.

Syntax. Grammar, Word organization to form sentences.

Task switching. Ability to focus attention on different cues or demands between two tasks.

Temporal-amygdala-orbitofrontal network. Network involved in linking outcome and emotional response to behavior/situation.

Ventral stream. Bilateral system linking anterior temporal lobe components to posterior middle temporal and inferior temporal gyri to support language understanding.

Ventromedial prefrontal cortex (VMPFC or VMPC). Another name for the OFVMC; involved in motivational decision-making and social awareness.

Wernicke's area. Temporal lobe site originally thought to be the locus for speech recognition/reception.

Word deafness. Inability to distinguish words from other sounds due to bilateral damage of the superior temporal gyri.

Working memory. Ability to retain and/or manipulate information cognitively for immediate use.

ABBREVIATIONS

ACC	anterior cingulate cortex
DLPFC	dorsolateral prefrontal cortex
EF	executive function
LDP	long-term depression
LTP	long-term potentiation
OFC	orbitofrontal cortex
OFVMC	orbitofrontal ventromedial cortex
PGSD	post-traumatic stress disorder
VMPFC/VMPC	ventromedial prefrontal cortex

Child Development

Deborah S. Nichols-Larsen

OBJECTIVES

1) Identify typical development associated with any given age across each developmental domain: gross motor, fine motor, oromotor/language, socioemotional/cognitive

2) Integrate the progressions of development with the underlying changes in the nervous system

3) Explore the influences of environment and experience on development

● INTRODUCTION

For any therapist, it is an expectation that they understand typical sensorimotor development to effectively identify atypical development and to understand some of the movement patterns demonstrated by patients with neurologic disorders. This chapter will introduce the reader to typical sensorimotor development in relation to the maturation of the nervous system, beginning during the fetal period and extending through adolescence, when mature movement patterns have been achieved. Although physical therapists aren't typically responsible for evaluating fine motor skills, and language, social, or cognitive skills, typical development in each of these areas is described to afford the practitioner with the knowledge to develop suitable activities for therapy as well as to provide a basis for subsequent referral to appropriate practitioners, when a delay is suspected. However, it should always be kept in mind that children develop at different rates, depending on environment, experience, maturation, and personality, so ages of behavior are averages with some children acquiring certain skills earlier or later than others.

Development can be divided into five domains: (1) gross motor – large muscle movements; (2) fine motor – small dexterous movements of the hand that support activities of daily living; (3) language – the acquisition of verbal and nonverbal expressive and receptive communication skills; (4) cognitive – the ability to reason, problem-solve, and remember; and (5) socioemotional/behavioral – the development of attachment to others, the ability to regulate behavior (self-regulation), and to interact in many environments with others.[1] For the discussion of early development, we have added oromotor development to language, as the two are related and eating is critical for adequate nutrition and overall development. We will also include some discussion of maturation of the special senses in the infant.

While the development of the neural tube and the nervous system are described in detail in Chapter 19 in relation to neural tube disorders, and developmental neuroplasticity is described in more detail in Chapter 9, we will just introduce some general concepts as they relate to behavioral development in this chapter. Brain development occurs as a process of neural and glial cell proliferation, migration of these cells to the appropriate target region, axonal growth, and synapse proliferation, followed by pruning of synapses, based on usage with those underutilized dying and those utilized most strengthening their connections. Our discussion of behavioral development will include the underlying neurologic changes, supporting these behaviors.

● FETAL STAGE

Motor Development

Fetal movements are first noticeable via ultrasound imaging about week 7 of gestational age (GA); these early movements are so small that they are referred to as **"just discernable" movements**. These early movements are initially characterized by slow bending of either the head or pelvis laterally in isolation or together; within days, the lateral bending of these two segments is accompanied by lateral arm and/or leg movement. Eventually, this lateral bending will incorporate both the arm(s) and leg(s).[2] Emergence of these early slow movements coincides with synapse development in the spinal cord, thought to relate to the development of central pattern generators (see Chapter 4) that will later control rhythmic movements such as locomotion.[3]

By GA week 9, single, quicker, isolated extension of either the arm, leg, or trunk can be seen, followed shortly by extension of both the arm and leg (week 11); these extensor movements increase in speed and become *twitches*. Thus, the slow bending movements disappear as these more generalized movements (GM) appear.[3] GMs are spontaneous and characterized by more variability in speed, direction, and amplitude, eventually incorporating multiple body parts.[4] Also between 10 and 12 weeks, isolated movements of the neck are seen: first extension (**retroflexion**), then flexion (**anteflexion**), and lastly rotation.[2] During this same time period, initial movement of the hands to the face can be seen; interestingly, thumb sucking has been observed by 15 weeks' GA. The frequency of hand-to-face movements increases over the remainder of the gestational period with the ability to slow the movement velocity, when approaching the eyes rather than the mouth noted; however, the amount of reaching is equally distributed between the upper and lower parts of the face.[3]

Other behaviors progressively emerge between weeks 9 and 14, including breathing, hiccups, and startle (9 weeks); jaw opening, sucking, and swallowing (10 weeks); stretch (11 weeks); yawning (12 weeks); isolated finger movements (11-13 weeks); and stepping-like movements (14 weeks). These complex GMs occur simultaneously with synapse development of immature neurons, originating in the subcortical plate of the developing cortex.[3] While these many movements occur from 9 to 14 weeks, most mothers report feeling their babies move between weeks 16 and 18. Fetal movement occurs up to 100 times per hour but demonstrates wide variability throughout the day and between babies. The size of the baby, the position in the uterus (e.g., breech less than head down), and gender (male more than female), as well as environmental noise, maternal glucose levels, and consumption of some substances (e.g., alcohol, caffeine), effect fetal movement. Diminished fetal movement can be a sign of fetal distress.[5]

GMs characterize movement throughout the remainder of gestation and into the first months of infant movement. Over these months, they increasingly become more forceful, incorporate a wider variety of muscles, including co-contraction of agonists and antagonists, and, thereby, become more complex. At the end of the gestational period (GA 36-38 weeks), GMs are characterized as **writhing**, referring to the larger forceful but slow movements of the extremities expressed with little trunk movement. Also noted in this time period, the neonate transitions from a posture of extension to one increasingly characterized by flexion, beginning in the legs but followed closely by the arms.[3]

Oral Motor Development

Between 15 weeks, when fetal thumb sucking is first observed, and 38 to 40 weeks GA, the fetus demonstrates increasingly complex movements of the mouth and tongue. Sucking and swallowing movements become more frequent. Initial jaw and tongue movements are simple, but by 28 weeks of gestation, repetitive mouth opening and closing as well as forward and backward tongue movements and fetal sucking in response to face touching are present. The **rooting reflex** has been reported to emerge at the same time as early fetal sucking (12-15 weeks) and continues for the first months of life. This involves head turning and mouth opening in response to touch to the side of the face. These early oral behaviors and their mature counterparts are controlled by neural networks in the brainstem (central pattern generators), which are modulated by higher centers and mature through experience (plasticity). During the latter part of gestation, complex facial movements are noted, characteristic of facial expressions of emotion (e.g., smiling, crying, and distress).[3]

Sensory Development

Sensory system development also occurs in a predictable order during gestation, beginning with the cutaneous system and followed by progressive development of the other sensory systems: smell and taste; vestibular and hearing; and finally vision. For cutaneous sensation, there is also a predictable order with responsiveness to perioral stimulation (7-8 weeks GA) preceding hand and foot palmar surfaces (10 weeks GA), followed by the abdomen (15 weeks GA). The spinothalamic tract is apparent by week 19 and myelinated by week 29; thalamocortical projections are evident by 26 weeks and are functional by week 29. Taste buds are present by 8 weeks, taste pores by 14 weeks such that some taste discrimination is likely by this stage; this system appears mature by the 4th month with changes in swallowing noted to injections of sweet (increased swallowing) or sour (decreased swallowing) to the amniotic fluid by 34 weeks (GA). Similarly the olfactory system (smell) is fairly mature by the end of the second trimester. On the other hand, the development of the ear begins at week 4 but all of its components to support vestibular function and hearing aren't complete until the 8th month. Yet, by week 18, some vestibular reflexes are evident; the auditory startle can be elicited by week 24; and hearing is reactive by week 29 and attuned to the mother's voice by week 34. The cornea is apparent by the 8th week but the retina isn't formed until week 24; however, eye movement is visible between weeks 16 and 20 with consistent pupillary reflexes by week 34.[6]

At birth, the central nervous system is quite immature in comparison to other organ systems; the processes of axonal growth, synapse formation, and pruning are continuing and the process of myelination is just beginning (see Box 8-1). Maturation of the nervous system continues until young adulthood. Thus, behavioral development over the first 20 years of life results from a combination of neural maturation and experience, including the environment, in which the child develops, and the opportunities to explore that environment. There are also periods of development, called **sensitive periods**, where the brain seems particularly ready for a given area to mature, and for some neural components, it is critical that they experience certain stimulation to assure complete maturation (see Box 8-2).[7,8]

Box 8-1 Myelination as a Correlate for Behavioral Maturation

At birth, the structures of the brain have been formed; however, the brain is far from mature. After birth, there continues to be additional axonal expansion, deepening of the sulci, further pruning and synapse formation, and initiation of the myelination process.[7] Myelination progresses in a systematic manner with sensorimotor systems completing their myelination by about 4 years of age. By age 6, the brain has reached about 90% of its adult size. The areas of the parietal and temporal lobes, supporting language and spatial awareness, are myelinated by about age 10. Areas of the brain that support higher level executive function (problem-solving, attention modulation, sensorimotor integration) mature last with myelination completed in adolescence (16-18 years). Completion of myelination correlates with improved performance of skills and abilities controlled by these developing areas; however, further training is necessary for each newly myelinated system to mature to adult levels of performance. This maturation involves additional strengthening of relevant synapses and pruning of irrelevant ones.[8]

Sensitive periods are time-limited stages of neurodevelopment, during which the brain is particularly influenced by the environment, leading to stimulation-induced plasticity (synaptic and structural change of neurons). A critical period is a very specific type of sensitive period, wherein the child must experience a specific type of stimulation to induce brain development or the development will not occur to the same degree. In humans, these critical periods can last years. The neural environment must demonstrate the appropriate balance between excitation and inhibition to create the optimal milieu for neural remodeling; when this balance changes, the critical period closes.

The neurologic changes induced, during a critical or sensitive period, are relatively permanent and involve structural modification of the nervous system, including synapse formation or elimination; sprouting of axons and dendrites or resorption; and enhanced rigidity in the extracellular matrix. (The extracellular matrix is a collection of macromolecules [e.g., proteins, collagen], which provides structural support to the cells of the nervous system [neurons and glia].)

THE FIRST 3 MONTHS (THE FIRST QUARTER)

Neural Maturation

At birth, all brain structures and white matter tracts are evident[12]; however, the corpus callosum is very thin in the newborn but begins to thicken at the genu over the first 2 to 3 months of life.[13] Initial myelination is seen in the dorsal pons, superior cerebellar peduncles, the ventrolateral thalamus, and the posterior limb of the internal capsule; these are all components of the motor system. Over the first quarter of life, the myelination proceeds in these areas to include the cerebral peduncles, more of the internal capsule, and portions of the pre- and post-central gyri. There is also some myelination within the hippocampus.[7,13] One means of identifying activity within brain areas is to measure glucose metabolism. In the newborn, the greatest level of glucose metabolism is seen in the primary sensory and motor cortices, the thalamus, brainstem, and central cerebellum (vermis); these are areas associated with cutaneous sensation and movement as well as primitive reflexes and vital functions. Similarly, there is greater metabolic activity in the amygdala and cingulate cortex, areas involved in emotion, to support the emergence of attachment to care providers. Other brain areas demonstrate minimal glucose usage initially consistent with a reliance on reflexive function. By 2 to 3 months, increased metabolic activity is seen in the primary visual cortex, associated with improved visuomotor skills, and the parietal and temporal lobes, associated with enhanced visuomotor and sensorimotor integration. In addition, the basal ganglia and the cerebellar hemispheres increase their activity, coinciding with increased movement and the onset of early postural reactions.[14] This time period is considered a **critical period** in primary sensory development, especially for the visual cortex.[15]

Gross Motor

Posture: The newborn's posture is one of flexion and asymmetry with the head turned to the side. This flexion, referred to as **physiologic flexion**, is thought to result from a change in muscle elasticity secondary to confinement in the uterine environment in the last months of gestation. It results in a resistance to extension in the newborn and a predominance of flexion in all postures. The head also appears large for the body and is often misshaped at birth due to skull compression during the birth process; this compression is facilitated by soft spaces between the cranial bones, called *fontanelles*, which allow the bones to slide over each other during birth.[16]

In prone, the neonates flexed hips and knees along with an anterior pelvic tilt shift their weight forward to the chest and head, often with the arms trapped under the chest. Despite their larger head-to-body relative size, even newborns have the capacity to lift their head momentarily to turn it to the side, so that the airway is clear. In supine, the legs are flexed at the hip, knee, and ankle with the feet off of the support surface, but physiologic flexion keeps the head somewhat in midline for the first few weeks. Also, the newborn is slightly less flexed in supine than in prone due to the **tonic labyrinthine reflex**, which enhances flexion in prone and extension in supine, caused by activity in the inner ear labyrinthine receptors. Over the first 2 months, physiologic flexion decreases, and the baby will lay flat on the surface in prone with the legs extended, externally rotated, and abducted at the hip; the knees and ankles remain partially flexed. In supine, the head lags more to the side and the decrease in lower extremity flexion allows the feet to rest on the support surface. With the head lagging to the side, there is considerable influence of the **asymmetrical tonic neck reflex** (ATNR) on the posturing of the arm and leg of the 2- to 3-month-old with greater flexion on the skull-side extremities and less on the face-side extremities (see Table 8-1). The ATNR is just one of many primitive reflexes that influence movement in the first months of life (see Box 8-3).[17,18]

Head control: At birth, the neonate can hold his head erect for just a few seconds, when the trunk is well supported (e.g., when held in sitting or at the caregiver's shoulder); otherwise the head flexes and bobs forward. In supported sitting, the back is rounded with the head forward and bobbing up and down, associated with brief extensor muscle activity. It is critical for infants to spend time in prone to achieve early motor milestones and prevent a flattening of the posterior aspect of the head, so parents should be advised to place infants on their tummies periodically throughout the day, targeting at least 30 minutes daily, but not for sleeping to avoid sudden infant death syndrome.[16] By 1.5 months, infants begin to lift their head briefly, when their stomach touches a support surface (prone body on head righting, see Table 8-2), and by 2 months, the infant will briefly lift their chest from the support surface while lifting their head in prone.[1] However, when pulled to sit, the infant's head lags behind the shoulders (Figure 8-3).

By 3 months, an infant has achieved the ability to keep the head stable and in line with the trunk, when the trunk is supported in sitting or when held upright at the caregiver's shoulder.[3] Over the first 3 months, the infant increases the frequency

TABLE 8-1 Primitive Reflexes[17]

REFLEX	DESCRIPTION	AGE SEEN
Asymmetric tonic neck reflex (ATNR)	Lateral head turning leads to flexion of the extremities on the skull side and extension (less flexion) on the face side	0-3 months
Crossed extensor reflex	Passive flexion of one leg is associated with extension of the other leg	0-6 weeks
Extensor thrust	Pushing on the foot elicits strong extension of the leg	0-2 months
Flexor withdrawal reflex	A tap to the heel or pulling of the great toe results in leg flexion away from the stimulus	0-2 months
Galant (truncal incurvation)	Stroking the lateral part of the trunk produces trunk flexing away from the stimulus (e.g., right stroke – convexity of trunk incurvation to the right)	0-4 months
Moro	Loss of balance backward toward the support surface from a sitting position, elicits abduction of the arms (away from midline), followed by adduction of the arms (toward midline) and trunk flexion	0-6 months
Palmar grasp	Applying pressure to the palm of the hand elicits grasping (baby will hold the tester's finger)	0-6 months
Plantar grasp	Pressure on the ball of the foot will elicit toe flexion as if to grasp with the toes	0-15 months
Positive support (primitive standing)	Placing an infant in a standing position results in leg and trunk extension	0-2 months
Rooting	Stroking the cheek elicits head turning, as if to find a nipple	0-4 months
Stepping	Placing an infant in a standing position and leaning them forward, will elicit stepping	0-2 months
Suprapubic reflex	Pressure above the pubic bone elicits bilateral extension and internal rotation of both lower extremities with plantarflexion of both feet	0-1 month
Symmetric tonic neck reflex (STNR)	Neck flexion leads to UE flexion and LE extension; neck extension leads to UE extension and LE flexion	0-4 months
Tonic labyrinthine reflex	Prone – increased flexion throughout Supine – extensor influence throughout (less flexion in the very young infant)	0-4 months

Box 8-3 Primitive Reflexes[17,18]

Primitive reflexes are controlled by networks in the spinal cord and brainstem, which are active at birth (Table 8-1; Figure 8-1). As the nervous system matures, these reflexes integrate into more complex patterns of movement under higher motor center control (e.g., cortex) but are no longer elicited as a reflexive response. One example of this involves head movement that elicits stereotypical body movements: (1) ATNR – lateral head turn elicits flexion (or more flexion) on the skull-side extremities and extension (less flexion) of the face-side extremities; and (2) symmetrical tonic neck – neck flexion elicits arm flexion and leg extension while neck extension elicits arm extension and leg flexion. **Infantile stepping** is another example of a primitive reflex; when the infant is suspended and tilted slightly forward with the feet on a solid surface, the newborn will step repeatedly. This stepping ability typically disappears by 2 to 3 months as the infant increases in size and weight, referred to as **abasia** (the inability to walk; see Figure 8-2A), until about 4 to 5 months, when the infant begins supported standing. Training of these stepping movements in 2- to 5-month-olds, through supported treadmill experiences, has been able to maintain

them through this period; however, most infants experience several months during which stepping and standing are not observed. It appears that the disappearance of stepping is largely due to the inability of the legs to support the infant's body weight rather than a loss of this movement pattern. Infantile stepping is characterized by excessive hip and knee flexion as well as more activity in their antagonists (extensors); it's postulated that this movement pattern is the product of an immature central pattern generator. Similarly, newborns stand when their feet are placed on a supporting surface, characterized by extensive extension in the legs and trunk. By 3 months, this primary standing has also disappeared, and the infant demonstrates leg flexion when held upright on a support surface; this is referred to as **astasia** (no stance) and will last until month 4 or so.[3]

and magnitude of head lifting in prone, which often includes chest lifting, and the beginning of weight-bearing on forearms briefly (**prone propping**). In supine, as the neck flexors increase in strength, the head is seen increasingly in midline,[18] and infants can lift their legs off the supporting surface via active hip flexion. Early postural adjustments can be seen to external

TABLE 8-2	**Righting, Protective, and Equilibrium Reactions**[17,19,20]	
RIGHTING REACTIONS	**ORIENT HEAD TO THE BODY**	
Rotational Righting	Turning a segment of the body (e.g., head) elicits rotation of the rest of the body in a "log roll" fashion	Present up to 6-12 months
Body on Head	Touching the body to a support surface elicits lifting of the head	
	Prone	Emerges 1.5-4 months
	Supine	Emerges 4-6 months
Vertical Righting	Orients head to vertical position	
Optical Righting	Holds head erect when tilted to the side, using visual input	Emerges 2.5-6 months
Labyrinthine Righting Reaction	Holds head erect when tilted to the side when vision is occluded	Emerges 3-6 months
Prone Vertical Righting (Landau)	Hold child in a supported prone position (arms under stomach and hips)	
	Partial – head up to 45 degrees	Emerges 2.5-4 months
	Mature – head up to 90 degrees	Emerges by 10 months
Protective Responses	Protect infant from falling	
Prone (parachute)	The child extends the arms when quickly moved from upright toward the support surface (face down)	Emerges 6-7 months
Sitting	Arm extends when the child falls in a given direction	
	Forward	Emerges 6-11 months
	Lateral (to the side)	Emerges 6-11 months
	Backward	Emerges 9-12 months
Tilting/Equilibrium Reactions	When destabilized the child will right themselves through muscle activity in the neck, trunk, arms, and legs; elicited by moderate perturbations that are insufficient to elicit a protective reaction.	
Prone	On an unstable surface (e.g., rocker board), the child will curve the trunk and extend the arm and leg away from the downward slope	Emerges 5-9 months
Supine	In supine on an unstable surface, the child demonstrates trunk incurvation away from tip with accompanying arm reach	Emerges 7-11 months
Sitting	In sitting, the child can right themselves to a loss of balance (first forward, then lateral and finally backward)	Emerges 7-8 months
Quadruped	While child is in quadruped, disturb balance to the side, will curve trunk to opposite side to return to stability	Emerges 8-12 months
Standing	With child in standing, disturb balance in any direction; extreme disturbance may elicit a step	Emerges 12-21 months

perturbations that are direction specific as early as one month of age; by 2 months, anticipatory postural reflexes are emerging such as increased trunk co-contraction prior to being lifted.[3]

Movement: Writhing movements are still noted in the early postnatal weeks but are replaced by **fidgety** movements by 6 to 8 weeks; these are smaller, more irregular movements. The onset of fidgety movements coincides with active synapse activity between the corticospinal projections and motor neurons in the spinal cord. Fidgety movements increase until 11 to 16 weeks of age and then disappear as the infant develops more

purposeful movements, fading out completely by 5 months or so.[3,4] Interestingly, in these early months, hyperkinetic movements like those seen in movement disorders are commonly seen: dystonic – twisting repetitive movements; myoclonic – sudden quick jerks; choreatic – slow, writhing-like movements.[4] Myoclonic twitches result from bursts of activity in spinal cord neurons, activated by brainstem centers.[21] It is likely that the other hyperkinetic movements also result from bursts of activity in the immature nervous system. These hyperkinetic movements disappear as the nervous system matures over the first

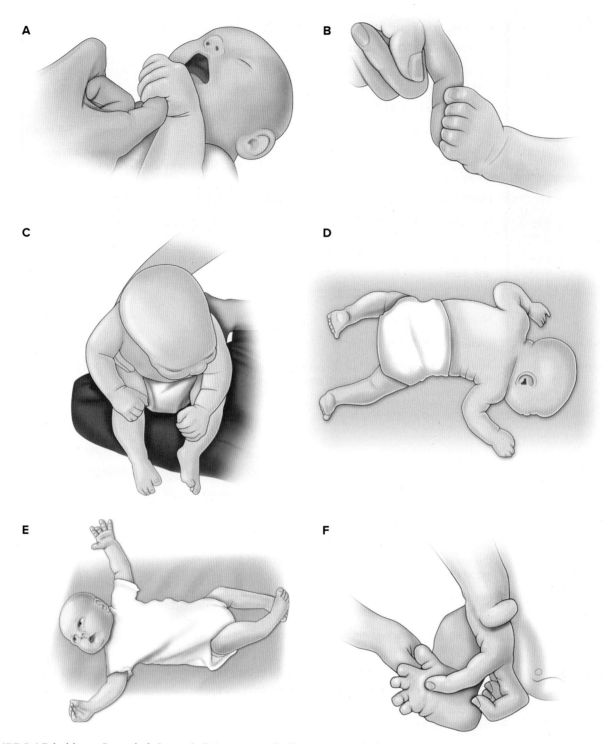

FIGURE 8-1 Primitive reflexes in infants. A. Palmar grasp. **B.** Plantar grasp. **C.** Symmetrical tonic neck in prone – flexion of neck is associated with UE flexion and LE extension. **D.** Asymmetrical tonic neck – head turn to side elicits extension (less flexion) of face-side extremities and more flexion of skull-side extremities. **E.** Moro – quick drop of head backward elicits abduction of arms (shown), followed by adduction as though reaching toward the holder. **F.** Babinski – splaying of toes and hallux extension to stroking the bottom of the foot.

three months, associated with increasing connections between the cortex and other motor areas; persistence of these hyperkinetic movements can be a sign of abnormality.[4]

Motor development in the first 3 months involves the exploration of movement through variable arm, leg, trunk, and head movements. Motor control proceeds in a **cephalocaudal** (head to toe) and proximal to distal manner; it also proceeds from generalized (large whole extremity or body movement) to differentiated (smaller single segment or extremity) movement patterns. For example, newborns kick with the joints of the leg coupled together (flexion then extension in all joints), quickly alternating between legs for up to 80 kicks per minute when

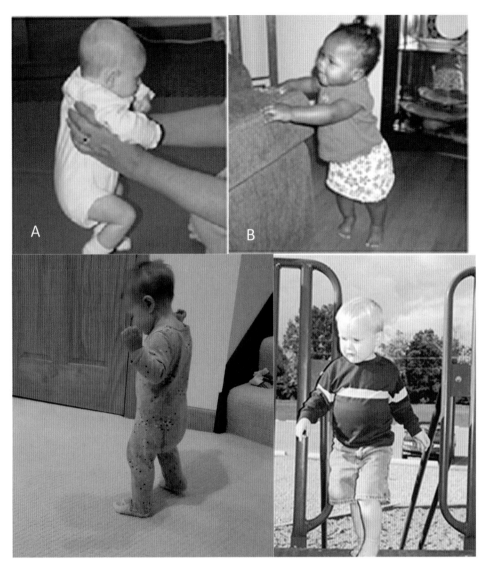

FIGURE 8-2 Development of walking. A. Astasia/abasia – infants flex legs when feet are touched to a surface. **B.** Cruising – 9- to 11-month-olds walk sideways while holding onto furniture, often on toes. **C.** Initial walking with arms in high guard position and wide base of support (10-15 months). **D.** Mature walking with arm swing and narrow base of support (18-24 months).

awake and active. Over the first 2 months, there is an increase in single-leg kicks and the tight coupling of the joints of the limb begins to fade. Some infants will show a preference for kicking one leg over the other, but they are able to kick both legs.[22] Early on, the infant also demonstrates what is called rotational righting, where turning of a body segment results in the entire body following (e.g., the care provider rotates the baby's right leg to the left side and the whole body follows); this will continue up to 6 months of age. The diminishing of primitive reflex influences over the first quarter allows for increasing variability of movement as the quarter ends.[17] Table 8-3 outlines gross motor skill acquisition over the first year of life.

Fine Motor

Physiologic flexion affects the arms as well as the legs and results in the arms being adducted at the shoulder and flexed at the elbows with hands fisted in the newborn when prone; similarly, in supine, the shoulders are retracted, the elbows flexed, and the hands fisted. Yet, in both postures, frequent hand opening is seen.[18] Arm movements in the newborn are ineffective but can be directed toward objects; however, these movements are synergistic, such that arm extension occurs with hand opening and flexion with fisting. Thus, the infant can't grasp an object even if contacted with the extended arm. Further, the fisting of the hand typically occurs with the thumb inside the fingers (palm). Infants demonstrate reflexive grasping (another primitive reflex) to objects placed in the palm but quickly drop the object as the arm moves.[16]

Over the first 3 months, there is an increase in hand opening, and the infant begins to coordinate visual gaze to an object with head turning and directional reaching toward the object. Head movement now accompanies visual tracking of objects.[16] The hand-to-face exploration, seen in utero, continues through the first 2 to 3 months with increasing frequency of hand-to-mouth exploration as this early time period ends; by 2 months of age, infants will bring hands to midline.[1] Toward the 3rd month,

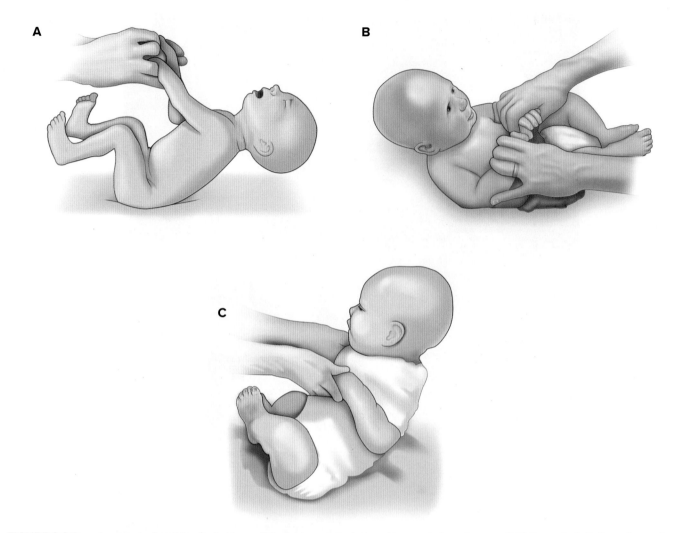

FIGURE 8-3 Development of pull to sit. A. Young infants demonstrate head lag and absent arm pull (0-3 months). **B.** 3- to 4-month-olds keep head in line with trunk and begin to pull with arms. **C.** Mature — head precedes trunk with strong arm pull (4-6 months).

TABLE 8-3	Gross Motor Skills: Birth to 24 Months[18–20]	
SKILL	**DESCRIPTION**	**AVERAGE AGE OF ACQUISITION**
Head Control		
Upright (held)	Bobs up and down Steady and in line with trunk	0-2 months 2-3 months
Prone	Able to turn head to clear airway Able to lift head and chest briefly Able to keep head in line with trunk, lifting head and trunk from bed Lifts head 60° with weight on forearms Lifts head 90° with weight on extended arms	0-2 months 2-2.5 months 2.5-3 months 3-4 months 4-6 months
Supine	Head lags to side Head in midline Neck flexion to lift head from surface	0-2 months 2-3 months 4-6 months
Pull to sit	Head lags behind body Head held in line with body some arm pull Head leads the trunk with strong arm pull and hip flexion	0-3 months 3-4 months 4-6 months

TABLE 8-3	Gross Motor Skills: Birth to 24 Months[18–20] *(continued)*	
SKILL	**DESCRIPTION**	**AVERAGE AGE OF ACQUISITION**
Rolling		
Rolls to Sidelying	Log roll from prone or supine to side, often initiated by reaching or looking	2-4 months
Log rolling both directions	Supine to prone; prone to supine – roll as a unit (no trunk rotation)	5-7 months
Mature rolling	Can lead with head, arm, and/or leg with trunk rotation	7-9 month
Sitting		
Sits when placed Sits with one-hand support Sits independently (15 min) Independent sitting	Trunk is flexed forward with weight on forearms Sits upright and is able to free one hand to play Trunk is erect and can free hands to play Able to assume sitting & reach in all directions	4-5 months 5-6 months 6-7 months 8-9 months
Mobllity/Locomotion		
Pivoting in prone Crawling Creeping Cruising Plantigrade walking Walking	Moving in a circular fashion while in a prone prop position Move on belly, first moving arms together followed by legs and eventually alternating arms and legs (arms do more work) Movement on hands and knees Lateral movement while holding onto furniture Movement on hands and feet Independent locomotion with hands in high guard, hips and knees slightly bent, and a wide base of support	6-8 months 3-6 months 9-11 months 9-11 months 10-12 months 10-15 months
Transitional Movements		
Sit to prone	Initial – fold forward over their legs, sliding their legs into extension; mature – rotation to the side to place hands on the floor and extend legs	6-9 months
Prone to sit	Initial – push upward into quadruped and then backward into sitting with limited trunk rotation and hip flexion and external rotation Mature – may assume sidelying and pushup or assume quadruped and rotate through the trunk and hips to sit	8-11 months
Sit to quadruped	Similar to sit to prone, initial sit to quadruped transitions are completed with limited trunk rotation but rotation and flexibility in patterns used increases with maturity	9-11 months
Pull to stand	Infants typically assume a kneeling position in front of a support and use both hands to pull to standing, moving both legs into extension simultaneously	9-12 months
Pull to stand with ½ kneeling	Pull to kneeling and then assume ½ kneeling (one knee up with foot flat on the floor) and then pull to stand; this requires less arm pull and more active knee extension in the forward leg	11-13 months
Standing to sitting (controlled)	Lowers himself to the floor with graduate knee flexion and arm support	11-13 months
Floor to standing without pull	Assumes weight-bearing on feet and hands, shifts weight backward, and rises	15-18 months
Squat and return to standing	Flexes at hip and knees into squat and uses leg extension to return, initially with trunk extension	15-18 months

TABLE 8-4	Fine Motor Skills in the First 24 Months[18–20]	
AGE (MONTHS)	**FINE MOTOR SKILL**	**DESCRIPTION**
0-2	Hand fisting	Hands are closed most of the time
	Palmar grasp	Grasp of any object placed in hand, typically holds for <10 seconds
2-4	Hand opening at rest	Increasing time spent with hand open and not fisted (or loosely fisted)
	Shakes rattle	Will shake rattle when held in hand for <20 seconds
4-6	Plays with hands	Brings hands together and to mouth
	Grasps objects	Will reach for and grasp objects within arm's reach in supine, prone, and supported sitting (whole hand grasp)
	Brings toys together	Will bang blocks or other items within each hand together, briefly
6-8	Grasps block	Uses thumb, index, and middle finger (3 jaw chuck grasp)
	Brings toys to mouth	Toys are typically brought to mouth to chew or "experience"
		Begins transferring items from one hand to the other
8-10	Grasps smaller objects	Will grasp small items (e.g., cereal) with a raking motion of all fingers (thumb will move from middle to lateral over this 2-month period)
	Removes pegs	Will remove peg from pegboard and explore opening with isolated finger
	Claps	Begins clapping hands together in imitation
10-12	Pincer grasp	Will grasp a small item (e.g., cereal) with pad of thumb and index finger
	Places objects	Will place block or other small objects in a container
12-14	Places pegs	Places up to 3 pegs in pegboard
	Puzzles	Begins placing simple shapes in a puzzle (circle, square)
	Feeding	Feeds finger foods to self
14-16	Scribbling	Begins scribbling with crayon, no hand preference; holds crayon with thumb and first finger
	Stacks blocks	Can stack 2-3 blocks
	Utensils for eating	Begins to play with utensil but still primarily uses fingers
16-24	Turns book pages	Can turn pages in books (may tear paper page)
	Vertical drawing	Can draw or imitate drawing a vertical line (still no hand preference)
	Utensil	Improved feeding with fork and spoon – scoops and stabs food

the hand is open at rest more than fisted.[3] Initial grasping at 3 months occurs with the lateral aspect of the hand (**ulnar palmar grasp**) and is often achieved with a raking motion.[23] The infant will shake a rattle or other toy by 2 to 4 months (see Table 8-4 for the progression of fine motor skills).[19]

● ORAL MOTOR/LANGUAGE

At the time of full-term birth, neonates demonstrate tongue movements, during sucking, that are very similar to adults; however, they have to perfect the timing of their breathing to their sucking and swallowing. The coordination of these activities takes months until they master swallowing at the transition between inspiration and expiration (the cusp), as is seen in adults; there is considerable variability between infants in the time needed

to develop this mature pattern, extending from 1 to 12 months. Often, early sucking is characterized by bouts of sucking and swallowing interspersed with bouts of respiration; not unusually, the neonate has episodes of sucking/swallowing during respiration, which can induce aspiration and coughing. Maturation of sucking is associated with increased milk intake.[3] In addition, newborns are able to make a number of sounds, separate from crying, that expand in variety and frequency over the first few months, characterized mostly by vowel-like sounds (oohs and aahs; cooing) with some squeals evident by 2 to 3 months.[1,3,24]

Sensory

The newborn has one-third the cones within the retina than an adult, and the fovea (the central part of the retina with the greatest cone density) is particularly immature, contributing to blurred vision in newborns. In addition, the eyeball is shorter, which results in the visual image being projected "beyond" the retina (hyperopia); immaturity in the optic nerve and visual cortex also contributes to the immaturity of vision in the very young newborn.[25] However, at birth, infants will visually orient to sounds and will startle to unexpected voices or sounds[1,26]; they can also see objects within inches of their face and will track slow-moving objects, but this occurs with repetitive saccades rather than smooth movements.[1,27] By 2 months, infants track with smooth horizontal eye movements[27] and make connections between sensations and things heard or seen (e.g., will look longer at an object that they have held in their hand).[28] By 3 months, they track objects that are moved in circles.[1]

Socioemotional/Cognitive

The facial expressions, noted in gestation, are observed in the newborn randomly and with increasing variability. Very early, the neonate will imitate sticking out the tongue, when observed in another person, which is a fun thing to do with any newborn. By 2 months, they will open their mouth when a bottle is sighted. However, by weeks 6 to 10, most infants will smile in response to observing a smile in another (social smiling) and in response to seeing their primary caregiver(s), and by 3 months begin to chuckle.[1] At birth, newborns also demonstrate a preference for their mother's voice over others and prefer to look at faces over other objects, tracking them as they move.[1,3,24] By 2 months, they visually recognize their primary caregiver(s).[1]

● MONTHS 3 TO 6 (THE 2ND QUARTER)

Neural Maturation

The second quarter is a time of extensive pruning in the sensorimotor system with the networks between the cortex and the basal ganglia and cerebellum active, supporting more goal-directed movements.[4] The splenium of the corpus callosum thickens to match the size of the genu by 7 months.[13] Myelination of the sensorimotor cortex continues, and now the anterior limb of the internal capsule and the anterior portion (splenium) of the corpus callosum show initial myelination by 4 months along with the corona radiata.[7,13] By 6 months, the genu of the corpus callosum shows myelin.[13] Glucose metabolism starts to increase in the frontal cortex, beginning at 6 months, to support the development of early cognitive skill.[14]

Gross Motor

Infants 3 to 6 months of age demonstrate an increasing variability in movement and progressive increase in strength. At 3 months, infants are able to volitionally lift both legs from the support surface in supine with weight-bearing on the upper gluteals, which strengthens the abdominal muscles[16]; similarly, by 5 to 6 months there's increased variability in kicking behavior with simultaneous bilateral kicking most frequent.[22] Over the next 2 months, they will increasingly bring hands to feet and will attempt to bring the feet to the mouth; they also begin to bridge in supine and may scoot this way, pushing forward toward the head.[18] The beginning of anticipatory postural adjustments are seen in the trunk in preparation for lifting or prior to arm lift in supported sitting at 4 months.[3]

Head control matures over this time period with gradual strengthening of neck muscles and the ability to co-contract flexors and extensors for stability. While at 3 months, infants are able to maintain their head in line with the trunk in prone and upright for brief periods, over the second quarter, they progress to hold their head at 60 degrees upright from the trunk, begin propping on their elbows (prone prop), may lift both arms and legs from the mat as though swimming (**pivot prone**), and may begin to inch forward on their belly.[3] By 6 months, they can maintain the head at 90 degrees and begin to weight bear on hands with elbows extended and on one arm to reach for objects; crawling may be initiated with arms moved first then legs (inch worm style).[1,16] *Note: crawling refers to movement on the stomach; creeping involves movement on hands and knees; while the lay public refers to the latter as crawling, this is a critical difference for pediatric therapists. This distinction is not used unanimously around the world or by various assessment tools, so it may be best to refer to belly crawling and quadruped* **creeping** *for clarity.* Reaching in prone initiates elongation of the trunk on one side (dissociation) as well as strengthening of the scapular adductors and trunk muscles.[18]

Supine neck flexion similarly increases over this 2nd quarter as reaching across midline emerges, incorporating head lifting and rotation. When the caregiver lays the baby down in supine, touching of the back elicits neck flexion and head lifting (supine body on head righting) by 4 to 6 months. When pulled to sit from supine, head lag is gone by 4 months, and the head is held in line with the body. By 6 months, the infant begins to pull with the arms and the head leads the trunk (Figure 8-3C).[1] As head control matures, the infant also starts to demonstrate vertical righting reactions (see Table 8-2) that help align the head when the body is tilted or repositioned.

By 4 months most infants will be rolling to their sides, and by 6 to 7 months, most are rolling supine to prone and prone to supine. Historically, most infants rolled prone to supine first, triggered by tracking or reaching for an object from a prone prop position with subsequent falling over. Repeating this activity led to rolling prone to supine. Supine to prone rolling typically occurred slightly later (within weeks) due to the more active antigravity nature of this movement. However, with infants spending more time in supine due to concerns with prone sleeping, rolling supine to prone may proceed prone to supine rolling, or they may occur almost simultaneously.[1,29] Notably, infants initially roll with the whole body aligned (log rolling), facilitated by the head-on-body reaction (described in Table 8-2) and won't demonstrate mature rolling with trunk rotation, in which they can lead with the head or the leg, until closer to 8 months.[29] The earliest protective response is also noted in this quarter with the infant extending their arms and hands when they are quickly moved toward a support surface in a prone position (**parachute response**).[17]

Infants will also resume standing when held upright during the 4th month and will enjoy bouncing in this position when supported; in standing, the legs are abducted, knees often flexed, and feet flat. The 5-month-old is beginning to sit, when placed with the trunk in a forward flexed position, hips widely abducted, flexed and externally rotated, and weight on their forearms, but quickly this transforms into upright sitting with extended arms for support; they will start to free one arm for reaching and play within weeks and by 6 months can sit independently without arm support for 15 to 20 minutes. The 6-month-old has a more erect posture, bearing weight on the buttocks, but their base is still wide with hip external rotation and abduction, called a *ring sitting* posture. During this progression; reaching may disturb their balance, and they may resume weight-bearing on the forearm or the extended arm to maintain balance. This is the beginning of forward and lateral protective responses (arm extension to loss of balance forward or to the side noted at 6 months).[18]

Fine Motor

The 3-month-old is actively reaching to grasp objects and the sense of touch has matured sufficiently to allow them to sense object characteristics; by 4.5 months, they are beginning to reach across midline for objects, eventually pulling themselves into a sidelying position (the beginning of rolling).[16] Reaching is characterized by multiple submovements in this early stage to correct the movement trajectory, with more submovements noted in reaching for smaller objects.[3] The hand often closes before contacting the object at 4 months,[10] but by 5 months, infants demonstrate effective goal-directed reaching.[28] Commonly, objects are brought immediately to the mouth for oral exploration, but infants also begin to shake objects to make noise (e.g., rattles).[1] Often, they will mouth and shake new objects to explore their capabilities. Five-month-old infants initiate grasping with a radial palmar grasp with the index and middle fingers and the thumb pressing the object into the palm of the hand. Release initially is involuntary, as if the infant forgets to continue holding the object, but by 6 months release is voluntary as the infant begins placing objects.[10] Also, by 6 months, the infant is grasping things with each hand, is attempting to hold their bottle, and uses a raking movement to grasp small objects; they will also bang toys together, when held in each hand.[1]

Sensory

While at birth, infants demonstrate attention to voices; by 3 months, they orient to a voice and other sounds. By 5 months, they will turn their head to find a sound out of sight. Similarly, infants recognize their parents visually by 3 months and will track objects horizontally and vertically by 5 months; also by 5 months, they start to respond to facial expressions.[1,27]

Oromotor/Language/Cognitive/Socioemotional

Piaget, a developmental psychologist, proposed a theory of cognitive development that captured the means by which children learn at different stages of life (Box 8-4). Learning in the first two years occurs through sensorimotor exploration and the repetition of activities, resulting in the understanding of cause and effect relationships.[30] The 3- to 6-month-old is playing with sounds, demonstrating increased vocalizations, and will enjoy turn-taking with caregivers, repeating sounds that they are already making and attempting new sounds. By 4 months, they are starting to make consonant sounds, using their lips (b, m, and p), and will say them repeatedly.[1,31] Social

---

| Box 8-4 | Piagetian Stages of Cognitive Development[30] |

1) **Sensorimotor Period** (birth to 18-24 months): learning is achieved through circular repetition of movement and manipulation of objects, including the sensations they experience through these movements. This begins simply as the infant moves and experiences a result, and then moves again, experiencing the same outcome. Eventually, the infant progresses from just body movements to exploration of objects, repeating object manipulation (e.g., shaking new objects to determine if they rattle) first with familiar objects and then with unfamiliar objects to explore their characteristics. Finally, they begin to manipulate objects not just with their body but with other objects (pulling a toy by the string). At the highest level of this stage, toddlers begin to manipulate novel objects, after observing other's manipulation of the object. The final component of sensorimotor learning is the development of object permanence, the awareness that objects and people continue to exist when out of sight; this includes the understanding that they are *separate* from others and objects.

2) **Preoperational Period** (ages 2-7 years): this period focuses on the development of representational thought, which includes language acquisition, imaginative play, mental imagery, the understanding of signs and symbols (letters, logos), drawing, and the ability to assimilate information to recount events. Pretend play is a key component of this stage of cognitive development where the child demonstrates mental imagery that allows him to create novel scenarios. However, preoperational period children remain egocentric, having difficulty seeing others' perspectives.

3) **Concrete Operations** (ages 7-11 years): in this stage of development, children begin to apply logic to their interactions with objects and are acquiring factual information. This includes learning the concepts of conservation (quantity, mass, and volume), reversibility (that if a taller slender container holds the same amount of sand as a shorter container, the shorter container must be fatter), and classification (categorization by shape, color, or type). They begin to use inductive logic, the ability to apply a principle (conservation of mass) to another problem (conservation of volume). At this stage, children are very literal and expect rules to be strictly followed; they often rigidly impose rules on others. However, they are less egocentric, initiating the ability to empathize with others.

4) **Formal Operations** (adolescence): teenagers begin to think abstractly and are able to apply logic to abstract concepts. This includes deductive reasoning, hypothesis testing, and the ability to manipulate multiple variables to determine the answer to a complex question. This stage is characterized by enhanced ability to see other's perspectives and "both sides" to a problem or discussion.

While there are many theories of development beyond Piaget, these stages provide a nice basis for the understanding of cognitive abilities in children.

---

interactions expand with the infant initiating verbal turn-taking by 6 months, and the infant begins to laugh in association with tickles and other interactions.[1] This maturation in oral musculature is also associated with munching behavior (upward and downward jaw movement), which prepares the infant for initial introduction of soft foods that usually occurs around 6 months of age.[32] The 6-month-old also brings most items placed in the hand to the mouth to explore them as the mouth is highly sensitive for not just eating but also for identifying object characteristics.[23] At this time, they become wary of heights and respond to gestures such as raising their arms when someone reaches to lift them; they also begin to respond to their name (5 months) and to "no" (6 months) but may only stop momentarily.[1]

● MONTHS 6 TO 9 (THE 3RD QUARTER)

Neural Maturation

While there is little change in the areas myelinated in the third quarter, this is a time of myelination thickening within the sensorimotor systems and corpus callosum that initiated myelination in the 2nd quarter.[7] By 8 to 9 months, the corpus callosum has an adult appearance, supporting increased bilateral activities.[13]

Gross Motor

The 6- to 8-month-old is maturing in the ability to sit; initially, when sitting without upper extremity support, the arms are held in a **high guard position** (elbows at shoulder height, scapula retracted) to control posture and add stability; the legs are typically externally rotated and abducted, assuming a ring position (ring sitting) to create a wide base of support. While the 6-month-old is exploring this "no hands" sitting, they quickly return the hand(s) to the floor when trying to play or reach and will still fall over when they reach too far. By 8 months, they are reaching forward and upward for toys and forward and lateral protective responses emerge (Figure 8-4), and the infant is able to rotate to reach for things to either side. This reaching and sitting behavior helps create the cervical and lumbar spinal curves.[18] Quickly (by 9 months), the infant is able to assume a sitting position (Table 8-2), typically by pushing up from prone to all fours (quadruped) and then backward into sitting with rotation of the trunk or pushing up from sidelying.[16] They also explore different sitting postures – half-ring sitting (one leg extended, one flexed and abducted), long sitting with both legs out in front, or w-sitting with the bottom between the heels. Some infants will scoot in a sitting position as a form of mobility.[18]

Infants of this age are spending more time in prone prop with arms extended, pivoting in all directions to explore their environment. Prone protective responses emerge (Table 8-2). **Crawling** (commando crawling or belly crawling) becomes the preferred movement pattern with the inchworm style giving way to a diagonal movement pattern of opposite arm and leg.[3] At this same time, they are pushing up into quadruped (all fours) from prone prop, rocking and bouncing. This pattern of assuming a position, bouncing and playing with weight-shifting, and then moving is repeated in prone prop, quadruped, and in standing. By 9 months, most infants are getting into and out of sitting and are demonstrating early creeping (crawling on all fours); similar to the belly crawling of the 6-month-old, initial creeping may involve movement of both arms before legs with a gradual emergence of a diagonal pattern of limb movement; some infants will also push up into a weight-bearing position on hands and feet.[18] Infants at this age moreover love to be in standing, often on tiptoes with legs in a wide stance and hips and knees bent. They enjoy bouncing in this position, playing with the feel of being upright.

Fine Motor

The more functional **radial palmar grasp** (thumb, index, and middle fingers) or **superior palmar grasp** (same fingers but object grasped from the top) is the preferred grasping method of the 6-month-old, also referred to as a three jaw chuck grasp, but by 7 months an **inferior pincer grasp** emerges (thumb against side of index finger). This initially requires stabilization of the forearm on a support surface but allows the infant to pick up smaller objects (e.g., cereal or snack foods). By 8 months, infants are expanding their bimanual activities, switching objects from one hand to the other, and now adjust the shape of the hand to match the object to be grasped. They will also pull a large peg from a pegboard or take a block from a bowl or cup and can bring their hands together to clap.[1,10]

Oral Motor/Language

In this third quarter, infants increasingly babble, adding more consonants and stringing them together; this strengthens their oral musculature to support eating and additional vocalizations. They also begin to make different sounds, playing with their tongue in their mouth, including making the raspberries sound by projecting air while their tongue protrudes from their mouth[24]; spitting is not uncommon. Additionally, they attempt new sounds that they've heard (see Table 8-5 for language milestones).[24,31]

In association with their oromotor maturation, infants at 6 months are usually eating soft foods by spoon, often trying to take the spoon away from the caregiver, but continue to get most of their nourishment from breastfeeding or a bottle. The protrusion reflex is stimulated by pressure on the tip of the tongue from the spoon or the food, which elicits tongue protrusion. In addition, the infant initially uses the same forward and backward movements of the tongue that are used for managing liquids; these things together result in a lot of food being pushed out of the mouth, but by the end of the third quarter, most infants will cleanly take food off of a spoon without much loss,[33] demonstrating a vertical chewing pattern (jaw up and down), and rake foods with their fingers from the tabletop or highchair tray to their mouth easily.[34]

Socioemotional/Cognitive

Receptively, infants begin to respond to "no" and associate names with common objects and people (e.g., a sibling's name).[35] They begin to point to desired objects and play peek-a-boo.[23] They also enjoy seeing themselves in a mirror and will interact with their image by smiling and babbling. Some anxiety toward strangers (*stranger anxiety*) may manifest by 6 months and will increase over this time period.[1] Infants, in the 3rd quarter, also start to use referential gestures (e.g., lift the arms to "ask" to be picked up).[3] They begin to respond to "come here" or to look for caregiver(s) when asked (e.g., where's dada).[1]

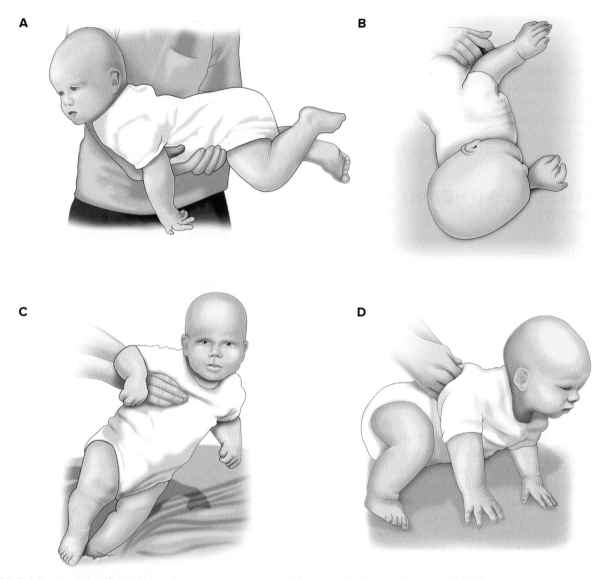

FIGURE 8-4 Postural reactions. A. Landau – prone support with head to 60 degrees (immature). **B.** Body-on-body reaction – log roll in association with rotation of the hip. **C.** Optical righting – head up to vertical when body is tipped laterally. **D.** Parachute response – forward movement toward mat elicits arm extension in protection manner.

• MONTHS 9 TO 12 (THE FOURTH QUARTER)

Neural Maturation

Over the first year of life, gray matter volume doubles with comparable increases in subcortical volume, associated with expansion of cortical surface area. Brain regions associated with sensory processing are particularly enlarged, including those associated with cutaneous sensations (post-central gyrus, parietal, and superior temporal regions). Cortical white matter also increases as myelination occurs; the corpus callosum and internal capsule have significant amounts of myelin by 12 months; however, there are many unmyelinated fibers in the temporal and frontal lobes (areas of memory and executive function).[13,36] During this 4th quarter, there's a further increase in metabolism of the frontal cortex, beginning with the dorsomedial cortex; simultaneously, there's an increase in dendritic projections

and capillary density. By 12 months, glucose metabolism in the infant mirrors that of adults, indicating activity throughout the cortex; however, the rate of metabolism is still significantly different than that of adults.[14]

Gross Motor

The fourth quarter is characterized by increased mobility and a focus on exploring the environment. Most 9- to 10-month-olds are pulling to knees and from there to standing by pulling up with their arms; the legs move in synchrony with no half-kneeling posture used (one knee up and the other on the floor). In standing, they have a wide base and flexed hips and knees; they often continue to be on tiptoes but also are flat-footed (see Figure 8-2B). The ability to pull to stand precedes the ability to get down from standing, so they may cry for assistance to get down initially. By 12 months, they will easily squat to the ground and pull back up, holding on with one hand. Within a month of pulling to stand, most will start to sidestep, still holding on with both hands, known as *cruising*; within a few weeks, they are able to do this while holding on with only one hand and will briefly stand without holding onto anything.[1] While the infant is frequently exploring their ability to stand, the primary mode of mobility for most infants, in the fourth quarter, is creeping on hands and knees (quadruped), rapidly increasing the speed at which they can move, and they can easily get into and out of sitting from quadruped. They also will pivot in circles while sitting. Some infants will continue to scoot in sitting as a means of mobility. In sitting, they demonstrate equilibrium and protective responses in all directions (Table 8-2), including posteriorly by 12 months. Equilibrium responses in quadruped also emerge by 12 months. Some infants will attempt movement on hands and feet, referred to as **plantigrade walking** *(bear walking)*, at this stage; however, many infants never use this method of mobility. Finally, most infants will take their first steps very near their first birthdays (range for first steps 10-14 month); in early walking, they are flat footed with a wide base and feet externally rotated; the arms are held in *high guard* (hands above shoulders); and the knees and hips are still flexed (Figure 8-3C).[1,16,18]

Fine Motor

Reaching in the 4th quarter is smoother than in the 3rd with only 1 to 2 submovements for most reach-to-grasp attempts.[3] While they are easily grasping objects, they often fling the object to release them at 9 months but demonstrate a graded object release to place an object in a container by 12 months. They are also able to take items apart (e.g., snap together beads/blocks), clap their hands repeatedly, and bang toys together.[23] This increased functional hand use is accompanied by a decrease in hand-to-mouth and oral exploration of objects.[31] At 9 months, they are able to poke with a single finger, and by 12 months, they demonstrate a mature pincer grasp, easily picking up a raisin or cereal between the tips of the index finger and thumb.[1,24] By 12 months, they also begin to hold a crayon and scribble.[1]

Oromotor/Language

By 10 months, most children are eating a variety of foods with increasing textures (lumps) and eating finger foods without gagging. By 12 months, they are eating firmer foods and keeping most of the food in their mouths.[34] By the beginning of the 4th quarter, infants know their name and respond to it by looking toward the individual calling them,[37] and by 10 months they understand up to 50 words.[38] **Babbling** is at its peak with consistent repetition of sounds (e.g., baba, dada, mama) without reference to objects or people. They also begin to point and gesture to make needs known and respond to simple commands.[23] The first "official" word usually emerges close to the first birthday, commonly "mama," "dada," or another noun (e.g., "baba" for bottle). There is considerable variance in whether "mama" or "dada" comes first, depending on the report read, with some suggesting the "dada" is easier to say and others that "mama" is easier to say; there's some suggestion that babies tend to say whichever they hear most from their parents. Nonetheless, "mama" and "dada," or their equivalent, are typically among each infant's first words, regardless of the language. This is likely the result of parental reinforcement of the spontaneous babbling of these syllables.[39]

Socioemotional/Cognitive

Infants in the 4th quarter demonstrate an increased interest in others, especially their peers. This is the earliest stage that differences in attachment behavior can be noted (see Box 8-5) with preference for primary caregivers observed. They are also aware of adult emotions and may even try to soothe an upset caregiver.[37] The 10-month-old will play peek-a-boo and wave

Box 8-5	**Social Development**

Social behaviors include social competence, attachment, emotional competence, **self-perceived competence**, and temperament/personality. More than any other aspect of development, social development is greatly impacted by the environment in which the child is raised. *Social competence* refers to the ability to interact with others.[37] **Attachment** is the development of a strong emotional positive relationship with caregivers, which impacts their ability to develop similar relationships with others. Studies have demonstrated four "types" of attachment, related to the responsiveness of caregivers and the infant's ability to use the caregiver as a secure base from which to explore: (1) *Secure* infants have responsive, loving caregivers and, thus, have learned to count on the caregiver's responsiveness and feel comfortable exploring their environment and other people, returning to the comfort of the caregiver when afraid or to seek comfort after a separation; (2) *Anxious/ambivalent* (resistant) infants have caregivers who are inconsistent, overwhelmed, or overly emotional; these infants are reluctant to explore, regardless of the caregiver's presence, are extremely upset when the caregiver leaves but show a mixture of contact seeking and avoidance, when frightened or the caregiver returns after separation (e.g., continued crying, hitting); (3) *Avoidant* infants have caregivers who are likely to ignore or become annoyed when the infant is distressed; these infants find exploration, even with the caregiver present, difficult, may be extremely upset when the caregiver leaves but do not seek out the caregiver when frightened or when (s)he returns after separation (avoid contact); and (4) *Disorganized* infants have caregivers that demonstrate aberrant or distorted behavior (e.g., frightening) and thereby demonstrate unusual behavior when the caregiver leaves (e.g., freezing or self-stimulating behavior [hand flapping]) but appear fearful when the caregiver returns; this is considered disorganized because it is inconsistent and doesn't help soothe the infant.[40] The three latter groups are considered to be insecurely attached, but anxious and avoidant infants are thought to use organized (consistent) behavior to deal with novel situations and caregiver separation. Notably, infants can develop strong attachment to multiple caregivers but may have a preference when highly distressed.[41] **Emotional competence** refers not only to the ability to understand one's own emotional state and to regulate it but also the ability to understand the emotional state of others and to provide a supportive response. **Self-perceived confidence**, as the name implies, is the ability to evaluate one's abilities in relation to the performance of others. **Temperament** refers to behavioral tendencies that emerge into personality, including emotionality, reactivity or self-regulation, and sociability; while temperament seems to have some biological origins, it also appears to be modifiable through the child's experiences and environment.[37,42]

good-bye; by 12 months, they can follow one-step commands, and begin to put an arm or leg out to assist with dressing.[1,23]

Infants begin to demonstrate imitative play in the fourth quarter, such as picking up a play phone and babbling, an activity commonly witnessed by the average infant.[31] Children also begin to develop **object permanence** as they near 12 months. In the earliest stage, infants will uncover a partially covered object to reveal the whole, but by 10 months, they will pull a cloth off of a completely covered toy that they've seen hidden; by 12 months, they will look briefly for objects that move out of sight (e.g., when a parent places a toy behind their back or inside a box). An 11-month-old will bring a toy to the caregiver for assistance, but by 12 months, will bring a toy to "share"; they will also point to an object that they desire.[1] While infants at this age enjoy social interactions and are interested in peers, they are mostly solitary in their play.[24]

● THE 2ND YEAR

Neural Maturation

The second year of life is a time of rapid gray matter growth; it is also a time of considerable synaptic pruning, which peaks at about 24 months.[4] The arcuate fasciculus, which connects the language areas of the temporal and frontal cortices shows myelination, greater on the left than the right, consistent with that hemisphere's dominance in language skills for most people.[36] Myelination is present within all brain regions but is still developing in the inferior frontal and temporal lobes.[13]

Gross Motor

As stated previously, the average toddler begins taking independent steps about the time of his/her first birthday; thus, gross motor function in the second year of life focuses largely on gait maturation. Early walkers have been found to take up to 14,000 steps per day with an average of 100 falls[3]; the good news is that they don't have far to fall and they have the padding of a diaper to cushion their landing. Over the year, the base of support narrows, and the arms move from a high guard to a low guard position, eventually maturing to an arm swing by the second birthday (Figure 8-2C). As the arms move downward from high guard (Figure 8-2D), the toddler begins to carry objects, typically by 15 months[1]; they also begin to demonstrate anticipatory balance reactions prior to pulling or pushing a toy in standing.[27]

Also by 15 months, toddlers demonstrate a stiff-legged run, but by 24 months, their run is much more mature with an emerging flight phase. In standing, the toddler is playing with his balance, squatting and returning to stand, stopping and starting, and turning around. Climbing is also initiated, both climbing up onto furniture and climbing stairs, first up (12-13 months) and then down (13-15 months). As this timeframe illustrates, the child is able to climb up onto things before he masters climbing down, so this is another time of many falls, demanding parental diligence in monitoring the child's activities. Within a few months of walking, toddlers will begin walking up stairs with one hand held or by using a railing and a step-to pattern (both feet to each step [16 months]), and follow with walking down stairs by 16 to 20 months, also using a step-to pattern.[1] By 22 to 24 months, most toddlers will walk up and down stairs with an alternating pattern, jump down from a step or up from the floor (just clearing their feet), and can initiate kicking a stationary ball by sort of walking into it (limited single limb stance). They can also throw a ball, while standing.[1,18–20]

Fine Motor

The second year is also one of rapid fine motor skill acquisition. By 12 to 13 months, most toddlers will begin using a superior (mature) **pincer grasp** (tips of thumb and index finger touch the object) to feed themselves finger foods; they will also put together toys with a few pieces (e.g., Legos™). By 15 months, they will stack 2 to 3 blocks and place a circle in a form board, by 20 months place a square, and by 24 months complete the form board or place shapes in a shape sorter as well as single puzzle pieces into a puzzle, orienting the object or piece to the slot.[1] By 20 months, they can build a 5-6-block tower, and by 24 months, will lay the blocks into a long straight line. Toddlers' reaching is smooth and coordinated, similar to that of an adult, as they approach their second birthday. This flexibility in hand function also supports initial self-feeding with a spoon and early cup drinking by 14 to 16 months, and by 24 months, toddlers are fairly proficient at these self-feeding skills. Coloring (scribbling) is also initiated, typically around 16 months, and toddlers are able to draw a vertical line by 24 months.[3,10,18–20,23,27,31,33,43] Also, by 24 months, they are able to unzip their jacket or pants and will attempt to put on shoes.[1]

Oromotor/Language

There is considerable variability in language acquisition, but on average, by 16 months, toddlers understand up to 170 words (range 92-321). While the first word is commonly uttered close to the first birthday, by 14 months most children have 2 to 10 words and then accelerate their rate of speech production, adding 10 words/month up to the first 50 and then, 30 words per month over the remainder of the second year.[24,38] By 24 months, they are putting together two-word phrases, understand you versus me, refer to themselves by name, and ask for more.[1,23,43] They will also point to familiar items in a book, and point to 5 to 6 body parts as well as items of clothing. Speech at this age is referred to as **telegraphic** – two-word bursts of speech that include a noun and verb consistent with the order of the child's primary language.[1]

Around 18 months of age, toddlers start to demonstrate rotary jaw movements while chewing, which allows for eating tougher foods (e.g., meats); this movement typically matures by 24 months.[32]

Socioemotional/Cognitive

In the second year, toddlers should have gained sufficient confidence in their attachment to begin moving away from caregivers to explore new environments; they are interested in playing with peers, but continue to primarily play in parallel but not interactive modes (stand next to another child while playing but aren't playing with the other child). Some group play is initiated by the end of the second year.[37] In addition, the 18- to 24-month-old child will begin to initiate imaginary play

TABLE 8-5	Log of Language Milestones, Birth to 6 Years[1,24,38]
AGE	**LANGUAGE SKILL**
Language Production	
0-2 months	Cries Vocalizations other than crying, beginning with vowel sounds such as "ooh" and "aah"
2-4 months	Increased variability in sounds, cooing, some squeals Responds to heard vocalization with sounds of their own
4-6 months	Babbling – playing with sounds, eliminates sounds not heard in their native language; adds consonants mama, dada without meaning; laughs
9-12 months	Increased babbling, stringing different sounds together with more consonants; makes "raspberry" sounds Associates names with common objects and points to access objects
12-15 months	Initial first word ~ 12 mo. Single words to express sentences (at least 3 words with meaning), expanding vocabulary; animal sounds (up to 20 words by 15 months)
15-18 months	Vocabulary increases by 10 words/month up to 50 words
18-24 months	Rapid vocabulary expansion (30 words per month); two-word (telegraphic) sentences initiated (noun + verb; e.g., dada away); naming pictures initiated; refers to self by name
24-30 months	270-400-word vocabulary, 50% of production is understandable; adds pronouns; begins imitating words heard
30-36 months	Beginning use of adjectives (big, little); 900-word vocabulary; understandability increases to 75%; sentence length of 4-5 words
3-4 years	Naming of colors, defining of words begins; sentence length increases to 5-8 words; begins asking questions; incorporating appropriate grammar;
4-5 years	Answering "why" questions; tells complex stories; uses adjectives and rhyming
5-6 years	100% understandable by others; uses future tense; 2500+ words
Language Reception	
0-2 months	Responds to loud noises with startle or awakening
2-4 months	Responds to familiar voice by calming
4-6 months	Turns to sounds/voice; begins to distinguish sounds, especially mother's voice; initiates verbal turn-taking
6-9 months	Changes vocalizations to those that are heard
9-12 months	Responds to simple words (bye-bye, no, food items); follows a one-step command; knows name and up to 50 words; begins to point to named picture and gestures to make needs known
12-18 months	Begins to follow commands and points to body parts
18-24 months	Expanding identification of body parts and understanding of words and commands
24-30 months	Can point to at least six body parts; listens to short story (5-10 minutes)
30-36 months	Begins to follow two-step commands (e.g., get the toy and bring it to me)
3-4 years	Begins to answer questions (e.g., who, where)
4-5 years	Shows understanding of longer stories (>short stories); recognizes common store and restaurant signs

(e.g., food preparation at toy kitchens, putting a doll to bed) and may include others in this play. By 16 months, toddlers begin to develop self-consciousness and may become "shy" when observed, a sign of embarrassment; by 18 months, they start to demonstrate "shame," when they have misbehaved.[1] This is the beginning of their understanding of the concepts of good and bad. They also start to demonstrate some self-soothing when upset and to identify ownership with statements like "mine."[37]

The 2nd year is a time of increased awareness of and play with objects, including problem-solving with objects. A 14-month-old will dump a raisin or pellet from a small bottle, after seeing the movement demonstrated; by 16 months, they can do this without a demonstration. By 18 months, they can match object pairs, and by 24 months, they begin sorting objects by characteristics (color, shape) and matching objects to pictures.[1]

At this time, most toddlers are becoming aware of bowel and bladder fullness, so potty training can be initiated. The timing of successful potty training is highly variable and can extend through much of the preschool years.[23,24]

AGES 2 TO 5: THE PRESCHOOL YEARS

Neural Maturation

Myelination is complete and similar to appearance to that of adults by the age of 3. Brain volume approaches 90% of adult size by the age of 5,[24] so the preschool years are a time of rapid brain growth, associated with thickening of the cortex, especially in the temporal and prefrontal cortices. However, it should be noted that some areas actually decrease in volume, specifically in the visual and somatosensory cortex, which likely indicates enhanced efficiency of neuronal processing in these areas.[36] During these preschool years, glucose metabolism increases dramatically, reaching twice the level of that for adults; this higher metabolic rate occurs in association with intense proliferation of synapses, supporting the rapid development of motor, language, and cognitive skills.[14]

Gross Motor

The preschool years continue the rapid skill acquisition seen in the first two years but focused on improved mobility and the acquisition of play skills (see Table 8-6). Two-year-olds mature in their walking and running skills, initiating walking on tiptoes and backward (28 months) as well as running with a flight phase and arm swing (30 months); then, over the next two years, preschoolers increase the velocity of the run and overall agility; by 5, running is well-coordinated and controlled (stop, starts, and turns).[18,23] Balance skills also improve over this time period with a 2½-year-old able to stand briefly on a balance beam and walk its length with one foot on and one off; by 3, they are able to walk heel to toe on the floor and by 5 are able to walk backward heel to toe. Stair climbing improves with the alternating of feet by age 3 without the need for holding onto a rail, allowing the child to begin carrying toys up and down.[1,19,20]

While the 2-year-old is just beginning to jump, by age 3, most children can jump forward by about 2 feet as well as repeatedly jump up and down or forward; in addition, they can perform a single hop on one foot, and kick a rolled ball with a leg swing. Initially, jumping occurs with a limited squat and no arm swing, but by 5, children incorporate a squat and an arm swing sufficient to move them several feet. The enhanced coordination of legs and arms allows the 3-year-old to begin pedaling and steering a tricycle; the speed and confidence in this skill will allow many to ride a bicycle without training wheels by their 6th birthday. Improved ball skills also develop during the preschool years with a 3-year-old catching a ball by scooping it into their chest; a 4-year-old is able to catch a large ball with their hands, no longer curling into their chest, and also begins to throw a small ball overhand; and by 5, they have a forward weight shift when throwing along with much better accuracy. Other skills mastered by the age of 5 are galloping (similar to skipping, only one foot remains forward [no alternating pattern]), repeated hopping on one foot up to 10 times, a forward somersault, and the ability to propel a swing.[44] As they near 5½, most children will convert their gallop into a skip as their ability to hop on either foot matures (see Table 8-3 for overview of gross motor skills).[1]

Fine Motor/Self-Care

The preschool years are also a time of rapid improvement in hand dexterity (see Table 8-4); by 2, most children can stack 4 blocks.[23] By 2 ½ they begin to draw a horizontal line; by age 3 a circle; by age 4, a cross; by 5, a square; and by 5 ½, a triangle. Similarly, preschoolers improve in their ability to construct toys (e.g., blocks, Legos™) and complete puzzles, from simple to fairly complex over this time period (20 to 60 pieces).[43] A 3-year-old can cut awkwardly with scissors, pour liquids, string beads, draw a person with 3 body parts, unbutton clothes, and put on shoes. Three-year-olds also begin turning pages in a book, pushing buttons, and turning knobs. By 4, they initiate writing their name and draw a person with 4 to 6 body parts, are independent in toileting, can wash their hands afterward, and can brush their teeth. By 5, they demonstrate improved cutting with scissors and draw a person with 8 to 10 body parts.[1,23]

Two-year-olds are able to feed themselves with utensils, but it's not until 4 that they are competent with a fork, and at age 5 that most children begin to use a knife to spread butter on a piece of bread; they cannot yet cut food with the knife.[1]

Self-dressing is typically accomplished by the age of 3 with some assistance in identifying front and back when donning clothes; they can't yet button, zip, or snap but can unbutton and unsnap. By 4 most children can button, and by 5, most children are independent in dressing, including buttons, snaps, and zippers.[1,23]

Oromotor/Language

By 2, oral motor development is largely complete with children able to chew most foods and drink from a cup, although many will continue to use a sippy cup to avoid spills; there is some increased lip closure strength up to 5 years of age, which supports drinking from a straw.[34]

Language development accelerates in the preschool years with the 2½-year-old verbalizing over 270 words, including verbs and pronouns (some only understood by caregivers but 50% is understood by strangers),[23] and combining them into 2-3-word sentences; this includes stating their first and last names and repeating familiar parts of stories. By 3, they express over 900 words into 4-5-word sentences with up to 75% understood by strangers; they also count to 3 and use plurals. Four-year-olds begin singing songs and telling stories, start incorporating appropriate grammar in their speech, and use words that connote feelings; they can also identify some colors and numbers. By 5, they can define simple words, answer "why" questions, and tell complex stories; they also know right and left of themselves, use adjectives in speech, and like to rhyme words. By 6, children know more than 2500 words, are using future tense, and are understandable to everyone.[1,23,24,45]

TABLE 8-6 Advanced Motor Skills[1,19,20]

SKILL	DESCRIPTION	AGE (IN MONTHS)
Stair mobility/Climbing		
Creeps up and down stairs	Typically goes up first; alternates hands and knees	12-15
Walks up stairs	Holds rail, brings both feet to each stair (step-to pattern)	15-16
Walks down stairs	With rail or hand held, step-to pattern	16-20
Walks up and down stairs	Alternating pattern (one step/tread) with rail	26-28
Walks up and down with toy	Alternating pattern, no rail, able to carry toy	34-36
Ladder climbing	Climbs 2-3 stairs of toy slide	12-16
Small ladder	Climbs vertical slide, step-to pattern	40-48
Vertical ladder	Climbs vertical ladder, alternating pattern	60-72
Jumping/Hopping	Begins jumping up from ground or down from stair	22-28
	Jumps forward up to 24 inches	30-32
	Jumps 2 inch hurdle	32-34
	Single hop in one foot	30-36
	Begins hopping multiple times on preferred foot	46-48
Advanced walking skills	Walks backward	24-26
	Walks straight line one foot in front of other (not heel to toe)	26-30
	Walks on tiptoes	28-30
Advanced movement		
Running	Stiff-legged, no flight phase	14-16
	Flight phase and arm swing	24-36
	Well-coordinated and controlled	50-60
Galloping	Forward movement with one foot ahead of the other at a fast pace	48-52
Skipping	Alternating feet with hop on each foot	57-64
Somersault	Forward somersault	57-64
Ball skills		
Catches large ball	2 handed with arms straight out in front of body, scoops to chest	26-34
	2 handed with hands on sides of ball and elbows flexed	40-42
Catches small ball	2 handed catch with hands together	50-52
Kicks ball	Kicks stationary ball	15-24
	Kicks rolled ball	36-40
Throws ball	Flings ball without directional intent	12-14
	Throws underhand	24-30
	Throws overhand	38-40
	Throws with step and weight-shift forward	55-65

Socioemotional/Cognitive

This is a time period of increasing interest in peers and the onset of friendships; preschoolers enjoy social interactions and should easily separate from parents, especially as they near their 5th birthday. While 24 to 36 months are often known as the terrible "2s," it is really a time for children to establish a sense of autonomy[37]; however, this increased interest in independence is also associated with an increased usage of "no" in response to many requests. This may also be a time of temper tantrums, as the two-year-old pushes the boundaries of their environments and caregivers.[24] The 3-year-old is beginning to share, first when prompted and then by choice. By 4, preschoolers have preferred friends, understand and label emotions (sadness, anger), engage in group play, and enjoy "tricking" and being tricked by others.[1]

The preoperational period, as described by Piaget, begins at 2 and extends to the age of 6.[30] While the 2-year-old is just beginning to show imaginative play, this is a hallmark of the preschool years with increased incorporation of peers and family members over this time period.[24,45] However, by 5, children begin to understand the difference between pretend and reality. Uniquely, at the beginning of the preschool period, children perceive their world through their own perspective so don't realize that others see things differently. An easy example of this is when an adult is driving and the child is in the back seat; they might ask a question about something that they can see but is behind the adult without realizing that it's beyond the adult's visual perspective. The ability to understand the perspective of others is beginning as the preschool period ends. Similarly, two-year-olds can't compare their skills with others, which allows them to think that they are "great" at everything, but as the preschool years progress, some ability to compare skills to those of others develops. However, most children continue to have a very positive perception of themselves.[37]

The ability to attend to an activity increases from 5 to 15 minutes over the preschool years, but preschoolers remain easily distracted. This is a time of learning through trial and error, which may include trying motor behaviors beyond their ability, resulting in many falls. However, they are learning to obey common rules (e.g., holding mom's hand in a parking lot, being quiet in restaurants), understand turn-taking, and are developing memory for basic information (full names of family members, names of animals, shapes, and colors).[45] Three-year-olds understand some relationship concepts (e.g., big/little; older/younger) and can match some letters and numbers. By 4, they begin to recognize common store and restaurant signs, can count items up to 5, and answer simple analogy questions (e.g., mommy is a girl, daddy is a_____?).[1] By 5, children are able to solve problems with a single variable (e.g., who's taller or older), identify coins, count to 10, and name colors. Many 5-year-olds are beginning to read (<25 words).[1,24]

● AGES 6 TO 11: MIDDLE CHILDHOOD

Neural Maturation

Gray matter volume reaches its maximum in the parietal lobe by age 10 for girls and 11 for boys while frontal lobe gray matter reaches its maximum by 11 and 12 for girls and boys, respectively.[46] Similarly, cortical surface area has been reported to increase up to the age of 12; however, there are areas that increase in size, followed by a decrease, as the child ages. This is thought to relate to enhanced efficiency of neuronal activity and pruning of unnecessary synapses. For example, improvement in executive function and memory occurs between the ages of 5 and 10; this is associated with a decrease in volume of fronto-parietal networks thought to be associated with changes in synapses (pruning), yet myelin in these areas is increasing, which also leads to efficiency of neural transmission.[36] Interestingly, dendritic density peaks at a level that is almost twice that of adults in this time period,[47] associated with a continued elevation in glucose metabolism that is twice as high as adults, and is accompanied by a 30% increase in oxygen utilization. These illustrate the excessive connectivity and synapse development between cortical areas that are

occurring in school-aged children.[14] Notably, some areas, such as the basal ganglia, begin to see a decline in synapse formation by 7 to 9 years, while others will wait until adolescence.[47]

Gross Motor

Skipping is a common mode of mobility for the 6-year-old; however, this is much more common in girls than boys. Boys may use galloping in place of skipping. Throwing accuracy improves with a small ball, and they can incorporate a run into the throw; 6-year-olds also are able to adjust their hands for catching balls of various sizes.[18,44] Jumping increases with the ability to jump up a foot and forward 3 feet. Gender differences are also noted in skill ability with boys, in general, out jumping and throwing girls but girls demonstrating better balance and catching. Most 7-year-olds have mastered riding a bicycle, and by 8, are demonstrating some competence in sports activities. The next few years are characterized by quick gains in these skills such that by 10 to 11, the fundamentals of most motor skills have been acquired, and they are able to anticipate the arrival of a thrown or kicked ball. Yet, sensory integration (the ability to use visual, auditory, vestibular, and cutaneous information in motor planning and execution) is not yet mature, so balance and movement continue to improve over this time period and into adolescence.[44]

Fine Motor

Handwriting is a focus of the early school years with a gradual increase in speed and clarity. The 6-year-old is just beginning to write, including their first and last names, but between 7 and 8 there's rapid improvement in handwriting ability; by the age of 9, handwriting is fairly mature and has become relatively automatic. Between the ages of 9 and 11, the speed of writing increases. Boys tend to lag a bit behind girls in the acquisition of handwriting. Knife use is typically mastered by 7 to 8 as is the ability to use a fork and knife together to cut food.[1,43]

Language

The primary school years are also a time of enhanced language skills. Most 6-year-olds use up to 10,000 words in sentences of 8 to 10 words and will ask the meaning of unfamiliar words. They are able to describe sequential events. By 7 to 8, children demonstrate adult articulation, yet grammar and vocabulary will continue to expand throughout the school years.[24]

Socioemotional/Cognitive

In Piagetian terms, the school years are a time of concrete thinking, including the ability to order, number, and classify things; 6-year-olds begin to understand the concept of conservation of mass and weight, and by 8, children understand the concept of volume. Yet, there is limited ability to think futuristically; they operate in the "now." School-aged children also have a strong sense of right and wrong with limited ability to see the "gray" in situations or evaluate the influence of other factors on a decision; they tend to be rule followers and also to impose rules on others. This is a time of factual information acquisition and the development of inductive reasoning. Increased problem-solving and critical thinking develop with increased attention span for learning activities; children remain somewhat distractible but are developing better selective attention (the ability to tune out some distractions). School-aged children are increasingly interested in playing games and sports but are also more tolerant to losing. While the preschool years are a time of pretend play, the primary school years are a time of increased fantasy thinking and imagination but less pretend play.[24,30,44]

The primary school years are also a time of body image development and awareness of and comparison to others; children are more realistic about their own skills. It is also a time of personality development, stronger friendships, and decreased aggression.[44]

● ADOLESCENCE (12-18)

The adolescent years can be divided into early (10-13), middle (14-16), and late (17-20) time periods. In general, it is a time of increasing gender differences and sexual maturation. Boys tend to increase in height and weight simultaneously while girls tend to grow in height first and then add weight. This may result in girls achieving their mature height before boys.[48]

Neural Maturation

Adolescence is a critical developmental period for the systems that support socioemotional and cognitive development. While gray matter volume peaks in the frontal and parietal lobes in mid-childhood, it doesn't peak in the temporal lobes until age 16. White matter demonstrates a linear increase from age 4 to 20, increasing on average by 12% over this developmental period.[46] The elevated glucose metabolism seen in preschool and school-aged children also diminishes to adult levels by 16 to 18 years of age.[14] Also in adolescence, areas of neural maturation are focused in the prefrontal cortex to support maturity of executive function (memory, inhibition, and higher level concept formation).[15] Yet, the teenaged years are also a time of synapse elimination, based on activity such that pruning occurs in relatively unused networks and synaptic stabilization in highly used areas.[14] This is associated with a thinning of the cortex in many areas but also an increase in white matter overall volume and density. This can be a time of vulnerability of the cortex, which can be heavily influenced by social and behavioral experiences; not surprisingly, it can be a time of dysfunctional development yielding psychopathological disorders (substance abuse, schizophrenia).[15]

Gross Motor

From early to middle adolescence, there's a continued increase in muscle mass, strength, and cardiopulmonary endurance that contribute to increased coordination and speed; however, many adolescents experience periods of rapid growth that result in phases of incoordination. By the end of adolescence, most have achieved adult height and physical skills but some increase in cardiopulmonary capacity and strength continues into early adulthood.[48]

Language

Adolescence is a time of formal operations (abstract thought); in terms of language development, teens increasingly use symbols and codes within their language skills as well as increased complexity of sentence structure and word usage. They also demonstrate enhanced understanding of verbal and written language.[48]

Socioemotional/Cognitive

Adolescence is a time of increased independence from parents associated with increased influence of peers. In early adolescence (10-13), strong friendships are developed with peers of both genders but parents continue to have a significant influence; pre-teens demonstrate a better understanding of other's emotions and enhanced regulation of their own. It is also a time of increased self-awareness that results in self-consciousness. Their adult personality is emerging. Middle adolescence begins deeper emotional relationships with peers, including intimate relationships, with increased emotional independence from parents. This is a time for acceptance of masculine or feminine social roles as well as one's physical characteristics. Late adolescence merges with adulthood as emotional independence from parents is achieved, preparation for adult life (career, marriage) is pursued, and an adult ideology is developed, including a set of values and principles that will guide one's adult life.[37]

According to Piaget, adolescence is the time of formal operations, when teenagers begin abstract thought, deductive reasoning, and the ability to manipulate multiple variables to solve a problem. This allows them to challenge themselves with coursework that builds on these developing skills.[30]

● ENVIRONMENTAL INFLUENCES ON BRAIN AND SKILL DEVELOPMENT

While the preceding sections have provided average and ranges of ages that typically developing children acquire various skills, there is also substantial variability in development between children. Development, both skill acquisition and brain maturation, can be altered, negatively and positively, by the environment to which the child is exposed.[30]

Negative Influences

Prenatally, maternal *environmental stress* can alter both brain development and epigenetics (the way various genes are expressed) in the developing fetus. Similarly, postnatal environmental stress (e.g., violence in the home or neighborhood) can have a similar effect on the developing child. Exposure to various substances in utero has been associated with altered brain development as well. For example, nicotine exposure in utero has been associated with later hyperactivity and/or learning disabilities; exposure to alcohol and many other drugs (marijuana, opiates, amphetamines) can affect overall brain development and has been associated with decreased gray matter in both the cortex and subcortical nuclei (e.g., basal ganglia). Children, who experience delayed attachment, such as those raised initially in orphanages and later adopted, have been reported to have smaller brains, characterized by decreased cortical volume and alteration in electrical activity; these changes were associated with unresolved delays in cognition and social skills. This may also be related to decreased stimulation in their early environment, which can impede overall development, especially if it extends through critical periods of development for specific brain regions. Similarly, infants and children, who experience inadequate diets during development, have been found to experience deficits in brain development coinciding with the time periods when food insufficiency is experienced.[11] While obesity has not been found to alter brain development, it can significantly delay gross motor development, especially for whole body movements; no effect on fine motor and other skills has been noted.[49]

Positive Influences on Brain and Behavioral Development

There have been a number of both animal and human studies that have documented enhanced neural maturation, including increased cortical thickness and dendritic spine density, associated with exposure to enriched environments. Enrichment has been characterized by greater exposure to language, toy variety, and books. For infants and children raised in such an environment, they are likely to demonstrate earlier skill acquisition, especially language and cognitive skills. For example, it's been reported that children raised in high socioeconomic environments (SES) have been exposed to over 11 million words by the age of 3, as parents are constantly talking to them, using an expanded vocabulary; conversely, lower SES children have been exposed to less than a third the number of words at the same age. This exposure resulted in a two- to threefold difference in the number of words used by the children at the start of first grade. Even more disturbing, this difference increased by ages 9 to 10 even though both groups were in school, suggesting that the school environment was unable to help the lower SES group to "catch up" to their higher SES peers. These differences in language skills were also associated with significant differences in cortical volume in the frontal, temporal, and parietal cortices.[11] Of course, there are many differences in school quality between public schools in higher and lower socioeconomic neighborhoods that likely confound these results.

REFERENCES

1. Scharf RJ, Scharf GJ, Stroustrup A. Developmental milestones. *Pediatr Rev.* 2016;37(1):25-38.

2. Luchinger AB, Hadders-algra M, Van Kan CM, De Vries JIP. Fetal onset of general movements. *Pediatr Res.* 2008;63(2):191-195.

3. Hadders-Algra M. Early human motor development: from variation to the ability to vary and adapt. *Neurosci Biobehav Rev.* 2018;90:411-427.

4. Kuiper MJ, Brandsma R, Lunsing RJ, et al. The neurological phenotype of developmental motor patterns during early childhood. *Brain Behav.* 2019;9:e01153.

5. Nowlan NC. Biomechanics of foetal movement. *Eur Cell Mater.* 2015;29:1-21.

6. Borsani E, Vedova AMD, Rezzani R, Rodella LF, Cristina C. Correlation between human nervous system development and acquisition of fetal skills: an overview. *Brain Dev.* 2019;41:225-233.

7. Barkovich MJ, Barkovich AJ. MR imaging of normal brain development. *Neuroimaging Clin N Am.* 2019;29:325-337.

8. Casey BJ, Tottenham N, Liston C, Durston S. Imaging the developing brain: what have we learned about cognitive development? *Trends Cog Sci.* 2005;9(3):104-110.

9. Knudsen EI. Sensitive periods in the development of the brain and behavior. *J Cogn Neurosci.* 2004;16(8):1412-1425.

10. Cioni G, Sgandurra G. Normal psychomotor development. *Handbook Clin Neurol. Vol III, Pediatfric Neurology Part I*: 2013:3-15.

11. Kolb B, Harker A, Gibb R. Principles of plasticity in the developing brain. *Dev Med Child Neurol.* 2017;59(12):1218-1223.

12. Dubois J, Dehaene-lambertz G. Kulikova S, Poupon C, Huppi PS, Hertz-Pannier L. The early development of brain white matter: a review of imaging studies in fetuses, newborns and infants. *Neuroscience.* 2014;276:48-71.

13. Branson HM. Normal myelination: a practical pictorial review. *Neuroimaging Clin N Am.* 2013;23:183-195

14. Chugani HT. Section 1: critical importance of emotional development – biological basis of emotions: brain systems and brain development. *Pediatrics.* 1998;102-1225-1229.

15. Dow-Edwards D, MacMastr FP, Peterson BS, Niesink R, Andersen S, Braams BR. Experience during adolescence shapes brain development: from synapses and networks to normal and pathological behavior. *Neurotoxicol Teratol.* 2019;76:106834.

16. Kobesova A, Kolar P. Developmental kinesiology: three levels of motor control in the assessment and treatment of the motor system. *J Bodyw Mov Ther.* 2014;18:23-33.

17. Zafeiriou DI. Primitive reflexes and postural reactions in the neurodevelopmental examination. *Pediatr Neurol.*2004;31:1-8.

18. Aubert EJ. Motor development in the normal child. In: Tecklin JS, ed. *Pediatric Physical Therapy.* 5th ed. Baltimore MD: Lippincott, Williams & Wilkins; 2015.

19. Bayley N, Aylward GP. *Bayley Scales of Infant and Toddler Development.* 4th ed. Pearson Products; 2019.

20. Folio MR, Fewell RR. *Peabody Developmental Motor Scales.* 2nd ed. Pearson Publishing; 2000.

21. Ben-Ari Y. The developing cortex. *Handb Clin Neurol.* 2013;111:417-426.

22. Heathcock JC, Bhat AN, Lobo MA, Galloway JC. The relative kicking frequency of infants born full-term and preterm during learning and short-term and long-term memory periods of the mobile paradigm. *Phys Ther.* 2005;85(1):8-18.

23. Misirliyan SS, Huynh AP. Developmental milestones. In: *StatPearls.* Treasure Island, FL: StatPearls Publishing; 2020. Available at: https://www.ncbi.nlm.nih.gov/books/NBK557518/?report=classic.

24. Goldson E, Angulo AS, Reynolds A, Raz DM. Child development and behavior. In: Hay WW, Levin MJ, Abzug MJ, Bunik,eds. *Current Diagnosis and Treatment: Pediatrics.* 25th ed. New York, NY: McGraw Hill; 2020.

25. Bremond-Gignac D, Copin H, Lapillonne A, Milazzo S. Visual development in infants: physiological and pathological mechanisms. *Curr Opin Ophthalmol.* 2011;22 (Clin Update 1):S1-S8.

26. Lickliter R. The integrated development of sensory organization. *Clin Perinatol.* 2011;38(4):591-603.

27. von Hofsten C, Rosander K. The development of sensorimotor intelligence in infants. *Adv Child Dev Behav.* 2018;55:73-97.

28. Ritterband-Rosenbaum A, Justiniano MD, Nielsen JB, Christensen MS. Are sensorimotor experiences the key for successful early intervention in infants with congenital brain lesion? *Infant Behav Dev.* 2019;54:133-139.

29. Darrah J, Bartlett DJ. Infant rolling abilities: the same or different 20 years after the back to sleep campaign? *Early Hum Dev.* 2018;89:311-314.

30. Scott HK, Cogburn M. Piaget. In: *StatPearls.* Treasure Island, FL: StatPearls Publishing; 2020.

31. Iverson JM. Developing language in a developing body: the relationship between motor development and language development. *J Child Lang.* 2010;37(2):229-261.

32. Wilson EM, Green JR, Yunusova Y, Moore CA. Task specificity in early oral motor development. *Semin Speech Lang.* 2008;29(4):257-267.

33. Carruth BR, Ziegler PJ, Gordon A, Hendricks K. Developmental milestones and self-feeding behaviors in infants and toddlers. *J Am Diet Assoc.* 2004;104:S51-S56.

34. Delaney AL, Arvedson JC. Development of swallowing and feeding: prenatal through first year of life. *Dev Disabil Res Rev.* 2008;14:105-117.

35. Werker JF, Tees RC. Influences on infant speech processing: toward a new synthesis. *Annu Rev Psychol.* 1999;50:509-535.

36. Walhovd KB, Tamnes CK, Fjell AM. Brain structural maturation and the foundations of cognitive behavioral development. *Curr Opin Neurol.* 2014;27(2):176-184.

37. Denham SA, Wyatt TM, Bassett HH, Echeverria D, Knox SS. Assessing social-emotional development in children from a longitudinal perspective. *J Epidemiol Community Health.* 2009;63(Suppl I):i37-i52.

38. Fenson L, Dale PS, Reznick JS, Bates E, Thal DJ, Pethick SJ. Variability in early communicative development. *Monogr Soc Res Child Dev.* 1994;59(5):1-173.

39. Locke JL. Structure and stimulation in the ontogeny of spoken language. *Dev Psychobiol.* 1990;232(7):621-643.

40. Benoit D. Infant-parent attachment: definition, types, antecedents, measurement and outcome. *Paediatr Child Health.* 2004;9(8):541-545.

41. Voges J, Berg A, Niehaus DJH. Revisiting the African origins of attachment research – 50 years on from Ainsworth: a descriptive review. *Infant Ment Health J.* 2019;40:799-816.

42. Coffman S, Levitt MJ, Guacci-Franco N. Infant-mother attachment: relationships to maternal responsiveness and infant temperament. *J Pediatr Nurs.* 1995;10(1):9-19.

43. Feder KP, Majnemer A. Handwriting development, competency, and intervention. *Dev Med Child Neurol.* 2007;49:312-317.

44. Patel DR, Pratt HD. Child neurodevelopment and sport participation. In: Patel DR Greydanus DE, Baker RJ, eds. *Pediatric Practice: Sports Medicine.* New York, NY: McGraw-Hill; 2009.

45. Conti-Ramsden G, Durkin K. Language development and assessment in the preschool period. *Neuropsychol Rev.* 2012;22:384-401.

46. Giedd JN, Blumenthal J, Jeffries NO, et al. Brain development during childhood and adolexcence: a longitudinal MRI study. *Nature Neurosci.* 1999;2(10):861-863.

47. Patanjek Z, Judas M, Simic G, et al. Extraordinary neoteny of synaptic spines in the human prefrontal cortex. *Proc Natl Acad Sci U S A.* 2011;108(32):13281-13286.

48. Greydanus DE, Pratt HD. Adolescent growth and development, and sport participation. In: Patel DR Greydanus DE, Baker RJ, eds. *Pediatric Practice: Sports Medicine.* New York, NY: McGraw-Hill; 2009.

49. Newell KM, Wade MG. Physical growth, body scale, and perceptual-motor development. *Adv Child Dev Behav.* 2018;55:205-244.

Review Questions

1. **The first fetal movements apparent by week 7 of gestation are known as:**

   A. Generalized movements

   B. Just discernable

   C. Twitches

   D. Writhing

2. **Which sensory system matures first?**

   A. Cutaneous

   B. Taste

   C. Vision

   D. Vestibular

3. **Active neural maturation is associated with which of the following?**

   A. Decreased glucose metabolism

   B. Decreased metabolic activity

   C. Myelin thinning

   D. Synaptic pruning

4. **A primitive reflex that results in flexion of the skull-side extremities and extension of the face-side extremities when the head is turned to the side is known as:**

   A. Asymmetrical tonic neck reflex

   B. Galant reflex

   C. Symmetrical tonic neck reflex

   D. Tonic labyrinthine reflex

5. **A child is able to keep her head in line with her body when pulled to sit, reaches for toys but often closes her hand prior to reaching the toy, and is starting to make consonant sounds when babbling. She is most likely:**

   A. 2 months old

   B. 4 months old

   C. 6 months old

   D. 8 months old

6. **A child is noted to move around their home on his hands and feet; this is appropriately called:**

   A. Creeping

   B. Cruising

   C. Plantigrade walking

   D. Pivot prone

7. **A 9-month-old is able to sit when placed with one arm support, is belly crawling, uses a radial palmar grasp to pick up blocks, demonstrates a protrusion reflex when eating from a spoon, and is pointing to desired objects, playing peek-a-boo, and initially shy with strangers. Which of the following would be a correct statement about this child's development?**

   A. S/he is demonstrating age-appropriate skills across all domains.

   B. S/he is demonstrating delayed gross motor development but appropriate fine motor and feeding skills.

   C. S/he is demonstrating delay in all areas but socioemotional/cognitive skills.

   D. S/he is delayed in all areas.

8. **A 20-month-old infant freezes in place without any crying when the parent leaves the room but avoids the parent on their return, seeming fearful of the parent. This child is demonstrating which type of attachment.**

   A. Ambivalent

   B. Avoidant

   C. Disorganized

   D. Secure

9. At what age would one expect a consistent flight phase and arm swing while running by what age?
   A. 18 months of age
   B. 2 years of age
   C. 2 ½ years of age
   D. 3 years of age

10. Which of the following correctly describes the speech of a 24-month-old?
    A. 75% understood by strangers
    B. Babbling
    C. Single-word sentences
    D. Telegraphic speech

11. By what age is myelination of the sensorimotor system typically complete?
    A. 4 years of age
    B. 6 years of age
    C. 9 years of age
    D. 12 years of age

12. The age at which most children can ride a bicycle without training wheels is:
    A. 6 years of age
    B. 7 years of age
    C. 8 years of age
    D. 9 years of age

13. Which of the following gross motor skills are appropriately tied to the age at which they are achieved?
    A. Catches large ball with 2 hands – 18-20 months
    B. Galloping – 4-5 years
    C. Skipping – 7-8 years
    D. Walks backward initially – 3-4 years

14. Failure to experience a specific type of stimulation during a critical period may lead to failure in the development of a specific brain region.
    A. True
    B. False

15. The concepts of conservation of mass, quantity, and volume are achieved in what Piagetian stage?
    A. Concrete operations
    B. Formal operations
    C. Preoperational period
    D. Sensorimotor period

16. An infant is sitting, when he loses his balance backward, you see that his arms abduct and then adduct quickly, as he falls backward. This is evidence of what reflex?
    A. Extensor thrust
    B. Moro
    C. Symmetrical tonic neck
    D. Tonic labyrinthine

17. Your 5-year-old niece is visiting, and you notice that she climbs the ladder to the slide, alternating feet, skips around the yard, and can propel the swing without needing a push. Your niece is demonstrating:
    A. About a 1-year delay in her gross motor skills
    B. Advanced gross motor skills for her age – more like a 7-year-old
    C. Gross motor ability consistent with her age

18. By what age would you expect a child to demonstrate adult articulation?
    A. 5-6 years of age
    B. 7-8 years of age
    C. 9-10 years of age
    D. 11-12 years of age

19. Brain maturation is complete during what time period?
    A. Preschool years
    B. Middle childhood
    C. Adolescence
    D. Young adulthood

20. Protective responses in sitting are mature in all directions by what age?
    A. 6-8 months
    B. 8-10 months
    C. 10-12 months
    D. 12-14 months

Answers

1. B	2. A	3. D	4. A
5. B	6. C	7. C	8. C
9. C	10. D	11. A	12. B
13. B	14. A	15. A	16. B
17. C	18. B	19. D	20. C

GLOSSARY

Abasia. Without stepping.

Astasia. Without stance.

Anteflexion. Neck flexion.

Asymmetrical tonic neck reflex. Skull-side flexion and face-side extension of the extremities when the newborn's head is turned to the side.

Attachment. A strong emotional tie to a caregiver.

Babbling. Repetitive vocalizations of vowels and consonants.

Cephalocaudal. Head to toe.

Concrete operations. Piagetian period focused on developing logic around objects and acquiring factual information.

Crawling. Propulsion with the belly still on the floor.

Creeping. Propulsion in quadruped (all fours).

Critical period. Type of sensitive period, during which specific stimulation is necessary for brain development, and if not experienced, my limit that brain development.

Emotional competence. Ability to understand one's own or another's emotional state.

Fidgety movements. Small irregular movements that develop at 6 to 8 weeks.

Formal operations. Piagetian period focused on developing abstract thought and logic.

Gallop/galloping. Forward movement in standing with one leg ahead of the other (no alternation).

High guard position. Hands held above shoulders when sitting or walking.

Infantile stepping. Early stepping movements triggered by tilting a newborn forward in supported standing with the feet on a solid surface.

Inferior pincer grasp. Object held with thumb against side of index finger.

Just discernable movements. First noticeable movements in utero; slow bending.

Object permanence. The awareness that an object (or person) continues to exist when not visible.

Parachute response. Protective response of arm extension toward a support surface, when the child is tipped from upright toward the surface.

Palmar grasp. Raking an object into the palm of the hand.

Pivot prone. Lifting both arms and legs in a prone position (on belly).

Plantigrade walking. Walking on hand and feet (bear walking).

Primitive reflexes. Reflexes seen in newborns that become integrated into movement patterns as the brain matures.

Physiologic flexion. A newborn's predominantly flexed posture with resistance to extension.

Pincer grasp. Object is grasped with tips of index finger and thumb.

Preoperational period. Piagetian period where representational thought develops.

Prone propping. Weight-bearing on forearms or extended arms with the stomach on the ground.

Protective responses. Extension of the arm toward a support surface to prevent falling when sitting.

Radial palmar grasp. Grasping with the thumb, index, and middle fingers into the palm of the hand.

Retroflexion. Neck extension.

Rooting reflex. Head turning and mouth opening to touch on the cheek.

Self-perceived competence. The ability to evaluate one's performance in comparison to others.

Sensitive period. Stage of neurodevelopment when the brain is primed for experience-induced plasticity.

Sensorimotor period. Piagetian stage where learning involves sensorimotor experiences.

Skipping. Forward movement where the legs alternate in a step-hop pattern.

Superior palmar grasp (3 jaw chuck). Object grasped from the top with thumb, index, and middle fingers.

Telegraphic speech. Two-word bursts of speech (noun plus verb).

Temperament. Behavioral tendencies, including emotionality, reactivity, and sociability.

Tonic labyrinthine reflex. Enhanced flexion in prone and extension in supine in the newborn.

Ulnar palmar grasp. Grasp objects with lateral aspect of hand (ring and little fingers into palm).

Writhing movements. Slow forceful movements of the extremities.

ABBREVIATIONS

ATNR	asymmetrical tonic neck reflex
GM	generalized movements
STNR	symmetrical tonic neck reflex

9

Neuroplasticity

Deborah S. Nichols-Larsen and D. Michele Basso

OBJECTIVES

1) Differentiate neurogenesis and gliogenesis

2) Compare and contrast neurogenesis in development and adults

3) Examine mechanisms of injury to the CNS

4) Differentiate the mechanisms of plasticity in the intact and injured CNS

5) Differentiate adaptive and maladaptive plasticity

6) Examine the role of rehabilitation in plasticity post-CNS injury

● DEVELOPMENTAL NEUROGENESIS

As described in Chapter 19 ("Neural Tube Disorders and Hydrocephalus"), the nervous system arises from neural crest cells within the ectodermal layer of the developing embryo. Cell proliferation transforms the neural plate into the neural tube that is initially differentiated into three vesicles from rostral to caudal: prosencephalon, mesencephalon, and rhombencephalon. Further cell proliferation results in a five-vesicle structure: telencephalon (cerebral hemispheres), diencephalon (retina, hypothalamus, thalamus, epithalamus, and subthalamus), mesencephalon (midbrain), metencephalon (pons, cerebellum), and myelencephalon (medulla), which is contiguous with the remainder of the neural tube that forms the spinal cord. The lumen of the neural tube develops into the ventricular system and central spinal canal.[1,2]

Initially, the tissue of the neural tube expands into three layers (see Figure 9-1): ependymal layer, mantel layer, and marginal layer. The **ependymal layer** provides the border for the developing ventricular system and is cell rich with rapidly dividing cells. The **mantel layer** will become the gray matter (cortex and deep nuclei), and the **marginal layer** will be filled with axons (white matter). Within weeks, there will be six identifiable layers of cellular activity plus the marginal zone: (1) **ventricular zone** – area of rapid cell proliferation; (2) **subventricular zone** – second area of cell proliferation; (3) **intermediate zone** – developing

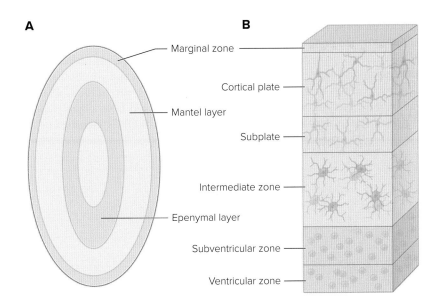

A
- Marginal zone
- Mantel layer
- Epenymal layer

B
- Marginal zone
- Cortical plate
- Subplate
- Intermediate zone
- Subventricular zone
- Ventricular zone

FIGURE 9-1 Cell proliferation in the developing CNS. A. Three layered neural tube with cell proliferation in the ependymal layer and cell poor mantel and marginal layers. **B.** Five layers of developing brain: ventricular and subventricular zones are areas of cell proliferation filled with neural stem cells; intermediate zone will be filled with glial cells and become the white matter; the subplate will house early neurons that will connect the cortex to the thalamus; the cortical plate will become the cortex; the marginal zone is cell poor but will contain axons and a few neurons. (Used with permission of Deborah S. Nichols Larsen, PT, PhD. The Ohio State University.)

white matter; (4) **subplate** – early neurons and glial cells that facilitate connections between the cortex and thalamus;[1] (5) **cortical plate** – developing cortex; and (6) **marginal zone** – cell poor with surface neurons and horizontal fibers.[2]

Cell Proliferation

Neurogenesis refers to the development of neurons, while **gliogenesis** is the development of glial cells; these are interrelated processes. **Neural stem cells** (NSCs) are progenitor cells for both neurons and glia that can be found initially in the ventricular zone, and then also in the subventricular zone, where they undergo rapid cell divisions; thus, they are also called neural progenitor cells (NPCs). While NSCs appear undifferentiated, they actually differ in their mitotic activity, cellular and molecular characteristics, transcription factor expression, and the types of cells that they produce.[3,4] One of the first cells to develop from the NSCs of the ependymal layer is the apical **radial glial cell** (a**RGC**). aRGCs extend a projection to the ependymal lining of the ventricle and another through the other cortical zones to the pial lining, which covers the outside of the developing neural tube.[5]

Radial glial cells replicate, initially forming neurons but ultimately forming glia – astrocytes and ependymal cells along with oligodendrocyte progenitor cells that proliferate to produce these crucial glia.[6] In addition, the aRGCs form a matrix that helps to guide the neurons to their ultimate settling point in the cortical plate[7] (see Figure 9-2). While aRGCs are the first progenitor cells to develop, eventually there are multiple progenitor cells, derived from ependymal cells, referred to as short neural precursors, intermediate progenitor cells, and basal radial glial cells.[3] As a group, these NSCs populate the neurons of the mature brain. Cell proliferation is stimulated and controlled by signaling **morphogens**; these are found within the cerebrospinal fluid and enter the ventricular and subventricular zones via the primary cilium (projection adhered to the ventricular lining). Morphogens include sonic hedgehog (SHH), growth factors (fibroblast and insulin), and bone morphogenic proteins (BMPs).[8] Within the VC and SVC, progenitor cells distribute themselves in distinct areas and generate unique neural cell types. Again, signaling from various morphogens and microRNAs trigger the migration of the progenitor cells to specific regions of the subcortical and cortical plates and apparently

play a role in the ultimate differentiation of neuronal cell type (e.g., excitatory or inhibitory).[9]

Developmental Neuroplasticity: Connectivity and Pruning

Following cell migration, networks of neurons develop that tie critical areas of the brain together through axonal growth to specific synaptic targets (e.g., corticocortical, thalamocortical). This process begins early in the second trimester of gestation. Axonal growth and the sprouting of terminal axon boutons are guided by neurotrophic and morphogenic factors, secreted by glial cells. For example, oligodendrocytes are known to secrete nerve growth factor and brain-derived neurotrophic factor (BDNF) that contribute to axonal outgrowth. Cell adhesion molecules on the surface of target neurons also appear to guide synapse formation.[10] Eventually, however, it is the activity within the neural circuits that fine-tunes ultimate synaptic connectivity; this second stage of axonal growth seems to be facilitated by neurotrophic factors (e.g., BDNF).[11] Initially, there is an overproduction of axon collaterals, and synaptic contacts, followed by remodeling that eliminates poorly connected axons, excessive synapses, and ultimately neuron overpopulation. The elimination of unnecessary axon collaterals is known as **pruning**, and the destruction of neurons is referred to as **programmed cell death**. One determinant of axonal pruning is the need for each axonal collateral to establish effective synapses with postsynaptic neurons; poorly connected axons are eliminated. This involves reabsorption of the axon fragment back into the proximal axon or disconnection of the distill axon component as a fragment that is then, phagocytized by surrounding microglia.[12] Figure 9-3 illustrates these changes.

Similarly, dendrites that do not establish connections are eliminated. Ultimately, neurons that are poorly connected or remain inactive go through programmed cell death so that effective neural networks remain. Microglia play a critical role in this process by phagocytosing the inactive synapses and junctions.[13] This process extends into the first 6 months of neonatal life.[10] In addition, myelination of developing neurons continues well into the second year of life, associated with developmental maturation. Myelin in the CNS is formed by oligodendrocytes that are derived from oligodendrocyte precursor cells (OPC); the density of OPCs increases or decreases, depending on the

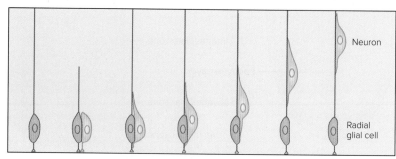

Radial glial cell division generates neurons   Neuronal migration on radial glial cells

Neuron

Radial glial cell

FIGURE 9-2 Neuronal migration along radial glial cells. Radial glial cells produce neurons and then guide them along their apical projection to the cortical plate. (Reproduced with permission from Kandel ER, Schwartz JH, Jessell TM, Siegelbaum SA, Hudspeth AJ. *Principles of Neural Science.* 5th ed. New York, NY: McGraw-Hill; 2013.)

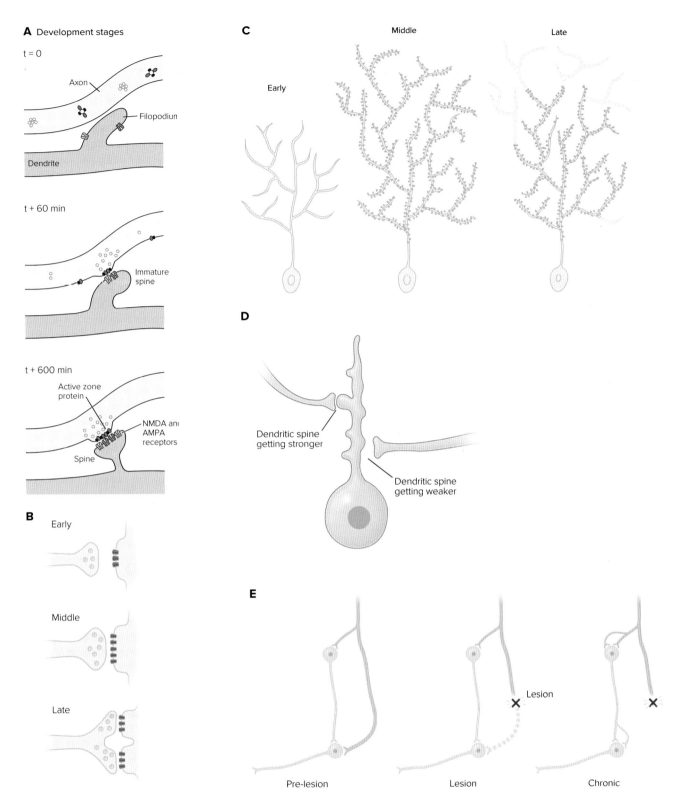

FIGURE 9-3 Synaptogenesis, pruning, and sprouting – mechanisms of neural development and injury repair. A. An axon passing by a cell can develop a new branch called a filopodium, which begins to form a synapse, and eventually becomes functional. The postsynaptic member begins to develop a synaptic spine. **B.** When a synapse strengthens over time, the presynaptic and postsynaptic elements can enlarge, and eventually, a second synapse can develop. **C.** As neurons develop, they initially lack synaptic spines. In the middle phase of development, they have an overabundance. As the connections mature, there is pruning, and some spines are eliminated. **D.** A dendritic spine can become stronger or weaker over time as the plasticity develops. **E.** In a circuit with alternative pathways, if one route is lesioned, the other can become stronger and replace the lost function. (A and C: Reproduced with permission from Kandel ER, Schwartz JH, Jessell TM, Siegelbaum SA, Hudspeth AJ. *Principles of Neural Science.* 5th ed. New York, NY: McGraw-Hill; 2013.) (B, D, and E: Used with permission from John A. Buford, PT, PhD.)

activity within the network that they support. Enriched environments in the neonatal period have been found to increase the number of OPC in the associated sensory or motor region and ultimately the number of oligodendrocytes, accounting for numerous myelin sheaths. Similarly, deprivation can result in a decrease in OPC, oligodendrocytes, and myelin. Interestingly, existing myelin sheaths were found to initially retract as training began, which seemed necessary for axon terminal sprouting to occur, which was then followed by sheath expansion.[14] OPC activation, resulting in new oligodendrocytes and myelin expansion, appears to be triggered by neurotransmitter release along the axon length; this is also related to the activity within the respective neuron.[15]

The efficacy of synapses, within the developing nervous system, is honed by long-term potentiation and depression (as described in Chapter 7). In the case of developing synapses, **long-term potentiation (LTP)** is associated with well-established connections, axon survival, and strengthening of the network; simply, continued excitation of a neuron by a presynaptic neuron results in a change in one or both neurons such that the presynaptic neuron can more easily excite the postsynaptic neuron (synaptic potentiation), thereby strengthening the connection and efficiency of the connection.[13] Conversely, **long-term depression (LTD)** results from poor connectivity and induces axonal pruning and potentially cell death. These two processes are commonly referred to as Hebbian changes and involve an increase or decrease in the number of dendritic spines or the number or density of synapses between the neurons.[16] Network remodeling in many neural networks occurs as a result of experience within sensitive periods; hence, inactivity, during a sensitive period, can result in loss of essential neurons. These changes occur through expansion of axon projections, elimination of dendritic spines, and creation of cross-linkages between the synaptic membranes, referred to as CAMs.[17] Importantly, critical periods are special sensitive periods, associated with a greater capacity for plasticity than at other times of development and are associated with increased GABA inhibition. BDNF is thought to play an important role in these critical periods through the stimulation of GABA neuron maturation. Other molecular changes, then, apparently impose a blockade to the critical period potentiation. Notably, premature birth or developmental trauma may block neural network formation within critical periods.[10]

● ADULT NEUROGENESIS

Interestingly, gliogenesis continues throughout the brain and spinal cord into adult life, while neurogenesis is largely confined to embryonic and early postnatal development. However, adult neurogenesis does exist in discrete areas of the nervous system, referred to as neurogenic niches; in humans, these appear localized in the subgranular and subventricular zones adjacent to the hippocampus, supporting new neurons for the dentate gyrus of the hippocampus and the olfactory bulb. Neurogenesis has also been described in the motor cortex in primates and the progenitor cells are thought to come from the subventricular zone.[18] It is important to remember that progenitor cells

in the embryonic period can produce both neurons and glial cells; thus, limitations in neurogenesis in adulthood likely stem from changes in the microenvironment necessary for the generation of neurons, including the absence of appropriate growth factors and the presence of cytokines, chemokines, and other signaling molecules that block the production of neurons.[4,19] Within the hippocampus, adult-born neurons appear to generate synapses and become active in the hippocampal networks; however, it is unclear what role these new neurons play in the functions of the hippocampus (learning, memory, emotion).[20] Neurotransmitters are also integral to the activation of NSCs to induce neurogenesis.[21] Further, neurogenesis is slower in the mature brain, fewer cells progress to neurons, and the survival rate of those that do become neurons is lower than seen in development.[22] Also, axonal projections typically target active synapses to insure viability; therefore, synaptogenesis in pathways damaged by disease is unlikely. However, synaptogenesis of bystander pathways, that is, pathways not directly damaged by trauma or disease, has been widely reported in animal studies.[23] There is also some indication that an enriched environment, exercise, and diet facilitate neurogenesis in adults, which, in turn, can be disrupted by aging and stress[19] as well as pathologic conditions such as seizures.[4] Aging appears to induce a state of quiescence (inactivity) in stem cells as well as moderate inflammation, resulting in limited cell proliferation.[4] In addition, the maturation of new neurons and their integration into existing networks is impaired in the aging brain even though the new cells appear normal. Factors that likely influence these findings with aging, include body system changes (decreased metabolism and overall activity level) as well as the neural environment, including decreases in neurotrophic factors, overall synaptic activity, and cellular energy production.[22]

● LEARNING-ASSOCIATED NEUROPLASTICITY

Similar to the earlier discussion of developmental plasticity, a significant body of evidence has emerged to support that the brain continues to be highly malleable throughout our lives, adapting and reorganizing in response to the level of activity it experiences. In Chapter 7, we discussed this in terms of memory; however, any skill acquisition is associated with neuroplastic changes within those neural networks activated during practice. For example, the motor area of the hand, in the primary motor cortex (precentral gyrus, M1), expands in response to specific training paradigms.[11] Multiple changes seem to support learning-induced plasticity: (1) *synaptogenesis* evident through new dendritic spines, changes in size and shape of the dendrites, and increased synaptic density per neuron[24]; (2) *oligodendrocyte precursor cell proliferation*, resulting in more oligodendrocytes and increased myelination in learning specific neurons; and (3) alterations in specific *gene expression* that seem to align with the changes in synapses and white matter. Neurotrophins such as BDNF and glial cell derived neurotrophic factor (GDNF) are proteins that are catalysts for cell signaling differentiation and other changes associated with neuroplasticity.[25] LTP occurs in two phases: (1) early, lasting

1 to 3 hours, which requires activation of *N*-methyl-D-asparate (NMDA) receptors and an influx of Ca^{2+}; and (2) late, lasting at least 24 hours, which requires protein synthesis induced by transcription factor activation and gene expression that results in structural change. In addition, LTP appears to involve activation of previously "silent synapses," which are inactive synapses that are unable to conduct impulses until provided with a sufficient stimulus. Maintenance of these synaptic changes, associated with LTP, requires the presence of BDNF to activate protein synthesis.[11,26,27]

LTP occurs in the presence of heightened neuronal activity, associated with skill acquisition. Of interest, tegmental dopamine projections to M1 seem to play a critical role in these mechanisms of learning-induced motor plasticity, and there is some speculation that naturally occurring differences in the density of these dopamine projections may underlie individual differences in motor ability.[11,27] Modulation of synaptic activity is mediated by multiple factors, including interleukin-1β (IL-1β) and tumor necrosis factor (TNFα). One method for synaptic modulation, known as synaptic scaling, is induced by TNFα and associated with an increase in the density of receptors at the synapse, specifically glutamate receptors (NMDA).[28] Other mechanisms of LTP include (1) increased calcium permeability; (2) dendritic spine enlargement; (3) increased protein synthesis; and (4) enhanced actin polymerization.[29] Calcium influx appears to trigger several different enzymatic cascades that enhance existing receptor function but also stimulate new receptor generation in postsynaptic neurons. Interestingly, different cascades respond to different stimulus characteristics (e.g., intensity versus frequency), suggesting that LTP likely involves different mechanisms at different synapses.[17] Actin polymerization is thought to be involved in early-stage LTP, providing reorganization of the cytoskeletal structure of active synapses, specifically to facilitate dendritic spine formation. Changes in actin are followed by the appearance of membrane attachment proteins that further consolidate LTP changes at the synapse.[30]

BDNF also appears to contribute to motor map reorganization and synaptogenesis, associated with motor learning, through stimulating protein synthesis to support synapse formation.[31] Neural reorganization increases the metabolic demands of the tissue and triggers the expansion of the capillary bed, known as **angiogenesis**. This involves either (1) the splitting of capillaries into two branches by a process called intussusception or (2) the projection of new vascular "sprouts" that connect to a second capillary. This results in increased vascular density and the ability to meet the oxygen and nutritional demand of the new synapses.[32] Angiogenesis is mediated by endothelial progenitor cells that migrate to areas of need and secrete VEGF and cytokines necessary for angiogenesis.[33]

Angiogenesis is important to motor skill learning in the intact CNS, but in the injured nervous system, it can lead to an altered cellular environment and delay or prevent neural plasticity. As new blood vessels form, they are leaky and allow the infiltration of white blood cells like neutrophils and macrophages into far-reaching areas of the brain and spinal cord.[34,35] These peripheral cells release inflammatory cytokines and create neuroinflammation in the neural environment. Barrier permeability and the accompanying inflammatory microenvironment

occur under stress, neuropathic pain, spinal cord injury, and amyotropic lateral sclerosis.[36–38] In terms of physical therapy, rehabilitation can increase barrier permeability, inflammatory cytokines, and metabolic dysregulation, which can impede motor relearning and recovery.[34,35,39,40] Interestingly, regular physical activity as part of a healthy lifestyle can have a protective effect on the barrier and reduce the neuroinflammatory response when it precedes CNS injury or the onset of neural conditions. Thus, the timing of when physical activity is administered warrants careful consideration and perhaps avoiding inflammatory periods. As discussed with developmental neuroplasticity, a second mechanism of plasticity with learning is LTD. In this case, synapses with limited activity levels can be eliminated; this may contribute to forgetting but is also a mechanism for honing neural pathways that are critical to function by eliminating those that are not as critical. This, in effect, is a method for achieving synaptic efficiency. Surprisingly, LTD is also characterized by an increase in calcium influx; however, in this instance, the increase is slow and prolonged. These two neural processes (LTP and LTD) occur simultaneously at adjacent synapses of the same neuron to maximize synaptic efficiency. LTD at some synapses can induce **microglial synaptic pruning**; this involves phagocytosis of the synaptic components in both the pre- and postsynaptic neurons of inactive synapses by resident microglia.[28]

● NEURAL RESPONSE TO INJURY

Focal Degeneration

Neural injury typically involves both focal damage (at the site of the injury) and secondary remote damage downstream from the initial injury. With **focal damage** there is disruption of cellular function within the soma (cell body) of neurons at the immediate site of injury, leading to cell death. Additionally, neurons that experience axon disruption (axotomy) will undergo either retrograde or anterograde degeneration or both. **Anterograde degeneration**, also known as **Wallerian** or **orthograde** degeneration, occurs in the distal segment or fragment that has been separated from the proximal component; since axonal transport is lost, this segment rapidly undergoes degeneration and is phagocytized by the circulating microglia. The proximal component may also undergo a series of intracellular changes that ultimately lead to degeneration of the axon (dying back), known as **retrograde degeneration**; this is dependent on the location of the injury and whether some axonal projections maintain functional synapses. If some projections remain, the axon may survive. However, completely axotomized neurons, in which no collaterals remain, undergo pronounced changes including swelling, chromatolysis, damage to cellular components, impaired protein synthesis among other mechanisms that disrupt endoplasmic reticulum function and cytoskeleton integrity, ultimately resulting in cellular shrinkage and cell death.[41] This loss of axons results in **synaptic stripping** on the somas and dendrites of postsynaptic neurons, to which the axotomized neurons project.[42] The release of intracellular components from damaged cells into the extracellular space attracts resident glial cells as well as peripheral immune cells to the site of injury and stimulates the production of chemokines, cytokines, and other excitotoxins, catalyzing an extensive immune reaction, designed to stabilize the injury site. Secondary disruption of the blood-brain barrier (BBB) follows in association with widespread neuroinflammation, altered cell metabolism, and abnormal glial activity, which may be accompanied by leakage of the neural capillaries, hemorrhage, and brain edema, resulting in generalized CNS hypoxia.[43] In association with neural loss, myelin sheaths also collapse and require removal by microglia; this myelin debris contributes to additional inflammation and microglial activation. Additionally, myelin damage on surviving neurons may impede neural conductivity or result in desynchronization.[44]

Remote Neurodegeneration

Secondary retrograde and anterograde degeneration can result from loss of connectivity with neurons lost at the site of the focal injury. Those neurons that project onto the lost neurons have lost their functional connections; thus, they may undergo **retrograde transneuronal degeneration**. Similarly, those neurons that typically receive axonal connections from the lost neurons have lost at least a portion of their activation source, and thus may undergo **anterograde transneuronal degeneration**.[41] This secondary neurodegeneration (e.g., retrograde and anterograde transneuronal degeneration) is common after neural injury, leading to loss of neurons in the area surrounding the focal injury and at sites distal to but functionally related to the injured area. While several factors impact the degree of remote cell death, including magnitude of the original injury, patient age, and connectivity characteristics of the damaged neuronal networks, several mechanisms contribute to cell survival or death.[41] In the subsequent sections, we will discuss the mechanisms of secondary cell damage.

Inflammation

Inflammation at the site of injury and in areas well away from the primary injury is mediated by both microglia and astrocytes that secrete pro-inflammatory chemokines and cytokines, attracting immune cells to the site of injury. The astrocytes function to reestablish the BBB, stimulate glutamate reabsorption, and limit the spread of damage. Once activated, astrocytes are called reactive, migrating to and proliferating at the injury site where they contribute to scar formation (glial astrocytosis) around the site of injury to limit the infiltration of inflammatory cells and toxic elements into adjacent healthy tissue, thereby serving a neuroprotective function[45]; yet this glial scar serves to block axon regeneration.[43] Astrocytes also control the permeability of the BBB and the extracellular ion concentration; post-injury, they can be hyperreactive and thereby deleterious to neurons.[43] In addition, microglia produce inflammatory mediators, including free radicals, glutamate, TNF-α, IL-1β, and nitric oxide, along with pro-inflammatory chemokines and cytokines, that function to initially remove damaged tissue but also contribute to a prolonged inflammatory period and exacerbate neural damage at the site of injury. Therefore, injury induces a battle between pro- and anti-inflammatory processes to regain homeostasis, yet multiple factors may prolong this inflammatory period, including the age and overall health of the individual.[46] Additionally, neuroinflammation can occur at sites remote from but anatomically connected to the initial injury site, also subsequent to an influx of microglia, astrocytes, and macrophages.[46] While most people consider that inflammation spreads slowly to remote regions over the course of 2 to 3 weeks, recent findings in the spinal cord showed profound microglial activation and inflammation within 24 hours of an injury at least 10 segments away. In these remote regions, changes in structural neural plasticity and dendritic spines can be seen within 7 days.[47] Further, this remote neuroinflammation can persist long after the inflammation at the initial site has declined, reportedly for years, exacerbating the dysfunction in the neural network.[47]

Excitotoxicity

Excessive release of glutamate, dopamine, and norepinephrine occurs as a result of CNS trauma or ischemia, as experienced with head injury, prolonged seizures (e.g., status epilepticus – see Chapter 20), or stroke. Reduced glial function may limit the scavenging of glutamate, also increasing its extracellular concentration. Excessive glutamate results in an influx of Na^+ and Ca^{++} into the cell with subsequent cellular edema and contraction of the extracellular space. Similarly, glutamate also stimulates reactive oxygen species production (see later section on oxidative stress).[48] Likewise, there is often an exaggerated release of dopamine and norepinephrine with a buildup of their toxic by-products. In addition, the loss and/or malfunctioning of inhibitory neurons can further exacerbate the excitotoxicity initiated by these excitatory neurotransmitters. Diminished functioning of GABAergic neurons can persist for weeks after the initial injury. Astrocytes are critical for the degradation of GABA and the production of glutamine, the precursor of GABA; this cycle is disrupted, post-injury, by the presence of TNFα and other pro-inflammatory mediators.[49] Together, these factors create a toxic environment and ultimately contribute to additional neuronal death.[48]

Apoptosis

Programmed cell death not only occurs as a process in neural development but also serves a maintenance function to assure homeostasis. Additionally, it occurs in response to neural injury and is known as apoptosis; in the case of a central nervous system injury or disease, a process of programmed cell death is initiated to help preserve the system. There are two pathways that induce apoptosis, which can both be activated by internal or external stimuli.[50] The first is known as the **external pathway** and involves surface receptors, known as death receptors that trigger a cascade of caspase activity.[41] **Caspases** are endoprotease enzymes that exist in an inactive form until neural damage transforms them into active molecules. The first caspases to be activated are known as initiators (caspases 8 and 9); these, in turn, activate executioner caspases (3, 6, and 7), which disrupt cellular structural proteins and other cellular components, leading to cell death. The second pathway also involves caspase activity, targeting the cell's mitochondria. Multiple factors can trigger this **internal pathway**, including loss of specific growth factors, cell membrane disruption, hypoxia, and certain hormones. This pathway is the one active in developmental programmed cell death.[51] Apoptosis works in conjunction with the immune system, eliminating target cells to achieve homeostasis. Apoptosis is distinguished from necrosis, which is trauma-induced cell death that is passive and results in inflammation; apoptosis is an active process ignited by a death signal. Interestingly, abnormal apoptosis is thought to contribute to neurodegenerative diseases such as Alzheimer's and multiple sclerosis.[50] After neural injury, calcium influx causes a series of cellular changes that disrupt neuron metabolism and eventually may trigger apoptosis as the cells are unable to reestablish the axonal membrane.[52]

Autophagy

Autophagy is a natural process to eliminate damaged proteins or organelles within the cell body to promote optimal cell functioning, whereby damaged intracellular components are phagocytized (encapsulated and degraded) by lysosomal enzymes[53]; it is triggered by multiple genes and complex cell signaling.[54] While autophagy, after focal injury, may initially be triggered to eliminate damaged organelles within injured neurons to promote homeostasis, it may actually determine cell survival and ultimately become a secondary pathway for cell death. Autophagy is also responsible for clearing glial cells, following neural injury.[54] Of interest, autophagy has been identified in remote neurons that are functionally connected to the injury site; however, the triggers for this occurrence remain elusive.[53] Autophagy and apoptosis may share common mechanisms and have been found to occur simultaneously; however, there is some suggestion that apoptosis occurs when autophagy is ineffective in achieving homeostasis.[41,54] Of note, autophagy has also been linked to multiple neurodegenerative disorders and cancers (e.g., amyotrophic lateral sclerosis).[55]

Oxidative and Nitrosative Stress

Following neural injury, there is also a proliferation of reactive oxygen species (ROS) and reactive nitrogen species (RNS); these are normally supportive of neural function but in excess can be hazardous. ROS are produced by mitochondria in the formation of ATP, and when mitochondria are damaged, there is excessive accumulation of ROS, which then attack the cell membrane and degrade other key cellular components (e.g., proteins), causing inflammation and disrupting the BBB. Similarly, nitric oxide (NO) is a signaling molecule that is active both intracellularly and extracellulary in multiple systems, including the nervous system. Following a brain injury, NO reacts with excess oxygen ions to produce RNS, which is toxic to neurons, leading to cell death by damaging key proteins and lipids.[41,56]

The mechanisms, discussed here, all contribute to secondary cell death after initial CNS injury; current treatment methods, both medical and rehabilitative, are focused on blocking this secondary cell loss to improve outcomes. Some of these methods will be discussed in the second half of this book, along with the disease processes; however, in the next section, we will review the general processes for neural plasticity associated with CNS injury or disease.

PLASTICITY AFTER CNS INJURY

Myelin Plasticity after CNS Injury

Most of what we know about plasticity during skill learning and in recovery from CNS injury or disease is focused on neural plasticity and is described below. However, recent discoveries point to an important role of myelin and myelin plasticity in recovery. Myelinated CNS neuronal axons are typically thought to be fully wrapped from the axon hillock to the presynaptic endings. However, it is now clear that gaps in myelination exist along some axons in healthy CNS, and these gaps slow neural conduction.[57,58] These large intermodal gaps hold the potential to improve motor learning, relearning, and recovery should new myelination occur in these regions. In fact, neuronal firing, as during skill learning or rehabilitation, releases neurotransmitters along the axon and triggers OPCs to become mature, myelinating oligodendrocytes.[59,60] When OPCs are prevented from maturing and therefore can't myelinate, complex motor learning fails, indicating that new myelin is required for skill acquisition.[61,62] Translation of these myelin-related effects recently occurred in animal and human SCI.[63] Using a challenging form of locomotor training in chronic SCI, greater myelin plasticity occurred in both animals and humans. Invasive techniques in animals with SCI proved that treadmill training was required to induce new myelin formation and axonal wrapping and contributed to greater locomotor skill.[63] Likewise, training-induced myelin plasticity plays a role in motor skill recovery of upper extremity function after stroke.[64] Some brain regions have greater myelin plasticity, during skill learning in both healthy controls and stroke, while other regions only reflect motor relearning in people with stroke. Also, reduction in myelin is a biomarker for other conditions treated by physical therapists, including the ipsilesional cortex post-stroke,[65,66] multiple sclerosis,[67] and traumatic brain injury.[68]

Neuroplasticity after CNS Injury

Sleep and Behavioral and Neural Plasticity

Sleep is considered to facilitate neuroplasticity.[69] Phases of greater sleep coincide with periods of heightened plasticity during memory consolidation, neural recovery, and neural reorganization in development. A particular part of sleep, rapid eye movement (REM) sleep, appears to play a primary role in plasticity. In infants, myoclonic twitches during REM sleep are considered part of a refinement process of sensory and motor cortical maps that will transition into mature coordinated movements. Episodes of sleep deprivation typically result in synaptic downscaling, via fewer new synapses and lower synaptic density, especially in the hippocampus, and results in memory deficits. An interesting new application in animal models uses sleep deprivation to eliminate synapses and maladaptive plasticity in post-traumatic stress disorder. For neurological conditions that require extensive rehabilitation, scientists are beginning to manipulate sleep to induce greater spontaneous plasticity. This plasticity reflects an optimal window to deliver activity-based training. Promising findings in animal studies are emerging for stroke.[70] Several other rehabilitation-intensive neural conditions are expected to have suboptimal plasticity due to recursive relationships.

Chronic pain or neuropathic pain interferes with sleep and sleep loss worsens pain. In spinal cord injury (SCI), sleep loss is severe and longstanding and limits activity-based plasticity. The causes of sleep disruption after SCI include apnea, night spasms and spasticity, neuropathic pain, bowel and bladder incontinence at night, and others.[71] Traumatic brain injury (TBI) induces opposite effects on sleep – insomnia/difficulty staying asleep or hypersomnia.[72] Prioritizing recovery of normal sleep patterns may increase the recovery potential for skill training, plasticity, and consolidation.

Plasticity Promoters

Neural changes, post-injury or during neurologic disease, target the salvaging and strengthening of survivor neurons and their synapses and facilitation of new axonal–dendritic connections. For example, after a SCI, astrocytes rush to the lesion, restoring blood flow, blocking the activity of peripheral leukocytes, and promoting revascularization.[23] Alternatively, after many types of neural injury, microglia stimulate the retraction of excitatory axonal boutons to protect surviving neurons from excessive excitation, known as **excitatory stripping**. There are several endogenous plasticity promotors, specifically **neurotrophins** (e.g., BDNF, NT-3), which are brain-derived proteins that are active in neurogenesis and activate complex signaling pathways post-injury to stabilize the BBB and limit the lesion size. Neurotrophins promote cell survival, strengthen synaptic connections, and promote axonal growth and sprouting,[73] yet following SCI, they are downregulated. Thus, research is targeting the application of these neurotrophins in the spinal cord to promote recovery, which in animal models of SCI has improved axonal regrowth around the lesion, prevented synaptic stripping, and protected against excitotoxicity by promoting inhibitory synapse connections.[42] Importantly, BDNF and NT-3 are regulated by exercise within the spinal cord and muscle. After SCI in rodents, treadmill training increased BDNF and was associated with resolution of neuropathic pain. Interestingly, static standing exercise or rhythmic non-weight-bearing swimming exercise did not produce the neurotrophin or sensory effects, and neuropathic pain remained.[74]

Spontaneous Recovery

Early spontaneous recovery is likely dependent on recovered activity of surviving neurons in the penumbra (area surrounding the lesion). Immediately following injury, a period of neural "shock" exists, known as diaschisis, whereby neurons in the penumbra and areas, connecting to the lesioned area, demonstrate limited conduction and metabolic activity. This resolves over a matter of weeks. During this time period, studies have demonstrated neurite outgrowth, local sprouting, synaptogenesis, and angiogenesis. Sprouting is a mechanism by which axons grow additional distal projections to fill vacated receptor sites. In animal models, improved motor performance has also demonstrated a reliance on compensation and expansion of motor maps, corresponding to the compensating muscle groups (e.g., trunk muscles compensating for shoulder muscles). Additionally, there is a bilateral change in NMDA and GABA receptors, with upregulation of the former and downregulation of the latter as well as sprouting of neurons that project to the peri-infarct area, including transcallosal projections from the non-lesioned hemisphere. Notably, interhemispheric connections likely play a greater role in recovery from larger lesions than smaller lesions.[11]

This **functional reorganization** occurs in areas that have synergistic functions to the damaged areas. This may involve adjacent areas of the cerebral cortex, such as an adjoining area within the primary motor cortex, within the premotor or supplementary motor cortices, or reorganization of brainstem and/or spinal cord networks, such as the rubrospinal, vestibulospinal, or tectospinal tracts in response to primary motor cortex damage.[75] These new projections to the peri-infarct area from the surrounding motor areas can completely replace the lost projections but may not be able to reproduce the same level of motor complexity.[5] Growth-promoting genes become present in the peri-infarct area and more distant areas that are functionally related to the recovering region; these facilitate axonal sprouting not just in the recovering area but also in the contralateral hemisphere. For example, motor cortex injury induces synaptic growth in the contralesional motor cortex and its projections to other areas such as the basal ganglia. Further, expansion of perilesional neuron projections into deafferented regions results in a reconfiguration of neural networks.[75] For example, damage of the primary motor cortex elicits expansion of premotor cortex, supplementary motor cortex, and motor area of the cingulate cortex. Similarly, spinal cord networks, especially those of the propriospinal neurons that link spinal cord levels, have been found to expand subsequent to SCI.[49] Such reorganization may involve not only axonal sprouting and dendritic arborization but also unmasking or potentiation of formerly silent synapses. However, such sprouting may change the excitatory-inhibitory balance within a given area; ultimately this can result in recovery of function, but the recovered function may not be the same as the pre-injury level of function.[76] There is some evidence that such neuroplasticity is associated with the presence of cytokines and other neurotrophic factors such as TNFα and, thereby, is limited to the time window when these mediators are present.[49] Multiple studies have examined the potential role of ipsilateral neural pathways in the recovery of function from a unilateral injury such as stroke; these pathways include the 10 to 20% uncrossed lateral corticospinal fibers, the anterior corticospinal tract as well as tracts originating in the brainstem – rubrospinal, vestibulospinal, reticulospinal. There is also a portion of the lateral corticospinal tract fibers that crosses again in the spinal cord, providing ipsilateral control. Imaging studies have demonstrated increased activation of contralesional primary sensorimotor, supplementary motor, and premotor cortices along with the cingulate cortex, thalamus, and red nucleus associated with gait post-stroke. The role of ipsilateral pathways in recovery is controversial as there is some suggestion that increased activity is associated with poorer outcomes. It may be that early contralesional (ipsilateral) activity is a predictor of poor recovery, but later activity may be associated with remodeling and recovery.[77]

Changes in neuronal phenotype have also been documented after CNS injury. One example of this is the apparent conversion of C fiber function in the spinal cord to assume Aδ function for the bladder. Typically, Aδ fibers convey bladder fullness while C fibers convey pain such as occurs with a bladder infection. Following a SCI, C fibers have been found to convey bladder fullness to initiate the voiding reflex.[49]

Remyelination begins within a few weeks of brain injury in surviving neurons, which is associated with an increase in OPCs and oligodendrocytes. Remyelination begins with rebuilding of the Nodes of Ranvier to allow conduction of action potentials; as myelin is reconstructed, it folds over itself, creating a double layer, and then wraps around the axon. When remyelination is incomplete, slower neural processing and desynchronization ensue.[44]

Cognitive reserve (CR) is thought to impact one's ability to recover from CNS injury. This refers to the complexity of the neural networks that have been created over one's lifetime; the greater the complexity, the greater the CR. This is similar to the effect training has on one's ability to run a marathon; the more training, the better prepared the body (muscles, cardiovascular and respiratory systems) is to complete the marathon. For the brain, it is also proposed that the more brain "exercise" that one does, the more CR is available to support recovery from an injury. This is supported by the finding that those with higher education levels often experience better recovery than those with less education.[75]

Experience-dependent Plasticity

Earlier in this chapter, we discussed the role of experience in the development of neural connections. Following neural injury, the nervous system demonstrates a remarkable capacity to repair and remodel itself. More important to the rehabilitation community, evidence over the last few decades has shown that this repair and remodeling responds to the experience of the patient following injury, and therefore is influenced by the therapy (or lack thereof) provided. Thus, experience-dependent plasticity is a critical process in the recovery of all patients with neurologic injuries/diseases. However, it should be noted that this plasticity can be adaptive or maladaptive, promoting recovery of lost function or preventing that recovery.

Maladaptive Plasticity

Perhaps the best example of maladaptive plasticity is the phenomenon that is known as **learned nonuse**. Briefly, this is a process whereby patients post-stroke experience negative feedback, when initially trying to use the paretic arm (e.g., limited success, pain); this feedback discourages subsequent use of the arm even as spontaneous recovery is occurring. Thus, patients fail to use retained function. Further, they are positively rewarded for developing compensatory strategies (e.g., trunk motion to achieve shoulder abduction) or using the non-paretic limb to achieve function, resulting in limited use of the paretic limb, despite greater movement ability than demonstrated. Interestingly, compensatory use of the non-paretic limb may disrupt plasticity in the peri-infarct area by targeting synaptogenesis within the contralesional hemisphere and decreasing neuroplasticity changes in the ipsilesional hemisphere.[11,75] Transcallosal projections from the contralesional hemisphere may also inhibit plasticity in the lesioned hemisphere, if early recovery focuses on compensatory use of the non-paretic limb.[75] These findings are critical for rehabilitationists, since they suggest that early treatment, which can be aimed at compensation

due to minimal motor ability in the paretic limbs, may, in fact, stimulate expansion of motor maps in the contralesional hemisphere rather than promoting plasticity changes in the lesioned hemisphere. Early in recovery some activity in the contralesional hemisphere is seen in patients who will go on to have good recovery; however, excessive activity in the contralesional hemisphere, as measured by functional magnetic resonance imaging (fMRI), appears to be maladaptive rather than adaptive, especially in the acute stage post-injury, where it has been linked to poorer recovery; however, many stroke survivors with good recovery demonstrate some contralesional control of the ipsilateral extremities as described in the spontaneous recovery section of this chapter.[77] Another example of maladaptive plasticity is the emergence of allodynia, following SCI, which seems to emerge from neural remodeling within the pain centers, responding to non-noxious inputs post-injury.[72] Similar to the previously described phenotypic change reported for afferent C and Aδ fibers, changes in Aβ fibers have been noted in the spinal cord such that they begin to function like C and Aδ fibers, contributing to allodynia post-SCI.[49] In addition, new evidence is emerging that spasticity may result from maladaptive plasticity within the gray matter of the spinal cord. An increased density of dendrites, combined with neuronal atrophy, leads to heightened excitability of neurons that produces hyperreflexia.[78]

Adaptive Plasticity

Adaptive plasticity is associated with functional recovery and is triggered by activity within the damaged networks. Rehabilitation is thought to promote adaptive plasticity through the same mechanisms described for spontaneous recovery – synaptogenesis, axonal regeneration, and functional reorganization. Importantly, exercise has been found to increase the presence of neurotrophins in damaged areas, supporting dendritic arborization and axonal regeneration, and to induce angiogenesis to support neuroplastic changes. Animal models have also demonstrated increased neurogenesis in response to exercise.[5]

Constraint-induced movement therapy (CIMT), which will be discussed in more detail in Chapter 11 ("Stroke"), is an evidence-based method to reduce learned nonuse and to expand the motor map of the paretic hand, as measured by TMS,[79] as well as to shift the locus of control of the hand back to the ipsilesional motor cortex as shown on fMRI.[80] Other rehabilitation techniques, including treadmill training and aerobic exercise, have also demonstrated enhanced neuroplasticity similar to that described for CIMT, characterized by stimulation of angiogenesis, upregulating the expression of neurotrophic factors, cell differentiation, greater integrity of white matter projections, and expansion of gray matter volume in cortical areas related to the training.[25,81] Recent research has also demonstrated that myelin plasticity occurs in targeted areas of training simultaneously with neuroplasticity and functional recovery post-SCI.[15] Similarly, following stroke, motor function was found to be strongly correlated with myelin integrity of the ipsilesional precentral motor area as measured by the myelin water fraction.[66] These findings illustrate the importance of focused training to promote neural and myelin plasticity to support better functional recovery post-injury.

Kleim reviewed multiple factors that seem critical to inducing adaptive plasticity in the injured CNS[82] (see Box 9-1).

Thus, as rehabilitation practitioners, physical, occupational, and speech therapists play a critical role in neural recovery through the implementation of targeted treatment programs. Notably, there is potentially a critical period post-injury, where the nervous system is maximally able to remodel itself, when protein and growth hormone upregulation peaks to promote neural regrowth and axonal sprouting. Thus, it is critical for us to identify that time period and provide therapy directed at promoting adaptive plasticity.[11] While specificity of training appears to be critical for new skill acquisition, there is evidence

---

Box 9-1 Critical Factors for Adaptive Neural Plasticity[82]

- Activity must target neural networks in which plasticity is desired.
- Activity can prevent secondary damage.
- Activity must target specific movements and skills that are salient to the patient to induce change in desired neural networks; saliency may activate critical emotional networks to facilitate plasticity.
- Neural plasticity requires repetition at an intensity that challenges the nervous system.
- The timing of activity is critical: (1) too much too early can exacerbate the lesion; (2) some early level of activity may be neuroprotective; (3) there may be a critical period or periods when plasticity is more likely; and (4) the window for plasticity is restricted and doesn't continue indefinitely.
- Older brains do not have the same capacity for remodeling that is available to younger brains.
- Plasticity in one neural network may facilitate (transference) or inhibit (interference) plasticity in other networks.

---

that aerobic activity (e.g., treadmill training or cycling) can raise BDNF, protein, and microRNA levels that support neuroplasticity mechanisms. Thus, this may also be an essential component of a rehabilitation program.[15,42]

METHODS OF MEASURING PLASTICITY IN VIVO

While much of what we know about neuroplasticity has been derived from animal studies, which allow the direct measurement of structural changes and the presence of neuroplasticity modulators, advances in multiple imaging techniques allow us to measure similar things in normal and clinical human subjects. **Structural imaging** typically uses magnetic resonance imaging (MRI) to measure overall brain size (total brain volume), the volume of given regions, or the thickness of the cortex in given regions, accomplished by specific analysis programs that allow targeted measurement of designated areas (see Figure 9-4). While this allows a gross measure of brain change, associated with neural injury or recovery, it does not provide specific information about what is causing the change in volume or thickness (e.g., dendritic or axonal expansion). Structural imaging, in conjunction with histological analysis, which can be done in animal models, allows clear examination of structural changes and changes in neuromodulators.[83] **Diffusion tensor imaging** (DTI) is another structural imaging technique that captures the direction of water diffusion within white matter structures. It is based on the concept that water diffuses along (parallel to) a white matter track rather than through (perpendicular to) it, referred to as anisotropic (single direction) diffusion. Thus, functional anisotropy (FA) is a measure of the consistency of water diffusion in a single direction and would be 1.0, if it was wholly in one direction. However, there is some diffusion between fibers and fiber tracts may cross; thus, FA is commonly less than 1.0 for a given spot within a white matter tract. Therefore, FA values

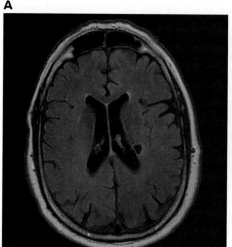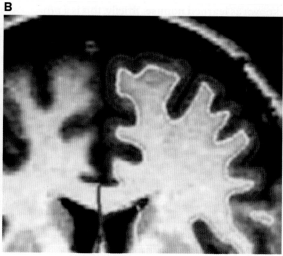

FIGURE 9-4 Structural imaging. A. MRI T1 scan allowing visualization of a small stroke (circled in red). **B.** An MRI FLAIR image, allowing segmentation and measurement of white and gray matter. (Used with permission from Deborah S. Nichols Larsen, PT, PhD. The Ohio State University.)

range from 0 to 1.0 for any give section (voxel) along a white matter tract. When white matter is damaged, the FA value also decreases further toward 0. DTI reconstructions, referred to as tractography, allow a visual depiction of white matter tracts, colorized to indicate direction so that **intrahemispheric** tracts (e.g., superior longitudinal fasciculus) can be distinguished from ascending/descending pathways (e.g., corticospinal tract) and **interhemispheric** tracts (e.g., corpus collosum) (see Figure 9-5A). While DTI allows visualization of white matter projections, it must be noted that these are reconstructions and not actual images of the white matter tract, yet, the relative size of the tract reconstruction does seem to correlate to the integrity of a specific tract.[84] Notably, changes in gray and white matter volume have been reported with skill acquisition and coincide with areas that are functionally tied to the skill acquired (e.g., visual and motor cortex with juggling).[83] In addition, early DTI after stroke has been found to be predictive of functional recovery,

based on the integrity of the corticospinal fibers (see Figure 9-5B).[66] DTI does not distinguish between changes in axons and changes in myelin; thus, a method to measure myelin plasticity is necessary. Functional magnetic resonance imaging (fMRI) and resting state fMRI are two methods used to examine the functional organization of neural networks. fMRI, also referred to as task-based FMRI (t-FMRI), captures the changes in blood flow that occur with brain activity to perform a task, referred to as the blood-oxygen-level-dependent (BOLD) signal; simply, areas of the brain that are active increase their metabolic activity, requiring increased blood flow to the active region (see Figure 9-6). Typically, studies involve comparing a period of activity to a period of rest and look for the change in blood flow across different brain regions between the two periods. Common parameters measured are the intensity and size of the change: the intensity is indicated by the color in an fMRI image (red = greatest intensity; yellow = least); size is measured

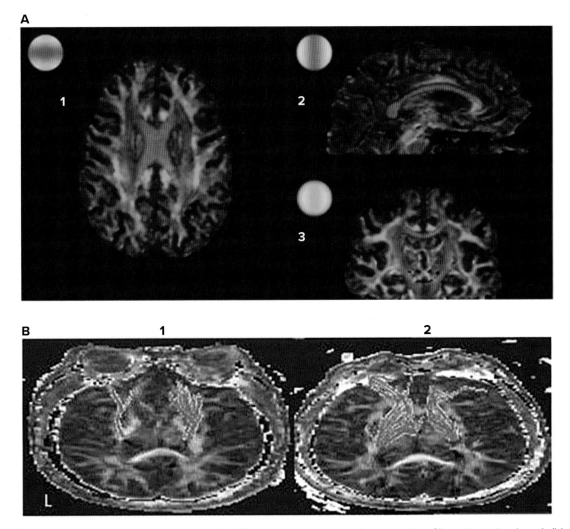

FIGURE 9-5 Measuring plasticity through imaging. A. Diffusion tensor imaging demonstrating fiber orientation (purple/blue = ascending/descending fibers; red = interhemispheric projections with the corpus collosum easily visible; green = intrahemispheric projections (e.g., superior and inferior fasciculi). 1 = transverse section; 2 = midsaggital section; and 3= coronal section.
B. Reconstruction of thalamocortical fibers conveying sensory information to the cortex post-stroke. 1 = Reconstruction is unable to capture many fibers in stroke hemisphere (left is much smaller than right), associated with poor sensory function; 2 = Reconstruction captures almost equal projections on right and left (stroke side), associated with good recovery of sensory function. (A: Reproduced with permission from Geyer JD, et al. Chapter 2. Neuroimaging in the Management of Neurological Disease. In: Carney PR, Geyer JD, eds. *Pediatric Practice: Neurology.* New York, NY: McGraw-Hill; 2010.) (B: Used with permission from Deborah S Larsen, The Ohio State University.)

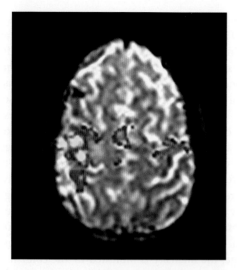

FIGURE 9-6 Functional magnetic resonance imaging (fMRI) post-stroke. Bilateral activity observed in sensorimotor cortex with greater activity on contralesional side during unilateral (hemiparetic) arm movement. (Used with permission from Deborah S. Larsen, The Ohio State University.)

by voxel number. The most intense point is referred to as the peak. Another commonly reported parameter is laterality. For most sensorimotor functions, the contralateral hemisphere demonstrates control, while the ipsilateral hemisphere is relatively silent. Laterality is analyzed, using a **laterality index** (LI = Contralateral voxel sum − Ipsilateral voxel sum divided by the sum of the contralateral and ipsilateral voxels.

$$LI = \frac{\sum C - \sum I}{\sum C + \sum I}$$

If a function is completely controlled by the contralateral hemisphere, the LI will be −1.0; if a function is completely controlled by the ipsilateral hemisphere, the LI will be +1.0. If a function is equally controlled by both hemispheres, the LI will be zero. Often, post-neural injury, the LI shifts toward the

ipsilateral hemisphere (less negative, 0, or a positive number); as recovery occurs, the LI should shift back toward −1.0, if the lesioned hemisphere resumes control of the function.[85]

Resting state fMRI (rs-fMRI) measures the spontaneous activity within neural networks during rest in the absence of a specific task. Again, it measures the BOLD signal; however, they are of much lower frequency than what is seen in t-fMRI. The goal of rs-fMRI is to establish functional connectivity between brain regions. This can be done by selecting a "seed" region and looking for simultaneous activity in the rest of the brain that indicates connectivity. Another method called independent component analysis looks for spontaneous fluctuations between brain regions that occur simultaneously, allowing identification of network connections. Multiple networks have been identified, including a default mode network, which is only active at rest and appears to contribute to introspection and mind wandering.[86]

Transcranial magnetic stimulation (TMS) uses magnetic stimulation to map activity in the motor cortex. Typically a figure of 8 coil is used, where the focus of the stimulation is at the intersection of the two rings of the eight. Activation produces a motor evoked potential (MEP) in muscles corresponding to the site of stimulation. The coil is moved over the scalp to define the area of activation of a specific muscle or muscle group (e.g., finger extensors), guided either with grids on a skull cap or a computerized image. The map size, location, and comparison between each hemisphere can be computed. Additionally, the amount of stimulation required to elicit the MEP can be compared between the two hemispheres (see Figure 9-7). This has been particularly useful in discriminating the integrity of the corticospinal tract post-stroke.[87]

Myelin Water Imaging is a novel, quantitative measure of myelin in vivo in animals and humans using MRI scanning. A T2 decay curve identifies three water components in the region of interest. The long component is a measure of cerebrospinal fluid. The intermediate component measures intra- and extracellular water molecules. The short component measures water molecules between the wraps of myelin. With thicker myelin,

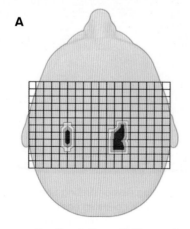
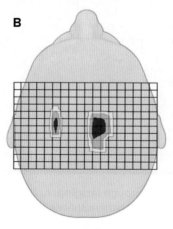

FIGURE 9-7 Transcranial magnetic stimulations. TMS mapping of the motor area controlling the extensor digitorum communis muscle. **A.** Pre-training with right lesioned hemisphere demonstrating larger area mapped but center is located at the same site as non-lesioned hemisphere. **B.** Post-training demonstrates expansion and posterior movement of mapped area for lesioned hemisphere (right) and no change on the non-lesioned hemisphere (left). (Used with permission from Deborah S. Nichols Larsen, PT, PhD. The Ohio State University.)

there is a greater water signal. The **myelin water fraction** (MWF) is calculated by dividing the short water component by the total water signal and is sensitive to demyelination, remyelination, and training-induced myelin during motor learning in healthy and injury conditions.[88] MWF has been found to be lower in several conditions described above (TBI,[66] the ipsilesional cortex following stroke,[66] and MS).[67] Within a specific brain region of interest, an MWF asymmetry ratio (MWF-AR) can be calculated: MWF-AR = MWF contralesional hemisphere/MWF ipsilesional hemisphere.[66]

REFERENCES

1. Hoerder-Suabedissen A, Molnar Z. Development, evolution and pathology of neocortical subplate neurons. *Nat Rev Neurosci.* 2015;16:133-146.

2. Kandel ER, Schwartz JH, Jessell TM, Siegelbaum SA, Hudspeth AJ. Chapter 53: differentiation and survival of nerve cells. In: *Principles of Neural Science.* New York, NY: McGraw Hill; 2013:1187-1208.

3. Laguesse S, Peyre E, Nguyen L. Progenitor genealogy in the developing cerebral cortex. *Cell Tissue Res.* 2015;359:17-32.

4. Urban N, Guillemot F. Neurogenesis in the embryonic and adult brain: same regulators, different roles. *Front Cell Neurosci.* 2014;9(article 396):1-19.

5. Xing L, Wilsch-Brauninger W, Huttner WB. How neural stem cells contribute to neocortex development. *Biochem Soc Trans.* 2021;49:1997-2006.

6. Dimou L, Gotz M. Glial cells as progenitors and stem cells: new roles in the healthy and diseased brain. *Physiol Rev.* 2014;94:709-737.

7. Tan X, Shhi SH. Neocortical neurogenesis and neuronal migration. *Wiley Interdisc Rev Dev Biol.* 2013;2(4):443-459.

8. Taverna E, Götz M, Huttner WB. The cell biology of neurogenesis: toward an understanding of the development and evolution of the neocortex. *Annu Rev Cell Dev Biol.* 2014;30:465-502.

9. Stappert L, Roese-Koerner B, Brüstle O. The role of microRNAs in human stem cells, neuronal differentiation and subtype specification. *Cell Tissue Res.* 2015;359:47-64.

10. Kiss JZ, Vasung L, Petrenko V. Process of cortical network formation and impact of early brain damage. *Curr Opin Neurol.* 2014;27:133-141.

11. Nudo RJ. Recovery after brain injury: mechanisms and principles. *Front Hum Neurosci.* 2013;7(article 887):1-14.

12. Shuldiner O, Yaron A. Mechanisms of developmental neurite pruning. *Cell Mol Life Sci.* 2015;72:101-119.

13. Presumey J, Bialas AR, Carroll MC. Complement system in neural synapse elimination in development and disease. *Adv Immunol.* 2017;135:53-79.

14. Xin W, Chan JR, Myelin plasticity: sculpting circuits in learning and memory. *Nat Rev Neurosci.* 2020;21(12):682-694.

15. Faw TD, Lakhani B, Schmalbrock P, et al. Eccentric rehabilitation induces white matter plasticity and sensorimotor recovery in chronic spinal cord injury. *Exp Neurol.* 2021;246:113853.

16. Barroso J, Herrara-Valdez MA, Galarraga E, Bargas J. Models of short-term synaptic plasticity. In: von Bernhardi R, Eugenin J, Muller KJ, eds. *The Plastic Brain Advances in Experimental Medicine and Biology.* vol 1015; 2017. Cham, Switzerland: Springer Cham. https://doi-org.proxy.lib.ohio-state.edu/10.1007/978-3-319-62817-2_.

17. Knudson EI. Sensitive periods in the development of the brain and behavior. *Cogn Neurosci.* 2004;16(8):1412-1425.

18. Gould E, Reeves AJ, Graziano MSA, Gross CG. Neurogenesis in the neocortex of adult primates. *Science.* 1999;286(5439):548-552.

19. Aimone JB, Li Y, Lee SW, Clemenson GD, Deng W, Gage FH. Regulation and function of adult neurogenesis: from genes to cognition. *Physiol Rev.* 2014;94:991-1028.

20. Cameron HA, Glover LR. Adult neurogenesis: beyond learning and memory. *Annu Rev Psychol.* 2015;66:53-81.

21. Matsubara S, Matsuda T, Nakashima K. Regulation of adult mammalian neural stem cells and neurogenesis by cell extrinsic and intrinsic factors. *Cells.* 2021;10:1145.

22. Kuhn HG, Toda T, Gage FH. Adult hippocampal neurogenesis: a coming of age story. *J Neurosci.* 2018;38(49):10401-10410.

23. Cotman CW. Axon sprouting and reactive synaptogenesis. In: Siegel GJ, Agranoff BW, Albers RW, et al., eds. *Basic Neurochemistry: Molecular, Cellular and Medical Aspects.* 6th ed. Philadelphia, PA: Lippincott-Raven; 1999. Available at: http://www.ncbi.nlm.nih.gov/books/NBK28183/.

24. Humeau Y, Choquet D. The next generation of approaches to investigate the link between synaptic plasticity and learning. *Nat Neurosci.* 2019;22:1536-1543.

25. De Sousa Fernandes MS, Ordonio TF, Santos GCJ, et al. Effects of physical exercise on neuroplasticity and brain function: a systematic review in human and animal studies. *Neural Plast.* 2020;2020:8856621.

26. Baltaci SB, Mogulkoc R, Baltaci AK. Molecular mechanisms of early and late LTP. *Neurochem Res.* 2019;44:281-296.

27. Heijtz RD, Forssberg H. Translational studies exploring neuroplasticity associated with motor skill learning and the regulatory role of the dopamine system. *Dev Med Child Neurol.* 2015;57(suppl 2):10-14.

28. Delpech JC, Madore C, Nadjar A, Joffre C, Wohleb ES, Layé S. Microglia in neuronal plasticity: influence of stress. *Neuropharmacology.* 2015;96(Pt A):19-28.

29. Baudry M, Zhu G, Liu Y, Wang Y, Briz V, Bi X. Multiple cellular cascades participate in long-term potentiation and in hippocampus-dependent learning. *Brain Res.* 2015;1621:73-81.

30. Kramár EA, Lin B, Rex CS, Gall CM, Lynch G. Integrin-driven actin polymerization consolidates long-term potentiation. *Proc Natl Acad Sci USA.* 2006;103(14):5579-5584.

31. Adkins DL, Boychuk J, Remple MS, Kleim JA. Motor training induces experience-specific patterns of plasticity across motor cortex and spinal cord. *J Appl Physiol.* 2006;101:1776-1782.

32. Thomas AG, Dennis A, Bandettini PA, Johansen-Berg H. The effects of aerobic activity on brain structure. *Front Psychol.* 2012;3(article 86):1-9.

33. Ma F, Morancho A, Montaner J, Rosell A. Endothelial progenitor cells and revascularization following stroke. *Brain Res.* 2015;1623:150-159.

34. Hansen CN, Norden DM, Faw TD, et al. Lumbar myeloid cell trafficking into locomotor networks after thoracic spinal cord injury. *Exp Neurol.* 2016;282:86-98.

35. Norden DM, Faw TD, McKim DB, et al. Bone marrow-derived monocytes drive the inflammatory microenvironment in local and remote regions after thoracic spinal cord injury. *J Neurotrauma.* 2019;36(6):937-949.

36. Weber MD, Godbout JP, Sheridan JF. Repeated social defeat, neuroinflammation, and behavior: monocytes carry the signal. *Neuropsychopharm.* 2017;42(1):46-61.

37. Montague-Cardoso K, Malcangio M. Changes in blood-spinal cord barrier permeability and neuroimmune interactions in the underlying mechanisms of chronic pain. *Pain Rep.* 2021;6(1):e879.

38. Waters S, Swanson MEV, Dieriks BV, et al. Blood-spinal cord barrier leakage is independent of motor neuron pathology in ALS. *Acta Neuropathol Commun.* 2021;9(1):144.

39. Arima Y, Harada M, Kamimura D, et al. Regional neural activation defines a gateway for autoreactive T cells to cross the blood-brain barrier. *Cell.* 2012;148(3):447-457.

40. Malkiewicz MA, Szarmach A, Sabisz A, Cubala WJ, Szurowska E, Winklewski PJ. Blood-brain barrier permeability and physical exercise. *J Neuroinflam.* 2019;16(1):15.

41. Viscomi MT, Molinari M. Remote neurodegeneration: multiple actors for one play. *Mol Neurobiol.* 2014;50:368-389.

42. Spejo AB, Oliveira ALR. Synaptic rearrangement following axonal injury: old and new players. *Neuropharmacology*. 2015;96(Pt A):113-123.

43. Zhou Y, Shao A, Yao Y, Tu S, Deng Y, Zhang J. Dual roles of astrocytes in plasticity and reconstruction after traumatic brain injury. *Cell Commun Signal*. 2020;18:62.

44. Armstrong RC, Mierzwa AJ, Sullivan GM, Sanchez MA. Myelin and oligodendrocyte lineage cells in white matter pathology and plasticity after traumatic brain injury. *Neuropharmacology*. 2016;110:654-659.

45. Hart CG, Karimi-Abdolrezaee S. Recent insights on astrocyte mechanisms in CNS homeostasis, pathology, and repair. *J Neurosci Res*. 2021;99:2427-2462.

46. Yang QQ, Zhou JW. Neuroinflammation in the central nervous system: symphony of glial cells. *Glia*. 2019;67:1017-1035.

47. Hansen CN, Fisher L, Deibert RJ, et al. Elevated MMP-9 in the lumbar cord early after thoracic spinal cord injury impedes motor relearning in mice. *J Neurosci*. 2013;33(32):13101-13111.

48. Brassai A, Suvanjeiev RG, Bán EG, Lakatos M. Role of synaptic and non-synaptic glutamate receptors in ischaemia induced neurotoxicity. *Brain Res Bull*. 2015;112:1-6.

49. O'Reilly ML, Tom VJ. Neuroimmune system as a driving force for plasticity following CNS injury. *Front Cell Neurosci*. 2020;14:187.

50. Xu X, Lai Y, Hua ZC. Apoptosis and apoptotic body: disease message and therapeutic target potentials. *Biosci Rep*. 2019;39(1):BSR20180992.

51. McIIwain DR, Berger T, Mak TW. Caspase functions in cell death and disease. *Cold Spring Harb Perspect Biol*. 2013;5:a008656.1-28.

52. Egawa N, Lok J, Washida K, Arai K. Mechanisms of axonal damage and repair after central nervous system injury. *Transl Stroke Res*. 2017;8(1):14-21.

53. Ray SK. Modulation of autophagy for neuroprotection and functional recovery in traumatic spinal cord injury. *Neural Regen Res*. 2020;15(9):1601-1612.

54. Mo Y, Sun YY, Liu KY. Autophagy and inflammation in ischemic stroke. *Neural Regen Res*. 2020;15(8):1388-1396.

55. Ghavami S, Shojaei S, Yeganeh B, et al. Autophagy and apoptosis dysfunction in neurogenerative disorders. *Prog Neurobiol*. 2014;112:24-49.

56. Salim S. Oxidative stress and the central nervous system. *J Pharmacol Exp Ther*. 2017;360:201-205.

57. Tomassy GS, Berger DR, Chen HH, et al. Distinct profiles of pyramidal neurons in the neocortex. *Science*. 2014;34(6181):319-324.

58. Hughes EG, Orthmann-Murphy JL, Langseth AJ, Berles DE. Myelin remodeling through experience-dependent oligodendrogenesis in the adult somatosensory cortex. *Nat Neurosci*. 2018;21(5):696-706.

59. Ziskin JL, Nishiyama A, Rubio M, Fukaya M, Bergles DE. Vesicular release of glutamate from unmyelinated axons in white matter. *Nat Neurosci*. 2007;10(3):321-330.

60. Hughes AN, Appel B. Oligodendrocytes express synaptic proteins that modulate myelin sheath formation. *Nat Commun*. 2019;10(1):4125.

61. McKenzie IA, Ohayon D, Huiliang L, et al. Motor skill learning requires active central myelination. *Science*. 2014;346(6207):318-322.

62. Kato D, Wake H, Lee PR, et al. Motor learning requires myelination to reduce asynchrony and spontaneity in neural activity. *Glia*. 2020;68(1):193-210.

63. Faw TD, Lakhani B, Schmalbrock P, et al. Eccentric rehabilitation induces white matter plasticity and sensorimotor recovery in chronic spinal cord injury. *Exp Neurol*. 2021;346: 113853.

64. Rubino C, Larssen BC, Chiu L, et al. Experience-dependent learning and myelin plasticity in individuals with stroke. *bioRxiv*. https://doi.org/10.1101/2022.02.17.480894.

65. Borich MR, Mackay AL, Vavasour IM, Rauscher A, Boyd LA. Evaluation of white matter myelin water fraction in chronic stroke. *Neuroimage Clin*. 2013;2:569-580.

66. Lakhani B, Hayward KS, Boyd LA. Hemispheric asymmetry in myelin after stroke is related to motor impairment and function. *Neuroimage Clin*. 2017;14:344-353.

67. Kolind S, Matthews L, Johansen-Berg H, et al. Myelin water imaging reflects clinical variability in multiple sclerosis. *Neuroimage*. 2012;60(1):147-154.

68. Russell-Schulz B, Vavasour IM, Zhang J, et al. Myelin water fraction decrease in individuals with chronic mild traumatic brain injury and persistent symptoms. *Heliyon*. 2021;7(4):e06709.

69. Weiss JT, Donlea JM. Roles for sleep in neural and behavioral plasticity: reviewing variation in the consequences of sleep loss. *Front Behav Neuroci*. 2022;15:777799.

70. Facchin L, Schone C, Mensen A, et al. Slow waves promote sleep-dependent plasticity and functional recovery after stroke. *J Neurosci*. 2020; 40(45):8637-8651.

71. Giannoccaro MP, Moghadam KK, Pizza F, et al. Sleep disorders in patients with spinal cord injury. *Sleep Med Rev*. 2013;17(6):399-409.

72. Aoun R, Rawal H, Attarian H, Sahni A. Impact of traumatic brain injury on sleep: an overview. *Nat Sci Sleep*. 2019;11:131-140.

73. Gilmore N, Katz DI, Kiran S. Acquired brain injury in adults: a review of pathophysiology, recovery, and rehabilitation. *Perspect ASHA Spec Interest Groups*. 2021;6(4):714-727.

74. Hutchinson KJ, Gomez-Pinilla F, Crowe MJ, Ying Z, Basso DM. Three-exercise paradigms differentially improve sensory recovery after spinal cord contusion in rats. *Brain*. 2004;127:1403-1414.

75. Hylin MJ, Kerr AL, Holden R. Understanding the mechanisms of recovery and/or compensation following injury. *Neural Plast*. 2017;2017:7125057.

76. Innocenti GM. Defining neuroplasticity. *Handb Clin Neurol*. 2022;184:3-18.

77. Cleland BT, Madhavan S. Ipsilateral motor pathways to the lower limb after stroke: insights and opportunities. *J Neurosci Res*. 2021;99(6):1565-1578.

78. Hansen CN, Faw TD, Kerr S, et al. Sparing of descending axons rescues interneuron plasticity in the lumbar cord to allow adaptive learning after thoracic spinal cord injury. *Fronti Neural Circuits*. 2016;10:11.

79. Sawaki L, Butler AJ, Leng X, et al. Constraint-induced movement therapy results in increased 30.motor map in subjects 3 to 9 months after stroke. *Neurorehabil Neural Repair*. 2008;22(5):505-513.

80. Liepert J, Hamzei F, Weiller C. Lesion-induced and training-induced brain reorganization. *Restor Neurol Neurosci*. 2004;22(3-5):269-277.

81. Pin-Barre C, Laurin J. Physical exercise as a diagnostic, rehabilitation, and preventive tool: influence on neuroplasticity and motor recovery after stroke. *Neural Plast*. 2015;2015:608581.

82. Kleim JA, Jones TA. Principles of experience-dependent neural plasticity: implications for rehabilitation after brain damage. *J Speech Lang Hear Res*. 2008;51:S225-S239.

83. Sampaio-Baptista C, Sanders ZB, Johansen-Berg H. Structural plasticity in adulthood with motor learning and stroke rehabilitation. *Ann Rev Neurosci*. 2018;41:25-40.

84. Douglas DB, Iv M, Douglas PK, et al. Diffusion tensor imaging of TBI: potentials and challenges. *Top Magn Reson Imaging*. 2015;24(5):241-251.

85. Reid LB, Boyd RN, Cunnington R, Rose SE. Interpreting intervention induced neuroplasticity with fMRI: the case for multimodal imaging strategies. *Neural Plast*. 2016;2016:2643491.

86. Smitha KA, Raja KA, Arun KM, et al. Resting state fMRI: a review on methods in resting state connectivity analysis and resting state networks. *Neuroradiol J*. 2017;30(4):305-317.

87. Hallett M. Transcranial magnetic stimulation: a primer. *Neuron*. 2007; 55:187-199.

88. MacKay A, Laule C, Vavasour I, Bjarnason T, Kolind S, Mädler B. Insights into brain microstructure from the T2 distribution. *Magn Reson Imaging*. 2006;24(4):515-525.

Review Questions

1. Cell proliferation in the developing nervous system begins in which area?
   A. Cortical plate
   B. Intermediate zone
   C. Subplate
   D. Ventricular zone

2. Which progenitor cells help to guide developing neurons to the cortical plate?
   A. Ependymal cells
   B. Intermediate progenitor cells
   C. Radial glial cells
   D. Short neural precursors

3. The overproduction of axonal projections is balanced by what process that eliminates some of these projections?
   A. Apoptosis
   B. Cell migration
   C. Pruning
   D. Programmed cell death

4. Adult neurogenesis differs from that in the developmental period by which of the following?
   A. It occurs only in the cortical plate of the mature brain
   B. It occurs only in neurogenic niches in the mature brain
   C. It occurs faster in the mature brain than in the immature brain
   D. It occurs more easily than gliogenesis in the mature brain

5. Long-term potentiation is associated with which mechanism?
   A. Decreased calcium permeability
   B. Enlargement of dendritic spines
   C. Decreased protein synthesis
   D. Diminished actin polymerization

6. Angiogenesis involves the creation of new blood vessels in the mature brain.
   A. True
   B. False

7. Microglial synaptic pruning is associated with
   A. LTD
   B. LTP
   C. Synaptic scaling
   D. Enhanced actin polymerization

8. Dying back of the proximal segment of the axon is known as:
   A. Anterograde degeneration
   B. Orthograde degeneration
   C. Retrograde degeneration
   D. Wallerian degeneration

9. The loss of neurons that normally synapse on neurons in the lesioned area is referred to as:
   A. Anterograde transneural degeneration
   B. Retrograde transneural degeneration
   C. Apoptosis
   D. Necrosis

10. The primary cause of excitotoxicity post-CNS injury is:
    A. Dopamine
    B. GABA
    C. Glutamate
    D. Norepinephrine

11. The internal pathway of apoptosis targets which organelle?
    A. Endoplasmic reticulum
    B. Golgi apparatus
    C. Mitochondria
    D. Ribosomes

12. Which of the following mechanisms is unlikely during early spontaneous recovery from a small ischemic lesion?
    A. Angiogenesis
    B. Interhemispheric functional reorganization
    C. Sprouting
    D. Synaptogenesis

13. Teaching a patient to get out of bed by lifting the paretic leg with the non-paretic leg is likely to lead to:
    A. Adaptive plasticity
    B. Maladaptive plasticity
    C. Synaptogenesis
    D. Apoptosis

14. To treat a patient, based on the critical factors for adaptive neural plasticity, it would be best to:
    A. Isolate joint activities to improve kinematics during gait
    B. Walk at the peak speed that the patient can tolerate
    C. Use an AFO to control ankle dorsiflexion
    D. Wait to ambulate until the patient can stand independently

15. **What substances stimulate and control cell proliferation and migration during neurogenesis?**
    A. Glial cells
    B. Morphogens
    C. Neurotransmitters
    D. Reactive oxygen species

16. **Which glial cells are responsible for reestablishing the blood-brain barrier after neural injury?**
    A. Astrocytes
    B. Microglia
    C. Macrophages
    D. Oligodendrocytes

17. **The elimination of damaged organelles within a neuron to promote homeostasis is achieved by what process?**
    A. Autophagy
    B. Excitotoxicity
    C. Nitrosative stress
    D. Oxidative stress

18. **Diaschisis refers to what?**
    A. A period of heightened cellular activity that contributes to excitotoxicity
    B. A period of shock following neural injury in adjacent and connected areas to the lesion
    C. A period of prolonged neurogenesis following neural injury
    D. A period of functional reorganization within the first 3 months after neural injury

19. **Early contralesional activation in the motor cortex is a positive sign for a good recovery.**
    A. True
    B. False

20. **Cognitive reserve is thought to result from what?**
    A. Changes in neural phenotype
    B. Double-folded myelin
    C. Enhanced network complexity
    D. Maladaptive plasticity

21. **The imaging method that looks to identify white matter projections using fractional anisotropy is:**
    A. Diffusion tensor imaging
    B. Functional magnetic resonance imaging
    C. Myelin water fraction
    D. Transcranial magnetic stimulation

22. **If an fMRI laterality index is +1.0, it indicates which of the following?**
    A. Control of the movement by the ipsilesional hemisphere
    B. Control of the movement equally by both hemispheres
    C. Control of the movement by the contralesional hemisphere

23. **How does activity-based rehabilitation induce white matter plasticity?**
    A. By increasing alpha motor neuron activity
    B. By causing neurotransmitter release from axons
    C. By reducing water molecules between the wraps of myelin
    D. By reducing astrocytic activity

24. **Motor learning of complex skills requires which of the following?**
    A. Synaptic stripping by microglia
    B. Collateral sprouting of corticospinal axons
    C. Angiogenesis of capillaries
    D. Mature myelinating oligodendrocytes

25. **Sleep disruption causes which of the following?**
    A. Fewer new synapses
    B. Better memory consolidation
    C. Greater long-term potentiation
    D. Less neuropathic pain

Answers

1. D	**2.** C	**3.** C	**4.** B	**5.** B
6. B	**7.** A	**8.** C	**9.** A	**10.** C
11. C	**12.** B	**13.** B	**14.** B	**15.** B
16. A	**17.** A	**18.** B	**19.** B	**20.** C
21. A	**22.** C	**23.** B	**24.** D	**25.** A

GLOSSARY

Adaptive plasticity. Plasticity that supports functional recovery in limbs or systems affected by neural damage.

Angiogenesis. New blood vessel formation, typically in capillary beds.

Anterograde degeneration (Wallerian or orthograde). Degradation of distill component of axon.

Anterograde transneuronal degeneration. Degeneration of neurons that have lost input from their presynaptic neurons.

Apoptosis. Programmed cell death.

Autophagy. Degradation of damaged proteins or organelles within a cell.

Caspases. Endoprotease enzymes involved in apoptosis.

Cognitive reserve. Greater complexity of neural networks that support functional recovery after neural damage.

Diffusion tensor imaging. A technique that measures the diffusion of water and allows white matter tracts to be visualized.

Excitatory stripping. Retraction of excitatory axonal buttons to protect neurons.

Excitotoxicity. Excessive excitation following neural injury secondary to the release of excitatory neurotransmitters.

Experience-dependent plasticity. Neuroplasticity that is triggered by activity/inactivity.

Fractional anisotropy. A measure of the consistency of water diffusion in a single direction.

Functional reorganization. Changes in the organization of cortical areas or projections to achieve function.

Gliogenesis. Development of glia.

Intrahemispheric. Within a hemisphere.

Interhemispheric. Between the two hemispheres.

Laterality index. Comparison of ipsilateral to contralateral activation, using fMRI, ranges from −1.0 to +1.0.

Long-term depression. Changes in neurons that lead to decreased connectivity between the neurons.

Long-term potentiation. Changes in neurons that strengthen the efficiency of a connection.

Maladaptive plasticity. Plasticity that decreases recovery in the damaged area but increases activity in compensatory neural areas.

Morphogens. Signaling compounds that stimulate cell proliferation.

Myelin water fraction. Calculation of the water within the myelin sheaths in comparison to the water in intracellular and extracellular space.

Neural stem cells. Progenitor cells for neurons and glia.

Neurogenesis. Development of neurons.

Neurotrophins. Proteins that catalyze changes associated with neuroplasticity.

Nitrosative stress. Damage to neurons caused by reactive nitrogen species.

Oxidative stress. Proliferation of reactive oxygen species that can damage cells.

Programmed cell death. Elimination of unnecessary cells.

Pruning. Elimination of unnecessary axon collaterals and dendrites.

Radial glial cell. One of first cells to develop from NSCs.

Resting state fMRI. A measure of the spontaneous activity within brain regions at rest.

Retrograde degeneration. Dying back of proximal component of axon after damage.

Retrograde transneuronal degeneration. Loss of neurons that project onto lost neurons.

Structural imaging. Imaging that allows the measurement of brain size and structures.

Synaptic stripping. Removal of synapses and dendrites on postsynaptic neuron after degeneration of presynaptic neuron.

Synaptogenesis. Changes in synapses that support plasticity.

Transcranial magnetic stimulation. The use of magnetic stimulation to activate motor neurons used to map a cortical area associated with a single muscle or muscle group control.

ABBREVIATIONS

aRGC	apical radial glial cells
BDNF	brain-derived neurotrophic factor
DTI	diffusion tensor imaging
fMRI	functional magnetic resonance imaging
Il-1β	interleukin-1β
LTP	long-term potentiation
MEP	motor evoked potential
MRI	magnetic resonance imaging
MWF	myelin water fraction
MWF-AR	myelin water fraction asymmetry ratio
NO	nitric oxide
OPC	oligodendrocyte progenitor cell
RGC	radial glial cells
RNS	reactive nitrogen species
ROS	reactive oxygen species
Rs-fMRI	resting state fMRI
TMS	transcranial magnetic stimulation
TNFα	tumor necrosis factor
FA	functional anisotropy

Neurologic Conditions — Neuropathology and Physical Therapy Management

SECTION

11

NEUROLOGIC CONDITIONS —
NEUROPATHOLOGY AND
PHYSICAL THERAPY
MANAGEMENT

Neurologic Exam

Deborah A. Kegelmeyer,
Jill C. Heathcock,
and Deborah S. Nichols-Larsen

10

OBJECTIVES

OBJECTIVES _____

1) Understand the parts of the neurologic examination and how they are performed

2) Determine when the systems review indicates the need for further evaluation

3) Determine which evaluative methods to use for the appropriate system

4) Choose appropriate outcome measures based on both the individual characteristics of the client as well as the measurement characteristics of the tool

5) Determine how to adapt and modify the neurologic examination based on the individual characteristics of the client

OVERVIEW OF THE NEUROLOGIC EVALUATION AS A PROCESS

An examination of the neurologic system is an essential component of a comprehensive physical examination for every client that a physical therapist sees. The examination may be limited to a screening as described under the System Review section, or in those clients who have sustained damage to any aspect of the neurologic system, it should be a comprehensive and systematic examination that surveys the functioning of nerves delivering sensory information to the brain and those carrying motor commands to muscles and organs (peripheral nervous system) as well as neural networks that support high-level multisystem processing and coordination of sensorimotor function (central nervous system). A careful neurological examination can help to determine impairments and their possible cause(s), functional loss, and focus of treatment.

For a PT neurologic exam, the therapist examines the patient in detail to determine if there are deficits in areas of body system and function, activity, and participation levels of the ICF while considering environmental and personal factors as part of the examination. The PT neurological exam is made up of a systems review, assessments, and appropriate outcome measures. The systems review is a cursory look at each system to assess whether the system is intact. If the system is not intact, the examination should include a more thorough assessment of that system. Assessments are completed to provide detailed information regarding how the individual's system is functioning. Both deficits and areas of strength are determined by performing assessments. Outcome measures can provide objective information regarding deficits in any of these areas and/or allow

comparisons to normative levels but are specifically selected to provide a measurement of therapeutic need and efficacy.

The examination begins with a history that helps the clinician to localize the problem and its onset. For example, symptoms that occur unexpectedly might suggest a blood vessel or seizure problem. Those that are not as sudden might suggest a possible tumor. Symptoms that have a variable course with recurrences and remissions but worsen over time suggest a disease that destroys nerve cells. Others that are chronic and progressive indicate a degenerative disorder. In cases of trauma, symptoms may be evident upon inspection, and causes may be explained by third-party witnesses. The history assists the clinician to diagnose conditions and focus the examination.

The examination is an ongoing process and continues throughout the course of treatment. While this chapter will attempt to lay out the path of the evaluation in a more step-by-step manner, it is actually more of a cyclical process. As the clinician generates hypotheses, based on the examination, they then design the intervention to address these hypotheses. After trying the intervention and observing the response, the original hypothesis is modified, and the impact on activity limitations is reassessed. Thus, the examination informs the intervention, which in turn informs the examination (Figure 10-1).

COMPONENTS OF THE ADULT NEUROLOGIC EVALUATION

History

A careful history will allow you to prioritize the examination. A well-done history should be brief yet comprehensive and

---

CASE A, PART I

Trisha is a 50-year-old female who is complaining of increasing weakness in her legs along with problems with falling and tingling in all of her limbs. Her history includes multiple ear and sinus infections, hypertension, two pregnancies with vaginal birth (children are 15 and 17), and diabetes for 15 years. She manages her diabetes with diet and her most recent A1C was 12. She lives in a two-story home with her husband, children, and dog; she enjoys knitting and hiking.

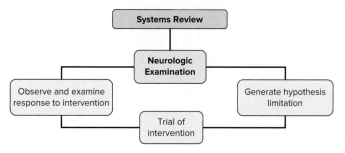

FIGURE 10-1 Diagram of the relationship between evaluation and treatment.

result in the generation of several hypotheses as to why the client is experiencing the symptoms and functional limitations that have brought her to the clinic. The role of the clinician is to be open and receptive to receiving information and to put the client at ease so that she is comfortable providing an adequate history. Secondarily, the clinician must be skilled at guiding the process so that it remains focused, does not stray off course nor take up unnecessary time from that allotted for the examination.

A history starts with personal information, such as name and age, and then moves on to the past and current medical history. It is important to gather this information from both the client and the medical record, if available; information on the home environment and support system is also critical to obtain (Box 10-1). The medical record provides an objective report of the condition(s) other professionals have identified, while the client's report provides insight into their health status as the patient is considered the expert of their symptoms. In addition, the client may provide critical information that has been left out of the medical record. Identification of medications and supplements that have been prescribed, as well as what is being taken, is critical as medication side effects are common and should be ruled out before moving on to other potential causes of the present change in health status. This initial history is essential as it provides the therapist with an indication of any precautions or limitations that may impact elements of the neuromuscular examination, such as weight-bearing limitations or cardiac precautions.

Box 10-1   Home Assessment

An area of the history that is often neglected is the assessment of home. The type of living environment and support system available to the patient will play a large role in discharge planning and goal setting. Therefore at a minimum the following questions should be addressed:

- Does the client live alone or with a spouse or companion? If alone, do they have assistance from neighbors or family?
- What architectural barriers exist at home? Are there stairs inside or outside the home? Where is the bathroom location and how is the shower set up (grab bars, in a tub, seat or not), etc.?
- What equipment does the client have?
- What is the client's occupation? What is their role in the home?
- What are their community or leisure activities?

Finally, and most importantly, the therapist needs to find out what the client hopes to achieve through their therapy – their goals. If their goals seem too easy, then the therapist should encourage them to be optimistic and not aim too low, based on their present status. The therapist must also be realistic and consider the client's status, prior to this current situation, and set goals in collaboration with the client that are appropriate and individualized to the unique needs of each patients. At times, clients have difficulty identifying what activities they are or will have difficulty participating in. There are tools that can help both the therapist and client get a better grasp on this such as the OPTIMAL scale (APTA)[1] and the Physical Self Maintenance scale.[2] These are used to determine activity level limitations and assist in goal setting.

CASE A, PART II

Trisha has revealed in her history that she has diabetes. Based on her A1C, is her diabetes well managed?

No – normal A1C is between 4.5% and 6%; for diabetics, the goal is to keep A1C below 7%. Given that Trisha's diabetes is not well managed, we might suspect that she has peripheral neuropathy, leading to weakness and tingling. We cannot rule out an upper motor neuron lesion, however, as cardiovascular disease and stroke are often secondary complications of poorly managed endocrine disease. We know that her functional goals will likely include fine motor skills, since she enjoys knitting, and we know that she needs adequate lower extremity strength and power to ascend stairs in her home and hike. With her history, we know that a careful systems review will be necessary as endocrine disorders can impact every system in the body.

Systems Review

A neurological screening is an essential component of every comprehensive physical examination. In cases of neurological trauma, disease, or psychological disorders, patients are usually given an in-depth neurological examination which is preceded by this screen. The examination is best performed in a systematic manner, which means that there is a recommended order for procedures.

Elements of the Systems Review (Screening)

The systems review is a general review of each of the body systems and is a guide for what areas should be investigated more thoroughly, dictate referral to another medical professional, or may impact the PT plan of care, as indicated by an impaired item. Each item on the systems review is marked as impaired or not impaired, meaning within normal limits. On documentation templates, either paper-based or as part of an electronic medical record, there is typically a small space available for brief comments under each system. At a minimum, the system's review should include a brief assessment of all of the following:

- Mental status: Are they alert? Are they alert to: Person? Place? Time? Situation? Do they remember recent events? Are they able to do simple problem-solving, such as figuring out how to lock a wheelchair?

- Cranial nerves should be screened by observing eye and facial movements.
- Sensory: Screen for adequate vision and hearing to participate in therapeutic activities. Also screen the ability to sense light touch and location of limbs.
- Integumentary: Examine for the presence of incisions, wounds, burns, inflammation.

  Note: Screening of the integumentary system is especially critical when diseases of the endocrine system are diagnosed or suspected because of their impact on the skin; similarly, pulmonary dysfunction may also affect the integumentary system (e.g., bluish nail beds).

- Cardiopulmonary: Vitals – heart rate, blood pressure, respiration rate.
- Endocrine: Endocrine disorders can cause neurologic symptoms and should be considered when examining for neurologic symptoms. Some symptoms associated with endocrine disorders are headache, altered mentality (diabetic coma, severe hypothyroid, hyperthyroid), muscle weakness (endocrine myopathy: thyroid, parathyroid, adrenal), **hypotonia** (hypothyroid), movement disorders such as chorea, athetosis, and tremor (hyperthyroid, Addison, hypoparathyroid).[3,4]
- Musculoskeletal: Rule out contraindications for further evaluation and treatment, such as a pre-existing joint limitation. Is the patient capable of doing examination activities? (Gross screen of strength and range of motion [ROM]).
- Neuromuscular: Screen for muscle tone, strength, and functional movement/coordination by observing mobility as the patient enters the evaluation area (e.g., gait and transfers) and performs gross movements; screen for coordination, using the finger-to-nose test or heel-to-shin test. Deep tendon reflexes (DTRs) should be checked along with screening for the presence of clonus at the wrist and ankle and upper motor neuron signs, using the Babinski and Hoffman tests (see Box 10-2).

Box 10-2 Upper Motor Neuron Screening Tests

Babinski (plantar reflex) – Stroke bottom of foot from heel to toes, using your thumb or the end of a reflex hammer, this should elicit flexion of the big toe and perhaps the other toes (negative sign); in very young infants (<24 months) and those with upper motor neuron injuries (stroke, brain injury, etc.), the big toe will extend and the other toes will splay out (positive sign).

Hoffman test/reflex – Flick the fingernail of the middle finger by squeezing the tip of the finger between your thumb and index finger and then rapidly releasing their finger in a flicking motion; watch for flexion of the thumb or index finger. This should be done on both sides. If flexion occurs, this is a positive Hoffman sign and can be an indication of upper motor neuron disease. However, some people without neurologic injury will have a positive Hoffman sign, so the tester should look for asymmetry in this reflex or the emergence of it after a neurologic injury, when it suggests corticospinal disruption.

- Genito-urinary systems: Ask about continence, urgency of voiding, and any recent changes. Ask about age-related changes. Also inquire about a history of bladder or urinary tract infections, which can be signs of incomplete voiding.
- Gastrointestinal, hepatic, and biliary: Ask about regularity, frequency, nausea, recent changes. Do they have issues such as heartburn when assuming supine?

In individuals who have a known neurologic disorder or are found to have deficits in the neuromuscular system during the systems review, the clinician should progress to the neurologic examination, targeting those areas of concern from the screening.

NEUROLOGICAL EXAMINATION: BODY STRUCTURE AND FUNCTION

The neurologic examination should be performed on any individual suspected of having any neurologic disorder or psychological disease. This examination is performed in a systematic and comprehensive manner and consists of several thorough and in-depth assessments of mental status, cranial nerves, motor examination, reflexes, sensory examination, and posture and mobility analysis.

Mental Status Examination

The first item to be examined is mental status. It is not possible to conduct the rest of the examination without determining how the individual is interacting with the environment and whether or not he/she is able to follow directions partially or completely. There are two types of mental status examination: informal and formal. The **informal mental status exam** is usually done while clinicians are obtaining historical information from a patient when a neurological problem is suspected. For the informal assessment, the client is commonly asked the following: his/her name (person); the location of the testing (place); the day of the week and date (time); and why she is there (situation). This is typically documented as Alert and Oriented × 1, 2, 3, or 4 (A & O × #). The numbers 1–4 stand for person, place, time, and situation. If it is documented that a patient is O × 2, then the area(s) of disorientation are indicated (e.g., "not oriented to place, person, or time"), or conversely, if O × 1, the area of **orientation** is stated (e.g., "oriented to person"). This is a very basic assessment of mental status and does not give an indication of ability to follow directions or problem-solve. Therefore, mental status should be assessed in more detail in individuals suspected of a neurologic disorder, even when orientation × 4 is present. This should include:

- **Retentive memory capability and immediate recall** – assessed by determining the number of digits that can be repeated in sequence from a string recited by the examiner;
- **Recent memory** – typically examined by testing recall of a series of three to five objects immediately, then after 5 and 15 minutes with intervening activities (e.g., other parts of this exam);
- **Remote memory** – assessed by asking the patient to review in a chronological fashion, his or her illness or personal life

events that the patient feels comfortable talking about (e.g., dates of birth of children and where they currently live);

- **General knowledge** – assessed by asking the patient to recall common historical or current events;
- **Higher functioning** (referring to brain processing capabilities) – assessed by spontaneous speech and repetition, reading, naming, writing, and comprehension of written and oral information. The patient may be asked to perform further tasks such as identification of fingers, whistling, saluting, brushing teeth motions, combing hair, drawing, and tracing figures. These procedures will assess the intactness of what is called dominant (left-sided brain) functioning or **higher cortical function**, referring to the portion of the brain that regulates these activities.

Other areas for assessment of mental function are delineated in Table 10-1 with their potential for providing information

TABLE 10-1	Mental Function Assessment for the PT	
AREA TO BE EXAMINED	**WHAT TO LOOK FOR**	**INSIGHT**
Appearance	Clothes, posture, grooming, alertness	Ability to take care of themselves; mood/affect
Behavior	Impulse control, fidgeting, overall movements	
Speech	Volume/Rate	Mood (e.g., loud and fast speech related to mania; soft and slow – related to depression)
	Coherence	Indication of higher level processing
Mood/Affect	Flat – minimal or absent affective response to situation	Signs of mental illness or cortical disease
	Labile – shifting emotional outbursts (e.g., crying/laughing)	
	Blunted – some emotional response but less than would be expected for the situation	
	Constructed/Inappropriate – responses that are inconsistent with the situation (e.g., laughing at a sad situation)	
Thought processing	Word usage	Language issues (agnosia, expressive aphasia)
	Thought stream	Slow versus overabundant gives an indication of mood and cognition
	Continuity – coherence of thought and idea association	Ability to follow the discussion and respond accordingly – Higher level cognition or receptive language problems
	Content – complete/incomplete responses	Higher level cognition/language issues, delusions suggest mental disorders
Perception	Screening of vision, hearing, touch, taste, and smell	General system integrity/dysfunction; potential medication side effects
Attention/Concentration	Ability to stay focused on a task	Frontal lobe dysfunction; anxiety
Memory	Long-term and current episodic memory (client's history and current events); immediate memory (naming three objects immediately and then in 5 and 15 minutes)	Temporal and frontal lobe function/dysfunction
Judgment	Decision-making in complex situations (safe versus unsafe)	Executive function (frontal lobe function)
Intelligence	Requires specific testing but a general sense can be obtained by responses to questions, general language used, etc.	Overall ability to participate in treatment/cortical deficits
Insight	Understanding of the current illness and potential limitations	Executive function

about mental function and possible areas that may be involved when dysfunction is seen. Box 10-3 describes two easy measures to objectively assess mental function.

Communication

While physical therapists are not the primary practitioner to evaluate communication disorders, it is important that we have an understanding of the presentation and consequences of these disorders in our patients. First, it is important to assess hearing ability very early in the examination and to adjust your communication appropriately, if the individual has hearing deficits. This can easily be done, while taking the history, by noting the patient's ability to hear questions and respond to what was asked. At a minimum, physical therapists should report the patient's comprehension and ability to express himself verbally or nonverbally. Assessment should answer the following questions (specific descriptions of these disorders are discussed in Chapter 11, "Stroke"):

- Can the client speak? Does he have word-finding problems consistent with **Expressive Aphasia** or trouble enunciating consistent with **dysarthria**?
- Note voice quality – is volume adequate?
- Does the individual understand language or show signs of **receptive aphasia**?

Autonomic Nervous System

The exam should include questions and tests designed to determine if the autonomic nervous system is functioning normally. Clients with diseases such as Parkinson's disease and many other neurologic disorders have impairment of the autonomic nervous system. During the history, ask if they have noticed decreased or absent sweating (anhidrosis) or have disturbances of bowel, bladder, or sexual function. Analysis of autonomic function should also assess the presence of postural (orthostatic) hypotension, which is lowered blood pressure when moving from supine or sitting to standing (drop $\geq$ 30 mm Hg

systolic or $\geq$ 15 mm Hg diastolic), and heart rate changes in response to the Valsalva maneuver. For this, the patient is asked to perform forced expiration against resistance for 15 seconds. The test is invalid if the forced expiration is not held for at least 7 seconds. In autonomic dysfunction, blood pressure declines progressively for as long as forced expiration can be maintained and heart rate does not increase.[8,9] Pupillary changes such as pupillary constriction can also indicate autonomic dysfunction, especially when accompanied by anhidrosis.

Motor Examination

The motor examination assesses the individual's muscle strength, tone, and shape; passive versus active ROM; and sustained postures versus functional movement. Findings will give an indication of whether the presenting disorder is muscular, neural (lower motor neuron, upper motor neuron), perceptual, or associated with the motor control system. It is important to look for abnormal movements (tics, myoclonus) as well as to observe the patient in multiple positions and activities.

Muscles could be hypertrophied (enlarged), due to overuse or some neurologic disorders, or atrophied (wasted), secondary to weakness, inactivity, or tissue destruction; asymmetry in muscle size suggests a unilateral problem (e.g., neuropathy, stroke), while bilateral changes are more likely associated with a more systemic disorder (e.g., Multiple Sclerosis, Parkinson's). It is important to look for twitching or abnormal movements, which are best observed while the individual is at rest, yet are characteristic of specific conditions (e.g., amyotrophic lateral sclerosis). Additionally, muscle activity can be abnormal during maintained postures in neurological disorders such as Parkinson's disease. Muscle tone is usually tested by performing passive motion of a relaxed limb first at a slow speed and then at a faster speed to determine the impact of speed of movement on tone. Decreases or increases in muscle tone can help the examiner localize the problem.

Strength (Force Production)

The examination of strength in individuals with neurologic disorders can be challenging as they often have impaired trunk control that can negatively impact their ability to stabilize themselves, while undergoing a manual muscle test. Therapists should be sure to set up the test so that sufficient support is provided to stabilize the trunk for the client during strength testing. Individuals who have significant motor impairments will attempt to substitute motions during strength testing (e.g., trunk extension to assist shoulder flexion). It is especially important to be cognizant of this in individuals with neurologic disorders and to take steps to prevent substitution. Notably, **the manual muscle test** can be invalidated by the presence of limited ROM, synergies, or disturbances of tone; when these are present, a functional test of strength should be used and any modifications to the test should be noted. Strength is first assessed by asking the client to move the limb through the ROM against gravity (fair grade), and then by determining the amount of resistance, against which the individual can maintain a mid-range position. If the individual is not able to move the limb against gravity, they should be placed in a position that allows movement through the ROM with gravity eliminated (e.g., side-lying).

When testing strength, document the following:

- What range did the individual move through?
- Was gravity eliminated or not?
- Did synergy (see description later in this chapter) influence the movement? If so, how?

The manual muscle test does not test the individual's ability to perform functional activities, and for strength grades above fair (3/5), it only examines the ability to produce an isometric contraction at one point in the ROM. Therefore, the manual muscle test does not fully inform us about the force production capabilities of the individual within functional activities. Individuals with upper motor neuron disorders often have difficulty developing consistent force over time such that force production may vary throughout the ROM. Methods for examining isotonic strength are standard manual muscle testing (Daniels and Worthingham method[10]), use of equipment such as a dynamometer, and functional muscle testing. Power is an important aspect of strength that relates to the ability to maintain force and speed to move a limb or an object (resistance), which is difficult to assess unless the clinician has access to isokinetic equipment.

Functional muscle testing involves evaluating the muscle's performance as the client performs activities or maintains postures consistent with normal daily conditions. The therapist then documents by describing the ROM that key joints moved through, in what position the activity was performed, and what was the relation of the limb to gravity. Some examples of things to consider when functionally testing the upper extremity are:

- Does the individual use both arms equally? If not, does the individual use the weaker/paretic arm at all or for what tasks? For support? For reaching?
- Does the individual have functional grasp bilaterally? If not, what was observed (e.g., fisting during the attempt to grasp)?
- Can the individual manipulate objects?
- Does the individual have fine motor coordination in their fingers (e.g., can they touch the fingertips of the thumb to each)?

Tone

Abnormal tone is a common finding in individuals with neurologic disorders. It can be hypertonic or hypotonic. Tone is assessed by performing passive ROM, in which the limb is moved through the ROM in a slow manner, while noting the resistance to the motion. If this is not painful, the limb is then moved through the ROM more rapidly. An increase in tone, **hypertonicity**, is present when the examiner notes an increased resistance to passive movement. There are two types of hypertonicity: spasticity and rigidity. **Spasticity** is characterized by increased resistance to passive movement, as the velocity of the movement is increased (velocity dependent), with **hyperreflexia** (exaggerated monosynaptic reflexes). The most common method for objectively documenting hypertonicity is the Ashworth Scale[11] (Box 10-4). While there are some issues with inter- and intra-rater reliability for the Ashworth Scale, this remains the only clinically accessible means of objectively measuring tone at this time. **Rigidity** is increased

Box 10-4	Modified Ashworth Scale[11]
0	No increase in muscle tone
1	Slight increase in muscle tone, manifested by a catch and release or by minimal resistance at the end of the range of motion when the affected part(s) is(are) moved in flexion or extension
1+	Slight increase in muscle tone, manifested by a catch followed by minimal resistance through the remainder of the range of motion but the affected part(s) is(are) easily moved
2	More marked increase in muscle tone through most of the range of movement, but the affected part(s) is easily moved
3	Considerable increase in muscle tone, passive movement difficult
4	Affected part(s) is (are) rigid in flexion or extension

Reproduced from Mutlu, A., Livanelioglu, A. & Gunel, M.K. Reliability of Ashworth and Modified Ashworth Scales in Children with Spastic Cerebral Palsy. *BMC Musculoskelet Disord* 9, 44 (2008). https://doi.org/10.1186/1471-2474-9-44.

resistance throughout the ROM that is independent of the velocity of the movement; reflexes are typically normal with rigidity. The causes of spasticity and rigidity are different and will be discussed with the conditions that are associated with them (e.g., stroke, Parkinson's disease). A limb that feels heavy or "floppy" is **hypotonic**, demonstrating limited resistance to passive movement and poor ability to sustain power or maintain a given posture. Because hypotonia can be caused by both central and peripheral nervous system disorders, reflexes can be decreased (hyporeflexia), normal, or exaggerated (hyperreflexia), depending on the cause of the hypotonia. Since tone can fluctuate over the course of the day and due to other factors, such as level of stimulation and room temperature, the assessment should always be performed at the same time of day, in the same room, and, if possible, by the same person. The examiner needs to be aware of things that can influence tone such as:

- Infections or fevers
- Stress and anxiety
- Volitional effort and movement
- Medications
- General health
- Environmental temperature
- State of central nervous system arousal or alertness
- Position interaction of tonic reflexes (see pediatric evaluation later in this chapter)

Additionally, the examiner should observe how the individual "holds" herself. An arm that is held in an antigravity position may indicate the presence of hypertonicity. Movement can also be impacted by tone, and the examiner should observe movements for signs of high tone, such as moving through a more limited ROM than is typical for the activity.

Synergistic Movement Patterns (Synergies)

It is common for individuals who have had an upper motor neuron lesion to exhibit movements that are highly influenced by or bound in synergistic movement patterns, which refers to multi-joint movements that occur simultaneously when trying to move an isolated joint (e.g., finger, wrist, elbow, and shoulder flexion when bringing the hand to the mouth to stifle a yawn). In Chapter 11, a description of synergy patterns seen after stroke is provided. To look for the presence of synergy patterns, the examiner should watch the client while they perform active ROM as well as functional movements (e.g., grasping, walking). If the client is able to achieve movement only through one rigid movement pattern, then they are said to be bound in synergy. When synergistic movement patterns are noted, the examiner should ask the client to move out of these patterns such as asking them to flex the shoulder while extending the wrist and elbow, and observe whether or not the client can perform movements out of the synergy pattern. The Fugl-Meyer[12] is the most common assessment tool for objectively examining synergistic movement patterns.

Reflexes

The patient's DTRs are tested by using a reflex hammer. The clinician will tap the rubber triangular-shaped end over key tendon insertions, in the arms (biceps, triceps, brachioradialis), knees (quadriceps, hamstrings), and heals (Achilles). If there is a difference in response from the left to the right, there may be an underlying problem that merits further evaluation. A difference in reflexes between the arms and legs usually indicates a lesion involving the spinal cord. Depressed reflexes in only one limb while the other limbs demonstrate a normal response usually indicates a peripheral nerve lesion. Hyperactive reflexes indicate a lesion in the central nervous system. DTRs are reported on a numerical scale (Table 10-2), and at a minimum, the biceps, triceps, quadriceps, and Achilles reflexes should be tested. In addition, the examination should include the Hoffman and Babinski reflex testing, for an upper motor neuron lesion, and

examination for clonus at the wrist and ankle. Clonus refers to a repetitive oscillating response to reflex testing (multiple beats). In general, the presence of clonus is indicative of an upper motor neuron lesion, although there are rare muscle disorders that can also lead to clonus.

Cranial Nerves (CN)

Cranial nerves are specialized nerves that originate in the brainstem and innervate the muscles of the face and eyes, innervate sensory receptors throughout the head and internal organs, and support the special senses (vision, hearing, smell, taste, vestibular function). The Physical therapist should always grossly screen these nerves by observing facial and eye movement as well as eye reflexes (response to light or turning of the head). Table 10-3 provides general screening methods for the CN.

Sensory Examination

Although an essential component of the neurologic examination, the sensory examination is the least exacting since it requires patient concentration and cooperation. Five primary sensory categories are assessed: vibration (using a tuning fork), joint position and awareness (examiner moves the limb side-to-side and in an upward or downward position), light touch, pinprick, and temperature. Individuals who have sensory abnormalities may have a lesion at any level of the sensory pathways (see Chapter 3). Spinal cord lesions or disease can possibly be detected by pinprick and temperature assessment. Sensation must always be screened; depending on the individual's problem and reason for therapy, you may or may not do a more detailed exam of any or all of the sensory modalities. For instance, in SCI during the acute stage, sensation by dermatome is assessed to both touch and pain to determine initial lesion level and subsequent recovery.

Tests of Proprioception

Movement Sense (Kinesthesia) – The examiner has the client close their eyes and then move the extremity through a small ROM; the client is asked to indicate verbally the direction of movement while the extremity is in motion. Prior to performing the test, the examiner and client should discuss the terminology that will be used to describe the direction of the motion so that it is clear that any discrepancies are due to actual deficits

TABLE 10-2	**Deep Tendon Reflex Grades**[13]	
REFLEX GRADE	**EVALUATION**	**RESPONSE CHARACTERISTICS**
0	Absent	No visible or palpable muscle contraction
1+	Hyporeflexia	Slight or sluggish muscle contraction with little or no joint movement. Reinforcement may be required to elicit a reflex response
2+	Normal	Slight muscle contraction with slight joint movement
3+	Hyperreflexia	Clearly visible, brisk muscle contraction with moderate joint movement
4+	Abnormal	Strong muscle contraction with one to three beats of clonus. Reflex spread to contralateral side may be noted
5+	Abnormal	Strong muscle contraction with sustained clonus. Reflex spread to contralateral side may be noted

TABLE 10-3	Cranial Nerve Function and Screening Methods[14]		
CRANIAL NERVE	**NAME**	**FUNCTION**	**SCREENING**
I	Olfactory	Smell	Have patient identify familiar smells (vanilla); there are vials that can be purchased or therapists can make their own
II	Optic	Vision	Reading close and distant items
III	Oculomotor	Eye movement, pupillary reflexes	Eye tracking in all directions, pupillary response to light; at rest, eye will be slightly depressed and rotated toward the nose, when damaged
IV	Trochlear	Superior oblique eye muscle innervation	Observe eye position at rest; will be elevated if there's a problem
V	Trigeminal	Muscles of mastication and sensation of the face	Observe jaw motion (resistance to motion, opening, side-to-side mobility), temporalis muscles can be palpated
VI	Abducens	Lateral rectus of the eye innervation	Look at eye movement; if damaged, there will be an inability to look outward (abduct the eye)
VII	Facial	Muscles of facial expression, taste for the anterior 2/3 tongue	Look for facial asymmetries, observe motions (raising eyebrows, wrinkling forehead, closing eyes, frowning/smiling, lip pursing, etc.). Taste with common liquids (lemon juice, honey) can also be tested
VIII	Vestibulocochlear	Hearing and Vestibular	Can use the "rub test" – rub thumb and forefinger together next to the ear. Ask the patient to point to which ear they hear it in. Check both. Look for differences. You can use a tuning fork, which tests for air conduction and structural problems that can occur inside the ear – strike tuning fork on your hand and place behind the ear on the bony surface. Observe balance
IX	Glossopharyngeal	Sensation and taste for posterior tongue and pharynx	Ask about swallowing, which may be impaired, have them say "ahh" and watch for palatal-uvula movement; unilateral nerve damage can yield asymmetric motion; absent gag reflex is also a sign of damage (stimulate with tongue depressor)
X	Vagus	Innervates epiglottis and larynx, parasympathetic innervation of internal organs	Voice hoarseness with increased heart and respiration rate are signs of CN X damage
XI	Accessory	Trapezius and sternocleido-mastoid muscle innervation	Observe ability to shrug shoulders and turn head to both sides
XII	Hypoglossal	Tongue muscles	Observe tongue protrusion and mobility; unilateral lesions will result in lateral movement when protruding tongue

and not due to miscommunication. Simple terms such as "up," "down," "out," and "in" should be used.[15] The most accurate areas to perform this test are on the hallux, wrist, and fingers. The examiner should use a light touch and grasp the limb at a joint space on the medial and lateral aspects of the joint, in order to minimize cutaneous input. There are also more objective tests, such as the Brief Kinesthesia Test,[16] that will provide measurable errors, if a problem is indicated.

Position Sense – The extremity is placed in a position and the individual is then told to verbally report the position. Another method is to have the client place her opposite extremity (e.g., right) in the same position as the examiner has positioned the tested extremity. This method can only be used in individuals who have full antigravity active movement in the opposite extremity.[15]

Vibration testing is the most reliable and valid way to test dorsal column–medial lemniscal system integrity. Since this tract carries sensory information, including position sense and kinesthesia, vibration testing can be a highly reliable and valid way to test for deficits in these sensory modalities. The most commonly used tuning forks are 64 or 128 Hz[17]; strike the fork against the palm of your hand or a solid surface and place it on a bony prominence (e.g., lateral malleolus) and ask the patient "what do you feel."

Cutaneous Sensation is commonly tested by: (1) **monofilament testing** for sensory threshold; (2) pinprick for pain; and (3) water vials for hot and cold modalities. The examiner should screen for the ability to sense touch as well as to locate the touch. For a screening exam, a light touch is often applied across the surface of both upper/lower limbs, and the individual is asked if she "can feel it" and "does it feel the same." Then, the patient should be asked to close their eyes and identify the location of randomly applied touch along each extremity. If deficits are found, a more thorough sensory exam, including pinprick and temperature, should be conducted. Temperature is typically examined using a vial with cold water and a vial with hot water that are randomly touched to the skin, while asking the client to identify the temperature. Additional tests can be performed, including identification of common objects or shapes (Stereognosis) via manipulation of the object in the hand.[18] See Table 10-4 for a listing of some common sensory disorders and methods for testing for each of them.

Coordination and Balance

Coordination is the ability to execute smooth, accurate, controlled movements. It is characterized by appropriate speed, distance, direction, rhythm, muscle tension, and synergistic movements accomplished via orchestrated reversals of opposing muscle group activations. For well-coordinated movements, the

> **CASE A, PART III**
>
> Her verbal history indicates that Trisha is experiencing paresthesias (abnormal sensations like tingling), dysesthesia (painful abnormal sensations like burning), and pain in both feet and lower legs of 2 years' duration that has worsened lately, especially at night; she has similar but much milder symptoms recently starting in her hands. Light touch, measured by monofilaments, is diminished on both feet (>2 SD above normal thresholds for the testing kit used), lower leg (1 SD above normal), and thumb and index fingers (1 SD above normal thresholds) consistent with carpel tunnel; all other areas are normal. Muscle strength is 3/5 in the anterior tibialis but still 5/5 in other muscles, her anterior tibialis reflex is 1+ but all others are 2+ (normal). These are typical symptoms for the most common form of diabetic neuropathy – symmetrical sensorimotor polyneuropathy (see Chapter 16).

individual must be able to achieve proximal fixation that allows for distal motion or maintenance of a posture. Coordination can be divided into nonequilibrium (does not require upright balance) and equilibrium (requires upright balance). Generally, nonequilibrium tests are completed first, followed by the equilibrium tests. Attention should be given to carefully guarding the patient during testing; use of a safety belt may be warranted. During the testing activities, the following questions can be used to help direct the therapist's observations and the results documented.

TABLE 10-4	**Common Sensory Impairments and Assessment Methods[18]**	
NAME OF SENSORY IMPAIRMENT	**DEFINITION OF SENSORY IMPAIRMENT**	**ASSESSMENT**
Abarognosis	The inability to recognize weight	Hold objects of varying weights in each hand and state which is heavier (or the same)
Allodynia	Pain is caused by non-painful stimuli such as light touch	Uncovered in the sensory exam when light touch or other non-painful stimuli elicit pain
Analgesia	A complete loss of pain sensitivity	Lack of pinprick sensation along with findings from the history
Astereognosis	The inability to use touch to recognize the shape or form of an object	Have the client identify shapes of objects while eyes are closed. Use common shapes like square and ball
Atopognosia	The inability to localize a sensation	During light touch testing ask to localize the touch with eyes closed
Dysesthesia	Abnormal touch sensation that may be experienced as unpleasant or painful	Typically determined during cutaneous testing (touch localization)
Hyperalgesia	Increased sensitivity to pain	Senses pinprick as being more painful than is typical and discovered through the history
Hyperesthesia	Increased sensitivity to sensory stimuli	Noted throughout the exam as an increased sensitivity to stimuli as compared to normal
Hypoalgesia	Decreased response to pain	Identified with the pinprick testing
Paresthesia	Abnormal sensation such as prickly or burning feeling that has no apparent cause	Noted during the history or when asked if they have any burning or prickling sensations

1. Are the movements direct, precise, and easily reversed?

2. Do the movements occur within a reasonable or normal amount of time?

3. Does increased speed of performance affect quality of the motor activity?

4. Can continuous and appropriate motor adjustments be made if speed and direction are changed?

5. Can a position or posture of the body or specific extremity be maintained without swaying, oscillations, or extraneous movements?

6. Are placing movements of both upper and lower extremities exact?

7. Does occluding vision alter the quality of motor activity?

8. Are the problems greater with movement proximally or distally? On one side of the body versus the other?

9. Does the patient fatigue rapidly? Is there a consistency of motor response over time?

Nonequilibrium testing involves repetitive motions as described in Box 10-5. Equilibrium testing begins with observing the ability to perform quiet stance and then progresses to more difficult standing balance tasks, as described in Box 10-6.

Box 10-5 Nonequilibrium Coordination Tests

Most of these tests should be performed first with eyes open and then with eyes closed to examine the influence of vision on the individual's coordination. After doing each test at a comfortable pace, instruct the client to move faster and examine the influence of speed on coordination:

1. *Finger to nose:* With shoulder in a flexed position, bring the finger to the tip of the nose and back out to the examiner's hand or just straight out in front, repeating several times.

2. *Finger to therapist's finger:* Therapist sits in front of the client and has them alternately touch the therapist's fingertip. The therapist places their fingertip at nose height, arm's length away from the client. The movement is alternated. The therapist can also try moving their own finger so that the client has to make contact with the finger in different locations and can also move their finger, while the client is reaching, to observe how easily and smoothly he can change the trajectory of this movement in response to a moving target.

3. *Opposition of fingers:* The thumb is touched to the tip of each finger on the same hand, moving in order from the index finger to the pinky and back down to the index finger. Be sure that the client is instructed to fully abduct the thumb after each digit is touched.

4. *Grasp:* The hand is opened and closed with gradually increasing speed. Encourage the client to fully open the hand with each repetition. Failure to fully open the hand or progressive shrinking of movement may be indicative of basal ganglia disorder.

5. *Alternating pronation and supination:* The client is asked to alternately pronate and supinate with the arms held at the sides and elbows flexed (hands can be placed on legs while seated so that palms and back of hands alternately touch the thighs).

6. *Tapping (hand and/or foot):* The arm is placed on a table or on the client's leg and they are instructed to tap the hand on the table or on his knee. For the foot, the client is seated with the knee flexed and foot flat on the floor; then, ask him to tap his toe on the ground.

7. *Rebound test:* The client is positioned with the elbow in 90 degrees of flexion and the therapist applies resistance to elbow flexion. The client is instructed to maintain the flexed posture. The therapist then suddenly releases their resistance and observes the response; since the elbow flexors are active, the arm will begin to flex, when the resistance is released. A normal response involves the opposing muscle group (triceps) rapidly checking the flexion movement with little motion occurring. Abnormal tests involve a large flexion of the elbow or a loss of trunk control in response to the sudden change in resistance.

8. *Heel on shin:* In supine or sitting, the client is asked to slide the heel up the shin from the ankle to the knee and back down again. Any movement off of the shin is considered a coordination deficit.

9. *Toe to examiner's finger:* Examiner holds their finger out and the client is asked to point to it with their great toe. This motion can be alternated

10. *Drawing a circle:* The client is asked to draw a circle on the floor with the big toe. A figure of eight can also be used. In supine, they can be asked to draw the figure in the air. This test can also be done with the upper extremity, using the finger to draw an imaginary circle in the air.

Box 10-6 Equilibrium Coordination Tests

Tests are listed from least to most difficult

1. Standing in normal, comfortable posture

2. Standing, feet together (narrow base of support)

3. Standing, with one foot directly in front of the other in tandem position (toe of one foot touching heel of other foot)

4. Standing on one foot

5. Arm position may be altered in each of the above postures (i.e., arms at side, over head, hands on waist, and so forth)

6. Displace balance unexpectedly (while carefully guarding the patient, wearing gait belt)

7. Standing, alternate between forward trunk flexion and return to neutral

8. Standing, laterally flex trunk to each side

9. Standing; eyes open to eyes closed; inability to maintain an upright posture without visual input is referred to as a **positive Romberg sign**

10. Standing in tandem position eyes open to eyes closed – **Sharpened Romberg**

11. Walking, placing the heel of one foot directly in front of the toe of the opposite foot (tandem walking)

12. Walking along a straight line drawn or taped to the floor, or place feet on floor markers while walking

13. Walk sideways, backward, or cross stepping

14. March in place

15. Alter speed of ambulatory activities; observe patient walking at normal speed, as fast as possible and as slow as possible
16. Stop and start abruptly while walking
17. Walk and pivot (turn 90, 180, or 360 degrees)
18. Walk in a circle, alternate directions
19. Walk on heels and then on toes
20. Walk with horizontal and vertical head turns
21. Step over or around obstacles
22. Stair climbing with and without using handrail; one step at a time versus step over step
23. Agility activities (coordinated movement with upright balance); jumping jacks, alternate flexing, and extending the knees while sitting on a Swiss ball

Table 10-5 outlines common movement and coordination abnormalities and their assessment methods.

Balance

Balance is a complex concept that is tied to limb and body movements. Clinicians typically examine static and dynamic balance within functional activities such as seated and standing reaching, transfers, and walking. The examination of balance is commonly done through the use of measures such as the **Berg Balance Scale** (BBS),[20] the Sensory Organization Test (SOT),[21] the Functional Reach Test,[22] and the **Romberg test**.[23] Each of these tests incorporates standing, assessment of limits of stability, and transfers from sitting to standing. Gait activities, which are a form of dynamic balance, can also give an indication of balance function. These include the Timed Up and Go test (TUG), the **Tinetti Mobility Test** (TMT), the **Dynamic Gait Index** (DGI), **Functional Gait Assessment** (FGA), and the BEST test or mini-BESTest.[24] Clinicians have many measures to choose from and should base their choice not only on the reliability and validity of the measure but also on the goals of the client with whom they are working. Measures can serve many uses including to screen risk, diagnose, provide insight into the person's condition or function, and objectively measure change over time. Many measures can be used for more than one purpose. For example, the Berg Balance Test can be used as a screen for fall risk, as a way to gain insight into a person's balance function and/or as an objective measure of change in balance over time. When a measure is used to assess change over time, it is referred to as an **outcome measure**.

TABLE 10-5	**Assessment of Movement and Coordination Impairments[19]**	
IMPAIRMENT	**DEFINITION**	**SAMPLE TEST**
Dysdiadochokinesia	Impaired alternating movements	Finger to nose Alternate nose to finger Pronation/Supination Knee flexion/Extension Walking, alter speed or direction
Dysmetria	Uncoordinated movement, characterized by over or under shooting intended position	Pointing to a target Drawing a circle or figure eight Heel on shin Placing feet on floor markers while walking
Dyssynergia	Movement decomposition and loss of coordination	Finger to nose Finger to therapist's finger Alternate heel to knee Toe to examiner's finger
Hypotonia	Diminished muscle tone	Passive movement DTRs
Tremor (resting)	Oscillating movements at rest	Observation of patient at rest Observation during functional activities (tremor will diminish or disappear with movement)
Tremor (intentional)	Oscillating movements with movement	Observation during functional activities Alternate nose to finger Finger to finger Finger to therapist's finger Toe to examiner's finger
Tremor (postural)	Oscillating trunk movements	Observation of steadiness of normal standing posture
Bradykinesia	Slowness of movement and loss of associated movements (e.g., arm swing)	Walking, observation of arm swing and trunk motions Walking, alter speed and direction Request that a movement or gait activity be stopped abruptly Observation of functional activities; timed tests

CASE A, PART IV

Trisha has reported a history of falls. Based on this, an examination of balance should be included in her assessment. Assessments at the body structure and function level might include the SOT and Romberg tests. These will help elucidate whether or not the balance problem is related to the vestibular or somatosensory systems. If the lesion is in the cerebellum, examination of coordination and equilibrium would likely yield positive findings. In addition, the clinician may wish to choose one or two outcome measures to better determine baseline function and document progress. The BBS, TUG, TMT, DGI, and BEST all give valid and reliable data, regarding functional balance status, and inform the clinician about fall risk. Given that Trisha has already had one or more falls, it is already known that she is a fall risk but measuring improvement with tools such as these would still be important. Choice of the tool to use should be based on the underlying cause of Trisha's balance problems, as some tools work well in older adults while others may be more appropriate for individuals with a neurologic disorder. In addition, age, level of function, and situation(s), in which falls typically occur, are all factors to consider in choosing the right measure to be used with Trisha.

In the SOT, she is unstable in both conditions where her eyes are closed (Conditions 2 and 5), falling within the first few seconds; she was able to assume a Romberg position but fell when attempting to maintain it with her eyes closed. Both of these findings indicate a strong reliance on vision and a strong likelihood of proprioceptive loss. Her Berg score was 50/56 with deductions for standing with feet together and eyes closed (could only hold for 3 seconds before falling), turning 360 degrees in each direction, which was very slow, and placing alternating feet on a low stool (only being able to complete four steps in 2 seconds). When reviewing her falls, each has taken place in dim light with tripping over a change in surface height or a throw rug in the house.

• NEUROLOGICAL EXAMINATION: ACTIVITY AND PARTICIPATION

The Academy of Neurologic Physical Therapy has developed a Clinical Practice Guideline on outcome measures in neurologic physical therapy.[25] Six core measures were identified and resources have been developed to help clinicians apply these measures, including pocket cards and a free online course. The six core outcome measures are the BBS, FGA, **Activities-Specific Balance Confidence Scale** (ABC), **10 Meter Walk Test** (10MWT), **5 Times Sit to Stand** (5TSTS), and the **6 Minute Walk Test** (6MWT). Ideally, therapists would incorporate these six measures in all patients' examinations so that the profession can begin to examine common data across time and settings to better determine therapeutic effectiveness. In cases when a patient cannot complete one or more core set outcome measures (e.g., a patient who is unable to walk; thus, cannot complete the 10mWT or the 6MWT), a score of 0 should be documented. Clinicians should continue to choose assessments that provide the best data for assessing individual clients. The core set are to be used for measuring outcomes and supplemented with measures specific to the individual's condition, goals, and potential for improvement in function.[25]

At the core of physical therapy practice lies expertise in the movement system. The movement system is defined as an integration of body systems that generates and maintains movement at all levels of bodily function.[26,27] Physical therapists examine the movement system to diagnose movement disorders and provide an individualized plan of care to meet the individual's goals.[26] In neurologic physical therapy there are six recommended core tasks for movement observation (Table 10-6).[27,28] These tasks can be regressed or progressed by doing things like increasing or decreasing the base of support, changing speed, adding perturbations, altering vision, or changing the cognitive demands of the task. Every physical therapy exam includes an assessment of movement, which should be completed in a formal manner so that it can be replicated across time, therapists, and patients. We use the six stages of the movement continuum as a framework for performing movement analysis (Box 10-7).[28,29] Movement analysis begins with the initial conditions such as the environment in which the movement is occurring, and the starting posture. The next stage of movement is preparation for movement, which includes stimulus recognition, response selection, and movement planning, but is not observable. We draw inferences about preparation from observations of the other stages of movement. You can assess whether or not the individual is able to identify the stimulus for movement by ascertaining if the patient understands the instructions. Initiation, execution, and termination all make up the observable part of the movement and should be carefully assessed and documented. Initiation should occur immediately after the stimulus for movement is given. If cognition is intact and the individual is able to identify

Box 10-7	Movement Analysis across the Continuum and Ways to Modify

Stage	Description
Initial Conditions	Conditions in which the movement is initiated, including both the environment and the patient position
Preparation	Includes stimulus identification, response selection, and programming of the response. This occurs rapidly prior to actual movement
Initiation	Instant when the displacement of the relevant body part begins
Execution	Period of actual movement
Termination	Instant when motion stops
Outcome	Was the goal of the task reached?

TABLE 10-6	Observation and Assessment of Core Movement Tasks[27]		
CORE TASKS FOR MOVEMENT OBSERVATION*	**STARTING CONDITION**	**REGRESSION EXAMPLES**	**PROGRESSION EXAMPLES**
Sitting	Stable surface with feet on the floor in a quiet environment. No back or armrests and arms are crossed so that they cannot provide support. No manipulation with hands and patient is allowed to focus on the task	Addition of trunk support Allow patient to use arms to support trun	Raise surface so that feet do not touch floor. Use a soft surface. Patient is asked to hold or manipulate an object. Patient is asked to focus on a cognitive task such as counting backward.
Standing	Stable, smooth surface in a quiet space without distractions. No external support provided. Feet shoulder width apart	Allow to use external support. Allow to widen base of support	Alter or remove vision. Change surface to be soft or uneven or sloped.
Sit to stand	Seated on a firm surface without arm rests in a quiet space	Raise sitting surface. Firmer seat. Allow to use arms to assist	Lower sitting surface Softer seat Combine with manipulation Combine with a cognitive task
Walking	A smooth surface in a quiet space. No external support	Provide external support	Rough or uneven or soft surface Change slope of surface. Alter vision Combine with manipulation Combine with a cognitive task
Step up	Standing on a smooth surface in a quiet space. Step is 7" tall and stable	Lower step height	Rough or uneven or soft surface Alter vision Combine with manipulation Combine with a cognitive task
Reach, grasp, and manipulation	Seated upright in a quiet space		Alter vision Combine with standing, transfer and/or walking Combine with a cognitive task

*Based on the article by Quinn et al. 2021[28]

and understand the stimulus, a delay in initiation of movement can be indicative of damage to the basal ganglia. We discuss execution for each of the selected tasks in more detail in the following segment. A detailed movement analysis of execution should be conducted for each patient. Termination is examined for timeliness, smoothness, and coordination of body segments. The final phase of movement, according to Hedman,[29] is the outcome, which is measured by whether the goal of the movement was reached.

Sitting

Sitting should be examined with the person seated on a firm surface with feet on the floor and hips and knee flexed to 90 degrees. First, assess the ability to sit without support for a prolonged period of time such as 30 to 60 seconds. If the individual cannot sit unsupported, assess ability to maintain upright using upper extremities for support. If the individual can sit unsupported for at least 30 seconds begin to incrementally increase the task challenge by altering vision or alter the stability of the surface. Other ways to increase the challenge of sitting are to add perturbations, starting with gentle nudges in all directions and increasing the force of the nudge. Adding in arm movement or marching also adds challenge to the task. Whenever you engage in conversation with the individual while they are doing the task you are adding in a cognitive challenge by asking them to dual task. You can purposefully do this by minimizing conversation unless you wish to assess ability to dual task, and then when assessing dual tasking, ask the individual to perform specific tasks such as counting backward by 3's. A final aspect of assessing any static position is to examine posture and document in detail. If assistance is needed to maintain a seated posture, document level of assistance. Refer to Table 10-7 for descriptions of assistance levels.

Transfers

The examination of transfers includes an assessment of the individual's ability to make position changes in the bed, go from a seated position to standing, go from standing to sitting, and transfer to and from surfaces that are of differing heights and softness.

TABLE 10-7	Levels of Assistance Terminology[30,31]		
BASED ON THE FUNCTIONAL INDEPENDENCE MEASURE (FIM)		**BASED ON THE GG CODES OF THE CENTERS MEDICARE & MEDICAID SERVICES**	
Level of Assistance	*Definition*	*Level of Assistance*	*Definition*
Independence Level 7	Completes the activity with no assistance and is safe while doing it.	06 Independent	Complete activity independently (no helper assistance)
Modified independence Level 6	Completes the activity with no assistance and is safe but requires the use of an assistive device or orthosis.		
		05 Setup/ Clean-up Assistance	Assistance only for set up or clean-up. Independent performance.
Supervision Level 5	Completes the activity with no assistance but is not safe <50% of the time. The level of safety risk is minimal. Assistance provided is that of the therapist being in close proximity, in order to assist if needed, but not touching the client.	04 Supervision/ touching assistance	Completion requires verbal or touch cues or contact guard assistance.
Contact guard assist (CGA)	Completes the activity with no assistance but there are consistent safety concerns or periodic losses of balance requiring light assistance to regain balance.		
Minimal assistance (Min) Level 4	Assistance is required but no more than 25% of the work is done by the person helping, during times of assistance.	03 Partial/ Moderate assistance	Requires assistance with support or movement but helper does less than 50%.
Moderate assistance (Mod) Level 3	Assistance is required but no more than 75% of the work is done by the person helping, during times of assistance.		
Maximal assistance (Max) Level 2	The majority of the work is done by the person helping (>75%).	02 Substantial/ maximal assistance	Helper provides more than 50% effort for task completion to lift, hold or support trunk/limb.
Total assist Level 1	The patient does not do anything and all work is done by the person(s) helping.	01 Dependent	Helper provides 100% of effort or two or more helpers are required.

Additional items to document: Number of helpers should be included. Typically this is documented as +1 Min assist meaning only one person helped. +2 Mod assist would mean that two people helped. Any assistive device that is used should also be documented. Ie: +1 Min assist with walker.

The level of assistance should be described, including any relevant details such as how the assistance is best provided (i.e., guard left knee from buckling during stance phase). Refer to Table 10-7 for descriptions of assistance levels. Bed mobility, including rolling side-to-side and the ability to go from seated to supine and supine to sitting, should be described. Movements should be attempted with and without assistive devices, if possible. Additional details that should be documented include:

- Movement strategy description
- Whether all extremities are used equally (e.g., one arm more than the other?)
- Presence of involuntary or uncontrollable movements
- Level of independence or assistance required (how much, what type, assistive device). Are any assistive devices typically used?

- Description of the quality of movement and environment/situation, whether skilled and efficient, or if not, the measurements of the movement for documenting progress.

Sample Movement Description: Sit to stand with use of armrests. Required vigorous rocking, six to seven times, followed by pushing off with (R) UE and LE. (L) UE and LE were not incorporated.

Walking (Gait)

Normal walking is a complex process and requires the use of many elements such as power, coordination, sensation, and balance working together in a coordinated fashion. The examination of gait can assist in detecting a variety of disease states. A slow velocity gait with short stride length and decreased arm swing could indicate Parkinson's disease, while a wide-based gait with ataxic movement may be indicative of disorders involving the cerebellum. The gait pattern should be carefully observed and documented by gait phase: initial contact, stance (early, mid, and late), push-off, and swing. It is essential in the neurologic patient that we determine in which phase(s) of gait the primary problem is occurring so that we can better direct our treatment. Some areas to document under gait analysis include:

- Can the individual ambulate independently? With or without assistive devices? What level of assistance is required from the therapist?
- What gait pattern is used? Be sure to describe what happens at each phase of gait. Describe both lower extremities. Be thorough and clear with this description and make sure that the descriptive terms are measurable.
- Can the individual turn and maneuver around objects? Do they choose a specific direction to turn (e.g., always to the right)?
- Can he walk backward and sideways, in both directions? Describe the pattern used.
- Can he walk on uneven surfaces like grass and thick carpet, or go from a linoleum floor to a carpeted floor? Does he change speed when approaching a different surface?
- With any of the above, is there a loss of balance? Is it consistently in a certain direction? Do the client self-correct or need assistance to prevent a fall?

The use of orthotic and assistive devices needs to be assessed and documented. Consider:

- What assistive devices and/or orthosis is the client presently using and when are they used?
- Observe gait with and without the use of the orthosis. Does the orthosis improve the client's gait pattern?
- Can the client walk without it?
- Is the client using any assistive devices for the upper extremity? If so, what and when? Are the devices effective?
- Are any orthosis and assistive devices in good working order? Would adjustments improve their performance?

Many researchers are now recommending that gait speed become the sixth vital sign.[32] Gait speed has been shown to correlate with measures of health, and therefore, can be a valuable tool for measuring activity status. Studies have shown that a gait speed of .8 m/s is necessary to be a community ambulator while gait speeds less than .4 m/s put individuals at highest risk for negative health outcomes (Figure 10-2). Fortunately, there are many easy-to-use measures that examine gait. Some of these tools focus on endurance (6MWT), many examine both gait and balance (DGI, TMT,[24] **Rivermead mobility test**[33]) while others examine both gait and transfers (timed up and go).

Assessment of stair climbing is performed by asking the individual to climb up and down stairs. Optimal stair climbing is the ability to independently ascend and descend in a foot over foot manner without the use of a handrail, and therefore, determining whether or not the individual can do this or how they deviate from this is the goal of the assessment. If the individual cannot climb foot over foot, then assess the ability to utilize a step-to pattern, and note which extremity is used to step up and which leads on descent. Optimally, the individual should be encouraged to try to ascend/descend the stairs without using the handrail, if this is not possible, note which handrail is used or that both handrails are needed. For individuals who use an assistive device, note whether or not they are able to use the assistive device on the stairs. Speed of climbing may also be measured as a means of tracking progress. You can assess the quality of stair climbing using the **Step Test Evaluation of Performance on Stairs** (STEPS) Tool developed by the Mobility and Exercise in Neurologic Disorders (MEND) laboratory at The Ohio State University. This tool rates elements of stair ascent and descent such as stepping pattern, foot placement, use of handrail, trunk stability, and balance on an ordinal scale.[34] The tool can be found at https://hrs.osu.edu/research/research-labs/mend-laboratory/steps

For individuals who will need to use a wheelchair for mobility, assess the ability to propel the chair. Some individuals find propelling the chair with their feet easier than using their arms; this is common in individuals with Huntington's disease. Other individuals may not be able to propel a standard wheelchair due to hand weakness or coordination problems. Modifications to the wheel or drive mechanism may be necessary for these individuals (this will be discussed related to appropriate disorders in later chapters). Still, other individuals are unable to self-propel due to significant deficits in the upper extremities or cognitive limitations and will, therefore,

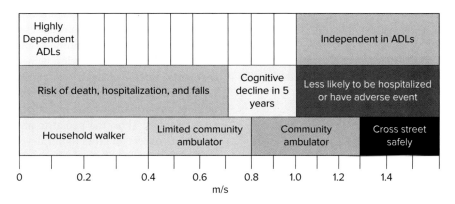

FIGURE 10-2 Gait speed correlation with health and function.

require a power wheelchair. Once a means of propulsion has been determined, examine the ability to propel on different surfaces, such as linoleum or carpet and ramps, and to change direction.

CASE A, PART V

Case Report: Trisha remains independent in her walking with only a slight increase in knee flexion, associated with a mild foot drop bilaterally; this likely contributes to her falling in low light situations when encountering a change in surface height (tile floor to carpet) or obstacle (throw rug). On the TUG, her time was 15 seconds or "mostly independent"; there was obvious slowing when she was turning around to walk back to the chair.

EVALUATION

This is your thought process and should discuss how you have confirmed or refuted your hypotheses regarding the cause of the movement disorders that you as a physical therapist are going to address in treatment. This includes:

- Synthesis of all data and findings gathered from the examination, highlighting pertinent factors
- Various forms of documentation such as a problem list, statement of general assessment with key factors influencing status

---

CASE A, PART VI

Case Report: *What do you think that Tricia's diagnosis should be?* Trisha's symptoms are consistent with bilateral symmetrical peripheral neuropathy secondary to diabetes.

Diagnosis

The diagnosis should describe how the identified limitations in body structure/function (impairment) and activity (functional limitation) restrict the client's desired participation role(s) and whether or not physical therapy can have a beneficial effect. Provide a movement system diagnosis and the relevant **International Classification for Disease 10 Code (ICD 10)**.[35]

CASE A, PART VII

Case Report: *What ICD-10 code and movement system diagnosis would you give Trisha?* Trisha's diagnosis is consistent with an ICD 10 Code of E11.42 (type 2 diabetes with diabetic polyneuropathy). The movement system diagnosis would be impaired walking.

Prognosis (Goals and Outcomes)

It is very important to consider and state the long-term functional prognosis as well as identify the short- and long-term goals for this episode of care (level of care). By focusing on the long-term functional prognosis, it assists the therapist in prioritizing and considering things such as impact on neuroplasticity and negative consequences of compensation techniques on long-term functional prognosis. The prognosis statement should address the following:

1. What is the potential for function or participation for the long term?
2. What specific motor functions should the patient be prepared for at this time (this level of care)?
3. Identify the positive factors that will contribute to the achievement of the goals.
4. Identify the attributes that might prevent or delay the acquisition of the goals.
5. Identify the likely time frame for achieving the long-term goals (include this in the prognosis).

Do NOT say "Good potential for rehab." This statement fails to provide useful information. Say something like "Trisha has good potential to learn knitting within 2 months because she is highly motivated and retains full strength in (B) hands. Her skill acquisition will be slowed by her sensory loss in (B) hands." Goal setting will be discussed more in the following chapters, in association with the different clinical case studies.

Short-Term and Long-Term Goals

Be sure that the goals are **measurable** and **functional**. Body structure/function (impairment) related goals are acceptable as short-term goals. If underlying impairments are not addressed, the client will not reach her full rehabilitation potential, and therefore these elements are important to consider in setting goals and designing a treatment plan. Be sure that the long-term goals come from the activity problem list and/or the recorded participation restriction on the examination notes.

COMPONENTS OF THE PEDIATRIC EVALUATION

Although the evaluation of children with developmental disorders is similar to that of adults, it is complicated by the interplay between the developmental processes of neurologic maturation, engagement with the environment, and neuroplasticity precipitated by an insult to the developing nervous system. As physical therapists, we are charged with not only identifying impairments (ROM, abnormal tone, etc.) but also the relative impact of these impairments on the typical acquisition of developmental milestones. Thus, the pediatric physical therapist must not only be an expert on gross motor development but also have an understanding of psychological, social, language, and fine motor development as these are tightly entwined as the child matures.

CASE B, PART I

Hayley is a 2-year-old Caucasian female born full-term at 38 weeks. She has a history of altered motor and cognitive skills, after a possible incidence of shaken baby syndrome (SBS) 6 months ago. Besides the recent "incident," she has an unremarkable medical history. Hayley lives in a two-story house with two steps to the front door. Hayley's father is an elementary school teacher, and her mother is a chiropractor. Hayley attended a daycare program until the "incident" but is currently being cared for by a babysitter in the home.

History

The evaluation of the pediatric client includes unique aspects because young infants and most children are not able to answer questions about their medical history or their reasons for coming into the clinic. To begin, the role of the clinician is to be receptive to the expertise of the parent in order to obtain a meaningful and adequate history. Allowing the parents a few minutes to talk candidly about their concerns may give you unique insight into the medical and functional needs of the child. A pediatric history starts with baseline data such as date of birth and due date plus the current concerns of the parents and child. It is useful to include the child in this line of questioning if they are able to respond. Some questions that could be asked in addition to the parents' concerns are: What would you like your child to be able to do? And, what is the latest thing your child has learned to do?

The medical history may be available in the medical records of the child, but in some clinical or educational settings, this information must be acquired from the parent, but the referring physician may be contacted to confirm the parent's report or obtain missing information. A clear understanding from the parent and physician regarding any precautions or contraindications to handling or positioning is necessary, so the clinician is aware of potential limitations in positioning, during the physical examination. Handling precautions could include things like restricted lower extremity weight-bearing because of a possible hip dislocation or avoidance of pulling to sit (a common physical test to evaluate head and trunk control) after cardiac surgery.

In addition to medical history, **demographics** include information about the child that is not medical, such as contact information, the best way to communicate with the family about appointment times, race, religion, occupation of the parents, and any general family information pertinent to the child or potential treatment implementation (e.g., number of siblings in the home). **Medical history** includes current and previous medical diagnosis and concerns, clinical tests that have been completed and their understanding of them (e.g., genetic, imaging, laboratory), medication(s) with dosage and adherence, previous and current diseases, illnesses, and surgical procedures. **Developmental history** includes pre- and postnatal information such as gestational age at birth, pregnancy, or post-delivery complications that could affect the child (e.g., a fall during pregnancy, feeding issues); timeline for developmental milestones that have been achieved; growth history (e.g., small for age);

adaptive or other equipment used by the child; and previous developmental evaluations. **Family history** includes a general overview of family medical issues, including developmental problems in other family members, especially siblings of the child (e.g., motor, learning, or cognitive impairments). Questions related to the **living environment** and the **support system** available will play a large role in goal setting, prescribing therapeutic exercises for developmental improvement, and designing a meaningful home exercise program (see Box 10-8).

The last question on the list in Box 10-8 (What are the daily activities of the family in the home and in the community?) leads nicely into the next section of the history – **Programs or related therapy services**. If the child is in a daycare program or school, further information about related therapy services available in either setting, including PT, OT, SP, adaptive physical education, dance, etc., will be helpful. If these programs exist in a currently utilized program, the PT can advocate for related therapy services, if needed. If the child is receiving supportive services, details about the setting, type, frequency, and goals of the treatments are necessary.

Functional Status describes the current functional activities that the child can perform. It is helpful to ask about functional

Box 10-8   Necessary questions to evaluate the living environment and support system:

- In what type of household does the child and family reside – two-story house, a walk-up apartment, etc.? *In some cases, an evaluation of the home might be done to determine assistive technology needs (e.g., before the child receives a wheelchair or for an assessment of where to place a ramp).*

- What is the entry way into the home, does it have stairs or an elevator, and how does the child get in and out – carried, wheeled, ambulates?

- Who lives in the household with the child, including the number of adults and ages of other children?

- Where does the family eat meals (at a table, kitchen counter, etc.)? Does the child sit with the family? How and what does the child eat?

- Where is the child's bedroom and bathroom?

- What adaptive equipment does the child have (e.g., adaptive toilet seat, stander, tub chair)?

- For older children, does the child participate in home chores, like setting the table?

- How is the child transported within the community – car, van, bus; include assessment of car seat or wheelchair, if used?

- What kinds of toys or play equipment outside of specific adaptive therapy equipment are available?

- What is the support system for the caregivers?

- What types of play activities/toys does the child like?

- What are the daily activities of the family in the home and in the community? Does the child attend daycare or school? Does the (older) child have a job? *Asking the caregiver/parent to describe a typical day may be the easiest way to obtain much of this information.*

CASE B, PART II

Hayley is an only child, conceived after multiple fertility treatments. Mother reports her pregnancy was uncomplicated and delivery occurred 18 hours after labor onset, aided by an epidural. Her parents also report an uncomplicated medical history, confirmed by the pediatrician's report. Prior to the "incident," she was at the 40th percentile for height, weight, and head circumference. She is currently having eating difficulties so has dropped to the 20th percentile for weight in just the last 4 months. Parents report that she rolled over by 6 months, sat independently at 8 months, walked at 11 months, and was saying multiple words (mama, dada, hi, bye, up, "ba" for bottle, dog, and cat) by 18 months when the incident occurred. They describe that they picked their daughter up from daycare, and she was unusually sleepy. After inquiring of the daycare provider (a mother of grown children, providing care in her home), she indicated that Hayley might have fallen as they found her on the floor behind a couch during "free play" time, acting sleepy. They were apologetic but did not seem overly concerned. The parents immediately took her to the Emergency Room, where she was found to have retinal hemorrhaging and a mild frontal subdural hematoma and associated mild cerebral edema on magnetic resonance imaging (MRI). She remained hospitalized for 4 days, when the subdural hematoma had resolved. The police investigation did not find sufficient evidence to charge anyone with shaking Hayley, but SBS was suspected; as SBS is difficult to diagnose, they could not rule out that Hayley had fallen (although there was no "bump" evident on her head). On discharge, Hayley was still able to walk, although seemed a little "wobbly" at first; since that time, she seems not to be progressing as she should with little change in motor skills. She is still crawling up and down stairs, does not catch or kick a ball, and is not using a fork or spoon to feed herself (she does feed herself finger foods as she did before the incident). She has acquired a few more words but is not putting two words together yet. Her parents state they can see that she is not progressing the same as others in their "play group." Their goals are for her to get "back on track" with her developmental progression.

Box 10-9   Questions about Learning

Questions about learning can be included during the history interview with the child and caregiver, and modified, if needed, after interacting one on one with the child.

- Does the child learn best with vision, pictures, hearing, or demonstration?
- Can the child read? Can the child understand what is read to them?
- Are there any language needs, including the need for an interpreter, if English is not the child's primary language?

The same questions are repeated about how the adult caregiver learns. During the examination note whether the child is attentive, responsive, cooperative, and what mode of communication is most effective.

pediatric clients. Either tool can also be used for examination of self-care and home management.

Systems Review

The systems review, for the child, contains many of the elements of the adult exam and some novel elements, specific to children. Here, we will focus on the elements that might be different from the adult exam or specific to children:

- Integumentary System review: Although the integumentary review for children mirrors that for adults, the skin areas around pressure points from clothing, braces, and weight-bearing surfaces, especially in children with limited movement, should be carefully evaluated. If skin issues are identified, careful review of any adaptive equipment must be completed to determine points of potential pressure.
- Musculoskeletal systems review: Gross ROM, Strength, and Symmetry in sitting and standing are screened and assessed during functional activities, since infants and young children don't typically understand or comply with standard adult-like testing methods. Presence of symmetry or asymmetry should be noted and further examined in the musculoskeletal assessment, as described in the next section.
- Cardiovascular/Pulmonary system review: No specific differences from adults.
- Gait, primary form of locomotion, balance, transitions, coordinated movements, proprioception, motor control, and motor learning are part of the Neuromuscular Systems review. Remember during this level of the review the indication for each item is impaired or not impaired.
- Other systems review: Standard testing for vision, hearing, and the other special senses is not feasible in infants and young children. However, tracking visually (following an object with the eyes laterally and vertically) and to sound (turning in the direction of a sound out of the visual field) can be screened even in young infants, using common toys; also, very young infants will blink to a light focused on the eyes. Taste is typically not tested in young children, but the other CNs may be screened by observing eating and facial expressions as well as shoulder movements.

status in a variety of conditions such as at school, in the home, on the playground. Qualify these activities with the type of assistive device that is used. In addition, questions about learning style can be included (Box 10-9) to determine how best to present information.

The **Pediatric Evaluation of Disibility Index** (PEDI)[36] and **PEDI-Computer Adaptive Test** (PEDI-CAT)[37] are survey-based tools that may be beneficial in assisting caregivers and families in identifying their child's current level of function and help identify areas of need. One advantage to these tools is the wide age range they encompass (PEDI: 6 months-7.5 years; PEDI-CAT: birth-21 years), so they can be used with a variety of

CASE B, PART III

The system review of Hayley is negative for any disturbances of the integumentary, cardiovascular/pulmonary, or other systems. Observation indicates a need for a comprehensive musculoskeletal and neuromuscular examination, as her movements are slow, she walks on her toes with hands at mid-guard position, and she requires an external support to pull to stand.

Examination

Like the methods for screening, examination of strength and ROM occurs through structured observation of functional motor skills and some passive handling/positioning. For example, kicking a ball in sitting can assess antigravity quadriceps strength, while squatting to the ground and returning to standing is an indication of good quadriceps strength. If she can also lift an object, during squat to stand (e.g., a large ball), normal strength is likely. Prone extension over a ball is a nice way to examine antigravity shoulder, back, and hip strength; the length of time the position can be held can suggest good or normal strength. Many of these skills are included in standardized tests with increasing time for maintaining the position as an indicator of developmental age. In Box 10-10, standard questions that the therapist should consider in each position, in which the child is observed, are delineated.

Box 10-10	Questions to be answered while observing a pediatric client:

(A similar framework is used in the Alberta Infant Motor Scale (AIMS),[20] a common scale of infant development.)
- What is the weight-bearing position?
- What are the antigravity movements, required by the position?
- Is the position/movement symmetrical or asymmetrical?
- What is the midline behavior while in the position?

The answers to these questions give information about strength, ROM, balance, and coordination.

In addition, the following overall questions should be addressed:
- What are the abilities of the child?
- What are the strengths of the child's functional movements?
- What is the quality of the movement?
- Can the child sustain the position?
- Can the child sustain a position and stabilize in order to play or perform ADLs with the arms and hands?
- Is there sufficient variability in the number of postures and positions, or does the child adopt only one position, putting them at risk for a secondary impairment or overuse injury?
- What positions and activities cannot be performed?
- Is the alignment, posture, or movement typical or atypical?
- What type of assistance is required to assume a position or perform a skill or task?

Muscle Tone: Muscle tone is objectively measured with the modified Ashworth, as described for the adult assessment, despite limited evidence of validity or interrater reliability. Commonly, pediatric assessments only describe tone as normal, hypotonic (low tone, floppy), hypertonic (high tone), or mixed (combinations of normal, high, and low tone), which is common in some developmental disorders. Tone should be assessed in all position; at rest; and during passive, active, and challenging (stressful) movements. Tone can impede acquisition of motor milestones, limit function, and interfere with the assessment of strength and muscle power.

CASE B, PART IV

Upper extremity tone is normal, but Hayley demonstrates mild hypertonia in her gastrocs and hip adductors (Ashworth = 1, DTR = 3+).

Range of Motion: Passive and active ROM is assessed while playing with the child or through the observation of functional movements; if there are any contractures or orthopedic deformities, goniometric measurements should be attempted, with help from the caregiver/parent to distract the child.

CASE B, PART V

Hayley has full ROM in her UE, but active dorsiflexion is neutral when her leg is straight (observed when asking her to touch the examiner's fingers with her toes, while her legs were straight; if external support was not provided, she would flex her knee, when dorsiflexing). She prefers w-sitting to tailor-sitting, assuming this position frequently, consistent with adductor tightness. Abduction with knees flexed is approximately 60 degrees but should be near 90 degrees.

Strength: Observation of movement against gravity and with resistance in functional activities or during activities that use muscle power is the primary method for assessing strength and power for infants and young children; fairly good reliability has been found with manual muscle testing in and dynamometry in children as young as 5, but it is important to be sure that the child to be tested understands and can follow directions.[38] Dynamometers are frequently available in a pediatric clinical setting. The Biodex offers options for measuring more advanced examination and outcome values of isometric, isokinetic strength, especially in the lower extremity, but are not common in pediatric clinics.

Anthropometrics: Body weight, length/height, and head circumference are commonly measured indicators of growth, and important for monitoring growth and development of the body due to nutritional concerns. Head circumference is also an indirect measure of brain growth and can indicate microcephaly and associated lack of brain growth within an expected trajectory. Head circumference may also be needed to monitor hydrocephalus and shunt function (see Chapter 19). Other less routine anthropometrics include limb lengths and circumference, which are used to evaluate asymmetrical growth, identify secondary joint dislocations, and fit assistive devices and braces.

CASE B, PART VI

Hayley demonstrates antigravity muscle strength in all major muscle groups. However, she still requires an external support to pull to stand and is not squatting to the ground and returning without an external support, suggesting some LE muscle weakness (Fair+/Good−). She can walk on her hands in a wheelbarrow position, which is indicative of good UE muscle strength.

Anthropometrics are unremarkable except for the recent failure to gain weight.

Sensory Integrity: Many aspects of sensory function are observed simultaneously with motor function and during play. Response to touch can be determined by looking for a withdrawal of the trunk, limb, or digit to a light tickle or pinch but formal sensory testing can't typically be done until the child is at least 5 years of age.[38] Proprioception can be grossly assessed by moving the limb into an awkward position and watching to see if the child moves it (e.g., place the arm under the child). Balance is typically assessed by observation of the child's ability to assume, maintain, and move within a given posture (sitting, standing, supine, prone) during play. Further, there are many reflexes that are present in the infant that come under higher nervous system control with maturation (primitive reflexes) and others that emerge as the child matures (protective, equilibrium, and righting reactions). Primitive reflexes were described in Chapter 8 (see Figure 8-1). While **primitive reflexes** (the historical name) are less obvious in the older infant/child/adult, they are often integral parts of coordinated movement patterns or become obvious when we are under stress. For example, while the crossed extensor reflex can't be elicited via the typical testing method after the second month of life, it is often apparent in our response to stubbing our toe or stepping on something. The first response to hitting your toe is to rapidly flex the injured leg with strong extension of the other (stance) leg to maintain an upright posture (often with some hopping and yelling) indicative of a crossed extensor pattern. Thus, primitive reflexes don't truly disappear; they just become part of our motor program repertoire, and their integration is a sign of nervous system maturation. However, failure to integrate these reflexes at the appropriate age is often a sign of central nervous system dysfunction; similarly, reemergence of these reflexes to their initial stimulus often occurs with central nervous system damage.[39] **Righting, protective,** and **equilibrium reactions** are mature responses that develop over the first 2 years of life that maintain our body alignment and balance (Table 10-8 describes the testing method and response for primitive reflexes and righting, protective, and equilibrium reactions; Figure 10-3 illustrates some of these testing methods.

CASE B, PART VII

Hayley has a mild Babinski in both feet but otherwise demonstrates integration of all primitive reflexes; a Babinski at this age is indicative of an upper motor neuron injury. She demonstrates normal protective and equilibrium reactions in sitting and quadruped; however, her equilibrium reactions in standing are delayed and not effective to a moderate disturbance (Hayley will fall or reach for a support).

TABLE 10-8	Primitive Reflexes and Righting, Protective, and Equilibrium Reactions Assessment[39]	
REFLEX	**DESCRIPTION**	**AGE SEEN**
Asymmetric Tonic Neck Reflex (ATNR)	Observe the child in supine when the head is turned to the side or manually turn the head to the side, look for extension of the face side extremities (less flexion) and increased flexion of the skull side extremities	0-3 months
Symmetric Tonic Neck Reflex	In prone prop or quadruped, encourage the child to look down, look for flexion of the arms with extension of the legs; encourage the child to look up and observe for extension of the arms and flexion of the legs	0-4 months
Moro	Carefully drop the child from an upright supported sitting position backward several inches toward the support surface, catching them as they start to fall backward. Look for abduction of the arms (away from midline), followed by adduction of the arms (toward midline) and trunk flexion	0-6 months
Rooting	Stroke the cheek; watch for head turning, as if to find a nipple	0-4 months
Galant (truncal incurvation)	Stroke the lateral part of the trunk; look for trunk flexing away from the stimulus (e.g., right stroke – convexity of trunk incurvation to the right)	0-4 months
Palmar grasp	Apply pressure to the palm of the hand; observe if the child grasps your finger (baby will hold the tester's finger briefly)	0-6 months
Plantar grasp	Press on the ball of the foot to elicit toe flexion as if to grasp with the toes	0-15 months
Stepping	Place the infant in a standing position and lean them forward to elicit stepping	0-2 months
Positive support (primitive standing)	Place the infant in a standing position; observe for leg and trunk extension	0-2 months

(Continued)

TABLE 10-8	Primitive Reflexes and Righting, Protective, and Equilibrium Reactions Assessment[39] (*Continued*)	
REFLEX	**DESCRIPTION**	**AGE SEEN**
Flexor withdrawal reflex	Tap the infant's heel or pull the great toe; watch for leg flexion away from the stimulus	0-2 months
Extensor thrust	Push the bottom of the foot; observe for strong extension of the leg	0-2 months
Crossed extensor reflex	Passively flex one leg; watch for extension of the other leg	0-6 weeks
Righting Reactions	Orient head to the body	
Rotational Righting	Turn a segment of the body (e.g., head; pelvis); watch for rotation of the rest of the body in a "log roll" fashion	Present up to 6-12 months
Body on head	Touch the body to a support services; watch for lifting of the head	
	Prone	Emerges 1.5-4 months
	Supine	Emerges 4-6 months
Vertical Righting		
Labyrinthine righting reaction	Hold the child upright and tilt laterally with vision occluded (blindfold), head will be maintained upright or return to upright	Emerges 3-6 months
Optical Righting	Tested same as LRR but with vision; head is maintained upright	Emerges 2.5-6 months
Prone Vertical Righting (Landau)	Hold child in a supported prone position (arms under stomach and hips)	
	Partial – head up to 45 degrees	Emerges 2.5-4 months
	Mature – head up to 90 degrees	Emerges by 10 months
Protective Responses		
Prone (parachute)	Support the child under the trunk in prone and quickly but carefully tip them forward toward a mat; the child should extend their hands	Emerges 6-7 months
Sitting	While the child is sitting, gently push them in a given direction (can be done on an equilibrium board by tipping the board)	
	Forward	Emerges 6-11 months
	Lateral (to the side)	Emerges 6-11 months
	Backward	Emerges 9-12 months
Tilting/Equilibrium Reactions	Typically tested with the child on an equilibrium board (tilting reaction) or by gently pushing the child to destabilize in a given direction (equilibrium):	
Prone	With the child prone, tip board to one side, trunk should curve away from the tip with arm reach toward the top of the board	Emerge 5-9 months
Supine	Tip board with child supine, trunk incurvation away from tip with arm reach toward top of board	Emerges 7-11 months
Sitting	In sitting, the child can be tipped forward/backward and to the side or while sitting on the floor, gently pushed in each direction	Emerge 7-8 months
Quadruped	While child is in quadruped, disturb balance to the side, will curve trunk to opposite side to return to stability	Emerges 8-12 months
Standing	With child in standing, disturb balance in any direction; extreme disturbance may elicit a step	Emerge 12-21 months

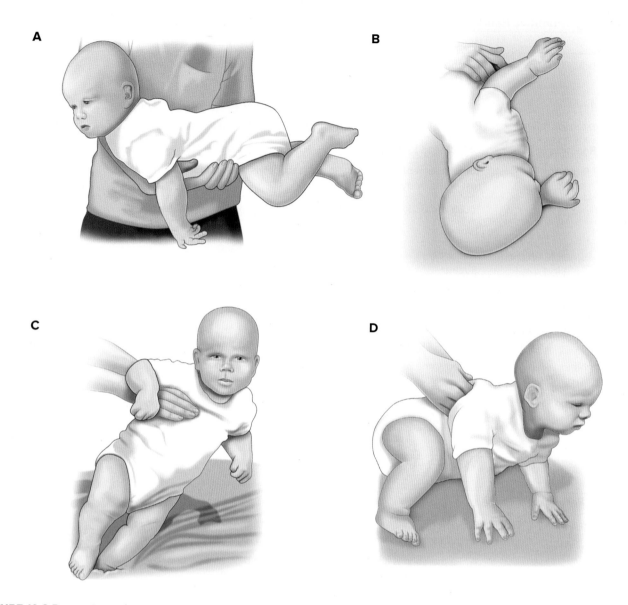

FIGURE 10-3 Postural reactions. A. Landau – support the infant under the abdomen and watch for leg and head extension; **B.** Body on body – turn the shoulders or hips and watch for rotation of the rest of the body; **C.** Optical righting – hold the child under the arms and tilt to the side, watch for head righting to upright; **D.** Parachute response – hold the child by the abdomen and bring quickly toward mat, watch for arm extension to protect from hitting the mat.

Developmental Assessment and the Examination of Movement

Pediatric evaluation for infants, toddlers, and children with apparent neurological dysfunction include a thorough examination, requiring observation and interaction with the child, usually in the context of play, in four body positions: supine, sitting, prone, and standing. In many settings, standardized assessment tools such as the **Bayley Scales of Infant and Toddler Development**[40] (BSIDT-3; birth-42 months), the **Peabody Developmental Motor Scales** (PDMS; birth-72 months),[41] or the **Alberta Infant Motor Scale** (AIMS; birth-18 months)[42] are used in conjunction with observation skills of the physical therapist to obtain a comprehensive evaluation. A systematic review that included these three measures found cultural differences in motor development in comparison cultures, especially from birth to 2 years, thus indicating that children outside of the United States and Canada may have different developmental trajectories than those used to develop these assessments. This must be taken into consideration when evaluating children of different cultures.[43] It should also be noted that an adjustment is made for any child born prematurely (<37 weeks) from birth up to age 24 months (Box 10-11). The **Gross Motor Function Measure** (GMFM)[44] is a common tool used to measure motor function and change in motor function in infants and children with cerebral palsy and has high psychometric properties; in addition, the GMFM-88[44] is validated in other populations, including Down syndrome. There are five domains on the GMFM: lying and rolling; sitting; crawling and kneeling; standing; and walking, running,

Box 10-11	Adjustment for Prematurity		
	Year	**Month**	**Days**
Due date	2020	4(3)	15(45)
Date of birth	2020	2	23
Prematurity correction		**1**	**22**
Date of testing	2021 (2020)	1(13)	30
Date of birth	2020	2	23
Uncorrected age	0	11 (10)	7 (37)
Correction		1	22
Corrected age		9	15

Almost every mother will remember her due date and the date of birth of the child. Subtracting the date of birth from the due date will give the prematurity adjustment (in **red**). An uncorrected age at testing is determined by subtracting the date of birth from the date of testing (this age would be used for any child that is over 2 or not born prematurely). The corrected age is then computed by subtracting the prematurity adjustment from the uncorrected age at testing.

Note, in this instance the due date was April 15, 2020, with a birthdate of February 23, 2020; to subtract the 23 days from the 15 days of the due date, one must add a month (30 days) to make this 45 and then subtract a month to make the 4 (April) a 3. This results in a correction factor of 1 month 22 days. When determining the corrected age at the time of testing, a year (12 months) must be added to the months to subtract 2 from 1, which subtracts 1 year from the 2021, making it 2020. Thus, the corrected age would be 9 months 15 days instead of 11 months 7 days, so the child should be meeting 9-month motor skills, not 11-month skills.

and jumping. Motor function for pediatric patients with neurological disabilities should be measured in all positions and in a functional context similar to those described and measured by the GMFM. When using a specific assessment tool, incorporate appropriate additional items that you would like to observe, while the child is in a given position (e.g., head movement, reaching, etc., while in prone), so that you are not requiring too many forced changes between positions. The more naturalistic the play and observation, the more accurate the examination will be, and the child will demonstrate better compliance. Older children or children with advanced motor skills need not be tested in every position. For all positions, the child should be observed for symmetry of movement to discern unilateral or asymmetrical abilities/deficits (see Box 10-11). To elicit movements, the therapist will need to make each activity fun, using toys, pictures, family members, or other types of stimulation to entice the child to look, reach, and move.

Table 10-9 describes movements and skills that should be evaluated in each position (supine, side-lying, prone, sitting, quadruped, and standing).

Mobility

In Table 10-9, posture, mobility, and function in supine to standing are discussed in association with the structured observation of the young child to limit the need for many position changes. In the mobile child, the therapist must use their observation skills and creativity to assess the quick transitions and gait of the child (see Box 10-12 for suggestions in movement observation). **Transitions** refer to the movements that children (and adults) use to go (transition) from one position to another, as described in Chapter 8. Some transitions elicit new postures for the child that they may maintain during play (e.g., ½ kneeling); transitions should be evaluated as part of the assessment while observing the child at play or in response to directions.

TABLE 10-9	Movement Observations by Position
POSITION	**OBSERVATIONS/SKILL TESTING**
Supine	Weight-bearing on the head, back, pelvis, posterior legs, and feet
	Spontaneous movements of arms and legs (frequency, vigor, pattern of leg kicks [unilateral, parallel, alternating])
	Ability to assume and maintain the head in midline (the position of the nose between the nipple line is a good reference for a midline head position) and tuck the chin (neck flexor control)
	Arm movement – length of movement (short or long), antigravity ability, ability to bring arms to midline (on belly or chest), extend to reach a toy, to mouth (self-soothing or toy-mouthing)
	Hand position – open or closed
	Visual tracking of a toy (cephalic, caudal, circular directions) – observe eye and head movements
	Orientation and tracking to sound (mother's voice, toy)
	Passive ROM – determine limitations, feel for tone restrictions (e.g., spasticity), screen for hip dysplasia (see Chapter 18)
	Antigravity movement of legs and pelvis (e.g., bridging) as an indication of abdominal and leg muscle strength
	Pull to sit – observe head position, arm pull and leg movement (see Figure 8-3, in the Development Chapter for an illustration and Box 10-13 for descriptions)

(Continued)

TABLE 10-9	Movement Observations by Position
POSITION	**OBSERVATIONS/SKILL TESTING**
	Rolling to prone – a toy can be used to stimulate this, if not done spontaneously; move a toy laterally in the child's line of vision and encourage reaching; assistance can be provided at the shoulder, hip, or leg, if the child needs assistance. If the child rolls on her own, look at the type of roll (log rolling, segmental – note which body part leads the roll)
Prone	Weight-bearing can be on the head, chest, belly, or hands and knees (in quadruped)
	Antigravity head control – sufficient to turn head and clear airway; distance lifted in degrees (e.g., 45 or 90 degrees for 10 seconds)
	Ability to lift in midline with nose between the nipple lines (harder than asymmetrical lifting with head turned slightly to side)
	Ability to turn the head to track a toy or sound
	Upper extremity weight-bearing – on elbows or hands; elbows flexed or extended; chest on or off the ground; ability to shift weight to reach (controlled or unsteady)
	Rolling to side-lying and supine – initially initiated with the head in a log roll (hip and legs in line) fashion; later led by the shoulders or legs in a segmental fashion (hip or shoulder ahead of the other)

	Movement in prone:
	    Pivot prone – ability to turn in a whole or partial circle
	    Commando crawling – ability to move forward, using arms and/or legs, often initially with bilateral motion and later alternating reciprocal motion

Side-lying	Note weight-bearing on the lateral trunk, head, legs, and arm. (*The child can be placed in side-lying, roll into side-lying on their own, or go through side-lying when transition to another position*)
	Midline and functional play of the arms should be noted, and the position of the legs
	Antigravity movements of lateral head flexion, trunk flexion and rotation
	Upper extremity weight-bearing – ability to prop on elbow
Sitting	Note whether weight-bearing is on the bottom, legs, and/or hands
	Trunk control (antigravity movement with the trunk), needed assistance or support to assume/maintain a sitting position. How the child supports himself – on elbows, hands with elbows flexed or extended, or without arm support, using trunk muscles (*note position of arms, if sitting without arm support – high with shoulder retraction, called a* **high-guard** *position, at the sides [ready to stop a fall] or free to reach and play*)
	Position of the pelvis – anterior tilt/posterior tilt; relation to trunk

	Position of the legs and width of the base of support
	  • Ring-sitting: legs are flexed with feet together, forming a circle or ring
	  • ½ Ring – sitting: one leg straight, the other flexed with foot toward midline
	  • Tailor-sitting: knees bent and hips externally rotated with one leg in front of the other and feet near the opposite knee
	  • W-sitting: legs are internally rotated with heels wide and the bottom between the heels

	Ability to assume and maintain
	Ask the caregiver/parent, whether he can leave the child in sitting when they leave the room; this is a good indication of the child's stability in sitting.
	Ability to weight shift (rotational or planer movements), reach to the side with trunk rotation or above the shoulder for a toy
	Ability to reach for and play with toys, switch objects from hand to hand, and bring hands or toys to midline

	Head righting, protective responses, and equilibrium reactions – elicited by tipping the child, a gentle to firm push, or reaching outside of the base of support, developed over first year of life
	  • Head righting – ability to maintain or return the head to upright when the trunk moves
	  • Protective responses – arm extension to stop a fall
	  • Equilibrium responses – trunk movement to avoid loss of balance

(Continued)

TABLE 10-9	Movement Observations by Position (*Continued*)
POSITION	**OBSERVATIONS/SKILL TESTING**
Quadruped	Weight-bearing is on the hands, knees, and occasionally feet (or foot). *The belly and chest are not on the ground, indicating antigravity movement of the trunk and abdominal control.* Movement in quadruped is observed by noting the coordination and pattern of the arms and legs, such as reciprocal movements, and measuring how far the child can move, if they can perform upper extremity object manipulation, and how they achieve functional play in this position. Weight shits might be cephalic or caudal resulting in rocking in this position, and lateral as infants reach for toys and move forward to creep
	Position of the pelvis (e.g., increased lumbar lordosis – indicates decreased abdominal control)
	Position of the hip relative to the knee and shoulder relative to the elbow
	Ability to maintain (how long)
	Ability to shift weight (laterally, cephalic–caudal), rock, reach for toys, functional play
	Ability to assume the position from prone and sitting and resume prone or sitting
	Movement – creeping • Reciprocal – alternating opposite arms and legs • Symmetrical (bunny hop) – moving both arms and then both legs
Standing	Weight-bearing position on the feet. (*In older children, a weight-bearing position on the toes can indicate some spasticity in the gastrocnemius, or dorsiflexion ROM deficits*)
	Independent or assisted: note how much weight (if any) is taken through the legs, and whether support is needed to assume/maintain (how much)
	Trunk control – upright or bending forward with UE support (elbows, hands) or resting chest against a support
	Alignment of the head, shoulders, and hips
	Ability to weight shift from one foot to the other, lift a foot off the ground
	Position of the arms, in independent standing: • High guard: hands above shoulders • Mid-guard: arms out to the side • Low guard: arms down by their sides
	Functional activities – maintain for play, reaching in all directions, including to the ground and returning to upright

Box 10-12	Targeting Quality and Maturity of Movement

During any assessment, the examiner should consider the quality of motor function and movement, including:
* Maturity of the movement
* Speed of the movement
* Influence of abnormal (primitive) reflexes on the movement
* Coupling and decoupling of the joints during a movement

Other questions to be answered during observation of movement in the child are:
* Can the child play or accomplish a task during a dynamic activity?
* Are there any missing or abnormal components of the movement?
* Is each joint moving through the available ROM needed for the activity?

Box 10-13	Pull to Sit

Observing the child's response to being pulled to a sitting position, with the examiner pulling at the hands, elbows, or shoulders, can tell the examiner many things about the child's strength and maturity at the neck, shoulders, and legs.

1. Head lag – head remains behind shoulders (ears posterior to shoulders) – normal in young children; abnormal after 4 to 6 months; persistence is often seen in children with cerebral palsy and other developmental disorders
2. Concentric neck flexion – initially keeps head in line with shoulders at approximately 4 months, but eventually the head will lead the shoulders, usually by 6 months
3. Arm pull and leg movement accompany the pull to sit by 6 months to assist in moving toward sitting
4. Lowering the child from sitting to supine, again by holding the hands, arms, or trunk, can give additional information about muscle activity and enable the therapist to determine at what point in the movement the child loses control for the child with hypotonia or immature head control

Primary form of mobility – There are several forms of independent mobility that allow infants and children to explore their environment. Rolling, belly/commando crawling, creeping in quadruped, bottom scooting, cruising on furniture, and walking are all meaningful ways of mobility and exploration. Assessment of these skills includes observation of the posture, weight-bearing positions of the limbs, movement pattern, symmetry of the movement, and ability to use the position for play. It is helpful to consider why the child is using a certain form of mobility as their primary form (e.g., scooting in sitting rather than creeping due to hemiparesis). When the child is moving, it is critical to observe whether the movements are performed selectively or as a mass movement (e.g., segmental versus log rolling). Is the child purposefully initiating movements, or are they not purposeful? The timing and sequencing of movements should also be considered. It is important to consider if the form of mobility can be used to maneuver around the child's environment, on uneven surfaces or hills, or contributes to functional play and development of new skills.

Walking (gait) is the motor milestone that defines the transition from infancy to toddlerhood; however, it is a skill that is achieved gradually. The average age for taking a few independent steps is 12 months. However, the infant achieves this early stepping ability after spending considerable time in standing. Initial movement in standing begins with bouncing and weight shift, first while supported (4-6 months) and then while holding onto a support (7-9 months); then, cruising around furniture is initiated with side-stepping (8-10 months), progressing to forward stepping with one hand on the support (9-12 months), and at the same time, the child is likely beginning to walk with first both hands held and then one hand (11-12 months). Finally, the first independent steps are achieved with hands in a high-guard position. Generally, if a child is 18 months or older without taking any steps, he/she is considered delayed in walking. The primary stepping patterns of alternating, step-to, and side-stepping can be observed in a variety of contexts. Young children take shorter steps, have a wide base of support, keep their arms in a high-guard position, and fall a lot. Over the second year of life, gait matures toward an adult-like pattern as different gait parameters, such as toe off, heal strike, and arm swing emerge and gait speed increases. Observation of weight acceptance can be helpful to assess the walking pattern, impairments, and identify asymmetries, as many children will fail to develop a heel strike and will initiate contact with their toes. Notably, children with more distal neurological impairment may use a hip strategy primarily for stepping, while those with less impairment may be able to use both a hip and ankle strategy. A complete gait assessment should evaluate heel strike, stance time, weight shifts, knee and hip positioning during swing, forefoot placement and position (pronation/supination), tibial torsions, genu varus/valgus, femoral anteversion/retroversion, pelvic tilt (anterior/posterior) or obliquities, scapular protraction/retraction, and positioning of arms. Further, gait observation should include assessment of postural control, balance, and the ability to use gait for play.

Advanced motor skills – An identical framework of weight-bearing position, antigravity movements, symmetry or asymmetry, and midline positions can be used for advanced motor skills. For some children with neurological impairments, like hemiplegic CP, advanced motors kills may be the only type of motor skills that are delayed or impaired. These tests of motor function should be adapted to the abilities of the child, but include play skills, such as throwing and kicking a ball, advanced mobility, such as running, hopping, and skipping, and playground skills, such as climbing a ladder. Common ages for the acquisition of some of these milestones are included in Chapter 8 (Table 8-5).

Fine motor skills – Toy manipulation with the hands should be examined in each position mentioned above; this observation should include unilateral and bilateral reaching in a variety of directions, bringing the hands to middle, crossing midline, and manipulating and transferring objects. Grasping skills using a raking, thumb-to-forefinger, and pincer grasp (thumb pad to index finger pad) can easily be evaluated using a small toy or piece of food and are typically evaluated in sitting (with or without support); fine motor skills for the first 24 months are listed in Table 8-4 in Chapter 8. It should be noted that hand preference typically isn't consistent until age 5, but most children begin to show some preference by age 3 or so. Fine motor assessment is typically done by an occupational therapist, but it is important for pediatric physical therapists to have some knowledge of fine motor skill development, for which most motor assessments include a fine motor or visuomotor assessment (e.g., the PDMS and Bayley). Examining fine motor skills for the older child with neurological disorders can follow the section in the adult examination (Box 10-5) for coordination. Self-care activities that involve arm and hand control like brushing teeth, eating, or object manipulation can be tested or mimed in the clinical assessment or addressed in the history.

Adaptive Equipment

Many children with developmental disorders will have been prescribed adaptive equipment. Any subsequent evaluation should include a check of this equipment, including mobility devices, orthoses, and protective devices, as growth can be a critical factor in their fit and usability. Thus, the fit of equipment and appropriateness (rationale for use, and age-appropriateness) should be assessed, including whether the equipment will grow with the child and is durable given the activity level of the child. Finally, the PT must determine the need for additional equipment. This will be discussed further in the chapters on neural tube disorders (Chapter 19), cerebral palsy (Chapter 20), and developmental disabilities (Chapter 21).

CASE B, PART VIII

Hayley was evaluated using the PDMS; her age at the time of testing was 2 years, 3 months (27 months). She received a score of "0" for walking (due to her wide base), walking up stairs, walking fast, and walking backward. She was able to throw a tennis ball with shoulder extension but not overhand or underhand; she was not able to kick or catch a ball. Her ceiling for her gross motor scale was 15 to 16 months. She was able to place two shapes in a shape board (not the triangle) and stack six cubes but couldn't remove the top from a bottle, make a vertical mark with a crayon, or snip with scissors, giving her a ceiling of 22 months on the fine motor scale. Thus, she's showing a moderate gross motor delay and a mild fine motor delay. She should be referred for a speech and occupational therapy evaluation, since she is presenting with global delays (see Chapter 21).

REFERENCES

1. Guccione AA, Mielenz TJ, DeVellis RF, et al. Development and testing of a self-report instrument to measure actions: outpatient physical therapy improvement in movement assessment log (OPTIMAL). *Phys Ther.* 2005;85(6):515-530.

2. Physical Self-Maintenance Scale (PSMS). Self-rated version. Incorporated in the Philadelphia Geriatric Center. Multilevel Assessment Instrument (MAI). *Psychopharmacol Bull.* 1988;24(4):795-797.

3. Yu J. Endocrine disorders and the neurologic manifestations. *Ann Pediatr Endocrinol Metab.* 2014;19(4):184-190.

4. Rodolico C, Bonanno C, Pugliese A, Nicocia G, Benvenga S, Toscano A. Endocrine myopathies: clinical and histopathological features of the major forms. *Acta Myol.* 2020;39(3):130-135.

5. Folstein MJ, Folstein SE, McHugh PR. Mini-mental state: a practical method for grading the cognitive state of patients for the clinician. *J Psychiatr Res.* 1975;12(3):189-198.

6. O'Caoimh RO, Gao Y, Gallagher PF, Eustace J, McGlade C, Molloy DW. Which part of the Quick mild cognitive impairment screen (QMCI) discriminates between normal cognition, mild cognitive impairment and dementia? *Age Ageing.* 2013;42:324-330.

7. Nasreddine ZS, Phillips NA, Bedirian V et al. The Montreal Cognitive Assessment, MoCA: a brief screening tool for mild cognitive impairment. *J Geriatr Soc.* 2005;53:695-699.

8. Pstras L, Thomaseth K, Waniewski J, Balzani I, Bellavere F. The Valsalva manoeuvre: physiology and clinical examples. *Acta Physiol (Oxf).* 2016; 217(2):103-119.

9. Weimer LH. Autonomic testing: common techniques and clinical applications. *Neurologist.* 2010;16(4):215-222.

10. Hislop H, Avers D, Brown M. Daniels and Worthingham's muscle *Testing.* 10th ed. Philadelphia: Elsevier/Saunders; 2019. ISBN: 9780323569149.

11. Pandyan AD1, Johnson GR, Price CI, Curless RH, Barnes MP, Rodgers H. A review of the properties and limitations of the Ashworth and modified Ashworth Scales as measures of spasticity. *Clin Rehabil.* 1999;13(5):373-383.

12. Fugl-Meyer AR, Jääskö L, Leyman I, Olsson S, Steglind S. The post-stroke hemiplegic patient: a method for evaluation of physical performance. *Scand J Rehabil Med.* 1975;7(1):13-31.

13. Boes CJ. The history of examination of reflexes. *J Neurol.* 2014;261:2264-2274.

14. Moya MJ, Menendez SM, Etessam JP, Vera JE, Fuertes MY. Cranial nerve disorders: clinical manifestations and topography. *Radiologia.* 2019;61(2):99-123.

15. Hillier S, Immink M, Thewlis D. Assessing proprioception: a systematic review of possibilities. *Neurorehabil Neural Repair.* 2015;29(10):933-949.

16. Dunn W, Griffith J, Morrison MT, et al. Somatosensation assessment using the NIH Toolbox. *Neurology.* 2013;80(11 suppl 3):S41-S44.

17. Lai S, Ahmed U, bollineni A, Lewis R, Ramchandren S. Diagnostic accuracy of qualitative vs quantitative tuning fork: outcome measure for neuropathy. *J Clin Neuromuscul Dis.* 2014;15(3):96-101.

18. Borstad AL, Nichols-Larsen DS. Assessing and treating higher level somatosensory impairments post stroke. *Top Stroke Rehabil.* 2014;21(4):290-295.

19. Bodranghien F, Bastian A, Casali C, et al. Consensus paper: revisiting the symptoms and signs of cerebellar syndrome. *Cerebellum.* 2016; 15(3):369-391.

20. Berg K, Wood-Dauphinee S, Williams JI. The balance scale: reliability assessment with elderly residents and patients with an acute stroke. *Scand J Rehabil Med.* 1995;27(1):27-36.

21. Cohen H, Blatchly CA, Gombash LL. A study of the clinical test of sensory interaction and balance. *Phys Ther.* 1993;73(6):346-351; discussion 351–344.

22. Duncan PW, Weiner DK, Chandler J, Studenski S. Functional reach: a new clinical measure of balance. *J Gerontol.* 1990;45(6): M192-M197.

23. Black FO, Wall CIII, Rockette HE Jr., Kitch R. Normal subject postural sway during the Romberg test. *Am J Otolaryngol.* 1982;3(5):309-318.

24. Langley FA, Mackintosh SF. Timed Up and Go test (TUG), the Tinetti Mobility Test (TMT), the Dynamic Gait Index (DGI) and the BEST test or mini-BEST test. *J Allied Health Sci Pract.* 2007;5(4):1-11.

25. Moore JL, Potter K, Blankshain K, Kaplan SL, O'Dwyer LC, Sullivan JE. A core set of outcome measures for adults with neurologic conditions undergoing rehabilitation. *J Neurol Phys Ther.* 2018;42:174-220.

26. Sahrmann SA. The human movement system: our professional identity. *Phys Ther.* 2014;94(7):1034-1042.

27. Hedman LD, Quinn L, Gill-Body K, et al. White paper: movement system diagnoses in neurologic physical therapy. *J Neurol Phys Ther.* 2018;42(2):110-117.

28. Quinn L, Riley N, Tyrell CM, et al. A framework for movement analysis of tasks: recommendations from the Academy of Neurologic Physical Therapy's Movement System Task Force. *Phys Ther.* 2021;101(9):1-8.

29. Hedman LD, Rogers MW, Hanke TA. Neurologic professional education: linking the foundation science of motor control with physical therapy interventions for movement dysfunction. *J Neurol Phys Ther.* 1996;20:9-13.

30. Dodds TA, Martin DP, Stolov WC, Deyo RA. A validation of the functional independence measurement and its performance among rehabilitation inpatients. *Arch Phys Med Rehabil.* 1993;74(5):531-536.

31. CMS Coding Section GG Self-Care and Mobility activities included on the post-acute care items sets. Available at: https://www.cms.gov/Medicare/Quality-Initiatives-Patient-Assessment-Instruments/HomeHealthQualityInits/Downloads/GG-Self-Care-and-Mobility-Activities-Decision-Tree.pdf. Accessed on 9/14/2022.

32. Fritz S1, Lusardi M. White paper: "walking speed: the sixth vital sign". *J Geriatr Phys Ther.* 2009;32(2):46-49.

33. Collen FM, Wade DT, Robb GF, Bradshaw CM. The Rivermead Mobility Index: a further development of the Rivermead Motor Assessment. *Int Disabil Stud.* 1991;13(2):50-54.

34. Kloos AD, Kegelmeyer DA, Ambrogi K, et al. The step test evaluation of performance on stairs (STEPS): validation and reliability in a neurological disorder. *PLoS One.* 2019;14(3):e0213698.

35. International Classification for Disease 10 Code (ICD 10). Available at: https://www.cdc.gov/nchs/icd/icd10cm.htm. Accessed on 7/21/21

36. Haley, SM, Coster WJ, Ludlow LH, et al. Pediatric Evaluation of Disability Inventory: Development. *Standardization and Administration Manual.* Pearson; available at https://www.pearsonassessments.com/store/usassessments/en/Store/Professional-Assessments/Developmental-Early-Childhood/Pediatric-Evaluation-of-Disability-Inventory/p/100000505.html.

37. Haley SM, Coster WJ, Dumas HM, Fragala-Pinkham MA, Moed R. PEDI-CAT: development. *Standardization and Administration Manual*. Available at: https://www.pearsonassessments.com/store/usassessments/en/Store/Professional-Assessments/Behavior/Pediatric-Evaluation-of-Disability-Inventory-Computer-Adaptive-Test/p/100002037.html.

38. Klingels K, DeCock P, Molenaers G, et al. Upper limb motor and sensory impairments in children with hemiplegic cerebral palsy: can they be measured reliably? *Disabil Rehabil*. 2010;32(5):409-416.

39. Zafeiriou DI. Primitive reflexes and postural reactions in the neurodevelopmental examination. *Pediatr Neurol*. 2004;31:1-8.

40. Bayley N. Bayley Scales of Infant and Toddler *Development*. 3rd ed. San Antonio, TX: Pearson; 2005.

41. Folio MR, Fewell RR. *Peabody Developmental Motor Scales: Examiner's Manual*. Austin, TX: Pro-Ed; 2000.

42. Piper MC, Pinnell LE, Darrah J, et al. Construction and validation of the Alberta Infant Motor Scale. *Can J Public Health*. 1992;83:S46-S50.

43. Mendonca B, Sargent B, Fetters L. Cross-cultural validity of standardized motor development screening and assessment tools: a systematic review. *Dev Med Child Neurol*. 2016;58:1213-1222.

44. Russell DJ, Rosenbaum PL, Avery LM, Hamilton ML Can Child Centre of Childhood Disability Research. *Gross Motor Function Measures (GMFM-66 and GMFM-88) User's Manual*. Hamilton, Ontario: Mac Keith Press; 2002.

Review Questions

1. **A trial of intervention is a part of the adult neurologic evaluation process (True or False).**
   A. True
   B. False

2. **If the client is not able to identify which activities they are having trouble with the therapist can facilitate the process by:**
   A. Determining best activities to focus on from their examination
   B. Utilizing an assessment tool to assist the client in identifying activities of interest
   C. Focusing on activities of daily living basic to all clients such as sit to stand from a couch
   D. Focusing on impairments that have been identified in the examination

3. **Which of the following would be included in a review of systems?**
   A. Detailed examination of range of motion
   B. Mental status assessment such as the mini-mental status exam
   C. Reflex testing for UMN lesion including the Babinski and the Hoffman
   D. Assess blood pressure during position changes from supine to sit to stand

4. **Which of the following is a method for examining remote memory?**
   A. Name three objects and have the client repeat them back to you
   B. Name three objects and ask the client to repeat them back to you 5 minutes later
   C. Ask the client to recall common historical events
   D. Ask for a chronological recall of the client's current illness

5. **Mrs. Smith is 4 weeks s/p CVA. On initial examination 1 week prior, her Ashworth scores in her right arm** were 2 throughout. On this day Mrs. Smith is tired and Ashworth scores in the right arm are 3–4. One possible cause of this increase in tone would be:
   A. Response to resistance exercise you performed the day before
   B. She has a urinary tract infection
   C. She has contractures in her arm
   D. Tone is increased when someone is sleeping or tired

6. **You are performing reflex testing and when testing the quadriceps with a reflex hammer the muscle exhibits a visible muscle contraction and the leg extends to 120 degrees then drops back down. The appropriate reflex grade to record would be:**
   A. 1+
   B. 2+
   C. 3+
   D. 4+

7. **Your client exhibits upward rotation of the eye and is complaining of double vision. Which cranial nerve is implicated?**
   A. CN III: Oculomotor
   B. CN IV: Trochlear
   C. CN V: Trigeminal
   D. CN VI: Abducens

8. **The most reliable way to evaluate position sense and kinesthesia is to:**
   A. Use a 250 mHz tuning fork on the bony prominence
   B. Have the client perform finger-to-nose testing
   C. Have the client perform alternating supination and pronation
   D. Move the limb up or down and ask the client what direction it moved

9. **You are working with a patient and note that this individual has difficulty recognizing objects simply by handling them. This indicates they may have which of the following impairments?**

A. Allodynia

B. Astereognosis

C. Dysethesia

D. Hyperesthesia

10. When performing finger to examiner's finger testing, your client exhibits jerky movements and his finger goes past the examiner's finger and sometimes stops short of the examiner's finger. This type of movement would be called:

A. Dysdiadochokinesia

B. Dysmetria

C. Tremor

D. Asthenia

11. I am evaluating a patient s/p stroke and ask them to reach for an object first at normal speed then more slowly and then moving as fast as they can. What domain am I testing?

A. Balance

B. Equilibrium

C. Nonequilibrium coordination

D. Sensation

12. To test balance in a new patient who has a diagnosis of vestibular hypofunction. Of the following which should be done first?

A. stand with one foot in front of the other

B. stand on one foot

C. Standing, perturb their balance

D. Standing, bend trunk to the side

13. Which of the following is a balance test that incorporates walking?

A. Romberg test

B. Mini-BESTest

C. Sensory organization test

D. Functional reach test

14. Which of the following measures is considered a core measure that should be done on every neurologic patient?

A. Dynamic Gait Index

B. Mini BESTest

C. Activities-Specific Balance Confidence Scale

D. Tinetti Mobility Test

15. Which of the following is one of the tasks that should be examined when performing a movement system evaluation?

A. Stand to sit transfer

B. Sit on a stable surface

C. Climb four steps

D. Roll supine to side

16. Mrs. Smith is unable to advance her right leg without some assistance to clear her foot. The therapist provides physical assistance for mid-swing to terminal swing to help the foot clear the floor. Mrs. Smith is able to balance herself, manage stance and her quad cane without assistance. Her assistance level should be documented as:

A. Modified independence

B. Contact guard assist

C. Minimal assistance

D. Moderate assistance

17. Other than level of assistance, what else should be included in the evaluation of movement?

A. presence of abnormal reflexes

B. tone

C. strength

D. quality of movement

18. The sixth vital sign is:

A. Temperature

B. Level of assistance

C. Gait speed

D. Capillary refill time

19. In examining an infant, how would you test for a Moro reflex

A. Stroke the bottom of the foot and watch for toe movement

B. With the infant in a sitting position, let them fall backward a short distance before catching them; watch for arm abduction, followed by adduction

C. Turn the infant's head to the side and watch for flexion of the skull side extremities and extension of the face side extremities

D. Stroke along the spine and watch for trunk incurvation

20. The most appropriate assessment to evaluate motor function for a 5-year-old child would be the?

A. AIMS

B. Bayley

C. PDMS

D. PEDI

21. The average age of independent walking (three steps) in typically developing children is

A. 6 months

B. 12 months

C. 18 months

D. 24 months

22. For most children, the first form of independent mobility is?

A. Belly crawling

B. Rolling

C. Scooting

D. Walking

23. **Which of the following are common concerns when completing an integumentary systems review in pediatrics:**

A. Abrasians from excessive limb movements

B. Integumentary checks are not performed in infants

C. Points of pressure (clothing, braces)

D. Tissue damage related to falling in young walkers

24. **In typical development, the transition of infant to toddler is around what milestone?**

A. Crawling

B. Creeping

C. Skipping

D. Walking

25. **The systems review in children includes which of the following?**

A. Determination of motor milestones

B. Completion of a developmental assessment

C. Screening of cardio/pulmonary function and special senses

D. Completing a thorough history from the parent

26. **How is strength measured in a toddler?**

A. Manual muscle testing

B. Biodex

C. Passive movement to feel for resistance

D. Observations of movement against gravity

27. **What is head lag?**

A. The head remains behind the shoulders in a pull to sit task

B. The inability to maintain the head in midline in supine lying

C. A roll that is initiated by the arm and not the head

D. Optical righting without labyrinthine righting

28. **A child was born at 28 weeks gestation; when performing a motor assessment at 4 years of age, it will be important to correct for prematurity**

A. True

B. False

29. **In your evaluation of a 7-month-old, you see evidence of a Babinski, the ATNR, and a palmar grasp. Which of the following would be consistent with the presence of these reflexes?**

A. The baby is exhibiting appropriate reflexes for age;

B. The baby is exhibiting reflexes beyond the time of their normal expression;

C. The baby is exhibiting reflexes in advance of their age.

30. **By 12 months of age, which equilibrium responses would you expect to be present?**

A. Prone but not supine

B. Quadruped in all directions

C. Sitting forward and lateral but not backward

D. Standing in all directions

31. **To examine proprioception in a very young infant, the easiest thing to do is:**

A. Move a limb and watch to see if the infant moves the other limb

B. Tickle the child and watch for withdrawal

C. Place a limb in an awkward position and watch to see if the infant moves it

D. Use the Bayley

Answers

1. A	2. B	3. C	4. D	5. B
6. C	7. B	8. A	9. B	10. B
11. C	12. A	13. B	14. C	15. B
16. C	17. D	18. C	19. B	20. C
21. B	22. B	23. C	24. D	25. C
26. D	27. A	28. B	29. B	30. B
31. C				

GLOSSARY

5 Times Sit to Stand (5TSTS). Core measure that assesses ability and time to sit and return to standing five times.

6 Minute Walk Test (6MWT). Core measure that assesses distance walked in 6 minutes.

10 Meter Walk Test (10MWT). Core measure of time to walk 10 meters.

Activities-Specific Balance Confidence Scale (ABC). Self-report core measure of perceived ability in performing various balance activities without loss of balance or unsteadiness.

Alberta Infant Motor Scales (AIMS). An observational assessment that examines posture and movement in prone, supine, sitting, and standing.

Anthropometrics. Measure of body weight, length/height, and head circumference in children.

Babinski (plantar reflex). Upper motor neuron screening reflex elicited by stroking bottom of foot; after 6 months of age, a negative response of hallux and toe flexion should occur; a positive response (before 6 months of age or with UMN damage) is hallux and toe extension.

Bayley Scales of Infant and Toddler Development. a Norm-referenced developmental assessment of cognitive, language and motor ability for infants birth to 3 years of age to identify developmental delay; also includes a caregiver report of social-emotional and adaptive behavior.

Berg Balance Scale (BBS). Core measure of static and dynamic balance.

Dynamic Gait Index (DGI). Assessment of fall risk in standing and walking with a variety of external demands (e.g., change in speed, step over and around obstacles).

Functional Gait Assessment. Core measure of gait performance; examines gait ability while performing a variety of activities (e.g., head turns, stepping over obstacles).

Functional muscle testing. Evaluating muscle strength by observing the client's activities and postures.

Gross Motor Function Measure (GMFM). Instrument to measure gross motor function in children with cerebral palsy.

Hoffman reflex. Flicking of the middle finger fingernail induces flexion of thumb and index finger in those with neurologic damage (positive Hoffman).

Hyperreflexia. Exaggerated deep tendon (monosynaptic) reflexes.

Hypertonicity. Increased resistance to passive movement; either spasticity and rigidity.

Hypotonia. Decreased muscle tone.

International Classification for Disease 10 Code (ICD 10). A standard diagnostic code used to track healthcare statistics.

Modified Ashworth Scale. Method of measuring spasticity.

Monofilament testing. A method to evaluate somatosensory function.

Orientation. Awareness of time, place, person, and situation.

Outcome measure. A measure that can be used to evaluate change over time.

Peabody Developmental Motor Scales (PDMS). A developmental assessment of fine and gross motor ability for children birth to 6 years of age.

Pediatric Evaluation of Disability Index (PEDI). A paper and pencil survey, completed by caregivers, to assess functional movement ability, independence in activities of daily living, and social skills, including levels of assistance or modifications needed, for children 6 months to 7.5 years.

PEDI. Computer Adaptive Test (PEDI-CAT) – a computer-based caregiver assessment of the PEDI, examining mobility, activities of daily living, social skills, and levels of assistance or modification.

Rigidity. Hypertonia that occurs throughout the range of motion and is independent of the velocity of the movement; not associated with hyperreflexia.

Rivermead Mobility Index. A self-report scale that evaluates bed mobility, sitting, standing, transfers, and walking/running.

Romberg test. Client stands with eyes open and then closed and feet together; test is positive if the client falls.

Sharpened Romberg. Tested with feet in tandem and eyes opened and then closed; positive if client falls.

Spasticity. A velocity-dependent increase in muscle tone associated with hyperreflexia.

Step Test Evaluation of Performance on Stairs (STEPS). A means of rating stair ascent and descent.

Synergistic movement. Multi-joint movements that occur in synchrony when trying to move a single joint (e.g., shoulder, elbow, wrist, and finger flexion).

Tinetti Mobility Test (TMT). A test that examines balance in sitting, standing, and walking ability.

Transfers. Position changes (e.g., sit to stand).

Vibration testing. Using a tuning fork to evaluate dorsal column medial lemniscal pathway integrity.

ABBREVIATIONS

5TSTS	5 Times Sit to Stand
6MWT	6 Minute Walk Test
10MWT	10 Meter Walk Test
ABC	Activities-Specific Balance Confidence Scale
AIMS	Alberta Infant Motor Scale
BBS	Berg Balance Scale
BSIDT	Bayley Scales of Infant and Toddler Development Test
CN	cranial nerve
DGI	Dynamic Gait Index
DTR	deep tendon reflex
FGA	Functional Gait Assessment
GMFM	Gross Motor Function Measure

ICD 10	International Classification of Disease
MoCA	Montreal Cognitive Assessment
Qmci	Quick Mild Cognitive Impairment Screen
PDMS	Peabody Developmental Motor Scales
PEDI	Pediatric Evaluation of Disability
PEDI-CAT	Computer Adapted PEDI
SOT	Sensory Organization Test
STEPS	Step Test Evaluation of Performance on Stairs
TMT	Tinetti Mobility Test (TMT)
TUG	Timed Up and Go Test

Stroke

11

Deborah S. Nichols-Larsen
and Deborah A. Kegelmeyer

CASE A, PART I

Richard Brown (ht. 6'1", wt. 245 lbs.) is a 62-year-old African American, former college football linebacker, who experienced a left ischemic cerebrovascular accident (CVA, or stroke) yesterday. He arrived in the emergency room per ambulance and was given TPA within 4 hours of symptom onset. He has a history of hypertension and was diagnosed as prediabetic 6 months ago. He takes atenolol for his hypertension, and a diet of lowered carbohydrates and fats has been recommended but inconsistently followed. He presents with moderate hemiparesis of the right arm and leg and non-fluent (expressive) aphasia. Comprehension of verbal and written language appears intact, and he is oriented to time, place, and person. Right hemianopia is present. He is married with two grown children, who live in town; he and his wife, Sheryl, live in a two-story house, where they raised their children. She is a teacher. He has also been a history teacher and football coach for the city schools for 30 years.

OBJECTIVES

1) Understand the pathophysiology of stroke

2) Relate the common risk factors for stroke to the cardiovascular changes created

3) Identify the typical symptoms of common stroke syndromes and the associated areas of brain damage

4) Identify assessment tools for use in individuals post-stroke across all settings

5) Identify and choose optimal treatment interventions for individuals post-stroke

● PATHOPHYSIOLOGY

What Is a Stroke?

Stroke, or cerebrovascular accident, is the leading cause of adult disability with an estimated 15 million people around the world experiencing a stroke each year. In the United States, nearly 800,000 people experience a stroke each year; of these, approximately ¼ are recurrent strokes, meaning the individual has had one or more prior strokes. It is estimated that more than 7 million people are living with disability post-stroke. A stroke occurs when there is interruption of blood flow within brain blood vessels; this can result from either blockage of the vessel (ischemia) or rupture of the vessel (hemorrhage). Ischemic strokes are about seven times more common than hemorrhagic strokes, accounting for 87% of strokes; conversely, hemorrhagic strokes typically produce much greater impairment than ischemic strokes and are more likely to result in death.[1] Notably, the incidence of stroke and death from stroke have decreased over the last several decades due to improved management of risk factors and improved emergency care. However, since the risk of stroke increases with age and we have an aging population, stroke incidence is expected to increase over the next decade.[1]

Ischemia can result from either an **embolism**, which is a clot that forms elsewhere, often in the heart, and then travels to the brain and lodges in one of the cerebral vessels, or a **thrombus**, which is a blockage of an artery that develops from a buildup of plaques, typically made up of fatty cells and cholesterol, within the wall of the vessel, which eventually slows blood flow substantially or blocks it all together (Figure 11-1A). Embolisms are most common in association with cardiovascular disorders such as arrhythmias, myocardial infraction, or valve disorders.[2] Ischemic stroke in a large blood vessel of the brain is referred to as a **thrombotic stroke** with neural consequences that relate to the vessel injured and the duration and extent (partial, complete) of the ischemia. Ischemic stroke in small vessels, referred to as **lacunar stroke**, may go undiagnosed until many such strokes have occurred and larger areas of brain damage, from these multiple strokes, have developed.[1] **Transient ischemic attacks** (TIAs) are the result of brief blockages with associated stroke symptoms that resolve quickly (typically <24 hours) and are not associated with an infarct (neuronal death) on imaging. However, TIAs are a sign of circulation disruption and the potential for subsequent stroke.[2]

Hemorrhagic strokes occur in cases of poorly controlled and typically long-term hypertension, resulting in leakage, or bursting of a small- or medium-sized vessel. Alternatively, they are the result of a weakening in the vascular wall, associated with an aneurysm or other vascular anomaly. Hemorrhage within the cerebral vessels is referred to as an **intracerebral hemorrhage**; if it occurs in a surface vessel within the pial lining of the brain, it is called a **subarachnoid hemorrhage** because the blood flows into the subarachnoid space (Figure 11-2). About 10% of stroke are intracerebral hemorrhages (ICH) and 3 to 5% are subarachnoid hemorrhages (SAH).[1,2]

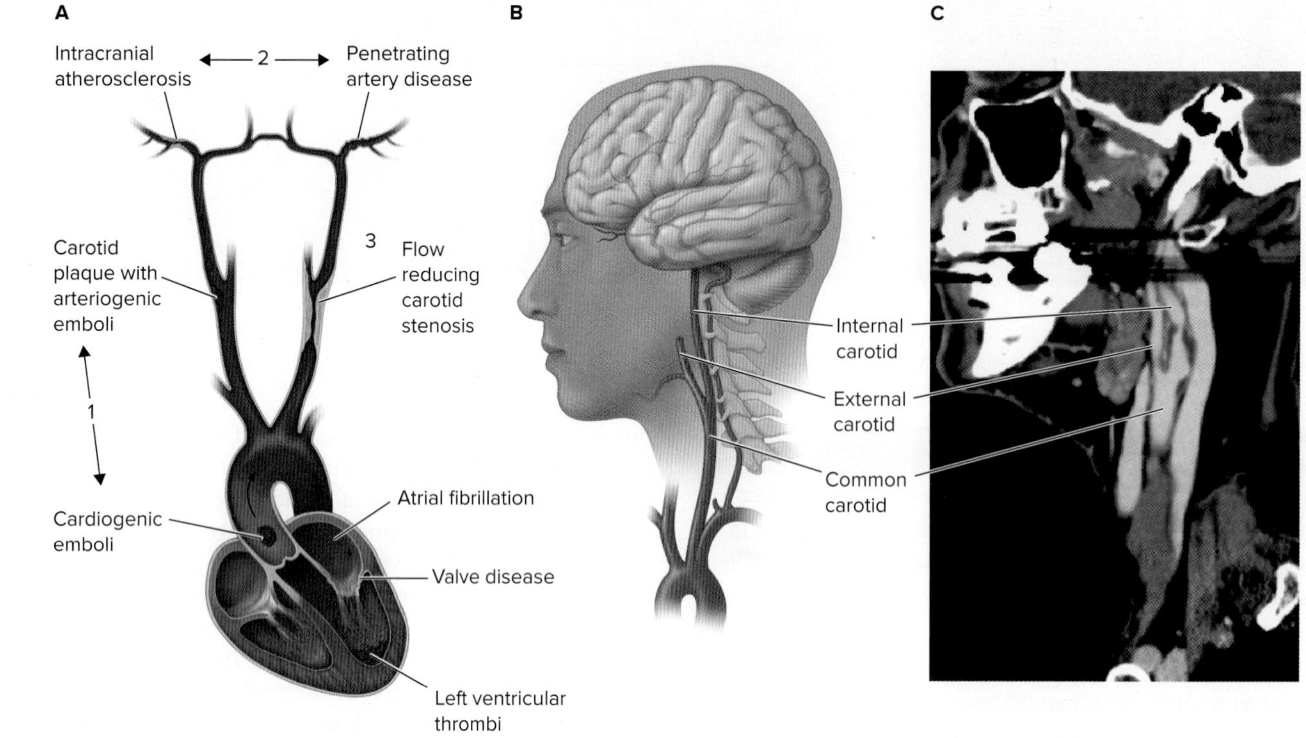

A   **B**   **C**

FIGURE 11-1 Ischemic stroke pathology. A. Right – Schematic of embolus from heart that enters cerebral circulation and is caught in the atherosclerotic cerebral artery. Left – Stenosis of the carotid artery can result in diminished cerebral blood flow and ischemia within the penetrating arteries of the cerebral hemispheres. **B.** Illustrates the division of the common carotid into the internal and external carotids. **C.** A CT image of the carotid arteries as they enter the cranium. (Reproduced with permission from Hauser SL (ED) *Harrison's Neurology in Clinical Medicine.* 3rd Ed. New York, NY: McGraw-Hill; 2013.)

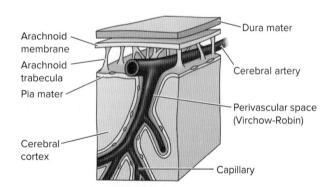

FIGURE 11-2 Illustration of cerebral artery within subarachnoid space. As illustrated, cerebral arteries lie within the subarachnoid space; thus, hemorrhage of one of the major vessels will result in bleeding into the space, referred to as a subarachnoid hemorrhage. (Reproduced with permission from with permission from Parent A. *Carpenter's Human Neuroanatomy,* 9th ed. Williams & Wilkins; 1996.)

● RISK FACTORS

Why Do Strokes Occur?

Risk factors for stroke include obesity, high cholesterol, heart disease (hypertension, atrial fibrillation, and congenital heart anomalies), atherosclerosis, diabetes, and substance abuse (smoking, alcohol, drugs – especially cocaine). Many of these risk factors are also associated with a sedentary lifestyle and are considered controllable, either by lifestyle change, medication, or both. Additionally, stroke is greater with advancing age, in certain racial/ethnic groups, and in people with a family history of cardiovascular disease or stroke.[3-5] See Table 11-1 for a discussion of risk factors and their relationship with stroke. However, it should be noted that strokes can occur in those without known risk factors and are referred to as idiopathic (without known cause).

● CEREBRAL CIRCULATION

Why Are the Symptoms and Outcomes of Strokes So Variable?

The brain is perfused by a complex system of arteries and their tributaries, originating from two ascending systems. The first is the **carotid artery system**, originating from the common carotid bilaterally, which bifurcates into the internal and external carotid arteries on each side (Figures 11-1B and C). The smaller external carotids are responsible for perfusion of the muscles and other tissues of the face. However, the **large internal carotid arteries** enter the cranium through the carotid canal bilaterally and then split on each side into a larger middle cerebral artery, the smaller anterior cerebral artery, and the even smaller posterior communicating artery. The **anterior cerebral arteries** supply the medial surfaces of the cerebral hemispheres, including the anterior portion of the corpus callosum, and the superior aspect of the lateral surface of the frontal and parietal lobes. The **middle cerebral arteries** supply most of the lateral surface of the frontal, parietal, and temporal

TABLE 11-1	Stroke Risk Factors and Their Cardiovascular Consequences
RISK FACTOR	**EXPLANATION OF RELATIONSHIP WITH STROKE[4,6–9]**
Age	With increasing age, the frequency and severity of many other risk factors increase, and multiple comorbidities are common, thus increasing the risk for stroke.
Gender	Men are more likely to have strokes at younger ages, but more women than men have strokes annually (NSA), likely due to more women living longer.
Race	Stroke is more common in African, Asian, and Hispanic Americans than in Caucasians. This partially reflects disparities in health care and the delay in diagnosis and treatment of risk factors in these racial groups. It may also relate to differences in diet or access to health literature.
Hypertension	Uncontrolled hypertension stresses blood vessels, decreasing their pliability and causing thickening of the arterial walls, which in turn, makes them susceptible to clot formation and hemorrhage. While the most common of the risk factors, hypertension can be treated with behavioral change (diet and exercise) and/or medication.
Hyperlipidemia	Cholesterol is an essential lipid for cell maintenance; cholesterol, specifically low-density lipoproteins (LDL), contributes to plaque formation in vessel walls. Manageable with behavioral change (diet and exercises) and/or medication (Statins).
Obesity	Stresses the cardiovascular system and is often associated with other risk factors.
Metabolic Syndrome	Characterized by at least three of the following: (1) hyperlipidemia; (2) elevated glucose (prediabetic or diabetic); (3) obesity; (4) hypertension; (5) elevated triglycerides. Since each is a risk factor for stroke, metabolic syndrome increases the overall risk. Behavioral change and/or medications to treat each symptom are used to manage this risk.
Atrial fibrillation	AF is associated with a high incidence of embolism formation and subsequent embolic stroke.
Congenital heart anomaly	A high incidence of stroke has been associated with a patent foramen ovale (PFO), which is the persistence of the fetal connection between the right and left atria that typically closes at birth. PFO is associated with embolitic stroke.
Atherosclerosis	Plaque buildup in blood vessels (atherosclerosis) throughout the body is associated with both embolitic and thrombotic stroke.
Diabetes	Vascular changes are common in type 2 diabetes, increasing the stiffness of the vascular wall and resulting in decreased capacity for vasodilation. Behavioral change is the initial treatment (diet, exercise, weight loss); medication may be required.
Alcohol abuse	Excessive alcohol consumption is associated with increased clotting and thereby stroke.
Smoking	Smoking increases the likelihood of blood clots and contributes to the development of atherosclerosis. Risk returns to normal after 10 years of abstinence.
Drug abuse	Many drugs (cocaine, LSD, amphetamines, heroin, opiates, Ecstasy, PCP) are associated with risk of stroke, often associated with induced hypertension, vasospasm with/without tachycardia. Heroin/opiates/LSD are more likely to induce stroke by cardioembolism.

lobes, including penetrating lenticulostriatal branches to the basal ganglia, internal capsule, and insular cortex. The **anterior communicating artery** connects the two anterior cerebral arteries and forms the anterior portion of the **Circle of Willis**. The **posterior communicating arteries** project back to the posterior cerebral arteries, completing the Circle of Willis (Figure 11-3).[2,10]

The second ascending arterial system is the vertebral artery system. The **vertebral arteries** are bilateral branches of the subclavian arteries and enter the skull via the foramen magnum. As they enter the skull, they each give rise to a small branch that merges to form the anterior spinal artery, which primarily supplies the spinal cord but also a small part of the distal brainstem. At the level of the medulla, the two arteries merge to form the large basilar artery. The **basilar artery** supplies most of the medulla and then gives rise to two cerebellar arteries (**anterior inferior cerebellar** and **superior cerebellar**) that supply the cerebellum and components of the brainstem, a series of **pontine arteries** to perfuse the posterior pons and midbrain, the **superior cerebellar artery**, and finally terminates as the **posterior cerebral artery** (Figure 11-3B).[11]

The **posterior cerebral artery** provides the blood supply for the occipital lobe and the inferior and partial medial surface of the temporal lobe, including part of the insular cortex and hippocampus; it also supplies the thalamus and ventral surface of the midbrain, including the cerebral peduncles. The **anterior inferior cerebellar artery** (AICA), as the name implies, provides circulation to the anterior and inferior cerebellum as well as the flocculus; it also gives off a branch that supplies the internal ear (**labyrinthine artery**). Other branches supply the inferolateral pons and middle cerebellar peduncle. It anastomoses with the posterior inferior cerebellar

A

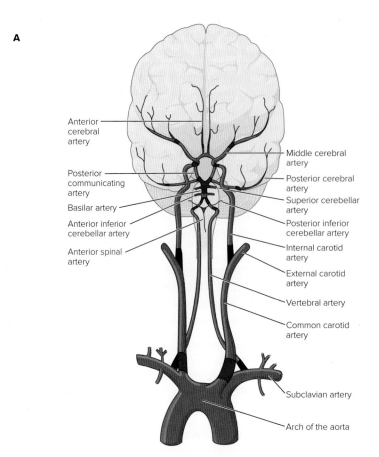

B

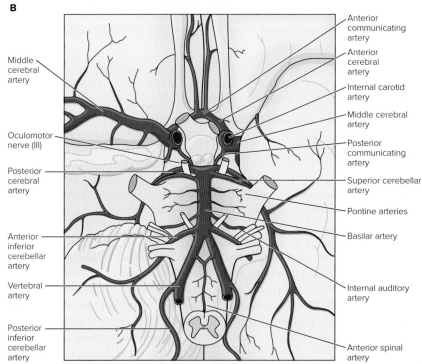

FIGURE 11-3 Schematic of the major blood vessels of the brain and the Circle of Willis. A. The brain is supplied by two networks, arising from the aorta: the internal carotid network, branching into the anterior and middle cerebral arteries that supply the anterior 2/3 of the cerebral hemispheres, and the vertebral artery system that supplies the posterior 1/3 and the brainstem and cerebellum. **B.** The Circle of Willis comprises the anterior cerebral arteries, the anterior communicating arteries, and the internal carotid arteries (components of the carotid artery system), as well as the posterior communicating arteries and the posterior cerebral arteries (components of the vertebral artery system). The vertebral artery distribution, illustrated on the dorsal surface of the brainstem, supplies the brainstem and cerebellum as well as the posterior cerebrum. (Reproduced with permission from Kandel ER, Schwartz JH, Jessell TM, Siegelbaum SA, Hudspeth AJ. *Principles of Neural Science.* 5th ed. New York, NY: McGraw Hill; 2013.)

artery such that the actual area supplied by these two arteries is highly variable between individuals. However, the **posterior inferior cerebellar artery** (PICA) typically supplies the posteroinferior cerebellum, including the vermis, and the inferior portion of the medulla. Strokes affecting the AICA or PICA are less common, in part, because of their anastomoses and, thereby, overlapping circulation. Finally, the **superior cerebellar artery** supplies the upper (superior) half of the cerebellum and components of the midbrain. It also anastomoses with the AICA and PICA, and strokes are also rare within this artery. Symptoms can be either cerebellar only or combined with midbrain dysfunction, depending on whether the terminal portion of the artery or its brainstem projections near its origin are the site of infarction.[11]

Multiple small arteries supply the thalamus and emanate from the posterior circulation; while the areas supplied by these arteries vary by individuals, the most common areas supplied are described here. The **tuberothalamic arteries** arise from the posterior communicating artery and supply the anterior, reticular, and intralaminar nuclei along with mamillothalamic and ventral amygdalofugal projections to the limbic system. Infarcts result in significant neuropsychological deficits, including personality changes, apathy, memory disturbances, and impaired learning. Right-sided lesions involve visual memory deficits while left-sided lesions commonly disrupt both verbal and visual memory. Left lesions can also result in anomia and impaired verbal comprehension. The **paramedian arteries** arise from the posterior cerebral arteries and supply the dorsomedial nucleus, some intralaminar nuclei, and the internal medullary lamina; infarcts of the paramedian distribution result in fluctuating consciousness, speech and language impairment (hypophonia, dysprosody, decreased fluency), as well as agitation, confusion, and other neuropsychiatric symptoms. The multiple **inferolateral arteries** also arise from the posterior cerebral artery and supply the geniculate bodies, lateral medullary lamina, and the ventroposterolateral (VPL) and ventroposteromedial (VPM) nuclei; the latter two nuclei are the primary somatosensory projection nuclei, so the primary consequence of infarcts in this area is loss of sensation (pain, temperature, vibration, proprioception, and touch) to varying degrees, depending on the magnitude of the infarct, referred to as pure sensory stroke, since motor function is maintained. When proprioception is disrupted, ataxia is present. For some, damage on the right results in what is called the thalamic pain syndrome. Lastly, the **posterior choroidal arteries** also arise from the posterior cerebral artery and supply components of the midbrain the subthalamic nuclei, part of the medial geniculate, and the pulvinar and posterior intralaminar nuclei. The most commonly reported symptom of infarct here is homonymous quadrantanopsia (defined later in the chapter) but cases of hemisensory loss, aphasia, and memory deficits have also been reported.[12]

Although rare (<1% of strokes), thrombotic stroke can also occur with occlusion of the venous system, often resulting in serious disability or death. The venous system includes the cerebral veins and dural sinuses. Cerebral veins differ from veins throughout the body as they don't have muscle within the vascular wall, making them thinner and allowing bidirectional flow.[13] In addition, small venous vessels and capillaries form a network of anastomosed collaterals, which compensate for focal disruption. However, when the collateral system is incapable of sufficient compensation for thrombus within the network, ischemia,

increased intracranial pressure, edema, and/or hemorrhage can result. Venous thrombosis is more common in younger adults (20-50) and women. Risk factors include oral contraceptive use and pregnancy, accounting for the increased occurrence in women, as well as cancer, inflammatory disorders, arteriovenous malformations, head trauma, and genetic thrombophilia.[14]

Stroke Consequences: How Do the Symptoms of Stroke Relate to Circulation Compromise?

Stroke, within a given artery, presents with symptoms indicative of the brain regions supplied by that artery and their respective functions (Figure 11-4). Variability in symptomology relates to the site of artery occlusion or hemorrhage – the main artery or its branches – and the relative length of time of the occlusion or severity of the hemorrhage along with individual differences in neuroanatomy. Common sites for large vessel thrombus are (1) bifurcation of the common carotid artery into the internal and external carotids; (2) origin of the middle cerebral artery; (3) the point of convergence of the vertebral arteries into the basilar artery; and (4) the point where the basilar artery forms the posterior portion of the Circle of Willis. Small vessels are often the earliest sites for arteriosclerosis, leading to vessel collapse and ultimately lacunar strokes; they can also be affected by vasculitis (inflammation of the vessel), associated with different types of infections.[2]

Hemorrhagic strokes are most common in small blood vessels due to the impact of long-standing hypertension, putting unrelenting pressure on the arterial wall and resulting in pathologic weakening of the endothelium. This, in combination with

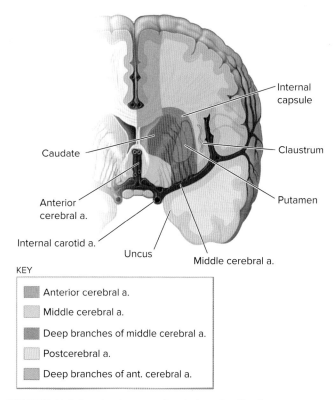

FIGURE 11-4 Cerebral artery circulation distribution. (Reproduced with permission from Hauser SL (ED). *Harrison's Neurology in Clinical Medicine*. 3rd Ed. New York, NY: McGraw-Hill; 2013.)

the progressive increase in arterial wall stiffness that occurs with aging, makes small lacunar strokes more likely as we age.[15] Other causes of hemorrhage include vasculitis, neoplasms, trauma, coagulation disorders, and malformation of the vessels. Deep hemorrhages are those that affect the thalamus or basal ganglia; hemorrhages affecting the cerebral hemispheres are referred to as lobar hemorrhages.[2]

Table 11-2 outlines specific stroke symptoms associated with the primary vasculature and common areas of damage. Figure 11-5 illustrates the complexity of impairments with disruption of brainstem circulation. It should be noted that patients will present with some or all of these symptoms, varying in severity, but can also present with a combination of symptoms from the different syndromes due to variability in individual circulation patterns.

Based on the symptoms, **what stroke syndrome has Mr. Brown experienced?**

MCA

What cortical areas are most likely affected to create Mr. Brown's symptoms?

Primary motor (hemiparesis), primary sensory (sensory loss), dorsal stream (non-fluent aphasia), optic radiations (upper and lower – homonymous hemianopia).

● MIDDLE CEREBRAL ARTERY (MCA) INFARCTION AS AN EXAMPLE OF STROKE

MCA strokes are the most common of the stroke syndromes, accounting for 51% of known stroke occurrences,[3] and their presentation is a good starting point for a discussion of stroke consequences, treatment, and outcomes. Onset of an MCA stroke is often associated with slurring of speech; tingling or numbness of the face, arm, and/or leg; loss of movement in corresponding body parts; or a combination of any of these. The acronym FAST has been initiated to expand stroke awareness and encourage people to get help quickly. It stands for Face drooping, Arm difficulty, Speech slurred, then Time to call 911.[18] Consciousness is typically maintained; however, when consciousness is lost, it is usually associated with a seizure or significant cerebral edema.

Motor Dysfunction

The motor consequences of an MCA stroke vary but can include early **flaccidity** (complete loss of movement and muscle tone) in the limbs contralateral to the lesion; this is referred to as **hemiplegia** (absence of movement) or when partial, **hemiparesis** (impaired movement). Corticospinal and corticobulbar projections are typically damaged with an MCA stroke, and often other stroke syndromes, either at the site of origin (the cortex) or as they pass through the internal capsule. Loss of corticospinal fibers, originating from the primary motor cortex, disrupts isolated muscle control in limb muscles. Loss of corticospinal fibers, originating in the premotor cortex, as well as corticobulbar fibers that project to brainstem nuclei, results in disruption of postural control, primarily within the trunk and proximal muscles. Some patients will have diminished movement and muscle tone early but not flaccidity. It is rare for the

limbs to remain flaccid, so the use of the term hemiplegia is an inaccurate representation of the movement abilities of most people post-stroke even though it is often used; hemiparesis is really the better term.

Motor recovery is complex and may be characterized by either return of isolated muscle control (partial or complete) or synergistic motor control. **Synergistic motor control** refers to activation of flexors or extensors in combination or synergy. For example, flexion of the shoulder is associated with elbow and wrist flexion and hand closing; conversely, extension of the shoulder is accompanied by elbow and wrist extension with hand opening. Similar flexion and extension patterns may be seen in the leg, described in detail in the treatment section of this chapter (Table 11-6). This type of movement is associated with brainstem-level motor control. **Isolated muscle control** is the ability to activate individual muscles to produce isolated movements in any combination (i.e., wrist flexion with finger extension) that is characteristic of typical motor control and requires motor cortex activation. Although some patients will progress from synergistic movement to isolated motor control, others will develop synergistic movements and fail to develop isolated movements. Despite regaining isolated muscle control, some stroke survivors will not have the variety of movement, dexterity, or force generation that they had pre-stroke even after years of treatment and recovery. **Ideomotor limb apraxia** is a complex condition that results in disruption of skilled movement, which can't be explained by loss of sensation, muscle weakness, or changes in tone. Patients with apraxia may be able to perform a given motion but may have difficulty incorporating that motion into a complex movement; as a consequence, their movements look clumsy, and they will often have trouble achieving the goal of the movement. This clumsiness involves disruption of the natural timing, sequencing, and/or spatial organization of the movement components, resulting from motor planning impairment, and is associated with damage to the premotor cortex (supplementary motor area and/or premotor area) but also likely involves multiple areas of the motor planning system, including the left inferior parietal lobule.[19]

Motor planning and control is a bilateral activity; for example during reaching, control of limb trajectory and segmental coordination is attributed to the left hemisphere, and limb impedance (resistance to control velocity), to minimize errors in the endpoint, attributed to the right[19]; both contribute to the accuracy of reaching. Not surprisingly, then, motor deficits often present bilaterally post-unilateral stroke. So, although post-stroke motor impairment has historically been referred to as contralateral, it is not uncommon to see subtle changes in motor control in the ipsilesional extremities that may not be apparent to the stroke survivor, or the novice clinician, but may impact recovery. These deficits are greater with more severe lesions, when contralateral paresis is greatest.[20] Specific deficits have been noted in more complex tasks (e.g., reaching, writing) but not in grip strength or individual finger tapping.[21] **Apraxia** is one contributor to these ipsilesional deficits, but ipsilesional deficits are found in the absence of apraxia.[20,21] These deficits may relate to loss of ipsilateral (uncrossed) corticospinal fibers or disruption of bilateral cortical networks, associated with motor planning and control. Also, loss of cortical projections from the lesioned hemisphere to the non-lesioned hemisphere results in lowered inhibition of the intact motor cortex that may disrupt fine motor control.[22,23]

TABLE 11-2   Stroke Syndromes and Associated Symptoms[10,11,16,17]

ARTERY		AREAS OF DAMAGE	COMMON SYMPTOMS
Anterior cerebral* A**		Frontal lobe	Apathy/lack of spontaneity
		Medial surface	Contralateral motor dysfunction of the lower leg and foot
		Anterior and superior aspect of primary motor area	Bladder incontinence
			Gait apraxia
		Anterior and superior aspect of premotor cortex	
		Parietal lobe	Contralateral sensory dysfunction of leg and foot
		Medial surface	
		Superior aspect of lateral surface	
Middle cerebral B***		Lateral surface of frontal lobe	Contralateral hemiparesis (UE > LE)
		Primary motor area	Apraxia
		Premotor area	Expressive aphasia (left)****
		Inferior Frontal and ventral precentral gyri	
		Lateral surface of parietal lobe	Contralateral hemisensory loss
		Parietal lobe projections to frontal lobe and contralesional parietal lobe	Contralateral neglect syndrome (right)
			Bilateral sensory discrimination loss
		Internal capsule (posterior limb)	Contralateral hemiparesis and hemisensory loss
		Optic radiations	
		Superior (parietal lobe)	Inferior quadrantanopia
		Inferior (temporal lobe, "Meyer's loop")	Superior quadrantanopia
		Both	Homonymous hemianopia
		Temporal lobe (Wernicke's area)	Receptive aphasia (left)****
Carotid artery		Distribution of both anterior and middle cerebral arteries	Combination of anterior and middle cerebral artery symptoms

(Continued)

TABLE 11-2 Stroke Syndromes and Associated Symptoms[10,11,16,17] *(Continued)*

ARTERY	AREAS OF DAMAGE	COMMON SYMPTOMS
Posterior Cerebral	Occipital lobe	Contralateral hemianopia or quadrantanopia
		Cortical blindness (bilateral)
		Visual agnosia, agraphia (dominant)
		Prosopagnosia – loss of facial recognition
	Thalamus	Contralateral hemisensory loss
	Hippocampus (temporal lobe)	Memory loss (dominant hemisphere)
	Cerebral peduncle/midbrain	
	Lateral geniculate	Hemianopia/quadrantanopia
	Cranial nerve III	Ophthalmoplegia:
		Ipsilateral gaze deviation – down and out (unopposed pull of superior oblique and lateral rectus)
		Double vision, lack of accommodation
Vertebral artery (Medial medullar syndrome of Dejerine)[Toyoda]	Medullary pyramids above decussation Medial lemniscus Cr N XII	Contralateral hemiparesis of limbs (face unaffected) Hemisensory loss Ipsilateral tongue paresis
Basilar	Medulla	Death is common due to loss of medullary centers associated with respiration control
	Reticular activating system	Loss of consciousness, coma
	Cr N IX and XII	Tongue paresis, loss of taste, swallowing deficits (dysphagia)Vocal loss (dysphonia)
	Pons	Ipsilateral/bilateral
	Cr N III	Dilated pupil(s) – ipsilateral/bilateral
	Cr N V and VII	Facial muscle paresis and sensory loss (dysarthria) – ipsilateral/bilateral
	Cr N VI	Horizontal gaze paresis – bilateral eye turns in – ipsilateral

Artery	Structure affected	Symptoms
	Descending motor fibers	Contralateral hemiparesis or quadreparesis (pure motor stroke)
	Ascending sensory fibers	Contralateral hemisensory loss
	Cerebellum	Ipsilateral/bilateral ataxia, vertigo, nystagmus (ipsilateral/bilateral)
	Distribution of posterior cerebral artery	Same symptoms as above
Anterior inferior cerebellar	Lateral Pontine syndrome	
	Vestibular nuclei	Vertigo, nystagmus, nausea, ipsilesional falling
	Cochlear nucleus	Ipsilateral tinnitus and deafness
	Trigeminal nucleus	Ipsilateral sensory loss to face; ipsilateral paresis of muscles of mastication (dysarthria, dysphagia)
Posterior inferior cerebellar	Wallenberg syndrome (lateral medulla)	
	Cerebellum/peduncles	Ipsilateral limb and gait ataxia
	Vestibular nuclei	Vertigo, nystagmus, nausea
	Cr N IX	Dysphagia
	Cr N X	Dysphonia
	Labyrinthine artery disruption	Ipsilateral hearing loss
	Horner's syndrome	
	Postganglionic sympathetic neuron damage	Ipsilateral ptosis, miosis, and anhidrosis
	Cr N V – sensory portion	Ipsilateral facial sensory loss
	2nd order spinothalamic neurons	Contralateral loss of pain and temperature in extremities
Superior cerebellar	Cerebellum/peduncles	Ipsilateral ataxia (mild trunk, severe limb, and gait), vertigo/dizziness, nausea, vomiting, dysarthria, dysmetria, optokinetic nystagmus
	Medial lemniscus/spinal lemniscus (midbrain)	Contralateral sensory loss (touch, pain, and temperature)
	Corticospinal fibers (pons)	Contralateral paresis

*Strokes of the anterior cerebral artery are uncommon, most likely due to the redundancy of circulation from the right and left systems.
**A (Reproduced with permission from Afifi AK, Bergman RA. *Functional Neuroanatomy*, 2nd ed. New York, NY: McGraw-Hill; 2005, Fig. 28-2, p. 361.)
***B (Reproduced with permission from Afifi AK, Bergman RA. *Functional Neuroanatomy*, 2nd ed. New York, NY: McGraw-Hill; 2005, Fig. 28-1, p. 360.)
****Damage to both areas results in Global aphasia (both expressive and receptive).

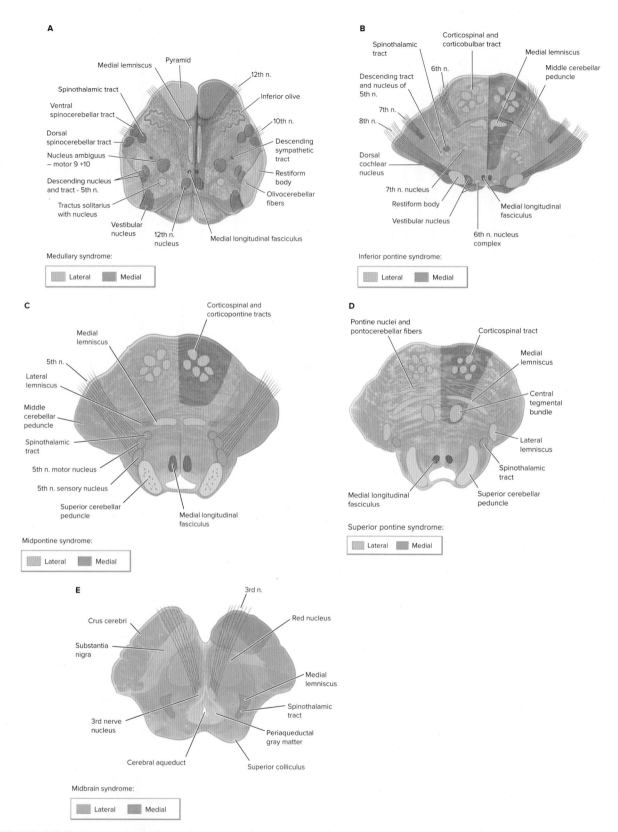

FIGURE 11-5 A-E. Brainstem circulation and stroke syndromes. Ascending syndromes A-E, from the medulla (A) to the midbrain (E), illustrate the complexity of structures damaged with lateral and medial stroke syndromes at each level. Damage to the corticospinal tracts, medial lemniscus, and spinothalamic tract results in loss of function contralateral to the lesion; damage at the level of the lower medulla often results in bilateral loss of corticospinal and medial lemniscal function because of the decussation of these fibers at this level. Typically, cranial nerve, spinocerebellar or cerebellar peduncle, or medial longitudinal fasciculus symptoms are ipsilateral to the lesion. Thus, brain stem syndromes often present with contralateral or bilateral changes in the limbs, ipsilateral or bilateral changes in balance/proprioception, and ipsilateral or bilateral changes in cranial nerve function. (Reproduced with permission from Hauser SL (ED) *Harrison's Neurology in Clinical Medicine*. 3rd ed. New York, NY: McGraw-Hill; 2013.)

Notably, the literature has included a number of terms to describe the extremities contralateral to a unilateral lesion post-stroke, including terms like "affected/more affected," "involved/more involved," and "paretic." The limbs ipsilateral to the stroke are referred to as "non-affected/lesser affected," "noninvolved/lesser involved," or "non-paretic." Since paresis best characterizes the contralesional extremities and has not been found in the ipsilesional extremities post-stroke, this chapter will use that label; the term "non-paretic" will be used to refer to the ipsilesional extremities. It should be noted that this does not mean there is no change in function; only that there is no paresis.

Sensory Dysfunction

Sensory dysfunction post-stroke is complex, involving multiple areas of the parietal and frontal lobes, and often goes undiagnosed because of that complexity. Sensory function includes touch perception, vibration, proprioception, pain, and discrimination of hot/cold, texture, weight, and shape. Often clinical evaluation of sensation focuses on touch, pain, and proprioception only. These may be impaired post-stroke on the limbs, face, and trunk contralateral to the lesion, sometimes referred to as **hemianesthesia**. This term is misleading, in that it suggests complete loss of sensation, yet sensation is rarely completely absent. It is much more common to have diminished sensation of varying degrees in different parts of the hemiparetic side. Sensory discrimination is less likely to be evaluated but more likely to be impaired; further, the sensory networks supporting sensory discrimination abilities are bilateral and include areas in the parietal and frontal cortices. Thus, sensory discrimination abilities are likely to be impaired bilaterally, especially when sensory discrimination loss ipsilesionally is moderate to severe.[24,25]

There are also two complex conditions associated with sensory disruption post-stroke: pusher and neglect syndromes. **Pusher syndrome** (contraversive pushing) is a confusing condition, in which the patient orients the head and trunk toward the hemiparetic side, resists attempts by careproviders to correct this orientation to upright, and pushes forcefully with the non-paretic extremities toward the paretic side. Contraversive pushing can occur with damage to either hemisphere but is slightly more common and longer lasting with right lesions.[26] When it occurs with right hemisphere damage, it is frequently associated with spatial neglect syndrome. When it occurs with left hemisphere damage, it is commonly associated with aphasia; thus, there has been much confusion about the origin of this disorder. However, the common site of damage seems to be the ventral posterolateral nucleus of the thalamus, which is a synapsing site for vestibular neuron projections, or parts of the insular cortex or postcentral gyrus. The consequence of this damage seems to be an impaired sense of upright (vertical); when tested, clients with pusher syndrome feel "upright" when shifted 18 to 20 degrees away from midline, so in pushing, they are really trying to "right" themselves.[27]

Unilateral spatial neglect syndrome (USN) is another complex disorder, characterized by failure to attend to things on the hemiparetic side of the body or, in other words, biased attention toward the non-hemiparetic side and/or disruption in mental representations of space. It is most common with right stroke (nearly 50% in the acute phase), since the right hemisphere is predominant in spatial attention and body representation.[28,29]

However, it also occurs with left CVAs, but when it occurs on the left, it is typically less severe. **USN** can manifest as multiple subtypes, involving visual, auditory, somatosensory, perceptual, and motor systems.[28] A variety of terms are used to describe this condition and to differentiate its subtypes. First, it can be characterized as **personal**, associated with one's own body, **peripersonal**, associated with things close to the body, and **extrapersonal**, associated with things far from the body.[30] Specifically, **personal neglect** presents as a lack of awareness of the paretic side of the body with attention focused on the non-paretic side of the body; it can present as a lack of awareness of the involved body parts (asomatognosia) or even the almost delusional misinterpretation of the paretic body part(s) as belonging to someone else (somatoparaphrenia). These extreme manifestations of unilateral neglect are associated with large lesions of the temporoparietal cortex as well as frontal lobe damage with the right medial frontal damage associated with asomatognosia and right orbitofrontal damage with somatoparaphrenia. There are likely other contributing factors as not all large lesions of these areas result in these manifestations of unilateral neglect.[30] Peripersonal and extrapersonal neglect are specific to objects nearer or father from the individual, respectively. In addition, neglect can occur within different sensory or motor systems. **Visual neglect** refers to focused attention on the non-paretic side with inattention to the visual environment on the paretic side. Multiple anatomic regions have been linked to visual neglect, including the temporoparietal junction, premotor cortex, basal ganglia, and thalamus as well as white matter projections that connect these areas. Similarly, **auditory neglect** to sounds from the environment on the paretic side and/or impaired sound localization can result from damage to the ventral and dorsal auditory streams, respectively. **Somatosensory neglect** can present as failure to detect sensory stimulation to the paretic limbs and/or a lack of awareness of limb position, involving lesions to the posterior parietal or premotor cortex. Motoric manifestations include lack of automatic or voluntary movement not explained by paresis or hypertonia and in the absence of a primary sensorimotor lesion. Lesions, resulting in **motor neglect**, have been identified in the posterior parietal and prefrontal cortices, motor association cortex, internal capsule, and putamen as well as the thalamus. **Allocentric neglect** refers to the inability to perceive the contralesional aspect of objects independent of their position relative to the patient (object-focused), which can result in the drawing of one side of familiar objects (see Figure 11-6). **Egocentric neglect** refers to a lack of attention to the contralesional space, based on the patient's position, and is characterized by a shift of the perceived center of the body toward the non-paretic side such that the individual will point off center toward the non-paretic (right) side, when asked to point straight ahead. Lastly, **representational neglect** is the inability to describe one side of an imagined but familiar space (e.g., the left side of their living room) from a specified vantage point but, interestingly, can describe that same side, if asked to do so from the opposite side of the room. Representational neglect commonly occurs with visual neglect and is associated with lesions in the prefrontal dorsolateral cortex or thalamus.[28,30] The presence of USN is associated with poorer functional outcomes and a greater chance of discharge to a nursing facility.[29]

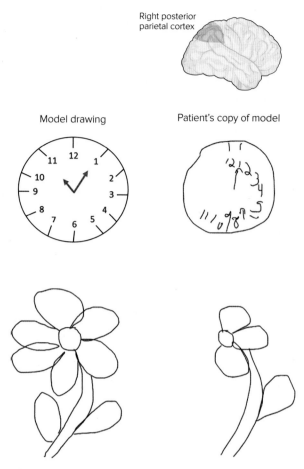

FIGURE 11-6 Unilateral spatial neglect syndrome paper and pencil testing outcomes.

Visual Field Disruption

The visual system disruption with an MCA stroke can result in a visual field loss. Mr. Brown presents with a **homonymous hemianopia**, which refers to the loss of the visual field contralateral to the lesion (or in Mr. Brown's case, to the right) and results from damage to the optic fibers (radiations) at some point after they leave the optic chiasm or the occipital cortex. It occurs most commonly with MCA stroke but can be seen with posterior cerebral artery stroke, affecting the occipital cortex. **Quadrantanopia** is the loss of a quadrant, or quarter, of the visual field; again, this occurs contralateral to the side of the lesion. When only the parietal fibers are damaged, the superior retinal fibers are disrupted, resulting in loss of the lower visual field; when Meyer's loop in the temporal lobe is damaged, the inferior retinal fibers are disrupted, resulting in loss of the upper visual field.[31] It is important to remember that visual fields are projected to both eyes and that the upper part of our visual field projects to the lower part of the retina, subsequently projecting to the occipital lobe through Meyer's loop in the temporal lobe, while the lower part of the visual field projects to the upper part of the retina and then to the occipital lobe through the parietal lobe. See Figure 11-7 for an illustration of these visual field deficits. Fifty percent of patients with a visual field deficit spontaneously recover within the first 3 to 6 months; the remainder continues to have a long-term deficit. Left

homonymous hemianopia may be accompanied by hemianopic alexia, which is a reading deficit associated with insufficient right to left eye movement.[31] See Figure 11-7 for an illustration of these visual field deficits.

Language Dysfunction

Mr. Brown also presents with expressive aphasia, or the absence/disruption of verbal expression. **Aphasia**, which refers to language impairment, presents primarily in three forms: expressive, receptive, or global. Since there is a left hemispheric bias for language processing in 95% of right-handed individuals and 78% of left-handed individuals,[31] aphasia is most common with a left MCA stroke. In **expressive aphasia** (also called non-fluent aphasia), there is damage to the frontal lobe, inclusive of Broca's

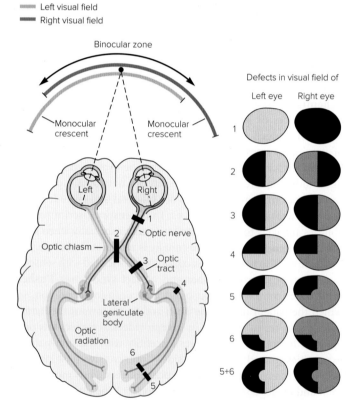

FIGURE 11-7 Visual field deficits associated with damage to visual projections. 1 = Unilateral blindness associated with optic nerve damage; 2 = bitemporal hemianopia due to damage of crossing nasal fibers at the optic chiasm; 3 = homonymous hemianopia due to optic tract damage; 4 = superior contralateral quadrantanopia due to damage of Meyer's loop; 5 = superior contralateral quadrantanopia with preservation of the macular vision duplicated in the parietal radiations; 6 = lower contralateral quadrantanopia due to damage of the parietal radiations with sparing of the macular vision due to duplication in Meyer's loop fibers; 5+6 = homonymous hemianopia, typically with macular sparing, which results from the large representative area for central vision in the occipital lobe that is rarely completely disrupted with a posterior cerebral artery occlusion. (Reproduced with permission from Kandel ER, Schwartz JH, Jessell TM, Siegelbaum SA, Hudspeth AJ. *Principles of Neural Science.* 5th ed. New York, NY: McGraw-Hill; 2013.)

area, and/or the projection systems of the dorsal stream, as described in Chapter 7, that impedes the ability to form words. Patients will understand what is said to them and often can produce single words or simple phrases but not complete sentences (syntax disruption). Frustration often occurs, since they are aware of what they want to say but unable to say it. Often writing ability is intact but limited because of the associated hemiparesis. Expressive aphasia should not be confused with **dysarthria**, which is associated with paresis of the oral musculature secondary to damage to the primary motor cortex, resulting in speech that is difficult to understand because of poor oral musculature control. **Speech apraxia** can also result in poor speech formulation due to disruption of the motor planning process to produce speech but results from premotor cortex damage and not damage to the dorsal stream. **Receptive aphasia** (fluent aphasia) is associated with damage to the ventral stream within the temporal lobe, or what some call the Wernicke complex (BA47, 45, 37, 38, 21, and/or 22); it is an impairment not only in the ability to understand what is said but also in the ability to create and monitor the verbalizations that are uttered. When we talk, we first must determine what we want to say and then listen to monitor the accuracy of what is verbalized. In receptive aphasia, the ability to select the right words and monitor one's speech is impaired, so although speech can be produced, it is likely gibberish. Plus, the survivor is unable to monitor their speech, so they are unaware that their utterance doesn't make sense. They also don't understand the listener's confusion with their statements. Frustration is, again, common. Finally, large strokes that impact both the ventral and dorsal streams can result in a devastating loss of the function of both, referred to as **global aphasia**.[32,33] Survivors of such a stroke have difficulty understanding or producing speech. A less common speech anomaly is **conductive aphasia**, which presents as an error in putting the syllables of words or the words within a phrase together (a phonological error) as well as deficits in repetition and naming. An example of such an error would be facemat or plantmat for placemat; the client is likely to make multiple attempts to select the right combination of syllables or words. This deficit has been historically thought to result from disruption of the arcuate fibers, connecting Wernicke's area with Broca's area; however, overlapping lesions within a small posterior aspect of the parietal lobe (posterior temporal region), which is a sight for sensory integration, may be the primary location of this aspect of speech (Figure 11-8).[34] Other abilities, associated with language, including writing, reading, and arithmetic, can also be disrupted post-stroke, referred to as **acquired dyslexia** or **alexia** (reading)**, agraphia** or **dysgraphia** (writing), and **acalculia** (arithmetic), respectively. These occur most commonly with dominant hemisphere stroke and may occur together or in isolation. When dysgraphia and dyslexia occur together, they are usually associated with damage to the angular gyrus of the dominant parietal lobe and often associated with acalculia and aphasia; this damage also disrupts the ability to spell or understand spelled words. When alexia occurs without agraphia, it is most commonly associated with occipital lobe damage secondary to a posterior cerebral artery infarct and damage to the

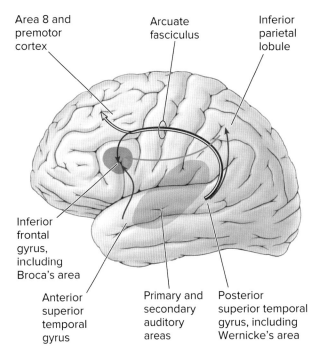

FIGURE 11-8 **Areas of the cerebral hemisphere supporting language function.** Regions of the temporal, parietal, and frontal lobes are linked via the arcuate fasciculus to support the complex components of language function, typically in the left hemisphere. (Reproduced with permission from Martin JH. *Neuroanatomy Text and Atlas.* 4th ed. New York, NY: McGraw-Hill; 2012.)

splenium of the corpus collosum; concurrent homonymous hemianopia is common. Spelling and the ability to interpret spelled words remain intact. Damage to the frontal lobe can also result in acquired dyslexia, **acalcula**, and agraphia in association with non-fluent aphasia; in this case, individuals may retain the ability to read short or common (sight) words but lack reading comprehension and the ability to spell or recognize spelled words.[35] It is always important to distinguish true agraphia and alexia from the consequences of aphasia, hemiparesis, or pre-existing reading, arithmetic, or writing disorders.

Cognitive Dysfunction

Cognitive dysfunction is common post-stroke with an estimated incidence of 40 to 60%; the incidence is greater in older survivors, and the outcome confounded by concurrent neural degeneration from Alzheimer's disease or other dementia (i.e., multi-infarct).[36] Dementia and stroke have common risk factors, including sedentary lifestyle, hypertension, diabetes, hyperlipidemia, and smoking as well as aging; thus, there is a strong link between the occurrence of these two conditions. Specific cognitive deficits post-stroke relate closely to the size and location of the lesion; however, the disruption of memory post-stroke appears to be much more complex, since memories are stored in many neural locations. First, damage in the area of the hippocampus within the temporal lobe rarely occurs with any of the common stroke syndromes; however, this temporal region is highly connected to many other areas of the brain that may be affected by stroke and support memory function. A decreased level of activity in the medial temporal lobe has been found to be associated with impaired short-term memory; it is thought that this change likely relates to a disruption of the networks of projections to that area, when lesions were not present in the temporal lobe. **Working** or **episodic memory**, which is important for many daily activities, including sensory discrimination, is most commonly affected.[37] Cognitive impairment post-stroke can be categorized as mild (subjective awareness of minor issues but with no effect on activities or participation), moderate (affects complex activities but not ADLs or routine activities), or severe (difficulties in all aspects of daily living). Obviously, stroke within the frontal lobes is most likely to disrupt executive function. Despite the frequency of post-stroke cognitive deficits, they often go undiagnosed, and therefore, untreated due to the complexity of the post-stroke symptoms and the focus on recovery of sensorimotor function and activities of daily living. Even survivors that score within the normal range on the Mini Mental exam© (a common test of orientation and memory) have been found to have some level of cognitive deficit when more comprehensive testing is conducted. Yet, early cognitive impairment has been found to persist with little improvement; in severe cases, progression to dementia is likely.[36] About 10% of stroke survivors develop dementia within the first year post-stroke; for those with recurrent stroke, this increases to 30%.[37] Cardiovascular disease is a contributing factor for both stroke and dementia, so there is likely a complex interaction contributing to the risk of dementia post-stroke.[38] Therapists should be aware of this and watch for the ability of clients to follow directions and retain information from one session to the next. If a problem is noted, referral to a neuropsychologist for evaluation and treatment may be beneficial. Restructuring of the treatment sessions, focusing more on procedural rather than declarative knowledge, may facilitate the relearning of motor skills in those with severe cognitive dysfunction. However, there is a paucity of information on treatment methods that facilitate learning in those with post-stroke cognitive deficits, but therapists should borrow from the literature on Alzheimer's disease to structure their treatment activities.

● ACUTE MEDICAL MANAGEMENT OF STROKE

Ischemic Stroke

The 2019 stroke guidelines reflect that transport by Emergency Medical Service (ambulance) to a stroke center results in earlier arrival at the emergency room, quicker assessment, and better outcomes.[39] Early care focuses on reperfusion, collateral blood flow optimization, and avoidance of additional injury due to secondary sequelae.[40] Initial medical management of stroke must include a comprehensive history; the most important component of this history is to determine the last moment that the client was neurologically normal, or in other words, to pinpoint the onset of stroke symptoms. This, along with careful clearing of exclusionary criteria, will determine the ability to use intravenous thrombolysis, such as **recombinant tissue-type plasminogen activator** (rTPA or TPA, medication name is Alteplase), to assist in clot

breakdown. Exclusion criteria for TPA include current or previous cerebral hemorrhage (intracerebral or subarachnoid); severe head injury within 3 months; uncontrolled high blood pressure; intracranial neoplasm or arteriovenous malformation; intracranial or intraspinal surgery within 3 months; CT/MRI evidence that the stroke involves multiple lobes of the brain; and bleeding tendency (diathesis) with or without use of anticoagulant. TPA is only effective if given within the first 4.5 hours post-stroke onset, but is most effective within the first 3 hours, so identification of the stroke onset is crucial for determining that critical application window. If the onset timeframe cannot be determined, TPA will currently not be administered; however, studies are in process around the world to determine benefits of TPA administration beyond 4.5 hours.[41] IV rtPA has been found to improve 3-month outcomes by 30%.[40] CT or MRI is required to rule out intracranial bleeding prior to application; ischemic changes are typically not evident until at least 6 hours post-onset, so imaging at admission may not allow visualization of the hypoperfusion, characteristic of ischemic stroke. For patients with large occlusions in the internal carotid or MCA that present within 6 hours of symptom onset, mechanical thrombectomy is the treatment of choice; this involves inserting a catheter into either the femoral artery or aortal arch and threading it into the internal carotid system to the point of the clot. A stentretriever is extended into the catheter to capture and retrieve the clot; this can also be done with aspiration, suctioning the clot through the catheter.[42] A series of clinical trials found that mechanical thrombolysis resulted in greater levels of independence than medical treatment alone; however, it can be combined with TPA administration. It has also been attempted in the posterior circulation for basilar artery strokes with some success but not as favorable as in the anterior circulation.[43] Sonothrombolysis (ultrasound-facilitated thrombolysis) has been found to enhance the effects of TPA without increased risk and may be administered in some stroke centers. Since stroke and cardiac events often occur together, a 12-lead electrocardiogram (ECG) is recommended. When TPA is applied, antihypertensive control is delayed unless the systolic pressure exceeds 220 mmHg, and then it is very slowly reduced by no more than 15% in the first 24 hours.[44]

Hemorrhagic Stroke

Brain hemorrhage is associated with a pooling of blood (hematoma) that results in cerebral edema and potentially hydrocephalus as debris and blood infiltrate the ventricles and impede/impair CSF flow and production. About 30% of patients will experience an expansion of the hematoma in the first 24 hours,[45] and nearly 40% will die within 30 days of onset.[46] Loss of consciousness and breathing impairment are much more common with hemorrhagic stroke; therefore, it is more likely that intubation and mechanical ventilation are needed on ER admission.[46] Post-stroke hypertension is thought to be a contributing factor to hematoma expansion; thus, the control of this hypertension has been the target of medical intervention in the early stages of acute hospitalization, aimed at decreasing systolic blood pressure to <180 mmHg or in some cases <140 mmHg. However, the effect of lowering blood pressure remains equivocal with some reporting enhanced recovery while others reporting negligible differences.[45] Methods to reduce intracranial pressure associated with hemorrhage include elevation of the head of the bed by 30 degrees, administration of analgesics or sedatives, hyperventilation (increasing CO_2 levels to 30–35 mmHg), minimizing hypoglycemia and hyperglycemia, maintaining normal temperature (treat fevers), and/or administering hypertonic saline to avoid hyperosmolarity.[46] Hemorrhage frequently occurs in individuals already receiving anticoagulant therapy and, thus, necessitates a reversal of the effect of the anticoagulant medications; although this includes discontinuation of the medication, other pharmacologic interventions are required to hasten the reversal of the anticoagulating effects. Hemorrhage can be a consequence of rtPA administration in 6% of those with initial ischemic stroke that receive it; when this occurs, there is typically lesion expansion, resulting in poorer outcomes and greater chance of death.[46]

Surgical intervention to remove the hematoma is only advised for those whose condition begins declining as a lifesaving attempt. In some who develop hydrocephalus, a shunt can be placed to drain cerebrospinal fluid and blood from the ventricles. In conjunction with thrombolytic administration, this has shown improved outcomes and lesser mortality.[46]

Measuring Stroke Severity

Physicians commonly assess stroke function in the acute period with the **NIH Stroke Scale (NIHSS)** or its modified version, the **mNIHSS**. The modified version was developed to eliminate components that were redundant or had demonstrated poorer reliability; it also rescaled the sensory component.[47] Both are used in the clinic (Table 11-3). On both scales, a zero is associated with normal function, and, therefore, a lower total score is associated with better (more normal) function. It should be noted that survivors with very different stroke symptoms can obtain equivalent total scores, so the individual component scores will provide better clarity.

Other scales that may be used by medical professionals to describe stroke outcome include the Modified Rankin Scale and the Glasgow Outcome Scale. Both characterize outcomes, based on the level of disability. The **Modified Rankin** is a 6-point scale: 0 = no symptoms and 6 = death; the magnitude of disability is ranked in the intermediate scores (1 = symptoms with no significant disability, 2 = slight disability, 3 = moderate disability,

TABLE 11-3 NIHSS versus mNIHSS Scales[47]	
NIHSS	**MNIHSS**
1. Consciousness 　1a. General (0-3); alert – unresponsive 　1b. Responds to 2 questions (0-3) 　　What month is it? 　　How old are you? 　1c. Responds to 2 commands (0-3) 　　Open and close eyes 　　Grip and release with non-paretic hand	Eliminated 1a; 1b and 1c are the same.
2. Gaze (0-3): normal, palsy, forced deviation	Gaze – Same
3. Visual (0-4): normal, partial hemianopia, complete hemianopia, bilateral hemianopia	Visual – Same
4. Facial palsy (0-3): normal – complete paralysis	Facial palsy – Excluded
5. Motor arm: 　5a. – Left (0-4) Normal – no movement 　5b. – Right (0-4) Normal – no movement	Motor arm – Same
6. Motor Leg: 　6a. – Left (0-4) Normal – no movement 　6b. – Right (0-4) Normal – no movement	Motor leg – Same
7. Limb ataxia (0-2s): absent, 1 limb, 2 limbs	Ataxia – Excluded
8. Sensory (0-2): normal, mild–moderate, severe	Sensory modified (0-1): normal, abnormal
9. Best language (0-3): normal, mild–mod, severe, mute	Language – Same
10. Dysarthria (0-2): normal, mild–mod, severe	Excluded
11. Neglect (0-2): none, inattention, profound hemi-inattention	Neglect – Same
Total score = 0-45	Total score: 0-35

4 = moderate disability, and 5 = severe disability).[48] The **Glasgow Outcome Scale** (GOS) is a similar 5-point scale: 1 = good recovery (mild lasting effects), 2 = moderate disability (independent but with disability), 3 = severe disability (dependent but conscious), 4 = persistent vegetative state, 5 = death.[49] Obviously, these are somewhat subjective ratings, and, therefore, don't provide a clear picture of the individual stroke survivor.

Initial Stroke Outcomes

Of those admitted to an acute care hospital with a diagnosed stroke, about 10.5% will die from the initial event or a complication within the first 30 days; the likelihood of death from stroke also increases with age.[1] The average length of stay in acute care is 6.5 days and nearly 90% of those admitted receive inpatient rehabilitative services (Occupational, Physical, and/or Speech Therapy). After the initial acute hospitalization, 25% of patients will be discharged to a skilled nursing facility (SNF), 30% to an inpatient rehabilitation facility (IRF), and 45% will be discharged home with (11-12%) receiving home health or outpatient rehabilitation and 32 to 34% receiving no follow-up rehabilitation. Medicare policy designates that transfer to a rehabilitation unit can only be made if the survivor will soon be able or is able to participate in 3 hours of therapy (OT, PT, Speech) per day, 5 to 6 days per week, to qualify for coverage; other health insurance has largely adopted this policy as well. If the survivor is medically unstable or progressing too slowly for this level of treatment, transfer to a SNF or home, with nursing and therapy at a lesser frequency, occurs. Subsequent admission to a rehabilitation facility can occur, if the survivor's stamina and recovery progress to the level of meeting the 3 hours/day of treatment with further improvement likely. IRF length of stay (LOS) averages 15 days post-stroke in the United States while LOS in SNF averages 38 days; this is not surprising since those transferred to SNF are typically older, with more comorbidities and longer hospital stays.[50] Rehabilitation services (PT, OT, ST) are also provided in a SNF with a frequency that may approach that of inpatient rehabilitation; however, the frequency and duration of treatment are matched to the tolerance level of the individual client. It is also common for those who transition first to IRF or SNF to receive some rehabilitative services either in outpatient centers or their home upon discharge from these facilities; a few patients will transfer from SNF to IRF.[50] Reportedly, up to 25% of stroke survivors have a second stroke within 5 years of the first, and this increases to 75% by 10 years; mortality after the second stroke is much higher.[51]

● ACUTE NEUROPLASTICITY POST-STROKE

How Does the Brain Try to Heal Itself in the First Hours/Days Post-stroke?

Neurologic insult, such as stroke, induces a cascade of events aimed at neural repair and return to homeostasis, often referred to as **spontaneous reorganization**. The initial impact of stroke is a loss of blood flow to the impacted areas with a central portion of cell death (**necrosis**), surrounded by an area of cell dysfunction

known as the **penumbra**. The stroke insult catalyzes an ischemic cascade, mediated by multiple signaling molecules and resulting in glutamate accumulation and excitotoxicity as well as oxidative stress; these things in combination can result in greater cell death in the penumbra. Early reorganization focuses on reperfusion of surviving tissue in the penumbra, often through **angiogenesis** (small blood vessel or capillary proliferation), and an infiltration of inflammatory cells to begin the healing process; if reperfusion is unsuccessful, due to extensive blood vessel damage, there will be a spread of necrotic tissue into the penumbra. However, successful reperfusion is associated with removal of necrotic tissue, a decrease in edema, and receding inflammation infiltrates. There is a gradual stabilization of remaining functional neuronal networks. Yet, neuronal loss at the infarct site results in disruption of networks distant from the actual infarct site, both those that project to the site and those to which the site projects. Thus, this cascade of events necessitates a dying back of lost neuronal axons as well as a change in synaptic organization at local and distant projection areas. These synaptic changes can include the unmasking of latent synapses; a proliferation of synaptic receptors, axon terminals, and dendritic branches; changes in membrane excitability; and changes in neurotransmitter production, release, reuptake, and/or degradation, resulting in enhanced or diminished activity within a synapse. It should be remembered that there are usually competing influences (excitatory or inhibitory) at any synapse. Reorganization is dependent on the activity of surviving neurons; thus, if only inhibitory neurons survive, these changes may result in exaggerated inhibition at a given synapse. Obviously, the opposite can occur in the presence of the survival of only excitatory projections. Optimal recovery is most likely dependent on a balance in remaining systems between inhibitory and excitatory projections. While neurogenesis is possible in mature brains, it is very limited in older adults and most of these new cells die without maturing; in addition, axon regrowth is limited by the glial scar that forms in the area of necrosis, which is made up of extracellular matrix proteins. Thus, neural recovery is largely dependent on other mechanisms and not neurogenesis.[52]

● PHYSICAL THERAPY MANAGEMENT IN THE ACUTE CARE FACILITY

General Concepts

Mr. Brown is in the acute stage of recovery from stroke and the primary focus is on medical and physical issues related to saving his life. The therapy staff serves a dual role, in this early time point, focused on assessment and treatment for the acute phase of stroke as well as prevention of common complications that might impede full potential for recovery. The initial hospitalization for stroke typically lasts 24 to 72 hours with subsequent discharge to a SNF, inpatient rehabilitation hospital/unit, or home. Findings of the AVERT study strongly discourage high-intensity rehabilitation in the first 24 hours post-stroke; however, more recent research suggests that getting patients up between 12 and 24 hours post-stroke rather than maintaining bedrest for greater than 24 hours results in fewer incidents of pneumonia, shorter LOS, and better functional outcomes. Thus, early stroke treatment for those with small ischemic strokes should include sitting and/or standing activity of less than 15 minute duration within the first 24 hours.[53]

It is important to keep the goals for long-term rehabilitation in mind even in the acute period. Studies have shown that early intervention is key to long-term improvement. In addition, this focus on rehabilitation prevents **learned nonuse**. This concept originated from Taub's work (1994) with sensory deafferentation in monkeys, achieved through severing the dorsal roots to one upper limb. Following this procedure, he noted that the monkeys failed to use the limb despite the fact that their motor function remained intact; he coined the term "learned nonuse" for this phenomenon. Their initial clumsy movements, without sensory input, were unsuccessful in achieving the goal of the movement; as a result, the monkeys stopped using the limb. Taub hypothesized that this was similar to people post-stroke, when not only sensory input but also motor control is impaired; thus, when stroke survivors initially try to move, they are met with failure, and even as their motor ability improves, they may fail to use the arm in meaningful ways. To prevent learned nonuse, it is critical to incorporate active movement of the paretic limbs in all activities; to do so, activities need to be well conceived and appropriate assistance be provided to assure success.[54]

In an environment focused on efficient care that optimizes use of funds, there is a great deal of pressure to return patients to the setting with the lowest level of care, and if possible, home as quickly as possible. This means that therapists, in the acute care setting, must focus on returning the client to the highest level of independent function possible as quickly as they can. This early focus on return to function can result in an emphasis on compensatory treatment techniques. **Compensatory treatment techniques** are those that encourage use of the non-paretic extremity to perform functional tasks independently while allowing the paretic extremity to be ignored. Teaching the client to eat and dress with the non-paretic hand and providing tools that allow return to function with only one hand are compensatory techniques for the UE. The use of walking devices that promote minimal weight-bearing on the paretic LE allows a gait pattern that is essentially using only the non-paretic LE and, thus, is a compensatory technique. Transfers that are done with the majority of weight born through the non-paretic LE are also compensatory. Early **compensation** has been shown to lead to learned nonuse and failure to recover use of the limb to its full potential. Therefore, the therapist must strike a balance between rehabilitation for the long-term benefit of the client and speedy return to function to allow a return to home or lower level of care. The therapist should keep in mind that they are the professional who is responsible for advocating for the client's long-term rehabilitation potential. Research provides evidence that therapy in the acute stage can lead to better outcomes at the 1-year mark. Treatment plans shown to be effective focus on the following key objectives:

1. Assessment
2. Early Intervention and Prevention of Complications
3. Task-Oriented Practice
4. Intensive Repetitive Practice

The Assessment

The neurologic assessment, outlined in Chapter 10, should be followed for the acute client post-stroke. When strength testing, fatigue should be avoided and position changes minimized by completing all testing possible in each position, before changing positions. (This principle can be continued once treatment is initiated to minimize position changes.) See Table 11-4 for a description of ROM and exercise suggestions by positions. Strength testing is usually initiated at the level of 3/5, testing to see if the individual can move the joint through the ROM against gravity. If not, then that joint is tested in a gravity-eliminated position. If the joint can be moved through the full ROM antigravity, then resistance is added to determine the strength grade. Many individuals with CVA are bound in synergy patterns. Strength testing should not be done within synergy patterns. If the only movement is within a synergy, then a description of the strength should be noted but a numerical grade cannot be given. Consider using relevant parts of the Fugl-Meyer assessment to better describe movement capabilities of each limb.[55]

TABLE 11-4	Joint Motions by Position for Use in Testing AROM and Doing Bed Exercises in the Acute Care Setting	
POSITION	**MOVEMENTS GRAVITY ELIMINATED**	**MOVEMENTS AGAINST GRAVITY**
Supine	Hip abduction Hip adduction Hip external rotation Knee flexion Knee extension Ankle dorsiflexion	Hip flexion Hip internal rotation Knee extension (hip flexed and leg supported on a pillow) Ankle dorsiflexion
Side-lying	Hip flexion Hip extension Hip internal rotation Knee flexion Knee extension Ankle dorsiflexion	Hip abduction Hip adduction Hip external rotation
Prone		Hip extension Knee flexion Ankle plantarflexion

CASE A, PART II

After determining that Mr. Brown is able to hear and see the therapist as well as understand instructions, strength should be assessed in the bed starting with AROM. To optimize Mr. Brown's ability to follow instructions, the therapist stands on his left side so that he can both see and hear the therapist without interference due to hemianopia. Mr. Brown is able to actively elevate the right shoulder and actively flex and extend the elbow. Strength grades are as follows: shoulder elevation 2/5, elbow flexion 2/5, elbow extension 2/5, wrist and finger flexion 2/5, wrist and finger extension 1/5. In the lower extremity hip flexion is 3/5, hip abduction 2/5, knee flexion 3/5, knee extension 2/5, and plantarflexion 2/5. During MMT he did not exhibit any active dorsiflexion. Since Mr. Brown does not exhibit active dorsiflexion in supine or side-lying, during the MMT he should then be placed in supine with the head of the bed elevated so that he can see his foot. When asked to dorsiflex his foot, while flexing the hip and knee, the therapist notes that his ankle moves into dorsiflexion through partial ROM. This would be documented as "able to dorsiflex through partial ROM against gravity within the flexor synergy." At times, dorsiflexion may not be noted until the client attempts to ambulate.

Mr. Brown's Ashworth scores in the UE are 1 in the shoulder elevators and elbow flexors and 2 in the wrist and finger flexors; in the LE scores are 0 in the hip, 1 in the knee flexors, and 2 in the plantarflexors.

Box 11-1 Stroke Outcome Measures from the Stroke EDGE II Task Force

ACUTE CARE	REHABILITATION (INPATIENT AND OUTPATIENT)
Orpington Prognostic Scale	Postural Assessment Scale for Stroke Patients
Postural Assessment Scale for Stroke Patients,	Stroke Rehabilitation Assessment of Movement
Stroke Rehabilitation Assessment of Movement	Fugl-Meyer Assessment Functional Independence Measure Stroke Impact Scale

In those clients, who do not exhibit any active dorsiflexion during strength testing, be sure to begin ambulation by encouraging dorsiflexion and have someone palpate and carefully observe the ankle to note any activity. Also, keep in mind, during the evaluation and early treatment sessions, that motions such as dorsiflexion, finger and wrist extension, and shoulder protraction are not strong parts of any of the synergy patterns but are commonly resisted by hypertonic muscles, often leading to more difficulty in activating and regaining use of these muscle groups. Special attention to these muscles, during evaluation and treatment, will be critical to assure recovery of function in these muscle groups. Also, to minimize position changes, keep in mind what position Mr. Brown will be placed in at the end of therapy and plan the session to finish in that posture.

Standardized outcome measures are an integral component of the examination and should be utilized in the acute care setting. This can be challenging as there are limited measures available for this setting. Stroke EDGE task force recommendations are made by setting (Box 11-1). In addition, when possible the core measures of gait, balance, and transfers recommended for all adults with neurologic disorders should be included. Additional measures that are appropriate for this setting can be found on the Academy of Neurology Physical Therapy website.[56]

CASE A, PART III

Mr. Brown is not yet able to ambulate without assistance, so the measure most appropriate for him would be the Orpington Prognostic Scale and the Postural Assessment Scale for Stroke Patients. Utilizing the Orpington Prognostic Scale will assist the therapist and other team members in developing discharge goals based on his prognosis. It is best if used 14 days after admission or when the patient's neurologic condition has stabilized. It should not be given to Mr. Brown until immediately prior to discharge. At this time he would likely score a 4.0 if we assume he would score a full 10 on cognition. This score indicates moderate impairment and that he is likely to discharge to a rehabilitation unit from the hospital.[57] Trunk control and posture are expected to improve during the acute care stay and should be objectively measured and documented. The Postural Assessment Scale is an objective measure of trunk control and will be valuable in providing an objective measure of therapy progress. Mr. Brown scores a 14 on the PASS indicating he is likely to regain function overall and the ability to ambulate.[58,59] Following the guidelines from the core measures clinical practice guideline of the Academy of Neurologic Physical Therapy, Mr. Brown should be scored on the core measures regardless of his level of function, At this time he would receive a 0 on the 10-meter walk test, 6-minute walk test, Berg Balance Test, Functional Gait Assessment, and 5 times sit to stand. This provides a baseline that can be used as he makes progress in his rehabilitation in other settings. He can be assessed on his balance confidence using the Activities-Specific Balance Confidence Scale; since he is unable to walk without assistance he rates himself as no confidence that he can balance while performing any of the listed activities.

Early Intervention and Prevention of Complications

Individuals who suffer complications during the acute and sub-acute stages of recovery tend to have lower functional status at 1 year post-CVA. Early activity and upright posture (sitting or standing) can prevent complications such as deep vein thrombosis, pulmonary emboli, pneumonia, and falls.[60] In addition to these risk factors, progression of the lesion has been found to occur in 11% of patients,[61] after leaving acute care, and this is one of the major predictors of a change to a lower level of functioning or death after discharge. Monitoring vitals and systematic progression of activity is particularly necessary to ensure patient safety during the acute and sub-acute phases of rehabilitation.

Based on the evidence and these considerations, Mr. Brown's vital signs (blood pressure, pulse, and respiration rate) should be evaluated by the therapist, before, during, and after each session for signs of any abnormal response to activity such as a rapid rise in pulse, abnormal rise or fall in blood pressure, or new arrhythmia. Therapy should be mildly exerting, consistent with the **Borg Exertion Scale** (e.g., <12) (Box 11-2). During the acute stage, the goal is to get Mr. Brown sitting upright and working on active movement without stressing the cardiovascular system. Cardiovascular fitness training is not initiated until the sub-acute phase of rehabilitation.

In addition, studies in animal models of stroke have shown that intensive, early exercise can lead to increased inflammation, neuronal death, and increased motor dysfunction.[63–65] In these studies the animals were either forced to exercise at a high intensity or were forced to use their paretic limb immediately after the injury. Taken together, studies indicate that individuals post-stroke should be encouraged to pay attention to and use their paretic limbs as they are able as soon as possible post-stroke. Exercise and forced use should be reserved for the post-acute stage, approximately 3 to 5 days post-stroke. Initiation of exercise should be graded with careful attention paid to vitals and to neurologic signs.

Box 11-2 Borg Exertion Scale[62]

EXERTION DESCRIPTION	BORG RATING	ACTIVITY EXAMPLES
None	6	Sitting
Very, very light	7–8	Washing hands
Very light	9–10	Washing dishes
Fairly light	11–12	Leisurely walking
Somewhat hard	13–14	Brisk walking
Hard	15–16	Maintained exercise to elevate heart rate
Very hard	17–18	Sustained activity at highest level possible
Very, very hard	19–20	Extreme burst of activity at maximum capacity

Data from Borg G.A. Psychophysical bases of perceived exertion. *Medicine and Science in Sports and Exercise.* 1982;14:377-381.

The acute period focuses on preventing complications, including contractures, infections such as pneumonia, thrombi in the extremities, skin breakdown, and postural hypotension. Clients should be encouraged to move all of their joints through the full ROM, three to five times a day, to maintain tissue extensibility and prevent contracture. One session per day of passive range of motion exercises with a therapist is minimally effective in maintaining normal tissue extensibility. Encourage the patient, family, and all healthcare workers to assist the client in moving his extremities on a regular basis and at least three times a day.

Skin breakdown is prevented through frequent position changes (at least every 2 hours), proper positioning to prevent pressure areas (see Table 11-5), and maintenance of healthy,

TABLE 11-5 Positioning in Bed for CVA: Need Images, Supine Needs to Show Ankle Supported in Neutral and Not Plantarflexed

SUPINE	SIDE-LYING ON INVOLVED SIDE	SIDE-LYING ON UNINVOLVED SIDE
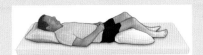	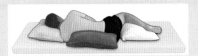	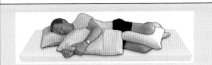

Keys to positioning

Involved shoulder should be in midline for abduction and flexion

Involved elbow, wrist, and fingers in extension

Involved forearm in neutral or supinated

Hips and knees slightly flexed

Hip neutral for rotation and slightly abducted

Involved foot on foot board or in orthotic to maintain neutral ankle and prevent from going into plantarflexion

Place pillows or padding at joints where there are bony prominences dry skin. Thrombi and postural hypotension are also prevented through active movement and frequent changes in position. Use of an upright posture, as soon as is medically possible, can prevent the occurrence of postural hypotension. If upright postures are not feasible, then active muscle contraction of the lower extremities encourages blood flow and reduces the risk of thrombi and hypotension. Activities that encourage deep breaths and increase the respiratory rate will assist in maintaining air flow throughout the lung tissue and are an effective means of preventing pneumonia. When doing activities with patients in the acute care setting, take time to instruct them to breathe deeply and monitor them to ensure that they are filling their lungs fully. Position changes that include upright postures of the trunk also assist in lung motility and prevent infections of the lung. Having the patient perform AROM as well as position changes throughout the day allows for intensive repetition during the acute phase of rehabilitation. The use of intensive repetition as a key to successful rehabilitation post-stroke will be discussed in more detail when the sub-acute and chronic phases of rehabilitation are discussed.

Hypertonicity of muscles may lead to contractures in these muscle groups (Table 11-6), and thus, positioning and ROM activities should focus on elongating potentially hypertonic muscle groups in order to prevent contracture and improve long-term prognosis, especially the ankle plantarflexors and hip flexors. Plantarflexors should be closely monitored for tone, and if increased tone is noted, the feet should be placed on a foot board, in an ankle contracture boot or static foot drop orthosis to prevent plantarflexion contracture and promote good ankle movement for transfers and mobility. Hip extension beyond neutral is a key component of normal gait. During the acute and sub-acute stages of rehabilitation, clients typically spend most of their day positioned in hip flexion, since they are sitting or lying down much of the day. Therapy should be designed to include

---

CASE A, PART IV

Mr. Brown should be encouraged to actively participate in all movements, whether he is able to do the movement or not. The therapist should provide assistance as needed and encourage Mr. Brown to look at the extremity, while it is moving, and to think about how it feels. Sensory stimulation of rubbing or a firm touch can also augment his ability to sense the extremity and better focus on activating the muscles. Imagery and visualization are effective means of improving motor control and should be utilized with Mr. Brown in the acute stage, when he is least able to tolerate rigorous exercise programs but can tolerate these types of therapeutic regimens.[66]

PROM and AROM into hip extension. This can be done in side-lying or prone positions.

Task-Oriented Practice

Therapy should be meaningful and encourage the use of activities or tasks to retrain motor control.[67] Early acute therapy, in the bed, should include active-assistive ROM to increase strength and motor control as well as initial rolling from supine to side-lying. Since AROM exercises are performed in both supine and side-lying, therapy should start with supine exercises and then move to side-lying where more exercises will then be performed. Intermingling strengthening exercises with functional activities minimizes unnecessary position changes and the impact of fatigue on therapy. Evidence shows that early trunk exercises, such as bridging, rolling in supine, and seated pelvic tilts, reaching and balancing activities on unstable surfaces, lead to improvement in not only trunk function but also standing balance and mobility in acute and sub-acute stroke.[68]

TABLE 11-6	Common Areas of Hypertonicity and Synergy Patterns after CVA		
	HYPERTONIC MUSCLE GROUPS	**FLEXOR SYNERGY PATTERN**	**EXTENSOR SYNERGY PATTERN**
Upper extremity			
Shoulder	Scapula retractors Adductors Internal rotators Extensors	Flexion Adduction Internal rotation	Extension Adduction Internal rotation
Elbow	Flexors	Flexion	Extension
Forearm	Pronators	Supination	Pronation
Wrist	Flexors	Flexion	Weak extension
Fingers	Flexors	Flexion	Weak extension
Lower extremity			
Hip	Flexors Adductors	Flexion Abduction External rotation	Extension Adduction Internal rotation
Knee	Flexors	Flexion	Extension
Ankle	Plantar flexors	Dorsiflexion	Plantarflexion Inversion

CASE A, PART V

If on initiating therapy, Mr. Brown is in supine and is not able to move the right extremities through the ROM against gravity, he should be encouraged to perform gravity-eliminated shoulder and hip abduction in supine. The therapist should provide him with a sliding board or assist to minimize friction between the extremity and the bed. In supine, he can also be assisted into a bridge position and to perform active bridging with the therapist helping to keep the pelvis level and to facilitate gluteal activation on the right, as needed. Facilitation of the gluteals is usually accomplished by applying a quick firm pressure into the lateral buttock with the fingertips. For an example see the video associated with our Laboratory Manual for Neurologic Rehabilitation, video 7-1 supine to sit. He can also work on exercises for the left upper and lower extremity.

Rolling/Bed Mobility

Rolling is an activity that can provide a great deal of benefit to the acute care client. It allows them to become more independent in pressure relief and position changes. Any independent movement is helpful in giving acute stroke clients a feeling of regaining control over their body and their lives and can be emotionally uplifting. When teaching bed mobility, the client should be encouraged to actively participate at all times, even if

CASE A, PART VI

Mr. Brown has been lying in supine for 2 hours; therefore, he should be placed in side-lying at the end of therapy to prevent skin breakdown due to pressure, especially given his diagnosis of prediabetes. He wishes to read or watch TV after therapy and would be better able to utilize the call button and manipulate books and TV controllers, if placed on his right side with his stronger left side unimpeded. The therapy session would end with Mr. Brown being taught to assist in rolling from supine onto his right side. Mr. Brown should be encouraged to actively roll, and the therapist should not provide any more assistance than is absolutely necessary. Positioning can be utilized to help Mr. Brown to obtain success with less therapist assistance, such as making sure that the right arm is flexed so that it does not end up trapped under the body and assisting Mr. Brown to cross his left leg over his right leg for rolling. The therapist can then place hands at shoulder and pelvis and assist Mr. Brown to use momentum to rock two times and then roll over on the third try. He should also be encouraged to use his head by turning it with the roll for additional momentum. He should be instructed as to where the call button, bed controls, and TV controller are located. Verify that he understands how to use them and position him appropriately in side-lying at the end of the treatment session (Table 11-5). Nursing should be told the time of the position change and what position he was placed in so that they know to reposition Mr. Brown within 2 hours.

they aren't able to provide meaningful help. The therapist should choose key points for hand placement that minimize therapist contact but allow optimal assistance to areas that are most impaired. Typically, placing the hands at the shoulders and hips is most helpful for bed mobility training. In addition, passive positioning can be used to preposition the client so that they are able to perform the transfer with minimal assistance from the therapist. It should be noted that handling always changes the motor output of the client and should be minimized in any way feasible, while keeping safety as a top priority.

Upright Activities

Once the client is cleared to begin upright activities, including transfers and gait, and is feeling able to participate in these activities, therapy should immediately initiate them; this typically occurs by day 2, barring extensive medical complications. See Box 11-3 on the use of imagery to facilitate movement and Box 11-4 for transfer and early gait activities. Examples of clients performing these activities can be seen in videos 7-1, 10-1, 10-2, 10-3, and 11-4 and detailed instructions are in Chapters 10 and 11 of the *Laboratory Manual for Neurologic Rehabilitation*. Arm function can be addressed in supine, side-lying, and sitting. Eccentric activation may be the easiest place to start for clients with profound weakness. To perform a low-level eccentric exercise for the elbow extensors, place the client in supine with the shoulder in 90 degrees of flexion and the elbow extended. The therapist supports the arm to prevent elbow flexion and instructs the client to slowly lower their hand to their mouth. The therapist provides assistance to slowly lower the hand and can provide sensory stimulation over the triceps to assist the client in developing an active contraction of this musculature. This activity allows the client to visualize the movement within a meaningful task; plus, the eccentric contraction, which slows the descent of the arm, will typically be regained prior to the ability to perform concentric activation of the muscle. Once the client successfully achieves an eccentric contraction, it is likely that they would be ready to progress to gravity-eliminated active movements.

Box 11-3   Motor Imagery

Motor imagery is done by instructing the individual to visualize how it feels to do a specific task. The therapist can have the client focus on certain aspects of the task such as visualizing how it feels to place equal weight through the feet for a sit to stand transfer or to bend forward with "nose over toes" during sit to stand. Studies have shown that adding motor imagery to conventional therapy can improve outcomes in post-stroke clients.[69] In order to ensure efficacy, the Movement Imagery Questionnaire – Revised, 2nd edition (MIQ-RS) should be used to ensure that the client is able to utilize imagery.[70] Some clients with poor sensory function have been found to have difficulty imagining motor movements, and therefore, would not be expected to respond to a motor imagery intervention. The benefit of motor imagery, in the acute stage of therapy, is that it provides an opportunity for intensive practice without adding physiologic demands and requires no additional time from the therapy staff.

Box 11-4   Techniques for Teaching Transfers and Gait in the Acute Setting

Keys to working on transfers

- Encourage the individual to be an active participant.
- The therapist should not provide any more assistance than is absolutely necessary.
- Positioning of the extremities in positions that lead into the movement can be utilized to help obtain success.

Supine to side-lying

- Utilize passive positioning to minimize therapist assistance: make sure that the bottom arm is flexed so that it does not end up trapped under the body; if moving onto the non-paretic side, cross the paretic leg over non-paretic leg to position for rolling (the client should be encouraged to assist with this positioning, as able).
- The therapist can then place hands at shoulder and pelvis to assist the client to use momentum to rock twice and then roll over on the third try.
- Encourage head turning with the roll for additional momentum.

Side-lying to sitting on the edge of the bed

- Roll to side-lying facing the edge of the bed, using the techniques above.
- Drop the legs off of the side of the bed, once in side-lying. Encourage the client to use the non-paretic leg to assist in getting the paretic leg off of the bed but with as much active movement of the paretic leg as possible.
- To make the move from side-lying to sitting easier, the head of the bed may be placed in a slightly elevated position.
- Instruct to push on the bed with both arms as the legs are dropped over the edge of the bed.
- The therapist should provide assistance at the shoulder and pelvis only as needed.
- If the paretic arm is "on top," the therapist may wish to assist by placing the hand in a weight-bearing position.
- The therapist then places a hand on the client's hand to stabilize it in weight-bearing and places their other hand on the posterior aspect of the elbow to encourage active weight-bearing through the paretic arm.

Sit to stand from bed

- First, ensure that the feet are both flat on the floor with the hips and knees flexed to 90 degrees (or elevate the bed and place with hips and knees in a less flexed posture to make the transfer easier).
- Both arms should be placed in a position of weight-bearing during the transfer to encourage active movement and provide proprioceptive input in the early stages of recovery.
- The bedside table can be utilized to provide a stable surface for weight-bearing through bilateral arms. Bedside tables allow you to start with the table at a lower level and raise the table, as the client comes to standing, and then provide a stable surface for standing activities that allows for use of both arms.
- If there is reasonable function in the paretic hand, then the client can push off of the bed with bilateral UEs and then place the hands on a walker. Unilateral assistive devices should not be used for standing activities, as they encourage learned nonuse of the paretic UE and LE and do not promote equal weight-bearing bilaterally.

Early gait activities: acute care

- Equal weight-bearing and use of the paretic leg should be a focus at this stage in rehabilitation.
- During gait, devices that allow for use of bilateral UEs post-CVA are parallel bars, wheeled walkers with arm trough attached, and the bedside table.
- Early gait and standing activities should focus on upright trunk control, encouraging use of the paretic limbs, during gait, and use of a step-through pattern bilaterally.
- Therapist assistance with the paretic extremities can be provided, as needed, to advance the leg and brace the extremities for weight-bearing support.
- Regardless of ability, the client should attempt to actively take part in all movements to encourage recovery of movement, even in flaccid extremities.

CASE A, PART VII (DAY 2)

The order of activities practiced should be based on where Mr. Brown is when therapy begins (lying or sitting in bed) as well as his goals. Transfer activities, including supine to sit and back, come to sit on the edge of the bed, and sit to stand, are initiated first and followed by early ambulation activities. In this case, Mr. Brown has a wife who will assist him at home and has set a goal of returning to his home. Therefore, assisted transfers and gait are reasonable goals for discharge from acute care. Given his moderate paresis of the arm and leg, he is likely to require moderate to maximal assistance for upright activities initially. Having a second person to assist, on the first day of upright activities, would allow for the incorporation of more challenging activities. Mr. Brown would begin this session by working on supine to sit on the edge of the bed (Table 11-7). To prevent learned nonuse, Mr. Brown is instructed to try to use his right arm and leg for all activities. If he cannot use the extremity, the therapist positions it in weight-bearing and assists in holding the limb so that Mr. Brown uses it appropriately throughout all activities. Additionally, he is directed to be aware of his paretic limbs through sensory inputs such as looking at the extremities and sensory cues such as light touch and/or pressure applied by the therapist. Detailed instructions on the application of sensory cueing can be found in Chapter 11 of the *Laboratory Manual for Neurologic Rehabilitation*.

Remember that during the acute stage of recovery, it is important to focus on preventing learned nonuse. This is accomplished by focusing on appropriate weight-bearing bilaterally, during all activities, and incorporating the paretic extremities into all activities. While canes and hemi-walkers provide the most viable assistance for functional ambulation on return to home, these devices do not function as the most appropriate assistive device for retraining a normal gait pattern. Utilizing devices that require or allow for bilateral UE support encourages

TABLE 11-7	Bed Mobility and Trunk Activities
POSITION	**ACTIVITY**
Supine: feet flat, hips and knees flexed	Bridging – if weak the therapist can assist on the weak side. Therapist can also provide sensory cueing to the gluteals to assist in activating the musculature. • Purpose: Strengthen trunk and hip musculature
Supine going to side-lying	Reach with arm in direction of roll • Purpose: Strengthens flexors of the trunk Pull on bedrail with UE • Purpose: Strengthens shoulder girdle musculature and biceps
Side-lying	Pelvic tilts • Purpose: Gravity eliminated trunk and hip musculature strengthening
Sitting edge of bed	Therapist pushes on the client at the shoulders while client works to maintain sitting balance. Therapist should provide pushes in the anterior, posterior, and side to side planes. • Purpose: Isometric coactivation of postural trunk musculature for stabilization Reaching up and down and side to side in front of body. Always have client reach for something such as a cup or other object as this encourages the neural system to activate the hand. • Purpose: Strengthens trunk musculature, reaching higher activates trunk extensors, reaching to the side activates the trunk rotators Reach laterally on bed • Purpose: Strengthens the muscles for trunk side-bending Place hand on ball and roll ball away from body and back toward body using either arm • Purpose: Provides support during trunk activities for individuals with balance problems or extremely weak trunk musculature

equal weight-bearing and involves the paretic UE and LE in functional activities. During therapy, devices such as a wheeled walker with an arm trough, parallel bars, or the bedside table should be used to encourage the use of bilateral UEs in equal weight-bearing. Discharge timing and location will determine when it is necessary to teach the individual to utilize a unilateral device, such as canes and hemi-walkers. These devices should not be introduced until it is necessary for return to independent function, such as a discharge to home, for a higher functioning client, as they utilize a compensatory method of gait training rather than rehabilitating the client to optimal long-term function. A short session with these devices at the end of each therapy session could be used to ensure that the client will be able to use a unilateral device for function, while focusing the majority of therapy time on bilateral UE weight-bearing with a natural gait pattern that incorporates both LEs. The therapist should strike a delicate balance between the need to quickly move the client to independence in function and the need to rehabilitate for optimal neuroplasticity and full potential functional recovery. See Box 11-5 for key rehabilitation principles. The challenge

---

Box 11-5 Keys to Rehabilitation of Function

1. Begin by making the task less physically demanding and within the ability level of the client by doing things such as the following:
   a. Placing the extremity in a gravity-eliminated position or raising seat heights for transfers
   b. Progression involves making the task more physically demanding until the client is doing the task as it occurs in the natural environment
   c. Adding variability to task practice will strengthen the learning process and make it more generalizable to "real-life" situations
2. Begin by using the task that demands the movement pattern you are training and does not allow for success with compensatory patterns, such as the following:
   a. When training sit to stand with a focus on weight-bearing through the paretic leg, seating the client on an elevated surface will lower the physical demands and improve the likelihood of success; also, placing a soft object such as an egg carton or foam under the **non-paretic** foot will further force weight-bearing through the paretic leg.
   b. To progress the task, change the setup to increasingly allow more choice by the client. For example, in the scenario above, the goal is to work on weight-bearing with the paretic leg by restricting the ability to weight-bear through the non-paretic extremity. Progressions would allow the client more choice as to how much weight to bear through the paretic limb. One progression might be:
      i Egg carton under non-paretic foot – forcing weight-bearing on paretic leg
      ii Use of an assistive device such as a pole or table on the paretic side – forces the client to lean over the paretic side with some weight-bearing through the non-paretic leg
      iii Use of an assistive device such as a pole or table in front of the client – allows the client to choose how much weight to bear on each leg. The goal is to have equal weight-bearing through the legs.

for therapists is functioning within the healthcare environment, while focusing on what is in the best interest of the client, who is s/p CVA. Compensatory techniques achieve fast results for return to function but impede neuroplasticity and full recovery of function.

Assistance Levels

When documenting, it is important to accurately depict the amount of assistance required by the client during each activity. The appropriate method for identifying level of assistance is described in Chapter 10. The key to good therapy practice is to first and foremost set up the practice session in a way that ensures patient safety. A goal is to minimize the amount of help that the therapist has to provide and to optimize active involvement of the patient. For Mr. Brown to work on a sit to stand transfer it would be ideal to start from an elevated plinth with a firm surface. The plinth would be elevated to a level that enables Mr. Brown to do the sit to stand transfer with as little help as possible, ideally CGA. Since his right arm remains paretic, it should be incorporated into the transfer by placing it in a position of weight-bearing, both during the transfer and once standing.

CASE A, PART VIII (DAY 2)

Mr. Brown comes to sitting on the edge of the bed with instruction and moderate assist of the therapist. He then works on his sit to stand transfer and standing balance using the bedside table for bilateral UE support. With a gait belt on and a wheelchair close at hand, he can attempt a few steps, using the bedside table as a wheeled walking device. The bedside table is beneficial for these activities, at this stage, because its height can be rapidly changed as Mr. Brown goes from sit to stand and returns to sitting from standing. Another option is the wheeled walker. Mr. Brown's hand can be placed on the walker and assisted to grasp by the therapist. He can then walk with the therapist helping to guide the walker and to advance his right leg. Ambulation should be initiated by having Mr. Brown take a step with his non-paretic (left) leg so that he immediately assumes weight-bearing on the paretic, right leg. This also places his right hip in extension, which will facilitate initiation of stepping (swing) on the right. The main peripheral drivers for activating the gait pattern generator involve hip extension, during stance, and alternately loading and unloading the lower limbs.[71] Since Mr. Brown is being discharged to a rehabilitation unit in 2 days, it is determined that working on ambulation with the wheeled walker is the most appropriate course of action for optimizing neuroplasticity and return to function. If he were returning home, gait training would be broken into two parts: (1) gait with the walker to work on relearning an appropriate and functional gait pattern and (2) gait with a hemi-walker or cane to learn a functional gait for use in the home environment with his wife.

CASE A, PART IX (INPATIENT REHABILITATION)

Mr. Brown was transferred to the inpatient rehabilitation hospital on his fourth day post-stroke. His intake reveals mild spasticity developing in his ankle plantarflexors with 3/5 strength in quads, hams, and hip flexors, 2/5 strength in dorsiflexors, plantarflexors, and gluts. His arm has 3/5 strength in the shoulder, 2/5 in flexors, and 1/5 in extensors of the elbow, wrist, and hand. He has moderate subluxation (grade 2) of the shoulder. Expressive aphasia persists, but he is able to utter single-word responses to some questions. He is able to come to sitting at bedside, by rolling to his left and pushing up with left arm, and performs a standing pivot transfer into the wheelchair with minimal assistance. Weight-bearing is asymmetrical, but he is able to stand, using a quad cane, and walked 12′ × 2 with moderate assist of 1, during his first treatment session.

Spasticity: What Is It and How Is It Medically Managed?

Spasticity is a sign of an upper motor neuron lesion and presents as both an increase in muscle tone (**hypertonia**) and exaggeration of tendon reflexes (**hyperreflexia**). Hypertonia in spasticity is a resistance to stretch that is velocity dependent, which means the faster you stretch, the greater the resistance to that stretch. This is referred to as the **tonic stretch reflex**. The cause of spasticity has received extensive research and is ongoing; however, there are multiple components at both the neurological and muscular levels. First, loss of corticobulbar projections results primarily in a loss of inhibitory control within the brainstem, creating some degree of unopposed excitation in remaining neural networks. This unopposed excitation has historically been referred to as a **release phenomenon**. The pontine reticular formation's descending pathway is known to facilitate upper extremity flexion (shoulder adductors and flexors, biceps, and wrist and finger flexors) and lower extremity hip flexors, hamstrings, and ankle plantarflexors. This facilitation is typically balanced by corticobulbar (cortex to medullary reticular formation) and corticospinal (cortex to the alpha motor neuron) inhibitory control and facilitation of opposing muscles via motor neurons in the spinal cord. Following stroke, corticospinal and corticobulbar fibers are often damaged. Thus, the reticulospinal fibers are "free" to produce unopposed excitation of the respective muscles in the extremities, leading to low-level muscle fiber contraction that is perceived as increased resting muscle tone. This hypertonia is accompanied by hyperreflexia of both the tonic and phasic stretch reflexes in spasticity. The **phasic stretch reflex** is the monosynaptic reflex, often referred to as a tendon reflex or tendon "jerk," and elicited by tendon tapping that activates Ia fibers from the muscle spindle that synapse directly on alpha motor neurons in the spinal cord, eliciting a quick responsive muscle contraction of the associated muscle. Hyperreflexia of the phasic stretch reflex also results from the loss of inhibitory influences, not in the brainstem, but in the synaptic junction between muscle spindle Ia fibers and alpha motor neurons. This allows the reflex activation to occur without descending inhibition (Figure 11-9). Whether or not spasticity develops and the magnitude of the spasticity, when it occurs, appears related to the location of the lesion and the degree of corticospinal and corticobulbar fiber damage; rehabilitation programming that focuses on recovery of isolated muscle function is important to maximize functional recovery and minimize spasticity development.[70,72,73]

Twenty to thirty percent of stroke survivors with hemiparesis will develop spasticity with onset typically in the first 3 months post-stroke. In only about 4% of survivors is the spasticity severe.[72] Spasticity is commonly measured by the original Ashworth Scale or modified Ashworth Scale[74] as described in Chapter 10. Although changes in neuronal activity are a primary influence in spasticity development, spasticity is also associated with changes in the muscle. These changes include loss of sarcomeres, infiltration of the muscle with collagen, changes in muscle fiber type, especially the ratio of fast to slow twitch muscle fibers, and, thereby, changes in the contractility and passive elasticity of muscle fibers.[73] There is much debate over the relationship between neurologic changes and muscular changes, especially as to whether the neurologic changes induce the muscular changes, but this has yet to be determined. Neither the Ashworth nor the

Modified Ashworth Scale effectively distinguishes the neural contribution from the muscle contribution to spasticity.[74]

Early management of spasticity typically includes range of motion activities with stretching, potentially fitting with braces or splits to provide passive elongation and facilitate movement, and functional activities to improve muscle strength and improve mobility. Neuromuscular electric stimulation has also been used to decrease spasticity when applied to the antagonist of the spastic muscle.[72]

PHYSICAL THERAPY MANAGEMENT IN THE REHABILITATION SETTING

During the first few days in the rehabilitation setting, clients are often still in the acute stage of recovery. This means that they remain medically fragile and easily fatigable, adding to the challenge of achieving optimal function in the short time frame that is reimbursable. Neuroplasticity remains a crucial element of the recovery process and must be considered alongside the pressures to regain independence in order to send the client to home or a lower level of care. Rehabilitation is focused on relearning functional tasks with impairments addressed within the practice of the functional tasks, when possible, and if not, then separately. It is often reasonable for clients to work on impairment-level therapy tasks on their own, such as ROM and strengthening exercises.

Intensity, Duration, and Frequency

When prescribing physical activity or exercise as an intervention it is important to consider intensity, duration, and frequency. While these are key components of exercise prescription, it is only recently that studies have begun to explicitly examine these factors. In recent years intensity has become a focus of clients, clinicians, and researchers. Early studies indicated that intensity matters, and the higher the intensity the better.[75] Yet, what do we mean by intensity? It is important that we define intensity clearly when deciding on the best evidence-based intervention for our clients. Exercise **intensity** refers to how hard the body is working. We can challenge the cardiovascular, pulmonary, muscular, sensory, or cognitive systems. When prescribing exercise it is important to challenge the system you are working to improve. It is also important to consider safety when working to provide an intervention that challenges the body. For the cardiovascular and pulmonary systems this means we need to consider the recommendations of the American Heart Association. In a recent statement, they raise safety concerns related to long-duration, high-intensity aerobic exercise in sedentary individuals and those with pre-existing cardiovascular disease; this is likely to apply to many of our clients post-stroke. They state that long-duration, high-intensity exercise can lead to potential cardiac maladaptations such as accelerated coronary artery calcification, myocardial fibrosis, and atrial fibrillation.[76] There are some who believe that the dose-response relationship is reversed J-shaped rather than curvilinear, resulting in potential loss of health benefits at the highest intensities of exercise, especially if it is longer duration exercise such as seen in things like triathlons.[73] Indeed, recent studies in patients with heart failure and stroke showed

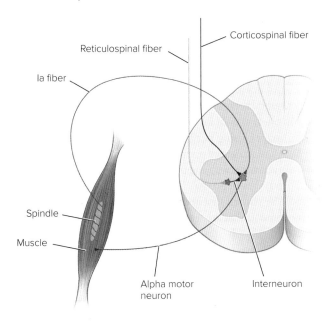

FIGURE 11-9 Illustration of hypertonia and hyperreflexia mechanisms. Loss of upper motor neuron fibers within the corticospinal tract removes inhibition from the reflex circuit within the spinal cord, creating increased excitability of the alpha motor neuron to Ia fiber activation. Further upstream, loss of corticobulbar fibers to the brainstem allows a net increase in facilitation to the monosynaptic reflex circuit from reticulospinal neurons, primarily through interneurons within the ventral horn. It should be noted that both inhibitory and excitatory interneurons are located within the ventral horn to modulate reflex activity. These interneurons are activated by many descending motor systems (corticospinal, reticulospinal, vestibulospinal), but when a stroke damages both corticospinal and corticobulbar fibers, the hypertonia that emerges seems driven by reticulospinal influences on alpha motor neurons to upper extremity flexors and lower extremity extensors. Secondary changes in muscle fibers emerge over time because of changes in innervation and contribute to the hypertonia and hyperreflexia seen, especially in more severe stroke.

Corticospinal fiber

Reticulospinal fiber

Ia fiber

Spindle

Muscle

Alpha motor neuron

Interneuron

no benefit of high-intensity exercise over guideline-based physical activity in peak VO$_2$.[77,78] Recent studies have begun to appear that question whether or not high intensity is always superior to moderate or light intensity. Many studies investigate aerobic intensity, defining high intensity as $\geq$60% of peak heart rate or $\geq$14 Borg rating of perceived exertion.[79] In the clinical setting, reaching these high intensities can be difficult with only 38% of total sessions in a hospital-based, acute stroke population reaching RPE of $\geq$14 or 85% of HRmax.[80,81] Importantly, when therapists focused on challenging their clients to work at the highest feasible intensity they were able to achieve, improvements in gait speed and endurance (6MWT) occurred, and participants tolerated the intervention well with no adverse events.[82] Exercise can also be continuous or interval (exercise period alternating with a rest period). High-intensity interval training or HIIT has become popular due to the potential to provide exercise at an appropriate intensity in a shorter duration.[75] There are also some early indications that it may be better accepted than high-intensity continuous exercise. Interval training also appears to be able to provide the same benefits as moderate-intensity continuous exercise. Clients who are post-CVA have tolerated these trials with no increase in adverse events, but it should be noted that these are younger individuals with mean age typically in the mid-50s, who have been cleared by their physician as safe to undertake this intense exercise program. Number of steps taken during gait training has been identified as an important consideration in gait training with HIIT protocols, providing more steps per session than standard therapy and significant improvements in locomotor outcomes.[80,82] There are studies that examine high-intensity protocols for strengthening. It is also possible to moderate intensity of effort by challenging balance and cognitive load (dual task) with perturbation during treadmill training, achieving better results than treadmill training alone.[83] Studies have not yet addressed the impact of level of intensity on these parameters. In studies of upper extremity function, the intensity is typically measured by number of repetitions. A recent randomized controlled trial of high-intensity training as compared to low-intensity resistance training in the upper extremity poststroke showed that both groups improved arm function with no superiority of high-intensity training.[84] A final consideration is compliance. Compliance with physical activity recommendations in individuals post-stroke is very low. Any intervention needs to be clinically feasible for the individual and result in long-term participation in physical activity.[85] **A key concept for any intervention is that it has to safely challenge the individual whether it be cognitive, aerobic, balance, or strength.**

Intensive Practice: Upper Extremity

Based on evidence from both basic science and clinical studies, learned nonuse is a negative outcome of poor rehabilitation of individuals post-stroke; it is recommended that early therapy encourage meaningful use of the paretic UE, which is often more impaired than the LE. Again, the paretic arm should be included in all activities and compensatory techniques should be avoided. In the case of a flaccid UE, the therapist should place it in a position of weight-bearing and then support it throughout transfers and gait so that weight is born as it would normally be, during all functional activities. In addition, the client should be encouraged to try to actively move the extremity during all PROM activities. An essential component of early therapy is to provide assistance as needed but no more than needed. In this way, the client experiences success in completing meaningful, active movement. Passive movement without actively engaging the client has not been shown to maintain range of motion but not to improve active movement of the paretic arm. Thus, robotic training that provides only passive limb movement is unlikely to improve motor function but may maintain range of motion; robotic training that adjusts to the volitional movement of the patient may improve movement within the limited repertoire of the robot's directional motion.[86]

Notably, the intended use of the hand shapes the activation of the musculature throughout the UE.[87] If a client is to perform a reaching task, they must have a meaningful end goal for the hand in order to appropriately shape UE movement. If the intent is to do an open-handed push or slap, such as giving a high five, the activation patterns will be much different than if the end goal is to pull a thumbtack from a bulletin board. A high five involves hand and finger opening and primarily gross motor control of the arm, while pulling out the thumbtack requires fine motor control of the fingers and little to no finger extension. The force output and coordination required of these two tasks also differ with one being a highly coordinated, low force movement while the other allows for more error in both force production and aim of the hand. Clients who lack finger extension can benefit from performing reaching tasks with an end goal of grasping a large object that requires finger extension in order to grasp it successfully, such that hand opening is a natural goal of the movement. This encourages neural reorganization to recover the function of hand opening. The task should be relatively easy, and the therapist can assist with finger closing periodically to allow for positive reinforcement. A task-oriented approach focused on performance of normal daily activities with the paretic hand can be highly beneficial and encourages neuroplasticity as well as functional return. Tasks should be chosen that are meaningful to the client and that involve movements that are feasible for the client but have not yet been mastered. The physical demands can be altered to enhance performance, such as placing the hand on a smooth table to practice elbow flexion/extension, during a reaching task in a gravity-eliminated position. This positioning also minimizes the degrees of freedom by supporting the arm such that the shoulder and trunk musculature does not have to provide this support. See Box 11-6 for a summary of the keys to the rehabilitation of the UE.

Bilateral training is another method that is successful in returning function to the UE after CVA. This type of therapy involves performing the same task with both hands at the same time but independently.[88] Both fine motor and gross motor tasks can be utilized during bilateral training.

This method is thought to normalize interhemispheric inhibition and improve lesioned hemisphere activity.[89] Many tasks can be practiced, such as stacking blocks, erasing a blackboard, flipping cards. It has been found to improve both ipsilesional and contralesional arm function.[89,90]

Techniques to Improve Motor Activation and Control in the UE and LE

The use of **functional electrical stimulation (FES)** has also been shown to be helpful both with unilateral and bilateral training

---

Box 11-6 | **Keys to the Rehabilitation of the UE**

1. The hand shapes the activation of the entire UE
2. Use meaningful tasks
3. Lower physical demands by
   a. Placing the extremity in a gravity-eliminated position for the key musculature
   b. Provide support to the trunk and proximal musculature to minimize degrees of freedom and focus on one joint motion
4. Choose functional tasks that will produce the movements that are the focus for that client's therapy session. Examples:
   a. For hand opening, have them reach for a 12-ounce soda can or small ball to encourage finger and wrist extension with a goal of lifting a relatively light object. This activity can also focus on the use of elbow extension in combination with shoulder flexion (moving out of synergy patterns).
   b. For coordination, have the individual reach for a small target and push on it.
   c. For fine motor control, have the client reach for a small object and remove it and then place it in another location. Example: remove thumbtack from bulletin board and place in small container for storage.

---

and in the UE and LE. Studies using functional electrical stimulation (FES) on the wrist and finger extensors during bilateral wrist extension activities demonstrated functional return of active wrist and finger extension.[91,92] The study by Sasaki et al. provides evidence that FES impacts areas of the brain related to sensory afferents indicating a role of the sensory system in recovery of function that appears to be positively impacted by the addition of FES during functional hand activities.[92] FES has been shown to improve gait speed when in conjunction with conventional therapy and alone.[93,94] Similarly, **mirror activities** benefit UE recovery.[95,96] Mirror activities involve placing a mirror between the limbs such that the client sees the non-paretic limb in the mirror. When the non-paretic limb is moved, it gives the illusion of normal movement in the affected limb. It is hypothesized that observing mirrored movements causes additional neural activity in motor areas located in the affected hemisphere, which should lead to cortical reorganization and improved function.[97-99] It is believed that mirror neurons, which are active both while performing and when observing an action, play a key role. Two systematic reviews have concluded that mirror therapy has significant effects on upper and lower extremity function.[98,99] The key to all of these therapeutic activities is that they involve active participation of the client in attempting to move the paretic extremity in a meaningful way.

Intensive Practice: Gait

As the client stabilizes, it now becomes feasible to focus on the concept of intensive practice for gait. Intensive practice is well supported by the literature and means a high number of repetitions are required to learn or relearn a skill. The literature on constraint-induced therapy and treadmill training leads us to believe that the number of repetitions needed is in the range of hundreds to thousands. This number can be difficult to achieve

using traditional therapy methods. Delivery that occurs only when the therapist is present limits the total time spent practicing the skill as well as the number of repetitions that can be feasibly accomplished. Therefore, clinicians and researchers have been investigating methods for providing practice opportunities on a frequent basis throughout the day. One very effective means of doing this is to utilize a team approach such that each team member knows how the client performs motor skills and activities of daily living. In this way, the client will be performing the learned tasks in the same manner, no matter who is with him, so that every repetition practices the correct and most beneficial means of doing the task. If the client is allowed to do tasks in an inappropriate manner, using poor motor control or only the non-paretic extremity, then they will end up doing many more repetitions of the wrong technique than of the prioritized technique emphasized in therapy. Therefore, it is imperative that skills be practiced not only in therapy but also when outside of therapy, in order to ensure that the number of repetitions of correct motor patterns exceeds the repetitions of incorrect motor patterns.

Another method of gait training that allows for intensive practice is **treadmill training** with a harness. Utilizing a treadmill with a harness can minimize therapist assistance and allow for gait training with fewer staff. The treadmill also allows for the consistent practice of a symmetrical gait over hundreds and thousands of repetitions. The harness can be used for body-weight support (BWS), if the client has difficulty maintaining upright posture without assistance. Relatively few studies have examined the benefits of BWS treadmill training in the acute–sub-acute phase of recovery, for individuals who require assistance from a therapist to ambulate, but, in the few studies that have provided early body-weight-supported treadmill training, a positive benefit has been reported.[100-102] Treadmill training using a high-intensity interval training paradigm results in improvements in gait speed, endurance, and balance.[80,82] HIIT involves alternating activity and rest for either short (30-60 second) intervals or long (4-minute) duration intervals with equal rest at a lower intensity.[75] Studies in spinal cord injury and stroke indicate that treadmill training should be augmented with or rapidly progressed to over-ground gait training due to the impact of task-specific training parameters (Box 11-7). The LEAPS trial provides evidence that, once an individual can ambulate independently with a device, it can be equally effective to train gait over-ground.[103] In addition, studies into neuroplasticity indicate that the impact of treadmill training on neuronal changes differs between individuals in the acute stages and those further into the sub-acute stage of recovery.[104] Combined, these findings further support the need to retrain a reciprocal and symmetrical gait pattern early in the recovery process.

Box 11-7 | **Parameters for Treadmill Training in the Post-stroke Population**

- Start with an initial velocity of 0.25 m/second and 30% BW in non-ambulatory patients[28]
- Treadmill speed should be increased incrementally as soon as possible
- Body-weight support should be reduced incrementally as soon as possible

Case Example

Mr. Brown is ambulating over-ground with a quad cane and moderate assist of one person. This does not afford him intensive practice of gait nor does it allow or promote a reciprocal gait pattern. It may be that Mr. Brown would be a good candidate for treadmill training to allow for more repetitions of a reciprocal gait pattern with less therapist support. He could continue to practice over-ground gait after each treadmill session, and as his gait and distance improve, he would be weaned off of the treadmill and onto a more task-oriented over-ground gait training program.

Both over-ground and treadmill training should focus on a reciprocal gait pattern that involves fully loading and unloading the paretic limb as well as taking a full step length; this will allow swing to be initiated from a position of hip extension. The treadmill is a very effective means of encouraging equal weight-bearing, symmetrical stepping, and the use of hip extension at terminal stance. Research has established that the gait central pattern generator is triggered when these components are present.[105] When doing over-ground training, it is suggested that early in the training process these components can be facilitated by instructing the client to take the first step with the non-paretic limb. A step, large enough to place the non-paretic foot in front of the paretic foot, should be encouraged to facilitate loading of the paretic limb and an extended hip position just prior to swing. This would activate the gait pattern generator, which will further assist in achieving a reciprocal gait pattern. Any assistance provided should be kept to a minimum and faded as quickly as possible. FES can also be beneficial during gait training. It can be used to assist with any muscle group but is most commonly applied to the tibialis anterior, often during both over-ground and treadmill-based gait training. Mr. Brown has significant weakness in his right dorsiflexors and would be a candidate for the use of FES on the tibialis anterior, during gait training.

Case Example

Clients should be encouraged to self-assess their performance and correct errors, based on this assessment. Mr. Brown has significant expressive aphasia, which would make it difficult for him to describe his performance to his therapist. This does not mean that he cannot perform self-assessment. He should be instructed to think about how the motor task felt and then asked some yes/no questions about his performance such as: "do you think you were putting equal weight on your right and left legs?" It may be appropriate to say something like, "that seemed to take a lot of effort, do you think you can do it in a way that would be less effortful?" If Mr. Brown indicates he is able to identify the difficulties in the activity, then have him try again and watch to see if he makes appropriate modifications. If he does not appropriately modify his movement, it would be appropriate to provide feedback as to what you are seeing and how to perform the activity in a way that will result in better overall coordination and motor

control. A common example would be that Mr. Brown may be attempting to transition from sit to stand with most of his weight on his left leg, while reaching for the assistive device with his left hand. After self-assessing, he places his left hand on the chair and pushes off from the chair with this hand but continues to place most of his weight over the left leg. The therapist would then tell him, "that was good that you used your arm to push up from the chair, this time also use your right arm to push and try to also stand up on your right leg." Mr. Brown's communication could be augmented with the use of a writing pad and a picture board so that he can point to pictures, depicting common areas of communication, such as a restroom and food. If the client has receptive aphasia demonstration is the most appropriate method of instruction.

Another method for enhancing time to practice and, therefore, intensity of practice is the use of group therapy.[106] This can be effective if common pitfalls are avoided. The common pitfalls are allowing individuals to practice a task using poor technique or compensatory strategies and failure to adequately supervise for safety. It is important that the leader be trained to watch for and identify errors and to intervene, by pointing these errors out to the client and assisting him in correcting them. Group therapy should not replace individual therapy time, as clients require one on one time to develop the skills necessary to effectively practice skills before performing them in a group setting. Safety must be ensured for all clients in the group. If adequate staffing is not provided for the task practiced, this can result in unsafe situations or limited practice for members of the group that are unable to perform all skills, due to safety concerns.

Task-Oriented Therapy: Sit to Stand to Sit Transfers

A key functional activity is the sit-to-stand (STS) and stand-to-sit (SIT) transfer. Being able to complete these transitional movements is a critical gateway skill between seated activities and standing and walking activities. If unable to independently transfer in and out of chairs, toilets, and beds, the person will be unable to live alone. STS requires skills, such as coordination between trunk and lower limb movements, muscle strength, control of equilibrium, and stability.[107] The goal of transfer training is to teach the client to develop the ability to transition from STS and SIT in a manner that is safe, efficient, and allows subsequent motion to occur. Clients with hemiplegia tend to perform the STS transfer with incoordination of the hip and knee, characterized by full knee extension occurring while the hips are still extending.[108] The trunk leans toward the less affected side. Placing the paretic foot behind the non-paretic foot corrects this trunk asymmetry.[109] In addition, when leaning forward, clients with hemiplegia do not displace their center of pressure as far anteriorly as do healthy controls due to the use of upper trunk flexion and limited anterior pelvic tilt.[110] Performing focused practice of STS and SIT from different surfaces in the rehabilitation setting an extra 3 times a week, 3 sets of 5 repetitions minimum, resulted in more clients attaining independence and attainment of independence more rapidly than those in standard care.[111]

Task practice is set to provide a setup that is appropriately physically demanding and includes variability. In addition, the task setup initially limits the client's ability to use compensation and progresses to a task setup that requires the client to use their motor planning to choose the best way to complete the activity. Refer back to Box 11-4 for training strategies. Clients with hemiplegia tend to perform transfers without fully incorporating the paretic extremities. A focus of task-oriented practice is getting the client to incorporate the paretic extremities in the transfer. In addition, clients may have difficulty with balance and weight shifts. One example would be the client who goes from standing to sitting by falling backward onto the surface. Training would involve raising the surface so that the transfer is appropriately physically demanding and teaching correct kinematics of hip and knee flexion with eccentric control of descent. One task setup that encourages appropriate kinematics for SIT is to have the client perform a forward reaching task while doing the SIT transfer.

Research studies examining best interventions for STS and SIT are limited to date but have supported the beneficial impact of training on time to complete and lateral symmetry.[112]

Gait

Over-ground gait training should include training to maneuver around obstacles, walk on different surfaces (rough, smooth, soft, hard, sloping), change speeds, and perform dual tasks (talking, carrying something). The use of task-oriented gait training can assist in promoting a more normal gait pattern. This task-oriented approach works by encouraging the client to solve the motor problem while minimizing assistance and feedback from the therapist. It is also meaningful in that everyday tasks that the client wishes to perform, after returning home, are utilized for this training process.[113] Suggested task-oriented activities for gait and transfers are given in Table 11-8 and an example therapy session is described in Box 11-8.

TABLE 11-8	Task-Oriented Approaches to Training Transfers and Gait Post-CVA	
ACTIVITY	**MOVEMENTS ENCOURAGED**	**MOVEMENTS DISCOURAGED**
Transfers		
Transfer sit to stand with an egg carton or other "soft" object under the uninvolved LE	Weight-bearing on the paretic LE	Unilateral weight shift onto the non-paretic side
Transfer sit to stand with a bedside table in front and utilized for bilateral UE weight-bearing	Equal weight-bearing in bilateral UEs and LEs Forward weight shift for transfer initiation	Discourages posterior weight shift when straightening up to stand
Transfer sit to stand with a pole positioned in front and to the paretic side with both hands on the pole, non-paretic hand holding paretic hand on pole	Forward weight shift for transfer initiation Weight shift to the involved side Weight-bearing on involved LE Upright trunk, position hands high on pole to get upright trunk	Discourages posterior weight shift when straightening up to stand
Gait		
Walking while repetitively stepping with the paretic LE over a low board that extends 12″ laterally	Swing with hip, knee, and ankle flexion Facilitates dorsiflexion	Swing with abduction as the primary means of advancing the leg
Walking up a slope	Hip flexion – to advance the leg Dorsiflexion – to clear the ground Muscle activity is increased in the hip, knee, and ankle extensors to propel the body uphill	Knee hyperextension
Walking down a slope	Knee extensors Encourages trunk extension to hold the person upright Requires eccentric gluteal activation and can increase strength in these muscles Also requires eccentric activation of the dorsiflexors to control for foot slap and can be used to strengthen these muscles	
Repetitively stepping over small objects with the non-paretic LE	Weight-bearing on the paretic LE	Decreased stance on the paretic LE
Walking with the paretic side next to a wall	Encourages the use of hip flexion for swing	Discourages circumduction for swing
Walking on uneven and soft surfaces	Encourages dorsiflexion Challenges balance	

Box 11-8	Circumduction/Circumducted Gait Pattern

One type of common gait deviation occurs when there is difficulty advancing the foot, typically due to a foot drop, resulting from lack of activation of the dorsiflexors. This often results in a **circumducted/circumduction** gait pattern, characterized by abduction of the hips and movement in a circular fashion to advance the leg. If there is 2/5 or greater strength in the dorsiflexors and a 3/5 or greater strength in the hip flexors, the use of small obstacles can provide a means of eliciting dorsiflexion in stepping over the obstacle, rather than circumduction, and facilitating neural reorganization to achieve a more normal gait pattern. Another activity, to address circumduction, is to place a long low board in front of the client such that they have to step over the board with their paretic LE, repeating for as many consecutive steps as necessary to change the pattern. The board should be long enough that it will block circumduction. The height of the board will encourage the use of hip, knee, and ankle flexion to clear the board. By using this technique the client has to problem-solve how to get over the board and the task has been constrained in such a way as to block the use of abnormal movement patterns and only allow the motor pattern that the therapist wishes to retrain. Table 11-8 lists a number of common gait deviations and some examples of tasks that can be utilized to encourage use of a more functional and appropriate motor pattern for that task.

After UMN injury, it is common for individuals to have difficulty with dual-tasking, such as walking while talking. To reintegrate into the community, the individual needs to be able to not only walk and talk at the same time but also to walk while reading directions on a map or carrying and manipulating objects. Studies have noted that the ability to dual-task often remains impaired after formal rehabilitation has ended. To regain and improve this skill, therapy should incorporate activities that involve dual-tasking, such as carrying a cup of water while transferring and ambulating, walking and talking, and reading signs and navigating while walking.[114] There are several outcome measures given in the appendix that are designed to assess dual-tasking skill, and these should be used to determine if there is a deficit in this area and to assess for mastery at the end of therapy.

Assistive Devices

The use of devices with wheels or over-ground harness support allows for a more normal step-through gait pattern. Studies utilizing treadmill training have demonstrated the importance of practicing gait with a step-through pattern to allow for the hip to go into extension just prior to swing.[105,115] This positioning is a trigger to initiating swing, even in spinalized animals.

Case Example

If you are not able to keep Mr. Brown's hand on the walker, the use of a wheeled walker with a trough may be necessary. It may be sufficient to place his hand on the walker with the therapist's hand over it to hold it in place. The therapist can then assist in guiding the walker. Pushing the wheelchair can provide good support that is heavier and won't tip over. Another method, when available, is to use harness support during over-ground gait training to assist the client with trunk control during gait. This method of training minimizes demands on the client for maintaining upright stance, allowing the client to focus on the stepping pattern. Studies have demonstrated that over-ground gait with partial body-weight support is an effective means of improving gait initiation, speed, and symmetry.[116,117]

Unilateral devices such as the cane and hemi-walker encourage a compensatory gait pattern with minimal weight-bearing and a shortened stance phase on the paretic side; usually, a step-to-gait pattern is used. This pattern is not normal, and thus,

could negatively impact neuroplasticity, during this early stage of recovery. The more time the client spends utilizing a gait pattern that encourages use of the paretic limb, the more likely the client is to recover to their full potential. If the client is able to use a unilateral device independently, they may do so in their room, but this does not preclude the use of bilateral devices during therapy to retrain gait with a more symmetrical gait pattern.[118]

Another common issue is the lack of dorsiflexion and ensuing foot drop during gait. This can be successfully managed with an orthotic device or FES.[119] Caution should be used in providing an orthotic device too early in the rehabilitation process as this too could impede neuroplasticity and full recovery of function. If the ankle is fully supported in dorsiflexion, then the normal triggers to activate the dorsiflexors are removed, and this may result in learned nonuse of this muscle group. The use of an ace-wrap can provide a low-cost alternative that enhances safety and the ability to work on ambulation, while allowing normal sensory and neural inputs to the ankle musculature. Individuals, wearing ace-wraps to assist in maintaining dorsiflexion, still sense the need to activate the dorsiflexors and can still fire both the dorsi- and plantar-flexor muscle groups. If available FES is a good option as it will assist with foot clearance and has been shown to stop muscle fiber conversion and promote neuroplasticity.[119] An additional issue, related to orthotic prescription, is reimbursement. Once an orthotic has been purchased, the client is no longer eligible to receive insurance reimbursement for a new orthosis for an extended period of time (at present it is 2 years). It is highly likely that the client will continue to make rapid and meaningful changes in strength, ROM, tone, and function for weeks to months after discharge from the rehabilitation setting. This is likely to lead to the need to obtain a different orthosis than was indicated in the rehabilitation setting. Therefore, every attempt should be made to wait as long as possible to obtain a definitive ankle orthosis so that the client will be encouraged to make optimal progress in rehabilitation of this musculature and, thus, assure the appropriate insurance coverage to assist in purchasing their final, optimal orthotic that matches their long-term functional abilities.

Spasticity: Medical Management in the Chronic Phase

Chronic spasticity is a challenge to manage and may be unresponsive to physical therapy interventions (stretching, splinting, NMES/FES, or strengthening). For those with localized spasticity in one or a few muscles/joints, they may benefit from botulinum toxin (botox) intramuscular injections; the most common type of botox used is botulinum toxin type A,[120] which has several varieties. These injections are applied within the spastic muscle and have a relatively localized effect; therefore, botox is not recommended when spasticity is widespread. Botox works by disrupting the release of acetylcholine, the neurotransmitter at the neuromuscular junction, which diminishes both tonic and phasic motor reflexes and, thereby, reduces spasticity. Changes in sensory neuron excitability, following injection, are thought to also have upstream implications in the spinal cord and brainstem that may contribute to the decrease in spasticity observed. Enhanced physical therapy, following injection, is thought to improve function through its ability to strengthen opposing muscles and maximize functional use of the extremity, while the botox is active. The effect of botox is transient, lasting 12 to 20 weeks before spasticity returns; repeated injections, up to three applications, have been found to continue the effect. There is some concern that repeated injections might induce immunological resistance; however, no such reaction was found with three sequential injections, spaced 12 to 16 weeks apart.[121]

Widespread spasticity can be most effectively treated through **intrathecal baclofen** infusion. Baclofen is a gamma amino butyric acid (GABA)-β receptor agonist, which means that it functions like the inhibitory neurotransmitter, GABA. When given orally, baclofen has trouble crossing the blood-brain barrier, and therefore must be given in large doses to affect peripheral spasticity; these doses can also cause headaches, sedation, and lethargy, which limit its desirability as a treatment method. Other oral medications, such as diazepam, dantrolene, and tizanidine, are also sometimes used but similarly induce side effects of sedation and lethargy that limit their use post-stroke.[122] However, intrathecal infusion is applied directly into the subarachnoid space of the spinal column, between the arachnoid and pia maters, with much better focal spinal effects and fewer central effects such as sedation. It is most commonly applied via an implantable pump that can deliver continuous infusion or periodic boluses. Often a single bolus infusion will be tried to determine effectiveness prior to a pump implantation; the effect of a single bolus is relatively short (hours) but can give some idea of what change in tone might be expected. Implantation at the level of T2–T4 has been found to maximize effectiveness for those with both upper and lower extremity spasticity, compared to the typical site of implantation at T11–T12,[123] where the effect is maximal for lower extremity spasticity. Progression from a continuous infusion to a periodic bolus may optimize effectiveness. Physical therapy intervention after implantation is critical to maximize the effectiveness and minimize side effects, as tone decreases, with emphasis on increasing the range of motion, strength, and function. Outcomes from baclofen infusion include not only decreased spasticity but also improved function, including mobility, walking speed, self-care, UE function, and work production; further, improvements have occurred years after stroke onset.[122,123] Initially, there was concern that baclofen infusion might result in diminished muscle strength on the non-paretic side due to the bilateral impact of baclofen infusion; however, this has not been documented in multiple trials. Notably, a common side effect is an initial decrease in function, following implantation. This results from the unmasking of weakness in spastic muscles or learned movement patterns

---

CASE A, PART X

Mr. Brown returned home 4 weeks after his stroke and was referred to home health physical therapy and after 8 weeks to outpatient therapy. He is walking independently for short distances with a quad cane and right AFO. Stairs require the use of the railing and the quad cane and +1 min assist of his wife in a step-to pattern. He requires +1 mod assist to do curbs or walk on inclines or uneven surfaces. Transfers from firm surfaces at least 18 inches tall are independent but he requires assist for couches and standard-height toilets. He uses a tub bench in his shower for bathing. Car transfers require +1 mod assist. He now has 2–3/5 strength in his elbow and shoulder muscles but limited hand movement. Spasticity in the fingers is noted, and the hand is partially fisted at rest; however, he can open the hand when reaching to touch a target. Grasp is facilitated by the spasticity, which makes release of objects difficult. He is using his left hand for all self-care activities; he has not resumed driving, due to the hemianopia. The aphasia is clearing with some continued word-finding problems. Despite his significant progress, he is depressed at his inability to drive and return to work.

---

that "use" the spasticity for function. Thus, this is a critical time for rehabilitation to address increasing strength and function. The methods for such rehabilitation are consistent with those described in the following sections.

PHYSICAL THERAPY MANAGEMENT IN THE HOME HEALTH AND OUTPATIENT ENVIRONMENTS

Mr. Brown is now medically stable and has become proficient enough in his basic activities of daily living that he is able to return home with the assistance of his wife. He is dealing with the psychological impact of his life-altering experience, and once in his home environment, the changes in his bodily function and ability to participate are more evident to him and his family. It is at this time that many of our clients face issues of depression and anxiety as they are beyond the crisis and now face life-altering changes on a daily basis. Recovery has slowed at this point and improvements will now be more a function of Mr. Brown's work than natural recovery. He continues to have the potential to improve his mobility and upper extremity function and should be encouraged to choose realistic short-term goals and acknowledge the weekly gains that he will be making as he works toward his long-term goals. His depression should be assessed and monitored and appropriately followed by the team, which should, at a minimum, include his physician and any nursing staff involved in his care and may involve a psychologist or counselor.

In the home environment, an intensive task-oriented training program is the most feasible approach. Once Mr. Brown can be transported to outpatient therapy without undue fatigue or hardship, therapy moves to that environment. Home-based therapy has the advantage of allowing the practice of functional tasks in the environment in which Mr. Brown will be functioning, while outpatient therapy has the benefit of allowing the use of more equipment and encourages Mr. Brown to begin moving about in the community environment. The LEAPS trial has demonstrated that ambulation and lower extremity function will respond well to a home-based approach while other studies involving circuit training and constraint-induced movement therapy have supported the use of these outpatient-based therapy programs.[103] Other issues to be tackled are Mr. Brown's increasing issues with spasticity and higher-level functional activities.

Task-Oriented Training: Uneven Surfaces

Mr. Brown has achieved modified independence in ambulation but continues to have difficulties with uneven surfaces such as curbs and steps. Early step training is beneficial both functionally and as a way to work on underlying impairments. Use of a low step can strengthen the paretic leg both concentrically (when stepping up with the paretic leg) and eccentrically when stepping down with the non-paretic leg. Stepping with the non-paretic leg encourages weight-bearing on the paretic leg. This activity should be started as early as possible. Many individuals develop a compensatory step-to pattern on the stairs that does not utilize the paretic leg. In addition, this pattern of stair climbing is slow and does not return the individual to normal community function. While it may be beneficial for expediting independence for a return to home, this method does not promote long-term return to participation goals. Practice of a reciprocal stair climbing pattern should be initiated when step training is started and continued until it becomes functional. Use of the compensatory step-to pattern should be utilized sparingly and only when necessary for safety. If the client is too weak to do standard height steps, the task can be made less physically demanding by using lower step heights, railings, and FES.

Task-Oriented Training: Transfers Low Surfaces

Mr. Brown is having difficulty with transfers onto surfaces that are low and/or soft as well as those that require maneuvering in order to approach them (e.g., car). Clients who have difficulties with these types of transfers generally require work on underlying impairments, such as strength, as well as on motor control. Functional practice that progresses from higher to lower and firmer to softer surfaces and is initiated early in rehabilitation leads to the development of flexible strategies for transferring in many different situations rather than a rigid motor plan that limits the individual to transferring from only a firm seat with armrests. It may take longer to develop independence when utilizing this approach, but the payoff in the end is a higher level of functioning.

Intensive Task-Oriented Training: Other Paradigms

Once the client is able to transfer in and out of the car in a functional manner, outpatient therapy can be initiated. The benefit of outpatient therapy is the access to equipment such as FES, treadmills, and perhaps even robotics or virtual reality. In addition, this environment allows for the use of training paradigms such as circuit training and constraint-induced movement therapy (CIMT). Circuit training as well as standard and modified CIMT have been shown to be effective in rehabilitating both motor impairment and function.[124–126]

Circuit Training

Circuit training is a method that involves setting up stations to practice specific skills or work on specific impairments. The client moves through a circuit, moving from station to station, and performing the activity or exercise at each station. The stations are set up such that the exercise or activity is individualized to each client as they move through that station. An example would be a station to work on sit to stand transfer training and lower extremity strengthening. At the station, there might be a standard height chair with a firm cushion or surface that can be placed in the chair to elevate the surface as well as a stool for a lower surface. Based on each client's physical capabilities and motor control, he/she would practice sit to stands from the chair that is appropriate for them. They would then progress, usually to the next lower surface, as their physical abilities and motor control improve. Progressions should challenge both motor control and physical limits. This training has been successfully utilized in an acute rehabilitation hospital setting (90-minute sessions, 5 days per week) and in sub-acute to chronic stroke in the outpatient setting. The stations can be supervised by staff or the clients can move through the stations in pairs. The use of pairs allows the partner to watch and give feedback on performance as well as document performance. Performance from the session is then used to motivate the individual at the next session. Examples of these programs can be found in the studies published by van de Port (outpatient)[124] and Rose (acute inpatient rehabilitation).[125]

Case Example

Circuit training for Mr. Brown would need to focus on both arm and leg function with stations that encourage grasp and release as well as control of grip force. In addition, he should do stations for transfers to low surfaces and surfaces that require maneuvering (car seat) as well as stations that encourage work on gait speed and gait over uneven surfaces such as curbs, slopes, and rough terrain. Mr. Brown was an athlete and might enjoy working with a partner who is also s/p stroke as this would encourage teamwork that he has enjoyed in the past. He might also have enjoyed and seen the benefits of a strength training program previously, and so, might appreciate the incorporation of some traditional strength training equipment into his circuit work. Other clients may not respond well to traditional strength training with weights or other equipment and would then be encouraged to do a strength training program that is based on functional activities such as sit to stand for quads and gluteals or toe tapping for the dorsiflexors.

Strength training can be done with traditional weights or through the repetition of functional activities.[127] If proper strength training protocols are followed (i.e., working to fatigue with 10 or fewer repetitions), then activities such as step-ups or sit to stand can be used to strengthen the hip and knee extensors. Tapping the foot to music may be sufficient to strengthen extremely weak dorsiflexors. The therapist has to set up the activity in a manner that works the key muscle groups to fatigue within the allotted number of repetitions, generally less than 10. The key to this therapy is the ability of the therapist to listen to the client and design an individualized program that incorporates meaningful activities for that client. This requires creative thinking skills as well as a strong understanding of the kinematics of movement across tasks and activities.

Constraint-Induced Movement Therapy (CI or CIMT)

CIMT, initially referred to as forced use, is a treatment paradigm focused on increasing the use of the paretic hand after stroke. This technique was initially described by Taub,[128] from his work with monkeys, and first implemented by Wolf in a clinic population.[129] For the monkeys, Taub found that restricting movement of the intact arm "forced" the monkey to use the deafferented arm, and by 2 weeks, it was impossible to differentiate the function of the arm from its pre-surgical state. This early work was verified in a large multi-site clinical trial, known as the EXCITe (extremity constraint-induced therapy evaluation) trial (2006) in sub-acute and chronic post-stroke participants.[130]

CIMT has traditionally been applied as a 2-week intervention with 6-hour practice sessions daily, 5 days per week; participants wear a sling or mitt that precludes use of the non-paretic limb for most of their waking hours so that the client focuses on using their paretic limb for most daily activities. A behavioral contract, signed by the participants, outlines exceptions to the mitt wear as well as activities to practice at home. Treatment is focused on high-intensity repetition of tasks (massed practice) with the paretic limb, following motor learning principles and shaping strategies. In other words, tasks are used that challenge the individual's current level of performance but can be made incrementally more difficult. Practice is varied, and feedback is provided in a variable manner but includes both knowledge of performance and results.

Some tasks that are commonly used include stacking blocks, placing shapes in a shape sorter, erasing lines on a chalkboard, playing checkers, or completing dot-to-dot tracings. Some household tasks such as folding or hanging up clothes, ironing, or dusting may be included. Tasks can be chosen to emphasize shoulder or elbow motion, hand opening/closing, individual finger motion, or some combination of movements, based on the participant's needs. Obviously, this form of treatment requires the participant to have some degree of hand and arm function; in fact, initial participants were required to have 90 degrees of active shoulder and elbow flexion with at least 10 degrees of wrist and finger extension at each joint. More recently, this method has been used with individuals with less function but some degree of hand and arm function needs to be present.[131] Also, multiple clinical trials have demonstrated that CIMT can be provided with less time in the clinic (as little as two 30-minute sessions weekly) and improves hand mobility; however, the traditional methodology seems most effective in changing self-care and participation post-stroke, based on a meta-analysis.[132] A more recent study found that CIMT provided to a group of 4 participants simultaneously was as effective as that provided to individuals.[105] Research needs to continue to evaluate alternative implementation methods, including telemedicine, to provide CIMT in a manner that more easily fits with insurance coverage and time for therapy post-stroke.

CIMT has also been administered to children with hemiparetic cerebral palsy from ages 18 months to the teenage years. Restriction of the non-paretic arm has included using gloves or hand splints,[133] slings,[134] and casts[135] for 2 hours/day to 24 hours/day; the CIMT protocol has been provided in intervals of 2 weeks, consistent with the traditional model, to 6 weeks, and in doses of 9 hours per week to 6 hours per day. In one study, using a uni-valved cast for 3 weeks and comparing dosages of 3 hours to 6 hours per day, equivalent upper extremity improvements were found for both doses, suggesting that 3 hours per day is sufficient to achieve improvement in hand mobility and use in daily activities.[134] Similar to the adult protocol, massed practice of age-appropriate play activities follows the principles of shaping and motor learning.

Sensory Training Post-stroke

Too often, sensory dysfunction, and its impact on motor recovery, is ignored. In the last decade, it has become evident that sensory dysfunction is much more common than previously thought, especially if sensory dysfunction across modalities (texture, weight, shape) is evaluated. Further, sensory function has been found to predict motor[136,137] and quality of life outcomes,[138] yet is rarely a focus of physical therapy intervention. There is some evidence that sensory function can be improved with high-intensity training protocols that are focused on sensory discrimination abilities.[25,139] There is also some suggestion that a training protocol that includes sensory discrimination activities that require active hand manipulation may improve motor function as well.[139] It is recommended that this type of treatment use training parameters consistent with shaping and motor learning principles, as described for CIMT; occluding vision, through the use of a curtain or other obstruction, allows for hand manipulation of items in tasks designed for sensory discrimination. Too often, vision allows compensation for sensory deficits, and thus, practice with vision may not force use of the sensory discrimination neural network. These same considerations should be applied to the lower extremity. While the foot is not used for manipulation it is important to train the use of sensory modalities for balance and coordination. Examples of tasks that can be used in sensory training for the upper extremity are: finding all of the puzzle edge pieces in a cloth bag, placing items in a shape sorter behind a curtain, and matching a texture felt with the non-paretic hand by manipulating match objects with the paretic hand.[25] A study that provided targets on the floor for foot placements as electrical stimulation was provided to the median plantar nerve found improved foot placement, during stimulation trials that was maintained after stimulation was removed.[140] Other tasks for the lower extremity would be walking while keeping the eyes up and ahead and not on the ground in front of the person, walking in dim light, and walking with head turns to challenge the postural control system. It should be noted that sensory discrimination dysfunction is often bilateral, so the non-paretic extremity may not have intact sensation for these types of comparisons.

Ankle Foot Orthotics: Clients who continue to have deficits in ankle dorsiflexion may require some type of external support to assist in clearing the foot during swing phase. Both AFOs and FES can improve walking speed, step length, and ankle dorsiflexion.[141] AFO prescription must be based on the client's biomechanical deficit and on clearly identified functional objectives and the client's prognosis. A critical consideration is to avoid over-prescribing control. AFOs should encourage recovery of function when possible and allow the individual to use their remaining function. Other considerations are listed in Box 11-9. Box 11-10 provides a list of types of AFOs currently in use and the key factors related to choosing between types of AFOs. A guiding principle is that the AFO should provide only the control that is necessary to obtain improved function. When assessing a client for an AFO and while using an AFO one must watch gait mechanics to assure that the AFO is having an overall positive impact on gait parameters. In addition, it is important to consider the energy cost of ambulation with and without an

Box 11-9	Orthotic Considerations

Orthotic Considerations
- Avoid over-prescribing control
- Device should not impede other functions
- Consider position of mechanical joints relative to anatomical joints
- Consider the weight of materials
- Compliance increases with comfort, cosmesis, and convenience
- Consider energy requirements
- Consider biological response (i.e., biomechanical and neurologic)
- Acute versus chronic condition

Box 11-10	Types of AFOs	
TYPE OF AFO		**CONSIDERATIONS**
SOLID		
		1. Solid AFO with trimline anterior to malleoli limits all foot and ankle motion. A broader posterior shell provides improved medial-lateral control. With the trimline placed anterior to the malleoli this AFO provides control of inversion and eversion of the ankle. As the trimline moves posterior to the malleoli control of inversion and eversion is lost.
		2. Posterior leaf spring – allows for greater motion with minimal limitation. Dorsiflexion assistance is achieved through flexion of the upright during early stance, allowing a minimal amount of plantarflexion. The upright acts as a spring. As the individual enters swing phase, the upright recoils, returning to its resting position and lifting the foot. Thinner, lighter plastic allows for relatively greater motion. Less control at the fore, mid, and hind foot.
		3. Spiral AFO – limits but does not eliminate motion in all planes. Also provides dorsiflexion assist through flexion of the upright during stance.
		4. Ground floor reaction AFO ("anti-crouch") – provides knee extension moment in stance to limit excessive flexion. Not commonly used in adults.

HINGED

Hinged AFOs provide support for frontal and transverse motion at the foot.

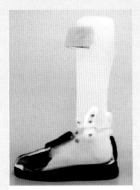

Plantar Stop (PS)

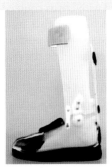

Dorsi Assist/Stop (DA-DS)

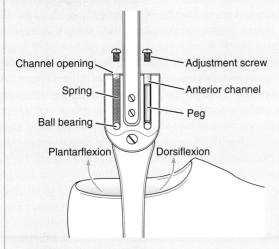

Channel opening — Adjustment screw

Spring — Anterior channel

Ball bearing — Peg

Plantarflexion — Dorsiflexion

1. Plantarflexion stop – placed posteriorly in the hinged AFO to prevent plantar flexion and support the ankle in dorsiflexion during swing.

2. Anterior dorsiflexion stop – involves the addition of a posterior strap to a hinged AFO to prevent knee buckling in terminal stance. These are not as common.

3. Dorsiflexion spring assist – spring assistance to dorsiflexion is added within each stirrup.

4. Double action ankle joint – also known as bi-channel adjustable ankle locks. These are adjustable to provide a locked ankle, dorsiflexion stop, plantar flexion stop, and dorsiflexion assist.

OTHER STYLES OF AFO

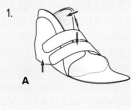

1.

A

B

MATERIALS

1. **Supramalleolar orthosis** (SMO) – designed to maintain a vertical, or neutral heel while also supporting the three arches of the foot. These are not commonly used in adults.
   - Thermoplastic materials – like polyethylene and polypropylene (plastics), are customizable and lightweight.
   - Carbon fiber – this is lighter, thinner, and stronger than plastic "off the shelf" AFOs. The spiral AFO is often made of carbon fiber.
2. Metal – used in older models of AFOs, it is heavier and bulkier. May be useful in heavier clients for whom the lighter weight materials do not function well.

AFO and across different types of AFOs. Do not forget to consider function during other activities including sit to stand to sit transfers and stair climbing. The sit to stand transfer requires ankle dorsiflexion and so can become more difficult with placement of an AFO that limits dorsiflexion. Sit to stand transfers are easier with a more flexible posterior column, such as the posterior leaf spring AFO. This is also true of stair descent, which also requires that the ankle move into dorsiflexion.

Robotics and Virtual Reality: Cochrane reviews and systematic reviews on robotics and virtual reality show that there is evidence to support further study of these interventions, but at this time, there is not sufficient evidence to state that they lead to improvements in upper extremity function.[142] Studies remain limited, small in scale, and diverse in methodology making it difficult to combine them for analysis across studies. A recent meta-analysis concluded that virtual reality has led to greater improvements in gait speed and stride length than conventional therapy.[143] Robotics has been used for rehabilitation of the arm and leg with the most promise for improving underlying impairments such as weakness and spasticity. This technique had the greatest impact on distal arm function (wrist and hand) and regaining ambulation in those who are non-ambulatory. Evidence for the use of virtual reality and video games is positive but its benefit over conventional therapy appears small; however, they may help to increase the intensity and amount of therapy delivered.[142–145]

Neglect Syndrome and Pusher Syndrome

Rehabilitation of individuals, who have developed either the neglect or pusher syndrome, can be challenging. Both of these syndromes typically require a longer duration of rehabilitation to ensure safety and independence in daily activities.

Neglect Syndrome. The goal in rehabilitating this client is to assist the client to develop awareness of the paretic side and the environment on that side of their body. The first step is to assess for the type and severity of the neglect and its impact on daily activities and function. No one test can determine if an individual has unilateral neglect. There are some common screening tools that are quick and easy to do in the clinic, it should be noted that these tests screen for visuospatial neglect in the peripersonal space and may miss neglect in the personal and extrapersonal spaces and neglect in other domains such as motor neglect. The line bisection test (illustrated in Figure 11-10) is a quick and easy test that is done using either paper and pencil

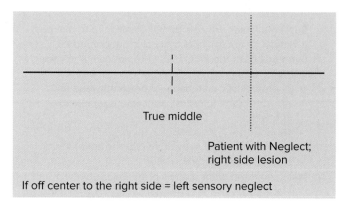

True middle

Patient with Neglect; right side lesion

If off center to the right side = left sensory neglect

FIGURE 11-10 Example of the line bisection test in an individual with neglect syndrome.

or a computer, involving indicating the middle of a line or lines drawn on the paper. The star and letter cancellation tasks are more sensitive and reliable than the line bisection test and involve finding a target item among distractors. Both of these tests screen for visuospatial neglect in the peripersonal space.

The Catherine Bergego Scale allows therapists to objectively assess the impact of motor neglect on functional activities such as grooming, eating, and navigating while walking. It includes items that require attention to the personal, peripersonal, and extrapersonal spaces. The therapist rates the individual's performance on tasks such as grooming the face, looking to the paretic side, and navigating around objects on the paretic side.[146–148] The wheelchair obstacle course is a lesser known test with limited psychometric data, that provides an objective measure of the impact of neglect on motor performance in the extrapersonal space. The test involves having the client navigate through a specifically designed obstacle course and is timed with errors counted.[149,150]

Treatment involves the use of techniques that incorporate visual scanning, sensory awareness, and spatial organization training and should be individually designed based on the evaluation. Visual scanning involves visually engaging the client within the space where they are comfortable and then drawing their vision slowly to the neglected side. Upon reaching the boundary of their ability, keep the object, to which they are visually engaged, at the boundary and encourage them to maintain their focus on the object. This task is more engaging if the client has to interact with the visual target in some way such as having to read text. Sensory awareness training should involve both proprioception and the many cutaneous senses (touch, object recognition). Activities that include weight-bearing on the paretic side along with explicitly focusing the client's attention on the feeling of the weight-bearing are thought to be especially beneficial. It is also recommended that therapists provide sensory stimulation of different types (soft, rough, hot, cold) to the paretic limbs while having the client watch as the stimulus is applied and describe how it feels and where it is being placed. Studies have found that combining visual exploration with either TENS or vibration to the paretic upper trapezius are effective means of treating neglect syndrome.[151] The use of prisms combined with an active pointing activity is also supported by research.[152] If the client is not eating well or otherwise severely impacted by the neglect, a compensatory technique is to turn the body so that the sternum faces the neglected space. The trunk is the internal representation of the body, and therefore, it appears that individuals with neglect are "neglecting" the space relative to the center of the trunk. If they are not eating food on the left side of the plate, turning their chair such that their sternum faces the left side of the plate will allow them to perceive the food from the left side of the plate to the right, and they will typically eat everything. This technique works well for seated activities but is generally not feasible for activities involving mobility. In addition, this technique is compensatory, and as such, does not aid in neuroplasticity nor resolution of the syndrome, so it should be used sparingly and only for issues where safety is a concern.

Pusher Syndrome. Individuals with pusher syndrome have a severely altered sense of their position in space. This results in their pushing strongly toward the paretic side in all positions and resisting any attempt at passive correction of their posture. Their head is turned to the non-paretic side and they are unable to relax their neck so that the head can be turned to the paretic side. They have a reduced ability to perceive stimuli coming in on the paretic side and their tactile and kinesthetic sensation may be severely impaired. These individuals often do not see or hear things on the paretic side. They lack facial expression and have a monotonous voice. During movement, they tend to keep their weight on the non-paretic side, while pushing their center of mass over the paretic side. This results in their falling over, both in standing and sitting. Even after falling, you will note that they appear to continue to be pushing onto the paretic side. It is also common for these individuals to push backward, and thus, appear to be resisting or fighting staff during transfers and gait training. In standing, the center of gravity is shifted to the paretic side, and they show no fear even when on the verge of falling. The legs are adducted and the paretic leg is flexed taking little weight with the non-paretic leg held in exaggerated extension. During stand to sit transfers, they often sit too soon, and they tend to talk a lot, offering lots of "explanations" for why things go wrong. These explanations are usually not appropriate to the situation. Due to the constant pushing motion, they are likely to develop skin breakdown and contractures. Pushing can be measured objectively using the Scale for Contraversive Pushing (SCP)[153] or the Burke Lateropulsion Scale.[154] The Scale for Contraversive pushing allows clinicians to numerically rate the extent of the pushing behavior in the seated position. The Burke Lateropulsion Scale is based on observation of lateropulsion, or pushing, in supine, sitting, standing, and walking. It is the only scale that incorporates assessment in supine and walking so could be useful across the spectrum of care from acute to outpatient therapy. It also has higher sensitivity (100%) but lower specificity (67%) than the SCP but is likely to be more useful in detecting small changes in pushing behavior.[155]

Treatment. The key to working with individuals who have pusher syndrome is to ensure they have visual information on vertical and use active movement to get vertical, followed by functional activities while in vertical. Patients who have contraversive pushing need to learn the following in sequential order:

1. Realize the disturbed perception of erect body position

2. Visually explore their surroundings and their body's relation to the surroundings. Use visual aids that give feedback about body orientation

3. Learn movements necessary to reach a vertical body position

4. Maintain vertical body position while performing other activities

It is important to be vigilant in guarding these clients to ensure their safety as they can be impulsive and the lateropulsion increases their instability in all positions. A key to working with these clients is to be sure that you do not allow the client to push into you and that you do not "fight" the pushing. In some situations, it may be appropriate to have a clinician on the non-paretic side to encourage the client to move toward them and thereby actively move out of the pushing behavior.[156]

The therapist should also structure the treatment such that there are visual cues available as to where vertical is situated. You might instruct the individual to look at a door frame, or you may put a stripe on a mirror in front of them. The key is to provide the client with a visual orientation to vertical. While utilizing the visual orientation, instruct the individual to actively move themselves into a more upright position. It is counterproductive to try to forcefully push them into upright. Rather, the therapist should provide activities that encourage actively moving out of the pushing posture. For example, have the client sit in front of a mirror. Place an object off to the non-paretic side and ask the client to reach for the object with either hand. Adjust where you place the object to ensure that the reaching activity results in a weight shift to neutral or even onto the non-paretic side. If the client is also slumping, move the object up higher to promote appropriate trunk extension and upright posture during the reaching activity.

If the client expresses a strong fear of falling, which is common, the therapist could place a large Swiss ball on the mat on the non-paretic side of the client and place the client's non-paretic arm on the Swiss ball. The instruction is to push on the ball. Again, the client is in control and is actively moving out of the pushing behavior. By allowing the client to stay in control and providing appropriate support, they will have less fear of falling and be better able to work through the sense that they are falling, while moving out of the pushing behavior.

Standing activities can initially be quite difficult. Safety can be enhanced by placing a knee brace on the paretic limb, so it is in a position to assume weight-bearing. In addition, the non-paretic upper extremity should be in a position that does not allow pushing but does allow it to weight bear. Use of a table that is at chest height can be helpful for standing activities as it allows the client to weight bear through the forearms, and thus, discourages pushing, while encouraging an upright posture and a very stable support surface. Once again, the therapist would instruct the client to lean to the non-paretic side, cueing an active movement out of pushing. Reaching activities to the non-paretic side provide a means of practicing actively moving out of pushing. When gait is initiated, stepping over objects with the non-paretic leg encourages weight-bearing on the paretic side. Typically, devices that allow the client to use the non-paretic arm to push are discouraged. At times, the therapist may even hold the client's non-paretic arm in a position of shoulder adduction and internal rotation with full elbow flexion to prevent pushing. Once the pushing begins to subside, the therapist should wean away from preventing use of the non-paretic arm.

Gait training may be done with the non-paretic side next to a wall and instructing the individual to keep their shoulder on the wall. Another method is to walk around a plinth that is set at hip height. Instruct the client to keep the non-paretic hip against the table while walking around it. The table also provides a means for upper extremity support that is low enough that the arm is not able to engage in pushing behavior. While walking, an obstacle course can be used to encourage appropriate weight shift to the non-paretic side by placing objects on the floor that are low enough to step over, then have the client walk and step over the obstacles with the paretic extremity.[155]

If the client has progressed to exhibiting a high level of cognitive functioning and good self-recognition of the pushing, the therapist can work on sitting by having the client close their eyes and assume what they perceive to be upright sitting. Then, ask the client to let you place them in true upright. This is followed by asking them to think about how this posture feels to them, while giving them feedback that they are truly in an upright posture. This is done with eyes closed because these individuals tend to stop resisting postural correction, when their eyes are closed.

SUMMARY

All therapeutic techniques that lead to improved daily function for individuals who are post-stroke involve intensive, task-oriented practice of functional activities. Clinicians should focus on ensuring that their clients are provided opportunities to perform task-oriented practice that involves numerous repetitions of a functionally appropriate activity. Compensatory training may lead to a faster return to independence but ultimately negatively impacts neuroplasticity and results in poorer long-term functional outcomes and motor recovery.

Neuroplasticity: How Does Treatment Induce Plasticity?

Neuroplasticity, as described in Chapter 9, refers to the natural change in synaptic function that is associated with behavioral change, including learning new motor skills or a decrease in the amount of use of a given body part. Therefore, physical therapy interventions naturally induce neuroplasticity with long-lasting implications. Too often, early therapy post-stroke focuses on improving function through use of the non-paretic limbs (i.e., lifting the paretic limb with the non-paretic limb). Therapists should keep in mind that limiting use of the paretic limb may result in loss of neural projections in the hand/arm or leg areas of the motor cortex, especially in the vulnerable penumbra; further, increased use of the non-paretic arm or leg will result in neuroplastic changes that expand the neuronal networks associated with these body parts. To preserve the neural networks and/or induce positive neural change within the lesioned hemisphere, it is imperative that therapy focus on increasing sensorimotor activity in the paretic limbs. Kleim outlined key principles that should guide physical therapy interventions to maximize neuroplasticity: (1) rehabilitation should focus on limb usage because failure to use the limbs will result in additional neural loss; (2) the plasticity induced will be specific to the treatment provided; (3) plasticity requires high intensity (rate and amount of practice) and many repetitions; and (4) early plasticity may improve or impede subsequent plasticity.[157] Too often, therapy sessions provide one or two repetitions of any given activity; it is unlikely that this is enough to produce plasticity or functional change unless the client is able to continually perform additional repetitions throughout the day. Home programs and involvement of family members or other health care professionals to encourage continuous activity are essential for assuring sufficient practice to induce plasticity.

What Kinds of Plasticity Are Found After Stroke and How Are They Identified?

Plasticity, in vivo, has largely been evaluated using imaging methods such as anatomical and functional magnetic resonance imaging (fMRI), positron emission tomography (PET), or diffusion tensor imaging/tractography (DTI or DTT). Findings from anatomical imaging (MRI or CT) suggest that lesion location and volume, comparing different regions, are poor predictors of stroke outcome,[158] but when comparing the same vessel territory may be moderate predictors of outcome[159]; however, these methods do allow for the location of damage to be documented and measures of lesion volume as well as whole brain or component brain volume (i.e., cortex) to be analyzed. Notably, high-intensity post-stroke training can increase cortex thickness in areas related to improved function,[160] as measured through MRI anatomical scanning methods. fMRI, which allows the visualization of changes in blood flow during a given activity (i.e., finger tapping), has shown that early motor recovery is often characterized by diffuse bilateral activation, compared to unilateral, typically contralateral, activation in non-stroke participants; however, good recovery is most often associated with a return to unilateral ipsilesional activation similar to non-stroke activation patterns. Plus, physical therapy training that is of high intensity can induce activation that is more similar to non-stroke activation, with the magnitude of activation correlated with the magnitude of recovery. Post-stroke survivors with poorer sensorimotor recovery often maintain a bilateral and more diffuse activation pattern, suggesting that this pattern of activation is inconsistent with effective neuroplasticity. Diffusion tractography (see description in Chapter 9) focuses on the evaluation of white matter projections and has revealed a strong relationship between the degree of white matter integrity, especially within the corticospinal projections, and functional motor outcomes.[161,162] However, the ability of training to increase white matter in the lesioned hemisphere has had limited study; in one such study, fractional anisotropy (FA), a measure of white matter, in the non-lesioned supplementary motor area increased, following robotic-assisted gait training, but FA in the lesioned hemisphere decreased. This suggested a compensatory plasticity in the non-lesioned hemisphere that supported enhanced function.[104]

Neuroplasticity within the sensory system appears to be more complex. First, although sensory perception, the ability to localize touch to a given body area, seems to be a unilateral process, involving the primary sensory cortex (S1) in the contralateral parietal lobe, sensory discrimination is a bilateral process, involving contralateral S1 and bilateral S2 (secondary sensory cortex) as well as bilateral areas of the prefrontal cortex. It is not surprising, then, that damage to this sensory discrimination network often results in a bilateral disturbance, which is greater in the contralesional (paretic) hand. Sensory discrimination recovery seems to, in part, mirror motor recovery in that activation patterns that are similar to non-stroke patterns are associated with better recovery, suggesting that the best recovery is associated with plasticity within the S1 and S2 areas of the lesioned cortex. Further, it appears that the degree of integrity in the superior thalamic radiations (the sensory projections from the thalamus to the parietal cortex) is strongly related to the degree of sensory discrimination ability post-stroke.[158] However, there is some suggestion that the bilateral nature of sensory discrimination may allow for fairly effective sensory discrimination through increased use of the contralesional hemisphere. To date, there have been no clinical trials that have evaluated the ability of sensory discrimination training to induce neuroplasticity within this bilateral network.

CASE B: BASILAR ARTERY ANEURYSM

Jennifer is a 36-year-old, Caucasian, female, who presented to the ER with what she termed was "the worst headache of her life." She complained of associated neck stiffness. CT scan revealed a large aneurysm at the basilar-vertebral artery junction that was leaking blood into the subarachnoid space. She was rushed to the OR and the aneurysm was successfully clipped. Post-surgery, she presents with complex symptomology, characterized by quadriparesis, right facial muscle paresis, diplopia, ptosis, nystagmus, vertigo, dysarthria, and dysphagia.

The symptoms described in this case most closely align with which stroke syndrome?

Basilar artery syndrome

Aneurysms: What are they? What causes them? And how are they medically managed?

An aneurysm is a weakening in a blood vessel wall that allows the wall to balloon out and presents a risk of rupture. Cerebral aneurysms are often asymptomatic and, therefore, undiagnosed with an estimated presence in 2 to 5% of the population[163]; however, the occurrence of rupture into the subarachnoid space or surrounding brain tissue is about 1 in 10,000 people annually.[164] Up to 60% of those experiencing an aneurysm rupture into the subarachnoid space die within the first 6 months, often before getting to the hospital[163]; the majority of those that survive will have some permanent neurologic deficit[165] consistent with the area of the rupture and damage to the surrounding tissue. Aneurysms are more common in women and with increasing age; however, pediatric occurrences are documented. Risk factors are similar to those for stroke and include hypertension, drug (especially cocaine) or excessive alcohol use, and smoking.[164]

Aneurysms are most common in the junctions between the vessels within the Circle of Willis, especially in the anterior and posterior communicating arteries (see Figure 11-11). Other common sites are at the carotid bifurcation and the basilar artery tip (the point of bifurcation into the posterior cerebral arteries) as well as within the middle cerebral and posterior inferior cerebellar arteries.[165] Aneurysms are much more common in the anterior circulation with approximately 85% presenting there. Although most aneurysms are asymptomatic unless they rupture, some will present with neurologic symptoms, if they enlarge to the point that they compress the adjacent brain tissue. However, it is much more common for aneurysms to remain "silent" until a small leak or full rupture occurs. Small leaks may present with headache, cranial nerve changes, nausea, photophobia (sensitivity to light), or neck pain; these may precede an actual rupture by hours or days and are referred to as **sentinel hemorrhages**. Rupture commonly presents with what is known as a "**thunderclap**" headache, referring to a rapid onset severe headache, which results from blood flowing into the subarachnoid space or brain tissue. Consciousness may be lost as the bleeding progresses. Aneurysms can be detected by CT or MRI scans; however, cerebral angiograms are commonly used to confirm the diagnosis and guide treatment.[163]

Medical management of an aneurysm that is leaking first focuses on stabilization of the patient and then prevention of a rupture, including administration of antifibrinolytic medications and managing hypertension[166]; treatment is surgical, using coiling with or without a stent/balloon, or clipping. **Coiling** involves advancing tiny coils into the aneurysm to obstruct blood flow from the main vessel into the aneurysm; coils are inserted via a catheter, typically guided through the femoral artery to the site of the aneurysm. A **stent** is a wire mesh tube that provides a shell for the coils and is more commonly used for fusiform aneurysms (those with wide oval openings).

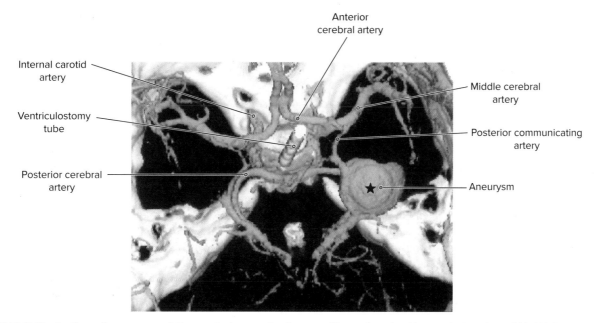

FIGURE 11-11 Illustration of aneurysm of the posterior cerebral artery. (Reproduced, with permission, from Afifi AK, Bergman RA. *Functional Neuroanatomy,* 2nd ed. New York, NY: McGraw-Hill; 2005, Fig. 28-5, p. 364.)

An alternative to a stent is a balloon, which blocks the neck of the aneurysm while the coil is inserted into the aneurysm sac, helping to hold the coil in place; balloons are used with smaller aneurysms. More recently, flow diversion has been implemented to improve the outcome for large aneurysms. In this method, a stent is placed in the vessel at the site of the aneurysm, providing a scaffold that incites endothelial growth, which eventually occludes the aneurysm. For even larger aneurysms, a pipeline embolization device (PED) may be used; this is a braided mesh that is used to occlude the aneurysm from the parent vessel.[167] In some instances, repair requires a craniotomy and clipping of the aneurysm, which simply uses a small clip across the aneurysm's neck to prevent blood from entering the aneurysm; clipping is most common for MCA aneurysms or for aneurysms in younger patients. Treatment for an aneurysm rupture is the same as for one that is leaking; both coiling and clipping are used. The outcomes of aneurysm repair are dependent on the management of complications and the amount of brain damage, resulting from the initial bleed, if the aneurysm ruptured. Common complications after an aneurysm rupture and repair are rebleeding, edema, hydrocephalus, vasospasm, and hyponatremia (low sodium). Each of these needs to be carefully managed.[163,164,166]

Rebleeding is most common in the first 24 hours after initial rupture and prior to repair in up to 15% of those presenting with initial hemorrhage. Thirty-five to forty percent of those that survive the first 24 hours will experience rebleeding. In those with successful coiling or clipping of an initially ruptured aneurysm, up to 19% will experience rebleeding due to insufficient occlusion. The most common result of rebleeding is death, occurring in up to 40% of patients. Thus, antifibrinolytic drugs that promote blood clotting are typically administered, following hemorrhage, to prevent rebleeding.[163]

Hydrocephalus may occur within 3 days of surgical repair, considered acute (20% of patients) or much later after discharge (10% of survivors). In acute hydrocephalus, up to 40% spontaneously recover; therefore, early treatment may focus on monitoring. Progression of the hydrocephalus may require shunting to control cerebrospinal fluid buildup and further brain damage. This may be done by placement of an external ventricular drain (placed into the lateral ventricle and shunted externally), a lumbar drain, or repeated lumbar punctures. Of course, these treatments carry with them risk of their own complications, so initial monitoring is critical to assure the need for shunting.[163]

Hyponatremia refers to a dramatic decrease in sodium in the brain. There is controversy over the cause of this condition post-aneurysm repair. It may result from abnormal secretion of antidiuretic hormone, resulting in retention of water in the cells, or it may be the result of a condition known as cerebral salt wasting, which occurs with increased salt in the urine and appears associated with sympathetic nervous system disruption. Treatment focuses on maintaining salt and fluid levels.[164]

Vasospasm, post-aneurysm, can induce a subsequent CVA or delayed ischemic deficit, so it is critical to prevent this complication. Notably, this complication is most common 5 to 14 days after rupture and presents with deterioration of the patient's condition, including additional neurologic deficits. Prevention has focused on pharmacologic management with the use of a calcium channel blocker, nimodipine, the most common method. Research is focused on identifying other, and perhaps better, medications to manage vasospasm.[164,166]

Brainstem Stroke: Why Are the Symptoms So Confusing? What Is Locked-in Syndrome?

The brainstem is a complex structure that houses cranial nerve nuclei as well as the nuclei of the reticular and vestibular systems. In addition, it is an area of fiber passage for ascending sensory fibers, originating from all body parts and conveying sensory information to the thalamus and cortex, and descending fibers (corticobulbar, corticospinal), traveling to brainstem structures and the spinal cord. Therefore, damage within the brainstem can produce upper motor neuron syndrome, presenting with hemiparesis and spasticity, due to damage of corticospinal and corticobulbar fibers, or lower motor neuron syndrome, associated with damage of alpha motor neurons within the cranial nerve nuclei that innervate the muscles of the eyes, face, mouth, tongue, and palate. Further, symptoms can be ipsilateral, contralateral, or bilateral, depending on the structures damaged and the size of the respective lesion. (Refer to Figure 11-5 and Table 11-2 for potential structures associated with brainstem levels and possible clinical presentations.)

Changes in sensory function similarly relate to the site of damage. Damage below the level of the cuneate and gracilis nuclei results in ipsilateral loss of somatosensory function, while damage at the level of these nuclei, as projection fibers cross, will produce bilateral somatosensory loss, and above this level will produce contralateral loss. Again, large lesions that impact both sides of the brainstem structures can also produce bilateral sensory loss. Since pain and temperature are conveyed in the anterolateral pathway's spinothalamic tract and not the dorsal column-medial lemniscal pathway, localized damage may result in the loss of one pathway and not the other below the merging of these sensory projections in the upper medulla. Damage to the lateral medulla is likely to disrupt the spinothalamic tract; while medial damage is likely to disrupt the medial lemniscal fibers. It should be noted that spinothalamic damage within the brainstem always yields contralateral dysfunction, so it is possible, but uncommon, to have ipsilateral loss of somatosensation and contralateral loss of pain and temperature with unilateral low-level medullary strokes. At the levels of the pons and midbrain, these projection pathways are collocated and damage will typically disrupt both, producing contralateral damage.

Cranial nuclei house the alpha motor neurons that innervate the muscles of the eyes (extraocular muscles), eyelids, face, tongue, and throat. Damage to motor cranial nerve nuclei produces ipsilateral lower motor neuron symptoms in the muscles innervated, presenting as weakness or flaccidity with hyperflexia/areflexia. Similarly, the sensory cranial nerves receive ipsilateral projections from the eyes, ears, face, and oral structures, so damage to these nuclei results in ipsilateral loss of sensory function (somatosensory, pain, and temperature).

There are four vestibular nuclei (lateral, medial, superior, inferior) located bilaterally in the upper medulla and lower pons that function with the inner ear and cerebellum to maintain the body's orientation in relation to the environment. Strokes that impact the medulla and pons will also disrupt the function of the vestibular nuclei, which include (1) antigravity muscle control to maintain upright posture (lateral vestibulospinal tract); (2) reflexive control of head position with visual orientation (medial vestibulospinal tract); (3) vestibular-ocular reflexes (nystagmus); and (4) integration of inner ear and cerebellar projections for motor control. The afferent and efferent projections of the vestibular nuclei are largely unilateral, so damage to these nuclei presents with ipsilateral symptoms. Similarly, cerebellar damage results in ipsilateral symptoms. It is difficult to differentiate the symptoms of vestibular nuclei and cerebellar damage, in part, because they often coexist. Nonetheless, damage within the vestibular network commonly results in ipsilesional nystagmus or ocular oscillations, vertigo, ataxia, or gaze paresis. When damage is localized to the vestibular nuclei, the ataxia produced is gravity dependent, absent when lying down but present in upright positions; due to the adjacency of the cochlear nucleus, vestibular damage also frequently presents with changes in auditory function (tinnitus, hearing loss). With cerebellar damage, ataxia is not gravity dependent and typically is associated with hypotonia, incoordination, and dysmetria (overshooting of intended targets).[168]

Locked-in Syndrome (LIS)

LIS is a complex condition, involving the posterior circulation, resulting from infarction that disrupts the ventral aspect of the pons, which can be the result of basilar artery ischemic stroke or deep penetrating pontine arterial hemorrhage as well as brain trauma. It involves (1) loss of the corticobulbar and corticospinal tracts, resulting in quadriplegia, with intact sensation (dorsal pons preserved); (2) loss of the ability to speak (anarthria) and bilateral oral motor paralysis due to damage of the nuclei for cranial nerves V, VII, and IX; (3) impaired horizontal eye movements, double vision (**diplopia**), and nystagmus (Cr N VI, paramedian pontine reticular formation); and (4) preserved consciousness (intact midbrain reticular activating system), upper eyelid control, and vertical eye movements (Cr N III, IV, midbrain vertical eye center).[169–171] Other features can include respiratory disruption (pontine tegmentum damage), vertigo (vestibular nuclei), and pathologic laughing or crying, which occurs to inappropriate stimuli and is related to damage to an effector system in the upper pons at the border of the midbrain that coordinates facial muscles and respiration for these reactions. This center is typically inhibited by higher centers in the amygdala and the premotor cortex.[172]

Control of vertical eye movement and the eyelids is typically maintained along with cognitive function. Communication can be achieved through vertical eye movement; however, the presence of nystagmus and other visual disturbances (diplopia, impaired accommodation) may complicate acquiring information through vision. For most, hearing remains intact.

Most of those surviving with LIS will initially require a tracheostomy and respiratory assistance via a ventilator. In about 1/3 of patients, a tracheostomy may be required long term but most can be weaned from the ventilator, relying on an involuntary ventilation pattern, controlled by a center in the medulla that triggers inspiration, followed by passive expiration.[173] Recovery from LIS, after basilar stroke, is poor and mortality high, yet outcome data are not well documented. However, intensive rehabilitation has been found to improve motor recovery and decrease mortality. The use of communication devices and other assistive technology is necessary to maximize function. Death, associated with LIS, most commonly results from respiratory complications.[174]

Assessment and Interventions Following Basilar Artery Aneurysm

Assessment, following basilar artery stroke, requires that the therapist incorporate more detailed examination of coordination, balance, visual, and vestibular function. Some outcome measures that may be appropriate include the Dynamic Gait Index, the Sensory Organization Test, Timed Up and Go, and the Dizziness Handicap Inventory. A full assessment of cranial nerve function should be conducted on anyone with a stroke in this region of the brain. In addition, coordination and balance assessment should be completed as outlined in the Evaluation (Chapter 10) and vestibular and cerebellar (Chapter 17) chapters.

Treatment for strokes that involve posterior circulation typically requires that the therapist address the significant balance deficits that can result from damage to structures of the cerebellum and vestibular nuclei. These treatments are outlined in the chapter on vestibular and cerebellar disorders (Chapter 17). In addition to these issues, it is likely that these individuals may have damage to one or more of the cranial nerves and will require muscle reeducation for the facial, oral, and throat musculature. While physical therapists can make a valuable contribution to therapy for facial motor weakness, speech therapy should be incorporated, and the client should be managed with a team approach.

Functional retraining utilizing the motor learning concepts covered earlier in this chapter is also used after basilar artery stroke. These clients will also require that activities focus on postural control, balance, and coordination associated with vestibular system disruption. Examples of interventions for these conditions can also be found in Chapter 17.

Case Example

Jennifer has diploplia, vertigo, and quadriparesis. An assessment tool that would give valuable objective outcomes for Jennifer and is valid in stroke and vestibular disorders is the Dynamic Gait Index.[59] Jennifer has a complex presentation, including many visual impairments. These will impede her ability to utilize vision for both balance and motor function feedback. Therapists should assess how her vision is interacting with her motor function and encourage her to learn to utilize her somatosensory feedback system for movement. In addition, objects that are used for functional training should be large and in strong, contrasting colors to simplify visual tracking. Vertigo secondary to cerebellar damage can be resistant to rehabilitation, but slow progress can be made through the use of accommodation exercises (see balance/vestibular Chapter 17). Jennifer will likely need to work on gaze stabilization and accommodation exercises prior to being able to fully benefit from an intensive task-oriented approach. Once she has begun to accommodate the changes in her vision and balance systems, she should respond to an intensive task-oriented approach as outlined earlier in this chapter. To accommodate her diplopia therapists should use large widely spaced print and simple line pictures for educational materials and home exercise programs. Jennifer's right facial paresis should respond to NMES and active exercise. Vision may be further impeded by the ptosis, and treatment focused on the levator muscle of the eye should be included in the therapy plan.

Therapy may involve interventions for lower and upper motor neuron injury. An appropriate therapy for both types of damage, as long as the lower motor neuron is intact, is the use of electrical stimulation. The unit can be set up for functional neuromuscular reeducation, or on flaccid muscles, may be set up to stimulate muscle activation in an attempt to promote neurologic recovery. If functional neuromuscular electrical stimulation (FNMES or FES) is used correctly, it can help to promote neuroplasticity. The key is to encourage the use of visual and proprioceptive feedback, while using the unit to assist in movement. Use of FES assists in producing a more normal movement and can allow the individual to complete more repetitions. Thus, the individual can achieve intensive task-oriented practice of complicated movement patterns such as walking. A common use of FES is on the tibialis anterior during gait. The typical setup is to utilize a unit with a switch that goes under the heel of the shoe. As the individual walks, the switch triggers the stimulator to assist with dorsiflexion at the appropriate times during gait. The individual can then ambulate more steps with a proper gait pattern. There is also some evidence to suggest that use of electrical stimulation can slow or stop muscle fiber type conversion from type II to type I that is common following stroke. In addition, FES has been shown to be effective in rehabilitating hand, shoulder,[175,176] and ankle[177] function post-stroke.

Locked-in syndrome presents many challenges to the rehabilitation team. The key to a successful rehabilitation program is establishing communication with the individual. Initially, watching eye movements and asking yes/no questions may be used, but speech therapy is typically involved immediately and will often incorporate a communication device. Physical and Occupational therapists should focus on moving the limbs and encouraging active movement where possible. Electrical stimulation is suggested for use in this population to enhance motor recovery. Upright positioning remains important to prevent secondary complications and to promote interaction with the environment. Therapists should assess for and provide a chair for upright positioning.

CASE C: SICKLE CELL STROKE

Amelia is a 3-year-old, born of immigrant parents from Senegal, who was diagnosed with sickle cell disease at 9 months of age, following an initial episode of **dactylitis** (inflammation) of the 3rd digit of her right hand. She takes daily doses of folic acid and penicillin to manage her disease. She was rushed to the ED by her parents with slurring speech, listlessness, and mild left hemiparesis. CT identified an area of hypoperfusion in the right frontoparietal cortex. Sickle Cell disease is associated with abnormal red blood vessels that are more likely to clot and place the individual at risk for stroke as well as clotting within other organs (Figure 11-12 and Box 11-11).

What Are the Causes of Pediatric Stroke?

Strokes that occur prior to or within the first month after birth are referred to as perinatal strokes; for some, they will initially present in the acute stage, often with seizures, while others won't be diagnosed until later in the first year but will be presumed perinatal, based on imaging. Strokes that occur after the first month are called childhood strokes. The causes of pediatric stroke are quite different than those for adult stroke. For perinatal stroke, contributing factors include intrauterine growth deficiency, gestational hypertension, pre-eclampsia, complicated labor or delivery, infections, thrombus originating from the placenta, and asphyxia. Other conditions that may lead to stroke in the perinatal or childhood period are congenital heart defects (septal defects such as patent foramen ovale) or cardiomyopathy and their diagnosis and/or treatment, vascular anomalies in the cerebral vascular system (i.e., Moyamoya syndrome), infections (meningitis, encephalitis, human immunodeficiency virus), metabolic conditions (hyperlipidemia), cancer, and some genetic syndromes (neurofibromatosis, fibromuscular dysplasia, SCA, inborn errors of metabolism, inherited thrombophilia).[180,181]

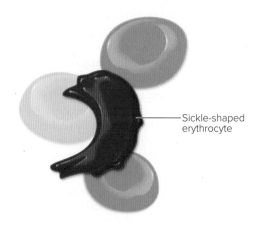

FIGURE 11-12 Sickle-shaped erythrocyte illustration. A single sickle-shaped red blood cell (erythrocyte) shown within a group of normal red blood cells.

Box 11-11	What Is Sickle Cell Anemia and Why Is It Associated with Stroke?

Sickle cell anemia (SCA) is an inherited autosomal recessive disorder that affects red blood cell formation, resulting in a sickle or crescent-shaped red blood cell (erythrocyte) instead of the typical circular shape (see Figure 11-12). This method of inheritance requires that both parents be carriers of the gene in order for a child to have the disorder. SCA is most commonly found in families with origins in Africa, the Mediterranean, Central and South America, the Caribbean, and the Middle East. The red blood cells are not only different in shape but are also weaker, more likely to rupture, and carry an abnormal hemoglobin protein, known as hemoglobin S, which is less effective in carrying oxygen. Remember, hemoglobin is the protein in red blood cells that carries oxygen.[177] Diagnosis of SCA can be made by a blood test, in which hemoglobin S can be identified.

The fragility of the sickle cell red blood cells in combination with the decreased amount of oxygen carried by hemoglobin S results in chronic anemia and subsequently, chronic fatigue. Notably, the red blood cells, in SCA, are also likely to stick together in clumps, thereby blocking smaller blood vessels throughout the body, including in the internal organs, extremities, and brain. When such a blockage occurs, especially in the internal organs, it results in severe pain, referred to as a "crisis" in SCA. The dactylitis, in Amelia's case, refers to a crisis occurring in the finger, creating pain and inflammation. Crises may occur with varying frequency in those affected. Organ damage, especially in the spleen, is common; spleen damage increases the chance of infection in those with SCA, which can, in turn, cause other problems.[65] Stroke is also a common problem in children with SCA, affecting 8% of those with the disorder by the age of 14.[178,179]

How Do Pediatric Strokes Present?

In infants and young children, it is more common to see impaired consciousness or seizures than motor symptoms at stroke onset; sometimes irritability may be the initial symptom. Of course, it may be difficult to "see" early motor changes in a very young infant, and therefore, early signs may be overlooked. Thus, stroke may go undiagnosed in very young children. For up to 50% of children who experience stroke, neurologic deficits, much like those in adults occur, with changes in speech/vocalization, coordination, or localized sensory or motor symptoms. Amelia, in the case description, presents with common symptoms of listlessness, mild hemiparesis, and slurring of speech. Diagnosis requires a complete history of symptom onset, blood work to rule out other causes and look for potential stroke causes, and imaging. MRI scans provide a better likelihood of lesion identification than CT scans in young children with even better clarity at an earlier stage found with single photon emission computed tomography (SPECT), but MRI is more likely to be done. Sedation is often required to image young children and infants.[180,181] Notably, recent work suggests that kinematic analysis can identify asymmetries in arm movements in infants as young as 2 to 3 months, which may be a future method for identifying those that don't present acutely.[182]

Medical Management of Pediatric Stroke

The medical management of pediatric stroke is not very different from adult management. Early stabilization is critical. rTPA has not been approved for use in children, in part, because the onset of symptoms is rarely clear, and its effectiveness is maximal in the 3–4½ hour window after onset.[183] Similarly, endovascular treatments are controversial in the pediatric population. However, anticoagulants, such as heparin or warfarin, are used to decrease blood clotting. Inducing hypothermia has also been found to be neuroprotective in infants/young children and may be used. Also, antiepileptics may be used to prevent further brain damage secondary to post-stroke seizures. Some congenital malformations, such as Moyamoya, can be treated by surgical revascularization.[183-185] Pediatric stroke, since it occurs during the developmental period, may have profound effects on subsequent development and acquisition of age-appropriate milestones across domains – cognitive, emotional, sensorimotor. Physical therapy intervention will mirror that provided for children with cerebral palsy and, therefore, will be discussed in that chapter.

Treatment of SCA

Treatment of SCA is largely focused on prevention of crises and stroke, including monitoring for stroke potential, using transcranial Doppler ultrasound to identify potential areas of blockage, in which stroke could occur; chronic blood transfusions may also be given to replace the damaged blood cells. However, chronic blood transfusions are not without risk, including the complications of too much iron (iron overload), alloimmunity (an immune response to the transfused blood), and infection. Other pharmacologic management may include (1) folic acid to increase iron in the blood; (2) prophylactic antibiotics to minimize infections; (3) pain medications in the event of crisis; and (4) hydroxyurea to stimulate red blood cell formation.[177]

REFERENCES

1. Virani SS, Alons A, Benjamin EJ, Bittencourt MS. Heart disease and stroke statistics – 2020 update: a report from the American Heart association. *Circulation*. 2020;141:e139-e596.

2. Pare JR, Kahn JH. Basic neuroanatomy and stroke syndromes. *Emerg Med Clin North Am*. 2012;30:601-615.

3. Diener HC, Hankey GJ. Primary and secondary prevention of ischemic stroke and cerebral hemorrhage. *J Am Coll Cardiol*. 2020;75(15):1804-1818.

4. Guzik A, Bushnell C. Stroke epidemiology and risk factor management. *Continuum (Minneap Minn)*. 2017;23(1):15-39.

5. Van Alabeek ME, Arntz RM, Ekker MS, et al. Risk factors and mechanisms of stroke in young adults: the FUTURE study. *J Cereb Blood Flow Metab*. 2018;38(9):1631-1641.

6. Ihle-Hansen H, Thommassen B, Wyllar TB, Engedal K, Fure B. Risk factors for and incidence of subtypes of ischemic stroke. *Funct Neurol*. 2012;27(1):35-40.

7. Roda L, McCrindle BW, Manlhiot C, et al. Stroke recurrence in children with congenital heart disease. *Ann Neurol*. 2012;72:103-111.

8. Esse K, Fossati-Bellani M, Traylor A, Martin-Schild S. Epidemic of illicit drug use, mechanisms of action/addiction and stroke as a health hazard. *Brain Behav*. 2011;1(1):44-54.

9. Parry CD, Patra J, Rehm J. Alcohol consumption and non-communicable diseases: epidemiology and policy implications. *Addiction*. 2011;106:1718-1724.

10. Nowinski WL. Stroke atlas: a 3D interactive tool correlating cerebrovascular pathology with underlying neuroanatomy and resulting neurological deficits. *Neuroradiol J.* 2013;26:56-65.

11. Schulz UG, Fischer U. Posterior circulation cerebrovascular syndromes: diagnosis and management. *J Neurol Neurosurg Psychiatry.* 2017;88:45-53.

12. Schmahmann JD. Vascular syndromes of the thalamus. *Stroke.*2003;34:2264-2278.

13. Uddin MA, Haq TU, Rafique MZ. Cerebral venous system anatomy. *J Pak Med Assoc.* 2006:56(11):516-519.

14. Silvis SM, deSousa DA, Ferro JM, Coutinho JM. Cerebral venous thrombosis. *Nature Reviews: Neurology.*2017:13:555-565.

15. Ihara M, Yamamoto Y. Emerging evidence for pathogenesis of sporadic cerebral small vessel disease. *Stroke.* 2016;47:554-560.

16. Balami JS, Chen RL, Buchan AM. Stroke syndromes and clinical management. *QJM.* 2013;106:607-615.

17. Toyoda K, Imamura T, Saku Y, et al. Medial medullary infarction: analyses of eleven patients. *Neurology.* 1996;47:1141-1147.

18. FAST. American Stroke Association. Downloaded from www.stroke.org/en/about-stroke/stroke%20symptoms. 6/25/21.

19. Foundas AL. Apraxia: neural mechanisms and functional recovery. *Handb Clin Neurol.* 2013;110:335-345.

20. Jayasinghe SA, Good D, Wagstaff DA, Winstin C, Sainburg RL. Motor deficits in the ipsilesional arm of severely paretic stroke survivors correlate with functional independence in left but not right hemisphere damage. *Front Hum Neurosci.* 2020;14:Article 599220.

21. Wetter S, Poole J, Haaland KY. Functional implications of ipsilesional motor deficits after unilateral stroke. *Arch Phys Med Rehabil.* 2005:86:776-781.

22. Manganotti P, Acler M, Zanette GP, Smania N, Fiaschi A. Motor cortical disinhibition during early and late recovery after stroke. *Neurorehabil Neural Repair.*2008;22(4):396-403.

23. Mooney RA, Ackerley SJ, Rajeswaran DK, et al. The influence of primary motor cortex inhibition on upper limb impairment and function in chronic stroke: a multimodal study. *Neurorehabil Neural Repair.* 2019;33(2):130-140.

24. Williams PS, Basso DM, Case-Smith J, Nichols-Larsen DS. Development of the hand active sensation test: reliability and validity. *Arch Phys Med Rehabil.* 2006;87:1471-1477.

25. Borstad A, Bird T, Choi S, Goodman L, Schmalbrock P, Nichols-Larsen DS. Sensorimotor training induced reorganization after stroke: a case series. *J Neurol Phys Ther.* 2013;37(1):27-36.

26. Lafosse C, Kerckhofs E, Troch M, et al. Contraversive pushing and inattention of the contralesional hemispace. *J Clin Exp Neuropsych.* 2005;27:460-484.

27. Karnath HO. Pusher syndrome: a frequent but little-known disturbance of body orientation perception. *J Neurol.* 2007;254:415-424.

28. Rode G, Fourtassi M, Pagliari C, Pisella L, Rossetti Y. Complexity vs. unity in unilateral spatial neglect. *Rev Neurologique.* 2017;173:440-450.

29. Yoshida T, Mizuno K, Miyamoto A, Kondo K, Liu M. Influence of right versus left unilateral spatial neglect on the functional recovery after rehabilitation in sub-acute stroke patients. *Neuropsychol Rehabil.* 2022 Jun;32(5):640-661.

30. Feinberg TE, Venneri A, Simone AM, Fan Y, Northoff G. The neuroanatomy of asomatognosia and somatoparaphrenia. *J Neurol Neurosurg Psychiatry.* 2010;81:276-281.

31. Luu S, Lee AW, Daly A, Chen CS. Visual field defects after stroke. *Aus Fam Physician.* 2010;39(7):499-503.

32. Thiel A, Zumbansen A. The pathophysiology of post-stroke aphasia: a network approach. *Restorative Neurol Neuroscience.* 2016;34:507-518.

33. Fridriksson J, den Ouden DB, Hillis AE, et al. Anatomy of aphasia revisited. *Brain.* 2018;141:848-862.

34. Buchsbaum BR, Baldo J, Okada K, et al. Conduction aphasia, sensory-motor integration, and phonological short-term memory: an aggregate analysis of lesion and fMRI data. *Brain Lang.* 2011;119:119-128.

35. Barbosa ACD, Emmady PD. *Alexia. In StatPearls.* Treasure Island (FL): StatPearls Publishing 2021 Jan. Available at: https://www.ncbi.nlm.nih.gov/books/NBK557669/?report=classic.

36. Vakhnina NV, Nikitina YL, Parfenov VA, Yakhno NN. Post-stroke cognitive impairments. *Neurosci Behav Physiol.* 2009;39(8):16-21.

37. Snaphaan L, Rijpkema M, van Uden I, Fernandez G, de Leeuw FE. Reduced medial temporal lobe functionality in stroke patients: a functional magnetic resonance imaging study. *Brain.* 2009;132:1882-1888.

38. Lo Coco D, Lopez G, Corrao S. Cognitive impairment and stroke in elderly patients. *Vasc Health Risk Manag.* 2016.12:105-116.

39. Powers WJ, Rabinstein AA, Ackerson T, et al. A guideline for healthcare professionals from the American heart Assoc/American Stroke Association. *Stroke.*2019;50:e344-e418.

40. Rabinstein AA. Treatment of acute ischemic stroke. *Continuum (Minneap Minn).* 2017;23(1):62-81.

41. Campbell BCV, Ma H, Ringleb PA, et al. Extending thrombolysis to 4.5-9 h and wake-up stroke using perfusion imaging: a systematic review and meta-analysis of individual patient data. *Lancet.* 2019;394:139-47.

42. Leung V, Sastry A, Srivastava S, Wilcock D, Parrott A, Nayak S. Mechanical thrombectomy in acute ischaemic stroke: a review of the different techniques. *Clin Radiol.* 2018;73:428-238.

43. Munich SA, Vakharia K, Levy E. Overview of mechanical thrombectomy techniques. *Neurosurgery.* 2019;85:560-567.

44. Barrett KM, Meschia JF. Acute ischemic stroke management: medical management. *Semin Neurol.* 2010;30(5):461-468.

45. Bosel J. Blood pressure control for acute severe ischemic and hemorrhagic stroke. *Curr Opin Crit Care.* 2017;23:81-86.

46. Morotti A, Goldstein JN. Diagnosis and management of acute intracerebral hemorrhage. *Emerg Med Clin North Am.* 2016;34(4):883-899.

47. Meyer BC, Hemmen TM, Jackson CM, Lyden PD. Modified national institutes of health stroke scale for use in stroke clinical trials: prospective reliability and validity. *Stroke.* 2002;33:1261-1266.

48. Broderick JP, Adeoye O, Elm J. The evolution of the modified Rankin scale and its use in future stroke trials. *Stroke.* 2017;48:2007-2012.

49. Teasdale GM, Pettigres LEL, Wilson JTL, Murray G, Jennett B. Amazing outcome of treatment of severe head injury: a review and update on advancing the use of the Glasgow Outcome Scale. *J Neurotrauma.* 1998;15(8):587-597.

50. Hong I, Goodwin JS, Reistetter TA, et al. Comparison of functional status improvements among patients with stroke receiving postacute care in inpatient rehabilitation vs skilled nursing facilities. *JAMA Network Open.* 2012;2(12):e1916646.

51. Singh RJ, Chen S, Ganesh A, Hill MD. Long-term neurological, vascular, and mortality outcomes after stroke. *Int J Stroke.* 2018;13(8):787-796.

52. Dabrowski J, Czajka A, Zielinska-Turek J, et al. Brain functional reserve in the context of neuroplasticity after stroke. *Neural Plast.* 2019 Feb 27; 2019:9708905.

53. Silver B, Hamid T, Khan M, et al. 12 versus 24 hour bed rest after acute ischemic stroke thrombolysis. *J Neurol Sci.* 2020;409:116618.

54. Taub, E. Crago JE, Burgio LD, et al. An operant approach to rehabilitation medicine: overcoming learned nonuse by shaping. *J Exp Anal Behav.* 1994;61(2):281-293.

55. Fugl-Meyer AR, Jääskö L, Leyman I, Olsson S, Steglind S. The post-stroke hemiplegic patient: a method for evaluation of physical performance. *Scand J Rehabil Med.* 1975;7(1):13-31.

56. Stroke Edge Task Force. Academy of Neurology Physical Therapy; available at: http://www.neuropt.org/practice-resources/neurology-section-outcome-measures-recommendations.

57. Rieck M, Moreland J. The Orpington Prognostic Scale for patients with stroke: reliability and pilot predictive data for discharge destination and therapeutic services. *Disabil Rehabil.* 2005;27(23):1425-1433.

58. Mao HF, Hsueh IP, Tang PF, Sheu CF, Hsieh CL. Analysis and comparison of the psychometric properties of three balance measures for stroke patients. *Stroke.* 2002;33:1022-1027.

59. Huang YC, Wang WT, Liou TH, Liao CD, Lin LF, Huang SW. Postural assessment scale for stroke patients' scores as a predictor of stroke patient ambulation at discharge from the rehabilitation ward. *J Rehabil Med.* 2016;48:259-264.

60. Meijer R, Ihnenfeldt DS, van Limbeek J, Vermeulen M, de Haan RJ. Prognostic factors in the subacute phase after stroke for the future residence after six months to one year. A systematic review of the literature. *Clin Rehabil.* 2003;17(5):512-520.

61. Rocco A, Pasquini M, Cecconi E, et al. Monitoring after the acute stage of stroke: a prospective study. *Stroke.* 2007;38(4):1225-1228.

62. Borg GA. Psychophysical bases of perceived exertion. *Med Sci Sports Exerc.* 1982;14:377-381.

63. Kozlowski DA, James DC, Schallert T. Use-dependent exaggeration of neuronal injury after unilateral sensorimotor cortex lesions. *J Neurosci.* 1996 Aug 1;16(15):4776-4786.

64. Humm JL, Kozlowski DA, Bland ST, James DC, Schallert T. Use-dependent exaggeration of brain injury: is glutamate paretic? *Exp Neurol.* 1999 Jun;157(2):349-358.

65. Tamakoshi K, Maeda M, Nakamura S, Murohashi N. Very early exercise rehabilitation after intracerebral hemorrhage promotes inflammation in the brain. *Neurorehabil Neural Repair.* 2021 Jun;35(6):501-512.

66. López ND, Monge Pereira E, Centeno EJ, Miangolarra Page JC. Motor imagery as a complementary technique for functional recovery after stroke: a systematic review. *Top Stroke Rehabil.* 2019;26(8):576-587.

67. Jeon BJ, Kim WH, Park EY. Effect of task-oriented training for people with stroke: a meta-analysis focused on repetitive or circuit training. *Top Stroke Rehabil.* 2015;22(1):34-43.

68. Saeys W, Vereeck L, Truijen S, Lafosse C, Wuyts FP, Heyning PV. Randomized controlled trial of truncal exercises early after stroke to improve balance and mobility. *Neurorehabil Neural Repair.* 2012;26(3):231-238.

69. Guerra ZF, Lucchetti ALG, Lucchetti G. Motor imagery training after stroke: a systematic review and meta-analysis of randomized controlled trials. *J Neurol Phys Ther.* 2017;41(4):205-214.

70. Butler AJ, Cazeaux J, Fidler A, et al. The movement imagery questionnaire-revised Second Edition (MIQ-RS) is a reliable and valid tool for evaluating motor imagery in stroke populations. *Evid Based Complement Alternat Med.* 2012:497289.

71. Guertin PA. Central pattern generator for locomotion: anatomical, physiological, and pathophysiological considerations. *Front Neurol.* 2013;3:183.

72. Sommerfeld DK, Gripenstedt UK, Welmer AK. Spasticity after stroke: an overview of prevalence, test instruments, and treatments. *Am J Phys Med Rehabil.* 2012;91(9):814-820.

73. Trompetto C, Marinelli L, Mori L, et al. Pathophysiology of spasticity: implications for neurorehabilitation. *Biomed Res Int.* 2014:2014:354906.

74. Pandyan AD1, Johnson GR, Price CI, Curless RH, Barnes MP, Rodgers H. A review of the properties and limitations of the Ashworth and modified Ashworth Scales as measures of spasticity. *Clin Rehabil.* 1999;13(5):373-383.

75. Calverly TA, Ogoh S, Marley CJ, et al. HIITing the brain with exercise: mechanisms, consequences and practical recommendations. *J Physiol.* 2020;598(13):2513-2530.

76. Franklin BA, Tomppson PD, Al-Zaiti SS, et al. Potential deleterious adaptations following long-term exercise training: placing the risks into perspective—an update: a scientific statement from the American Heart Association. *Circulation.* 2020;141(13): e705-e736.

77. Mueller S, Winzer EB, Duvinage A, et al. Effect of high-intensity interval training, moderate continuous training, or guideline-based physical activity advice on peak oxygen consumption in patients with heart failure with preserved ejection fraction: a randomized clinical trial. *JAMA.* 2021;325(6):542-551.

78. Gjellesvik TI, Becker F, Tjonna AE, et al. Effects of high-intensity interval training after stroke (the HIIT-Stroke Study): a multicenter randomized controlled trial. *Arch Phys Med Rehabil.* 2020;101(6):939-947.

79. Luo L, Zhu S, Shi L, Wang P, Li M, Yuan S. High intensity exercise for walking competency in individuals with stroke: a systematic review and meta-analysis. *J Stroke Cerebrovasc Dis.* 2019;28(12):104414.

80. Hornby TG, Holleran CL, Hennessy PW, et al. Variable intensive early walking poststroke (VIEWS): a randomized controlled trial. *Neurorehabil Neural Repair.* 2016;30(5):440-450.

81. Fahey M, Brazg G, Henderson CE, et al. The value of high intensity locomotor training applied to patients with acute-onset neurologic injury. *Arch Phys Med Rehabil.* 2022;103(7S):S178-S188.

82. Moore JL, Nordvik JE, Erichsen A, Rosseland I, Bø E, Hornby TG. Implementation of high-intensity stepping training during inpatient stroke rehabilitation improves functional outcomes. *Stroke.* 2020;51(2):563-570.

83. Esmaeili V, Juneau A, Dyer JO, et al. Intense and unpredictable perturbations during gait training improve dynamic balance abilities in chronic hemiparetic individuals: a randomized controlled pilot trial. *J Neuroeng Rehabil.* 2020;17(1):79.

84. Högg S, Holzgraefe M, Drüge C, et al. High-intensity arm resistance training does not lead to better outcomes than low-intensity resistance training in patients after subacute stroke: a randomized controlled trial. *J Rehabil Med.* 2020;52(6):jrm00067.

85. Sammut M, Fini N, Haracz K, Nilsson M, English C, Janssen H. Increasing time spent engaging in moderate-to-vigorous physical activity by community-dwelling adults following a transient ischemic attack or non-disabling stroke: a systematic review. *Disabil Rehabil.* 2020:1-16.

86. Volpe BT, Ferraro M, Lynch D, et al. Robotics and other devices in the treatment of patients recovering from stroke. *Curr Neurol Neurosci Rep.* 2005;5:465-470.

87. Klatzky RL, Fikes TG, Pellegrino JW. Planning for hand shape and arm transport when reaching for objects. *Acta Psychol.* 1995;88:209-232.

88. Lee MJ, Lee JH, Koo HM, Lee SM. Effectiveness of bilateral arm training for improving extremity function and activities of daily living performance in hemiplegic patients. *J Stroke Cerebrovasc Dis.* 2017;26(5):1020-1025.

89. Whitall J, Waller SM, Sorkin JD, et al. Bilateral and unilateral arm training improve motor function through differing neuroplastic mechanisms: a single-blinded randomized controlled trial. *Neurorehabil Neural Repair.* 2011;25(2):118-129.

90. Waller SM, Whitall J, Jenkins T, et al. Sequencing bilateral and unilateral task-oriented training versus task oriented training alone to improve arm function in individuals with chronic stroke. *BMC Neurol.* 2014;14(1),236-245.

91. Chan MK, Tong RK, Chung KY. Bilateral upper limb training with functional electric stimulation iin patients with chronic stroke. *Neurorehabil Neural Repair.* 2009;23(4):357-365.

92. Sasaki K1, Matsunaga T, Tomite T, Yoshikawa T, Shimada Y. Effect of electrical stimulation therapy on upper extremity functional recovery and cerebral cortical changes in patients with chronic hemiplegia. *Biomed Res.* 2012 Apr;33(2):89-96.

93. Nascimento LR, da Silva LA, Araújo Barcellos JVM, Teixeira-Salmela LF. Ankle-foot orthoses and continuous functional electrical stimulation improve walking speed after stroke: a systematic review and meta-analyses of randomized controlled trials. *Physiotherapy.* 2020 Dec;109:43-53.

94. Prenton S, Hollands KL, Kenney LPJ, Onmanee P. Functional electrical stimulation and ankle foot orthoses provide equivalent therapeutic effects on foot drop: A meta-analysis providing direction for future re-search. *J Rehabil Med.* 2018 Feb 13;50(2):129-139.

95. Thieme H, Morkisch N, Mehrholz J, et al. Mirror therapy for improving motor function after stroke. *Cochrane Database Syst Rev.* 2018;7(7). CD008449.

96. Zeng W, Guo Y, Wu G, Liu X, Fang Q. Mirror therapy for motor function of the upper extremity in patients with stroke: a meta-analysis. *J Rehabil Med.* 2018;50(1):8-15.

97. Michielsen ME, Selles RW, van der Geest JN, et al. Motor recovery and cortical reorganization after mirror therapy in chronic stroke patients: a phase II randomized controlled trial. *Neurorehabil Neural Repair.* 2011;25(3):223-233.

98. Yang Y, Zhao Q, Zhang Y, Wu Q, Jiang X, Cheng G. Effect of mirror therapy on recovery of stroke survivors: a systematic review and network meta-analysis. *Neuroscience.* 2018;390:318-336.

99. Broderick P, Horgan F, Blake C, Ehrensberger M, Simpson D, Monaghan K. Mirror therapy for improving lower limb motor function and mobility after stroke: a systematic review and meta-analysis. *Gait Posture.* 2018;63:208-220.

100. Hesse S. Treadmill training with partial body weight support after stroke: a review. *NeuroRehabilitation.* 2008;23(1):55-65.

101. Lau KW, Mak MK. Speed-dependent treadmill training is effective to improve gait and balance performance in patients with sub-acute stroke. *J Rehabil Med: Official Journal of the UEMS European Board of Physical and Rehabilitation Medicine.* 2011;43(8):709-713.

102. McCain KJ, Smith PS, Polo FE, Coleman SC, Baker S. Excellent outcomes for adults who experienced early standardized treadmill training during acute phase of recovery from stroke: a case series. *Top Stroke Rehabil.* 2011;18(4):428-436.

103. Duncan PW, Sullivan KJ, Behrman AL, et al. LEAPS Investigation Team: body-weight-supported treadmill rehabilitation after stroke. *N Engl J Med.* 2011;364:2026-2036.

104. Yang YR, Chen IH, Liao KK, Huang CC, Wang RY. Cortical reorganization induced by body weight-supported treadmill training in patients with hemiparesis of different stroke durations. *Arch Phys Med Rehabil;* 2010;91:513-518.

105. Takakusaki K. Neurophysiology of gait: from the spinal cord to the frontal lobe. *Mov Disord.* 2013;28(11):1483-1491.

106. Doussoulin A, Rivas C, Rivas R, Saiz J. Effects of modified constraint-induced movement therapy in the recovery of upper extremity function affected by a stroke: a single-blind randomized parallel trial-comparing group versus individual intervention. *Int J Rehabil Res.* 2018;41:35-40.

107. Boukadida A, Piotte F, Dehail P, Nadeau S. Determinants of sit-to-stand tasks in individuals with hemiparesis post stroke: a review. *Ann Phys Rehabil Med.* 2015;58(3):167-172.

108. Ada L, Westwood P. A kinematic analysis of recovery of the ability to stand up following stroke. *Aust J Physiother.* 1992;38:135-142.

109. Lecours J, Nadeau S, Gravel D, Teixera-Salmela L. Interactions between foot placement, trunk frontal position, weight-bearing and knee moment asymmetry at seat-off during rising from a chair in healthy controls and persons with hemiparesis. *J Rehabil Med.* 2008;40:200-207.

110. Messier S, Bourbonnais D, Desrosiers J, Roy Y. Dynamic analysis of trunk flexion after stroke. *Arch Phys Med Rehabil.* 2004;85:1619-1620.

111. Barreca S, Siqouin CS, Lambert C, Ansley B. Effects of extra training on the ability of stroke survivors to perform an independent sit-to-stand: a randomized controlled trial. *J of Geriatr Phys Ther.* 2004;27(2):59-64.

112. Pollock A, Gray C, Culham E, Durward BR, Langhorne P. Interventions for improving sit-to-stand ability following stroke. *Cochrane Database Syst Rev.* 2014; 26(5):CD007232.

113. Winstein CJ, Stein J, Arena R, et al. Guidelines for adult stroke rehabilitation and recovery: a guideline for healthcare professionals from the American Hear Association/American Stroke Association. *Stroke.* 2016;47:e98-e169.

114. Liu YC, Yang YR, Tsai YA, Wang RY. Cognitive and motor dual task gait training improve dual task gait performance after stroke: a randomized controlled pilot trial. *Sci Rep.* 2017;7:4070.

115. Mao YR, Lo WL, Lin Q, Xiao X, Raghavan P, Huang DF. The effect of body weight supported treadmill training on gait recovery proximal lower limb motor pattern and balance in patients with subacute stroke. *Biomed Res Int.* 2015;175719.

116. Gama GL, Celestino ML, Barela JA, Forrester L, Whitall J, Barela AM. Effects of gait training with body weight support on a treadmill versus overground in individuals with stroke. *Arch Phys Med Rehabil.* 2017;98(4):738-745.

117. Gama GL, Celestino ML, Barela JA, Barela AMF. Gait initiation and partial body weight unloading for functional improvement in post-stroke individuals. *Gait Posture.* 2019;68:305-310.

118. Beyaert C, Vasa R, Frykberg GE. Gait post-stroke: pathophysiology and rehabilitation strategies. *Clin Neurophys.* 2015;45:335-355.

119. Knutson JS, Fu MJ, Sheffler LR, Chae J. Neuromuscular electrical stimulation for motor restoration in hemiplegia. *Phys Med Rehabil Clin N Am.* 2015;26(4):729-745.

120. Olvey EL, Armstrong EP, Grizzle AJ. Contemporary pharmacologic treatments for spasticity of the upper limb after stroke: a systematic review. *Clin Ther.* 2010;32(4):2282-2303.

121. Bakheit AMO, Fedorova NV, Skoromets AA, Timerbaeva SL, Bhakta BB, Coxon L. The beneficial antispasticity effect of botulinum toxin type A is maintained after repeated treatment cycles. *J Neurol Neurosurg Psychiatry.* 2004;75:1558-1561.

122. Dvorak EM, Ketchum NC, McGuire JR. The underutilization of intrathecal baclofen in poststroke spasticity. *Top Stroke Rehabil.* 2011;18(3):195-202.

123. Schiess MC, Oh IJ, Stimming EF, et al. Prospective 12-month study of intrathecal baclofen therapy for poststroke spastic upper and lower extremity motor control and functional improvement. *Neuromodulation.* 2011;14:38-45.

124. Van de Port IGL, Wevers LEG, Lindeman E, Kwakkel G. Effects of circuit training as alternative to usual physiotherapy after stroke: randomized controlled trial. *BMJ.* 2012;344:e2672.

125. Rose D, Paris T, Crews E, et al. Feasibility and effectiveness of circuit training in acute stroke rehabilitation. *Neurorehabil Neural Repair.* 2011;25(2):140-148.

126. Kwakkel G, Veerbeek JM, van Wegen EEH, Wolf SL. Constraint-induced movement therapy after stroke. *Lancet Neurol.* 2015;14(2):224-234.

127. Han P, Zhang W, Kang L, et al. Clinical evidence of exercise benefits for stroke. *Adv Exp Med Biol.* 2017;1000:131-151.

128. Taub E. Somatosensory deafferentation search with monkeys: implications for rehabilitation medicine. In: Ince LP, ed. *Behavioral Psychology in Rehabilitation Medicine: Clinical Applications.* New York, NY: Williams & Wilkins; 1980:316-401.

129. Wolf SL, Lecraw DE, Barton LA, Jann BB. Forced use of hemiplegic upper extremities to reverse the effect of learned nonuse among chronic stroke and head injured patients. *Exp Neurol.* 1989;104(2):125-132.

130. Wolf SL, Winstein CJ, Miller JP, et al. Effect of constraint-induced movement therapy on upper extremity function 3 to 9 months after stroke: the EXCITE randomized clinical trial. *JAMA.* 2006;296(17):2095-2104.

131. Taub E, Uswatte G, Bowman MH, et al. Constraint-induced movement therapy combined with conventional neurorehabilitation techniques in chronic stroke patients with plegic hands: a case series. *Arch Phys Med Rehabil.* 2013;94:86-94.

132. Peurala SH, Kantanen MP, Sjogren T, Paltamaa J, Karhula M, Heinonen A. Effectiveness of constraint-induced movement therapy on activity and participation after stroke: a systematic review and meta-analysis of randomized controlled trials. *Clin Rehabil.* 2011;26(3):209-223.

133. Eliasson AC, Shaw K, Berg E, Krumlinde-Sundholm L. An ecological approach of constraint induced movement therapy for 2-3 year old children: a randomized control trial. *Res Dev Disabil.* 2011;32:2820-3828.

134. Gordon AM, Chalres J, Wolf SL. Methods of constraint-induced movement therapy for children with hemiplegic cerebral palsy: development of a child-friendly intervention for improving upper extremity function. *Arch Phys Med Rehabil.* 2005;86(4):836-844.

135. DeLuca SC, Case-Smith J, Stevenson R, Ramey SL. Constraint-induced movement therapy (CIMT) for young children with cerebral palsy: effects of therapeutic dosage. *J Pediatr Rehabil Med.* 2012;5(2):133-142.

136. Si-Woon P, Wolf SL, Blanton S, Winstein C, Nichols-Larsen DS. The EXCITe Trial: predicting a clinically meaningful motor activity log outcome. *Neurorehabil Neural Repair.* 2008;22(5):486-493.

137. Rand D. Proprioception deficits in chronic stroke: upper extremity function and daily living. *Plos One.* 2018;13(3):e0195043.

138. Baumann M, Bihan EL, Chau K, Chau N. Associations between quality of life and socioeconomic factors, functional impairments and dissatisfaction with received information and home-care services among survivors living at home two years after stroke onset. *BMC Neurol.* 2014;14:92-104.

139. Byl NN, Pitsch EA, Abrams GM. Functional outcomes can vary by dose: learning-based sensorimotor training for patients stable poststroke. *Neurorehabil Neural Repair.* 2008;22:494-504.

140. Walker ER, Hyngstrom AS, Schmit BD. Sensory electrical stimulation improves foot placement during targeted stepping post-stroke. *Exp Brain Res.* 2014;232(4):1137-1143.

141. Nascimento LR, da Silva LA, Barcellos A, Teixeira-Salmela LF. Anle-foot orthosis and continuous functional electrical stimulation improve walking speed after stroke: a systematic review and meta-analyses of randomized controlled trials. *Physiotherapy.*2020;109:43-53.

142. Laver KE, Lange B, George S, Deutsch JE, Saposnik G, Crotty M. Virtual reality for stroke rehabilitation. *Cochrane Database Syst Rev.* 2017;11: Art ID: CD008349.

143. Ghai S, Ghai I, Lamontagne A. Virtual reality training enhances gait poststroke: a systematic review and meta-analysis. *Ann NY Acad Sci.* 2020;1478(1):18-42.

144. Clark WE, Sivan M, O'Connor RJ. Evaluating the use of robotic and virtual reality rehabilitation technologies to improve function in stroke survivors: a narrative review. *J Rehabil Assist Technol Eng.* 2019;6:2055668319863557.

145. Kim WS, Cho S, Ku J, et al. Clinical application of virtual reality for upper limb motor rehabilitation in stroke: review of technologies and clinical evidence. *J Clin Med.* 2020;9(10):3369.

146. Bergego C, Azouvi P, Samuel C, et al. Validation d'une échelle d'évaluation fonctionnelle de l'héminegligence dans la vie quotidienne: l'échelle CB. *Annales de Readaptation et de Medecine Physique.* 1995;38:183-189.

147. Azouvi P, Olivier S, de Montety G, Samuel C, Louis-Dreyfus A, Tesio L. Behavioral assessment of unilateral neglect: study of the psychometric properties of the Catherine Bergego Scale. *Arch Phys Med Rehabil.* 2003;84:51-57.

148. Azouvi P, Samuel C, Louis-Dreyfus A, et al. for the French Collaborative Study Group on Assessment of Unilateral Neglect (GEREN/GRECO): Sensitivity of clinical and behavioral tests of spatial neglect after right hemisphere stroke. *J Neurol, Neurosurg Psychiatry.* 2002;73:160-166.

149. Webster JS, Cottam G, Gouvier WD, Blanton P, Beissel G, Wofford J. Wheelchair obstacle course performance in right cerebral vascular accident victims. *J Clin Exp Neuropsychol.* 1989;11(2):295-310

150. Whitehouse CE, Green J, Giles SM, Rahman R, Coolican J, Eskes GA. Development of the Halifax Visual Scanning Test: a new measure of visual-spatial neglect for personal, peripersonal, and extrapersonal space. *J Int Neuropsychol Soc.* 2019 Apr 16:1-11.

151. Pernet L, Jughters A, Kerckhofs E. The effectiveness of different treatment modalities for the rehabilitation of unilateral neglect in stroke patients: a systematic review. *NeuroRehabilitation.* 2013;33:611-620.

152. Fortis P, Ronchi R, Senna I, Perucca L, Posteraro L, et al. Rehabilitating patients with left spatial neglect by prism exposure during a visuomotor activity. *Neuropsych.* 2010;24(6):681-697.

153. Baccini M, Paci M, Rinaldi LA. The scale of contraversive pushing: a reliability and validity study. *Neurorehabil Neural Repair.* 2006;20(4):468-472.

154. D'Aquila MA, Smith T, Organ D, Lichtman S, Reding M. Validation of a lateropulsion scale for patients recovering from stroke. *Clin Rehabil.* 2004;18(1):102-109.

155. Bergmann J, Krewer C, Rieß K, Müller F, Koenig E, Jahn K. Inconsistent classification of pusher behaviour in stroke patients: a direct comparison of the Scale for Contraversive Pushing and the Burke Lateropulsion Scale. *Clin Rehabil.* 2014;28(7):696-703.

156. Pardo V, Galen S. Treatment interventions for pusher syndrome: a case series. *NeuroRehabilitation.* 2019;44:131-140.

157. Kleim JA, Jones TA. Principles of experience-dependent neural plasticity: implications for rehabilitation after brain damage. *J Speech Lang Hear Res.* 2008;51:S225-S239.

158. Borstad A, Schmalbrock P, Choi S, Nichols-Larsen DS. Neural correlates supporting sensory discrimination after left hemisphere stroke. *Brain Res.* 2012;1460:78-87.

159. Schiemanck SK, Post MM, Kwakkel G, Witkamp TD, Kappelle LJ, Prevo AJH. Ischemic lesion volume correlates with long-term functional outcome and quality of life of middle cerebral artery stroke survivors. *Restor Neurol Neurosci.* 2005;23:257-263.

160. Gauthier LV, Taub E, Perkins C, Ortmann M, Mark VW, Uswatte G. Remodeling the brain: plastic structural brain changes produced by different motor therapies after stroke. *Stroke.* 2008;39(5):1520-1525.

161. Schaechter JD, Moore CK, Connell BD, Rosen BR, Dijkhuizen RM. Structural and functional plasticity in the somatosensory cortex of chronic stroke patients. *Brain.* 2006;129:2722-2733.

162. Loubinoux I, Brihmat N, Castel-Lacanal E, Marque P. Ceral imaging of post-stroke plasticity and tissue repair. *Rev Neurol.* 2017;173:577-583.

163. Steiner T, Juvela S, Unterberg A, Jung C, Forsting M, Rinkel G. European stroke organization guidelines for the management of intracranial aneurysms and subarachnoid haemorrhage. *Cerebrovasc Dis.* 2013;35:93-112.

164. Dupont SA, Wijdicks EFM, Lanzino G, Rabinstein AA. Aneurysmal subarachnoid hemorrhage: an overview for the practicing neurologist. *Semin Neurol.* 2010;30(5):545-554.

165. Grobelny TJ. Brain aneurysms: epidemiology, treatment options, and milestones of endovascular treatment evolution. *Dis Mon.* 2011;567:647-655.

166. Neifert SN, Chapman EK, Martini ML, et al. Aneurysmal subarachnoid hemorrhage: the last decade. *Transl Stroke Res.* 2021;12:428-446.

167. Jiang B, Paff M, Colby GP, Coon AL, Lin LM. Cerebral aneurysm treatment: modern neurovascular techniques. *Stroke Vasc Neurol.* 2016;1:e000027.

168. Lee H. Neuro-otological aspects of cerebellar stroke syndrome. *J Clin Neurol.* 2009;5:65-73.

169. Stalcup ST, Tuan AS, Hesselink JR. Intracranial causes of ophthalmoplegia: the visual reflex pathways. *Radiographics.* 2013;33(5):e153-e169.

170. Farr E, Altonji K, Harvey RL. Locked-in syndrome: practical rehabilitation management. *Am J Phys Med Rehabil.* 2021 Dec;13(12):1418-1428.

171. Smith E, Delargy M. Locked-in syndrome. *BMJ.* 2005;330:406-409.

172. Sacco S, Sara M, Pistoia F, Conson M, Albertini G, Carolei A. Management of pathologic laughter and crying in patients with locked-in syndrome: a report of 4 cases. *Arch Phys Med Rehabil.* 2008;89:775-778.

173. Heywood P, Murphy K, corfield DR, Morrell MJ, Howard RS, Guz A. Control of breathing in man: insights from the "locked-in" syndrome. *Resp Physiol.* 1996;106:13-20.

174. Schjolberg A, Sunnerhagen KS. Unlocking the locked in: a need for team approach in rehabilitation of survivors with locked-in syndrome. *Acta Neurol Scand.* 2012;125:192-198.

175. DeKroon JR, IIzerman MJ, Chae J, Lankhorst GJ, Zilvold G. Relation between stimulation characteristics and clinical outcome in studies using electrical stimulation to improve motor control of the upper extremity in stroke. *J Rehabil Med.* 2005;37(2):65-74.

176. Daly JJ, Ruff RL. Construction of efficacious gait and upper limb functional interventions based on brain plasticity evidence and model-based measures for stroke patients. *Sci World J.* 2006;7:2031-2045.

177. Quinn CT. Sickle cell disease in childhood: from newborn screening through transition to adult medical care. *Pediatr Clin North Am.* 2013;60(6):1363-1381.

178. Mazumdar M, Heeney MM, Sox CM, Lieu TA. Preventing stroke among children with sickle cell anemia: an analysis of strategies that involve transcranial Doppler testing and chronic transfusion. *Pediatrics.* 2007;120:e1107.

179. Hirtz D, Kirkham FJ. Sickle cell disease and stroke. *Pediatr Neurol.* 2019;95:34-41.

180. Grunwald IQ, Kuhn AL. Current pediatric stroke treatment. *World Neurosurg.* 2011;76;(6S):S80-S84.

181. Felling RJ, Sun LR, Maxwell EC, Goldenberg N, Bernard T. Pediatric arterial ischemic stroke: epidemiology, risk factors, and management. *Blood Cells Mol Dis.* 2017;67:23-33.

182. Mazzarella J, McNally M, Chaudhari AMW, Pan X, Heathcock JC. Differences in coordination and timing of pre-reaching upper extremity movements may be an indicator of cerebral palsy in infants with stroke: a preliminary investigation. *Clin Biomech.* 2020;73:181-188.

183. Amlie-Lefond C. Evaluation and acute management of ischemic stroke in infants and children. *Continuum (Minneap Minn).* 2018;24(1):150-170.

184. Steinlin M. A clinical approach to arterial ischemic childhood stroke: increasing knowledge over the last decade. *Neuropediatrics.* 2012;43:1-9.

185. Fan HC, Hu CF, Juan CJ, Chen SJ. Current proceedings of childhood stroke. *Stroke Res Treat.* 2011;43:28-39.

Review Questions

1. **You have your client in supine with hips extended. You are testing active range of motion. Which of the following motions can be tested with gravity eliminated in this position?**

   A. Ankle dorsiflexion

   B. Hip abduction

   C. Hip flexion

   D. Knee extension

2. **When providing range of motion in the acute care setting for an individual who is post-stroke and developing typical patterns of hypertonicity, which of the following muscle groups should be a focus through providing range of motion that moves the joint into _____**

   A. Elbow extension

   B. Forearm pronation

   C. Shoulder adduction

   D. Wrist extension

3. **Your client who is s/p CVA is having difficulty rolling from supine to side-lying. In order to work on this activity and improve his motor control and strength for the activity it would be advisable to:**

   A. Assist him to roll by placing your hands under his shoulder and hip and push him over into side-lying

   B. Cross his leg over the other leg in the direction he is rolling, then instruct him to use his arm and head to develop momentum and then roll over by flinging them to the side he is rolling onto

   C. Place a pillow between the legs to position them in abduction prior to initiating rolling

   D. Raise the foot of the bed and have him fling his arm and head side to side to develop momentum to move into the roll

4. **When rehabilitating for function the appropriate progression is to start with the task that is least physically demanding and use the task that**

   A. Allows for the most error in movement

   B. Avoids variability until the first form of the task is mastered

   C. Demands the movement pattern you are training

   D. Utilizes the non-paretic extremities to ensure the task is accomplished

5. **When working to retrain gait after a stroke the BEST choice of assistive device for the individual who continues to need a device during therapy sessions would be:**

   A. Parallel bars

   B. A quad cane or standard cane

   C. A standard walker

   D. A wheeled walker with arm trough

6. **Which of the following statements is true about best practice as related to the use of treadmill training with the individual post-stroke?**

   A. Is best used in the chronic stroke population

   B. Should be progressed to over-ground training

   C. Use 50% body-weight support

   D. Use velocity set at 1.0 m/s or greater

7. **When training gait which of the following setups would discourage knee hyperextension?**

   A. Stepping over small objects with the paretic extremity

   B. Transferring sit to stand with a soft object under the non-paretic foot

   C. Walking up a slope

   D. Walking while stepping with the non-paretic extremity

8. **Functional electrical stimulation (FES) can be used during gait to aid in dorsiflexion. Which of the following is a true statement regarding FES?**

   A. At present there is insufficient evidence to support the use of FES

   B. FES can slow or stop muscle fiber type conversion

   C. The stimulation is applied to the dorsiflexors throughout the gait cycle

   D. The use of functional electrical stimulation impedes neuroplasticity

9. **In the client with "locked in" syndrome the key to successful rehabilitation is to:**

   A. Establish a means of effective communication

   B. Position the individual in upright to aid in breathing

   C. Provide position changes at least every 2 hours

   D. Provide sensory stimulation to assist in bringing them out of their coma

10. **When working with an individual who has developed "pusher syndrome" post-stroke it is important to:**

    A. Set up training to obtain effective weight-bearing on the side they are pushing toward

    B. Set up training to obtain effective weight-bearing on the side that is doing the pushing

    C. Set up the environment so that all visual stimuli are on the paretic side and force the gaze to that side

    D. Set up the environment so that all visual stimuli are on the non-paretic side and force the gaze to that side

11. **Which stroke syndrome is likely to produce lower extremity paresis without upper extremity paresis?**

    A. Anterior cerebral artery stroke

    B. Basilar artery stroke

    C. Middle cerebral artery stroke

    D. Posterior cerebral artery stroke

12. **Loss of the upper left visual field is likely to occur with damage to which component of the optic projections?**

    A. Left temporal optic radiations

    B. Left parietal optic radiations

    C. Right temporal optic radiations

    D. Right parietal optic radiations

13. **A patient presents with the ability to understand speech but can only produce a few single words. What type of aphasia would present like this?**

    A. Conductive aphasia

    B. Expressive aphasia

    C. Global aphasia

    D. Receptive aphasia

14. **Overactivity of the pontine reticular formation is a major factor in what post-stroke phenomenon?**

    A. Clonus

    B. Hyperreflexia

    C. Hypertonia

    D. Phasic stretch reflex

15. **Your patient is experiencing localized spasticity in the thumb abductor; what would be the most likely medical treatment to decrease his spasticity?**

    A. Intrathecal baclofen

    B. Injection of botulinum toxin type A

    C. Oral baclofen

    D. Oral diazepam

16. **A patient presents with ipsilateral paresis of the facial muscles, ipsilateral sensory loss of the face, contralateral paresis of the trunk and extremities, and contralateral sensory loss in the trunk and extremities. A lesion of which area of the brain would produce these symptoms?**

    A. Cerebellum

    B. Medulla

    C. Midbrain

    D. Pons

17. **In newborns, which symptom is most likely to be noticed at stroke onset?**

    A. Absent speech

    B. Hemiparesis

    C. Impaired consciousness

    D. Sensory loss

18. **A client who is 2 days s/p stroke and has weakness in the right leg is being discharged home. He is taught to ambulate with a cane. Use of the cane could promote which of the following?**

    A. Decreased spasticity in the right leg.

    B. Development of abnormal reflexes.

    C. Learned nonuse of the right leg.

    D. Recovery of hip flexion in the right leg.

19. **Mr. Brown requires moderate assistance of one person and the use of a wheeled walker to ambulate 5 feet. Based on the recommendations of the ANPT clinical practice guideline how should gait speed be assessed and scored?**

    A. He would be unable to complete the 10-meter walk test so it should not be performed.

    B. He should be given a score of 0 on the 10-meter walk test and level of assistance should be recorded.

    C. Measure the time it takes him to walk 5 feet and record the time in seconds.

    D. He should be given the Timed Up and Go test.

20. If a patient who is s/p stroke is unable to actively move or be in an upright posture for 7 days which of the following is likely to happen when therapy first works on sitting on the edge of the bed?

A. The patient could become light headed or pass out.

B. Heart rate and blood pressure will initially increase to dangerous levels.

C. Respiratory rate will decrease with a concomitant increase in heart rate.

D. The patient will feel fine and can safely work on upright activities.

21. Mr. Brown is in supine with his arm elevated to 90 degrees. The therapist supports his arm at the wrist and upper arm. Mr. Brown is then told to slowly lower his hand to his nose. The purpose of this exercise is to:

A. Initiate early activation of the elbow flexors through gravity-eliminated movement.

B. Initiate early strengthening of the triceps with concentric exercise.

C. Initiate early activation of the triceps with an eccentric movement.

D. Provide eccentric strengthening of the triceps later in rehabilitation.

22. Your patient who is 2 days s/p CVA reports that she imagines moving her leg and walking as she did before her stroke when she is not in therapy. You realize that she is using motor imagery. Which of the following is a true statement regarding her use of this technique?

A. Motor imagery is not effective but is also not detrimental so she can continue if that is her wish.

B. Motor imagery should be used later in the rehabilitation process and should be discouraged during acute stages of recovery.

C. To be effective motor imagery must be paired with active movement of the extremity.

D. Motor imagery can be beneficial in the acute stage of care as it allows for practice without fatiguing the patient.

23. A client who is 5 days post-stroke and has no active movement in the hand or elbow is working on transferring sit to stand. The client should be instructed to do which of the following with the paretic upper extremity?

A. Place the paretic arm in a weight-bearing position with assistance from the therapist and push up into standing using both the non-paretic and paretic arms.

B. Place the paretic arm in a weight-bearing position but do not bear weight through it until there is fair or better strength in the elbow extensors.

C. Place the paretic arm in the client's lap; use the non-paretic arm to assist in pushing up to standing.

D. Place the paretic arm in a sling during all transfer and gait activities until there is active movement in the shoulder and elbow.

24. Mr. Brown is 5 days post-stroke and in an inpatient rehabilitation facility. He walks with decreased stance time and weight bearing on his paretic leg and he tends to take a short step with the paretic leg and then step to it with the non-paretic leg. He is set up with a rolling bedside table in front of him with both arms on the table for support. Which of the following is the correct way to initiate gait so that he is optimally set up to use a cyclical pattern that incorporates increased stance time on the paretic leg?

A. Initiate gait by stepping with the paretic leg first.

B. Initiate gait by stepping with the non-paretic leg first.

C. It does not matter which leg he steps forward with first.

25. When working on regaining motor control in the upper extremity it is important to include which of the following?

A. A goal for the position of the elbow as spasticity in the elbow flexors can overpower active movement into elbow extension.

B. Facilitation to the extensor muscles to ensure that they are active throughout the movement.

C. Feedback on performance as the movement is occurring to prevent errors during the movement.

D. Provide an end goal for the hand, as intended use of the hand shapes movement of the entire arm.

26. Which intervention technique is thought to work by normalizing interhemispheric inhibition while improving activation of the lesioned side of the brain?

A. Mirror therapy

B. Proprioceptive neuromuscular facilitation (PNF)

C. Bilateral training

D. Functional electrical stimulation (FES)

27. Mr. Brown is 3 weeks post-stroke and continues to exhibit foot drop during the swing phase of gait. He discharges home from inpatient rehabilitation in 3 days with recommendation to continue therapy as an outpatient. How should his foot drop be managed at this time?

A. Do not provide any assistance as walking without it will promote activation of the dorsiflexors.

B. Set him up with functional electrical stimulation to the peroneal muscles.

C. Refer to an orthotist to fit him with a solid ankle foot orthotic.

D. Refer to an orthotist to fit him with a hinged ankle foot orthotic.

28. The use of robotics is being investigated as an intervention in stroke. It has been most successful in improving which of the following?

A. Balance

B. Coordination

C. Distal arm function

D. Ambulation in chronic phase of recovery

29. **Which of the following is an effective intervention for resolving unilateral neglect?**
    A. Provide vibration to the paretic upper trapezius while doing visual exploration with a pointing activity.
    B. Position the client so that the trunk is turned to the left and everything the client needs to focus on is to the right of their sternum.
    C. Place TENS on the paretic extremity while doing a pointing task and visual exploration.
    D. Provide vibration to the quadriceps on the paretic side during the stance phase of gait.

30. **A blood clot, formed in the heart, is released and creates blockage in a small lenticulostriate artery. This would most likely result in what kind of stroke?**
    A. Hemorrhagic
    B. Lacunar
    C. Thrombotic
    D. Transient ischemic attack

31. **Which of the following rarely occurs in the ipsilesional extremities post-stroke?**
    A. Apraxia
    B. Paresis
    C. Sensory discrimination dysfunction
    D. Writing dysfunction

32. **You have a patient that fails to eat his food from the left side of the plate or notice the toothpaste on the left side of the counter to brush his teeth. This would correctly be referred to as:**
    A. Allocentric personal visual neglect
    B. Allocentric peripersonal visual neglect
    C. Egocentric personal visual neglect
    D. Egocentric peripersonal visual neglect

33. **A patient that presents with agraphia and alexia is most likely to have a stroke involving what area of the brain?**
    A. Frontal lobe
    B. Occipital lobe
    C. Parietal lobe
    D. Temporal lobe

34. **Cognitive deficits after stroke most likely occur due to what?**
    A. Loss of connections between the temporal lobe and the lesion
    B. Ischemic damage to the temporal lobe
    C. Loss of connections between the parietal lobe and the lesion
    D. Ischemic damage to the parietal lobe

35. **In patients with locked-in syndrome, what movement is typically maintained?**
    A. Lower extremity contralateral to the injury
    B. Finger tapping
    C. Speech
    D. Vertical eye movement

36. **A thunderclap headache is the common presentation for which of the following?**
    A. Aneurysm leakage
    B. Aneurysm rupture
    C. Ischemic stroke
    D. Transient ischemic attack

Answers

1. B	2. D	3. B	4. C	5. D
6. B	7. C	8. B	9. A	10. A
11. A	12. C	13. B	14. C	15. B
16. D	17. C	18. C	19. B	20. A
21. C	22. D	23. A	24. B	25. D
26. C	27. B	28. C	29. A	30. B
31. B	32. D	33. C	34. A	35. D
36. B				

GLOSSARY

Acalcula. Impaired mathematical ability due to damage to the angular gyrus or frontal lobe.

Acquired dyslexia (alexia). Impaired reading due to either damage in the occipital lobe, frontal lobe, or angular gyrus.

Agraphia (dysgraphia). Impaired writing due to damage to the angular gyrus or frontal lobe.

Allocentric neglect. Inability to perceive the contralesional aspect of objects independent of the patient's position.

Aneurysm. A weakening in a blood vessel, causing it to balloon out.

Ankle foot orthosis (AFO). Supports leg and foot from below knee to the toes; can restrict all motion (solid), assist with dorsiflexion (spring or spiral) or knee extension (ground floor reaction); and/or block plantarflexion (anterior or dorsal stops).

Anterior cerebral artery. Branch of the internal carotid; supplies the medial surface of the cerebral hemisphere.

Anterior communicating artery. Connects the 2 anterior cerebral arteries.

Anterior inferior cerebellar artery. Supplies the anterior and inferior portion of the cerebellum, cerebral peduncles, and inferolateral pons.

Aphasia. Language impairment.

Apraxia (ideomotor limb apraxia). Disruption of skilled movement due to impaired motor planning.

Auditory neglect. Impaired sound localization or awareness toward the contralesional side.

Baclofen. A GABA-β agonist that is used to treat spasticity, primarily through application to the subarachnoid space of the spinal column (intrathecal).

Basilar artery. Formed by the merging of the vertebral arteries; branches into cerebellar arteries and posterior cerebral arteries.

Bilateral training. Performing the same task with both hands or legs to promote paretic extremity use.

Borg Exertion Scale. A means of subjectively measuring exertion.

Botulinum toxin (botox). A drug that can be injected into single muscles to block acetylcholine activity and decrease hypertonia.

Circle of Willis. Formed by the anterior and posterior communicating arteries to link the anterior (internal carotid) and posterior (vertebral) blood systems.

Circuit training. Setting up practice stations for patients to practice specific tasks, moving from station to station.

Circumducted/circumducted gait pattern. Abduction at the hip and a circling pattern of advancing the limb secondary to hip flexor and dorsiflexor weakness.

Coiling. Insertion of a coil into an aneurysm to obstruct blood flow.

Compensation (compensatory movements). Use of the non-paretic extremity in place of the paretic extremity or alternate movement patterns in place of using the paretic muscles.

Conductive aphasia. Deficit in phonology due to damage in the posterior temporal lobe.

Constraint-induced movement therapy (CIMT). Focused practice with the paretic upper limb typically while use of the non-paretic limb is restricted.

Contraversive pushing (pusher syndrome). Impaired sense of upright secondary to ventroposterolateral nucleus damage and associated with pushing toward the hemiparetic side.

Dactylitis. Inflammation of a digit.

Diplopia. Double vision.

Dysarthria. Impaired speech due to poor oral muscle control.

Egocentric neglect. Lack of awareness of contralesional aspect of the environment dependent on the patient's perspective.

Embolism. Blood clot that forms elsewhere in the body and travels to the brain.

Expressive aphasia (non-fluent). Impeded ability to form words.

Flaccidity. Loss of muscle tone and movement.

Global aphasia. Receptive and expressive aphasia secondary to damage of both the ventral and dorsal streams.

Hemianesthesia. Impaired sensation on one side of the body, typically contralateral to the lesion.

Hemiparesis. Impaired movement on one side of the body.

Hemiplegia. Absence of movement on one side of the body.

Hemorrhagic stroke. Stroke caused by bleeding from a rupture of an artery or vein.

Homonymous hemianopia. Loss of the contralesional visual field secondary to damage beyond the optic chiasm.

Hyperreflexia. Exaggerated monosynaptic tendon reflexes (phasic stretch reflex).

Hypertonia. Increased muscle tone (spasticity or rigidity).

Inferolateral arteries. Branches of the posterior cerebral artery, supply ventorposterolateral and ventroposteromedial nucleis of thalamus (primary sensory nuclei).

Intensity. How hard the body is working.

Internal carotid artery. Originating from the common carotid off the aorta, primary blood supply to frontal, parietal, and temporal lobes; origin of anterior and middle cerebral arteries.

Intracerebral hemorrhage. Hemorrhage of cerebral vessel.

Ischemic stroke. Interruption in blood flow due to a clot or narrowing of the artery, resulting in neurologic damage.

Isolated muscle control. The ability to move individual muscles outside of synergistic patterns.

Labyrinthine artery. Branch of anterior inferior cerebellar artery; supplies internal ear.

Lacunar stroke. Ischemic stroke in a small blood vessel in the brain.

Learned nonuse. Failure to use the paretic arm even after there is a return of function secondary to early attempts at moving that failed.

Locked-in syndrome. Inability to speak or move secondary to a basilar artery or penetrating pontine arterial stroke or ventral pons brain damage; vertical eye movements and cognition are preserved.

Middle Cerebral artery. Branch of the internal carotid; supplies lateral surface of frontal, temporal & parietal lobes.

Motor neglect. Failure to move the hemiparetic side of the body not secondary to paresis.

Motor imagery. Visualizing the movement necessary to complete a task that functions like mental practice of the task.

Paramedian arteries. Branches of posterior cerebral arteries; supply part of thalamus.

Penumbra. Area of cell dysfunction surrounding the area of necrosis created by a stroke.

Posterior cerebral arteries. Terminal portions of basilar artery; supply occipital lobes and inferior and some of the medial temporal lobe.

Posterior Choroidal arteries. Branches of posterior cerebral artery and supply medial midbrain.

Posterior communicating artery. Terminal portion of internal carotid that connects to posterior cerebral arteries within the Circle of Willis.

Posterior inferior cerebellar artery. Branch of basilar artery; supplies posteroinferior cerebellum and inferior medulla.

Quadreparesis. Impaired movement in all extremities, typically due to brainstem stroke.

Quadrantanopia. Loss of ¼ of the contralesional visual field (upper loss of superior retinal fibers in **parietal lobe; lower** Loss of inferior retinal fibers in Meyer's loop).

Receptive aphasia (fluent aphasia). Impaired understanding of speech due to damage to the ventral stream and/or temporal lobe.

Recombinant tissue-type plasminogen (rTPA, TPA, altepease). Thrombolytic medication given to reverse the effects of an ischemic stroke.

Representational neglect. Inability to describe one side of a familiar space, based on the person's position.

Sentinel hemorrhage. Small leaks that precede a rupture of an aneurysm.

Sickle cell disease. Inherited autosomal recessive disorder affecting red blood cell formation and leading to increased chance of blood clots and stroke.

Somatosensory neglect. Failure to detect touch or limb position in the contralesional extremities.

Spasticity. Velocity dependent hypertonia (tonic stretch reflex) with associated hyperreflexia.

Speech apraxia. Disrupted motor planning for speech.

Stent. Wire mesh tube inserted into a blood vessel to wall off an aneurysm.

Subarachnoid hemorrhage. Hemorrhage of a surface vessel into the subarachnoid space.

Superior cerebellar artery. Branch of basilar artery; supplies upper half of cerebellum and the midbrain.

Supramalleolar orthosis (SMO). Orthotic that controls heel position; more commonly used in children.

Synergistic muscle/motor control. Activation of muscles in combination; in ability to activate isolated muscles.

Task-oriented practice. Focusing treatment on actual tasks rather than just movement patterns or strengthening.

Thrombotic stroke. Ischemic stroke in a large cerebral blood vessel.

Thrombus. Blockage of a cerebral artery, originating in the artery.

Thunderclap headache. Severe headache from an aneurysm bleeding into the subarachnoid space or brain tissue.

Transient ischemic attacks. Brief blockage of an artery in the brain producing transient stroke symptoms.

Tuberothalamic arteries. Branches of posterior communicating artery; supply components of thalamus.

Unilateral spatial neglect. Failure to attend to the hemiparetic side of the body or environment.

Vertebral arteries. Branch off subclavian artery to supply spinal cord, brainstem, cerebellum, and occipital lobe.

Visual neglect. Focused visual attention toward the ipsilesional environment and inattention to the other side.

ABBREVIATIONS

AFO	ankle foot orthosis
AIFC	anterior inferior cerebellar artery
BWS	Body Weight Supported
BWSTT	Body Weight Supported Treadmill Training
CIMT/CI	Constraint Induced Movement Therapy
CVA	cerebrovascular attack
FES	functional electrical stimulation
FNMES	functional neuromuscular electrical stimulation
GOS	Glasgow Outcome Scale
IRF	inpatient rehabilitation facility
LIS	locked-in syndrome
LOS	length of stay
MCA	middle cerebral artery
mNIHSS	modified NIHSS
NIHSS	National Institutes of Health Stroke Scale
NMES	Neuromuscular Electrical Stimulation
PASS	Postural Assessment Scale for Stroke
PED	Pipeline Embolization device
PICA	posterior inferior cerebellar artery
PROM	passive range of motion
rTPA	recombinant tissue-type plasminogen activator
SCA	Sickle Cell Anemia
SIT	stand to sit transfer
SNF	Skilled Nursing Facility
SOT	Sensory Organization Test
STS	sit to stand transfer
TIA	transient ischemic attack
TPA	tissue-type plasminogen activator
USN	unilateral spatial neglect syndrome

Brain Injury: Trauma, Anoxia, and Neoplasm

12

Deborah A. Kegelmeyer and Deborah S. Nichols-Larsen

OBJECTIVES

1) Differentiate anoxic from traumatic brain injury

2) Differentiate primary from secondary sequelae of brain injury

3) Examine the medical management of the patient with brain injury

4) Differentiate the evaluation and treatment methods of those with brain injury from those for other neurologic conditions

5) Structure evaluations and treatment sessions appropriate to the cognitive recovery level described by the Ranchos Scale to promote both physical and cognitive gains

6) Manage various behaviors as they arise during a treatment session with particular emphasis paid to agitation

7) Screen for mild traumatic brain injury/concussion

8) Recognize family adjustment issues and provide appropriate education

9) Recognize causes and unique features of anoxic brain injury and structure evaluation and treatment of these patients.

10) Review the presentation, pathology, and medical management of brain tumor in adults and children

11) Discuss the role of physical therapy in the management of patients with brain tumor

CASE A, PART I

Aaron is a 22-year-old Caucasian male brought by ambulance to the Emergency Department, following a motor vehicle accident (MVA), in which he was driving without a seatbelt, struck an electric pole, and flew through the windshield. His blood alcohol level is .20, and he is unconscious with multiple fractures, including his right femur, right clavicle, right radius and ulna, multiple ribs, and jaw. He has multiple **contusions** and a deep gash on the right side of his head, although the skull remains intact. He is not opening his eyes even to deep pressure on his palm or foot, is not verbalizing, and his intact left extremities are held in flexion.

● INTRODUCTION

Acquired brain injury has many causes. In this chapter we will focus on traumatic and anoxic brain injuries (BI) and neoplastic brain disorders. **Traumatic brain injury** (TBI) is thought to affect up to 10 million people worldwide[1] and is a leading cause of long-term disability with 1% of the population living with some long-term complication of TBI.[2] There are an estimated 2.53 million emergency room visits annually, of which nearly 300,000 result in hospitalization and nearly 60,000 result in death from TBI. Estimates of the cost of care, both acutely and long term, range from $56 to $221 billion annually,[2] yet that cost does not reflect the growing numbers of concussions (mild TBIs), for which medical attention is not typically sought.[1] In the United States, the incidence of occurrence averages 68.3 per 100,000[3]; in Europe, it averages 258/100,000.[4] The incidence of TBI is greatest for those over 75, followed by children under 4, and then by adolescents and young adults (15-24).[2] It is universally more common in men (55-80%), especially in those 15-24, becoming more gender neutral in older adults.[3,4] This commonly relates to the level of activity and degree of risk-taking displayed by boys/young men. The most common causes of TBI are falls, MVAs, assault, and self-harm. Sports-related injuries make up 10 to 15%; notably, sports-related concussions are more common in females (2:1 ratio), but there is concern that this may be due to decreased reporting in males.[2]

TBI can result from a blow to the head, when the head is struck or strikes an object, and/or sudden acceleration–deceleration or rotation of the head. As described in the case, many TBIs (often the most severe) occur as a result of a car accident, where the driver or passenger experiences a rapid forward movement of his body as the car hits an object or another car, stopped quickly by either the seatbelt, dashboard, or ground (acceleration–deceleration); in the worst situations, the car flips and there can be multiple head blows against the side window, roof of the car, and/or the dashboard along with rotational shear as the head and body roll, or the individual is thrown from the car with severe trauma to the head as it strikes the ground. Head injuries can be **open** or **closed**, referring to whether the skull is penetrated or intact. Penetrating injuries can arise from projectiles, like bullets, or are associated with skull fractures, where a piece of the skull itself penetrates the underlying brain tissue. Closed head injuries are much more common than penetrating injuries and result from MVAs (crash injuries), falls, and blows to the head from assaults as well as recreational activities, such as sports; blast injuries are common in military personnel, presenting as a closed head injury but internal brain injury.[5] Notably, falls are

TABLE 12-1	TBI Severity[1]		
SEVERITY LEVEL	**GLASGOW COMA SCORE**	**PERIOD OF UNCONSCIOUSNESS + AMNESIA**	**POTENTIAL OUTCOME**
Mild (concussion)	13-15	<30 minutes	High likelihood of survival with minimal long-term disability
Moderate	9-12	30 minutes-24 hours	Good likelihood of survival but with some long-term disability
Severe	3-8	>24 hours	Poor likelihood of survival and high likelihood of long-term disability

the most common cause of TBI, especially in young children and older adults. TBI is defined as mild, moderate, or severe, depending on the initial presentation and length of unconsciousness plus amnesiac period (see Table 12-1 and later section on amnesia), and this initial presentation is somewhat predictive of the potential outcome for the injury. Of note, some individuals with initially mild TBI have died and some with severe TBI recover and return to a normal level of participation and function. So, while these levels are somewhat predictive, they are not absolutely predictive, since site of injury, age, and co-morbidities also impact outcomes. The

Glasgow Coma Scale[6] (Box 12-1) is used almost exclusively to document initial presentation; however, increasing use of sedatives, anesthetics, and paralytics at the site of the accident is making its use more difficult by preventing the assessment of responsiveness acutely, while improving outcomes.[5] Other signs of TBI that may be evident on initial examination are noted in Box 12-2.

Based on the description of Aaron in Part I, how would he score on the GCS?

If you said 5, then you're correct.

Box 12-1   Glasgow Coma Scale

The Glasgow Coma Scale (GCS) was developed in the 1970s and assesses eye movements, verbal responses, and motor behavior, looking for spontaneous versus responsive activity, with each scale recorded numerically as indicated here.

SCORE	EYE OPENING	VERBAL RESPONSIVENESS	MOTOR BEHAVIOR
1	None	None	None
2	Opens in response	Makes sounds	Limbs in extension to deep pressure
3	Opens to verbal stimulation	Saying words	Limbs in flexion
4	Spontaneously opens	Confused but talking	Flexor withdrawal of limb to stimulus
5	N/A	Oriented	Localized response to stimulus
6	N/A	N/A	Moves to commands

Adapted from Teasdale G, Maas A, Lecky F, et al. The Glasgow Coma Scale at 40 years: standing the test of time. *Lancet Neurol.* 2014;13(8):844-854.[6]

Box 12-2   Signs of Traumatic Brain Injury[7]

1) Cerebrospinal fluid leaking from ears or nose
2) Confusion, altered mental status, or agitation that may worsen
3) Dilated or unequal pupils
4) Headache
5) Nausea or vomiting
6) Post-traumatic amnesia
7) Positive neurologic signs – Babinski, decerebrate, or decorticate posturing (see below)
8) Seizures
9) Sleepiness

Decorticate posturing defines a condition of upper extremity flexion, including fisting of the hands, and lower extremity extension with toe extension that results from damage to the brain at the junction of the midbrain and diencephalon, resulting in dominant descending control by the vestibulospinal and rubrospinal tracts, which stimulate the lower extremity extension and upper extremity flexion, respectively. In contrast, **decerebrate posturing** is characterized by excessive extension and internal rotation of the upper and lower extremities secondary to damage at the level of the midbrain below the red nucleus or severe damage to the frontal lobes, allowing disinhibition of the vestibulospinal tracts that activate extensor muscles.[8] Both conditions can be associated with brain herniation through the tentorial notch with patients demonstrating decorticate posturing as the upper midbrain is compressed, followed by decerebrate posturing as more distal areas of the brainstem are compressed; this is typically secondary to excessive brain swelling or an expanding **hematoma**. When trunk and neck extension accompany the decerebrate posture, it is called **Opisthotonus**.[8,9]

PATHOPHYSIOLOGY OF TBI

The typical TBI presents with two types of injury: focal and diffuse. **Focal injury** results at the area(s) of contact between the skull and the brain or from the projectile that penetrates the brain. In the typical acceleration–deceleration injury, there is a focal injury as the brain bumps into the skull as the body's momentum comes to a rapid stop, and then a **contra coup** (opposite side) injury as it "bounces back" into the opposite side of the skull. For example, Aaron's car hit an electric pole, causing his head to move rapidly forward, hitting the windshield on its way to the pavement and resulting in severe damage to the frontal lobe as the brain hit the anterior part of the skull; as he came to rest on the pavement, his brain would have quickly bounced back toward the posterior surface of the skull, creating a contra coup injury to the occipital lobe. The site of focal damage is characterized by (1) **contusions** – bruising of the brain surface, (2) **lacerations** – tearing of the pia or arachnoid matter or the brain tissue, and/or (3) **hematomas** – bleeding within the subdural or epidural spaces or within the brain tissue, referred to as **intraparenchymal**. These hemorrhages occur due to rupture of the blood vessels within these areas: (1) subdural – tearing of cerebral arteries or veins that bleed into the space between the dura and arachnoid matters, (2) epidural – tearing of meningeal arteries of the dura with bleeding into the space between the dura and the skull, (3) intraparenchymal – tearing of the penetrating intracerebral arteries with bleeding into the brain tissue, and (4) intraventricular – bleeding into the ventricles from intraparenchymal hemorrhage or subependymal vein rupture.[2,10]

The **diffuse axonal injury** (DAI) results from the tearing of axons that comprise the white matter due to inertial or rotational forces as the brain "bounces" within the cranium (see Figure 12-1). MVAs are associated with the greatest amount of DAI[6]; however, even relatively minor concussions, as are seen in athletes, whether professional or amateur, from **concussive events** (e.g., helmet–helmet or head–head contact) have been shown to create axonal injury, and repeated concussions can produce permanent and significant damage (discussed later in this chapter).[11] DAI is most common in the white matter of the brainstem, corpus callosum, and parasagittal projections in the lateral hemispheres. It can be quantified as **Grade 1** (mild) – microscopic changes noted in the white matter; **Grade 2** (moderate) – apparent damage to the corpus callosum; and **Grade 3** (severe) – damage to the corpus callosum and brainstem white matter.[11] Early imaging is used to determine the extent of the early damage; this is typically done with computed tomography (CT scan), which is effective in identifying skull fractures, hematomas, or the location of projectiles or bone fragments in penetrating injuries. Later, magnetic resonance imaging (MRI) is used to better characterize the brain injury and may include diffusion tensor imaging (DTI) that can visualize white matter integrity; this can help in determining the potential prognosis.[2,12]

The consequences of TBI are dependent on the areas of focal damage and the degree of white matter damage. However, the initial trauma is followed by a cascade of secondary changes that result in further loss of neurons. First, damage to the axon disrupts the **axonal transport** conveying nutrients through the

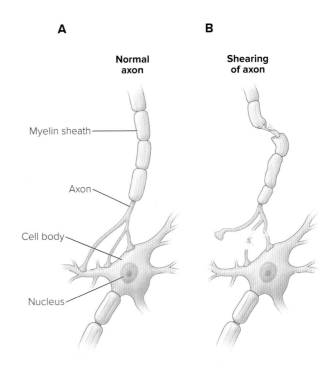

A   **B**

Normal axon   Shearing of axon

Myelin sheath

Axon

Cell body

Nucleus

FIGURE 12-1 Diffuse axonal injury: A. Normal neuron axon with connections to a postsynaptic neuron. **B.** Diffuse axonal injury is characterized by a twisting and tearing of the myelin and underlying axons; this will be followed by retrograde degeneration back to the cell body.

length of the axon, resulting ultimately in the loss of the distal segment of the axon. Second, there is a loss of ATP (adenosine 5'-triphosphate), disrupting the cellular mechanisms that maintain the sodium, calcium, and potassium cellular balance in the cell body and proximal axon, allowing calcium to rush into these components and resulting in disruption of intracellular function and cellular hypoxia. At the same time, there is an overproduction of oxidants, generating oxidative stress, and exaggerated release of glutamate and free radicals, which further disrupt cellular function in damaged and adjacent neurons. **Anterograde degeneration** occurs early, resulting in the death of the distal segment; this is followed by **retrograde degeneration**, or a dying back, of the proximal axon segment and ultimately the cell body. The brain transitions to glycolytic metabolism, lactic acid build-up, breakdown of the blood-brain barrier, and additional cell death.[2] These changes induce inflammation, trigger macrophages to invade the area, and further disrupt cellular function in adjacent neurons and glia.[11] These changes are present within the first 4-7 hours of injury. Notably, the loss of neurons and white matter disruption seems to continue for a considerable time after the initial injury, resulting in additional general brain atrophy, white matter abnormalities, and secondary loss of function[1] that can occur months after the initial injury such that the individual demonstrates improvement to a point of plateau, followed by a subsequent loss of function. These chronic changes, referred to as **negative or maladaptive plasticity**, appear related to amyloid and tau protein deposits and ongoing neuroinflammation, associated with reactive microglia (see Chapter 2).[13] Maladaptive plasticity may continue for years and is thought to result from the same processes that impact aging, including (1) decreasing activity levels within limited and often unstimulating environments; (2) disruption of sensory processing, referred to as noisy processing (see Chapter 18 on Aging), associated with decreased activity in the sensory cortices and less cognitive analysis of sensory information; and (3) decreased neuromodulation, stemming from lower levels of dopamine and acetylcholine that are critical for executive function and attention. Together, these maladaptive plasticity changes result in further deterioration of those functions already disrupted by the initial injury.[13] The concept of maladaptive plasticity opens the door for physical therapists, along with the rehabilitation team, to address and potentially prevent negative plasticity.

Pathophysiology of Anoxic/Hypoxic Brain Injury

Anoxic brain damage occurs when the brain is deprived of oxygen either due to decreased circulation or impaired respiratory function. Individuals can experience hypoxia, lowered cerebral oxygen levels, or anoxia, loss of oxygenation to the brain. **Anoxic brain injury** typically results in bilateral and diffuse injury that affects the "boundary zones" of the cerebral circulation with brain areas of high metabolic need manifesting greater likelihood of insult; these include the cerebellum, hippocampus, thalamus, basal ganglia, frontoparietal and parieto-occipital cortex.[14-21]

Hypoxia can be a chronic problem, stemming from conditions that prevent effective oxygenation of blood, such as pulmonary disease or severe anemia, or recurring disruption of respiration such as obstructive sleep apnea; brain damage secondary to these conditions occurs progressively over time. Acute onset of hypoxia/anoxia results from cardiac or respiratory arrest (see Box 12-3) with cardiac arrest the most common cause of anoxic brain injury; notably, respiratory arrest will result in cardiac arrest within minutes of breathing cessation. Hypoxic ischemic brain injury is one of the major causes of adverse outcome after cardiac arrest and contributes to the high mortality rate of those experiencing cardiac arrest[17]; it is also a common effect of failed suicide attempts.[14,15,19,20] Healthcare systems are seeing an increasing number of individuals who have survived an opioid overdose. Opioid overdose leads to respiratory depression which in turn can cause cerebral hypoxia and damage to brain areas sensitive to hypoxia, including the hippocampus and cerebellum.[18]

Studies show that hypoxic events lead to widespread damage in the brain. Once cerebral circulation is disrupted, independent of cause, oxygen depletion in the brain is present within 20 seconds, resulting in loss of consciousness. Within five minutes, loss of glucose and oxygen disrupts ATP production within brain cells, causing release of excitatory neurotransmitters (glutamate, norepinephrine) and rapid disruption of the cell membrane barrier. Secondary influx of calcium and sodium into the cells further disrupts cell function and triggers cell edema and oxygen-free radical production, triggering cell death.[20,21] Post-resuscitation, there is a rapid increase in cerebral oxygen metabolism that can lead to reperfusion injury within 30 minutes; over the next 1½ to 12 hours, a hypoperfusion state may emerge, associated with diminished cerebral blood flow and lower oxygen metabolism, altered blood glucose concentration and secondary brain injury (post-resuscitation encephalopathy).[20] Hyperthermia can occur secondary to pathophysiologic changes, triggered by widespread brain trauma; this increase in temperature can further exacerbate cerebral edema and blood-brain barrier disruption. Thus, imposed hypothermia or maintenance of body temperature below 36°C is recommended.[22] Anoxic brain injury has a 13 to 23% greater likelihood of death and is more likely to result in severe disability than TBI, since it is bilateral and generalized throughout the brain[23]; there is some suggestion that younger age is associated with better outcomes, yet this is confounded by cause of injury and duration of anoxic period.[15] Following anoxia, careful reoxygenation and monitoring of blood glucose levels, secondary intracranial pressure elevation, and blood pressure are critical to maximize recovery potential.[20]

Individuals who have experienced hypoxia may not be aware of the episode (e.g., sleep apnea), may not seek medical care or report the event to healthcare providers. Therapists must be alert to the possibility of a hypoxic episode in individuals who are at risk (Box 12-3) and include screening for neurologic damage. Areas of particular concern are cognitive function including memory (inclusive of **anterograde amnesia**), executive function, Parkinsonism, and coordination.[20,21] A key role of the physical therapist is to assess the movement system. In individuals with known or suspected hypoxia/anoxia, the assessment should include tests of movement initiation and speed to screen for basal ganglia involvement as well as tests of coordination to screen for cerebellar involvement. Screening to determine if the patient is alert and oriented is not sufficient to identify potential cognitive issues secondary to hypoxic events. Measures such as the Montreal Cognitive Assessment or the clock drawing test should be administered to screen for cognitive issues. If cognitive issues are suspected appropriate referrals are made for a complete workup. It is important for therapists to be aware of

Box 12-3	Individuals at Risk for Having Experienced Hypoxia/Anoxia[14-18]

Any history of:
- Cardiac arrest with resuscitation
- Opioid drug use and possible or confirmed overdose
- Carbon monoxide poisoning
- Severe blood loss
- Near drowning
- Attempted hanging
- Strangulation
- Anesthetic accidents

Diagnosis of:
- Chronic obstructive respiratory disease
- COVID-19 with hospitalization
- Severe asthma
- Severe anemia
- Acute respiratory distress syndrome (ARDS)
- Emphysema
- Pneumonia
- Pulmonary embolism
- Pulmonary fibrosis

the potential for hypoxia as these individuals may present to therapy without having previously sought medical care for the hypoxic event, or milder symptoms related to hypoxia may have gone undetected during an acute hospital stay due to the focus on life-saving measures. Individuals who experience a hypoxic event with coma will present with similar sequalae and will require similar treatment as those with TBI.

● BI CONSEQUENCES

Pre-hospitalization/Emergency Room

Stabilization of the patient and provision of adequate ventilation is critical for the survival of patients with severe TBI. Transfer to a level I trauma center via helicopter is recommended. Application of basic airway strategies to prevent hypoxia is critical but intubation by paramedics is not recommended. Once in the ER, caretargets ventilation and circulation to prevent hypoxia and hypotension. While hyperventilation has been used to prevent hypoxia and lower ICP, it can increase secondary brain injury, so must be used sparingly.[24] Similarly, after anoxic BI, patient resuscitation is critical to reestablish ventilation and cardiac rhythm.[20]

Infusing hypertonic saline may be initiated when brain edema is suspected. Administration of packed red blood cells is often used to increase systolic blood pressure above 90 mmHg, after TBI. For all BI, an initial neural exam is performed once ventilation and circulation have been addressed, focusing on pupillary responsiveness and initial GCS. For those with TBI, laterality differences should be noted as a sign of a hematoma, accompanied by a search for other injuries.[24]

Hematomas

With TBI, hematomas may be present in the epidural space, subdural space, or within the brain tissue (parenchymal). Early operative evacuation is recommended, based on the size of the mass, the degree of brain shift, and neurologic presentation of the patient (see Box 12-4); those with smaller masses or stable symptoms may be monitored for increased ICP, signs of herniation, or symptom exacerbation. Early evacuation within 4-6 hours is associated with improved survival rates, when surgery is indicated.[24]

Box 12-4	Operative Evacuation of Hematoma Criteria[24]

Surgical evacuation of hematomas is recommended when the mass size or symptoms meet the listed criteria.

1) Epidural: mass > 30 cm³ or mass thickness > 15 mm with midline shift > 5 mm with GCS < 9 or focal deficits
2) Subdural: mass > 1 cm or those with a midline shift > 5 mm and GCS < 8 with rapidly progressive symptoms or ICP < 20.
3) Parenchymal: frontal or temporal masses > 20 cm³ with .5 mm midline brain shift and GCS 6 to 8, or mass volume > 50 cm³ or declining neurologic scores

Coma, Post-Traumatic Amnesia, and Executive Dysfunction

As should be evident from the earlier discussion of the GCS, the first consequence of a BI is loss of consciousness; this can be so short that it goes unnoticed (seconds) or last for weeks. When the period of unconsciousness exceeds 6 hours, it is referred to as **coma**, characterized by a lack of responsiveness, volitional movement, and a sleep-wake cycle. Unlike in the movies, people in coma do not typically just "wake up," they gradually emerge from the coma into a state of confusion; however, in those with mild injuries, this stage can last a minute or minutes, while in those with more severe injuries, it can last for many months, and for some, they never fully emerge from this state. Some survivors of severe BI will enter what is known as an **unresponsive wakefulness syndrome (UWS),** formerly referred to as a vegetative state (Stage II of the Braintree Scale – see Table 12-2). UWS is characterized by (1) an emergence of a simulated sleep-wake cycle; (2) maintenance of brainstem function to control breathing and circulation; (3) intact pupillary reflexes but absence of focusing on and tracking of objects; (4) primitive chewing, sucking and swallowing; and (5) a generalized response to stimuli (Ranchos Scale – Level II, Table 12-2). When these clinical features are associated with an absence of cortical brain activity, it indicates a reliance on the brainstem centers that control the sleep cycle, respiration, and reflexive responsiveness and is most often a permanent condition, in which patients can survive for many years (**UWS**). Some move through this state to one of minimal consciousness, indicated by specific responses to stimulation (e.g., withdrawal of foot to touch of the sole), following simple commands, yes/no verbalization or gestures (may not be accurate), visual fixation and tracking of objects, reach and grasp of objects, and some intelligible verbalizations.[29,30] Emergence from minimally conscious state (MCS) requires the functional use of objects and/or communication.[30]

For those that emerge from coma, after a moderate to severe TBI, they progress through the **UWS** to a gradual reemergence of responsiveness and severe confusion, abnormal behavior (agitation, disinhibition, and altered mood), and memory disruption.[31] This period is referred to as **post-traumatic amnesia** (PTA), which disrupts memories prior to the accident as well as the formation of new memories, including the day-to-day activities within the hospital setting (see Box 12-5 for more information on amnesia). As PTA clears, the patient is left to deal with a myriad of deficits in multiple systems – sensory, motor, behavioral, and cognitive.[33] Ways to document recovery of behavior, memory, and responsiveness from TBI are the Ranchos Los Amigos Cognitive Recovery Scale,[8–25,29,30] Galveston Orientation and Amnesia Test (GOAT),[34] the Disability Rating Scale,[26] the JFK Coma Recovery Scale–Revised,[27] and the Braintree Scale of Neurologic Stages of Recovery from Brain Injury.[28] The GOAT is principally used to identify the clearing of PTA and asks the patient a series of questions to determine orientation to person, place, time, and circumstance, including details of what is remembered about the accident and how he came to be at the hospital. Errors are scored and subtracted from a total of 100.[34] Table 12-2 provides a comparison of some of these measures.

TABLE 12-2 Measures of Recovery in TBI[6,25–28]

GLASGOW COMA SCALE SCORE[6]	JFK COMA RECOVERY SCALE – REVISED (SCORE)[27]	RANCHOS LOS AMIGOS COGNITIVE SCALE[25,*]	BRAINTREE SCALE[28]	DISABILITY RATING SCALE[26**]
3	Unarousable (0); none responsive on all scales (0); may have abnormal posturing (1); total = 0-1	Stage I: Unresponsive	1. Coma – unresponsive	No response on any scale and totally dependent; total score = 29
4-8	Startles to auditory and visual stimuli (1 each); flexor withdrawal to noxious stimulus (2); reflexive oral responses (1); opens eyes to stimulation (1); no communication; total = 6	Stage II: Generalized response – whole limb or body response to touch, requires complete assistance	2. Vegetative state – begins sleep-wake cycle	Opens eye to pain (2); incomprehensible speech-groans/moans (3); extends (4) or flexes (3) limb to pain or withdraws (2); no awareness for feeding, toileting, grooming (3 each); totally dependent (5) and non-employable (3); total = 24-26
9-10	Localizes sound (1); object fixation – visual pursuit (2-3); localized response to noxious stimulus (3); vocalization/oral movement (2); intentional vocalizing (1); eye opening with or without stimulation (1-2); total = 10-12	Stage III: Localized response – moves part specific to site of touch/pinch, still requires total assistance	3. Minimally conscious – responds inconsistently, no speech	Opens eyes to speech (1) or spontaneously (0); incomprehensive speech (3); localized movement to stimulation (1); no feeding, toileting, or grooming (3 each); totally dependent (5); non-employable (3); total = 21-22
12-14	Moves to command inconsistently – consistently (3-4); reaches to object or recognizes object (4-5); object manipulation or automatic movement or functional object use (4-6); verbalizations understood (3); communication is functional (2); some attention to situation (3); total = 19-23	Stage IV: Confused and agitated, can be abusive and easily provoked, maximal assistance required Stage V: Confused with less agitation but still inappropriate behavior, requires maximal supervision	4. Post-traumatic amnesia	Spontaneous eye opening (0); confused speech (1); obeying commands to move (0); some awareness of feeding (2); some awareness of toileting needs (2); primitive ability to groom self (2); marked (4) assistance required; not employable (3); total = 17 Eye opening (0); confused speech (1); moving to commands (0); partial awareness of how to feed self, toileting, and grooming (1 each); marked assistance all of the time (4); not employable (3); total = 10

(Continued)

TABLE 12-2	Measures of Recovery in TBI[6,25-28] (Continued)			
GLASGOW COMA SCALE SCORE[6]	JFK COMA RECOVERY SCALE – REVISED (SCORE)[27]	RANCHOS LOS AMIGOS COGNITIVE SCALE[25,*]	BRAINTREE SCALE[28]	DISABILITY RATING SCALE[26**]
15		Stage VI: Confused but more appropriate behavior; requires moderate supervision	5. PTA resolution, increased independence	Eye opening (0); oriented speech (0); obeying movement commands (0); full awareness of feeding, toileting, grooming needs (0 each); moderately dependent – needs supervision in the home (3); not employable (3) or able to work in sheltered workshop (2); total = 5 or 6
		Stage VII: Automatic appropriate – can complete ADLs and routine activities if physically able with minimal supervision/assistance, but still have memory problems and difficulty with problem-solving		
		Stave VIII: Purposeful, appropriate – independent in many tasks, understands limitations, still some behavioral problems, requires standby assistance	6. Increasing independence and social skills with return to community activity, work, etc.	Same as above but with increasing ability to perform independently with some supervision (1) and likely can work either in a sheltered workshop (2) or selected jobs (1); total = 2 or 3

*The Ranchos Scale actually has two more levels: IX, which is associated with increasing ability to maintain focus and switch focus from one task to another but continued mild emotional/behavioral challenges that may require caregiver assistance to refocus, and X, which is associated with good goal-directed function, the ability to multi-task, but still with some attentional challenges and the need for more time to complete some activities. Therapists rarely see patients that are at levels VIII-X.

**The Disability Rating Scale has a final category of functioning = independent in all skills (0) and work = unrestricted work ability (0).

Box 12-5	Amnesia

Amnesia is typically divided into two aspects: retrograde amnesia and anterograde amnesia. **Retrograde amnesia** is associated with a loss of memory for prior events; this likely results from an inability to retrieve those memories from our memory storage, which may relate to an inability to identify appropriate cues for memory retrieval. Since memory storage is not localized to a given area, damage in multiple areas can be associated with retrograde amnesia. **Anterograde amnesia** is an inability to form new memories, likely as a result of damage to the temporal or frontal lobes or the white matter connecting them; this impedes the consolidation of new memories. For those with a moderate to severe TBI, the consolidation of the memory of the accident is usually disrupted by the head injury, so most survivors do not remember the actual accident and may not remember a period of time leading up to the accident. This time period varies with the severity of the injury but can include just minutes, hours, or days. **Post-traumatic amnesia** is a period of both retrograde and anterograde amnesia in those with moderate to severe TBI. The retrograde amnesiac component may prevent patients from knowing their family members, friends, and information that defines who they are – occupation, likes/dislikes, etc. However, procedural and semantic memories (discussed in Chapter 7) are typically unaffected or more mildly affected. The anterograde amnesia component prevents new memory accrual, including memory for those providing the patient's care, the location of care, and the ability to verbalize what events or activities occurred previously (earlier in the day or over preceding days). However, procedural learning can occur even though the patient will not be able to verbalize the process. The clearing of PTA is an important stage for the patient, as it indicates the ability to actively participate in their rehabilitation; early PTA recovery is characterized by the ability to remember the activities of the day and to begin to follow a schedule.[32]

It should be noted that recovery can stall at any level of these scales with no further progression or some delay (variable in length) between stage progressions.

After anoxic injury, prognosis is also related to the period of unconsciousness. Typically, those who gradually regain alertness within a few hours have a good prognosis; for those experiencing coma for longer than 6 hours, return of independent function is unlikely (estimated at 10%).[20] When brainstem dysfunction is noted (e.g., lack of pupillary reflexes), prognosis is also poor. The use of sedatives and paralytics may impede prognostication in the first 72 hours, but a motor response to pain within the 48 to 72 hour timeframe is a positive indicator of a favorable outcome. Many patients may experience seizures, either myoclonic, tonic-clonic, or focal (see Chapter 20 (Cerebral Palsy) for description) within the first few hours after resuscitation, especially during the re-warming process after imposed hypothermia. However, a condition known as status myoclonus, which manifests as repetitive myoclonic seizures that are unrelenting, may occur and is a poor prognostic sign; while antiepileptic medications are not recommended in this early timeframe, even when seizures are present, status myoclonus must be treated, usually with a combination of anti-epileptics and sedatives.[21]

Respiratory Distress Syndrome

Presentation

Respiratory compromise is associated with severe brain injury secondary to loss of consciousness and damage to medullary regions that control respiration. In addition, swallowing may also be impaired due to brainstem damage, and in TBI, facial and/or tracheal damage is common with secondary bleeding or hematoma formation in the throat.[35] A secondary complication of TBI can be **acute respiratory distress syndrome (ARDS)**, which occurs in up to 31% of TBI admissions, during their hospital course, and is characterized by inflammation of the lung lining, disruption of gas exchange, and hypoxia. This is a leading cause of death in those with TBI but can also result in secondary anoxic brain damage due to hypoxemia (low blood oxygen levels).[36] ARDS occurs most commonly in association with other secondary complications (sepsis, renal or heart failure, or hypertension).[37,38] There is no definitive test for ARDS, so it is diagnosed based on a combination of (1) a ratio of arterial oxygen partial pressure to inspired oxygen fraction that is <300 mm Hg, (2) a chest x-ray illustrating bilateral pulmonary edema, and (3) normal EKG (electrocardiogram).[37]

Treatment

In those with a GCS of ≤8 after TBI, respiratory support is required either by intubation with an oropharyngeal, nasopharyngeal, or an endotracheal tube with ventilator support.[39] This is typically done at the site of the accident. Some patients with moderate TBI may also need ventilator support, if orofacial injuries are present or they have disruption of respiratory function. For those that are able to breathe on their own, ventilation support, using continuous positive airway pressure (CPAP), provided through a mask, or positive pressure support, provided through a nasal cannula, may be enough.[12]

There is no definitive treatment for ARDS; in fact, the best treatment is prevention. Standard care for ARDS is to provide ventilator support that minimizes the stress on the lungs; this is typically done with what is termed **lung-protective ventilation**, which uses a lower inspiratory volume (tidal volume), to prevent over-stretching the weakened alveoli, in combination with an increased respiration rate. For some, this will require additional sedation to prevent dyssynchrony between the patient and the ventilator.[38] Prone positioning is effective in non-TBI patients with ARDS or TBI patients with normal or minimally elevated intracranial pressure (ICP); however, it is not used when ICP is significantly increased because it tends to produce a further increase. In the presence of high ICP, a 30 degree elevation of the head of the bed is recommended. Extracorporeal membrane oxygenation (ECMO) has also been effectively used for those with refractory ARDS.[36]

Intracranial Hypertension (ICH)

Presentation

Following BI, ICH arises from multiple causes. In TBI, the presence of hematomas may create increased pressure, shifting the brain tissue across midline or caudally into the brainstem compartment. The latter can occur either (1) medially, producing bilateral compression of cranial nerve III with unresponsive pupil dilation or (2) laterally with herniation of the uncus of the temporal lobe, associated with unilateral pupil dilation (see Figure 12-2). Edema of the brain tissue, compromise of cerebrospinal fluid (CSF) circulation, and disruption of the autoregulatory mechanisms that maintain ICP may further increase ICH days after the initial traumatic injury. In anoxic brain injury, cerebral edema also occurs secondary to vasogenic or cytotoxic mechanisms. Vasogenic-induced edema appears to result from an alteration of cell membrane proteins that allows fluid to leak into the interstitial space from cells or vessels. Conversely, cytotoxic edema results from intracellular fluid retention secondary to disruption of the cell membrane ion channels as the cells experience metabolic crisis.[22] Additionally, compromised blood flow may further impede perfusion and, thereby, exacerbate ICH; this can occur from dysfunction of the normal autoregulatory mechanisms that control cerebral blood flow.[22] Normally, ICP measures 10 to 15 mm Hg with cyclic increases and decreases, associated with cardiopulmonary rhythms; an increase to 20 mm Hg signals the need for treatment, so the goal is to maintain ICP below 20mm Hg. Signs of increased ICP include nausea, vomiting, papilledema (swelling around the optic disc) with retinal hemorrhaging, and drowsiness.[24,40]

Treatment

ICP must be monitored in patients with severe BI (GCS < 9) and any patient with an identified hematoma; this is typically done with a catheter placed in the epidural space or ventricle. Those placed in the lateral ventricles, called external ventricular drains, also allow drainage of CSF, either intermittently or continuously, to lower ICP. Subarachnoid screws, which are placed into the subarachnoid space through a bur hole in the skull, allow ICP monitoring without CSF drainage. Other implantable

microtransducers can also be used, which measure the pressure on the device, equating it to the ICP; these are typically placed within the brain tissue but can also be placed in the subarachnoid space, subdurally, or epidurally. Placement of any monitoring device can cause additional brain trauma and potentially hemorrhage and can also be a site for secondary infection, so careful monitoring for these issues is critical.[41] The first step in treating ICH is sedation to minimize arterial hypertension, agitation, and the potential for fighting the rhythm of the ventilator, which can lead to increased ICH and dislodging of the monitoring device. However, sedation can have detrimental side effects, including depressed heart function and blood pressure and additional risk for infection. The second step involves administration of hyperosmolar agents (mannitol or hypertonic saline) to increase osmolarity in the blood and draw fluid out of the brain tissues into the circulation, reducing brain volume. Herniation into the brainstem, which can occur with hematoma expansion or excessive brain edema, is a medical emergency, requiring immediate treatment to relieve ICH and potentially necessitating surgical intervention. In those, for whom sedation and hyperosmolarity treatment are ineffective, a decompression craniotomy may be performed to allow some brain expansion through the opening in the cranium. However, the benefit of this remains controversial.[24,40] Hyperventilation may also be used to increase cerebral perfusion to facilitate clearing of edema and hematomas; however, as mentioned earlier, this can result in greater secondary brain injury. For some patients with refractory elevated ICP, a phenobarbital-induced coma may be used to control ICP.[24]

Epilepsy

Presentation

Approximately 17% of patients with severe TBI will develop post-traumatic epilepsy (PTE) (see Chapter 20 for a description

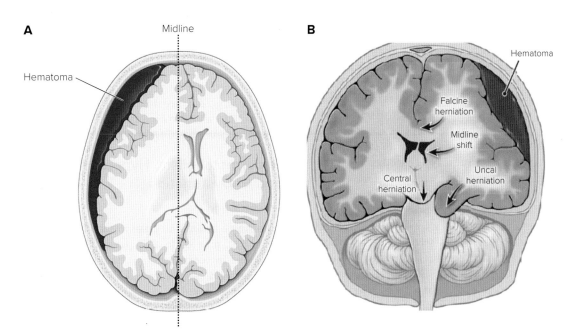

FIGURE 12-2 Brain shifts associated with traumatic hematoma: A. Frontotemporal hematoma compressing the lateral hemisphere with midline shift to the opposite side of center. **B.** Cerebral hematoma inducing herniation of the uncus and central white matter downward, compressing brainstem tissue.

of epilepsy); this can occur within the first week of the incident (5% of patients) or much later – within a year (5%) or more post-injury (another 7%).[42] The incidence of PTE, following a moderate TBI is lower and rarely occurs in the late stages; in contrast, the incidence of PTE is much higher for those that experience a penetrating head injury at almost 53%. For those with mild or moderate TBI, the risk is minimal at <0.1%.[43] Early PTE may exacerbate the original injury by contributing to the detrimental excitotoxicity that occurs post-injury; there is some suggestion that late PTE may also cause expansion of the initial brain tissue loss through a similar mechanism. The cause of these post-traumatic seizures remains elusive. One theory suggests that iron deposits left, as hematomas dissolve, trigger free radical formation that subsequently stimulates abnormal glutamate release and neuronal hyper-activation.[43] Another implicates pro-inflammatory cytokines in the development of lesion expansion and epilepsy onset.[44] The type of seizure is highly variable but includes generalized, focal, and focal that progress to generalized.[45] Focal seizures arise most frequently from the frontal or temporal lobes.[44] With anoxic encephalopathy secondary to cardiorespiratory arrest, seizures occur early in nearly 36% of patients; as described earlier in this chapter, these are most commonly myoclonic but can also be tonic-clonic or focal. When these occur within the first 24 hours, they are poor prognostic indicators.[46]

Treatment

Most patients with severe TBI and some with moderate TBI were historically placed on prophylactic antiepileptic medications, typically phenytoin, as soon as they are admitted to the hospital.[47] If the patient survived the first week without a seizure, this prophylactic application was weaned with careful observance for any indication of seizure emergence. More recently, findings suggest little benefit from this prophylactic administration, so it is not recommended.[47] There is some indication, however, that subclinical seizure episodes may take place without obvious symptoms, so even those that appear to be seizure free may, in fact, be having abnormal neuronal activation. Regardless of whether prophylactic antiepileptic medications are provided, many TBI survivors will develop epilepsy either during hospitalization, the first year or later. Long-term antiepileptic medications may control seizure activity with a variety of medications utilized (see Chapter 20 for potential medications). However, for those with focal epilepsy, surgical resection of injured tissue may be effective; this is more commonly possible with temporal than frontal lobe epilepsy, as the area is more easily accessed and typically the seizure site is more focal.[44] Since many patients post-resuscitation from anoxia are placed on a respirator, they are sedated and an antiepileptic may be added to suppress seizures, if they occur.[46] Status epilepticus or status myoclonus are related to greater mortality and disability. In some, the EEG pattern can indicate seizure activity in the absence of motor activity, referred to as subtle generalized convulsive status epilepticus; this has only been reported in those that remain in coma.[48] Seizures raise the metabolic demand and can exacerbate the metabolic crisis within brain tissue, resulting in greater brain injury, so control is critical.[49]

Inflammation: Systemic Inflammatory Syndrome and Multi-organ Dysfunction Syndrome

Presentation

CNS inflammation is a natural consequence of BI, both traumatic and anoxic; however, with severe injury there may be a systemic inflammatory response that can disrupt function in multiple organs. There is strong evidence that this systemic inflammation involves a disruption of the autonomic nervous system's centers in the hypothalamus, hippocampus, pituitary, and brainstem (nucleus tractus solitarii).[50] Systemic infection is characterized by cytokine diffusion through the blood-brain barrier (BBB) into the systemic circulation; this emergence of cytokines is accompanied by elevated plasma leukocytes plus alterations in circulating electrolytes, metal ions, excitatory amino acids, glucocorticoids, and free radicals.[51,52] Together, these changes trigger the liver to stimulate protein synthesis to achieve homeostasis, stimulate tissue repair, and decrease inflammation. However, with severe injury this acute response can be ineffective and transition to a condition known as **systemic inflammatory response syndrome** (SIRS) may occur; SIRS presents with fever, hyperventilation, and extreme elevation in white cell count that seems to result from injury-induced immunosuppression. The accumulation of circulating inflammatory cells in the organs can damage the liver as well as the lungs and kidneys, resulting in **multi-organ dysfunction syndrome** (MODS), which can ultimately lead to organ failure.[51,52]

Treatment

Recent evidence suggests that normalization of autonomic nervous system activity by administration of medications that block either parasympathetic activity or sympathetic activity may be effective in treating SIRS; however, there is currently no definitive way to determine whether SIRS is the result of exaggerated parasympathetic activity or sympathetic activity. Administration of anticholinergics (e.g., galantamine) has demonstrated the ability to diminish sympathetic hyperactivity, reducing SIRS; conversely, administration of β2-adrenergic agonists (e.g., dexmedetomidine) can block parasympathetic hyperactivity and also diminish SIRS.[50] Ultimately, 10 to 20% of those that develop MODS will die.[51,52]

Hypermetabolism, Hypercatabolism, and GI Dysfunction

Presentation

Following a brain injury, the metabolic demand of the patient is elevated, referred to as **hypermetabolism**; this results from elevation in corticosteroids, epinephrine, norepinephrine, glucagon, and cortisol as well as increased circulating inflammatory mediators (e.g., cytokines).[53,54] Increased levels of epinephrine and norepinephrine disrupt the normal control of metabolism by the sympathetic nervous system that seems to be further exacerbated by a systemic inflammatory process with energy demands as high as 200% of normal.[53,54] In some cases, this hypermetabolism progresses to hypercatabolism, which involves exaggerated glucose utilization and the breakdown of body proteins (e.g., muscle – both skeletal and cardiac), leading to substantial loss of skeletal muscle. The more severe the head injury (lower GCS), the greater the metabolic demand and likelihood of hypercatabolism.[54] The challenge of meeting the nutritional demands of the patient with a severe TBI can be exacerbated by orofacial injuries, dysphagia due to damage to the centers or cranial nerves that control swallowing, and disrupted gastrointestinal function. Gastrointestinal dysfunction is characterized by delayed or slower emptying of the GI tract and esophageal reflux secondary to diminished sphincter tone. The latter can result in aspirational pneumonia.[54]

A secondary complication of BI is gastric stress ulcers, which is found not only with acquired brain injury but also following craniotomy in association with brain tumor removal[55]. Multiple factors contribute to their development, including (1) the highly stressful nature of a severe head injury, impacting all major organ systems; (2) uninhibited parasympathetic activity, caused by damage to the hypothalamus and resulting in excessive gastric acid secretions; (3) diminished blood flow to the gastric mucosa, resulting from a cascade of post-traumatic changes; and (4) irritation or infection from enteral feedings.[56]

Treatment

Comprehensive nutritional support is critical to survival from severe brain injury. Initially, this is provided by IV, known as total parenteral nutrition (TPN); however, to meet the metabolic demands of the TBI survivor in coma or with severe orofacial injuries, enteral nutrition is commonly initiated within 24 to 48 hours of admission to the hospital. This requires placement of a nasogastric or orogastric tube.[53] If prolonged feeding support is required or orofacial injuries are severe, a percutaneous gastrostomy (PEG) tube is used, which is a tube placed directly into the stomach through the abdominal wall; when gastric dysfunction or reflux is severe or there is impaired gastric emptying, the tube may be placed into the jejunum (jejunostomy) to provide post-pyloric feeding.[54,57] To assist with ICH, a hyperosmolar formula is typically initiated early.[12] However, there remains uncertainty about the best other dietary components to provide, but there is some evidence to suggest a high-protein diet with zinc supplements and immune-enhancements may be beneficial.[53] Despite the controversy over the type of diet, it is critical to meet the high metabolic demand of the TBI survivor through appropriate nutrition therapy. As recovery progresses, it is also important to adapt the diet to meet the normalizing catabolic demand to prevent weight gain. There is no definitive method identified for gastric ulcer prevention or treatment, although histamine 2 receptor blockers and proton pump inhibitors have been used; in patients able to take medications by mouth, sucralfate or antacids can be given.[53,55,58]

Dysautonomia/Paroxysmal Autonomic Instability and Dystonia (PAID)

Presentation

Dysautonomia, more recently renamed PAID, is a dysregulation of autonomic function that presents in up to 34% of TBI admissions, especially in those with severe injury. It is most common in those with fractures, infections, or prolonged ventilation that had significant DAI, hypoxia prior to admission, and/or injury of the brainstem.[59,60] Although a definitive cause has not been identified, PAID likely results from damage to the connections between the cortex and hypothalamus, leading to a loss of inhibition and hypersensitivity to internal and external stimuli. As a result, episodes of tachycardia, hyperpyrexia (fever), elevated blood pressure, extensor posturing (decorticate or decerebrate), and copious sweating occur, lasting a few minutes to hours. While most common when patients are in the ICU, this condition can persist into the rehabilitation phase, and when it does, is disruptive to recovery.[59]

Treatment

Pharmacologic treatment is commonly used with a variety of medications attempted, including baclofen, beta blockers (e.g., propranolol), benzodiazepine, and morphine. Recently, intrathecal baclofen administration has been found to provide longer-term management; however, this may not be the first method of choice due to the need for surgical implantation of the administration catheter into the spinal epidural space.[60,61]

Neuropsychiatric Changes

Presentation

Behavioral/emotional dyscontrol: Perhaps the most debilitating consequences of BI are the neuropsychiatric changes that ensue. Two common behavioral syndromes, experienced by many BI survivors, are emotional and **behavioral dyscontrol**. **Emotional dyscontrol** manifests with agitation, irritability, restlessness, pathologic laughing/crying (pseudobulbar affect), and/or emotional lability. Pathologic laughing/crying appears as involuntary and sustained periods of these emotions can occur without provocation but disrupt function. In contrast, emotional lability is an exaggerated response to an appropriate trigger, so in this condition, there might be excessive crying to a somewhat sad situation (e.g., saying good-bye to a loved one that they will see again the next day). This condition is incredibly common and increases in frequency in the post-acute stages with up to 62% of survivors experiencing it to some degree. **Behavioral dyscontrol** is characterized by disinhibition and sometimes aggression; this can result in the pulling out of IV lines and feeding tubes, fighting and swearing early in recovery as well as hyper-sexual behavior and excessive risk-taking in later recovery. Minor manifestations include poor social awareness and impulsivity; however, even these can have a profound impact on the long-term outcome of BI, impeding social participation and employment. Notably, some BI survivors will also experience other psychiatric conditions, of which depression is the most common; this will require careful monitoring and treatment but also must be distinguished from the more common emotional and behavioral dyscontrol.[62] Of course, for those with ABI secondary to a suicide attempt, there is already a pre-existing psychiatric condition, which may continue, but in those with ABI from other causes, multiple psychiatric conditions have been reported post-injury, including depression, anxiety, and changes in personality.[19]

Cognition/Communication: BI, regardless of etiology, is associated with heterogenous changes in all aspects of higher-order brain function – memory, executive function, attention, communication, and processing speed.[60] The degree of dysfunction relates primarily to the extent of the damage rather than the etiology. However, in general, ABI produces greater deficits due to its bilateral nature than TBI, yet language disturbances are less severe.[14]

Treatment

The most critical treatment for the common neuropsychiatric consequences of BI is careful and consistent behavioral management and cognitive remediation. Both will be discussed within the physical therapy management section of this chapter, but behavioral management includes creating an environment to minimize excessive stimulation, maintaining a calm demeanor when working with clients, and preventing self-injurious behavior. In some cases, pharmacologic management is required; this can involve many forms but sedation to prevent self-injurious behavior early and antidepression medications to treat ongoing depression at later stages are common.[62]

For other cognitive deficits, treatment focuses on cognitive and adaptive strategies but some pharmaceutical interventions have been used with variable success. Methylphenidate (monoamine agonist) has been effectively used to improve attention and concentration. There is some suggestion that cholinergic agonists (e.g., rivastigmine or donepezil) may improve sustained attention and thereby working memory.[60]

Physical Therapy Management

The therapist, treating a client after a BI, must manage three core problem areas: physical, cognitive, and behavioral. Just as in our case study of Aaron, many clients have been involved in some type of accident that has led to multiple trauma. In the physical area, there are findings similar to those discussed in Chapter 11 (CVA); though in the case of BI, many of the problems may be bilateral and are often accompanied by musculoskeletal and peripheral nervous system injuries. For those with ABI, basal ganglia damage is more common than primary motor cortex damage, presenting with Parkinsonian symptoms or other involuntary movements, while damage to the cerebellum bilaterally may result in bilateral limb or trunk ataxia and impaired posture and gait.[63] Examination and treatment are conducted as outlined in Chapters 10 (Evaluation) and 11 with appropriate modifications for bilateral impairments. This chapter will discuss management of the cognitive and behavioral sequela of TBI.

Cognition/Memory

As discussed in Chapter 7, cognition is a complex function, involving the ability of the brain to process, store, retrieve, and manipulate information to solve problems. It includes:

- Attention – consists of selective attention, divided attention, and sustained attention.
- Memory – the ability to consolidate, store and retrieve facts, events, experiences, etc.
- Initiation – the ability to initiate action.
- Judgment – the ability to make considered decisions or come to sensible conclusions.
- Speed of processing – the rate at which directions can be processed into actions.

BI may impact any of these areas; therefore, the physical therapy assessment includes careful examination of the domains of cognitive function, and treatment is based on these findings. Assessment of attention is typically done by observing the client's ability to stay focused on the task at hand, during the therapy evaluation. The client should also be observed in situations where there are distractions to determine if selective attention is impaired. Divided attention is intact, if the client can talk while carrying out a task (e.g., performing an exercise). Sustained attention is measured by the length of time the client can stay on task, during their work with the therapist.

Memory loss is common, after even mild BI, and questions should be asked to assess the client's ability to retrieve old memories and acquire new ones. To identify the degree and recovery of retrograde amnesia, questioning about the period leading up to the injury, the time of the injury, and immediately after the injury will identify the window of memory loss. On subsequent therapy sessions, asking about events from the previous therapy session is a means to assess for the presence of anterograde amnesia. PTA, as described earlier in the chapter, is the inability to lay down memories reliably from one day to the next. This also includes orientation to time, person, place, and situation. The duration of PTA is a key indicator of injury severity and prognosis and is defined as the time from injury to regaining continuous memory for ongoing events (see Box 12-6). It is important to remember that other factors such as age, pre-morbid condition, and social support, all impact prognosis for return to independent function.[64–66]

For explanations of cognitive assessment for initiation, judgment, and speed of processing along with functional examples, see Table 12-3.

It is hypothesized that deficits in divided attention, executive function, and long-term memory are due to either impaired working memory or speed of processing deficits. A study by Ciarmelli et al. supports the hypothesis that deficits in these cognitive functions are primarily due to impairments in working memory.[67] Thus, progressively challenging working memory, during therapy, while allowing sufficient time to process information, should, hypothetically, lead to better functional outcomes.

CASE A, PART II

Differential assessment of Aaron's other cognitive abilities would be done as part of the physical therapy assessment as he is coming out of his coma. He is asked to wave good-bye to his mother. He is given time to respond, and it is noted that he waves after a 30-second delay. Also, during the evaluation, Aaron is asked to point to the red paper. After 2 minutes and a cue, he has not pointed to the paper. This assessment has shown that speed of processing is slow and that Aaron understands simple familiar commands, like "wave good-bye," but he is unable to cognitively process pointing to the red paper despite being given additional time to respond. Waving is limited by speed of processing, while the pointing task is limited by a higher-level cognitive dysfunction.

TABLE 12-3	Cognitive Function and Assessment	
	HOW IT IMPACTS FUNCTION	**ASSESSMENT**
Initiation	Closely related to apathy though the two are separate and distinct entities. Individuals who lack initiative are capable of solving the problem but are unable to initiate the process. It can be difficult to separate issues with initiative from depression, apathy, or severe cognitive disability.	Need to rule out apathy and depression with input from psychology services. Observe the client's ability to generate a new conversation where he must choose the topic or engage in an activity that he is not specifically told to complete. Initiation often becomes a larger problem when the client returns home.
Judgment	Impairs safety	Ask the client to make decisions requiring them to judge safety in a controlled environment (e.g., ask the client when it is safe to cross a street in a mock setup or while under close supervision of therapy staff).
Speed of processing	There's a slowing of processing, but individuals with slow processing can solve the problem, if given enough time.	Allow time for processing during the examination to determine what time frame each client requires to process information. Once the time needed for successful processing is determined, future sessions can be conducted based on this measurement.

Box 12-6	Prognosis Based on PTA[64–66]

Severity based on duration of PTA:

Mild = <1 hour

Moderate = >1 hour and <24 hours

Severe = >1 day and <7 days

Very severe = >7 days

Personality

The personality and behavioral changes that commonly occur after BI have a significant impact on the individual's sense of self and can be quite debilitating for both the patient and their family and friends. Personality changes are most difficult for individuals with mild BI as they are cognizant of the changes and the impact of those changes on their friends and family. Therapists should acknowledge these changes, when working with the patient and family, and recognize the need to modify therapy based on mood and negative behaviors.

Recognizing cognitive and behavioral deficits is important as these are most closely associated with long-term disability.[68] Common behaviors that occur after TBI include agitation, confusion, perseveration, and apathy among others. See Table 12-4 for a description of each behavior and ways to manage those behaviors in the clinic. This text will address specific behavior-management techniques throughout the rest of the chapter based on the time since injury and the stage of recovery.

Motor Learning

Motor learning may be intact, depending on the areas of the brain impacted by the BI, though it is common for some aspect of motor learning to be negatively impacted by BI. Usually, procedural learning remains intact while declarative learning is negatively affected. An individual with impaired declarative learning is unable to state how to do a task, but when presented with the task, can perform it, demonstrating intact procedural learning. For therapy tasks, such as sit to stand and transfer to walking with a rollator walker, BI survivors often demonstrate

intact procedural learning, but when asked to explain how to safely stand up, the client with a BI is not able to explain the steps of the transfer. With repetition, these clients continue to demonstrate procedural learning to be safe while transferring. However, they are limited in their ability to apply this learning to new situations, requiring the therapy staff and family to teach the task in each environment in which it will be performed.

Successful motor learning in individuals with cognitive, memory, or behavioral deficits requires many repetitions with consistent structure and feedback. The number of repetitions completed in studies that demonstrate neuroplasticity is far higher than that achieved in typical therapy. This highlights the need for therapists to be very cognizant of practice time and number of repetitions, if they hope to optimize neuroplastic changes after BI.[70] To date, research in the area of motor learning and BI is very limited due to difficulties in defining the population. One study demonstrated that gait adaptation to novel environmental demands is impaired in persons with chronic BI, and therefore, may be an important skill to target in rehabilitation.[71] There is also evidence that some individuals with BI can benefit from random (variable) learning methods, and that this type of learning improves transfer to novel conditions better than blocked practice, just as was found in non-BI subjects.[72]

Early Management

Immediately following BI, the focus of care is on saving the individual's life. Within the intensive care setting (ICU), therapists focus on determining the severity of the injury, preserving life, and prevention of further damage. Early PT intervention, during the ICU stage, has been associated with decreased ICU length of stay and hospital length of stay, fewer complications, and greater likelihood of discharge home; thus, early mobilization seems to prevent the negative physiologic complications of prolonged immobilization.[73] As recovery progresses and the patient becomes more stable, therapy can be progressed to include mobility, strength, and range of motion. The initial PT assessment focuses on state of arousal, cognitive level as defined by the Ranchos Amigos Stages, and identifying injuries to the neuromuscular and musculoskeletal systems.

TABLE 12-4	Common Behaviors s/p TBI and Their Management[69]	
BEHAVIOR DESCRIPTION	**KEY TO MANAGEMENT**	**MANAGEMENT STRATEGIES**
Agitation is common s/p TBI and is defined as excesses of behavior. Typical agitated behaviors include restlessness, inability to focus or maintain attention, irritability and, at higher levels of agitation, combativeness.	Prevent escalation of agitation and modify the environment and staff behavior to avoid the use of both physical and medical restraints.	• Be calm both verbally and in your physical and nonverbal actions. • Treatment session goals should be flexible to allow adjustment to the level of agitation. • Treatment environment should be quiet with minimal external stimuli. • Be aware of tension building up in the client, stopping the external stimulation before agitation becomes combative. • Redirect the patient's attention and move them to a location with less stimulating or frustrating activities, until agitation is reduced. • Do not attempt to discuss agitation logically or elicit guilt for the behavior. • Do not leave the patient unsupervised or alone during agitation. • Try to maintain consistency in the personnel who interact with the patient so as to promote familiarity and decrease novel stimuli. • To the extent possible, permit moving about or verbalization during periods of increased agitation.
Confusion results from the inability of patients to recall minute-to-minute, hour-to-hour, or day-to-day events in their life. As a result, they are unable to understand their current situation in light of what has or what will occur. Associated problems include diminished attention, learning, and orientation.	Increase and even provide the external structure for the individual, particularly in regard to time, place, and activities.	• Place calendars in client's rooms with a schedule of daily activities posted in their room; also have one that they can take with them throughout the day. • Post the steps for them to follow for their ADLs in their room. • At the start of each treatment session, review your name, what day and date it is, what time of day it is, and where they are. Use calendars, clocks, name tags, and building signage to reinforce this information. • Maximize consistency and establish routines within and between treatment sessions. • To increase client awareness, start each activity with a short and easy to understand explanation of what is expected of them. • At the end of the session, use the client's schedule to elicit from him or her the next activity, in which he/she will engage.
Impulsivity is a tendency to act without thinking. It is common in people s/p TBI and often seen along with agitation and confusion.	Provide consistency across caregivers and visitors, and have the client verbally rehearse strategies for each treatment activity.	• The entire team should attempt to use the same strategy with a patient; inconsistency will only create confusion. • Verbally review the steps for each activity, before allowing the patient to start. • Use a written list of steps that the patient reviews (out loud or to himself) before starting. • The patient verbally rehearses aloud the steps needed to complete the task. • The patient waits a few seconds, before beginning a task, and is instructed to think about how to complete the task, before doing it. • Aloud, verbal rehearsal should be consistently implemented, in all treatment sessions and throughout the day. As a patient demonstrates increased control, this can be gradually shaped into rehearsing to oneself and then simply pausing before starting the task.

(Continued)

TABLE 12-4	Common Behaviors s/p TBI and Their Management[69] *(Continued)*	
BEHAVIOR DESCRIPTION	**KEY TO MANAGEMENT**	**MANAGEMENT STRATEGIES**
Disinhibition is an inability to stop oneself from acting on one's thoughts. Sexually Inappropriate Behavior is a special case of lack of inhibition.	Remain calm and provide concrete feedback about the behavior.	• Initially, focus on addressing simple situations that may be easiest for patients to learn to manage. • Identify the issue as "self-control" and use this as the key word for cueing the patient, when they need to be controlling their behaviors. • When delaying gratification is the issue, start with short increments between the behavior and the reward, lengthening the increment as the patient improves. Using a watch or timer for specific cueing may be helpful in this regard. • It is important to provide the patient with feedback on the inappropriateness of sexual behavior, in this situation, and not to regard its presence with negative attention. • Avoid emotional responses such as anger or embarrassment; this can reinforce the behavior. • Ignoring the behavior or passing it off with a humorous comment also may reinforce its presence and not provide the patient with the adequate information to understand that the behavior is inappropriate. • The best approach is an immediate, unemotional, straightforward expression of the inappropriateness of the behavior. Be certain the patient knows what behavior is being referred to, such as "your sexual hand gesture is inappropriate and won't be appreciated by most women/men."
Perseveration is a person's repetition of certain behaviors, either actions or verbalizations. Some individuals perseverate on a consistent theme, while others repeat external stimuli or their own immediately preceding responses.	Use cueing and pacing to interrupt the repetitive behavior and provide a stimulus to move on to the next step.	• Pace interactions with the client to allow disengagement from one activity before proceeding to the next. • Provide a highly structured environment. • Use cues to redirect the client from the perseverative behavior to the next step. • Do not attempt to use logic to "discuss away" a repetitive theme.
Confabulation is the creation of false memories and is frequent in confused patients, sometimes reflecting the inability to find another explanation for what is happening.	It is important to keep in mind that confabulation may be serving a purpose for the patient, including reducing anxiety.	• For lower functioning, more confused patients, ignore the confabulation and do not challenge its veracity. • For higher functioning patients, provide nonthreatening feedback on the inaccuracy of the memory; then redirect attention to another task.
Inability to self-reflect is due to a lack of insight into the effects of ones behavior on others. The client is not aware of their capabilities or limitations and typically overestimates their ability to perform any given task. These patients will often blame others for their frustration and may exhibit paranoia.	Use concrete goals that are posted within easy access of the person with TBI, and note on the posted goal form as progress is made.	• Include the client in goal setting. • Goals should be concrete and progress should be recorded, where the client can monitor her own progress. • Consistently attempt to elicit the client's insight into their deficits. Be nonjudgmental and express expectations that the deficit will be overcome. • Videotape can provide concrete feedback. • Only make the client aware of deficits that can be worked on in rehabilitation and for which you expect to see improvement. • Continual reinforcement is necessary, after insight is accomplished, to change the behavior.

(Continued)

TABLE 12-4	Common Behaviors s/p TBI and Their Management[69] (*Continued*)	
BEHAVIOR DESCRIPTION	**KEY TO MANAGEMENT**	**MANAGEMENT STRATEGIES**
Apathy can be differentiated from resistance by the presence of lethargy with a bland affect, an absence of agitation, and low motivation. *Depression* is sometimes evident as a patient's self-awareness improves. It may show itself in tears, but also may be evident in social withdrawal, self-degrading comments, anxiety, irritability, and catastrophizing.	Treatment should target choices and acknowledge accomplishments.	• Staff and family should encourage participation. • You may need to remind them of the consequences of their injury and the impact of the lack of participation in rehabilitation. • Graphs or other concrete ways of showing progress may be useful to elicit motivation. • Be firm in presenting activities and do not present yes/no choices. Offer two or more alternatives for a given activity. • Working in conjunction with other patients may be motivating. • Activities that the patient spontaneously shows interest in should be used to meet rehabilitation goals. • Ask the client to choose the activity to elicit motivation. • Identify short-term goals and be explicit about the relationship between therapy activities and these goals. • Review progress to date. • Redirect the patient's attention from catastrophic or anxious thoughts. • Inform the psychology staff of the nature of the patient's depressive or anxious thoughts.
Lack of Initiation differs from apathy in that the patient is motivated to perform an activity but is unable to determine how to carry it out. Lack of initiation may be evident in problems determining the correct sequence of steps or simply not knowing the first step. It is important to keep in mind that the patient is not always aware of this shortcoming and may provide other excuses for why an activity is not initiated or carried out.	Cueing at the start of or next step in an activity is the key to facilitating initiation.	• Cueing is the primary means of assisting a person who lacks initiation. Cues should be external. • Do not perform or passively assist them to initiate the activity. • Verbal cues should be used initially. Using the same word to cue the same behaviors will assist the patient in moving to the next step. • As independence increases, replace verbal cues with other external cues that do not require another person to present the cue. Examples of external cues are lists posted in the room for ADL routines. External cues should be succinct, readily visible, and free of distracting content. • Client's whose improvement continues should be weaned from external cues to simple verbal statements that can be said aloud or thought to oneself as the patient completes the activity. These self-reminders should be succinct and easy to learn. • While in the inpatient setting begin to train the patient and family in techniques for establishing a daily routine.

The musculoskeletal and neurologic systems should be reevaluated periodically as it is easy to miss deficits in these systems in a comatose patient. Before standing and walking a client s/p TBI, the therapist must reassess the lower extremities for pain, ligamentous laxity, and signs of fracture. Minor injuries such as these can be missed in multi-trauma life and death situations. The therapist plays a critical role in monitoring the musculoskeletal system throughout the course of care.

What coma level is Aaron in?

He is in Ranchos level III since he is responding to stimuli and following simple commands.

Is it safe for the therapist to begin to work on rolling side to side in supine?

Yes, the therapist could put Aaron in supine and work on side-to-side rolling with physician clearance, since his ICP is normalized. If his vitals make any notable changes or if he were running a fever, therapy should not proceed.

Contracture Prevention

In the ICU, therapists utilize position changes, range of motion exercises, and splints to prevent contractures. The development of hypertonia often leads to severe contractures of the elbow and plantarflexors. Foot boards can be used to position the foot at 90 degrees but are only effective if the client is consistently positioned correctly on the foot board and knee flexion can be avoided. The use of a pressure relief ankle foot orthosis (PRAFO) that positions the ankle at 90 degrees and relieves pressure on the heel is the most effective means of preventing contractures of the ankle while in bed. Contractures of the forearm, wrist, and hand are best prevented with splints that typically require an occupational therapy consultation for fitting and construction.

In those individuals who develop contractures, the most common treatments are pharmacologic, stretching, dynamic splints, and serial casting. There is very little research examining the benefit of dynamic splints in individuals with hypertonia

CASE A, PART III

Aaron has been in the ICU for 10 days and remains in a coma. Physical therapy has been ordered, his ICP has normalized, and the intraventricular catheter has been removed and the skull closed. While performing ROM to the left UE, the therapist asks Aaron to help bend his arm into elbow flexion. On the third repetition, Aaron actively assists with elbow flexion. He is no longer posturing into flexion/extension and has been noted to open his eyes periodically, especially when his family is in the room. Aaron has a hard lump in his biceps muscle on the right and grimaces, during ROM to that arm. The therapist suspects that he has developed a **heterotopic ossification** (HO) in the biceps brachii (see discussion in latter section) and performs only active ROM to this muscle in the pain-free range to avoid further inflaming the tissue.

or those with BI. Studies have shown improved range of motion in the elbow after dynamic splinting, when combined with botulinum toxin and stretching.[74] No studies were identified that examined the use of dynamic splinting of the LE in individuals with spasticity. Static stretching, using serial casting, and botulinum toxin has been shown to improve range of motion in individuals who are s/p TBI and is well tolerated.[75] A study comparing serial casting with dynamic splinting of the elbow found both modalities to be equally effective, but three individuals, assigned to the dynamic splinting group, requested to be changed to the static – serial casting group. Dynamic splinting is more likely to lead to complaints of discomfort or pain. In agitated individuals, a possible benefit of serial casting may be that the cast is more difficult for the patient to remove. Effective contracture reduction is difficult and maintenance of increased ROM appears to depend on the individual's ability to use that range of motion functionally.[76,77]

Dynamic splinting involves a splint that has a spring that provides a constant, low-level stretch. Dynamic splints favor the elastic response of tissue. It is easier to monitor skin status while using this type of splint, and it can be taken off to clean and to perform ROM exercises. Caution should be used in the presence of hypertonia, as this type of splint can aggravate hypertonia. Since these splints are also easily removed, they may not be effective in clients with agitation or poor cognitive function. Care should be taken to apply the splint exactly at the anatomic

CASE A, PART IV

Aaron should be positioned with pillows under both UEs such that his elbows are in slight flexion, his shoulder is slightly elevated and abducted, and the forearm is in neutral. His right wrist and fingers are in a cast for the forearm fracture, which should be supported by the pillow on the right and kept in slight flexion on the left. Padded semi-rigid boots are placed on his feet to position the ankles in 90 degrees of dorsiflexion.

joint to avoid discomfort. This type of splint is also more likely to cause skin breakdown because it is not total contact.

Serial casting involves a prolonged low-level stretch that favors the plastic response of tissue and, thereby, results in a greater amount of permanent elongation with the least amount of trauma and weakening of tissue. When utilizing serial casting, the therapist performs range of motion to the joint, then takes it to the end range but not into a stretch. The limb is casted in this position, and the cast remains on for 7 to 10 days. When the cast is removed, ROM and joint mobilizations are performed. The joint is then taken to end range but no further, and a new cast is applied. Casts are changed every week for 3 to 6 weeks. Serial casts are effective and safe and are associated with a lower risk of skin breakdown, as they are total contact. The limb must be monitored for circulation status distal to the cast and for signs of swelling.[76]

Severe contractures that do not respond to therapy may be managed with **surgical release.** Typical sites of release are the heel cord (Achilles tendon), hamstrings, hip adductors, and the biceps brachii. Individuals undergoing lower extremity release are typically able to ambulate after the surgery. Not every patient, who exhibits toe walking or equino-varus, benefits from tendon lengthening surgery. Careful assessment should be performed to ensure that the individual is adopting this posture purely due to contracture. In some individuals, as discussed for the child with CP, tight muscles may provide stability for weight-bearing or to enhance stability in other joints of the leg. Therapists can provide valuable insight to the surgeon regarding the potential impact of tendon lengthening surgery on any given client. An alternative approach, specifically for ankle spasticity, is a selective tibial neurotomy, where the motor nerve fibers of the tibial nerve to the gastrocnemius are selectively resected.[78] This procedure has been used in the upper extremity for the flexor muscles of the elbow, wrists, and fingers as well as the lower extremity adductors, hamstrings, quadriceps, and soleus.[79]

Heterotopic ossification (HO) is the abnormal presence of bone in soft tissue and is most frequently seen with either musculoskeletal trauma, spinal cord injury, or central nervous system injury. Surgery to remove the bone cannot be done until the lesion is mature (typically 1.5 years) due to the high likelihood of recurrence.[80–82] Active motion is typically encouraged to minimize ROM loss. It remains controversial as to whether stretching leads to more inflammation and should be avoided. Until conclusive evidence is available, it is recommended that therapists provide active range of motion, in the pain-free range. If indicated, gentle passive range of motion can be undertaken, but stretching should be avoided.

Management of the Medically Stable Client S/P TBI

Once the client is medically stable, the task is to return them to society at the highest possible level of function. This is also the time when therapists may identify more minor musculoskeletal injuries that were not apparent during coma. At this time, the emphasis of management is based on level of cognitive functioning. One of the most common scales for cognitive and behavioral functioning after TBI is the Ranchos Los Amigos Levels of Cognitive Functioning (Ranchos Scale, as described in Table 12-2).[83] This scale sets rules for the language all professionals use to communicate regarding the care of the client with TBI. It equips you to treat for physical, cognitive, and behavioral sequela of TBI. The Ranchos Scale provides a means to guide goal setting, based on the level of recovery. The recovery process from TBI is sequential, but as mentioned earlier, the patient's progress can stop at any level.

● ASSESSMENT AND MANAGEMENT BASED ON RANCHOS LOS AMIGOS LEVELS OF COGNITIVE FUNCTIONING (LOC)[84,85]

Coma Levels

The first three levels, Ranchos Los Amigos levels I, II, and III, are often called the coma levels. In this stage of recovery, the individual is unresponsive and may be described as appearing to be asleep. In Stage I, the individual makes no response to stimuli, including painful stimuli. When the individual begins to make generalized responses to stimuli, they are said to be in Stage II. The responses in this stage are the same regardless of the type of stimulus presented. Responses may be physiologic changes, gross body movements, and/or vocalization. When the individual begins to withdraw from painful stimuli or blink when strong light crosses the visual field, they are making stimulus-specific responses and are said to be in Stage III. The individual may also follow simple commands like closing eyes or squeezing a hand. These responses are often inconsistent and may be delayed.

Management of TBI survivors, while in the stages of coma, focuses on maintaining the health of the individual with PT focusing on the musculoskeletal and neuromuscular systems. Learning is not possible while the client is in a coma. Proper positioning to prevent contracture is important and often must be done around tubes and wires. If the individual has elevated ICP, the head of the bed must be kept elevated to about 30 degrees[86] and should not be lowered until the physician clears the individual to go supine. It is important to note that lowering the head of the bed in stable patients improves brain oxygenation and circulation. Therefore, an individualized approach to head positioning is recommended.[87] Before performing any range of motion or positioning, the PT should check all lines and tubes and ensure that they are each out of the way for the intended movements. Specific positioning strategies are discussed in Chapter 11 (see Table 11-5).

It is important to talk to the person with TBI as you would talk to any other client. Studies have shown that individuals, who are in a coma, can hear, and it is believed that talking to them may help to arouse them and improve their responsiveness. In fact, a small study of ICU patients showed that time to arousal from coma was significantly shorter in individuals who spent 30 minutes a day listening to familiar auditory sounds on an MP3 player as compared to controls who did not.[88] A review of the literature found that family-centered sensory stimulation was more effective than nurse-implemented sensory stimulation. In addition, multi-sensory stimulation was found to be more effective than single stimulation.[89] The therapist should ask visitors for information about the person with TBI, and then talk to him about topics that would be of interest to him as well as greeting him, before starting therapy, and explaining what you are doing throughout therapy. Carefully observe the client for any indication of a response to sensory stimulation. When feasible, rolling the person side to side can help to stimulate the vestibular system, while raising the bed into reverse Trendelenburg with a foot plate for weight-bearing can stimulate the autonomic nervous system and the somatosensory system. Additional sensory stimuli can be used clinically to stimulate the patient, including familiar odors to stimulate the olfactory system and touch with different textures to stimulate the somatosensory system. Multimodal stimulation is an effective technique that involves health care professionals or the patient's family member(s) applying stimulation systematically to one or more of the patient's five senses, for the purpose of increasing patient responsiveness.[88,89] The rationale is that exposure to frequent and various sensory stimulation will activate the sensory systems and facilitate both dendritic growth and improved synaptic connectivity in those with damaged nervous systems[90–92] (see Box 12-7).

Box 12-7	Rules for Applying Multimodal Sensory Stimulation Program

- Before starting, check resting vital signs (heart rate, blood pressure, and respiratory rate). Monitor vitals throughout the treatment and stop treatment if vital signs change in a significant manner.
- Avoid or minimize stimulation programs with patients that have a ventriculostomy, who still have unstable or high intracranial pressure (ICP) and/or cerebral perfusion pressure (CPP); monitor ICP and CPP during and after treatment.
- Control the environment to eliminate as many distractions as possible. The environment should be simple and uncluttered, with a limited number of people around the patient, and with the TV off and the door closed, during treatment.
- Make sure the patient is comfortable before starting.
- Present the stimuli in an orderly manner and involve only one or two sensory modalities at a time. It is important to control how much and how often to provide stimulation, because patients can "habituate" or get used to the stimulation, in which case the stimulation can become less meaningful.
- Explain to the patient what is happening before and during stimulus presentation.
- Allow extra time for the patient to respond. Start by providing 1 or 2 minutes between stimulus presentations, until the length of response delay for that individual is established.
- Keep sessions brief – patients can usually tolerate 15 to 30 minutes.

- Conduct sessions frequently, allowing patients to respond several times daily, but alternating periods of stimulation with periods of rest.
- Select meaningful stimuli, such as the voices of family and friends, favorite music, smells of favorite foods, etc. Stimuli that have emotional significance to the patient are usually more likely to elicit a response.
- Provide verbal reinforcement for responses to increase the likelihood of getting responses in future sessions.

Motor examination becomes possible, once the individual enters Ranchos level IV. The examination and evaluation are conducted as outlined in Chapter 10 (Evaluation). The neurology section of the APTA convened a taskforce in 2013 to determine the most appropriate outcome measures for use in the TBI population.[93] Recommended measures are listed in Table 12-5. In addition, the therapist should utilize the core measures as described by the Academy of Neurologic Physical Therapy.[94]

Ranchos Level IV: Confused and Agitateds

The treatment strategy, for the Stage IV client, is a behavioral treatment strategy rather than a learning treatment strategy. For many therapists, this is a key philosophical shift. When employing a behavioral treatment strategy, the focus is on impairments and is more compensatory in nature. Cognitive learning requires that the individual can learn alternate ways to behave and can understand the consequences of their actions. The individual in this stage of recovery is not able to do either. To understand the consequences of one's actions, the individual must be able to discern between self and the environment, which individuals in Stage IV cannot. Cognitive learning first becomes possible in Ranchos Stage VI. The key to working with clients who are s/p BI is to be calm and controlled, flexible, and consistent. Specific guidelines for setting up sessions with a client who has behavioral problems are listed in Table 12-6.

Motor learning is not dependent on cognitive learning and can occur starting in Ranchos Stage IV, or when the individual is able to actively move. The ability to motor learn is also dependent on which areas of the brain have been damaged and the severity of that damage. At this stage in recovery, any motor learning would be implicit and from repetitive practice of the movement.

TABLE 12-5	TBI EDGE Recommendations[93]
ACUTE SETTING	**IN AND OUTPATIENT REHABILITATION**
Agitated Behavior Scale	High-Level Mobility Assessment*
Coma Recovery Scale*	Moss Attention Scale*
Revised Moss Attention Rating Scale	6-minute walk, 10-m walk, Berg Balance Scale
Rancho Levels of Cognitive Function	Community Balance and Mobility Scale
	Disability Rating Scale
	Functional Assessment Measure
	Modified Ashworth Scale
	Patient Health Questionnaire
	Quality of Life after Brain Injury
	Rancho Levels of Cognitive Function
Inpatient Rehabilitation Only	**Outpatient Rehabilitation Only**
Agitated Behavioral Scale	Action Research Arm Test
Barthel Index	Apathy Evaluation Scale
Cog-Log and Orientation Log (O-Log)	Balance Error Scoring Scale
Disorders of Consciousness Scale	Global Fatigue Index
FIM (functional independence measure)	Sydney Psychosocial Re-integration Scale
	Community Integration Questionnaire
	Dizziness Handicap Inventory

*Highly recommended measures.
Data from American Physical Therapy Association. TBI EDGE outcome measures for in- and outpatient rehabilitation.

CASE A, PART V

Aaron is now 5 weeks post-accident and has been moved to an inpatient rehabilitation facility. He has become very agitated. He tries to get out of bed and has torn off part of the cast on his right arm. He tends to yell, but the statements he makes are not relevant to the situation. A net bed has been put in place, and the staff has been instructed to keep their hair tied back as he has been grabbing and pulling on staff member's hair and arms. He is also spitting, cussing, and masturbating. Aaron's mother is in tears as she exits his room.

Aaron is in Ranchos Stage IV. Which features of his presentation tell us he is in this stage?

Agitation, tearing off the cast, trying to stand when he is unable to do so safely, inappropriate verbalizations, and the inability to recognize that staff and family member's hair and arms are not objects but belong to other people.

What should staff tell the mother when she becomes upset by his behavior?

Staff should explain that Aaron is in a state of confusion, in which he is being inundated with sensory stimuli but is unable to understand what is going on around him. His behavior is not aimed at any person, and he does not understand that his behavior is impacting other people.

Now that Aaron is in Ranchos Stage IV, his treatment will focus on reorienting him frequently, preventing self-harm, and getting him to participate in activities that are meaningful, familiar, and automatic, such as walking. Aaron continues to have PTA and will not remember previous therapy sessions. Therapy activities should be short, and the therapist should come prepared with plans for multiple potential activities. Activities will have to be changed every few minutes, since Aaron will have a very short attention span. In addition, the therapist should become familiar with the signs that Aaron exhibits, when he is becoming agitated,

TABLE 12-6	Guidelines for Treating Clients – with Agitation	
GUIDELINES	**STRATEGIES**
Provide a calm and controlled environment	• Treat the patient as an adult respecting them in your interactions even when they act childlike • Model calm and controlled behavior both verbally and physically
Be flexible in your planning and throughout the therapy session	• Redirect the patient physically and verbally rather than argue • Expect the unexpected • Plan several activities for each treatment goal and be willing to change activities when signs of agitation occur • End the treatment session on success for you and for the patient
Provide consistency from one session to the next	• Consistency occurs across all areas of care and requires interdisciplinary team management • Provide a structure and ensure that all members of the team will respond to behaviors in the same manner • Give as much control and responsibility as the patient can handle while maintaining that predictable and structured environment, as much as needed, to allow the patient to function optimally • Avoid over stimulation and chaotic stimulation as TBI patients are more sensitive to stress

so that activities can be changed at the earliest sign of agitation. Therapy should be highly structured, and it is best to have consistent staff work with Aaron to help him gain familiarity and comfort with his situation. Instructions should be simple and brief. Therapy should be conducted in a quiet environment with minimal distractions. Family members are asked to be part of therapy, whenever possible, to facilitate cooperation and to help keep the patient calm and comfortable. When agitation occurs, the activity is stopped, and the client is allowed to rest.

CASE A, PART VI

Aaron is allowed to walk with weight-bearing, as tolerated. He can ambulate with two-person assist and a rollator walker with forearm support on the right side because of his fracture. Therapists place the walker in front of Aaron and stand on either side with the person on the left, helping to advance the left leg. Aaron's mother is asked to stand across the room and call to Aaron to come to her. Aaron responds to his mother by beginning to walk toward her. Midway across the room he begins to vocalize in a loud voice, the therapist recognizes that this is an early sign of agitation for Aaron and so his wheelchair is brought to him, and he is told to "sit down" in a calm quiet voice. Aaron sits and continues to vocalize and pick at his cast on his right arm. His mother comes to him and talks to him in a quiet voice, while rubbing his shoulder, and he calms down. Currently, Aaron only tolerates 15 minutes of therapy, before he becomes severely agitated.

Examples of behaviors that typically indicate a client is becoming agitated are increased movements like wiggling or tapping the foot, vocalizations, or a shortening of the attention span. Each client will have a unique presentation, and staff should learn to recognize each client's signs of oncoming agitation and respond to them by taking the client to a quiet place and allowing them to rest. When Aaron spits, he is told that

this behavior is inappropriate in a calm and unemotional voice. The staff is told to be consistent, in managing this behavior, and to recognize that at this time Aaron is not able to learn to change the behavior. When he masturbates, staff tell him that this should be done in privacy, in his own room, and move him to his room. This is an example of an appropriate behavior in an inappropriate setting. As Aaron's cognitive skills improve, he will be taught to delay gratification, by asking him to stop behaviors such as masturbation, and wait a set amount of time until he goes to his room to engage in the behavior. The time to gratification is incrementally increased.

Agitation is a difficult behavior for staff and family. It can be very upsetting to family members to see their loved one acting inappropriately and out of character. For the individual in Ranchos Stage IV, agitation is the person reacting to their own internal confusion. In Ranchos Stages V-VIII, the individual is reacting to the environment. There are many misconceptions about agitation. Box 12-8 spells out some of these misconceptions and provides the correct explanation.

CASE A, PART VII

Aaron is now able to respond to simple commands fairly consistently. He requires external structure to function and to minimize agitation; thus, staff should follow the same schedule every day, and the same staff should work with him, whenever possible. He now demonstrates gross attention to the environment but is highly distractible and lacks the ability to focus his attention. He can converse on a social automatic level for short periods of time. For example, he will greet the therapist with "hello" and when asked "how are you?" he answers. If the conversation goes on too long, he becomes agitated and begins to hum loudly. His verbalizations are often inappropriate, and sometimes, he will make confabulatory statements such as saying he has pain in his leg because he was tackled, while playing football last week. His memory is severely impaired, and he has limited to no recall of previous therapy sessions. He is unable to learn new information at this time but demonstrates procedural learning improvements in therapy activities.

What Ranchos level is Aaron now in?
He is now in Ranchos level V. He remains somewhat agitated and has a short attention span, but he can converse in a social, automatic level.

During Ranchos level V, the staff work on extending the time that Aaron can stay on task and focus his attention. In physical therapy, they are working on walking without breaks for longer and longer periods of time. This serves to improve his endurance and his attention to task. When he begins to follow simple directions and demonstrates carryover of learning for tasks, such as dressing and sit to stand transfers, he is considered to have moved on to Ranchos level VI (the confused and appropriate stage). In level VI, he can complete goal-directed activities such as walk to the green chair and sit down, but he continues to require direction from staff to do the task safely. When asked what day it is, he answers incorrectly three out of five times, but he always answers with a day of the week, indicating his answers are appropriate to the situation. Aaron is still trying to remove his cast, but when staff explain that his arm is broken and he needs to leave the cast alone, he is compliant. He does require frequent reminders as he does not remember these instructions for more than a few hours.

> Usually there is something that is causing the client to get loud and yell; find out what it is and modify the environment accordingly.
>
> Can't benefit from treatment
>> Clients s/p TBI can benefit from treatment.
>> Short treatment sessions are most effective.
>
> Should be ignored until he calms down.
>> Being alone in an unfamiliar environment increases fear and agitation.
>> Human contact has a very calming effect.

In Ranchos Stages V and VI, individuals continue to exhibit agitation and other behaviors such as confusion, resistance to treatment, apathy, lack of initiation, inability to self-reflect, impulsivity, disinhibition, depression, perseveration, and confabulation. They may be resistant to treatment, and at this stage, are able to refuse. Often resistance is due to agitation and confusion. To manage resistance to treatment, the therapist can offer several choices for each activity to be practiced without any "yes/no" options. For these individuals, it is important to provide them with activity choices that offer a high likelihood of success and then provide positive feedback to reinforce their engagement in therapy.

Return to employment is one of the major goals for adults s/p BI, but up to 60% are not employed 2 years after injury.[95] The Functional Assessment Measure (FAM) was developed by clinicians to specifically address the major functional areas, including cognitive, behavior, communication, and community functioning. The FAM consists of 12 items and is intended to be used in conjunction with the FIM (FIM+FAM). Scores <65 on the FAM are predictive of long-term unemployment.[95]

Box 12-8 Misconceptions Regarding Agitated Behavior and Its Management

The person s/p TBI:

Is "mean" or angry at staff and visitors
> The person s/p TBI is confused and frightened.
> Agitation is a reaction to that fear and confusion.

Needs medication to "calm him down"
> Medication further reduces the person with TBI's ability to process stimuli and interpret what is going on around them, which compounds agitation and confusion.
> In addition, medications are often ineffective in calming the patient until the dosage is so high that the patient is lethargic and asleep.

Won't cooperate with treatment
> The person s/p TBI is cognitively unable to cooperate and is not capable of the motivation to participate.

Must be restrained at all times for everyone's protection
> Restraints result in increased agitation.
> People are calmer, if unrestrained.

Requires a large number of people to control them
> More people will increase agitation.

Is yelling and should be yelled at to "be quiet"

CASE A, PART VIII

Aaron, at 10 weeks post-injury, is now behaving appropriately in the inpatient rehabilitation setting and is able to go through his dressing and self-care tasks independently. He does this very automatically and follows a set routine every day. He is able to learn new skills such as how to use a walker and how to use adaptive equipment to feed himself. He exhibits poor judgment when confronted with situations such as maneuvering in a room full of obstacles or crossing the street.

What Ranchos LOC is Aaron now in?
Aaron is in Ranchos Stage VII. He is exhibiting behaviors that are automatic and appropriate but lacks the judgment and abstract reasoning that are found in Ranchos Stage VIII.

It is important to note that, while Aaron has progressed through the Ranchos Stages to level VII, progress can stop at any Ranchos level. Aaron has been in rehabilitation as long as his insurance will pay and his progress has slowed down substantially. At this point, he is discharged to home. He will continue therapy in the outpatient setting with a focus on community re-integration. Aaron may continue to progress through the Ranchos stages, or he may remain in Ranchos Stage VII. With his initial level of injury, his prognosis would indicate that he is unlikely to return to his previous level of functioning and could be expected to remain at a Ranchos Stage VII. In this stage, he is cognitively able to learn (see Box 12-7 for learning ability by stage of recovery). Aaron now has moderately decreased ability to learn and has carryover for new learning. He continues to require close supervision due to safety and judgment issues. Based on these difficulties, the recommendation is that he live with his parents. Were he to live on his own, it would need to be in a structured environment, and he would continue to require assistance with his finances, making appointments and getting to them, and any other higher-level daily activity. Someone would need to be available to take him grocery shopping and to check on him frequently. An Assisted Living setting would also be appropriate for Aaron at this time. If Aaron continues to make progress, he would first be appropriate for living alone with no supervision at Ranchos Stage VIII.

Agitation is no longer present every day but can be elicited, when Aaron is under a great deal of stress. In addition, he becomes impulsive, when he is with his old friends and/or in a highly stimulating environment. It is typical for individuals who are s/p BI to continue to manifest behaviors that were present in earlier stages, when they are fatigued or under stress. Alcohol is very likely to intensify safety and judgment issues and should be avoided.

Cognitive Qualifiers

When writing treatment plans for recovery of motor function, it is important to incorporate behavioral and cognitive modifiers into the plan of care. These modifiers allow the therapist to address all the issues associated with the brain injury. In addition, cognitive deficits have a profound impact on learning and time to meet mobility goals. Consider what it takes to safely ambulate in the community. The individual must be able to walk independently but also be cognitively able to find their way and to determine safety (e.g., to cross streets). Problematic behaviors also interfere with successful therapy interventions and influence independence and safety in mobility. In order to engage in therapy, the individual must be able to maintain attention long enough to walk a set distance and to respond to requests to walk with the appropriate action. Box 12-9 outlines the ability of individuals to learn across GCS levels, and Box 12-10 provides examples of qualifiers that could be used when writing goals.

Family Adjustment

"a brain injury isn't like death. You're in limbo. After death, you eventually get on with your life. This TBI goes on forever and you're dealing with it one stage or another for the rest of your life"

[family member[96], p3]

Box 12-9	Ability to Learn Cognitively by Ranchos LOC[25]

Stages I-V:	absent
Stage VI:	severely impaired; some carryover for things relearned
Stage VII:	moderately decreased; some carryover for new learning
Stage VIII:	minimally impaired; good carryover for new learning with no supervision required for performance once learned

---

Box 12-10	Cognitive and Behavioral Documentation Modifiers

Appropriateness of Response: Does the individual's response fit in the correct category and do they use equipment appropriately.

- Aaron will lock his wheelchair and use his left hand appropriately on the arm of the wheelchair to come to standing on four of five attempts.

Attention: Describe the duration of time the individual can attend to a particular task (e.g., repetitions, distance, time).

- Aaron will be able to walk 30 feet × 3 within 1 minute without becoming distracted and with appropriate movement of the walker and standby assistance.

Body Awareness: Define neglect, the individual's attention to their hemiparetic side, their care of the non-weight-bearing body part.

- Aaron will note when his left foot has fallen off the footrest and will place it back on the footrest, using only self-cueing.

Carryover: Does the individual exhibit retention of repeated activities and is there any evidence of new learning of skills, names, and places.

- Aaron will demonstrate carryover from the am session to the pm session for the sit–stand steps with only tactile cueing.

Cueing: Define the amount and type of cueing that is necessary to accomplish the task successfully (i.e., tactile, verbal, both).

- See above examples

Participation: Describe the number of activities, type of activity, is it easy or difficult, how long they participate in an activity, a treatment session, and will they participate in what you want them to do.

- Aaron was able to complete three consecutive activities within the am session without agitation or impulsivity, following single-step directions.

Orientation: Consider things like knowing the building, how to get to places, and how to get back, using a map, following a schedule, use of environmental cues (i.e., signs).

- Aaron is able to transport himself by wheelchair, using his right hand and foot for propulsion, on time, based on the schedule taped to his wheelchair tray.

Safety: This encompasses orientation skills, judgment, body awareness, environmental awareness, impulsivity, and carryover.

- Aaron is oriented × 2 (person and place) with improved awareness of avoiding weight-bearing on his broken arm and decreased attempts to remove his cast.

Social Interactions: Are they appropriate with peers and staff, sexually inappropriate, exhibit disinhibition, use effective communication.

- Aaron is greeting family and staff with appropriate "hi" and "good-bye" verbalization but is not remembering names from one meeting to the next.

"Almost all TBI survivors who have been comatose for more than a few days sustain irreversible alteration of some socially important aspect of psychological makeup"[97], p248

At the time of injury, the family's energy is focused on their loved one's survival. As the patient comes out of coma, the family is confronted with all the drastic changes that their loved one has undergone.[98] Changes in personality and behavior are often the most difficult for family and friends to understand. Families, who do well, learn to "let go" of the person, who was there before the injury, and figure out a way to incorporate the "new person" into the family system. The therapist's role is to educate the family on how to physically assist the person s/p BI but also on the effects of BI on the entire person. Also, therapists are often in frequent close contact with the family and may be the person they first talk to about their feelings and their struggles to deal with this situation. Therapists play a key role in referring family members to local support systems.

Mild TBI and Concussion

Historically, concussion and mild TBI (mTBI) were considered separate entities; in fact, concussion was defined as a disturbance of brain function without permanent physiologic or structural damage, while mTBI involved a brief loss of consciousness with mild structural damage that could result in permanent disability. More recently it has been acknowledged that concussion is the mildest form of TBI that can result in microstructural damage that alters brain activity and connectivity that is not detectable through imaging methods and may involve loss of consciousness. We will refer to both as concussion to remain consistent with recent publications such as the Clinical Practice Guideline for Physical Therapy Evaluation and Treatment after Concussion/Mild TBI.[99] Smaller axons are likely more susceptible to the overstretching (rather than tearing) thought to occur with a mild injury that, in turn, is followed by disruption of the sodium–potassium–calcium cellular balance and exaggerated metabolic cellular requirements with subsequent microstructural damage.[6] However, when multiple concussions occur, especially in close time proximity, they may have an additive effect on long-term cognitive ability, psychological health, and behavioral control (see later segment on second-impact syndrome).

BI occurs at an alarmingly high rate in athletes with sports-related TBI accounting for up to one-third of all TBI.[100] Other common causes of concussion and TBI include falls, domestic violence, MVAs, and blast injuries. More alarming, concussions/mTBI are increasingly common in adolescence, a time when the brain is still developing and potentially at greater risk for injury and/or poorer outcome from a mild injury. It also appears that symptoms in children and adolescents take longer to recover and may still be undergoing neural recovery even after symptoms have dissipated and neurologic testing is normal.[101] In general, younger school-age children show greater cognitive impairments than adolescents with mTBI. Children and adolescents have an exaggerated and longer lasting **pro-inflammatory response**, accompanied by atypical synaptic pruning and dendritic branching; possibly explaining their vulnerability to psychosocial disorders.[101] Identification of individuals with concussion can aid in primary prevention efforts, such as reducing risk for reinjury in high-risk groups. In addition, it can facilitate access to appropriate interventions that can reduce the long-term effects of concussion. Table 12-7 provides details on early symptoms of concussion. Notably, these may manifest some hours or even days after the initial injury.

In some individuals, repetitive concussive events have led to long-standing neural atrophy. Studies to date seem to indicate that executive functions including verbal fluency are most sensitive to multiple mTBIs[103,104]; however, studies in this area are varied and often conflicting. There is emerging evidence that multiple concussions can increase the risk of developing neurodegenerative diseases such as Alzheimer's later in life.[105] Due to these worrisome findings, screening for mTBI has taken on a new urgency in athletics and the military with more conservative management post-concussion recommended. It should be

TABLE 12-7	Symptoms of Concussion or mTBI[102]		
COGNITIVE	**PHYSICAL**	**EMOTIONAL**	**SLEEP**
Poorer concentration	Blurred vision/vision problems	Irritability	Trouble falling asleep
Memory disturbance	Headache	Depression	Hypersomnia or sleeping more than usual
Slower processing	Nausea/vomiting (early on)	Hyper-emotionality	Insomnia
	Noise and/or light sensitivity	Anxiety	
	Dizziness or balance problems		
	Feeling tired or fatigued		

noted that older adults are at higher risk for falls and thereby should be screened whenever they report a fall, which could be a potential concussive event. A concussive event is one in which there is a direct blow to the head, face, or neck or a force to the body that is transmitted to the head, followed by the onset of symptoms noted in Table 12-7.

When a therapist suspects the patient has had a concussive event, the therapist should screen the individual according to the clinical practice guidelines endorsed by the American Physical Therapy Association.[99] These guidelines include recommended screening, examination, and treatment methods for individuals with suspected or confirmed concussion along with detailed algorithms for each of these areas.[99] The guidelines, summarized here, apply only to post-concussion and do not apply to assessment on the field. Individuals may present to physical therapy without ever having been medically evaluated for diagnosis of a concussive event. Athletes and older adults are often reticent

to admit that a fall or injurious event may have led to a concussion. When an individual has had a suspected concussive event, the therapist screens for any indication of emergency medical conditions such as changes in orientation/cognition, reports of vomiting, seizure, or worsening headache. A full list is provided in Table 12-7. If emergent conditions are identified, the client should be referred for emergency medical assessment. In the absence of emergent conditions, continue with screening for indicators of concussion in Table 12-8. Instituting appropriate screening, examination, and interventions as early as appropriate is aimed at preventing the occurrence of persistent symptoms and improving recovery from concussion. If signs and symptoms are consistent with concussion, the therapist then uses the interview questions in Table 12-8 to determine if the patient is appropriate for a full physical therapy concussion examination. If answers to the questions indicate the possible presence of impairments in the following movement-related domains:

TABLE 12-8 Screening for Concussion[99]		
INDICATORS OF AN EMERGENT CONDITION	**CRITERIA FOR DIAGNOSIS OF CONCUSSION**	**PATIENT INTERVIEW QUESTIONS**
Decline in or loss of consciousness, cognition or orientation	Any period of decreased orientation or loss of consciousness	What are the type, severity, and irritability of concussion-related symptoms?
New onset of asymmetry of the pupils, seizures, vomiting, or other focal neurologic signs	Post-traumatic amnesia	What was the preinjury medical history with emphasis on previous concussions or BI, medical conditions that could result in/present with symptoms similar to concussion, history of personal or familial migraine, sleep quality history?
Severe or worsening headache	Any alteration in mental state or cognition, confusion, disorientation, slowed thinking, difficulty with concentration (attention)	Do they have any conditions or diseases that would limit or be a contraindication to a comprehensive physical therapy evaluation or therapy interventions?
Signs or symptoms consistent with skull fracture (swelling and tenderness at site of injury, facial bruising, bleeding from nostrils or ears)	Physical symptoms: headache, dizziness, balance disorders, nausea, vomiting, fatigue, sleep disturbance, blurred vision, sensitivity to light/noise, **tinnitus**, seizure, numbness, tingling, neck pain, exertional intolerance	What was the mechanism of injury and early signs and symptoms associated with the injury?
Serious cervical spine fracture, dysfunction, or pathology (cervical ligamentous instability, signs of central cord compression, vertebrobasilar insufficiency)	Emotional and behavioral symptoms including depression, anxiety, agitation, irritability, impulsivity, aggression	What treatment strategies have been used since the injury including pharmacological? Do any help? Are any making symptoms worse?
	Glasgow Coma Scale score of 13-15 within 24 hours	What are the patient's goals, priorities, and perceived limitations?
	Brain imaging is normal (if available)	Screen for mental health issues and substance use for referral needs.
	Symptoms are present that cannot be explained by preinjury history or drug, alcohol, or medication use or an exacerbation of symptoms from a pre-existing condition	

musculoskeletal, vestibulo-occulomotor, autonomic/**exertional intolerance**, or motor function, then a comprehensive physical therapy examination should be conducted. All patients with signs and symptoms consistent with a diagnosis of concussion should be educated about concussion and referred to other providers as indicated.

When examining the patient with concussion, the therapist should first determine the level of irritability and which movement-related impairments are likely. In concussion, the irritability refers to how easily symptoms are provoked or worsened by an activity. The order of examination should be based on types of impairments and irritability of those impairments (Table 12-9). It may be best to reserve performing exam activities that are likely to provoke symptoms until the end of the examination or skip them altogether. The cervical spine is cleared first, followed by examination of dizziness and/or headache (Table 12-10). Once neck pain, any potential cervical issues, dizziness, and headache have been addressed, the therapist then examines the patient for impairments in movement-related domains. Therapists are encouraged to carefully select outcome measures based on current evidence and the individual patient's presentation. Choice of tests and measures is based on irritability and disability of symptoms, patient's needs and preferences and their ability to tolerate the tests.[99] It is important to carefully document findings related not only to the outcomes of the tests and measures but also the influence that symptom irritability and disability had on patient response. Therapists should also carefully document how easy it is to provoke symptoms as well as severity and characteristics of symptom resolution (Table 12-4).

The physical therapy plan of care includes education, individualized interventions for any movement-related impairments and appropriate referral to other providers.[99] It is important to educate individuals with concussion about self-management and the importance to remain active while getting appropriate rest. A key to safe return to activity is appropriate pacing, based on individual symptom response. Patients should also be educated regarding potential signs that indicate the need for urgent follow-up care. Most individuals with concussion get good symptom resolution in two to four weeks and even those who take longer have a high probability for a good recovery.[99,106] Treatment of concussion is a rapidly evolving field where the physical therapist can play an important role in promoting the beneficial aspects of activity and providing expertise in dosing and progression of activity. While an initial period of rest is

TABLE 12-9	Impairments and Irritability Levels with Concussion
IMPAIRMENTS IN MOVEMENT-RELATED DOMAINS	**IRRITABILITY LEVELS**
1. Cervical musculoskeletal 2. Vestibulo-oculomotor 3. Autonomic dysfunction/exertional intolerance 4. Motor function impairments	• Frequency of symptom provocation • Vigor of movement required to reproduce symptom(s) • Severity of symptoms produced • How quickly and easily symptoms are provoked • How much, how quickly, and how easily the symptoms resolve

TABLE 12-10	Examination of the Person with Concussion[99]	
EXAMINATION	**RESULTS OF EXAMINATION**	
1. Clear the cervical spine	Neck pain is present with rest or movement then examine for cervical musculoskeletal impairments and provide interventions as indicated for pain relief before continuing with testing.	
2. No neck pain or cleared cervical spine Screen for dizziness and headache (rest or movement)	Dizziness and/or headache is present then examine for cervical musculoskeletal, vestibulo-oculomotor, and autonomic impairments (e.g., Orthostatic hypotension) that may contribute to dizziness/headache. • Perform this examination in order from least to most irritable system. • Provide basic interventions for symptom relief so that the individual can tolerate the rest of the examination. • If symptom relief is not adequate delay further testing until next session • Continue with motor function assessment based on patient tolerance.	
3. No dizziness or headache or have provided basic symptom relief for dizziness/headache Examine any movement-related impairment domains and administer appropriate outcome measures. Sequence based on: • Levels of irritability and disability • Patient's needs and preferences • Patient's ability to tolerate tests	Determine and document: • The patient's impairments and irritability levels (Table 12-9). • Potential type of headache. • Ability to self-manage and other psychosocial factors for recovery. • Need for follow-up testing. • Plan for outcome administration.	

Proceed to physical therapy plan of care

recommended (24-48 hours), a gradual return to activity with rest as needed should follow. However, clients should avoid high risk for concussion activities (e.g., sports). Treatment should target symptoms such as neck or other injuries, movement impairments or dizziness along with aerobic exercise[99], which has been found to counteract some of the pathophysiologic responses to injury.[101] Treatment of cervical dysfunction, vestibular, or oculomotor symptoms should follow guidelines for those conditions. When introducing aerobic exercise, it should be progressive and guided by symptom provocation with exercise terminated if symptoms exacerbate beyond a mild increase. Consensus is that aerobic exercise can be initiated within days of injury as tolerated by the patient and enhances recovery.[99]

Long-Term Outcomes from BI

As stated earlier, patients progress through the stages of recovery from TBI at different rates and may stall at any stage. For those that stall in a state of unresponsive wakefulness (Ranchos II) for at least 1 month, about one-half will regain consciousness by 1 year, most of these within the first 3 months. After 1 year, it is unlikely that a patient will emerge from unresponsive wakefulness. For those that stall at a Ranchos level III, there is a much better chance that they will recover with only minor disability than those that stall at level II, yet up to 40% will be severely disabled, if they remain in this MCS for at least 30 days. For those with prolonged UWS or MCS, about 50% have been reported to be discharged home and the other half to a skilled nursing facility at discharge from rehabilitation. Long-term follow-up for these patients found 25% improved to a level of mild or no disability; 25% continued to demonstrate severe disability; and the remainder (50%) displayed moderate disability, as rated on the Disability Rating Scale. Notably, 22% returned to work or school; however, about 5% of these, returned at a partial level.[28] Similarly, patient outcome has been found to relate to the length of time spent in prolonged PTA with those that returned to full or partial employment, school, or homemaking roles (productive) within 1 year distributed as follows: (1) moderate PTA (0-14 days) – 68% returned to productive lives; (2) moderately severe (15-29 days) – 41%; (3) severe (29-70 days) – 21%; and (4) extremely severe (>70 days) – 9%.[64] For many of those that fail to return to productivity, there is persisting behavioral (e.g., irritability/aggression, disinhibition/impulsivity) and executive dysfunction (e.g., impaired problem-solving, memory, and attention). Similarly, persistent problems with motor sequelae – balance problems, spasticity/dystonia – can impede function and return to productivity. In fact, tonal changes and balance deficits may worsen over time. This can be addressed by ongoing physical therapy to prevent contractures (splinting, stretching) and maximize function (therapeutic exercise, mobility training) long after the acute rehabilitation period. For some, medications may be required to control spasticity (e.g., baclofen or botulinum toxin).[107]

It should be noted that, given the same initial level of coma and length of PTA, anoxia has a worse prognosis than TBI.[108] Studies show that 27% of patients with post-hypoxic coma regained consciousness within 28 days, close to 9% remained in a coma, and 64% died.[107] Patients with ABI are, therefore, more likely to be discharged to a residential facility than those with TBI (33% versus 11%).[14]

> ### CASE A, PART IX
>
> For Aaron, he would likely fall into the severe group as described in the preceding paragraph as his coma lasted about 5 weeks and his PTA another 5 weeks (35 days). So, Aaron will likely return home, but it is relatively unlikely that he will be employed full-time 1 year post-injury.[28]

As mentioned in an earlier section of this chapter, the secondary neurologic consequences of BI (e.g., inflammation, excitotoxicity) may continue in the post-BI brain for a prolonged period after injury, resulting in secondary functional loss that may appear more than a year post-injury. Of interest, there is an increased incidence of both Alzheimer's and Parkinson's diseases post-TBI; while these prolonged neurodegenerative processes have been implicated in the development of these diseases, other factors (e.g., environment and genetics) likely contribute to their occurrence.[43] In addition, hypoxia has been implicated in the cognitive changes of aging due to cerebral hypoperfusion as well as the development of Alzheimer's disease and other neurodegenerative disorders such as Parkinson's disease. Thus, a hypoxic event may exacerbate the changes that naturally occur with aging.[109] Even in the absence of a degenerative disease, a moderate to severe BI has been found to decrease a survivor's life expectancy for a variety of reasons. Ongoing seizures or respiratory issues can impact longevity with death associated with seizure activity or aspiration pneumonia, respectively. Further, younger BI survivors are more likely to resume a high-risk lifestyle, including substance abuse that contributes to a higher mortality rate than non-injured controls.[110]

Interestingly, there are also multiple chronic changes that occur post-BI that impact long-term survival. For one, up to 80% of survivors demonstrate a change in neuroendocrine function, resulting in **hypopituitarism** and secondary loss of circulating hormones, specifically growth, sex, and thyroid hormones. Loss of these critical hormones can result in diminished bone density/osteoporosis, exercise capacity/endurance, and muscle strength (weakness) that further limit the survivor's physical fitness.[110,111] Additionally, there is an increased occurrence of **metabolic syndrome** (obesity, hypertension, elevated blood lipids, and insulin resistance) in BI survivors that likely stems from these hormonal changes in association with disturbance of the hypothalamic and thalamic satiety centers, limited mobility, and lack of initiation; in combination, these result in an inactive lifestyle, a propensity for weight gain, and risk of metabolic syndrome that increases susceptibility to heart disease, stroke, and diabetes.[111,112] Chronic hormonal changes along with the impact of loss of function, loss of income, and familial issues may contribute to the pervasiveness of **depression** and **anxiety** in BI survivors, especially younger survivors. Further, depression is difficult to treat in this population because of the common side effects of antidepressants, including sedation, slowing mentation, and the possibility of inducing seizures. Also, up to 50% of survivors experience chronic pain, most commonly headaches, that can contribute to depression and affect quality of life.[111] **Chronic pain** is also difficult to treat due to the high incidence of substance abuse in this population, and thereby, the need to avoid many pain medications. Yet, up to 72% of those with moderate and severe brain injury receive some opioid medication during their inpatient treatment, and nearly 30% have reported continued use up to 1 year post-injury to treat ongoing pain complaints. Ongoing use has been linked to increased suicide attempts as well as accidental overdoses. Of course, TBI and ABI are more common in those that are high risk takers, including illicit drug use, so this likely confounds the evidence for continued drug use after BI.[113] However, this is an opportunity for the physical therapist with some success reported from biofeedback, TENS, ultrasound, and dry needling among others in treating the chronic pain conditions of TBI survivors.[111,114] Other chronic conditions that impact TBI survivors include **sleep disturbance**, most commonly insomnia and sleep-wake cycle disruption, with secondary **fatigue**.[115]

While mTBI or concussion by their very names indicate minimal or no apparent damage to the CNS, there is a growing body of evidence that multiple incidents of even mild head injury can result in permanent disability. First, there is **second-impact syndrome**, where a second mild injury in a close timeframe to the first, can result in severe cerebral edema with potential brain herniation; this is thought to result from dysautoregulation of cerebral blood flow and exaggerated catecholamine release that induce extensive cerebral edema. In almost all cases, this secondary injury is associated with sports participation (e.g., football, boxing, and hockey) in adolescent or young athletes. There is some indication that juvenile head trauma syndrome is, in fact, a secondary-impact injury manifestation. For those that experience repetitive head injuries, there is almost a 20% likelihood of the development of a condition, known as **chronic traumatic encephalopathy**, previously known as pugilists' dementia, as it was first diagnosed in boxers; however, in recent years it has been diagnosed much more pervasively in football players, who experienced numerous concussions. This condition initially manifests with emotional or behavioral changes but eventually develops into progressive memory and cognitive deficits (dementia). These changes are associated with a general cerebral atrophy and secondary expansion of the lateral ventricles.[116]

• BRAIN TUMOR

CASE B, PART I

Alice is a 48-year-old woman, who was brought to the Emergency Department by the EMT, s/p grand mal-seizure in her home within the last 30 minutes. Her daughter, aged 17, reports that her mother seemed fine immediately preceding the seizure and that to her knowledge this is the first such episode experienced by her mother. Her mother is postictal but the neurologic exam that could be completed is unremarkable – pupils are reactive and equal, reflexes are 2+, muscle tone is normal, and Babinski and Hoffman tests are negative. She is awaiting a CT scan.

Types of Primary Brain Tumors (PBTs)

PBTs are relatively uncommon in adults with only about 6.4 per 100,000, diagnosed each year,[117] yet they are the most common tumors for children, with 5.5 per 100,000 population for those under 14 and 6.8 per 100,000 for those 15 to 19.[118] For adults, PBTs account for only 1.4% of deaths from cancer annually with a 33.4% chance of a 5-year survival rate overall; they are the most common cause of death from cancer for children. The brain is also a common site for metastases in adults but not children; however, we will focus on PBTs within this chapter.[119] Like tumors throughout the body, PBTs involve abnormal cell proliferation of neurons or glia within the brain or cells within structures of the brain – meninges (meningioma), vasculature, cranial or spinal nerves, or pituitary or pineal glands.[119,120] PBTs are named for their cell type (e.g., meningioma, glioma) and graded according to morphology (histological profile), pattern of growth (staging), and molecular profile[117,121].

Based on the primary cells within the brain tissue, the most common tumor type in both adults (77% of adult PBTs)[59] and children (up to 50% of PBTs)[118] is the **glioma**. These can be further differentiated into **astrocytomas** (most common; from astrocytes), **oligodendrogliomas** (from oligodendrocytes), **ependymomas** (from ventricular lining ependymal cells), and mixed gliomas, which typically involve both astrocytes and oligodendrocytes. In addition, there are neuronal-glial tumors that involve both neurons and glia. Gliomas are staged progressively from relatively benign (Stages I and II) to malignant grades (Stages III and IV; see Table 12-11), based on their rate of growth, differentiation, and infiltration of the surrounding brain tissue. See Table 12-12 for tumor descriptions. There is a tendency for some benign tumors to transition to malignant, so the initial staging may not reflect the ultimate stage. **Differentiation** is the ability to distinguish the cell types within the tumor under a microscope with better differentiation associated with more benign tumors. Increased severity is also associated with greater infiltration of the brain tissue. While **localized tumors** grow within the area of origin and are typically encapsulated, **infiltrating tumors** penetrate and become entwined with the surrounding neural tissue, making them much more difficult to remove. Yet, even localized tumors can damage surrounding brain tissue, resulting in permanent brain damage and even death, depending on their location. Other types of brain tumors have similar staging methods.[118,120]

Tumors are also distinguished by their location as (1) posterior fossa (**infratentorial**) – involving the cerebellum, vermis, or brainstem or (2) **supratentorial** (above the tentorium cerebelli) – involving the cerebrum, deep nuclei (basal ganglia), ventricular choroid plexus or ependymal cells (lining of the ventricles), optic track, hypothalamus, pituitary, pineal gland, or other structures.[118,120] Notably, children can present with a variety of tumors that are unique to the developing nervous system, of which the **medulloblastoma** is the most common with a 30% fatality rate; in the 70% that survive, there is often significant residual physical disability. These tumors occur in the posterior fossa, most commonly within the cerebellum, and are thought to develop from undifferentiated stem cells, originating in the germinal regions of the ventricular zone of

TABLE 12-11	Staging of Glioma Tumors[117,118,120–122]	
STAGE	**CHARACTERISTICS**	**REPRESENTATIVE TYPES**
Stage I	Benign, localized, well differentiated, slowest growing, removable, good outcome	Pilocytic astrocytoma Gangliocytoma or ganglioglioma Giant cell astrocytoma
Stage II	Benign but may become malignant, slow growing, less differentiated than Stage I (look more abnormal), non-infiltrating, removable but may recur	Diffuse fibrillary astrocytoma Oligodendrogliomas
Stage III	Malignant, poor differentiation, infiltrating, faster growing, treated by surgery plus chemotherapy and/or radiation, likely to recur as Stage IV tumor	Anaplastic astrocytomas or oligoastrocytomas
Stage IV	Malignant, undifferentiated, faster growing with greater infiltration than Stage III, generate angiogenesis, very difficult to treat	Glioblastoma • Multifocal – separate but connected foci • Multicentric -separate unconnected foci Diffuse midline glioma Medulloblastoma

TABLE 12-12	Tumor Types, Locations, and Characteristics	
TUMOR TYPE	**COMMON LOCATIONS**	**CHARACTERISTICS**
Ependymoma	Usually infratentorial but can be supratentorial (parietal or temporal lobe)	Arise from ventricular ependymal cells (lining of the ventricles); infratentorial tumors are typically Stage III while supratentorial tumors are typically Stage II.[118]
Gliomas	Anywhere	Arise from glial cells – astrocytes (astrocytoma), oligodendrocytes (oligodendrocytoma); can range from grade I to IV (see Table 12-11)
Glioneuronal	Temporal or frontal lobes; cerebellum	Tumor comprising both glial cells and neuronal components (neural or ganglion cells), arising from neuroepithelial tissues[62]; most common in temporal lobe. Ganglioglioma (ganglion cells and glial cells); Gangliocytoma (ganglion cells without glial cells); Glioneuronal (glial and neurons)[121] Associated with epilepsy that is pharmacologically resistant.[123]
Medulloblastoma	Cerebellum and vermis	Fast-growing malignant posterior fossa tumor in children <7; associated with hydrocephalus.[118]
Meningioma	Arachnoid matter	Stages I-III (most are stage I); multiple genetic contributions; Stages I and II are effectively treated with surgery and radiation.[124]
Neurocytoma	Lateral Ventricle	Stage II – comprises neural tissue without glial tissue without IDH mutation. May block CSF circulation, leading to hydrocephalus.[121]
Pituitary adenoma	Pituitary gland	Benign tumors of one of the six cell types of the pituitary, leading to abnormal secretion of the respective secretory hormones (adenocorticotropic, growth, prolactin, thyroid-stimulating, follicle-stimulating, and luteinizing) with associated symptomology. Tumor growth may disrupt pituitary function. Commonly treatable with gamma knife surgery.[125]
PNETs	Supratentorial – often within pineal gland	Metastasize easily so staged according to: 0 = no metastases; 1 = cells in CSF; 2 = supratentorial metastases; 3 = spinal metastases. Fatal in almost 50% (only 20% if in pineal gland), especially once metastasized. Treated with surgery and radiation, sometimes with chemotherapy.[126,127]

the fourth ventricle.[120] Similarly, primitive neuroectodermal tumors (PNETs) derive from cells, affect either the peripheral or central nervous system (see Chapter 19 for description of neural tube development), and when in the brain are referred to as CNS PNETS. CNS PNETs are similar to medulloblastomas but are genetically distinct,[122] and in adults they typically occur supratentorially, rather than infratentorially as commonly seen in children.[126,127] Further, the outcomes in adults are typically poorer than those for children.[126] See Table 12-12 for tumor types and characteristics.

CASE B, PART II

In the Emergency Department, once Alice was alert, a more complete history revealed frequent headaches of increasing severity over the last few weeks with associated nausea and some mild memory issues that Alice had attributed to insomnia. Alice underwent an unenhanced CT scan, which is typically the first type of imaging used to evaluate patients that present to the ED with initial seizure activity and can typically visualize the tumor and look for signs of hemorrhage or brain herniation. This was followed by a Gadolinium-enhanced MRI the next day to more fully characterize the tumor. This diagnosed a Stage IV glioblastoma in the left temporal lobe with projections into the parietal lobe.

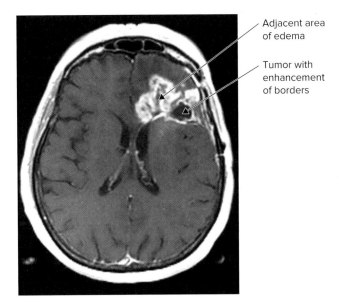

Adjacent area of edema

Tumor with enhancement of borders

FIGURE 12-3 CT scan of glioblastoma. In this T1-weighted image, the tumor appears dark with a surrounding area of high intensity that marks the border or external margin of the tumor. Also, infiltration of the surrounding area with edema appears as hyperintensity. (Reproduced with permission from Hauser SL. *Harrison's Neurology in Clinical Medicine*, 3rd ed. New York, NY: McGraw-Hill; 2013.)

Tumor Symptoms

Although many tumor symptoms are site-specific (e.g., ataxia with posterior fossa tumors), initial presentation can be general or focal. General signs of increased ICP are often the first indications of the presence of a tumor and include nausea, headaches, blurred vision secondary to papilledema and/or retinal hemorrhage, and drowsiness; as occurred with Alice, these symptoms may be attributed to other causes such as fatigue, stress, or a minor illness until they become more severe. A tumor-related headache is often described as worse in the morning and accompanied by nausea and vomiting.[117] In young infants, a tumor may present with irritability, sleep disturbances, protruding fontanelles, and poor feeding.[118] Also, many tumors induce seizures and ultimately epilepsy due to the irritation and eventual death of adjacent cells. Initial seizure activity is the first sign of the tumor in up to 50% of patients with brain tumors, and these can present as both generalized or partial seizures.[128] Seizure activity is most common in cerebral tumors, yet these are often the more treatable tumor types.[128] Focal changes can involve changes in sensory or motor function as well as cognition.[117] Memory or executive function changes are often associated with temporal or frontal lobe tumors; similarly, tumors of the posterior frontal/parietal lobe can present with contralateral sensorimotor disturbances similar to stroke. Of course, these tend to be mild at first and progress to more severe as the tumor grows. Tumors of the posterior fossa disrupt the cerebellum and brainstem; thus, they present with symptoms similar to a brainstem stroke or cerebellar disease, including incoordination, dizziness, ataxia, and cranial nerve disruption.[117]

Tumor Diagnosis

Imaging is usually the only required diagnostic tool for tumor identification with **CT scanning** often the first method used, since it is readily available in most emergency rooms and offers a quick analysis. Tumors appear as areas of hypointensity (lighter) than the normal surrounding tissue, with those that are most dense and of higher grade appearing brighter

on the scan. However, if a brain tumor is suspected, an MRI with and without gadolinium, which allows greater clarity, is the standard method for tumor identification. Gadolinium enhancement allows the determination of tumor characteristics, including cell differentiation, level of brain tissue infiltration, abnormal blood vessel development, and the degree of tissue necrosis and edema within and surrounding the tumor (see Figure 12-3). Depending on the MRI scan type, the tumor will appear either darker (T1 weighted) or lighter (T2 weighted) than the surrounding tissue. Additional imaging techniques, such as positron emission tomography (PET) can illustrate tissue metabolic activity and MR spectroscopy can elucidate blood vessel proliferation/compromise and clarify tumor tissue cellular composition.[129] Sometimes, functional magnetic resonance imaging (fMRI) is used to clarify sensorimotor and cognitive regions prior to tumor resection to minimize damage to these areas.[118] While some non-neoplastic disorders can appear like a tumor, advanced imaging is the best non-invasive tool available for tumor diagnosis. Distinguishing metastases from PBTs can also be challenging but some general differences exist: metastases tend to have a sharper contour and adjacent normal brain tissue while brain tumors tend to be less well defined and likely to extend into adjacent brain tissue.[129]

Tumor Pathogenesis

Some tumors, specifically gliomas and medulloblastomas, seem to arise from **abnormal neurogenesis**, which is the process by which neurons and glial cells are formed. While neurogenesis occurs in multiple areas during fetal development, in adults, only two areas of neurogenesis have been identified: (1) the subgranular zone of the hippocampus and (2) the subventricular zone of the lateral ventricles. Glioma formation is thought to result from abnormal cell differentiation, transforming normal stem cells into **tumor-producing stem cells**.[120] Similarly, medulloblastomas seem to arise from brainstem and fourth ventricle stem cells; since these neurogenic areas aren't active in adults, these tumors affect only children. While they may originate in the brainstem region, these tumor cells often enter the CSF and can, thereby, travel to areas of the forebrain or spinal cord. Other tumor types seem to result from abnormal cell proliferation within the specified tissue (e.g., ependymoma – proliferation of ependymal cells).[130]

So, what triggers this abnormal neurogenesis or cell proliferation? For normal neurogenesis, **transcription factors**, which are proteins that bind to DNA and control gene expression, promote or block cell proliferation. The abnormal neurogenesis, associated with tumor development, appears to result from a disruption of the natural neurogenic/gliogenic transcription factors. This disruption may be triggered by genetic anomalies, stemming from chromosome deletion or amplification.[130] Within our DNA, there exist genes, referred to as proto-oncogenes, that when mutated become **oncogenes** and trigger tumor development. Similarly, DNA includes natural **tumor suppressor genes** (TSGs; antioncogenes) that, when mutated, fail to suppress abnormal cell proliferation, thus, allowing tumor development via abnormal cell proliferation. While gliomas emerge from disruption of a natural cell proliferation process (neurogenesis of stem cells), other tumors appear to be the result of cell proliferation in normally non-replicating cells (e.g., meningioma). Oncogenes and the mutation of TSGs contribute to cell proliferation in most or all tumor types. Multiple genetic defects and changes in growth factors have been identified as triggers to these DNA changes with secondary changes in cell cycle regulation and cell metabolic processes identified. The cause of most types of brain tumors is likely multi-factorial and still under investigation. Further, environmental factors may contribute; however, only exposure to environmental radiation has been definitively linked to brain tumor development. In addition, immunosuppression, such as that associated with HIV infection, has been linked to brain tumor genesis.[120,121]

Medical Treatment of Brain Tumors

Brain tumors need to be aggressively treated to avoid secondary neural damage, resulting from their growth. Surgical resection is the primary initial treatment for most PBTs; to prevent damage to critical brain regions, surgery is typically conducted with the patient awake, using intraoperative cortical electrode stimulation to prevent damage to critical brain tissue. Surgical resection can also help clarify the molecular genotype for the tumor. Subsequent radiation therapy follows resection for most tumors.[129] Stereotaxic radiosurgery (STR, gamma knife) is the use of high-dose radiation from multiple angles simultaneously, guided by imaging (CT or MRI) and stereotaxic (three-dimensional) coordinates. This is particularly useful when the tumor is located within the brainstem or deep within the cerebral hemispheres and surgical resection is not an option; however, it is also effective in benign tumors, such as meningiomas, either as the initial treatment modality or as a secondary treatment after initial resection.[131] Chemotherapy may also be

implemented but is relatively ineffective for many tumor types. However, a combination of chemotherapy with temozolomide and STR, following primary resection of glioblastomas, has resulted in longer survival times.[129,131] Recurrence is likely for many higher stage tumors and most gliomas, often recurring at a more severe grade. Similar treatment methods are used when tumors recur.[129]

Other treatments that are receiving attention, include **gene-centered** treatments to correct the gene mutation, associated with the tumor growth; of course, identification of the appropriate genetic mutation will be key in developing these treatment methods. Viruses, nanomolecules, and stem cells have been used to insert genes into target cells. Other research is attempting to stimulate immune cells to attack cancer cells (immunotherapy) via monoclonal antibodies, cancer vaccines, and other methods.[129]

Physical Therapy Management of the Patient with a Brain Tumor

> ### CASE B, PART III
>
> Alice underwent surgical resection, followed by stereotaxic radiation with chemotherapy. Following these treatments, she entered an inpatient rehabilitation unit with a diagnosis of profound sensory loss with secondary motor dysfunction, characterized by incoordination and apraxia. In addition, she presented with receptive aphasia and apparent memory loss.

As the case illustrates, damage from a brain tumor and the methods used to treat it (surgery, radiation, and chemotherapy) can result in neurologic consequences similar to those of a stroke or focal brain injury. Initial damage may result from the tumor or the surgical resection: this damage is typically localized to the area adjacent to the tumor. Radiation encephalopathy is a secondary consequence of radiation treatment that can occur: (1) acutely – within 2 weeks; (2) early delayed (1-4 months post-radiation); or (3) late delayed (greater than 4 months after treatment). Radiation encephalopathy is characterized by generalized effects of fatigue, cognitive dysfunction with impairments in processing speed, working memory or attention, diminished respiratory capacity, or worsening of initial symptoms associated with the area of radiation: cerebral – motor, sensory, and cognitive changes; brainstem – ataxia, dysarthria, cranial nerve dysfunction. In children, radiation can disrupt endocrine function, resulting in long-term alteration of growth. Application of corticosteroids during radiation therapy is used to minimize radiation encephalopathy. Chemotherapy administration is also associated with similar side effects, including fatigue, hair loss (alopecia), headache, peripheral neuropathy, cardiac effects, and GI upset.[132]

Thus, a growing area for rehabilitation practitioners, especially physical therapists, is in the area of oncology rehabilitation in the acute care, inpatient rehabilitation, and outpatient settings. Primary reasons for referral include cognitive deficits, generalized weakness, and visuospatial dysfuction.[132] Therapy should focus on specific impairments and functional limitations as well as general physical conditioning. Early inpatient rehabilitation has been found to improve functional outcomes and decrease length of stay.[133] In addition, exercise post-radiation, especially when long-term corticosteroids are given, may ameliorate some of the devastating effects of this combined treatment, including fatigue, depression, and diminished physical conditioning, including muscle loss. For some, the onset of muscular wasting occurs weeks after the termination of treatment, so it is important to educate the patient on maintaining the exercise regimen beyond the initial treatment phase.[132] Notably, there is some evidence from animal studies that exercise may also facilitate improved cortical gliogenesis, allowing repopulation of microglia that are lost with radiation treatments and, thereby, improve the microenvironment for neural function.[134] Similarly, an aerobic exercise program was found to induce neural plasticity, manifested as cortex thickening in the sensorimotor areas, in children previously treated with radiation or chemotherapy.[135] Additional research is needed to determine timing, dosage, and intensity best suited to promote best outcomes in those recovering from PBTs.

CASE B, PART IV

For Alice, treatment focused on sensory retraining that included sensory stimulation with a variety of stimuli (e.g., hot/cold, textures, vibration, and electrical stimulation – TENS); this was progressed to sensory discrimination activities using manual manipulation with vision occluded by a curtain between handled objects and Alice. This allowed discrimination of temperature, texture, weight, and shape of objects, usually involving matching to a target object. In addition, her treatment focused on many object manipulation tasks, whereby she had to place a block into a shape sorter or slot by orienting her hand to the orientation of the targeted slot. She also had impaired sensation in her leg/foot that resulted in tripping and exaggerated step height, so treatment focused on sensory stimulation to her foot and gait training to improve safety with ambulation on a variety of surfaces and often in bare feet to facilitate her "feeling" the surface. Initially, she demonstrated marked improvements and was discharged to outpatient care. On a follow-up visit, 6 weeks later, the therapist noted motor weakness in her left biceps and deltoid. Alice was referred back to her physician for evaluation, where recurrence of her tumor into her frontal lobe was diagnosed. Within a week, Alice was transferred to hospice, where she again received physical therapy. At this time, the focus of care was on minimizing pain and management of physical symptoms.

Physical therapy management of the terminal cancer patient is also a growing area of practice. Common treatments include exercise and range of motion (active, active assistive, or passive) to prevent painful contractures, transfer techniques and activities of daily living as function diminishes, management of edema, relaxation techniques, and/or massage to manage pain and muscle cramping. In addition, physical therapists may be called upon to determine appropriate adaptive equipment – wheelchairs, ambulation aids – to maximize mobility and care for the terminal patient.[136]

REFERENCES

1. Sundman MH, Hail EE, Chen NK. Examining the relationship between head trauma and neurodegenerative disease: a review of epidemiology, pathology, and neuroimaging techniques. *J Alzheimers Dis Parkinsonism.* 2014;4:137.

2. Capizzi A, Woo J, Verduzco-Gutierrez M. Traumatic brain injury: an overview of epidemiology, pathophysiology, and medical management. *Med Clin North Am.* 2020;104:213-238.

3. Peterson AB, Thomas KE. Incidence of nonfatal traumatic brain injury-related hospitalizations – United States, 2018. *MMWR Morb Mortal Wkly Rep.* 2021;70(48):1664-1668.

4. Brazinova A, Rehorcikova V, Taylor MS, et al. Epidemiology of traumatic brain injury in Europe: a living systematic review. *J Neurotrauma.* 2021;38:1411-1440.

5. Robinson CP. Moderate and severe traumatic brain injury. *Continuum (Minneap Minn).* 2021;27(5):1278-1300.

6. Teasdale G, Maas A, Lecky F, Manley G, Stocchetti N, Murray G. The Glasgow coma scale at 40 years: standing the test of time. *Lancet.* 2014; 13:844-854.

7. Ganti L, Daneshvar Y, Bodhit A, et al. TBI ADAPTER: traumatic brain injury assessment diagnosis advocacy prevention and treatment from the emergency room – a prospective observational study. *Mil Med.* 2015;180(4):380-386.

8. Knight J, Decker LC. Decerebrate and decorticate posturing, 2021 Nov 30. In: *StatPearls [Internet].* Treasure Island, FL: StatPearls Publishing; 2022. PMID: 32644561.

9. Gilardi BR, López JIM, Villegas ACH, et al. Types of cerebral herniation and their imaging features. *Radiographics.* 2019.39(6)1598-1610.

10. Laleva M, Gabrovsky N, Naseva E, Velinov N, Gabrovsky S. Delated intraventricular hemorrhage in moderate-to-severe traumatic brain injury: prevalence, associated risk factors, and prognosis. *Acta Neurochir.* 2016;158:1465-1472.

11. Meythaler JM, Peduzzi JD, Eleftheriou E, Novack TA. Current concepts: diffuse axonal injury-associated traumatic brain injury. *Arch Phys Med Rehabil.* 2001;82:1461-1471.

12. Pasquina P, Kirtley R, Ling G. Moderate-to-severe traumatic brain injury. *Semin Neurol.* 2014;34:572-583.

13. Tomaszczyk JC, Green NL, Frasca D, et al. Negative neuroplasticity in chronic traumatic brain injury and implications for neurorehabilitation. *Neuropsychol Rev.* 2014;24:409-427.

14. FitzGerald A, Aditya H, Prior A, McNeill E, Pentland B. Anoxic brain injury: clinical patterns and functional outcomes: a study of 93 cases. *Brain Inj.* 2010:24:1311-1323.

15. Brownlee, Naomi N. M. et al. Neurocognitive outcomes in adults following cerebral hypoxia: a systematic literature review. *Neurorehabilitation.* 2020;47(2):83-97.

16. Lo CP, Chen SY, Lee KW, et al. Brain injury after acute carbon monoxide poisoning: early and late complications. *AJR: Am J Roentgenol.* 2007; 189(4):W205-W211.

17. Hoiland RL, Ainslie PN, Wellington CL, et al. Brain hypoxia Is associated with neuroglial injury in humans post-cardiac arrest. *Circ Res.* 2021; 129(5):583-597.

18. Winstanley EL, Mahoney JJ3rd, Castillo F, Comer SD. Neurocognitive impairments and brain abnormalities resulting from opioid-related overdoses: a systematic review. *Drug Alcohol Depend.* 2021;226:108838.

19. Hopkins RO, Bigler ED. Neuroimaging of anoxic injury: implications for neurorehabilitation. *NeuroRehabilitation.* 2021;31:319-329.

20. Nguyen KPL, Pai V, Rashid S, Treece J, Moulton M, Baumrucker SJ. Prognostication in anoxic brain injury. *Am J Hosp Palliat Med.* 2018;35(11):1446-1455.

21. Ramiro JI, Kumar A. Updates on management of anoxic brain injury after cardiac arrest. *Mo Med.* 2013;112(2):136-141.

22. Sekhon MS, Ainslie PN, Griesdale DE. Clinical pathophysiologyb of hypoxic ischemic brain injury after cardiac arrest: a "two-hit" model. *Crit Care.* 2017;21:90.

23. Shavelle RM, Brooks JC, Strauss DJ. An update on survival after anoxic brain injury in adolescents and young adults. *Brain Inj.* 2018;32(13-14):1879.

24. Vella MA, Crandall M, Patel MB. Acute management of traumatic brain injury. *Surg Clin North Am.* 2017;97(5):1015-1030.

25. Ranchos Los Amigos Cognitive Recovery Scale. Available at: https://www.jhsmh.org/LinkClick.aspx?fileticket=8hAd-OqTIQ0%3D&tabid=298. Accessed 3/5/2015.

26. Disability Rating Scale. Available at: http://www.tbims.org/combi/drs/DRS%20Form.pdf. Accessed 3/5/2015.

27. Kalmar K, Giacino JT. The JFK Coma Recovery Scale – revised. *Neuropsychol Rehabil.* 2005;15:454-460.

28. Katz DI, Polyak M, Coughlan D, Nichols M, Roche A. Natural history of recovery from brain injury after prolonged disorders of consciousness: outcome of patients admitted to inpatient rehabilitation with 1-4 year follow-up. *Prog Brain Res.* 2009;177:73-88.

29. von Wild K, Laureys ST, Gerstenbrand F, Dolce G, Onose G. The vegetative state: a syndrome in search of a name. *J Med Life.* 2012;5(1):3-15.

30. Bonsignore LT, Macri S, Orsi P, Chiarotti F, Alleva E. Coma and vegetative states: state of the art and proposal of a novel approach combining existing coma scales. *Ann Ist Super Sanità.* 2014;50(3):241-248.

31. Sherer M, Yablon SA, Nakase-Richardson R. Patterns of recovery of post-traumatic confusional state in neurorehabilitation admissions after traumatic brain injury. *Arch Phys Med Rehabil.* 2009;96:1749-1754.

32. Marshman LAG, Jakabek D, Hennessy M, Quirk F, Guazzo EP. Post-traumatic amnesia. *J Clin Neurosci.* 2013;20:1475-1481.

33. Andriessen TMJC, Jacobs B, Vos PE. Clinical characteristics and patho-physiological mechanisms of focal and diffuse traumatic brain injury. *J Cell Mol Med.* 2014;14(10):2381-2392.

34. Galveston Orientation and Amnesia Test (GOAT). Available at: http://scale-library.com/pdf/Galveston_Orientation_Amnesia_Test.pdf. Accessed 3/5/2015.

35. Keren O, Cohen M, Lazar-Zweker I, Groswasser Z. Tracheotomy in severe TBI patients: sequelae and relation to vocational outcome. *Brain Inj.* 2001;15(6):531-536.

36. Torre VD, Badenes R, Corradi F, et al. Acute respiratory distress syndrome in traumatic brain injury: how do we manage it? *J Thorac Dis.* 2017;9(12):5368-5381.

37. Rincon F, Ghosh S, Dey S, et al. Impact of acute lung injury and acute respiratory distress syndrome after traumatic brain injury in the United States. *Neurosurgery.* 2012;71:795-803.

38. Carlucci M, Graf N, Simmons JG, Corbridge SJ. Effective management of ARDS. *Nurse Pract.* 2014;39(12):35-40.

39. Franschman G, Peerdeman SM, Greuters S, et al. Prehospital endotracheal intubation in patients with severe traumatic brain injury: guidelines versus reality. *Resuscitation.* 2009;80:1147-1151.

40. Stocchetti N, Maas AIR. Traumatic intracranial hypertension. *N Engl J Med.* 2014;370:2121-2130.

41. Harary M, Dolmans RGF, Gormley WB. Intracranial pressure monitoring-review and avenues for development. *Sensors (Basel).* 2018;18:465.

42. Fordington S, Manford M. A review of seizrues and epilepsy following traumatic brain injury. *J Neurol.* 2020;267:3105-3111.

43. Bramlett HM, Dietrich WD. Long-term consequences of traumatic brain injury: current status of potential mechanisms of injury and neurological outcomes. *J Neurotrauma.* 2015;32:1-15.

44. Gupta PK, Sayed N, Ding K, et al. Subtypes of post-traumatic epilepsy: clinical, electrophysiological, and imaging features. *J Neurotrauma.* 2014;31:1439-1443.

45. Lowenstein DH. Epilepsy after head injury: an overview. *Epilepsy.* 50(suppl 2):4-9.

46. Beleza P. Acute symptomatic seizures: a clinically oriented review. *Neurologist.* 2012;18:109-119.

47. Szaflarski JP, Nazzal Y, Dreer LE. Post-traumatic epilepsy: current and emerging treatment options. *Neuropsychiatr Dis Treat.* 2014;10:1469-1477.

48. Khot S, Tirschwell DL. Long-term neurological complications after hypoxic-ischemic encephalopathy. *Sem Neurol.* 2006;26(4):422-431.

49. Topjian AA, de Caen A, Wainwright MS, et al. Pediatric post-cardiac arrest care: a scientific statement from the American Heart Association. *Circulation.* 2019;140:3194-e233.

50. Kiryachkov YY, Bosenko SA, Muslimov BG, Petrova MV. Dysfunction of the autonomic nervous system and its role in the pathogenesis of septic critical illness (review). *Sovrem Tehnologii Med.* 2020;12(4):106-116.

51. Anthony DC, Couch Y. The systemic response to CNS injury. *Exp Neurol.* 2014;258:105-111.

52. Lu J, Goh SJ, Tng PYL, Deng YY, Ling EA, Moochhala S. Systemic inflammatory response following traumatic brain injury. *Front Biosci.* 2009;14:3795-3813.

53. Costello LAS, Lithander FE, Gruen RL, Williams LT. Nutrition therapy in the optimization of health outcomes in adult patients with moderate to severe traumatic brain injury: findings from a scoping review. *Injury.* 2014;45:1834-1841.

54. Pepe JL, Barba CA. The metabolic response to acute traumatic brain injury and implications for nutritional support. *J Head Trauma Rehabil.* 1999;14(5):462-474.

55. Wifdicks EFM. Stomaching acute brain injury. *Neurocrit Care.* 2019;39:542-545.

56. Biteghe-bi-Nzeng A, Wang Y. Cushings ulcer in traumatic brain injury. *Chin J Trauma.* 2008:11(2):114-119.

57. Acosta-Escribano J, Fernandez-Vivas M, Carmona TG, et al. Gastric versus transpyloric feeding in severe traumatic brain injury: a prospective, randomized trial. *Intensive Care Med.* 2010;36:1532-1539.

58. Al-Mufti F, Mayer SA. Neurocritical care of acute subdural hemorrhage. *Neurosurg Clin N Am.* 2017;28:267-278.

59. Hendricks HT, Heeren AH, Vos PE. Dysautonomia after severe traumatic brain injury. *Eur J Neurol.* 2001;17:1172-1177.

60. Iaccarino MA, Bhatnagar S, Zafonte R. Rehabilitation after traumatic brain injury. *Handb Clin Neurol.* 2015;127:411-422.

61. Laxe S, Terre R, Leon D, Bernabeu M. How does dysautonomia influence the outcome of traumatic brain injured patients admitted in a neurorehabilitation unit? *Brain Inj.* 2013;27(12):1383-1387.

62. Arciniegas DB, Wortzel HS. Emotional and behavioral dyscontrol after traumatic brain injury. *Psychiatr Clin N Am.* 2014;37:31-53.

63. Hopkins RO, Haaland KY. Neuropsychological and neuropathological effects of anoxic or ischemic induced brain injury. *J Int Neuropsychol Soc.* 2004;10:956-961.

64. Nakase-Richardson R, Sepehri A, Sherer M, et al. Classification schema of posttraumatic amnesia duration-based injury severity relative to 1-year outcome: analysis of individuals with moderate and severe traumatic brain injury. *Arch Phys Med Rehabil.* 2009;90:17-19.

65. Walker WC, Stromberg KA, Marwitz JH, et al. Predicting long-term global outcome after traumatic brain injury: development of a practical prognostic tool using the traumatic brain injury model systems national database [published correction appears in *J Neurotrauma.* 2020 Mar 15;37(6):905]. *J Neurotrauma.* 2018;35(14):1587-1595.

66. Ponsford JL, Spitz G, McKenzie D. Using post-traumatic amnesia to predict outcome after traumatic brain injury. *J Neurotrauma.* 2016;33(11):997-1004.

67. Ciaramelli E, Serino A, Di Santantonio A, Ládavas E. Central executive system impairment in traumatic brain injury. *Brain Cogn.* 2006;60(2):198-199.

68. Ritter J, Dawson J, Singh RK. Functional recovery after brain injury: independent predictors of psychosocial outcome one year after TBI. *Clin Neurol Neurosurg.* 2021;203:106561.

69. Riedel D, Shaw V. Nursing management of patients with brain injury requiring on-on-one care. *Rehabil Nurs.* 1997;22(1):36-39.

70. Winstein C, Kim B, Kim S, Martinez C, Schweighofer N. Dosage matters. *Stroke.* 2019;50(7):1831-1837.

71. Vasudevan EV, Glass RN, Packel AT. Effects of traumatic brain injury on locomotor adaptation. *J Neurol Phys Ther.* 2014;38(3):172-182.

72. Giuffrida CG, Demery JA, Reyes LR, Lebowitz BK, Hanlon RE. Functional skill learning in men with traumatic brain injury. *Am J Occup Ther.* 2009;63(4):398-407.

73. Elkbuli A, Fanfan D, Sutherland M, et al. The association between early versus late physical therapy initiation and outcomes of trauma patients with and without traumatic brain injuries. *J Surg Res.* 2022;273:34-43.

74. Lai JM, Francisco GE, Willis FB. Dynamic splinting after treatment with botulinum toxin type-A: a randomized controlled pilot study. *Adv Ther.* 2009;26(2):241-248.

75. Leung J, King C, Fereday S. Effectiveness of a programme comprising serial casting, botulinum toxin, splinting and motor training for contracture management: a randomized controlled trial. *Clin Rehabil.* 2019;33(6):1035-1044.

76. Singer BJ, Jegasothy GM, Singer KP, Allison GT. Evaluation of serial casting to correct equinovarus deformity of the ankle after acquired brain injury in adults. *Arch Phys Med Rehabil.* 2003;84(4):483-491.

77. Moseley AM, Hassett LM, Leung J, Clare JS, Herbert RD, Harvey LA. Serial casting versus positioning for the treatment of elbow contractures in adults with traumatic brain injury: a randomized controlled trial. *Clin Rehabil.* 2008;22(5):406-417.

78. Jang SH, Park SM, Kim SH, Ahn SH, Cho YW, Ahn MO. The effect of selective tibial neurotomy and rehabilitation in a quadriplegic patient with ankle spasticity following traumatic brain injury. *Yonsei Med J.* 2004;45(4):743-747.

79. Madsen PJ, Chen HCI, Lang SS. Neurosurgical approaches. *Phys Med Rehabil Clin N Am.* 2018;29:553-565.

80. Shehab D, Elgazzar AH, Collier BD. Heterotopic ossification. *J Nucl Med.* 2002;43(3):346-353.

81. Hoyt BW, Pavey GJ, Potter BK, Forsberg JA. Heterotopic ossification and lessons learned from fifteen years at war: a review of therapy, novel research, and future directions for military and civilian orthopaedic trauma. *Bone.* 2018;109:3-11.

82. Teasell RW, Mehta S, Aubut JL, et al. A systematic review of the therapeutic interventions for heterotopic ossification after spinal cord injury. *Spinal Cord.* 2010;48(7):512-521.

83. Lin K, Wroten M. Ranchos Los Amigos. In: *StatPearls.* Treasure Island, FL: StatPearls Publishing; 2021.

84. Gouvier WD, Blanton PD, LaPorte KK, Nepomuceno C. Reliability and validity of the Disability Rating Scale and the Levels of Cognitive Functioning Scale in monitoring recovery from severe head injury. *Arch Phys Med Rehabil.* 1987;68(2):94-97.

85. Flannery J. Using the levels of cognitive functioning assessment scale with patients with traumatic brain. *Rehabil Nurs.* 1998;23(2):88-94.

86. Kose G, Hatipoglu S. Effect of head and body positioning on cerebral blood flow velocity in patients who underwent cranial surgery. *J Clin Nurs.* 2012;21(13-14):1859-1867.

87. Burnol L, Payen JF, Francony G, et al. Impact of head-of-bed posture on brain oxygenation in patients with acute brain injury: a prospective cohort study. *Neurocrit Care.* 2021;35(3):662-668.

88. Gorji MA, Araghiyansc F, Jafari H, Gorgi AM, Yazdani J. Effect of auditory stimulation on traumatic coma duration in intensive care unit of Medical Sciences University of Mazandarn, Iran. *Saudi J Anaesth.* 2014;8(1):69-72.

89. Zuo J, Tao Y, Liu M, Feng L, Yang Y, Liao L. The effect of family-centered sensory and affective stimulation on comatose patients with traumatic brain injury: a systematic review and meta-analysis. *Int J Nurs Stud.* 2021;115:103846.

90. Cossu G. Therapeutic options to enhance coma arousal after traumatic brain injury: state of the art of current treatments to improve coma recovery. *Br J Neurosurg.* 2014;28(2):187.

91. Megha M, Harpreet S, Nayeem Z. Effect of frequency of multimodal coma stimulation on the consciousness levels of traumatic brain injury comatose patients. *Brain Inj.* 2013;27(5):570-577.

92. Abbate C, Trimarchi PD, Basile I, Mazzucchi A, Devalle G. Sensory stimulation for patients with disorders of consciousness: from stimulation to rehabilitation. *Front Hum Neurosci.* 2014;8:616.

93. TBI EDGE outcome measures for in- and outpatient rehabilitation. Available at: https://www.neuropt.org/practice-resources/neurology-section-outcome-measures-recommendations/traumatic-brain-injury. Accessed 4/7/2022.

94. Core Measures. Available at: https://www.neuropt.org/practice-resources/anpt-clinical-practice-guidelines/core-outcome-measures-cpg. Accessed 4/7/2022.

95. Cuthbert JP, Harrison-Felix C, Corrigan JD, Bell JM, Haarbauer-Krupa JK, Miller AC. Unemployment in the United States after traumatic brain injury for working-age individuals: prevalence and associated factors 2 years postinjury. *J Head Trauma Rehabil.* 2015;30(3):160-174.

96. Mitiguy, JS. Coping with survival: headlines. 1990:228. In: Power PW, Dell Orto AE, eds. *Families Living with Chronic Illness and Disability: Interventions, Challenges, and Opportunities.* New York, NY: Springer Publishing Company; 2004.

97. Page TA, Gordon S, Balchin R, Tomlinson M. Caregivers' perspectives of the challenges faced with survivors of traumatic brain injury: a scoping review. *NeuroRehabilitation.* 2021;49(3):349-362.

98. Lezak MD. Psychological implications of traumatic brain damage for the patient's family. *Rehabil Psychol.* 1986;3(4):241-250.

99. Quatman-Yates CC, Hunter-Giordano A, Shimamura KK, et al. Physical therapy evaluation and treatment after concussion/mild traumatic brain injury. *J Orthop Sports Phys Ther.* 2020;50(4):CPG1-CPG73.

100. Theadom A, Mahon S, Hume P, et al. Incidence of sports-related traumatic brain injury of all severities: a systematic review. *Neuroepidemiology.* 2020;54(2):192-199.

101. Serpa RO, Ferguson L, Larson C, et al. Pathophysiology of pediatric traumatic brain injury. *Front Neurol.* 2021;12:696510.

102. Mejerske CW, Mihalik JP, Ren D, et al. Effect of cognitive activity level on duration of post-concussion symptoms. *Pediatrics.* 2014;133(2):e299-e304.

103. Honig MG, Dorian CC, Worthen JD, et al. Progressive long-term spatial memory loss following repeat concussive and subconcussive brain injury in mice, associated with dorsal hippocampal neuron loss, microglial phenotype shift, and vascular abnormalities. *Eur J Neurosci.* 2021;54(5):5844-5879.

104. Barkhoudarian G, Hovda DA, Giza CC. The molecular pathophysiology of concussive brain injury: an update. *Phys Med Rehabil Clin N Am.* 2016;27(2):373-393.

105. McAllister T, McCrea M. Long-term cognitive and neuropsychiatric consequences of repetitive concussion and head-impact exposure. *J Athl Train.* 2017; 52 (3): 309-317.

106. Langer LK, Alavinia SM, Lawrence DW, et al. Prediction of risk of prolonged post-concussion symptoms: derivation and validation of the TRICORDRR (Toronto Rehabilitation Institute Concussion Outcome De-termination and Rehab Recommendations) score. *PLoS Med.* 2021; 18(7):e1003652.

107. Synnot A, Chau M, Pitt V, et al. Interventions for managing skeletal muscle spasticity following traumatic brain injury. *Cochrane Database Syst Rev.* 2017;11(11):CD008929.

108. Lacerte M, Hays Shapshak A, Mesfin FB. Hypoxic Brain Injury. [Updated 2021 Aug 14]. In: *StatPearls [Internet].* Treasure Island, FL: StatPearls Publishing; 2022.

109. Pinilla LL, Ugun-Klusek A, Rutella S, De Girolamo LA. Hypoxia signaling in Parkinson's disease: there is use in asking "What HIF?" *Biology.* 2021;10:723.

110. Fuller GW, Ransom J, Mandrekar J, Brown AW. Long-term survival following traumatic brain injury: a population-based parametric survival analysis. *Neuroepidemiology.* 2016;47(1):1-10.

111. Murphy MP, Carmine H. Long-term health implications of individuals with TBI: a rehabilitation perspective. *NeuroRehabilitation.* 2012;31:85-94.

112. Morris TP, Tormos Muñoz JM, Cattaneo G, Solana-Sánchez J, Bartrés-Faz D, Pascual-Leone A. Traumatic brain injury modifies the relationship between physical activity and global and cognitive health: results from the Barcelona brain health initiative. *Front Behav Neurosci.* 2019;13:135.

113. Starosta AJ, Adams RS, Marwitz JH, et al. Scoping review of opioid use after traumatic brain injury. *J Head Trauma Rehabil.* 2021;36(5):310-327.

114. Fraser F, Matsuzawa Y, Lee YSC, Minen M. Behavioral treatments for post-traumatic headache. *Curr Pain Headache Rep.* 2017;21:22.

115. Bay EH, Chartier KS. Chronic morbidities after traumatic brain injury: an update for the advanced practice nurse. *J Neurosci Nurs.* 2014;46(3):142-152.

116. McKee AC, Daneshvar DH, Alvarez VE, Stein TD. The neuropathology of sport. *Acta Neuropathol.* 2014;127(1):29-51.

117. Perkins A, Liu G. Primary brain tumors in adults: diagnosis and treatment. *Am Fam Physician.* 2016;93(3):211-217.

118. Koob M, Girard N. Cerebral tumors: specific features in children. *Diagn Interv Imaging.* 2014;95:965-983.

119. Ostrom QT, Fahmideh MA, Cote DJ, et al. Risk factors for childhood and adult primary brain tumors. *Neuro Oncol.* 2019;21(11):1357-1375.

120. Kheirollahi M, Dashti S, Khalaj Z, Nazemroaia F, Mahzouni P. Brain tumors: special characters for research and banking. *Adv Biomed Res.* 2015;4:4.

121. Wang KY, Chen MM, Lincoln CMM. Adult primary brain neoplasm, including 2016 world health organization classification. *Neuroimaging Clin N Am.* 2021;31:121-138.

122. Dubois LG, Campanati L, Righy C, et al. Gliomas and the vascular fragility of the blood brain barrier. *Front Cell Neurosci.* 2014;8(418):1-13.

123. Park CK, Phi JH, Park SH. Glial tumors with neuronal differentiation. *Neurosurg Clin N Am.* 2015;26:117-138.

124. Miller R, DeCandio ML, Dixon-Mah Y, et al. Molecular targets and treatment of meningioma. *J Neurol Neurosurg.* 2014;1(1):1-15.

125. Hasegawa T, Shintai K, Kato T, Iizuka H. Stereotactic radiosurgery as the initial treatment for patients with nonfunctioning pituitary adenomas. *World Neurosurg.* 2015;83(6):1173-1179.

126. Lester RA, Brown LC, Eckel LJ, et al. Clinical outcomes of children and adults with central nervous system primitive neuroectodermal tumor. *J Neurooncol.* 2014;120:371-379.

127. Jakacki RI, Burger PC, Kocak M, et al. Outcome and prognostic factors for children with supratentorial primitive neuroectodermal tumors treated with carboplatin during radiotherapy. *Pediatr Blood Cancer.* 2015;62(5):776-783.

128. Giulioni M, Marucci G, Martinoni M, et al. Epilepsy associated tumors. *World J Clin Cases.* 2014;2(1):623-641.

129. Lapointe S, Perry A, Butowski NA. Primary brain tumours in adults. *Lancet.* 2018;392:432-436.

130. Swartling FJ, Cancer M, Frantz A, Weishaupt H, Persson AI. Deregulated proliferation and differentiation in brain tumors. *Cell Tissue Res.* 2015;359:225-254.

131. Kondziolka D, Shin SM, Brunswick A, Kim I, Silverman JS. The biology of radiosurgery and its clinical applications for brain tumors. *Neuro Oncol.* 2015;17(1):29-44.

132. Vargo M. Brain tumor rehabilitation. *Am J Phys Med Rehabil.* 2011;90(suppl):S50-S62.

133. Bartolo M, Zucchella C, Pace A, et al. Early rehabilitation after surgery improves functional outcome in inpatients with brain tumors. *J Neurooncol.* 2012;107:537-544.

134. Rodgers SP, Trevino M, Zawaksi JA, Gaber MW, Leasure JL. Neurogenesis, exercise, and cognitive late effects of pediatric radiotherapy. *Neural Plast.* 2013; Article ID 698528, 12 pages.

135. Szule-Lerch KU, Timmons BW, Bouffet E, et al. Repairing the brain with physical exercise: cortical thickness and brain volume increase in long-term pediatric brain tumor survivors in response to structured exercise intervention. *Neuroimage Clin.* 2018;18:972-985.

136. Jensen W, Bialy L, Ketels G, Baumann FT, Bokemeyer C, Oechsle K. Physical exercise and therapy in terminally ill cancer patients: a retrospective feasibility analysis. *Support Care Cancer.* 2014;22:1261-1268.

Review Questions

1. A young man experiences a closed head injury with a contusion of the right frontal lobe, from falling over the handlebars of his bicycle; the likely place for a contrecoup injury would be:
   A. Right temporal lobe
   B. Left temporal lobe
   C. Right parietal lobe
   D. Left occipital lobe

2. Which of the following correctly describes the demographic findings for acquired brain injury?
   A. Children under 4 have the highest incidence of acquired brain injury
   B. Teenage girls report concussion at a higher rate than boys
   C. MVAs account for the greatest number of acquired brain injury across all ages
   D. Older men have a higher incidence of brain injury than women

3. A Grade 2 diffuse axonal injury typically involves damage to which structure(s):
   A. Corpus callosum
   B. Corpus callosum and parasagittal projections
   C. Corpus callosum, parasagittal projections, and brainstem white matter
   D. Microstructural damage to the parasagittal white matter

4. Chronic neurodegeneration (>1 year post-TBI) likely results from which mechanisms?
   A. Anterograde degeneration
   B. Excitotoxicity
   C. Retrograde degeneration
   D. Negative plasticity

5. Which of the below descriptions, best describes the brain damage associated with an anoxic brain injury?
   A. Bilateral and diffuse damage to the boundary zones
   B. Diffuse axonal injury

C. Hyperperfusion of the cerebrum associated with reperfusion

D. Hypothermia exacerbation of excitotoxicity

6. **Which assessment is commonly used to determine the clearance of post-traumatic amnesia?**

    A. Braintree Scale of Neurologic Stages of Recovery from Brain Injury

    B. Galveston Orientation and Amnesia Test

    C. JFK Coma Recovery Scale

    D. Ranchos Los Amigos Cognitive Recovery Scale

7. **Amy is 14 weeks s/p a severe head injury; she does not remember anything about her accident. She is currently unable to remember what kind of job she held prior to the accident, anything about her 2 years of marriage to Matt, or details of her college years. She is able to remember her therapy schedules and transport herself to each session. Within sessions, she is able to remember some of the things learned from the preceding day and verbalize them. What kind of amnesia is Amy demonstrating?**

    A. Anterograde

    B. Post-traumatic

    C. Retrograde

8. **A patient that is receiving PT in the ICU, following a severe TBI, begins to vomit. The therapist should be most concerned about:**

    A. Dysautonomia

    B. Elevated intracranial pressure

    C. Multi-organ failure

    D. Seizure activity

9. **A patient, recovering from TBI, is watching a TV show, where one of the characters dies; in response, the patient begins to cry and continues to cry for almost an hour. This is likely a sign of what condition?**

    A. Emotional dyscontrol

    B. Emotional lability

    C. Pathologic crying

    D. Pseudobulbar affect

10. **While assessing a client who is s/p TBI a therapist asks the client to demonstrate how to safely perform a sit to stand transfer. The client takes a long time to initiate the activity but then performs the activity in a safe and correct manner. When a nurse rushes the client to stand up from the dining room chair after dinner the client is unsafe and requires cueing. Based on this description the two transfers look different due to which area of cognitive function?**

    A. Loss of memory

    B. Poor judgment

    C. Slow speed of processing

    D. Poor selective attention

11. **To improve function that is impaired by deficits in divided attention and executive dysfunction the therapist should progressively challenge which area of cognitive functioning?**

    A. Working memory

    B. Speed of processing

    C. Selective attention

    D. Initiation

12. **In an individual with elevated intracranial pressure the head of the bed should be in what position?**

    A. Flat

    B. Elevated to 10 degrees

    C. Elevated to 30 degrees

    D. In 5 degrees of Trendelenburg

13. **An individual post-TBI who is in Ranchos LOC Stage IV and agitated has left hemiplegia and is doing repetitive sit to stand transfers in all therapies and with nursing. After a week he remains in Ranchos LOC IV and has improved his transfer from moderate assist to CGA with cueing. This improvement is due to:**

    A. Hypertrophy of the quadriceps

    B. Explicit learning

    C. Implicit learning

    D. Improved memory

14. **Multimodal sensory stimulation programs should**

    A. Present stimuli in a random order

    B. Include monitoring of vitals

    C. Sessions can be up to 1 hour long

    D. Use standardized stimuli with no emotional overlay

15. **The team plans to spend time each day talking to their patient who is status post anoxic brain injury while showing them pictures. Which of the following would be the best way to apply this intervention?**

    A. Make sure to apply the intervention for at least 20 minutes a session

    B. Have both nursing and therapies apply the intervention when family is not visiting to ensure quiet space where patient can focus.

    C. Work to have the intervention applied primarily by family and good friends rather than staff.

    D. Apply one sensory modality, choosing either talking or showing pictures but not both.

16. **At which Ranchos LOC can you begin to expect explicit learning with carryover?**

    A. IV

    B. V

    C. VI

    D. VII

17. **In dealing with a client who is agitated which of the following is appropriate?**

   A. Restrain the individual to prevent self-harm and harm to others

   B. Medication improves time to recovery from agitation and confusion

   C. Be sure to bring at least three staff into the room to ensure that you can control the individual

   D. Try to figure out what is causing them to be agitated and modify the environment and agitation can be decreased

18. **For impulsivity which of the following is an appropriate intervention?**

   A. Use a written list of steps to be followed for each activity

   B. Encourage task completion without rehearsal

   C. Do not leave the client unsupervised

   D. Provide calendars of daily activities

19. **Physical therapists working in a brain injury unit should come prepared with which of the following?**

   A. A second person to help ensure safety if the individual becomes agitated

   B. The ability to be flexible and consistent

   C. A schedule for the session that is to be followed and consistent plan of care

   D. A means to restrain the patient if they become agitated.

20. **A patient who is Ranchos stage V is beginning to talk in a loud voice, yelling at the therapist, and demonstrating difficulty staying on task. This patient often becomes agitated, especially when facing a challenging or unfamiliar task. In response to these behaviors the therapist should:**

   A. Take the patient out of the therapy gym and place them in an empty, quiet room until they stop yelling.

   B. Restrain the patient and quietly ask them to lower their voice and calm down.

   C. Ignore the behavior and continue with therapy.

   D. Stop therapy, go to a quiet area, and speak to the patient in a calm voice. Remain with the patient.

21. **What is the impact of medicating a patient who is s/p TBI and exhibiting agitation while in the early stages of recovery?**

   A. It reduces their ability to process stimuli and slows recovery.

   B. It calms them down so that they can better participate in therapy.

   C. It improves safety of the patient and those around them.

   D. It calms them down so that they can mentally process and be less confused.

22. **Your patient is in Ranchos Stage VI and needs to use a wheelchair for mobility due to their injuries. Given the** stage of recovery what is the most likely scenario for learning wheelchair mobility?

   A. They will be able to learn to propel and manage the wheelchair but it will take longer and learning will be moderately impaired.

   B. Ability to learn to propel and manage the wheelchair will be severely impaired.

   C. They will learn to propel and manage the chair with minimum impairment.

   D. They will require supervision for safety but will learn wheelchair propulsion and management with little difficulty.

23. **Your patient who is recovering from a TBI has minimal physical deficits, exhibiting good to normal strength and range of motion throughout. This individual was in a coma for 3 weeks and has now been admitted to inpatient rehabilitation. The chart indicates they are in Ranchos Stage VII. What type of physical therapy is this individual likely to need?**

   A. No therapy will be required based on the lack of physical limitations.

   B. Minimal therapy to improve strength to optimal levels to enhance function.

   C. Likely will require therapy to work on safety, judgment, and ability to dual task during mobility.

24. **A teenage lacrosse player comes to therapy for neck pain. He reports it began two weeks ago after being hit in the head with another player's lacrosse stick. When performing the cervical screen he complains of dizziness and nausea. Which of the following statements is true regarding his screen for concussion?**

   A. The screening exam is negative and he has symptoms due to cervical injury.

   B. The screening exam has a positive finding without any emergent conditions indicated;

   C. proceed with physical therapy exam and treatment.

   D. He exhibits symptoms of an emergent condition, refer to emergency medical care.

25. **Which of the following systems should be examined first in the person with a concussion?**

   A. Autonomic function

   B. Cervical spine

   C. Cognitive function

   D. Vestibular system

26. **Recent research suggests that the best treatment for concussion is:**

   A. Absolute rest

   B. No physical activity but encourage a resumption of cognitive activity.

   C. A short period of rest with physical activity as tolerated to resolve symptoms faster.

D. High-level physical and cognitive activity are recommended.

27. For those with severe TBI, which long-term outcome is most likely?

A. Complete return to work, school, or homemaking activity

B. Return to supervised work and living environments

C. No return to work but able to live independently

D. Require total care at home and unable to work

28. An 80-year-old patient with long-standing and poorly managed chronic obstructive pulmonary disease presents to outpatient therapy due to recent falls. Which of the following tests should be included in her examination given her history of pulmonary disease?

A. Ability to stand with eyes closed

B. Gait velocity

C. Rapid alternating tapping of the feet

D. Timed Up and Go Test

29. Which of the patients has the worst prognosis?

A. 14-year-old with TBI secondary to motor vehicle accident. Coma 7 days.

B. 14-year-old with anoxic brain injury from near drowning. Coma 7 days.

C. 70-year-old with TBI secondary to motor vehicle accident. Coma 7 days.

D. 70-year-old with anoxic brain injury from near drowning. Coma 7 days.

30. An oligodendroglioma presents with fairly good differentiation, no infiltration, and is slow growing. This tumor would be staged as:

A. Stage I

B. Stage II

C. Stage III

D. Stage IV

31. Which tumor would correctly be classified as a glioma?

A. Astrocytoma

B. Medulloblastoma

C. CNS PNET

D. Pituitary adenoma

32. Which of the symptoms of a brain tumor is only found in young children?

A. Irritability

B. Fatigue/sleep disturbance

C. Seizures

D. Protruding fontanelles

33. For the patient, receiving radiation treatment for brain tumor, exercise should be avoided until treatment is complete?

A. True

B. False

34. In hospice, the primary focus of treatment should be?

A. Increasing aerobic capacity

B. Strengthening

C. Pain management

D. Walking endurance

35. A patient in ICU is in a coma s/p a suicide attempt by hanging. The patient demonstrates a sleep-wake cycle with eye opening but no tracking, a lack of cortical brain activity, and extensor posturing in all extremities. This patient can best be described by which of the following statements?

A. Unresponsive wakefulness with decerebrate posturing

B. Unresponsive wakefulness with decorticate posturing

C. Ranchos Level III with decerebrate posturing

D. Ranchos Level III with decorticate posturing

Answers

1. D	2. B	3. A	4. B	5. A
6. B	7. C	8. B	9. B	10. C
11. A	12. C	13. C	14. B	15. C
16. C	17. D	18. A	19. B	20. D
21. A	22. B	23. C	24. B	25. B
26. C	27. B	28. C	29. D	30. B
31. A	32. D	33. B	34. C	35. A

GLOSSARY

Acquired brain injury. Non-congenital injury to the brain.

Anoxic brain injury. Brain injury caused by loss of oxygenation of the brain.

Anterograde amnesia. Inability to form new memories.

Astrocytoma. Glioma originating from astrocytes.

Behavioral dyscontrol. Disinhibition of behavior.

Concussive event. One in which there is a direct blow to the head, face, or neck or a force to the body that is transmitted to the head, followed by the onset of symptoms such as changes in consciousness, alteration in mental state, vomiting, and sensitivity to light and noise.

Contra Coup. Injury opposite site of impact.

Contusion. Bruising of brain surface.

Decerebrate posturing. Excessive extension of all extremities.

Decorticate posturing. Upper extremity flexion; lower extremity extension.

Diffuse axonal injury. Tearing of axons due to stretching or rotation.

Dysautonomia. Paroxysmal autonomic instability and dystonia.

Emotional dyscontrol. Dysregulation of emotion.

Ependymomas. Glioma arising from ependymal cells.

Exertional intolerance. A condition where the person has an inability or decreased ability to perform physical exercise at the expected level or duration for people of and equivalent age.

Focal injury. Localized injury at site of impact.

Glasgow Coma Scale. Assesses eye movements, verbal responses, and motor behavior.

Glioma. Tumor originating from glial cells.

Hematoma. Pooling of blood.

Heterotopic ossification. Abnormal bone formation in soft tissue.

Hypercatabolism. Exaggerated glucose utilization and body protein breakdown.

Hypermetabolism. Exaggerated metabolism due to increased levels of epinephrine and norepinephrine.

Hypopituitarism. Loss of circulating hormones secondary to neuroendocrine dysfunction.

Hypoxic brain injury. Brain injury caused by decreased oxygenation of the brain.

Infratentorial. Posterior fossa tumors located within the cerebellum, vermis, or brainstem.

Intraparenchymal. Within the brain tissue.

Medulloblastoma. Brainstem tumor common in children.

Oligodendroglioma. Glioma originating from oligodendrocytes.

Opisthotonus posture. Extremity, neck, and trunk hyperextension.

Paroxysmal autonomic instability and dystonia. Dysregulation of the autonomic nervous system.

Post-traumatic Amnesia. Period of anterograde and retrograde amnesia following a BI.

Primary brain tumors. Tumors that originate in the brain.

Pro-inflammatory response. The immune system's response when triggered by the presence of a foreign material or injury to tissue. This response results in the release of cells that mediate the body's inflammatory response resulting in inflammation. The inflammation can be localized or systemic.

Retrograde amnesia. Loss of memory for prior events.

Supratentorial. Tumors above the tenorium cerebelli, within the cerebrum.

Tinnitus. Hearing sounds that are not produced externally, typically described as high-pitched or ringing.

Unresponsive wakefulness syndrome. Emergence of sleep-wake cycle with brainstem function.

ABBREVIATIONS

ABI	anoxic/hypoxic brain injury
ARDS	acute respiratory distress syndrome
BI	brain injury
DAI	diffuse axonal injury
GCS	Glasgow Coma Scale
GOAT	Galveston Orientation and Amnesia Test
HO	heterotopic ossification
ICH	intracranial hypertension
MODS	multi-organ dysfunction syndrome
mTBI	mild traumatic brain injury (concussion)
PAID	paroxysmal autonomic instability and dystonia
PBT	primary brain tumor
PRAFO	pressure relief ankle foot orthosis
SIRS	systemic inflammatory response syndrome
TBI	traumatic brain injury
TPN	total parenteral nutrition
UWS	unresponsive wakefulness syndrome

Spinal Cord Injury

D. Michele Basso

13

OBJECTIVES

1) Understand the pathophysiology of spinal cord injury (SCI)

2) Describe the neuroanatomical relationship and effect of SCI for the lungs, skin, bowel, bladder, and cardiovascular system

3) Examine the medical management of the most serious and common complications after SCI

4) Differentiate the sensory, motor, and reflex function for different types and levels of SCI

5) Identify and structure rehabilitation interventions for incomplete and complete SCI

6) Recognize adjustments of individuals with SCI and that of their families

CASE A, PART I

Jane Roberts is a 45-year-old African-American woman who entered the Emergency Department via ambulance with a self-inflicted gunshot wound to the neck at C2–3. She was intubated in the field and placed on a respirator when admitted to the hospital. Her blood pressure, 98/62, and heart rate, 60, were low and continued to fall. Radiographs show a projectile near C2, a vertebral fracture of C2, and a bony fragment within the spinal canal. She has a history of depression and mild obesity but takes no medications for these conditions. Ms. Roberts presented in the Emergency Department with no volitional movement in any of the extremities. The plantar reflex was present, but deep tendon reflexes (DTRs) in all extremities were absent. She is not married, works in a parts-assembly factory, and lives alone in a two-story home.

● PATHOPHYSIOLOGY

What Is Spinal Cord Injury?

The spinal cord is protected by the surrounding bone of the vertebrae, but in severe trauma, the vertebrae fracture or dislocate. In fact, fracture, dislocation, and/or subluxation of the vertebrae are the most common causes of SCI. The damaged bony segments impinge the spinal cord and immediately cause a lesion. This direct damage to the spinal cord is called the **primary injury**. It is important to note that the spinal cord is rarely completely severed; some spinal cord tissue is usually spared. Commonly, the fractured or dislocated bone compresses the cord or only partially pierces it. In most cases, the primary injury begins in the gray matter of the cord, when the blood vessels shear and rupture, directly damaging neurons. There is frank hemorrhage at the injury site and small petechial hemorrhages away from the injury over the next couple of hours. White matter axons may also be directly lesioned with the primary injury. These initial events set off a complex secondary cascade that causes the lesion to expand in size, over a long distance and over a long period of time.

The **secondary injury** events stem from a toxic environment created by the initial injury.[1,2] The opening of the blood-brain barrier allows red blood cells to flood the gray matter, and the iron and hemoglobin they contain are toxic to neurons that were not initially damaged by the trauma. As these bystander neurons die, they release neurotoxins and glutamate that go on to kill other neurons beyond the primary injury site. Other toxic substances are produced, including free radicals, reactive oxygen species, and peroxidases, which degrade cell membranes and cause further cell death. With this necrotic cell death, edema increases and the damaged blood vessels are sealed a few segments away from the primary injury, causing ischemia. Loss of oxygen results in expanding cell death, and even the cells that overcome this stress are often lost once blood flow returns to the area (reperfusion) as even higher levels of reactive oxygen species occur.

Another major contributor to secondary injury and lesion expansion is neuroinflammation.[1] Within the first few hours and days after the injury, resident microglia and infiltrating macrophages from the peripheral blood stream flood into the lesion center. Early on, they play an important beneficial role in sterilizing the wound and scavenging debris. However, the inflammatory response extends for very long periods of time, producing detrimental effects well away from the injury site. The activated microglia produce high levels of pro-inflammatory cytokines and chemokines, and these factors impair neuronal function up to 10 segments below the injury site. Additionally, oligodendrocytes are especially vulnerable to pro-inflammatory cytokines, leading to oligodendrocyte cell death and creating zones of demyelination many segments above and below the level of the injury. The notion that there is a localized site of SCI is being challenged, and it is important to start to understand that areas well away from the primary injury will also experience secondary lesion effects that will impact rehabilitation.

During this secondary injury phase, reactive astrocytes surround the primary lesion, creating a glial scar that acts as a physical barrier to regenerating axons. The astrocytes also produce chemical inhibitory barriers (i.e., chondroitin sulfate proteoglycans, known as CSPGs) that extend two or three segments above and below the primary injury. Reactive astrocytes extend well away from the injury site but likely do not create a scar. Some ideas are that they are providing metabolic support and helping to control edema in these remote regions. Astrocytes also adsorb excess glutamate, buffering the toxic environment and may help limit cell death away from the injury site.

Importantly, these secondary injury pathways offer the best target for treatment after SCI. By quelling some or all of these pathways, the severity of lesion and resulting motor impairments can be greatly reduced. Thus, neuroprotection has been a major focus of scientific investigation. Regeneration, growth promotion, and cellular replacement therapies have also shown some promise.[3,4] Any reduction of lesion size or effective cellular growth promotion will offer important substrates upon which to improve functional recovery after SCI.

Who Has a Spinal Cord Injury?

Each year about 17,000 people have an SCI. The most common cause of SCI is trauma from car accidents (38%), falls (32%), violence (14%), or sports (8%).[5] Although sports-related injuries used to be the highest cause, it has steadily declined while vehicular accidents and falls continue to rise. The changes in how people are injured result in an increase in age at the time of injury. In the 1970s, the average age at the time of SCI was about 27 years, but now, the average age is 43 years.[5] Still, about half of all SCIs occur in young people under the age of 30.[5] Spinal cord injuries also occur in men much more often than in women, at a rate of 75 to 80%. Recently, injuries in people who are non-Hispanic and Black have risen to much higher levels (24%) than expected based on the general population (17%). Moreover, adults who are Black were significantly more likely to have been hospitalized early (1 year) and later (5 years) after SCI and longer lengths of stay than Hispanic or white individuals.[6] In contrast, people of Hispanic descent had the lowest chance of hospitalization during this period, although hospitalization rates increased by 10 yrs.[6] Thus, adults who are Black may be more vulnerable to negative health consequences after SCI and warrant special attention to improve prevention approaches over the first decade after SCI.

Other causes of SCI include **transverse myelitis**, spinal stenosis, spinal abscess, or tumor. **Spinal stenosis** means that the spinal canal narrows to the point that the spinal cord becomes compressed. It most commonly occurs in the cervical or lumbar vertebrae. The narrow canal may not cause any neural symptoms until a minor trauma like a fall or neck hyperextension occurs. People with osteoarthritis are particularly at risk for hyperextension-type SCI. With this otherwise minor trauma, the cord is greatly compressed resulting in a primary injury of the gray matter. We will discuss the specific type of SCI observed

with spinal stenosis, called **central cord syndrome**, in a later section. Spinal stenosis-related SCI occurs in older individuals with a mean age of 64 years and affects women at a higher rate, about 40%, than in traumatic SCI.[7] The severity of the injury appears less than traumatic SCI in that **paraplegia** is more common than **tetraplegia** and rehabilitation is shorter.[7] In a large study of veterans, almost all men, falls accounted for 40% of SCI in those with diagnosed, pre-existing cervical stenosis.[8] As in women, SCI after stenosis was less severe (79% incomplete) and occurred in older individuals. Stenosis was more prevalent in African-Americans than Caucasians, possibly due to race-dependent differences in neural canal size.[9] Implementing fall prevention therapy for people with stenosis and Black individuals with fall-risk will be important to reduce SCI risk. Radiologic confirmation of stenosis in people with frequent fall history is warranted since low threshold motor impairments due to stenosis may be causing the instability and falls.

Transverse myelitis is pronounced inflammation across both sides of the spinal cord that typically occurs with a sudden onset over a few hours and worsens over a few weeks.[10] It isn't clear what initiates the inflammation, but viral infections are a strong candidate. Both children and adults can be affected with about 1400 people diagnosed each year with transverse myelitis. As in traumatic SCI, inflammatory cascades target oligodendrocytes and the resulting cell death produces regions of demyelination and axonal loss. The degree of recovery is highly variable with most individuals having long-term motor disabilities.[10] Recurrence is rare but not unheard of.

Differential Diagnosis – Could This be a Spinal Cord Injury?

Traumatic SCI is routinely diagnosed in the Emergency Department, but non-traumatic SCI is often misdiagnosed as a musculoskeletal condition; thus, physical therapists must be cautious when treating these conditions. In the case of abscess, tumor, transverse myelitis, or stenosis, the primary symptom is back pain, which can be localized or radiating pain. Because this type of pain is common in both musculoskeletal conditions and non-traumatic SCI, a thorough neurologic examination is needed to rule out SCI. The best indicators of SCI are changes in reflexes below the level of pain, a positive Babinski sign, and/or difficulty voiding the bowel or bladder.

With SCI, there are two areas of neuropathology at the injury site – the neurons in the gray matter and the long ascending and descending white matter tracks. Motor neurons in the ventral horn of the grey matter send their axons to innervate muscles in the body (see Chapter 4). They are often called the final common pathway because when damaged, the muscle is greatly weakened or fully paralyzed. Damage to motor neurons in a single segment or multiple segments of the spinal cord produces lower motor neuron (LMN) signs. When white matter tracks are lesioned in the spinal cord, it means that the neurons for these axons are above the lesion – primarily in the brain. The problems that emerge from damaged axons are called upper motor neuron (UMN) signs. Most of the time, SCI results in both UMN and LMN signs, since both gray and white matter are damaged.

LMN signs include **areflexia** and **flaccid paralysis** early after injury and extreme **muscle atrophy** within weeks or months. These signs are directly related to death of motor neurons that innervate muscles at the level of the injury and occur in other conditions. Regions of flaccid paralysis and areflexia are used to determine the level of injury but are difficult to examine in the trunk where DTRs are not available for testing. Any LMN signs observed in people with musculoskeletal conditions, like low back pain, require immediate referral to a neurologist. The **Beevor sign** of the umbilicus may help to identify motor neuron loss within the thoracic region (T10–12). This is evident when the upper rectus abdominus muscle is innervated but the lower part is poorly innervated and weak, so that only the upper rectus contracts forcefully. By raising the head from a supine position, the upper rectus contracts and pulls the umbilicus toward the head, identifying a lesion in the lower thoracic cord. Beevor sign is also diagnostic for other conditions.

UMN signs occur because information from the brain to the spinal cord is disrupted in the white matter tracks. **Hyperreflexia**, **spasticity**, **clonus**, and positive **Babinski** sign occur with UMN lesions, but unlike in stroke, these problems emerge because of damage to the *axons* of supraspinal neurons rather than to the *neuron cell bodies*. Any person being treated for a musculoskeletal condition that demonstrates UMN signs must be immediately referred to a neurologist.

● CLASSIFICATIONS OF SCI

Spinal cord injury is classified by the level and severity of the primary pathology using the **ASIA Impairment Scale** (AIS) and the **International Standards for Neurological Classification of SCI** (ISNCSCI).[11,12] The AIS was developed by the American Spinal Cord Injury Association; the ISNCSCI is a revised version, adopted by the International Standards Committee. There is an online training program to learn to administer the exam with reduced fees for students and residents.[13] The level of the injury refers to the segmental location of the primary lesion, based on radiographic and clinical symptoms. The designated level is the most distal, uninvolved segment with normal function. A patient with a C4 level injury means that dysfunction and impairments occur below C4. Cervical injuries result in impairments of the upper and lower extremities, called tetraplegia. When SCI occurs in the thoracic or upper lumbar regions, the lower extremities are affected, which is known as paraplegia.

The severity of SCI is classified into four categories, AIS A to AIS D, ranging from complete to incomplete SCI (Table 13-1). Normal is designated as AIS E. The AIS/ISNCSCI system examines each sensory dermatome of the body for perception of sharp versus dull, and light touch – one of three scores – 0 = no sensation, 1 = altered sensation, which can be either hyper- or hyposensitive, and 2 = normal sensation for a total score of 56 for each side. Motor function is assessed using manual muscle testing (MMT) of five key muscle groups in each upper extremity and five muscles of each lower extremity. Traditional MMT scores ranging from 0 to 5 are used for each muscle group bilaterally, which yields a maximum score of 50 for upper extremity

TABLE 13-1	Classification of SCI[11]
AIS A	Complete; no sensory or motor function below the level of the injury
AIS B	Incomplete; no motor function but some sensation below the injury, including in the anal sphincter region (S4–5)
AIS C	Incomplete; some sensory and motor function below the injury but most of these muscles score below 3 on MMT
AIS D	Incomplete; sensory and motor function with at least half of the muscle groups scoring 3 or higher on MMT
AIS E	Normal motor and sensory function

motor scores (UEMS) and 50 for lower extremity motor scores (LEMS).

There are several important clinical considerations for the AIS system. When the AIS classification is made at 72 hours after the injury, it can be a good predictor of whether people will go on to regain walking function. Some or intact pinprick sensation in the perianal region predicted ambulation in individuals with SCI.[14,15] During the first year after SCI, there is a high rate of AIS conversion to a higher classification.[16,17] Conversion from complete SCI (AIS A) to incomplete injury is about three times higher currently than a decade ago.[18] Clinically, we can expect higher conversion rates for cervical versus thoracic injuries, and sensory versus motor improvements.[18,19] Importantly, up to 28% of cervical SCI convert to motor incomplete (AIS C or D).[18] Predicting outcomes for patients in the acute setting suggest recovery of sensory or motor function in up to 30 to 50% of cases with cervical SCI and 15 to 23% with thoracic injuries.[18,19] Regaining some motor control below the injury likely confers benefits including more independence.[20] Regaining only sensory function (AIS B conversion) reduces length of hospitalization and lifetime costs.[21] This means that in the acute setting and during inpatient rehabilitation therapists should expect some sensory and motor recovery and use interventions that will encourage recovery. Traditionally, little change in AIS classification and motor scores have been reported between 1 and 5 years after SCI,[22] which has been used to focus rehabilitation within the first year of SCI. However, walking-based programs on a treadmill for AIS C or D injuries greatly increased motor scores for both the upper and lower extremities in people with subacute to chronic SCI.[23,24] Conversion to higher AIS classification was greater than expected, and people with both tetraplegia and paraplegia improved with treatment.[22-25] These findings suggest that motor recovery after SCI is highly responsive to the type of rehabilitation administered, even at chronic time points.

While the AIS system is the most widely used classification system for SCI, it has several limitations. It does not measure motor function in the trunk that can be a clinically important indicator of the type of physical therapy treatment to deliver. The sensory score of 1 can mean that sensation is below normal (hyposensitive) or well-above normal (hypersensitive), thereby, making it a poor measure of neuropathic pain.

An AIS A classification means the injury is *clinically complete* but postmortem studies of human SCI by Richard Bunge found that anatomical sparing occurred in a large number of AIS A cases.[26,27] Recently, Harkema and others implanted epidural stimulators below the level of SCI in people with AIS A or AIS B injuries.[28–31] Across these independent studies, individuals with SCI had no voluntary control of lower extremity muscles, prior to implantation, but on the first day of stimulation, each individual demonstrated voluntary movement of the leg, foot, or toe. Taken together with the work of Bunge, these studies indicate that even when an AIS A complete classification is assigned, anatomical sparing is highly likely. This sparing may be an important substrate for recovery of function, when task-specific training and/or electrical stimulation is delivered.

An SCI-specific assessment tool, the **Neuromuscular Recovery Scale** (NRS), was designed to classify SCI relative to normal, pre-injury motor performance. It uses 14 items or tasks for trunk, upper extremity, and lower extremity motor control. The items range from coming to sitting, sitting, coming to stand, walking, and unimanual and bimanual manipulation. The performance is scored in four broad phases (Phases 1-4) with higher phases reflecting greater return of normal movement. Each of these phases is further subdivided into three categories (A, B, or C) to better differentiate functional performance. The overall classification is designated by the Phase and subclassification (i.e., Phase 1A, Phase 4B, etc.). Lower phase means the person with SCI is performing only small parts of the task in a normal manner (e.g., using uninjured movement patterns). Likewise, the lower the subclassification of the phase (i.e., A),

the lower the ability to perform normal movements. The NRS can also be used to measure recovery of function by assigning one point for each subphase that is performed at a pre-injury level. A total of 161 points are available. The psychometrics of the NRS has been tested on people with AIS A–D SCI, in both the outpatient and inpatient rehabilitation settings. It has shown high inter-rater and test–retest reliability,[32,33] strong validity,[34] and better sensitivity to functional improvement over time than most other SCI outcome measures, including ISNCSCI motor and sensory scores, 10-minute walk test, 6-minute walk test, Berg Balance Scale, and modified functional reach.[35] Because normal, pre-injury function is the basis of the scale, the NRS classification system enables the therapist to identify areas of function that show specific deficits and target treatment interventions to these areas.

Relationship between Injury and Clinical Presentation

To effectively treat SCI, it is important to understand the relationship between the injury and the clinical presentation. Some aspects of the injury result in permanent loss of function while others may have the potential to recover. Distinguishing between these can be accomplished by diagramming the lesion. Review the ascending and descending tracks and their position in the cord in chapter 3 and chapter 4, respectively.

Brown-Sequard injury is an injury to primarily one side of the cord leaving the other side relatively intact (Figure 13-1). This type of injury can occur with fracture or dislocation but

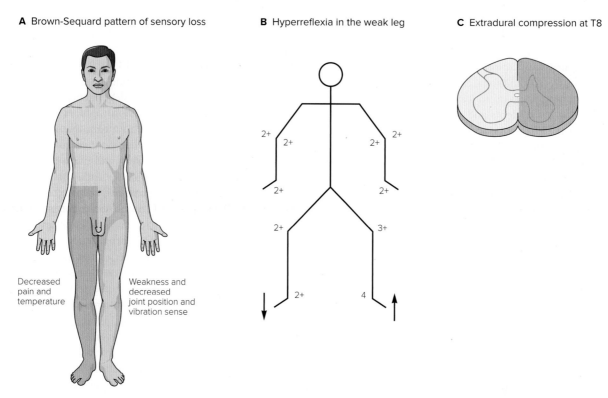

A Brown-Sequard pattern of sensory loss   **B** Hyperreflexia in the weak leg   **C** Extradural compression at T8

FIGURE 13-1 Brown-Sequard pattern of injury. The primary symptoms of a BS pattern are ipsilesional motor and somatosensory dysfunction with contralesional loss of pain and temperature (**A**); hyperreflexia in the ipsilesional leg (**B**); and a lesion confined to one side of the spinal cord (**C**). (Reproduced with permission from Kandel ER, Schwartz JH, Jessell TM, et al. *Principles of Neural Science*, 5th Ed, New York, NY: McGraw-Hill; 2013.)

is most commonly seen after a penetrating injury from broken glass, a knife, or gunshot. The clinical presentation is motor impairment on the side of the lesion, loss of gross touch and vibration on the side of the lesion, and impairment of pain and temperature on the opposite side of the injury. Hyperreflexia as measured by brisk tendon reflexes and an upward Babinski response occurs below the lesion on the side of the injury (Figure 13-1B). Sweating, piloerection, and flushed face, which are signs of autonomic dysfunction, occur on the same side of the injury.

Central cord syndrome is caused by a lesion of the center core of the gray matter and occurs with trauma especially falls that cause hyperextension of the neck, tumors, or syrinxes. Central cord syndrome presents with LMN signs (flaccidity and muscle atrophy) of the upper extremities and less severe impairments of the lower extremities (Figure 13-2). Often the loss of hand function is pronounced and permanent, while the legs retain or regain a great deal of function sufficient to support walking with relatively stable balance. The lesion is primarily localized to the gray matter of the cervical cord, leaving most of the descending motor systems intact. In this way, there are lower motor signs at the level of the injury due to loss of motor neurons, while descending input from the brain can initiate central pattern generators (CPGs) for locomotion, which are intact below the injury.

Anterior spinal cord syndrome is a lesion of the anterior two-third of the spinal cord and is caused by damage or infarction of the anterior spinal artery (Figure 13-3). Interruption of blood flow through the artery can occur due to a blood clot and is commonly referred to as spinal stroke. Other causes are bony fragments either blocking or cutting the artery, hyperflexion of the spinal column that compresses the artery, or clamping the

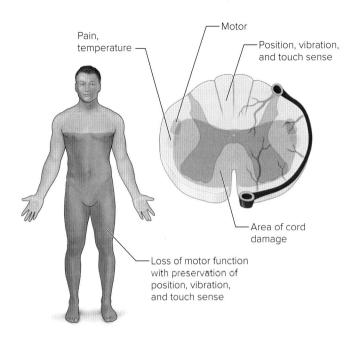

FIGURE 13-3 Anterior spinal cord injury. The lesion location in the ventral gray and white matter is shown on the right image of the cord. The shaded regions on the left show loss of motor function and pain and temperature sensation. Vibration and position sense remain.

descending aorta for abdominal surgery, which causes a delayed ischemic/reperfusion injury in up to 40% of surgical patients.[36,37] With anterior spinal cord syndrome, there is complete loss of volitional movement at and below the level of injury because the anterior and lateral corticospinal tracts are within the damaged area. Other descending motor systems, such as the vestibulospinal and reticulospinal tracts, also occupy these regions, resulting in a motor complete SCI. The ascending sensory tracts for pain and temperature also travel in the anterolateral white matter and are impaired at and below the level of the injury. However, the dorsal columns receive their blood supply from the dorsal spinal artery, so vibration and proprioception remain intact. This injury pattern is an example of an AIS B classification of SCI. Depending on the level of SCI, such as cervical or high thoracic injury, autonomic impairments may also occur.

Posterior spinal cord syndrome (Figure 13-4) – The posterior part of the spinal cord can be lesioned by a penetrating wound to the back or hyperextension that fractures the vertebral arch; however, this is a rare type of SCI but has a classic presentation. Proprioception and vibration sense are lost while pain and temperature sensation remain intact. Motor function is also intact.

Conus medullaris (Figure 13-5) – The injury to the conus medullaris occurs at the L1 vertebral level, which is where the spinal cord tapers to an end. Nerves that originate from this part of the cord and nerves that travel through this space are affected by the injury. These nerves control legs, genitals, bladder, and bowel. The most common symptoms are deep aching pain in the low back and numbness in the groin, thigh, leg, or foot. Urine retention, bowel dysfunction, and sexual impotence may also occur. These problems have a sudden onset and usually a bilateral presentation.[38]

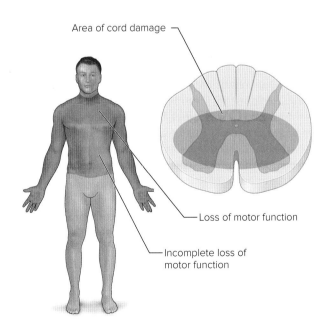

FIGURE 13-2 Central cord syndrome. This shows a lesion in the central gray matter, sparing a peripheral rim of white matter (right). The shaded areas (left) show the regions with complete loss of motor function (dark) and incomplete, mild loss of motor function (light).

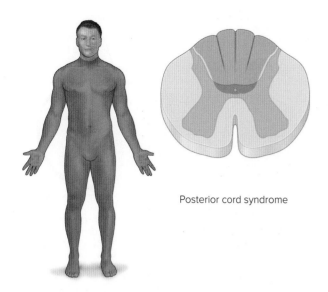

FIGURE 13-4 Posterior cord syndrome. The shaded region depicted in the right image of the cord shows the lesion located in the dorsal columns. The affected body regions are shown on the left which have loss of vibration and position sense.

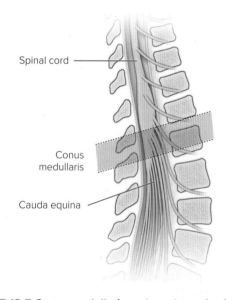

FIGURE 13-5 Conus medullaris and cauda equina injuries. The conus medullaris injury damages the distal portion of the spinal cord at L1; the cauda equina injury damages the spinal nerves, located in the spinal segments below the end of the cord.

Cauda equina syndrome – The term cauda equina translates to horse's tail and is named for the nerves that travel in the terminal spinal canal (Figure 13-5). It is difficult to differentiate Cauda Equina syndrome from a conus medullaris lesion because the nerves traveling down to their foramenal exit are often injured in both conditions.[39] The location of the cauda equina injury will be below the L2 vertebral level. With a cauda equina injury, back pain is typically severe and stabbing (radicular) along dermatomal patterns, and the symptoms will likely be unilateral.

● MEDICAL MANAGEMENT

The acute medical management of SCI begins in the community, when the injury is traumatic, or in the emergency department for other forms of SCI. If the injury is not of traumatic origin, then a thorough differential diagnosis should be undertaken with particular attention given to bowel and bladder function and reflexes below the area of concern so that someone with an abscess or tumor is not misdiagnosed or goes untreated.

An early decision will be made as to whether spinal decompression and stabilization surgery is needed. Conditions that necessitate surgery include progressive worsening of neurological symptoms, dislocated or locked facets, epidural abscesses, or cauda equina syndrome. The use of spinal decompression and stabilization surgery has been inconsistent and wasn't considered standard of care for SCI because the level of evidence to support surgery was not prospective or randomized.[40,41] The results of a well-controlled surgical trial are increasing surgical stabilization and decompression in SCI.[42] Importantly, 20% of people that received decompression within about 14 hours of SCI regained two AIS grades or more at the 6-month follow-up.[42] In contrast, this level of improvement occurred in only 9% of people who had delayed surgery (2 days after SCI). Thus, spinal decompression and stabilization surgery within the first day after SCI is increasing.[43] Therefore, physical therapists can expect greater gains in sensory and motor function in twice as many individuals who receive early surgery relative to later surgery.

The other early medical decision will be whether to administer steroids. Over the last 10 years, there has been a dramatic shift away from the use of steroids within 8 hours of non-penetrating SCI in the United States. Three randomized controlled trials called National Acute Spinal Cord Injury Studies (NASCIS I, II, and III) showed that high-dose methylprednisolone improved motor and sensory scores on the AIS/ ISNCSCI exam in both people with complete or incomplete SCI.[44,45] However, questions about scientific design, randomization, and data analysis emerged. Many physician groups changed their recommendations for steroid use for treatment of SCI, stating that any clinical gain may be heavily offset by serious side effects such as sepsis or pneumonia.[46] This means that the physical therapist will need to be a diligent member of the care team in any patient that receives methylprednisolone by checking for signs of sepsis, pneumonia, or other infections.

Once an SCI has been identified, the medical treatment focuses on several key factors that will continue to be carefully monitored throughout all phases of rehabilitation. Across the SCI treatment continuum, the physical therapist functions as part of a team. They are an extra set of eyes and hands to prevent life-threatening conditions, so it is important that the medical consequences and symptoms be familiar. The 5 areas of critical concern monitored by the SCI team acutely, and thereafter are: (1) Cardiovascular changes, (2) Hypotension, (3) Bladder and Bowel Dysfunction, (4) Respiration, and (5) Skin Integrity. Hypotension and other cardiovascular complications result from autonomic dysfunction. These systems demand close attention because they represent life-threatening conditions if unmanaged.

Autonomic Dysfunction

Neuroanatomical Relationships and Normal Function

As introduced in Chapter 1, the autonomic nervous system consists of the sympathetic and parasympathetic systems that are responsible for complex reflex integration between the central nervous system (CNS) and vital organs. Excitatory sympathetic signals from receptors in the heart, arteries, and skeletal muscles are sent to the solitary nucleus in the brainstem. Parasympathetic input from Barrow receptors in the carotid artery, aortic arch, and other vessels inhibit the solitary nucleus via cranial nerves IX and X. Control of the heart is provided by two regions in the brain – the hypothalamus and the paraventricular nucleus surrounding the third ventricle. The hypothalamus increases sympathetic activity in the heart and other organs. Sympathetic vasomotor drive to the medulla raises blood pressure, and input to the raphe nucleus increases heart rate. The paraventricular nucleus sends axons to the spinal cord to also increase heart rate and regulate the sympathetic system in the lower thoracic cord.[47] The autonomic nervous system plays a critical role in supplying blood to CNS tissues at high enough levels to meet metabolic requirements, even when low blood pressure exists.[48] Unfortunately after SCI, this regulation is disrupted and swings between low and excessively high arterial pressures. In acute SCI, mean arterial pressure is closely monitored in intensive care. In fact, raising blood pressure with fluids and drugs during this early stage improves neurological recovery, AIS grade, ambulation, and bowel and bladder function.[48–50] Given the complexity of the autonomic nervous system, a clinical evaluation tool was developed by International Standards for Autonomic Function after Spinal Cord Injury (ISAFSCI)[51] and online training modules are available.[52] Key systems impacted by autonomic dysfunction are described in detail below.

Effects of SCI

Cardiac and vasomotor changes – Injury at T6 or above interrupts supraspinal sympathetic control to the cardiac system, leaving the only control of the heart to parasympathetic innervation through the vagus nerve. Without sympathetic drive, the heart slows (**bradycardia**) and may beat at a fluctuating rate (**arrhythmia**). Problems with vasomotor responses also develop, including a decrease in vascular tone, which allows blood to pool in the vessels and organs thereby lowering blood pressure (**hypotension**). This sympathetic loss has been termed **neurogenic shock** and should not be confused with **spinal shock** described later. These cardiac and vasomotor effects last at least 5 weeks or longer. Blood pressure instability occurs throughout life and is greater in older individuals and in chronic SCI.[53] With BP instability, systolic and/or diastolic pressures shift more than 20 mmHg, and can be extreme, with 38 to 164 mmHg being reported.[53] Systolic pressures can rise to life-threatening levels as part of **autonomic dysreflexia** (see below). Intermittent swings into hypertension at lower thresholds or hypotension also impact daily life for people with SCI. When SCI is below T6, more brainstem connections to sympathetic thoracic neurons are spared and allow greater vasomotor

control. However, blood pressure instability exists even with lower thoracic SCI.[48]

Long-standing hypotension may cause fatigue, depression, and change in cognition, all-too-common symptoms after SCI. New areas of research are trying to find the cause-effect relationship between dynamic fluctuations in cerebral blood flow and these mood and cognitive disorders.[54,55] Unfortunately, even when hypotension is apparent in the medical record, diagnosis and treatment are quite rare.[56] Greater attention to reducing hypotension may have far-reaching beneficial effects, and the physical therapist can provide information about magnitude and frequency of fluctuations. It will be necessary to incorporate BP measurement prior to, during, and after each PT treatment across acute, inpatient, and outpatient rehabilitation and into chronic SCI because BP instability changes over time. The intensity of PT treatment can be adjusted to initial BP levels and reduce the risk of cardiovascular events. The other value of routine and standardized BP measures is to provide the medical team with necessary information to secure treatment for hypotension and BP instability. Additionally, effective treatment will likely lead to greater responsiveness to rehabilitation and improve the rate and extent of recovery after SCI.

Deep vein thrombosis – A deep vein thrombosis (DVT) is a blood clot in large veins below the level of SCI. A DVT can move proximally and produce a pulmonary embolism (PE) which can be suddenly fatal. The mortality rate due to PE is almost 10% in the first year after SCI.[57] Children develop DVT only when SCI occurs after age 12.[58] Loss of supraspinal sympathetic drive to the liver, spleen, and bone marrow may contribute to the development of DVTs. While stasis is one important factor in DVT, changes in blood platelets and fibrinogen have also been found in individuals with SCI who developed DVTs.[47,59–61] Another factor that contributes to DVT development is damage to the blood vessel itself due to additional trauma at the time of injury.[57] It is important for rehabilitationists to note that some people with SCI have silent DVTs, e.g., show no signs of DVT.[62] The risk factors for DVT include[63] bed rest (stasis); active smoker (hypercoagulability); obesity (stasis); estrogen treatment for gender-related care, menopause, or types of breast cancer (hypercoaguability); older age; paraplegia[64]; complete SCI (AIS A)[65]; **heterotopic ossification**; LE fracture; and flaccid paralysis. The symptoms of DVT are sudden pain and/or swelling in only one leg that is 2 to 3 cm larger in circumference. The other symptom is pain in the calf during dorsiflexion of the ankle known as Homan's sign; however, this may not be clear if sensory impairment from SCI is present. Ultrasonography is commonly used to identify DVTs in the extremity but has little efficacy with proximal thromboses.[66] Prevention procedures include the use of compression stockings or pneumatic devices as soon as possible, if there is no leg fracture; active and passive range of motion to reduce stasis; leg elevation in bed and wheel chair; and/or electrical stimulation of the calf to create a LE muscular pump of venous blood back to the heart. Anti-coagulant medications are also prescribed prophylactically. Should a DVT develop during the phases of rehabilitation, all strenuous exercise, movements, and electrical stimulation must be suspended because they can cause the DVT to migrate proximally and potentially become a PE. Resuming activities will be determined by the clinical team.

Autonomic dysreflexia (Figure 13-6) – This condition develops when the SCI is above T6. It is defined by a pronounced increase in blood pressure and rapid heart rate. Quite often after SCI the resting blood pressure resets to a "new normal" that is much lower than levels for uninjured people. Of critical importance in autonomic dysreflexia (AD) is remembering that serious, medically urgent BP levels triggered in AD can occur within ranges considered normal for people without SCI. An increase in systolic pressure >20 mmHg from the "new normal" baseline constitutes AD in people with complete SCI at T6.[67] Visible signs can be the first indicator of AD in the PT clinic and include sweating, piloerection (goose bumps), and facial flushing above the injury while cool, pale skin appears below the injury. During or before these visible signs, patients often report sudden, severe headache; blurred vision; anxiety; constricted pupils; nausea/vomiting; and/or stuffy nose.[68] Autonomic dysreflexia is a life-threatening condition, in which strong but not necessarily noxious sensory input below the level of the injury ascend in the cord (Figure 13-6A) and trigger a large sympathetic surge from the splanchnic nerves (Figure 13-6B). These signals cause vasoconstriction and hypertension. Baroreceptors in the neck signal the brain of this hypertensive crisis (Figure 13-6C) via cranial nerves IX and X, and two different reflexes are elicited to solve the problem (Figure 13-6D). First, greater descending sympathetic inhibitory drive is sent to the cord to stop the surge, but the signals are blocked by the injury. Second, parasympathetic input to slow the heart is conveyed through the vagus nerve, but the modest lowering of the heart rate does not compensate for the massive vasoconstriction. If left unchecked, seizures, pulmonary edema, myocardial infarction, stroke, and death can occur. Some common triggers for people susceptible to AD are shown in Table 13-2.

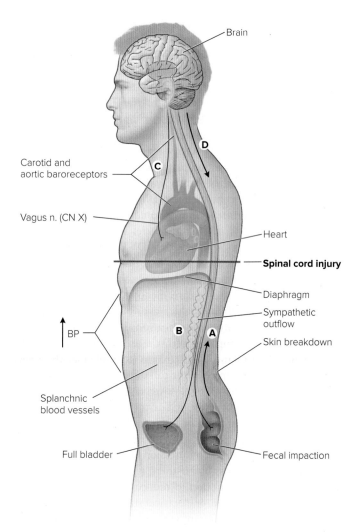

FIGURE 13-6 Autonomic dysreflexia. Autonomic dysreflexia occurs when stimuli below the injury cause an elevated blood pressure that cannot be inhibited because descending input from the brain is blocked by the injury.

TABLE 13-2	Autonomic Dysreflexia Triggers[67]
Bladder	Full bladder
	Bladder/kidney stones
	Blocked/pinched catheter
	Bladder Infection (pyocystis)
	UTI
Gastrointestinal Tract	Bowel impaction
	Bowel distention
	Bowel Management Techniques
	Rectal Fissures
Integumentary System	Tight clothing or shoes
	Pressure Injuries or wounds
	Blisters, burns, bug bites
	Ingrown/Infected toe nails
	Sun burn or frost bite
Reproductive System	Intercourse
	Ejaculation
	Pregnancy, Labor, Breast Feeding
	Menstruation
Other	Fracture
	Hip dislocation
	DVT
	Heterotopic ossification
	Intentional "boosting" for athletic benefit
	Medications like nasal decongestants, gastric ulcer drugs, etc.
	Exposure to hot environments

People with SCI can experience 40 or more episodes of AD a day and it commonly occurs before or during bladder and/or bowel management.[68] Surprisingly, many physical therapy patients report they do not experience AD and confirm they know how to recognize AD. However, in response to a follow-up question, they confirm sudden headache with each episode of bowel care. This inconsistency points to the need for physical therapists to ask about symptomology rather than the broader diagnostic category. It also suggests that AD is probably under-reported and under-diagnosed.

Quick and focused treatment to reduce or resolve AD is required by the physical therapist. The first goal is to lower the BP, using postural positioning. The person exhibiting AD should be placed upright in sitting with the feet dangling. Any tight clothing and compression stockings or therapy-related items like harnesses, gait belt, and/or abdominal binder should be loosened or removed. Place a BP cuff and monitor the BP at 2 to 5 minute intervals. Keeping the head above and the feet below the heart allows gravity to drain blood from the brain thereby reducing BP. Do **NOT** tilt the chair back to lower the head. This increases BP in the brain arteries and increases the risk of stroke. The next objective is to eliminate any possible physical triggers. The most common trigger in the rehabilitation setting is a pinched bladder catheter followed by folded/tight clothing or pinched skin by a strap, gait belt, or harness. Check for each of these conditions and correct them quickly. If the BP remains high, assess for ingrown toenails or infection, any unknown or unseen skin wounds like burns, insect bites, or blisters. Ask about the possibility of constipation/impaction and check for bowel distention. Assess body temperature to identify elevation secondary to systemic infection or inflammation, including urinary tract/bladder infection. Be aware that infection and inflammation are often accompanied by increased tone and/or spasticity. If you confirm any of these conditions or find they are likely, it will be necessary for the person with SCI to see a physician. If you can't identify a potential cause for AD and the BP remains high, then the person will need to receive quick medical care according to whether they are inpatients (hospital physicians and nurses) or outpatients (transportation to an emergency department).

Impact of Climate Change/Environment on Autonomic Dysreflexia: A consequence of complete SCI at T6 or above is the inability to prevent hyperthermia (e.g., a core body temperature above 100°F/37.8°C). When all other causes of fever have been ruled out (infection, inflammation, etc.), this is called **neurogenic fever**.[67] A neurogenic fever can occur when the room is too hot, while sitting in a hot car and/or when too many blankets or too much warm clothing is used. Since neurogenic fever is a trigger for AD, the excessive heat waves brought about by climate change present greater risk to individuals with T6 level and above injuries. Health care providers and the rehabilitation team will need to record the living environment of individuals at risk for or with a history of AD. Specific features like living on upper floors, availability of air conditioning, access to a dwelling-wide back-up power generator and the financial resources to use these electronics should be part of a standard assessment. Extreme environmental temperatures and severe storms threaten the power grid, so even those with air conditioning are at greater risk for overheating, developing neurogenic fever and/or AD due to power outages. To prevent or treat hyperthermia, the individual with SCI will benefit from wearing light clothing of light colors, maintaining hydration, drinking cool liquids, spraying cool water on the body, and having a fan blowing air over those wet skin regions.

New Roles of Autonomic Dysfunction in Immune Suppression with SCI

A series of human and pre-clinical studies after SCI established cross-talk between the autonomic nervous system and the immune system.[69–72] The peripheral immunologic organs, including the spleen, liver, adrenal gland, and kidney, have sympathetic innervation via mid-thoracic cord region T5-8. Gut lymph nodes and bone marrow are innervated from T9-12, while high thoracic sympathetic innervation to the lungs is T1-4. High thoracic SCI above T4 that is motor complete (AIS A or B) disinhibits the sympathetic efferents, creating maladaptive hyper-reflexia below the lesion. This prolonged sympathetic activity to lymphoid tissue causes lymphocytic cell death, deactivates monocytes, and induces significant spleen atrophy.[70] This profound immune deficiency syndrome can not fight off bacterial loads, causing pneumonia and wound infection in acute SCI in humans and pre-clinical models.[70] While the primary infection is a significant health risk, it has even more serious long-term consequences. People who develop infection after SCI have a significantly slower rate of recovery and lower sensory and motor function at discharge from rehabilitation, 1 year and 5 years after SCI. These infection-related limitations are associated with year-over-year high mortality rates up to 10 years after SCI.[71,72]

Bladder Dysfunction

Neuroanatomical Relationships

The bladder is made up of smooth muscle and retains fluid with two urethral sphincters – external and internal urethral sphincters. The **detrusor muscle** forms the wall of the bladder and the internal sphincter at the bladder neck. The bladder wall and internal sphincter are innervated by the **hypogastric nerve** (T11–L2), which is the post-ganglionic branch of the sympathetic nervous system and inhibits muscle contraction, while the bladder is filling (Figure 13-7). Of the two sphincters in the bladder, the **external urethral sphincter** is a true sphincter because it consists of striated muscle, innervated by the **pudendal nerve** (S2–4), and is under voluntary control. It is located at the urethral opening. The pudendal motor neurons are tonically active, which keeps the external sphincter closed and prevents bladder emptying until the time and place are appropriate. The internal **urethral sphincter** is considered a functional sphincter that contracts or tightens in response to increased pressure of urine within the bladder, which means it is under reflex rather than voluntary control.

Normal Function

The bladder has two functions – urine storage and emptying. To void the bladder, contraction of the bladder muscles must be precisely timed with sphincter opening. It requires the integration of parasympathetic, sympathetic, and somatic nervous systems.

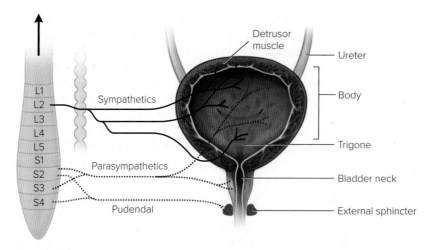

FIGURE 13-7 Sympathetic and parasympathetic innervation of the bladder and urethral sphincters. Sympathetic fibers promote relaxation of the bladder for filling and closure of the internal sphincter; parasympathetic fibers control detrusor muscle contraction and opening of the internal sphincter. The external sphincter is kept closed by the tonic activity in the pudendal nerve. For bladder emptying, this activity must be inhibited from higher brain centers. (Reproduced with permission from Hall JE. *Guyton & Hall Textbook of Medical Physiology*, 13th ed. Philadelphia, PA: Elsevier; 2016.)

Parasympathetic fibers control bladder emptying while the sympathetic fibers are active in bladder filling. Under normal conditions, the internal and external sphincters are closed and the urine collects in the bladder. When the bladder is full, bladder afferents in the wall send signals to the sacral spinal cord and to the micturition center in the brainstem. The brainstem sends inhibitory input to pudendal and hypogastric motor neurons, which allows the external and internal sphincters to relax. At the same time, the parasympathetic fibers in the pelvic nerve cause the detrusor muscle to contract, and urine is expelled.

Effects of SCI

With SCI, the ascending signal to the brainstem is typically impaired or lost completely, and the response of the bladder walls becomes either hyper- or hyporesponsive. A **spastic bladder** (hyperresponsive) means that the sacral reflex is overactive, causing the bladder to contract regardless of the amount of urine in the bladder. A **flaccid bladder** (hyporesponsive) occurs when the reflex response is blunted or absent entirely, and urine is not expelled from the bladder. With poor or absent afferent input to the brainstem, the coordinated control of the sphincters is lost, resulting in **sphincter dyssynergia**. This common problem occurs when the bladder contracts but the external sphincter does not open, which causes the bladder to distend. Pressure within the bladder becomes quite high, preventing the kidney from draining, so urine backs up in the kidneys, which is known as reflux. Reflux damages the bladder, ureters, and kidneys and can be life threatening. **Renal calculi** and renal stone disease also pose life-threatening conditions by blocking urine flow and damaging the kidneys. Formation of stones happens when calcium and other waste products are not fully emptied from the bladder. Other contributing factors include dehydration, urine with high pH, and/or bacterial infections especially associated with urinary tract infections. Individuals with tetraplegia have a higher risk of renal calculi and men have them twice as often as women.[73] About 38% of individuals with SCI develop renal calculi early and years after SCI, with the highest risk of calculi occurring in the first 3 to 6 months after injury.[73]

The most important goal of the bladder management program is to remove urine and prevent high pressures within the bladder. Another objective of bladder management is to prevent renal or bladder calculi (stones). There are several methods to accomplish these objectives, and the selection of the best bladder management depends on residual hand function, amount of support care available to the individual, and complications such as urinary tract infections and autonomic dysreflexia. In the acute stage of SCI, an indwelling catheter will be the most common method of removing urine from the bladder, and the transition to a long-term management program will occur during inpatient rehabilitation. Deciding between pharmacological treatment, non-invasive techniques, and those requiring invasive surgery for long-term use is based on the type of bladder dysfunction – urine retention or incontinence.[74] Each type of management will require different amounts of fluid consumption in order to reduce the risk of calculi formation and infection (see Box 13-1 for bladder management techniques).

Urinary Tract Infections

One of the most common complications of bladder dysfunction after SCI is urinary tract infection (UTI). The prevalence across patients ranges from 10 to 68% and often occurs with decubitis ulcers.[78] Such infections usually have elevated white blood cells and bacteria in the urine as well as some of the following symptoms: fever, chills, sweating, nausea, headache, greater spasticity, and autonomic dysreflexia in people with SCI at T6 or above. To diagnose UTI after SCI, a systematic review indicates that presence of fever and pyuria have high specificity and sensitivity, respectively.[78] Treatment with antibiotics and immediate medical referral will be needed, if a UTI is suspected. Most people with SCI have bacteria in the bladder that is carried in from the skin or urethra during catheterization. For some individuals, these bacteria "colonize" the bladder and eventually do not

Intermittent catheter – Moderate but not high water consumption of about 2 quarts (8-10 glasses) per day and catheterization every 4 to 6 hours during the day should occur. Sterile or "clean, aseptic" techniques can be used. Sterile catheter equipment has a one-time use and means that the insertion tube is not touched. It reduces the risk of bacteria entering the bladder. Clean technique means that a single-use catheter is cleaned after each use and is used multiple times. A recent systematic review endorsed the use of single-use catheters over reuse.[75] However, insurance coverage or living in developing countries may limit or prevent the use of sterile, single-use catheters. When clean intermittent catheterization (CIC) is the most feasible option, adherence to an effective cleaning program and low amount of reuse is important.[75] There is a lack of evidence about which cleaning technique and the number of uses are most effective at preventing infection. Most urological nursing associations ask patients to reuse catheters for only a week.[75]

Indwelling catheter – High water consumption of about 3 quarts (15 glasses) per day should be maintained in order to reduce the risk of bladder or kidney stones.

Foley – A urethral catheter that is held in place by a partially inflated balloon. It is typically changed monthly. This type of catheter may inhibit or impede sexual function.

Suprapubic – A surgically inserted tube through the abdominal wall and into the bladder. This type of catheter is often selected by females and is increasing in general because it does not have the problem of urine leakage like a urethral catheter. It also does not interfere with sexual function in males or females. There is also less burden on caregivers.

Condom catheter for males – Water consumption should be about 2 quarts (8-10 glasses) per day. It should be changed daily or every other day. There is no version of this system for females. This type of catheter is less effective if bladder contraction is weak or sphincter dyssynergia limits full voiding.

Botulinum toxin (Botox) injection into the urinary sphincter – Growing evidence suggests that Botox injection is becoming more widely used to improve bladder voiding and overcome sphincter dyssynergia, after SCI. Botox induces muscle paralysis of the sphincter, allowing urine to pass more easily. It loses its effectiveness over 3 to 6 months, requiring re-injection three times a year. A recent systematic review suggests that Botox injection improves continence, quality of life, and bladder urodynamics in people with SCI and other conditions.[76] While surgical options exist (see below), use of Botox may be the best first step, since the effects are reversible.

Sacral neuromodulation – Electrical leads are placed at the S3 nerve roots in a phased procedure to test the efficacy of bladder emptying. If efficacy is at least 50%, then an implantable pulse stimulator is placed in a second phase. It is typical for the implanted generator to be even more effective than the phase 1 testing. The approach is thought to restore balance between inhibitory and excitatory systems for the bladder. This neuromodulation procedure is not FDA approved but is used off-label in SCI.[76,77] Well-designed randomized controlled trials will add vital evidence to support FDA consideration.

Sphincterotomy – Surgical cutting of the external sphincter is an irreversible but effective way to treat dyssynergia. It is often restricted to males and used after all other treatment options have failed. A condom catheter is used to collect urine. This procedure is not typically done for women because it causes continuous leakage of urine and poses a serious risk of skin ulcers (see below).

Urethral stents – A mesh tube is inserted through the lumen of the sphincter so that it is held open, and urine will flow continuously. They are often used for failed sphincterotomy. Risks include migration of the stent into the bladder, becoming encrusted, or causing pain and autonomic dysreflexia.[74] Stents can be removed, if needed. A condom catheter is used to collect urine, making this procedure unavailable for women. Stents are considered a medium-term option because at least half of them are removed within the first 2 years.

Reflex and manual techniques – These techniques apply pressure over the bladder to either stimulate afferent drive and elicit detrusor contraction or push the urine through a flaccid sphincter. The **Crede method** involves pressing down on the lower abdomen and, thereby, the bladder. **Suprapubic tapping** provides intermittent pressure over the bladder. **Valsalva maneuver** creates pressure by bearing down and/or leaning forward to empty the bladder.

Pharmacological agents – Failure to store urine can be treated with anticholinergics to reduce detrusor hyperreflexia and alpha-adrenergics to promote greater sphincter control. For difficulty emptying the bladder, cholinergics (bethanechol) increase bladder reflexes, alpha-adrenergic blockers aid in sphincter relaxation, and CNS depressants, like valium and baclofen, reduce dyssynergia.

initiate an infection. For other individuals, frequent symptomatic infections occur each year.[79] A presumed cause of UTI was intermittent catheterization with clean but not sterile catheters, but until recently, there was no evidence to support this idea.[80] In this international study, individuals that reused catheters had four times the number of UTIs compared to individuals that never reused catheters. Due to cost and availability, single-use catheters were reused on average 34 times, but some individuals reused the catheter over 200 times. Thus, patient education to avoid catheter reuse may be an effective way to reduce UTIs. The incidence of UTIs was higher with indwelling catheterization than CIC.[81] There is no consensus on effective strategies for preventing UTIs, although a variety have been tested and shown some efficacy. Strategies showing promise include the use of cranberry extract tablets, competitive bacterial interference using non-pathologic bacteria, and long-term cyclic antibiotic use, but the studies are small, haven't been replicated, and/or carry risks of developing antibiotic resistance.[78]

Cross-Talk between Bladder and Blood Pressure Fluctuation

After SCI, many people have low storage capacity of the bladder and high detrusor pressure. These conditions can trigger autonomic dysreflexia with high injury above T6. New evidence shows that as the bladder distends there is an increase in blood pressure into ranges of autonomic dysreflexia.[82] Abnormalities of the autonomic nervous system seem to form a mechanistic network linking bladder distention to blood pressure and cerebral blood flow instability. This integrative network forms regardless of what type of catheterization is used.

Pulmonary Complication and Respiratory Dysfunction

Neuroanatomical Relationships

Respiration relies on descending neurologic drive from rhythm-generating neurons in the medulla. Both inspiratory and expiratory bulbar neurons reside in the medulla and send projections via the bulbospinal tract to the phrenic nucleus in the spinal cord. Some of the descending bulbospinal axons cross in the medulla, but the majority project ipsilaterally. The phrenic nucleus is located from C3 to C5 and innervates the diaphragm (Figure 13-8). The primary muscles of inspiration are the diaphragm and the scalenes, which are innervated from C2 to C7. Secondary muscles of inspiration are the sternocleidomastoid, innervated from C2 to C3 and the accessory cranial nerve, and intercostals, innervated from T1 to T11. Expiration is typically done passively, but the abdominal muscles, innervated by T7–L1, play an important role in forceful expiration (e.g., during coughing). Based on these innervation patterns, an SCI above C5 will impair most of the primary and secondary muscles for

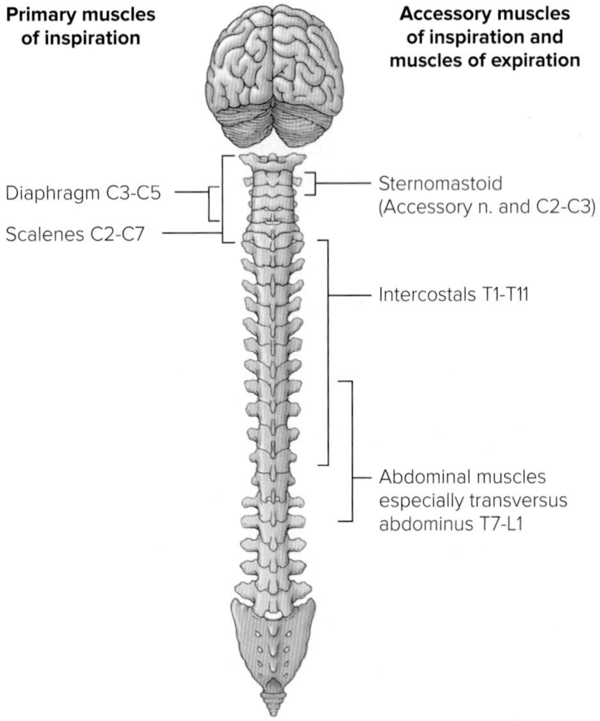

FIGURE 13-8 Levels of innervation for the primary and secondary respiratory muscles. The primary respiratory muscles (diaphragm and scalenes) and the sternomastoid (secondary muscle) are innervated from cervical spinal levels. Intercostal and abdominal muscles are secondary muscles, innervated from thoracic levels.

inspiration and expiration. Even lower injuries in the mid-thoracic region will reduce pulmonary function.

Normal Function

Typically, contraction of the diaphragm causes it to flatten out and pull the thorax down, while the scalenes, intercostals, and sternocleidomastoids contract to raise the thorax. In this way, the thorax expands pulling air into the lungs. The secondary muscles become active only with greater ventilatory demand, as during running or exercise. When the diaphragm relaxes, the lungs and muscle tissue recoil, which passively pushes air from the lungs and causes expiration. Strong contraction of the abdominal muscles also helps drive air out of the lungs.

Effects of SCI

The degree of respiratory dysfunction, after SCI, depends on the level of the injury with the most severe effects occurring with high cervical SCI, but even low thoracic SCI can impair respiration. Partial or complete loss of neural drive to respiratory muscles is the most common cause of respiratory dysfunction and is termed **restrictive ventilator impairment** (see Box 13-2). Restrictive impairment also occurs in acute SCI of traumatic origin when the chest wall or lungs are injured at the same time. This damage can be a serious complication with long-lasting effects.

Obstructive ventilator impairment also contributes to SCI-related respiratory problems. Acute SCI, at T6 or above, causes autonomic dysfunction as described above. For the lungs, this means that excessive bronchial secretions and mucus are produced. Impaired sympathetic input allows unopposed parasympathetic drive, which causes bronchial spasm, vascular congestion, and ineffective ciliary activity to clear the mucus. The excess mucus builds up in the lungs, the cilia do not move the mucus out of the lungs, and although the cough reflex may be intact, the cough itself is weak and ineffective.

Box 13-2	Restrictive Ventilator Impairment

- Paralysis of the diaphragm due to lesion of bulbospinal axons, loss of phrenic motor neurons, or damage to the phrenic nerve. Cough is absent. This occurs with complete cervical SCI at C4 or above and requires a ventilator. Complete paralysis of the diaphragm results in a **paradoxical breathing** pattern, in which the abdomen retracts on inspiration and protrudes during exhalation. This pattern is caused by poor intercostal activation and weak abdominal contraction.

- Paresis of the diaphragm due to incomplete injury of bulbospinal tract, phrenic motor neurons, or phrenic nerve. Cough is weak and ineffective. This occurs with incomplete cervical SCI from C2 to C4/5. A ventilator may be required, if vital capacity, inspiratory pressure, or CO_2 levels worsen.

- Paralysis/paresis of intercostal and abdominal muscles. Cough is weak, especially with upper thoracic injuries above T5. This occurs with complete or incomplete SCI from C5 to T11. A ventilator is typically not required unless complications arise.

These conditions place the patient at risk for **atelectasis** (collapse of alveoli), pneumonia, and respiratory failure.[83]

In individuals with tetraplegia, who do not require a ventilator, body position will affect respiration. In a seated posture, the weak or flaccid abdominal muscles allow the abdominal contents to protrude forward, which flattens the diaphragm and holds the thorax in an expanded position. With the inspiratory muscles already weak from the SCI, they are ineffective at overcoming this mechanical disadvantage. However, if the patient is placed in a supine position, gravity pulls the abdominal contents back, allowing even weak contractions of the diaphragm to expand the thorax and create inspiration. Greater respiratory capacity typically occurs in a supine position, during acute SCI, because the abdominal contents do not protrude and the diaphragm mechanics are more effective.[84]

Use of an abdominal binder to compensate for abdominal laxity can produce immediate improvements in respiratory function, for people with tetraplegia. Increased lung volume and cough mechanics have been reported in an upright position when binders are used.[85]

Pressure Injury and Skin Integrity

Neuroanatomical Relationships and Normal Function

The skin is the largest organ of the body, serving as a protective barrier and maintaining thermoregulation. To cool the body, blood passes through vascular networks just below the skin surface. On cold days, receptors in the skin help to raise the body temperature by constricting the vessels near the surface. The autonomic nervous system controls blood flow and, thus, contributes to temperature regulation. The outer layer of the skin is the epidermis, where cells sluff off and new cells replace them. The dermis lies below and contains sensory receptors, sweat glands, lymphatic vessels, and blood vessels. Below the dermal layer, lies an adipose layer, a muscle layer, and bone.

Effects of SCI

After SCI, light touch, pressure, pain, and thermal sensation from areas below the injury are impaired, so signals to the brain telling you to move and relieve pressure are lost. Also, the neural control of blood flow is disrupted, making it difficult for people with SCI to control body temperature in extreme cold or heat conditions. A pressure injury develops when prolonged pressure is applied to the skin, usually over a bone, and injures the skin and deep tissues. The amount of pressure and the length of time the pressure is in place will increase the severity of the wound. High pressures for short periods and low pressures for long periods can both cause a pressure injury. The pressure crimps small blood vessels and prevents oxygen from reaching tissues under the area of pressure. Ischemia and cell death occur within the deeper tissues, while the superficial layers and skin may only show changes in skin blanching, initially. The wound begins below the skin and expands upward creating a pyramid-shaped lesion with a small wound at the skin and a wide lesion at deeper levels. Note that the term pressure ulcer has been changed. Ulcer means that there is an open wound but there are pressure wounds and stages that are not open wounds, so the term pressure injury avoids any confusion.

There are several systems to stage the type and severity of pressure injuries, but newer recommendations are to categorize rather than stage the wound. Staging implies that the wound develops and heals sequentially through each level (i.e., Stage 1 to Stage 2 to Stage 3 and the reverse with healing), but this isn't necessarily the case. An international panel of experts developed and revised a universal system that combines all of the different staging systems (Table 13-3).[86] Important assessment factors include color, depth of the wound, and presence of **slough**, which is stringy, soft moist tissue that is light in color, ranging from yellow, white, or green. **Eschar** is thick, hard tissue that is dark brown or black and attached to the wound bed or edges.

At-risk Areas

Areas of the body with little or no adipose tissue overlying bony prominences have the highest risk for pressure injury. The most common locations for pressure injuries, after SCI, are the sacrum/coccyx, ischium, heels, and trochanters. Other areas that are at risk include the back of the head, scapula, elbows, knees, and ears as these locations will be exposed to pressure in some positions, when lying in bed.

The risk factors for pressure injuries in the acute stage of SCI are related to medical conditions and medical procedures that restrict changing body positions. The risk of pressure injury is much higher for patients with a tracheostomy, prolonged recovery following surgical decompression, or low arterial blood pressure when arriving in the emergency department.[87] Factors that restrict mobility before arriving at the hospital, also increase risk for pressure ulcer development, including the length of time spent on the backboard, placement of a neck collar, and length of transportation time to the hospital.[87] Urinary incontinence poses less risk acutely because of the routine placement of an indwelling catheter in the emergency department. Risk factors, during inpatient rehabilitation, have not been well-studied and are confounded by a relatively high rate of pressure injuries coming from acute hospitalization, estimated to be 30% or higher.[87,88] At chronic time points after SCI, many factors have an impact like sociodemographic, behavioral, neurological, and medical issues.[89] Perhaps the most concerning is a history of a previous pressure injury. Estimates suggest that up to 90% of people with a pressure injury will go on to have another, and the new wound may not be in the same location (i.e., recurrence).[90] A recurrence means that pathological tissue changes from the initial pressure injury pose a serious risk. However, when the recurrent pressure injury occurs in a new location, it suggests that systemic factors may pose the greatest risk.

Pressure injuries are serious, lifelong burdens globally. In a large meta-analysis representing over 600,000 people with SCI from America, Europe, Asia, and Africa, the rate of pressure injuries was 32%.[91] Given this high incidence rate and the high risk of developing pressure injuries again, it is important that the rehabilitation team study and identify much more effective prevention strategies.

Pressure Injury Prevention

To prevent pressure injuries, during acute hospitalization, the patient's position must be changed every 2 hours, the heels

TABLE 13-3	Category of Pressure Injury[86]
STAGE	**DESCRIPTION**
Stage 1	Non-blanchable erythema • Intact skin • Localized non-blanchable redness • May be painful, firm, soft, warmer, or colder than surrounding tissue • May be difficult to detect in individuals with dark skin tones
Stage 2	Partial-Thickness Skin Loss With Exposed Dermis • Shallow open wound with a red pink wound bed • No slough • May also be a closed or open fluid-filled blister • No bruising
Stage 3	Full-Thickness Skin Loss • Subcutaneous fat may be visible but bone, muscle, and tendon are not. Bone or tendon is not directly palpable. • Slough, if present, doesn't obscure tissue loss • May have undermining or tunneling • Shallow ulcers and deep ulcers can occur depending on body location and the amount of adipose tissue. Areas without adipose tissue will be shallow
Stage 4	Full-Thickness and Tissue Loss • Bone, tendon, or muscle is exposed or directly palpable • Slough or eschar may be present • Undermining or tunneling likely • Depth varies by location • Ulcer may invade muscle, fascia, tendon, etc. likely leading to osteomyelitis or osteitis
Unstageable	Obscured Full-Thickness Skin or Tissue Loss • Depth obscured by slough or eschar and can't be determined until enough can be removed to see the wound bed • On the heel, stable eschar that is dry, adherent with no erythema is a good protective covering and should not be removed
Deep Tissue Injury	Suspected Deep Tissue Injury – Depth Unknown • Persistent non-blanchable deep red or purple/maroon area of intact or non-intact skin • Blood-filled blister from shear or pressure • Prior to discoloration/blister, area may be painful, firm, mushy, boggy, warmer, or cooler compared to intact tissue. • Evolution may be rapid and may have a blister covering a dark wound bed

should be raised off the bed, and the head of the bed should not be elevated above 30 degrees. Higher elevations of the head increase pressure over the sacrum, a high-risk region. The heels need to float above the bed by placing a pillow under the calf and/or using pressure-relieving boots. Be sure the knee is slightly flexed to avoid risking a DVT (see below). The important thing to remember about changing the position of the patient in bed is to avoid damaging the skin. Never drag the body across the surface as shear forces and friction can cause skin damage. Use any available assistive system to turn the patient such as sheets, grab bars, and/or overhead lift systems and other safe patient handling equipment. Placing the person at a 30-degree tilt between supine and full side-lying, allows the greatest blood flow and produces lower pressures over the trochanters than a 90-degree side-lying position. Pillows and foam, rather than towels, should be used to maintain each position because towels create greater pressure rather than reducing pressure on the skin. Be mindful that pillows or foam should be placed between body parts that rest on each other. If angled side-lying cannot be used because of surgical precautions, then reposition the patient every 2 hours from side-lying to supine and then side-lying on the opposite side. In some facilities, special beds to reduce pressure may be available, and new bedside pressure mapping systems are emerging technologies that may help with prevention, during acute hospitalization.[92]

A critical part of pressure injury prevention during inpatient rehabilitation, and thereafter, will be pressure relief and checking the skin regularly. Inspecting the skin for redness, swelling, hardness, or injuries like blisters, over at-risk areas, should be done daily. These areas include the sacrum, coccyx, ischial tuberosities, greater trochanters, heels, elbow, knee, ankle, and foot. Prolonged sitting in a wheelchair can result in pressure injury over the ischial tuberosities. Weight shifts, while seated in a wheelchair, should occur every 15 minutes, continue for 60 seconds, and the patient should be as independent as possible (Table 13-4). If a patient is not independent in lateral weight shifts or forward lean, a posterior tilt, either manually from a caregiver or a power wheelchair with a tilt-in-space option,

TABLE 13-4	Pressure Relief Techniques for SCI Levels	
SCI LEVEL	**METHOD**	**DIFFICULTY**
C4, C5, C6	Tilt-in-space wheelchair moved into posterior tilt Manual wheelchair – Lateral Trunk Lean Manual wheelchair – Hook the arm around the push handle of the wheelchair for balance and lean away to unweight the ischial tuberosity or remove the arm of the wheelchair	Most people will use tilt-in-space chair with this SCI level which poses little difficulty For manual wheelchairs, these are easiest to perform; requires less trunk control than other methods
C6 and below	Forward Lean Walk the hands down the legs to the floor if possible so the tuberosities are clear of the seat.	More difficult; requires more trunk control and balance Risk of shoulder injury if trunk position is poor
C6 and below	Wheelchair Push Up Place the hands on the arm rests or wheels and push down until the buttocks are lifted off the seat	Most difficult; person must have the strength to lift their own weight
C4	Tilt-in-space wheelchair moved into posterior tilt Be sure the legs are elevated to unweight the pelvis as much as possible	In a manual wheelchair assistance required; in a power chair, may be done without help

is necessary. Specialized seating including pressure-cushions should be utilized.

To prevent pressure injuries across the treatment continuum, it is important to understand who is at the greatest risk of developing one. People at risk are often male, older, have had SCI for more than a year, have tetraplegia, underweight, smoke, and/or do not have a lifetime partner.[91] Individuals that have one or several of these factors should have routine, thorough skin inspection and be diligent with pressure relief. They will also need a personalized prevention plan. New approaches used wearable sensors to improve repositioning for medical/surgery ICU patients and found that pressure injuries were three times lower than those without monitors.[93] Sensors attained better adherence to the repositioning schedule and used fewer resources than team rounds, charting, and paper records. The next steps will be to understand how effective wearable sensors are specifically in people with SCI. Poor nutrition is a major risk factor in pressure wound development and makes pressure injury healing difficult. It is important that good dietary habits be in place not only to prevent pressure injuries but also to ensure optimal participation in physical therapy. While there is no single nutritional factor that is associated with pressure wound, protein, albumin, and hemoglobin levels are commonly monitored after SCI as indicators of malnutrition. With insufficient protein consumption after SCI, the body catabolizes protein, resulting in poor collagen formation and a loss of lean body mass. A second factor is prolonged moisture on the skin. Two of the most common sources of moisture are sweating, in areas with skin-to-skin contact, and incontinence. Because urine and feces have high acidity, it is important to wash the exposed skin as quickly as possible before the skin becomes irritated. Regular, long-term exposure to moisture causes skin maceration or breakdown. A third factor is smoking because nicotine limits cutaneous blood flow and reduces tissue oxygenation. Because pressure injury risk and prevention involve the interaction of many complex factors, greater emphasis is being placed on adopting a healthy lifestyle rather than focusing on patient education for unweighting techniques alone (i.e., weight shifts, cushions).[94] Therapists should encourage good nutrition, regular exercise, and smoking cessation at all stages of rehabilitation. These lifestyle changes will not only lower the risk of pressure injuries but also reduce cardiovascular and other complications.

Neurogenic Bowel

Neuroanatomical Relationships

The colon extends from the small intestine to the anal sphincters at the end of the rectum (Figure 13-9). There are two sphincters: (1) an **internal anal sphincter**, made up of the inner, smooth muscle of the colon and (2) the striated, **external anal sphincter** which is under voluntary control. The internal sphincter is innervated by the hypogastric nerve (S2–S4), and the external sphincter is supplied by the pudendal nerve (S2–S4). The **puborectalis muscle**, innervated by roots from S1 to S5, encircles the rectum to hold it in a bent position, and along with the two sphincters, these three structures ensure fecal continence. While neural control of the colon includes the somatic and autonomic nervous systems, its primary innervation is the **enteric nervous system**, also called the intrinsic nervous system. The enteric nervous system is very interesting because it can function independently of the brain and autonomic nervous system and contains so many neurons that it is called the brain of the gut. This means that even after SCI and loss of communication with the brain, many of the functions of the colon remain intact. The enteric system is made up of (1) the myenteric plexus (Auerbach's), located between muscle layers of the colon and (2) the submucosal plexus (Meissner's plexus), lying between the mucosa and the inner layer of muscle. The parasympathetic system, acting through the vagus and pelvic (S2–4) nerves, causes contraction of the colon. The sympathetic system, through the mesenteric (T9–12) and hypogastric (T12–L2)

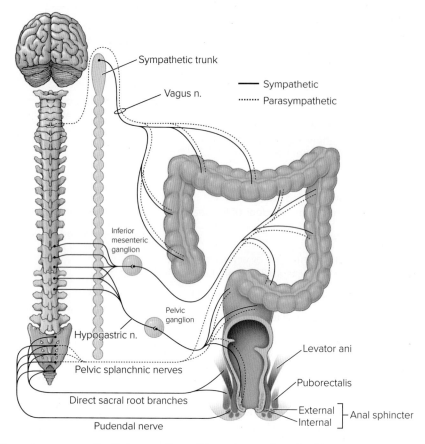

FIGURE 13-9 Sympathetic and parasympathetic innervation of the colon and anal sphincters.

nerves, produces relaxation of the colon and decreases motility through the gut. Excitatory enteric reflexes are inhibited and the sphincters contract.

Normal Function

The role of the colon is to extract water and nutrients while forming food products into stool and propelling it to the rectum and anal sphincters. Reflex contractions of smooth muscle in the wall of the colon help to mix the contents and then move the stool forward through an action called **peristalsis**. Stretch of the colon wall activates the myenteric plexus above the dilation, and the smooth muscle contracts, pushing the stool forward. At the same time, the plexus causes the muscles below the dilation to relax, allowing the stool to move into the next space. This motility occurs with only the enteric system and doesn't require brain or autonomic input. The gastrocolic reflex can also act solely through the enteric nervous system and initiates peristalsis in the small intestine and colon within minutes of food being eaten. These activities, driven by the enteric system, are coordinated with increased sympathetic drive to the internal anal sphincter, which increases tone, but once the rectum begins filling with stool, inhibition of the internal sphincter occurs. Sacral parasympathetics and the pelvic nerve add to the enteric activity to induce defecation. Stool in the rectum initiates stretch of the puborectalis muscle and the smooth muscle of the rectum. Defecation is under voluntary control and occurs when inhibition from the brain causes the external anal sphincter and puborectalis to relax. During coughing or a Valsalva maneuver, increased neural drive to the EAS and puborectalis prevent incontinence. Normal transit time of stool through the colon is 12 to 30 hours.[95]

Effects of SCI

After SCI, the autonomic and brain input is impaired or lost, but the enteric nervous system remains functional, resulting in **neurogenic bowel dysfunction** (NBD). This means that some motility will be present but control of the sphincters, especially the EAS will be greatly impaired. The transit time of stool is greatly prolonged to 80 hours or more,[96] which means there is more time for water to be extracted by the gut, resulting in dry, hard stool. The location of the SCI will produce either UMN or LMN bowel dysfunction[97] (Table 13-5).

NBD presents major challenges to health and quality of life for individuals with SCI and takes two forms – fecal retention and/or fecal incontinence. In the retention form, the much slower motility, sphincter dyssynergia, and constipation lead to a plethora of GI problems, including pain, abdominal distention, bloating, hemorrhoids, nausea, poor appetite, and gastroesophageal reflux. These complications can be even more severe, when the level of injury is above T6, because they trigger autonomic dysreflexia, which is life-threatening as discussed earlier in this chapter. Other serious complications include perianal abscess, stercoral perforation (a rupture of the intestinal wall), megacolon, and intestinal obstruction.

On the opposite end of the spectrum and perhaps even more disruptive to good quality of life is fecal incontinence.

TABLE 13-5	Bowel Management Program Based on Reflexic Dysfunction[97,98]	
CHARACTERISTICS	**REFLEXIC NEUROGENIC BOWEL DYSFUNCTION**	**AREFLEXIC NEUROGENIC BOWEL DYSFUNCTION**
Location of Lesion	UMN Lesion at and above T12 (i.e. above conus medullaris)	LMN Lesion below T12 at the conus medullaris and cauda equina
Dysfunction	EAS can't relax; IAS relaxation is intact if SCI is above T12	Lower motility, flaccid EAS, flaccid puborectalis
Frequency	3 times a week minimum to reduce constipation and overflow incontinence	Daily to avoid incontinence
Stool Quality	Avoid hard, dry, large stool. Return to or adapt Lifestyle Factors and Medications to achieve firm or smooth soft stool formation.	Avoid hard, dry, large stool. Adopt Lifestyle Factors and Medications to achieve firmer stool than Reflexic NBD to help promote some stool retention.
Approach	Digital Rectal Stimulation using a single finger in a slow, circular swipe along the rectal wall. Evacuate stool by hand; Stimulants like mini-enema or suppository may also be needed. Incontinence and constipation are correlated.	Suppositories for lubricant or irritant actions are often used. Manual stool removal. Incontinence and constipation are correlated.
Lifestyle Factors	Sufficient fluids and fiber consumption; engage in physical exercise; for Reflexic NBD, eat/drink 30 min before a bowel session to start gastrocolic reflex.	
Medications	Oral laxatives (stimulants, bulk forming agents, stool softeners) and pro-kinetics to increase colonic muscle activity. Check any new medications for risk of causing constipation.	
Autonomic Dysreflexia	People at risk for AD and/or had previous episodes should use a lidocaine lubricant during bowel sessions. If AD symptoms occur during a bowel session, stop the session and check for any potential causes	
	Physical Therapist Focus Areas and Decision Pathway	
	No	**Yes**
Does the person have enough sitting balance to be seated upright for 30-60 minutes? Can they do some weight shifts?	If NO, then sidelying in bed may be the best option. Training in bed mobility will be needed.	If YES, then evaluate skin break down risk.
Does the person have a current skin wound? Do they often have urine leakage or wet areas in the pelvic region? Do they have risk factors for skin breakdown?	If NO, they are at low risk. Being seated on commode chair may work well.	If YES, they are at high risk and side-lying in bed may be the best option.
Does the person have good arm and hand control to manage clothes? Can they reach the anal region? Do they have some wrist and finger control? Can they hold a finger rigid and long enough to apply pressure during rectal stimulation?	If NO to any question, then assistance will be needed to carry out part or all the bowel program. Consider training the patient and in-home care giver together.	If YES, then most or all of the program may be performed by the person with SCI.
Before the SCI, what was the typical time of day and frequency of bowel movements? Will care givers be available at this time daily or at least three times a week?	If NO, then the care giver and person with SCI will select a time that fits easily into their lifestyle or works best to avoid incontinence.	If YES, then select the pre-injury time frame.

Evaluate quality of the bowel program routinely and be prepared to adjust it. Gains in recovery, changes in lifestyle, different medications, and spasticity will impact effectiveness and efficiency.
Use the "NO" answers above to guide PT treatment goals, make bowel sessions easier/shorter, improve Quality of Life

This incontinence occurs under two conditions – hyperreflexic rectum contraction, causing uncontrolled defecation; or areflexia, which causes stool retention and impaction with fecal matter overflowing around the impaction. This means that physical therapists will need to assess the type and frequency of incontinence in people with areflexic and reflexic NBD. People at risk for overflow incontinence have low anorectal sensitivity, no voluntary EAS control, and current or past fecal compaction.[98]

Bowel dysfunction is quite disabling to individuals with SCI by causing anxiety, depression, and an inability to maintain activities and lifestyle.[99,100] If frequent or lasting complications become routine, formal evaluation for depression or anxiety is recommended.[98] Importantly, these serious and life-threatening complications can be lessened or prevented. At this time, the best approach is regular diagnostic screening for complications and an early, personalized bowel management program.[98] However, there is very little evidence available regarding NBD treatments and the few existing studies provide only low-level evidence. The absence of high-quality research and evidence may explain why hospitalizations and mortality due to GI issues remain an all-too-common problem in SCI.[98]

Bowel Management Program

The goal of the program is to achieve predictable, effective evacuation of stool to prevent unplanned or difficult eliminations and reduce GI complications. An effective bowel program takes about 30 minutes but should be no longer than 60 minutes. Unfortunately, as many as 14% of those living with SCI report taking well beyond this time frame.[100] The ideal program will be individualized to meet the person's: goals, best time of day, best quality of life, most access to care assistants (if needed), and ability to complete in the home and the community. The program will require diligent monitoring and adjustments over months/years by clinicians. The key to good results is starting early because the GI system can be trained to make repeatable, predictable responses. To entrain the enteric nervous system, it takes time, consistency, and dedication by the person living with SCI.

Developing the training program will first identify the new reflex functions after SCI. Injuries above T-12 are usually classified as UMN because the bowel and anal sphincter are hyperreflexic or spastic. For UMN hyperreflexic dysfunction, the objective of the program is to enable stool evacuation through digital rectal stimulation and formation of *soft* stool so it passes more easily through the colon. Typically, the bowel management program will occur every other day to maintain effective enteric reflex training. Injury below T-12 within the cauda equina and conus medullaris is classified as LMN because the bowel and sphincter are areflexic and flaccid. For LMN areflexic dysfunction, the objective is to reduce incontinence and unexpected voiding by increasing stool *firmness*, so it is retained in the rectum and can be manually evacuated. Individuals with LMN typically use a bowel program daily to reduce the risk of unexpected voiding. To individualize the bowel program, the following parameters must be identified: pre-injury bowel habits, type of bowel dysfunction (UMN, LMN), hand function, upper extremity strength and proprioception, sitting balance, musculoskeletal spasticity and spasms, risk or presence of pressure injuries, transfer skills, and feasibility of moving the program to the home and community settings. Nutritional intake and food preferences, fluid consumption, and medications must also be tracked as they all influence bowel function. The bowel program will begin in the acute hospital setting and adopt a routine time of day, regular intervals, and consistent preparatory procedures.

The role of the physical therapist in the bowel management program is to determine the type of program and location that is possible given the physical function of the individual living with SCI. The physical therapist will also provide a personalized education program to the individual and the caregiver or assistant. As recovery of function returns or lifestyle changes occur, adaptations to the program will be needed and an advanced education program developed. The ability to perform the bowel program in sitting rather than lying in bed depends on good sitting balance, less severe SCI, infrequent spasticity/spasms, ease of transfers, and low risk of pressure injuries. A seated program will use a toilet, roll-in upright shower/commode chair with padding, or a tilt-in-space shower/commode chair with padding. While a seated program improves evacuation and clean-up, it is difficult to access the anal region and poses pressure wound risk because of the long time spent sitting. To determine the best bowel management program at each point in recovery and phase of life, diligent monitoring of changes in physical function, injury progression/regression, reflexic bowel function, frequency of autonomic dysreflexia and reliance on assistants will be needed (Table 13-5).

Bowel programs require a multifaceted approach that make use of spared function, modulate fluid and food intake, and carefully consider the impact of medications on bowel function. In what seems counterintuitive, a high-fiber diet can actually reduce motility and lengthen colon transport time in individuals with SCI, thereby, requiring careful titration of fiber for each individual. Understanding the impact and amount of soluble and insoluble fiber in the diet will be important to optimize fluid intake, stool firmness and avoid constipation or incontinence. Attention to sufficient nutrition and water intake on days of physical therapy/active exertion will improve both exercise and bowel outcomes. The most common medications that can negatively impact bowel function by decreasing motility and increasing constipation include antidepressants, anticholinergics, anti-spasticity drugs, and narcotics. Most conservative approaches to bowel care will combine the gastrocolic reflex, **digital stimulation** of the colon, and a stool softener or enema to aid in evacuation.[97] Digital stimulation involves insertion of a gloved finger into the rectum and moving it in a circular motion to elicit peristaltic waves via the enteric nervous system. Eating a meal or sometimes drinking warm liquids like coffee also triggers peristalsis via the gastrocolic reflex; using digital stimulation, after consuming one or both of these, has an additive effect on motility. Suppositories such as bisacodyl, glycerin, and polyethylene glycol reduce the time and support needed for the bowel program.[98] A basic management program will commonly transition from using chemically potent suppositories like bisacodyl to gentler glycerin suppositories. The next transition is alternation between glycerin suppositories one day and only digital stimulation the next. At this point, elimination of glycerin is possible in many people with SCI so that only digital stimulation is needed for effective evacuation.

Some people living with SCI do not respond effectively to a basic bowel management program and more invasive procedures will be needed. Major complications with bowel management programs are a lack of flexibility when the program must be implemented, the interference of the program with other life activities such as work and recreation, lack of necessary attendant care, and loss of autonomy and privacy.[100,101] About 20% of individuals require full assistance with their bowel care program, and these individuals report lower life satisfaction. Women with SCI report more problems with bowel function and have more symptoms of abdominal distension, pain, constipation, and unplanned evacuations.[100] Autonomic dysreflexia can increase in frequency or severity based on dry stool, long transport time, strong chemical irritants, enemas, and digital rectal stimulation. If AD occurs regularly during the bowel program, lidocaine lubricant can be applied to the gloved finger prior to bowel care.

Advanced Bowel Management: If basic bowel management proves ineffective, then transanal irrigation (TAI), oral medications, and/or surgery may be necessary. TAI relies on a bolus of fluid pumped through a rectal catheter placed in the anus. The catheter is held in place until all the fluid has been delivered and the stool is evacuated into a toilet or commode. The benefits of TAI include management of both constipation and fecal incontinence, decreasing or eliminating pharmaceutical use for bowel management, and people with SCI reporting high satisfaction.[102,103] However, one reason people with SCI decide not to use TAI is that the catheter can be expelled frequently. There are also multiple medical contraindications that prevent the use of TAI.[98] Oral medications that stimulate intestinal motility and gastric emptying include metoclopramide, prucalopride, fampridine, neostigmine, and glycopyrrolate. Use of these pharmacological interventions improves expulsion after SCI.[97] If complications continue after pharmacological treatment, then several surgical options demonstrate efficacy. Because these are invasive and carry greater risk than the basic approaches and pharmaceutical options, surgery is a last resort. Malone antero-grade continence enema (MACE) requires a minimally invasive surgery to attach the appendix to the abdominal wall and place a stoma into appendicostomy. A catheter is placed into the stoma to irrigate the colon and rectum. An advantage of MACE is that waste is not collected externally. Disadvantages include leakage through the stoma, infection, and difficulty inserting the catheter. The most common surgical approach for bowel management is colostomy/ileostomy. The colo/ileostomy procedure opens the colon or intestine so stool flows into an external collection device, bypassing the rectum and anus. People that elect to have a colostomy or ileostomy report high satisfaction, greater independence, faster bowel care, and the desire to have had the procedure even earlier.[98,101,104] Complications arise when chronic pressure wounds and slow healing requires flap surgery. The colostomy may need to be diverted to improve wound healing. An important thing to remember is that these more invasive procedures have greater complications as they are used over years and increased decades of life. Careful, regular assessment for complications must become standard for all members of the rehabilitation team.

Physical Activity: From a physical therapy perspective, bowel function benefits from increased activity, less bed rest after SCI, or both. In fact, exercise and activity is a crucial part of a healthy lifestyle and promoting gut health.[105] Several forms of physical activity, including standing (with support if needed), electrical stimulation, exoskeleton-assisted walking (EAW), and body-weight supported treadmill training, have been shown to improve bowel function.[24,106–115] While the level and amount of evidence are growing, some are contradictory.[116] Still, taken together, it is critical for the physical therapists to assess the positive and/or negative impact of activity-based interventions for SCI on bowel function.

Several modes of electrical stimulation are being closely studied because of case series and pilot studies showing benefits to bowel function after SCI.[117] In general, stimulation can be used as a neural prosthesis to replace lost voluntary neural or muscle activity and/or to induce neural plasticity in sacral spinal cord segments.[107,108,118] Two studies used the compensatory, electrical stimulation approach and induced abdominal muscle contraction to enhance abdominal pressures during defecation. In both studies, improved motility and reduced colonic transport time occurred and are currently being studied in a clinical trial.[107,108,119] Several clinical trials are underway testing electrical stimulation to improve bowel and bladder function.[120–123] Taking a neuroplasticity approach, a small study of two individuals with incomplete SCI and fecal incontinence applied electrical stimulation to the posterior tibial nerve in order to activate sacral sensory and motor fibers (S1–3), which form the nerve.[109] Stimulation (30 min/day) occurred every other day for 4 weeks and then every 2 months. Improvement in rectal sensation, pudendal motor function, quality of life, and lower severity of incontinence occurred. With the large number of new clinical trials of electrical stimulation and existing evidence of benefit in small studies, greater clarity in clinical guidelines for bowel management after SCI is just over the horizon. Many of these approaches are mentioned in the new clinical practice guideline for bowel management but lack sufficient evidence at this time. Nonetheless, patients with SCI will seek out these options. The physical therapist will need to be knowledgeable in the benefits and adverse responses of each approach so their patients can make informed decisions. Importantly, many of these stimulation approaches also benefit functional performance, respiration, and cardiac function and should be incorporated in physical therapy treatments for patients that elect to use these systems.

● PHYSICAL THERAPY IN THE ACUTE SETTING

During acute hospitalization, the patient will have most, if not all, of these medically challenging conditions that will impact the type of and tolerance for therapeutic interventions. All rehabilitation interventions will need to be performed without worsening these medical conditions. At this stage of rehabilitation, the physical therapist must anticipate the type of functional recovery that is likely given the level and severity of the SCI. It will be important to assure that the current rehabilitation interventions facilitate the next phases of therapy, in the inpatient and outpatient settings. Keep in mind that the next therapists shouldn't have to spend valuable treatment time undoing deleterious factors like joint contractures. The role of physical therapy is to assess motor and sensory function, prevent complications, incorporate spared muscles into rehabilitation, promote plasticity to improve recovery of function, and continually monitor for and incorporate return of motor and sensory function.

The Physical Therapy Assessment

Use the standardized neural assessment, described in Chapter 10. If no ISNCSCI /AIS exam has been performed, you will need to complete a full exam. If an exam has been completed by the physician, then a quick confirmation of the below-lesion muscle and sensory effects should be done. Remember that we expect some return of sensorimotor function, and an early return may lead to more extensive recovery and better long-term prognosis. Perhaps greater attention should be directed at checking for trace muscle contractions, since it means that the motor neuron pool is not completely lost. Attention should also be focused on muscle groups not included in the ISNCSCI exam like shoulder abduction, shoulder depression, gluteus maximus and medius, hamstrings, and great toe extensors. These muscle groups are important for future actions like transfers, unweighting, and gait training. In the acute phase, the absence of muscle response or reflexes may not necessarily indicate the severity or location of the injury due to spinal shock.

Within minutes of SCI, widespread depression of neural activity in the spinal cord occurs and reflexes below the injury are absent or very weak (hyporeflexic). This pattern is called **spinal shock** or **diaschesis**. Spinal shock means that neurons and reflexes not directly damaged by the injury cease to function and over time return.[124] A classic example of spinal shock is early paralysis of both limbs after a unilateral hemisection or Brown-Sequard type injury. After a few days, motor activity returns in the contralateral limb. The return of uninjured function takes place over days, weeks, and months and progresses from hyporeflexia to hyperreflexia.[124] Reflexes appear in a sequential order: delayed plantar response, bulbocavernosus, cremasteric, ankle DTR, Babinski sign, and knee DTR[124] (see Table 13-6).

Many neurorehabilitationists consider the end of spinal shock to be when the cremasteric reflex returns, but keep in mind, that this reflex may be abolished by an SCI at the level of the conus medullaris or cauda equina. Some resolution of spinal shock will likely occur in the acute setting. As spinal shock resolves, not only do reflexes return, but also expect to see spared voluntary movement return. For a physical therapist, it is often impossible to tell whether gains in function are due to treatment or resolution of spinal shock, especially because the time period of shock can be up to a year after SCI.

Few physical therapy assessment tools for SCI are available for the acute hospital phase after SCI. The APTA (EDGE) Task Force highly recommends six outcome measures for the 0- to 3-month acute period after SCI. However, within this timeframe, both acute and inpatient rehabilitation will occur. Only two measures would be feasible in the acute hospital setting,

TABLE 13-6	Sequential Resolution of Spinal Shock[124]	
REFLEX	**ACTION**	**HYPO-HYPERREFLEXIA**
Delayed plantar response (L5–S2)	Strong deep pressure from heel along lateral border of sole of foot and across 3rd, 4th, 5th MT heads produces slow plantar flexion	Emerges within hours and worsens over first week; declines/absent after 1 week
Bulbocavernosus (S2–S4)	Squeezing glans penis or clitoris causes anal sphincter contraction	Emerges by 3 days; modest hyperreflexia develops within 4 weeks–1 year
Cremasteric (L1–L2 genitofemoral nerve)	Stroke of inner, upper thigh pulls up ipsilateral testicle	Emerges by 3 days; modest hyperreflexia develops within 1–12 months
Ankle Stretch reflex (S1–S2)	With foot dorsiflexed, tap of Achilles tendon causes plantarflexion	Emerges by 3 days; modest hyperreflexia develops within 1–12 months
Babinski (Corticospinal tract)	Pressure on sole of foot curving from heel up to MT heads causes big toe to lift, other toes to fan out; replaces delayed plantar response	Emerges by 3 days; modest hyperreflexia develops within 1–12 months
Flexor withdrawal (L2–S1)	Pinprick of sole of foot causes flexion of LE joints	Emerges by 3 days; modest hyperreflexia by 4 weeks, pronounced hyperreflexia by 1–12 months
DTRs Knee (L2–4) Biceps (C5–6) Triceps (C7–8) Brachioradialis (C6)	Tendon tap below the level of the injury causes brisk response	Emerges by 3 days; modest hyperreflexia by 4 weeks, pronounced hyperreflexia by 1–12 months

the AIS/ ISNCSCI exam described previously and handheld myometry. Handheld myometry uses a force transducer to objectively quantify muscle strength and has shown high reliability and greater sensitivity than MMT within the first week after SCI.[125,126]

CASE A, PART II

Ms. Roberts had an AIS/ISCNSCI completed 5 days after SCI, which confirmed the level of SCI at C2. The UEMS was 5 and the LEMS was 8. The motor scores were asymmetrical with higher motor scores on the left versus the right (Table 13-7). The pinprick scores were also asymmetrical with higher scores on the right versus the left. The S4-5 pinprick sensation appeared intact. The injury was classified as AIS C – Brown-Sequard injury due to the greater strength and impaired pain sensation contralateral to the major portion of the lesion. The poor pain sensation over the lower half of the body places her at high risk for pressure injuries, so a regular skin inspection and turning schedule must be followed. Some pain sensation, although impaired, has returned in the neck and shoulder region which may help protect her scapulae from developing pressure wounds. Spine stabilization surgery was not performed, and the neck was immobilized with a cervical collar. Ms. Roberts had the ventilator removed on day 6.

What other test should be performed by the physical therapist to diagnose Brown-Sequard syndrome?

Proprioception should be tested.

Babinski sign

What would you expect the results of the test to show to confirm Brown-Sequard syndrome?

Greater proprioceptive deficits on the right than the left side

Positive Babinski on the right foot only

TABLE 13-7 | **ASIA Motor Scores**

ASIA KEY MUSCLES	RIGHT	LEFT
C5 elbow flexors	0/5	2/5
C6 wrist extensors	0/5	1/5
C7 elbow extensors	0/5	2/5
C8 finger flexors	0/5	0/5
T1 finger abduction	0/5	0/5
L2 hip flexors	0/5	2/5
L3 knee extensors	1/5	2/5
L4 ankle dorsiflexors	0/5	0/5
L5 long toe extensors	0/5	0/5
S1 ankle plantar flexor	1/5	2/5

Acute Physical Therapy Management

Prevent Complications

The most common medical complications at the acute stage include pneumonia, pressure wounds, erratic blood pressure, and DVT. The physical therapist will reinforce the training provided to the patient and family for assisted coughing techniques, add breathing exercises to each treatment session, improve chest wall mobility through range of motion (ROM) of the trunk, and place an abdominal binder on all patients with SCI above T12.

Individuals with tetraplegia are at risk for future shoulder and elbow pain, injury, and contractures, which greatly compromise independence. Contractures cause reduced joint ROM and mobility and are attributable to spasticity of muscles that cross the affected joint, loss of sarcomeres in these muscles, lost compliance of tendons and/or tight joint capsules.[127,128] The goal of treatment, in the acute phase, is to prevent muscle, tendon, and capsule changes, using stretching and positioning Avoid placing the arms on the abdomen or chest because the elbow flexors, shoulder abductors, and external rotators will be in a shortened position, creating a new, restrictive resting length. After SCI, hip and knee flexion contractures are quite common because of all the time spent sitting. Although acutely, the patient will be lying in bed, it is important to target prevention strategies for the hips and knees early. If there are no surgical or medical precautions, place the individual prone as part of the rotation program to protect the skin. Prone position will maintain hip and knee extension, which will be critical for future walking rehabilitation, exoskeleton use, and active or passive standing programs. These rehabilitation activities contribute to overall health, benefit bowel management, and reduce the risk of pressure injuries.

ROM is a key determinant of function throughout rehabilitation and for return to home and full participation. In some muscle groups and joints, greater ROM will allow better function (i.e., hamstrings). However, in some muscles, shortened ROM will be beneficial. The tenodesis position is an important example. The finger flexors are allowed to shorten so that when the wrist is extended the fingers close, creating **tenodesis grip**. The optimal ROM for specific joints will enable independence in daily activities in the future, as provided in Table 13-8. The ROM activities will initially be largely passive due to spinal shock but should rely on active-assistive or active ROM for any voluntary muscle actions that the individual can produce. Even during passive ROM, the patient should attempt to perform the motions voluntarily. These brain-initiated commands engage the nervous system, may prevent synaptic disuse and potentially provide neural drive to weakly innervated muscles that falsely appear paralyzed. This cognitive engagement helps prepare the patient for the exertion and tasks during upcoming inpatient rehabilitation.

Stretching and ROM activities, especially in chronic SCI, have shown little efficacy in treating existing contractures in that little or no increase in joint motion occurred.[127,128] However, little research has been done on the role of these therapies in preventing contractures, the impact of early positioning to protect the shoulders and elbows from future injury, or the prevention of associated conditions like future development of severe spasticity or heterotopic ossification. Until prevention of contractures

TABLE 13-8	Physical Requirements for Functional Mobility	
OPTIMAL JOINT ROM/MUSCLE LENGTH	**ASSOCIATED FUNCTIONS**
Full elbow extension, full supination and 70-90 degrees wrist extension	WC propulsion; weight shifts; dressing; transfers
Neutral ankle dorsiflexion	Placing/maintaining feet on WC foot rest; important for future standing/walking
Hip and knee 90-degree flexion	Optimal WC use; dressing; transfers
Full external rotation and hip abduction	Dressing; putting on shoes and socks
Shortened finger flexors	A C6 SCI requires tight flexors to allow a grasp by extending the wrist – tenodesis grip
Long hamstrings	Attains 100+ hip flexion with knee extension; prevents falling backward in long sitting; must avoid stretching low back muscles
Shortened low back extensors	Improves stability in sitting

and joint protection has been fully studied, stretching and ROM remain a high priority in the acute phase and when spasticity beings to emerge. Relying on bed positioning to attain stretch and ROM has the advantage of longer duration stretch than therapist-applied stretch and can transfer to each care setting and home.

Incorporation of Spared Muscles into Rehabilitation

Muscle activation will fall into one of three categories: (1) unimpaired and fully activated; (2) partially innervated and weak activation; and (3) no observable activation. An unstable medical condition is typical, during this phase, so the individual will be unable to tolerate strenuous strength training activities due to large swings in heart rate and BP as well as respiratory challenges. In addition, resistance might be contraindicated for muscle groups attaching to or crossing a vertebral fracture. At this stage, active exercise of muscle groups with full or partial innervation is important to reduce the risk of contracture and secondary complications. This exercise should be done as part of meaningful tasks like moving in the bed, whenever possible, to facilitate new skill learning, ensure better carryover to daily activities, and improve cardiovascular and physical endurance.

CASE A, PART III

Ms. Roberts had passive ROM applied to all joints except the long finger extensors. Wrist extension was passively stretched with the fingers flexed to allow for the potential for a tenodesis grip in the future. She was encouraged to actively move each joint during the ROM exercise, and the therapist palpated for any muscle contraction. The ventilator connections restricted movement of the shoulder, so ROM of the shoulders was coordinated with changing her position in bed to protect the skin. When she was lying on her right side, ROM of the left shoulder was completed and vice versa. Once the ventilator was removed, Ms. Roberts was encouraged to perform deep breathing exercises, given an abdominal binder, and passive trunk rotation exercises were added.

Most individuals do not tolerate upright sitting early after SCI due to the cardiovascular changes and hypotension described earlier. Using heart rate, blood pressure, and medical concerns as your guide, individuals will begin a sitting program in the acute setting. Issues that would limit or prevent starting a sitting program include an erratic heart rate or blood pressure, an unstable fracture or dislocation, and existence or risk of a pressure wound over the sacrum or ischial tuberosities. An abdominal binder and compression stockings on the legs will help reduce dizziness by preventing blood pooling in the legs. Most hospital beds have a "chair" position also called **reverse Trendelenburg**, which can be used to elevate the head and lower the feet. Moving in and out of this position will train neural and cardiovascular systems to tolerate being upright. Raising the head angle near the threshold of dizziness for the patient and staying in that position for a few seconds to a few minutes, before lowering the head slightly helps improve upright tolerance. Each session attempts to move the threshold higher with a goal of tolerating a 60-degree incline, at which point, the individual can begin to use a tilt-in-space wheelchair (WC). The tilt-in-space WC moves the entire seat rather than reclining the backrest, so sitting posture is maintained in a head lowered, legs/feet raised position, and vice versa. Tilting the seat angle compensates for dizziness or other symptoms and provides pressure relief over the sacrum and ischial tuberosities. Once a WC can be used, pressure relief must be incorporated into the sitting program, by using different cushions, regularly changing the tilt angle, and beginning to train the individual to perform components of weight shifts. Most people will not be able to perform weight shifts at this early stage of rehabilitation but educating them to adjust position every 15 minutes and increasing their tolerance of common positions, used for unweighting, will facilitate the transition to independent weight shifts in the future.

CASE A, PART IV

Ms. Roberts was restricted from starting a sitting program for the first week in the hospital, while evaluation of the fracture site and attempts to stabilize an erratic heart rate were made. Because individuals with cervical SCI will have abnormal breathing patterns when the head is elevated, the abdominal binder was applied to improve diaphragm and chest wall mechanics. Raising the head of the bed from horizontal caused an increase in respiration, abnormal breathing patterns, and drops in blood pressure and heart rate at about a 20-degree incline, during the first session. Reducing the angle stabilized the symptoms, and she tolerated up to 30 seconds per bout. Over the next 5 days, the head of the bed was raised to 45 degrees, and she maintained this position for up to 60 seconds. Ms. Roberts will be discharged to inpatient rehabilitation now that her medical condition has stabilized. The fact that she progressed from complete paralysis to some motor and sensory function within 5 days of injury, suggests that some of the effects of spinal shock are resolving and greater return of muscle function may occur during inpatient rehabilitation. The presence of S4–5 pinprick sensation also points to further motor recovery over the next months. She also weaned from the ventilator in less than 7 days, which reduces the risk of complications and avoids long-term muscle weakness including the diaphragm.

MANAGEMENT OF THE PATIENT IN THE INPATIENT REHABILITATION SETTING

CASE A, PART V

Ms. Roberts was transferred to inpatient rehabilitation 16 days after her SCI. The AIS/ISCNSCI exam was performed within 3 days of admission to the rehabilitation hospital. Scores of the key muscle groups are shown in Table 13-9.

Testing for non-ASIA muscle groups had 2/5 strength for left shoulder abductors, 2/5 for the erector spinae and upper part of the rectus abdominus. Gluteus medius and maximus were 2/5 on the left and 1/5 on the right. The hamstrings were 3/5 on the left and 1/5 on the right. Proprioception on the left side was absent from C2 and below. DTRs were present for the biceps, brachioradialis, patella, and Achilles tendon bilaterally. The Babinski reflex was positive on the right and negative on the left. The delayed plantar response was absent. Tolerance of upright sitting had improved to 55 degrees. Ms. Roberts is dependent in all transfers, bed mobility, and daily activities, including dressing and eating.

General Approach

The focus of inpatient and outpatient rehabilitation is moving beyond a compensatory approach and seeks to promote neuroplasticity and recovery. Compensation in SCI uses functional body parts, braces, or equipment to replace the impaired actions. There is a delicate balance between these approaches. Some

TABLE 13-9 | **ASIA Motor Scores**

ASIA KEY MUSCLES	RIGHT	LEFT
C5 elbow flexors	0/5	4/5
C6 wrist extensors	0/5	3/5
C7 elbow extensors	0/5	2/5
C8 finger flexors	0/5	0/5
T1 finger abduction	0/5	0/5
L2 hip flexors	1/5	3/5
L3 knee extensors	1/5	3/5
L4 ankle dorsiflexors	0/5	1/5
L5 long toe extensors	0/5	0/5
S1 ankle plantar flexor	1/5	3/5

Impaired pinprick sensation was noted on the left but intact on the right.

compensatory techniques will likely be needed during periods of spinal shock or absent muscle activation to accomplish daily activities, like transferring, eating, dressing, or toileting. Given that inpatient rehabilitation stays are shorter than in the past due to insurance limitations, compensatory strategies may be necessary to ensure a safe discharge to home environment. However, reliance on compensation reduces the drive to those inactive neuromotor systems, thereby providing an opportunity for maladaptive plasticity to emerge. After SCI, spontaneous reorganization in the nervous system occurs by filling synaptic sites vacated by the damaged systems. Animal and some human studies show that activity-based therapies can induce functional neuroplasticity.[129–132] Another reason to place greater emphasis on activity-dependent plasticity, instead of compensation, is because compensatory techniques can be added at any time, like periods when plasticity and recovery have plateaued. However, using a majority of compensatory techniques may make it difficult to overcome maladaptive plasticity.

Three factors are important in using a neuroplasticity approach for rehabilitation. **First**, the individual should use maximal attention and effort in trying to perform the tasks. This will demand a high level of cognitive engagement because there will be a high rate of errors or lack of response early on. **Second**, the training must allow errors to be made for skill learning to occur. An interesting study, performed in rodents with SCI, proved this point very well.[133] After SCI, a robot was used to move the leg in a stepping pattern using precise control of the movement with no errors in one group and less control that allowed movement errors in the other group. When the robot was turned off and the groups generated stepping on their own, the error-free group demonstrated poor walking and greater disability. Likewise, in human robotic step training, poor learning occurred when errors or their magnitude were experimentally held low. Muscle EMG activation was much lower than when errors were magnified.[134] **Third**, a high number of repetitions will be needed in order for any training effects and recovery to emerge. In a rodent SCI model, a training dose of 100 steps during a treadmill session was compared to

1000 steps per session.[135] Only the high-repetition training paradigm improved walking, showing that the benefits of rehabilitation depend on thousands of trials.

Spasticity versus Flaccidity

After spinal shock has resolved, spasticity and hyperreflexia often develop in muscles supplied by motor neurons that have lost their descending motor drive (i.e., UMN lesion). **Spasticity** has traditionally been defined as an increase in the velocity-dependent stretch of muscle.[136] More recently an expanded definition has come into use because it captures and/or differentiates between clinical presentations like clonus, increased tone, and hyperreflexia.[137,138] The broad definition of spasticity is "disordered sensorimotor control, resulting from an upper motor neuron lesion, presenting as intermittent or sustained involuntary activation of muscles."[138] The DTRs below the level of the injury will be hyperexcitable, meaning they are easier to elicit and have a more robust response. Reflexes above the injury will be normal. Spasticity is a combination of limited or lost descending drive from the brain and greater input from the sensory afferents. The corticospinal system itself and/or imbalance between it and the reticulospinal system contribute to less inhibitory drive, which can manifest as spasticity.[139] Changes in the muscle fiber, collagen, and tendon also contribute to greater muscle tone.[140] When the motor neurons, the peripheral nerve, or the ventral root is damaged as part of the injury, the muscle and the reflex will be **flaccid**. This is considered a LMN injury. Most SCIs below T11 will have a LMN injury because the cord has tapered to a small cone shape or thick thread (filum terminale), surrounded by motor nerves. Therefore, spinal injury below T11 damages these motor nerves and is referred to as conus medullaris/cauda equina SCI.

The majority of people with SCI develop spasticity, and severe or problematic spasticity can be as high as 87% in cervical or thoracic SCI and over 50% in lumbar SCI.[139] People with incomplete AIS C injuries have the highest prevalence of long-term, problematic spasticity.[141] Spasticity-induced contractures at 1 year after SCI occurred at the shoulder in 43% of people, 33% elbow/forearm, 41% in wrist/hand, 32% hip, 11% knee, and 40% in ankle.[139] Spasticity fluctuates, varies greatly across individuals and presents as sudden, involuntary flexing or extending of the trunk or limbs; rhythmic jerking or bouncing of muscles or joints called clonus; muscle spasms from light touch; muscle stiffness/tightness at rest or during activity that doesn't relax.[137] Because of the heterogeneity and ever-changing spasticity profiles in SCI, fine grain assessment, including patient-reported quality of life, and direct testing of spasticity by the physical therapist will be needed to determine the best treatment options.[139,142] Recommended and/or validated spasticity measures for SCI[142-144] include Modified Ashworth Scale, Penn Spasm Frequency Scale, Patient Reported Impact of Spasticity Measure (PRISM), and SCI Spasticity Evaluation Tool (SCI-SET) (Table 13-10). While spasticity commonly creates negative impacts on caregiver burden, lower quality of life, more pain, and greater disability, it also has advantages. Spasticity often enables enough tone to allow standing or transfers, indicates the need for bowel/bladder care, and may signal the need for medical care due to infection, pressure injury, or fracture. It is

across this complex, changing, and difficult-to-assess condition that treatment must be determined by prioritizing the patient's goals and the risk of ever-greater debilitation in the future.

The most common medical treatment for spasticity and hyperreflexia is baclofen, a CNS inhibitor. It can reduce spasticity and flexor spasm, when given orally, but it carries many limiting side effects that can impede rehabilitation. These side effects include drowsiness, dizziness, weakness, and ataxia.[145] To overcome these side effects and enable more concentrated doses, baclofen can also be administered via an intrathecal pump directly over the spinal cord. It is important to note that use of baclofen, especially orally, will likely inhibit neural activation and limit the therapist's ability to promote activity-based neuroplasticity.

Botulinum toxin (Botox), a neurotoxin, is also commonly used to reduce localized rather than generalized spasticity. It is injected directly into the affected muscle which reduces acetylcholine release in the neuromuscular junction, thereby lowering muscle tone and causing some muscle weakness. The treatment effects last between 3 and 4 months and must be repeated to maintain the anti-spasticity effects. The Botox dose must be carefully titrated when treating major muscle groups so that paralysis and lost function do not occur. The complications with Botox may include allergic reactions or affecting unintended/non-spastic muscles. Side effects for LE injections include pain in the back, muscle, joint, and injection site as well as respiratory infection. Side effects for UE injections are nausea, tiredness, muscle weakness, UE pain, and bronchitis.[139]

Physical therapy procedures have been used to reduce spasticity either alone or in combination with pharmacological agents. The interventions showing efficacy based on clinic trials or systematic reviews are FES leg cycling in medically stable SCI; reflex down conditioning in incomplete SCI[146-148]; and Botox combined with stretching.[149] However, for FES cycling, the most effective intensity, duration, and pulse width remain unspecified.[150]

Other physical therapy interventions that show some benefit in treating SCI spasticity in systematic reviews but with much less evidence include **transcutaneous spinal cord stimulation** (tDCS)[151]; transcranial magnetic stimulation (TMS)[152]; and transcutaneous electrical nerve stimulation (TENS).[152] Notably, there appears to be benefit when using TENS in a prevention strategy – that is starting treatment early after SCI near the onset of spasticity.[153] Administration of TENS to the peroneal nerve during inpatient rehabilitation and prior to physical therapy treatment reduced muscle tone and clonus in a randomized control trial.[153,154]

Interventions with inconclusive evidence or no evidence for SCI spasticity, based on systematic reviews, are vibration, stretching alone, and passive ROM.[152] Muscle strengthening is also a clinical choice to reduce spasticity, but there is no evidence from randomized clinical trials for its efficacy in SCI.[155] An important benefit is that strength training doesn't appear to worsen spasticity, which had been a concern for several decades. Some clinical trials are underway that will add greatly to the role of strength training on SCI-induced spasticity,[156-158] but at this point resistance training appears to impact strength and is not a first line choice for spasticity treatment. Bracing, taping, and casting can

TABLE 13-10	Assessment measures of SCI spasticity			
	PROPERTIES	**RELIABILITY**	**VALIDITY**	**WEAKNESSES**
Modified Ashworth[139,341]	Subjective Tone assessment by PT for catch/release, resistance or rigidity to passive movement	Inter-rater Fair to Good Test/retest Fair to Good	Poor validity for UE; fair validity for resistance to passive movement	Scores Fluctuate by time of day, prior activities, different raters, inconsistent speed of passive movement. Can't separate spasticity from other tone disorders
Penn Spasm Frequency[139,341]	Patient report of number of spontaneous and/or triggered muscle spasms	Test/retest Good	Construct Validity Good to Excellent	Concerns about Interpretability; some difficulty comparing scores across groups; best used in conjunction with Modified Ashworth Scale
PRISM[142,144]	Patient report; 44 items for SCI spasticity's impact on quality of life	Internal consistency good Test/retest Fair	Content validity Good Construct Validity Fair generalizable	Concerns about interpretability; Doesn't assess sleep; limitations in positive aspects of spasticity Only available in English and Serbian
SCI-SET[142,144]	Patient report; 35 items to assess the impact of spasticity in daily life over 7 days; captures both positive and negative aspects of spasticity	Internal consistency fair to poor Test/retest Fair to Poor	Content validity Good Construct Validity Fair Generalizable but some concerns Assesses sleep Discriminates positive aspects of spasticity	Concerns about interpretability; Available in English, Persian, and Turkish

PRISM: Patient Reported Impact of Spasticity Measure; SCI-SET: Spinal Cord Injury Spasticity Evaluation Tool

be used to maintain or attain normal joint positions due to SCI-induced spasticity. Enabling typical positions and posture enables better respiration, weight-bearing training, and more effective splints for daily activities like eating and dressing. Evidence to support the use of splints relies primarily on clinical experience.

Using the strongest evidence available, it appears that formerly standard physical therapy treatments for SCI like passive ROM and stretch have only short-term effects and produce no lasting reduction of spasticity after SCI. On the other hand, different forms of electrical or magnetic stimulation alone or in combination with activity-based training offer at least moderate efficacy in treating spasticity. Notably, greater emphasis on using these more effective treatments early after SCI, before spasticity starts, seems warranted, especially for treatments with low risk and low need for resources like TENS during inpatient rehabilitation.

Emerging rehabilitation treatments that reduce spasticity in initial studies should be tracked as possible treatments once more evidence is available. Interventions for gait that neuromodulate and/or neuroregulate motor control, during swing phase, reduce tone and hyperreflexia and improve gait.[148,159] Operant conditioning of reflexes in the LE is an effective, long-term intervention after SCI in both animal and human studies.[146-148] Using focused attention on neuromuscular activity readouts,

people with chronic, incomplete SCI have been operantly trained to inhibit spasticity and hyperreflexia during standing. The neuromuscular activation is a read-out of motor neuron excitability, and evidence shows that training promotes greater inhibitory synapses on the motor neurons. This reflex down conditioning lowered hyperreflexia and improved walking speed and motor control of the knee and ankle.[147] Recently, a new operant conditioning intervention was applied during a complex, dynamic task rather than standing.[148] The operant down conditioning training targeted the abnormally large soleus reflex during the swing phase of walking and was highly effective. A greater magnitude of reflex inhibition occurred during walking and within a shorter training period. Improvements in gait and locomotor EMG also resulted. Most importantly, lower hyperreflexia was maintained for at least 6 months after the training ended. These studies show that people with SCI can be trained to modify neuroplasticity, leading to long-term reduction of spasticity and hyperreflexia. A more effective approach is training under task-specific conditions and dynamic rather than static conditions.

A systematic review of powered exoskeleton training for overground walking found three of seven studies significantly reduced spasticity and may suggest that some types of exoskeletons, and at specific times, are more effective than others.[160-162]

The treatment pathway for spasticity starts by finding out from the patient with SCI whether spasticity is a debilitating problem by using PRISM or SCI-SET.[139,143,163] After confirming a spasticity problem, detailed information about the location, types, and frequency should be collected. Discuss with the patient if they recognized any triggers for spasticity. Use MAS and other rating scales to document severity, so any treatments can be assessed for reducing symptoms. Remember, that the spasticity profile changes, so routine assessment will be important.

The first line of treatment is to relieve or resolve potential triggers such as pressure injuries, bowel constipation, which is an unfortunate side-effect of anti-spasticity medication, and bladder complications like UTI. Any infection can trigger greater spasticity including oral, respiratory, and skin infections. Skin irritation caused by tight clothing, hot or cold weather, anxiety/depression, and bone fracture should also be screened if there is a sudden increase in spasticity. Many of these triggers may need medical treatment and are first detected during physical therapy treatment.

Should problematic spasticity continue or worsen, physical therapy, Botox injections, and drugs, either together or alone, will be the next line of treatment. Ideally, treatments that specifically address the patient's symptoms and have the strongest level of evidence should be the first treatment. Generalized or multisegmental spasticity as well as severe side effects from oral medications may be best treated by a baclofen pump rather than an oral administration. If all treatment options fail, a non-reversible surgery may be the only option to meet the patient's quality of life and functional goals.[139] The surgical approaches damage the nerve near the muscle or spinal cord to disrupt the reflex arc. These procedures often cause loss of sensation and can weaken the muscle but may be the only way to improve function such as reducing adductor tone and giving access for perineal hygiene.

Heterotopic Ossification

Heterotopic ossification (HO) is pathological bone formation within muscle and soft tissue and occurs in 10 to 78% of individuals with SCI.[164,165] It usually develops within the first 2 months of injury and is associated with other factors, including spasticity, pneumonia, smoking, and UTI.[166] While the mechanisms that cause HO are not fully understood, evidence shows that stem cells differentiate into bone-forming cells rather than muscle, ligament, or fat cells.[167] The signals that drive the stem cells down an osteogenic path are unknown, but once the process has started, calcification occurs within a few weeks.[167] In the initial stages of HO, nonspecific signs of inflammation may appear. When it has more fully developed, the primary clinical symptoms will be joint and muscle pain with swelling in the region and a low fever. When the SCI is above T6, HO can cause autonomic dysreflexia, so HO must be considered when dysreflexia with an unknown cause emerges. The presence of HO severely limits ROM and can result in ankyloses (fixation) of the joint that can prevent daily activities, such as dressing, transfers, and WC use. Prevention of HO may be possible by nonsteroidal anti-inflammatory drugs, prescribed early after SCI, before HO has started.[164] Once HO is diagnosed, surgical resection is considered to restore the lost ROM, but some individuals do not sustain long-term gains, possibly due to recurrence of HO.[168]

Bone Health and Osteoporosis

Within a few days after SCI, bone resorption begins, which results in high levels of calcium in the urine. The injury greatly disrupts the balance between bone formation and resorption with rapid resorption being the primary function early on. This resorptive process continues for months, years, decades, and potentially throughout the life of the individual.[169] As the years after SCI increase, the rate of bone formation is markedly slower below the level of injury. It results in bone mineral loss of up to 50-60%, especially in the hip and knee. The primary cause appears to be prolonged bed rest, absence of muscle function, no weight-bearing activities, and profound vitamin D deficiency.[169] Clinical guidance often encourages people with acute and subacute SCI to avoid dairy intake of vitamin D, under the assumption that the calcium will further increase hypercalciuria. However, there is little or no evidence of a nutritional contribution. Given the progressive, prolonged impact of SCI on bone health, interventions must be considered by acute/subacute or chronic times after injury.

Mechanisms that threaten and worsen bone health have been targets for physical therapy and pharmacological interventions. Increasing weight-bearing and muscle contraction activities may quell bone loss. However, a systematic review of FES cycling, treadmill training, electrical stimulation, arm crank, and standing exercise found the evidence was inconsistent and of very low quality for acute SCI.[170] The same findings occurred for chronic SCI in two large systematic reviews, and no recommendations could be made for these therapeutic exercises and bone health.[170,171]

The frank bone loss increases the risk of fracture. The following factors predict a fracture: under the age of 16 years, high alcohol use, low body mass index, SCI of 10 years or more, being female, motor complete SCI, paraplegia, prior fracture, family history of fractures, and use of anticonvulsants, heparin, or opioids.[172] The presence of five or more of these factors reflect a high fracture risk. Bisphosphonates are the first line of treatment to prevent bone loss in acute/subacute periods after SCI, including tiludronate, clodronate, and etidronate.[169,173] Stronger evidence from a recent systematic review showed that zoledronic acid prevents bone mineral density loss in acute SCI.[171] Low-quality evidence in studies of chronic SCI prevent any recommendations but zoledronic acid and vitamin D supplements may be suitable.[171] Importantly, bisphosphonates do not seem to protect the knee from bone loss in people that are fully dependent on a WC for mobility.[169] In the future, studies that not only account for time since injury but also SCI level and completeness will be needed to define the most efficacious treatments across the heterogenous SCI profiles.[174]

Physical Therapy Management in the Inpatient Rehabilitation Setting

The level and the completeness of SCI provide a guide for the expected function that will be available once spinal shock has resolved (Table 13-11). It is important to remember that these characteristics are a general guideline, and most individuals with SCI show unique rates, extents, and patterns of recovery. This means the physical therapist must be vigilant in checking

TABLE 13-11	Prediction of Mobility and Outcomes by Level of SCI		
SCI LEVEL	**EXPECTED ACTIVE MUSCLES**	**POTENTIAL FUNCTIONAL OUTCOME**	**REQUIRED EQUIPMENT**
C1–4	Neck and facial muscles Diaphragm – C4	*Bed mobility*: dependent *Transfers*: dependent *Pressure relief*: independent with power WC *Eating*: dependent *Dressing*: dependent *Grooming*: dependent *Bathing*: dependent *WC propulsion*: independent with power WC *Standing*: dependent *Walking*: not expected	Hospital bed Transfer board and/or lift Tilt or recliner WC; WC cushion – – – Rolling shower/commode chair Tilt table; standing frame ventilator
C5	Muscles listed for C1–4 Biceps, brachialis, brachioradialis Deltoid Infraspinatus Subscapularis	*Bed mobility*: min–mod assist *Transfers*: min assist *Pressure relief*: independent with power WC *Eating*: min assist *Dressing*: dependent *Grooming*: min assist *Bathing*: dependent *WC propulsion*: independent with power WC *Standing*: dependent *Walking*: not expected	Hospital bed Transfer board; lift Tilt or recliner WC; WC cushion Splints and equipment to assist eating, dressing, and grooming Rolling shower/commode chair Tilt table; standing frame
C6	Muscles for C1–5 Extensor carpi radialis Serratus anterior	*Bed mobility*: min assist *Transfers*: min assist *Pressure relief*: independent with power WC *Eating*: independent *Dressing*: independent upper body; min–mod asst lower body *Grooming*: independent *Bathing*: independent upper body; min–mod asst lower body *WC propulsion*: independent with power WC; manual: independent indoors; min–mod asst outdoors *Standing*: dependent *Walking*: not expected	Hospital bed Transfer board; lift Tilt or recliner WC; WC cushion Splints Splints Splints Rolling shower/commode chair Tilt table; standing frame
C7–8	Muscles for C1–6 Triceps, flexor carpi ulnaris, finger extensors Finger flexors C8	*Bed mobility*: independent *Transfers*: independent *Pressure relief*: independent with power WC *Eating*: independent *Dressing*: independent *Grooming*: independent *Bathing*: independent upper body; min asst lower body *WC propulsion*: manual independent indoors and outdoors *Standing*: min asst *Walking*: not expected	Hospital bed or standard bed With or without Transfer board WC cushion Adaptive devices Adaptive devices Adaptive devices Shower/commode chair Tilt table; standing frame
T1–9	Muscles for C1 to level of injury; Intrinsics of hand Intercostals Erector spinae Abdominals T6	*Bed mobility*: independent *Transfers*: independent *Pressure relief*: independent *Eating*: independent *Dressing*: independent *Grooming*: independent *Bathing*: independent *WC propulsion*: manual independent *Standing*: independent *Walking*: not functional	Standard bed With or without transfer board WC cushion Shower/commode chair Standing frame

(Continued)

TABLE 13-11	Prediction of Mobility and Outcomes by Level of SCI (*Continued*)		
SCI LEVEL	**EXPECTED ACTIVE MUSCLES**	**POTENTIAL FUNCTIONAL OUTCOME**	**REQUIRED EQUIPMENT**
T10–L1	Muscles C1 to level of injury; Intercostals, external and internal obliques; Rectus abdominus; L1 partial hip flexor	*Bed mobility*: independent *Transfers*: independent *Pressure relief*: independent *Eating*: independent *Dressing*: independent *Grooming*: independent *Bathing*: independent *WC propulsion*: manual independent *Standing*: independent *Walking*: functional; independent to min assist	Standard bed WC cushion Padded tub bench Standing frame Walker, forearm crutches, braces
L2–S5	Muscles C1 to level of injury; Iliopsoas; quadratus lumborum; priformis; obtruators	*Bed mobility*: independent *Transfers*: independent *Pressure relief*: independent *Eating*: independent *Dressing*: independent *Grooming*: independent *Bathing*: independent *WC propulsion*: manual independent *Standing*: independent *Walking*: functional; independent to min assist	Standard bed WC cushion Padded tub bench Standing frame Forearm crutches, braces

for atypical gains and incorporate these into interventions. Given the short length of stay for inpatient rehabilitation, about a month, the primary goal is to prepare the individual for the next transition, typically to home. The individual will need to be able to manage bowel and bladder care, transfers, skin protection, components and use of the WC, and daily activities like eating and dressing. For some of these tasks, the individual with SCI may be independent or nearly so. For other tasks, the individual will need to be able to instruct others in how to assist or carry them out. The priorities of this phase of rehabilitation are as follows:

- Gain appropriate strength, mobility, balance, and endurance for expected functions;
- Educate the patient and caregivers to perform functional tasks in bed mobility, transfers, pressure relief, and WC use; and
- Assess the home, work, and social environments in which the individual will live after discharge from rehabilitation.

Most patients will have a goal of returning home, when discharged from inpatient rehabilitation. To determine the focus of physical therapy interventions in this phase, the team will determine or predict the realistic living arrangements. Factors that are associated with a return to home include being married/significant other, high participation in physical therapy, and the ability to use equipment effectively.[175] People who are unmarried, older, Black, or Hispanic with a more severe SCI were more likely to be discharged to a nursing facility or location other than home.[175] Racial disparities are evident in surgical intervention, discharge to inpatient rehabilitation and the extent of improvements during inpatient rehabilitation.[176,177] Race predicts surgery for cervical SCI with Black and Hispanic races having lower odds of surgery compared to Caucasians.[177]

Moreover, Black individuals with cervical SCI are significantly less likely to be favorably discharged to home or to inpatient rehabilitation than other races and Caucasians.[177] For people with SCI that receive inpatient rehabilitation, those of Black race have lower mobility and self-care scores at discharge than white and Hispanic individuals.[176]

Factors that can predict motor performance at discharge from inpatient rehabilitation are age, body mass index, and delayed admission to inpatient rehabilitation[178-180] Greater injury severity and need for ventilator support on entry to the emergency department predicted low motor function at rehabilitation discharge.[181] In contrast, physiological factors of heart rate, oxygen saturation levels, and systolic blood pressure had no predictive value.[181,182] The physical therapist and rehabilitation team should expect a longer length of stay for inpatient rehabilitation among people with SCI who are overweight or obese.[179] While this longer dose initially increases medical costs, it results in significantly greater improvement in motor performance by discharge.[179] In fact, evidence from computer simulations suggests that longer treatment sessions will also improve outcomes regardless of type of injury or personal factors like obesity.[183] Increasing therapy intensity by having 50% longer sessions per day predicts a faster more efficient rate of motor recovery and lower medical care costs.[183] Extended length of stays also result from medical complications such as UTIs and pressure injuries and could limit motor recovery rather than improve it, given the role of early infection on 5- and 10-year outcomes.[72,184] Unfortunately, there is no established threshold for time in physical therapy to produce effective, efficient gains in motor performance. Insurance payers and the Center for Medicare and Medicaid Services (CMS) stipulate that 3 hours of therapy a day must be delivered over 5 to 7 days in inpatient rehabilitation facilities in order to receive payment for services.

However, compliance with the 3-hour rule didn't result in shorter length of stay or greater gains in recovery across a variety of diagnoses.[185] While it is easy to track PT, OT, and speech therapy treatment time toward the rule, the successful treatment of patients with complex conditions often require advanced medical care by skilled physicians and nurses in order to participate in these therapies, but this care is not considered toward payment, based on the 3-hour rule.[185]

All people with SCI have the potential for inpatient rehabilitation regardless of type of injury, complications, race, or personal factors. However, little is known about which physical therapy interventions are most effective in individuals with SCI because of the complexity of the injury. Neurorehabilitationists developed physical therapy taxonomies to begin to examine the most effective treatments and to better specify the treatments administered to ensure continuity of care.[186–189] The 10 common treatment areas that are deemed most relevant by international experts are muscle strength, walking/pre-gait, arm and hand use for daily activities, standing and balance, wheelchair mobility, bed mobility, transfers, muscle tone management, and bathing.[187] To increase strength, endurance, and skill learning, starting with simpler tasks before moving to more difficult tasks is typical. Evidence shows that the more time spent on musculoskeletal treatments (e.g., ROM/stretching, upright activities) was associated with greater reliance on others for motor function (i.e., lower FIM motor scores) 1 and 5 years after SCI.[175,190] In fact, ROM activities have very low priority in this phase of treatment because they don't produce lasting changes in joint contractures.[187] Importantly, strength training and walking training progressively matched motor recovery as it occurred and produced benefits regardless of AIS or neurologic level of SCI.[191] Therefore, the physical therapist will want to progress to functional tasks like bed mobility, transfers, WC mobility, and upright, gait activities as soon as possible. Using strength and gait training across AIS classification early, during inpatient rehabilitation, is supported by a large European multicenter SCI study; although in the U.S., gait training is used primarily in AIS D injury and rarely with AIS A, B, or C injuries (25%).[191,192] A recent clinical practice guideline for acute, inpatient management of SCI, developed by an international multidisciplinary group of SCI experts, also supports beginning rehabilitation as soon as medically stable and using body weight support treadmill training when available.[193–195]

Strength Training

Two approaches of strength training can be used during inpatient rehabilitation – progressive resistance exercises and in-task performance. A recent meta-analysis of resistance training in SCI specifically included studies that administered training for at least 6 weeks and directly measured force, power, or endurance in isometric or concentric contractions.[196] The amount of resistance used in training was determined as a percentage of 1 repetition maximum, 10 maximum repetitions or a maximal isometric contraction. Intensity of training across the studies was typically 3 to 4 sets of 10 to 12 repetitions. There is clear evidence that resistance training significantly increased strength relative to controls by as much as 244% and within a short course of treatment. However, large-scale

adoption of these training parameters is limited to people who do not require assistance to complete the resisted range, and it is unclear what the optimal time frame for training should be. The included studies either didn't specify time since injury or appeared to deliver training during inpatient rehabilitation, outpatient rehabilitation or years after SCI. Indeed, a clinical guideline to improve fitness, which included strength training, found insufficient high-quality evidence for early intervention.[170,197] Interestingly, manual resistance training during inpatient rehabilitation increased isometric force of the trained leg relative to the contralateral, control leg.[155] While the authors questioned whether the improvement was clinically meaningful, it must be noted that using the opposite leg as a control jeopardizes this interpretation. It is well known that strength training of one limb produces a cross-over benefit to the untrained, opposite limb in healthy people.[198,199] It seems likely that training one limb early after SCI improved strength in both limbs, resulting in less difference between the two sides. An overview of many systematic reviews for resistance training presented similar training guidelines as outlined recently, including the lack of evidence for what to use during inpatient rehabilitation.[196,200] The recommended strengthening parameters from the culmination of systematic reviews and meta-analyses are 3 sets of 8 to 10 repetitions at 50 to 80% of 1-repetition maximum, using either conventional resistance (weights, elastic bands, cables) or in combination with electrical muscle stimulation.[200]

Resistance training within tasks and natural movements offers improved motor learning of skills, relies on movements across multiple joints, and has higher efficiency by accomplishing two goals during a single training activity. Resistance training in healthy individuals often takes place within tasks such as lunges to increase gluteal and quad strength. Similarly, performing sit to stand transfers and back, during inpatient rehabilitation, also provides resistance training. To modulate resistance, the height of the seating surface can be lowered to increase strength training. Also, overhead body weight support systems can be set to provide low support, which requires greater strength training, while challenging motor skill learning. For in-task UE resistance training, moving from supine to short or long sitting and back can be used by starting from different supine heights with wedges. As with most strength training studies, in-task functional strength training evidence is limited to chronic, thoracic SCI.[201] Nevertheless, significant gains occurred in strength in terms of anaerobic power, WC agility, and quality of life.[201] Strength training using progressive resistance during inpatient rehabilitation does not appear to worsen spasticity.[155] Some benefits include less shoulder pain, improved overall quality of life, and improved perception of physical and social functioning.[202,203]

Demanding physical exercise that requires intense exertion can lead to concerning blood pressure changes, during inpatient rehabilitation and later after SCI. Strength training of the UE muscles can cause orthostatic hypotension when it is performed above the level of heart. Paralysis or paresis causes poor muscle pumping of blood back to the heart. Loss of sympathetic neural input at a level that affects the heart will also cause a drop in blood pressure. Resistance training can also induce autonomic dysreflexia in people with SCI above T6.

Another negative consequence of strength training is overuse injuries, especially in the shoulder and wrists. Overuse complications can take two forms. One form causes inflammation, pain, and stiffness, and when the shoulder and wrists are affected, it severely limits daily activities and manual WC use. The other form is hypertrophy of anterior muscle groups in the chest and shoulders, which can pull the shoulders forward into a rounded position and cause impingement. Poor thermoregulation combined with high exertional exercise can raise body temperature, cause overheating, and may trigger autonomic dysreflexia. Cool ambient temperatures and additional fans will be needed during rehabilitation. High exertion exercise outside on a hot day may need to be avoided in individuals with poor thermoregulation or autonomic dysreflexia. Lastly, resistance training can cause skin sheering or pressure injuries as the person tries to stabilize themselves to overcome the resistance. Support straps to reduce sheering movements and added cushioning can prevent these skin complications.

Bed Mobility

The importance of good bed mobility can't be underestimated because dressing, bowel management, and skin protection are performed within this environment. Activities on mat surfaces will be easier than in the bed, and a hospital bed is easier than a bed in the home. Transitioning physical therapy training from the mat to bed surfaces will be necessary to promote the greatest functional attainment by the individual with SCI or the caregiver. People with high cervical SCI will depend on care attendants for bed mobility, and the role of the therapist will be to educate the patient and caregiver. The person living with high cervical SCI will need to be able to direct the training of future care providers on completion of repositioning, using low-risk techniques to avoid injuries to limbs and skin sheering.

Independence in bed mobility will require skills in rolling and moving in and out of different positions. People with injuries at the lower cervical and thoracic levels should be able to achieve independence with equipment. Mat and bed activities can be structured to promote activity-dependent plasticity or for compensation. The choice, of which to use, will depend on the anticipated functional outcomes for the SCI level (Table 13-12), time since injury, and completeness of the injury. If the SCI is low cervical or below and incomplete, task-specific training should be part of the training program to promote neural drive and plasticity. In terms of unsupported sitting, there is a weak recommendation to avoid additional training due to lack of proven benefits beyond the sitting training given in standard rehabilitation.[194,204] It is likely that this therapy time could better be used on training tasks, mobility, and strength, given their reported benefits to endurance and motor control.

CASE A, PART VI

Ms. Roberts is now able to perform some trunk muscle activation on the left side, but it is minimal and inconsistent. Part of treatment will be spent on strengthening these muscles and incorporating them in bed mobility. Ms. Roberts should be placed in side-lying. Rolling out of side-lying is the easiest form of rolling. She should be encouraged to initiate rolling using the shoulders and pelvis. Initially, she will have little success, so angling slightly out of side-lying will allow her to

---

TABLE 13-12	Bed Mobility Training Designed for Plasticity or Compensation	
FUNCTION	**VOLUNTARY ATTEMPTS AND FUNCTIONAL PLASTICITY**	**LITTLE OR NO VOLUNTARY MOVEMENTS**
Rolling 　Log rolling 　Segmental	• Focused attention • Begin in side-lying and encourage pre-injury pattern • Structure for success by allowing gravity to assist the movement	• Flex neck when moving supine to prone • Extend neck when moving prone to supine • Rocking or swinging extended arms to create momentum and carry pelvis over
Prone on elbows		• Use for stretching hip flexors • Used for changing position in bed
Prone on hands		• Stretch into hip and low back hyperextension • Prepare for gait
Come to sitting 　Hips and knees 　flexed, feet on 　the floor	• Use overhead lift or active assist to sit up from an incline or from supine • Train for success by starting nearly upright • Use mirrors to help correct body alignment if proprioception is impaired • Discourage using upper extremities	• Use hands behind, at the side or in front of pelvis to increase stability • Use upper extremities to assist in maintaining an upright trunk
Long sitting 　Hips flexed, 　knees straight 　out on the mat	• Use overhead lift or active assist to sit up from an incline or from supine • Train for success by starting nearly upright • Use mirrors to help correct body alignment if proprioception is impaired	• In tetraplegia, use shoulder hyperextension to passively extend the elbow • Side-to-side weight shifts on elbows in supine and shoulder hyperextension to assume long sitting

use gravity to assist the movement. Moving out of side-lying into supine will enable a transition to hook-lying – where the knees are bent and the feet are flat on the mat. Attempts to press down on the feet will try to recruit gluteal muscles and erector spinae. Lying prone on a wedge is an effective way to stretch the hip flexors. As upright tolerance improves, incorporate short and long sitting. She will require assistance when coming to short sitting and maintaining it with proper body alignment. Long sitting is important to enabling dressing, and hamstring flexibility will be needed. In both sitting positions, therapy should progress from having the hands behind the pelvis, to out to the sides to in front. Add dynamic activities, like lifting one hand slightly to add difficulty, and strength and endurance training. Continue to encourage active use of the right upper extremity. It may take thousands of attempts before any muscle activation occurs, so be persistent and consistent.

Transfers

Transfers refer to moving between two surfaces. Skill attainment will depend on balance, arm strength, ability to manage equipment, and body type/size. Skill progression will move from stationary sitting at the edge of bed/mat, to an assisted transfer to independent performance, and also move from easier to more difficult types of transfers. Transfer difficulty will progress from using a transfer board to seated transfers without a board to standing transfers, if feasible for the anticipated functional outcome (Table 13-11). The appropriate transfer type will pose the least risk to skin shearing and falling, while allowing as much independence as possible. As in bed mobility, the type of surface represents added difficulty and can be used to drive greater endurance as well as increase motor learning demands and in-task strengthening. Most importantly, transfer training will need to emphasize the surfaces the individual will encounter at home such as WC to sofa, bed, toilet, tub/shower, floor, and vehicle. For individuals with high cervical SCI or considerable body size, lift equipment may be necessary for the home to protect the caregiver from injury.

CASE A, PART VII

With the return of upright tolerance, Ms. Roberts will need to begin to incorporate strength gains into functional tasks. To promote neuroplasticity, structure the tasks to allow trial and error as well as success. While breaking the task into its parts may be helpful for some, shortening the range or allowing gravity to assist the movement may improve skill learning. For transfer training, use of a ceiling-mounted support system with adjustable levels of assistance will allow Ms. Roberts to practice the whole task. For each type of transfer, the level of support can be set to a range that allows her to move the weakest areas. To address her weak abdominals and erector spinae, use of the support system

will allow Ms. Roberts to work against gravity in these tasks: moving from supine to sitting and back, forward leaning and back in the WC, and trunk rotation and reaching in all directions while sitting at the edge of mat. Progression through these tasks will be based on her ability to maintain good alignment of the head and body and then by adding challenges via lowering the support provided and/or adding arm movements. Moving from sitting to standing and back can also be progressed by using a ceiling support system. Initially, the seat height should be elevated and the level of assistance increased to allow her to attempt and complete the whole task, that is, leaning forward and putting weight through the legs and standing. Through trial and error, she will learn where her center of gravity is and how to control it during all components of standing without the risk of falling.

WC Mobility

Upon entering inpatient rehabilitation, people with SCI will be assessed for a temporary WC that best meets their current needs.[205] Two overall types of WCs will be used after SCI – a power WC, for individuals who do not have sufficient arm strength or function to propel themselves, and a manual WC, for those that do have such strength and function. These temporary chairs are either loaned from the rehabilitation hospital or rented and can be exchanged for different types to best match recovery progression or to quickly resolve negative impacts like pain, too much skin pressure, or wrong size. The temporary chair will allow for concentrated WC mobility training and learning to manage the WC components. Late in inpatient rehabilitation or in outpatient rehabilitation, the person with SCI will decide on their permanent WC in conjunction with their PT, OT, primary care physician, and/or a WC seating clinic, if one is available.

The minimal physical criteria for propelling a manual WC, using standard push rims, include normal strength of the shoulder abductors, elbow flexors, and wrist extensors bilaterally. For individuals with less arm function, upper extremity pain, or poor endurance, power-assisted push rims will be beneficial. Power-assisted WCs have motors that boost propulsion while requiring less shoulder muscle activity.[206] Requirements for a power WC will be based on the following: bicep, tricep, and wrist extensor weakness; inability to effectively perform pressure relief; the living environment and community impede independent propulsion; and/or poor endurance that prevents home and community propulsions.[207]

To develop WC mastery, a hierarchy of WC mobility skills, from easiest to hardest, will be trained. Training starts with propulsion over level surfaces, and progresses to maneuvering in small spaces, mobility in crowded areas, moving over uneven terrain, moving up and down ramps/inclines, negotiating ridges and curbs, and descending stairs. Completing a formal WC skills training program, which moves through these progressive tasks, improves skills 13-23% more than typical rehabilitation over the short term, as shown by systematic review.[208,209] Persistence of these differences long-term are unclear. Importantly, the skill training program requires a total of only 2 hours over four sessions. To ensure that WC skills required for daily living are adequate, a newly revised assessment tool is recommended, the **Wheelchair Skills Test,** which is reliable, valid, and has normative values for SCI at different levels.[210-212] Additionally, training for the safe use of each component of the WC by the patient (when capable) or caregiver will be needed.

WC seating must reduce the risk of pressure injuries, while maintaining good body alignment and promoting better function.[207,213] With weakness of trunk muscles, gravity will pull the head and upper body forward, pulling the spine into a C-shape or exaggerated kyphosis.[213] A posterior pelvic tilt and flattened lumbar spine also occur. This posture creates greater pressure over the sacrum, limited diaphragmatic breathing, and hyperextension of the neck to maintain gaze on the environment. Angling the seat backward slightly allows gravity to extend the spine and reduces these risks. Goals for seating support differ for level of injury and associated physical limitations (Table 13-13). Asymmetrical spasticity or strength causes deviation from good body alignment. Strengthening for the weak side is a therapeutic objective to allow for greater functional mobility and less risk of pressure injuries. If asymmetry persists, then supports will likely improve seated posture.

CASE A, PART VIII

Early WC skills will focus on learning to manage the components of the WC, using only the left arm and hand. WC mobility training will focus on propulsion using the left upper limb and left leg as muscle strength of the hamstrings returns to 3 or higher and elbow extensors reach 4/5. For pressure relief, she will need to start using the lateral weight shift techniques because she doesn't have enough trunk control to perform forward leaning or bilateral arm strength to lift the body.

Care of the Upper Limb

Individuals with tetraplegia consider hand function to be as important or more important as sexual function or bowel and bladder management.[214-217] While treatment of the upper limb is a primary focus of occupational therapy, it is expected that physical therapists will also care for the upper extremity. It is a fundamental part of most mobility functions after SCI such as transfers, WC use, pressure relief, and ambulation. The primary rehabilitation objectives for the upper extremity are to prevent complications, optimize function within the expected limits of the SCI, and restore function when possible. These objectives will be addressed early, in the acute phase and through inpatient and outpatient rehabilitation. Here, we will discuss both the inpatient and outpatient approach, since the greatest difference will be in progression of difficulty.

The physical capacity of the upper limb and the ability to withstand fatigue will be addressed by strength training with high repetitions. Because overall prognosis depends on the ability to perform physical activity, gains in strength allow better engagement in activity-based rehabilitation, especially since less time is spent in inpatient rehabilitation. The theory is that an increase in the capacity to do work will translate in improvements in performing daily tasks, hand function, and gait. Strength training can utilize gravity or active assistance with electric stimulation. Strength training guidelines described above apply to the UE and should be used.

New approaches that are directed at increasing neuroplasticity have shown good effects and suggest that compensatory interventions might be able to be delayed or omitted entirely, in the future, for some people with tetraplegia.[218] Electrical stimulation is garnering more attention as augmenting rehabilitation procedures, especially in the UE, given its importance for daily living and quality of life. New evidence from the application of transcutaneous electrical stimulation over the cervical spine region greatly improved arm and hand function.[219] This study represents a major advance in tetraplegia because it produced benefits in very difficult-to-treat conditions – lowering spasticity, improving heart rate, thermoregulation, and bladder function. All gains outlasted the training by 3 to 6 months, which holds promise for very long-term retention simply by participating in half-yearly treatments in the clinic or at home. Other promising approaches by Field-Fote and colleagues combined motor learning theory and somatosensory stimulation with TENS to augment afferent drive to the spinal cord.[220-222] The theory is that the afferent stimulation will increase neural activity, and the intensive massed practice will shape the plasticity into long-term functional plasticity, rather than maladaptive plasticity. Individuals with incomplete SCI, who completed this combined treatment, had significant gains in pinch strength, movement speed, and hand function. They outperformed individuals that completed massed practice alone or somatosensory stimulation alone.[221] Additionally, sensory perception improved, and cortical excitability increased, supporting the idea that greater neural activation occurred with this treatment approach.

Splinting is a standard approach in individuals with tetraplegia to compensate for lost function and enable greater independence. The role of splinting is to prevent contractures, support and protect a weak joint, and reduce the risk of pain and overstretching.[223] Splints for the hands and at the elbow to prevent flexor contracture, due to denervated triceps, are common. Hands splints for night use to increase the web space didn't produce positive results,[224] but new 3-D printing of custom wrist-driven orthoses produced improved function in one person and worsened it in another.[225] Using splints as assistive devices during rehabilitation has taken several forms. New robotic, soft hand splints use electrical stimulation to promote active or passive ROM of the hand and wrist.[226] A different approach uses a new wearable sleeve with 150 embedded EMG surface electrodes on the forearm, wrist, and hand, called the NeuroLife EMG system, which is being tested in people with tetraplegia and stroke.[227] The sleeve can decode 12 functional hand, wrist, and forearm movements in real time which can be used as a controller to assist with movements that patients cannot perform on their own.[227]

One of the most serious and common long-term complications after SCI is the development of severe shoulder pain.[223] Shoulder pain can be seen within the first year of SCI and has been found in 81% of long-term WC users.[228] Elbow injuries are less common while carpal tunnel injuries lie in between.

TABLE 13-13	Wheelchair Seating Systems		
POWER WHEELCHAIRS	**FUNCTION**	**BENEFITS**	**DISADVANTAGES**
	Battery-operated seating system in which propulsion is achieved via motors electronically controlled by the user	Allows for independent mobility for those unable to propel a manual wheelchair due to upper extremity weakness, pain, or decreased endurance	Heavy, does not fold therefore increased difficulty with transporting, relies on battery, expensive
Base	**Function**	**Benefits**	**Disadvantages**
Rear-Wheel Drive	Drive (larger) wheels are behind the center of gravity with casters in the front	Predictable drive and stability	Large turning radius making it difficult in smaller spaces
Front-Wheel Drive	Drive wheels are in the front of the center of gravity with casters in the rear	Stable base and tight turning radius	Less of a smooth ride, difficult to maintain a straight line on uneven surfaces
Midwheel Drive	Drive wheels in line with center of gravity	Small turning radius	Less effective outdoors over uneven terrain
Controls	**Function**	**Benefits**	**Disadvantages**
Standard Joystick	Proportional drive control (speed/direction mirror the force/direction of the input). Typically located on either left or right arm rest but location can be altered	Most intuitive type of controller for injuries at C5 and below	May be difficult to position if spasticity or contractures are present
Alternative Joystick: Chin control, Goal Post/U-shape	Proportional drive control (speed/direction mirror the force/direction of the input)	Ability to use proportional drive with injuries above C5	Chin Control: May interfere with ADLs (grooming, eating), facial hair may affect accuracy, caregiver likely needed to adjust position throughout the day Goal Post/U-shape: May be more sensitive resulting in unwanted movements
Head Array	Pads on wheelchair headrest has switches to allow the user to control the wheelchair	Allows for increased independence for high cervical injuries	Caregiver may be required to assist in proper positioning to access head controls. Spasticity or uneven terrain may result in unintentional movements
Sip-and-Puff	User controls the wheelchair via a straw device accessible from user's mouth with positive pressure (puff) and negative pressure (sip). Duration of applied pressure indicates direction	Allows for increased independence for high cervical injuries. Caregivers can easily adjust position of the straw for access	May interfere with ADLs, communication (cannot talk while driving), may cause respiratory fatigue, increased maintenance for hygiene care
Positioning Features	**Function**	**Benefits**	**Disadvantages**
Recline	Allows for change in seat to back angle for a posterior recline while seat/lower extremities stay fixed	Allows for a more comfortable positions, helps prevent or accommodates for contractures, some pressure relief, better for caregivers with toileting needs and safer transfers, improves vasodilation (100 deg with 35 deg tilt)	Continued pressure on ischium and sacrum, risk of shearing

(Continued)

TABLE 13-13   Wheelchair Seating Systems (*Continued*)

POWER WHEELCHAIRS	FUNCTION	BENEFITS	DISADVANTAGES
Tilt-in-Space	Seat and back angle stays fixed while tilting posteriorly	Better pressure relief without shearing (30-45 deg), safer transfers are easier when using a lift, maintains back kinematic alignment in any position, reduces fatigue and discomfort by position change	Risk for backflow in indwelling catheter or leg bag leakage, if attached tray items may spill
Elevating Leg Rests	Allows for knees to be extended	Helps prevent knee flexion contractures, maintain appropriate positioning, helps prevent pooling in distal lower extremities and better management for orthostatic hypotension with tilt/recline	May be difficult if spasticity present, benefit in blood flow if combined with tilt/recline
Seat Elevation	Seat raises higher or lower while seat to back angle remains fixed	Allows for easier transfers and better shoulder mechanics by making surface levels even or downhill, can access community and home features (items in refrigerator/countertop, lightswitches), psychological benefits with being eye-level with others	Not always included on power chairs, foot rests may not elevate with seat resulting in poor positioning of ankles/feet
Power-Assist	A manual wheelchair with a motor that assists with propulsion	Allows for easier and faster propulsion, especially for longer distances, uneven surfaces, and ramps, especially for individuals with tetraplegia or shoulder pain; lighter and easier to transport than power chairs	Heavier/bulkier than manual chairs resulting in more difficulty for transport and maneuverability
Manual Wheelchairs	**Function**	**Benefits**	**Disadvantages**
	Typically used for mobility by individuals with injuries below C6 using push rims for propulsion, but will depend on fitness/strength, pain, and environment. Manual chairs with push handles also available for caregiver dependent mobility	Allows user to stay physically active with mobility, lighter weight, typically folds or easily dissembles for transport	Does not change height for easier transfers, can lead to overuse shoulder injuries
Frame	Folding: collapses by folding through the middle, typically "lightweight" (<34 lbs) Rigid: typically does not fold but parts can be removed for transport. Typically "ultralight" (<30 lbs) make up of titanium, aluminum, or carbon fiber features	Folding: less expensive, easier to transport without taking parts off Rigid/ultralight: customizable (size of seat and backrest, foot rest/plate position, types of arm rests, change in seat to back angle, wheel axle position, camber, material), lighter weight resulting in less risk for shoulder injury, better maneuverability	Folding: often not customizable, heavier than ultralight Rigid/ultralight: more expensive resulting in difficulty getting insurance coverage

(Continued)

TABLE 13-13	Wheelchair Seating Systems (*Continued*)		
POWER WHEELCHAIRS	**FUNCTION**	**BENEFITS**	**DISADVANTAGES**
Manual Wheelchair Features	Seating: Height should allow for optimal access to push rims and transfers, width should be wide enough to avoid pressure sores without sacrificing stability Slope (or dump) with front seat-to-floor height higher than rear height ideal for stability while seated in chair	Armrest: optional feature to support the upper extremities while at rest and can be customizable in length, height, swing-away or flip-back, and removable Footrests: support the feet ideally in neutral or slightly dorsiflexed position. Can be removable/swing-away or fixed foot plate	Wheels: *Locks* act as brakes to stabilize the chair while not moving or during transfers. Can push/pull to lock and positioned to user's preference *Axle position* should be as far forward as possible for improved shoulder mechanics without sacrificing WC stability resulting in tipping backward *Camber* refers to the ankle of the bottom of the wheel relative to the chair. Larger camber improves base of support and mobility but makes the WC wider limiting *Anti-tippers* prevent the wheelchair from tipping posteriorly *Casters* help assist with maneuverability *Tires*: Typically air-filled which are lighter weight and more ideal as opposed to solid foam inserts, however require more maintenance and have the risk of puncture
Cushions	**Function**	**Benefits**	**Disadvantages**
Foam	Provides structure and stability while conforming to body type	Lightweight, low maintenance, variable sizes, least expensive	Least pressure relieving, increased temperature and moisture retention, cannot be washed
Air filled	Allows for dispersed weight for improved pressure distribution. Consists of cells/chambers inflated with air	Conforms to users pressure as air travels between cells, provides shock absorption, amount of air can be adjusted	More expensive, frequent adjustment of air required, higher maintenance, instability results in increased difficulty with transfers and positioning
Gel	Gel pocket in areas of highest pressure within a foam base	Decreased pressure and shear, cooling, contours to user's body	Heavier, gel can leak, gel may need to be redistributed in areas needing the most pressure relief, difficulty with transfers
Hybrid (Air/Foam)	Air cells located in areas of most pressure within foam base	Addresses issue of stability allowing for easier transfers	Does not support individuals with pelvic asymmetry

These injuries are likely due to a combination of overuse and poor biomechanics, when performing transfers in/out of the chair and manual WC propulsion. In tetraplegia, shoulder joint instability may also cause shoulder injury. Therefore, improving body position, during all mobility tasks, may limit the severity or delay the onset of shoulder and upper limb injuries. Joint resting strategies might also be helpful, but be mindful, that as one joint is protected the joints nearby may develop overuse injuries. Adjustment of the WC rear axle to the most forward position without causing instability will help reduce shoulder pain. Seat height and camber of the wheel will also improve shoulder position during propulsion.[207] Patients may benefit from (1) changes in equipment to better match current functional capacity and changes in body weight to improve ergonomics; (2) avoiding or reducing transfers to non-level surfaces; and (3) ongoing assessment and changes to strengthening, stretching, and conditioning exercises.

CASE A, PART IX

Ms. Roberts might benefit from an FES program for the right upper limb since most of the muscles cannot be volitionally activated. The FES may help to facilitate muscle activity and strength, but it might also become an electrical splint that compensates for lost function. It will be important to have her attempt functional tasks with and without the FES system to promote skill development and reduce the risk of compensation early after SCI. Once upper limb motor control begins to return, use of somatosensory stimulation and massed practice may be more beneficial to long-term recovery. The tasks used for massed practice should be functional and graded for difficulty, so the training can progress as greater control develops. The therapist would expect to see functional gains and improvement in sensation, using somatosensory stimulation and massed practice, which would benefit her, since proprioception is impaired on the right.

CASE A, PART X: INPATIENT REHABILITATION DISCHARGE SUMMARY

Ms. Roberts made gains in strength, especially on the left (Table 13-14). Strength in non-ASIA/ ISNCSCI muscle groups also improved by one muscle grade for left shoulder abductors, erector spinae, left gluteus maximus, hamstrings, and the emergence of trace movement of the great toe extensors bilaterally was noted. Spinal shock continued to resolve, and with that bowel and bladder function returned. Spasticity increased during inpatient rehabilitation with hyperreflexia noted in the DTRs of the patella, Achilles, and biceps bilaterally. There was no clonus, but the Babinski continues to be positive on the right.

Neuropathic pain developed in the right cervical region, which limited her ability to participate in her rehabilitation.

Problems with focus emerged, and inconsistency in functional performance was noted. The motor scores of the right upper extremity likely do not reflect her true functional capacity. While she was unable to produce any muscle activation during the ASIA exam, later in the evaluation she was observed moving the right arm and hand. Despite a progressive return of function, she was lethargic, unable to focus, and having difficulty engaging in rehabilitation. Depression interfered with her progress during inpatient rehabilitation, and concern for her current and future well-being warranted inpatient treatment for depression in a psychiatric hospital.

TABLE 13-14	ASIA MOTOR SCORES	
ASIA KEY MUSCLES	**RIGHT**	**LEFT**
C5 elbow flexors	0/5	4/5
C6 wrist extensors	0/5	3/5
C7 elbow extensors	0/5	2/5
C8 finger flexors	0/5	0/5
T1 finger abduction	0/5	0/5
L2 hip flexors	3/5	4/5
L3 knee extensors	3/5	5/5
L4 ankle dorsiflexors	1/5	3/5
L5 long toe extensors	1/5	1/5
S1 ankle plantar flexor	3/5	5/5

● PHYSICAL THERAPY MANAGEMENT OF THE PATIENT IN THE OUTPATIENT REHABILITATION SETTING

In this phase of rehabilitation, the emphasis will be to promote as much recovery as possible and to optimize functional performance to attain the highest level of independence possible. During this phase, things like neuropathic pain, hyperreflexia/spasticity, and sexuality become more prominent. Depression is also a concern. The greatest change in motor ability occurs within the first year after SCI, and the first 6 months see the sharpest rate of improvement.[17] This is the period when spinal shock is largely resolved and the opportunity to induce functional neuroplasticity should not be missed.

Chronic Complications of SCI

Neuropathic Pain – How Is It Different from Acute Pain Related to Tissue Damage?

Pain is a complex problem that includes emotional, cognitive, physiological, and neural components and plays an important role in preventing serious, lasting body injury by alerting the individual to the noxious event. Recently, the International

Association for the Study of Pain revised the definition that existed for more than 40 years to better align with greater understanding of pain complexity and its impact on individuals. "Pain is an unpleasant sensory and emotional experience associated with, or resembling that associated with, actual or potential tissue damage."[229] The traumatic nature of most SCI means that body tissues will be damaged as part of the trauma and will create pain. This type of acute pain is a natural part of the injury and healing process, and typically goes away. However, after SCI, pain responses can become quite abnormal in intensity, can outlast the tissue damage itself, and can become permanent. This type of pain is called **neuropathic pain**.

Neuropathic pain develops due to direct trauma to the somatosensory system within the CNS and/or in the periphery. This means that the SCI itself changes the remaining nervous system and produces neuropathic pain. Also, remember that traumatic SCI typically includes peripheral nerve injury co-located to the trauma site, which contributes to neuropathic pain. Using pre-clinical SCI models and peripheral nerve injury models, growing evidence shows that both structural and physiological changes across the somatosensory system contribute to neuropathic pain. These maladaptive changes are not simply within the superficial dorsal horn pain pathways (e.g., Lamina 1) but also involve deep dorsal horn pathways (lamina 5) for touch, proprioception, and vibration. Maladaptive plasticity occurs within several CNS regions where pain projections and touch/proprioception projections are co-located, including within the dorsal root ganglion,[230–232] the ventral posterior lateral nucleus (VPL) of the thalamus,[233,234] and higher order processing in the anterior cingulate cortex, premotor cortex, and prefrontal cortex.[235,236] Furthermore, neuronal hyperactivity occurs within these regions causing or modulating neuropathic pain. Critical factors of the neuropathic pain phenotype include heightened glial responses[233]; disinhibition related to growth-promoting factors like BDNF and neurotransmitter availability[231,233]; greater synaptic plasticity producing thalamic hypertrophy and greater cortical grey matter volume[233–236]; and facilitation via neuroinflammation.[232,237–239] In summary, the mechanisms of neuropathic pain are receiving even greater research attention because of the difficult complexity of the glial, neural, and inflammatory systems involved and the realization that no single factor or intervention is likely to resolve this serious condition.

The clinical presentation of neuropathic pain after SCI is described as burning, stabbing, shooting, electrical shock, and/or crushing pain. It often emerges several months or years after the injury and greatly interferes with the daily lives of individuals just as they are moving on from their SCI and returning to a more normal lifestyle. Interference with mood, sleep, participation, and quality of life make SCI-induced pain the most difficult complication of the injury across many countries.[240–242] The prevalence of neuropathic pain is more than 80% one year after SCI in the United States[243] and lower worldwide at 53%[244]; although, these differences may depend on how neuropathic pain was defined.[245] Studies do not agree on whether neuropathic pain is more common in tetraplegia versus paraplegia, men versus women, young versus older age.[244,245] One remarkable challenge that continues, despite federal priorities and greater recognition in health care, is that racialized minorities experience greater pain severity, worse pain outcomes, and are under-treated for pain.[246] In people with SCI, physical therapists must advocate for equal treatment for pain of any kind and recognize that health care providers mistakenly ascribe biological differences between Caucasians and people of color when none exist.[247]

Two types of neuropathic pain exist. **Allodynia** is intense pain to a normally innocuous stimulus like the wind blowing on the skin or clothing softly touching the skin. **Hyperalgesia** is exaggerated pain to a noxious thermal or mechanical stimuli like hot water or a deep pressure or pinch. The body regions affected by neuropathic pain can be quite far reaching and can occur below, above, and/or at the level of the injury.

Evaluation of location, intensity, and frequency of pain helps to classify SCI-induced pain after SCI and a standardized Basic Pain data set has been endorsed by international SCI groups and organizations.[248] The **International SCI Basic Pain Data Set** (ISCIPBD) is sensitive, reliable, and valid, and differentiates musculoskeletal, visceral, and neuropathic pain, based on pain quality and location.[249] It also measures pain intensity and captures the impact of pain on activity, sleep, and mood. A version 3 of the ISCIPBD is under review, and training materials and cases are available at the International Spinal Cord Society (https://www.iscos.org.uk/international-sci-pain-data-sets). Clinically, the ISCIPBD has advantages over other scales due to its flexibility to assess overall pain, or multiple distinct pain problems, or worst pain at a single or several locations. It also uses a standardized time period for reporting pain data, i.e., the last 7 days. Collecting information over a consistent time period improves detection of changes from one assessment to the next. Also, a pain drawing or map can be used to better present pain locations, types, and intensities and how they differ over assessments. For detailed tracking of potential treatment efficacy, a standardized approach is available in the expanded pain data set.[250]

Treatment for SCI-Induced Pain

As a physical therapist, the approach to treating neuropathic pain after SCI comes with some harsh realities. First, patients with SCI-related pain typically experience severe intensity and multiple types of pain at the same time.[245,251] Second, despite important scientific advances (reviewed above), the neural mechanism of pain in general and neuropathic pain specifically remain largely unidentified. Third, medical treatment for pain primarily relies on pharmacological interventions, but these are ineffective.[252,253] Fourth, living with persistent, unresponsive neuropathic pain after SCI causes significant, negative impacts on quality of life, often leading to depression.[253,254] Therefore, the National Pain Strategy was developed to improve the care and treatment of people with pain and emphasizes multidisciplinary treatment strategies to optimally manage pain.[255] Consumers with SCI-induced neuropathic pain identified barriers to pain management as pronounced negative side effects of prescribed medication, limited or no access to SCI pain experts, and poor access to non-pharmacological treatment options.[253]

Pharmacological Treatment

Future treatment for neuropathic pain after SCI will likely be multimodal and include approaches that have failed as a single treatment.

Pharmacological Options

Antiepiletics: The antiepileptics Gabapentin and Pregabalin are first line medications for SCI-Induced Neuropathic pain. Gabapentin trials show mixed effects on pain[256] while a meta-analysis of pregabalin randomized controlled trials found reduced pain relative to placebo controls.[257] The negative side effects of drowsiness, constipation, nausea, loss of balance, peripheral edema, and dizziness can outweigh their usefulness.[258] More importantly, new guidance calls for caution when prescribing gabapentinoids for neuropathic pain in SCI due to extremely high rates of misuse at 70 to 80%; notably, more severe neuropathic pain is associated with misuse.[259]

Opioids: The use of opioids as a potent analgesic is commonly used for pain management but is controversial for SCI-induced pain due to significant adverse side effects, including addiction, need for escalating dose concentrations to maintain potency, extreme interference with cognitive acuity, and pronounced constipation which interferes with bowel management.[256] Additionally, caregivers and people with SCI often want to avoid opioids and seek non-pharmacological approaches instead.[253]

Tricyclic Antidepressants: Tricyclic antidepressants (TCA) change afferent pain signals within the CNS and have some efficacy in general pain management. However, only one study has been done in SCI-induced neuropathic pain, and the TCA amitriptyline had no benefit.[256]

Cannabinoids: The growing legalization of *cannabis* for medical use in 37 U.S. states and recreational use in 19 states provides people with SCI access its pain-relieving effects.[260] Analgesic effects of cannabis have been recognized in Europe and the United States since the 1800s but have been in use since before 5000 BC.[260] Despite the long-recognized medicinal properties for complex conditions common in SCI, there is little scientific research available because of past reluctance to use federal funds on a recreational and still illicit drug in some states. The FDA has approved five cannabinoid medications (Dronabinol capsule and its liquid formulation Syndros, Nabilone capsule, Epidiolex, Nabiximol oromucosal spray), but none of these were approved for pain relief. The available meta-analyses on cannabinoid effects rarely include SCI and instead reflect unrelated conditions like cancer pain, rheumatoid arthritis, multiple sclerosis, fibromyalgia, and diabetic neuropathy.[261] Currently, only one meta-analysis for cannabinoid effects on SCI-induced pain exists, but it was comprised of only four studies and considered very low level of evidence.[262] Two studies showed no benefit relative to placebo, and two studies significantly reduced pain ratings by at least twice as much as placebo.[262] Scientists and clinicians recognize the complex nature of this potential treatment for SCI and advocate widely divergent perspectives.[263-265] Nonetheless, Physical Therapists should recognize that patients with SCI pain may likely use cannabis and its synthetic derivatives to treat neuropathic pain. It is also common for these patients to deny usage to avoid jeopardizing their health insurance.

Non-Pharmacological Treatment

Non-pharmacological treatment for SCI-induced neuropathic pain is in greater demand by patients with SCI and their families given that pain medications have limited efficacy. Emphasis on understanding pain and **behavioral self-management** strategies is growing.

Behavioral Self-Management: Behavioral pain management typically includes cognitive behavioral therapy (CBT), relaxation, and body awareness strategies. The goal of behavioral self-management is for the person living with neuropathic pain to manage symptoms, treatment, and psychosocial conditions associated with SCI-induced pain. Effective management involves controlling cognitive, behavioral, and emotional responses in order to sustain satisfaction with life.[266] Core skills of self-management are problem-solving, decision-making, resource utilization, building partnerships, taking action, and self-tailoring. Importantly, delivery of training by a multidisciplinary team of a psychologist, physical therapist, and nurse facilitates greater pain improvement, less depression, better sense of control, improved coping strategies, and gains in socialization.[266,267] Of particular interest, self-management techniques are effective in improving quality of life even without directly changing pain intensity.

Physical Exercise/Rehabilitation: Exercise has shown promise in reducing neuropathic pain and even normalizing sensation in experimental SCI by modulating trophic factors, inflammation, and synaptic plasticity.[129,232,268,269] In these pre-clinical studies, rhythmic weight bearing via treadmill stepping was more effective at reducing allodynia than rhythmic non-weight bearing during swimming or static weight bearing in standing.[129] Initiating weight bearing and stepping early after SCI was more effective than later after neuropathic pain had fully developed.[232,268-270] Translating and testing the potential benefits of exercise/neurorehabilitation to people with SCI-induced neuropathic pain is growing. Forms of training that were shown to reduce pain rely on moderate or high intensity and bouts lasting 30 to 90 minutes. One study examined the effects of a single bout of training while others reported pain reduction after long training programs of 4 weeks to 9 months. Effective types of training that reduced neuropathic pain in chronic SCI included (1) Arm ergometry and resistance training,[271] (2) robot-assisted gait training (Lokomat) and resistance training,[272] (3) a double-poling arm ergometry that simulates cross-country skiing,[273] (4) arm ergometry alone,[274] (5) exoskeleton gait with treadmill training with body weight support,[275] and (6) transcutaneous direct current stimulation (tDCS) of the primary motor cortex, followed by arm ergometry, resistance training, and stretching.[276] One pilot study was inconclusive when combining exoskeleton with body weight support treadmill training in chronic SCI.[277] When using rehabilitation and physical activity to treat neuropathic pain after SCI, the exercise itself can produce pain and stress, which is known to interfere with staying on a regular training schedule.[278] Additionally, pain reduction can occur within 30 minutes of a training bout while other people experience the benefit 4 weeks after the end of the training program.[274,275] In fact, individuals with SCI and neuropathic pain report that the most effective treatment for pain was physical therapy.[279]

Non-invasive Stimulation: Forms of electrical or magnetic stimulation administered cranially or peripherally have shown mixed results in reducing SCI-induced neuropathic pain. The most well-studied pain interventions use transcranial electrical stimulation and rely on constant direct current, tDCS, and, for magnetic stimulation, two forms are used transcranial magnetic stimulation (TMS) and repetitive TMS (rTMS). A recent systematic review with meta-analysis focused on tDCS and rTMS for neuropathic pain after SCI.[280] It confirmed that rTMS over the motor cortex produced analgesic effects on neuropathic pain 2 to 6 weeks after stimulation ended but not early (1 week) after stimulation. Four studies with proper controls assessed the efficacy of tDCS over the motor cortex, but each study used different time courses so no conclusions could be made.[280] At least two studies found tDCS reduced neuropathic pain within a few days of stimulation, but studies relying on tests completed weeks later found no benefit. More studies are needed with tDCS to explore if early analgesic effects are routinely seen, how long the effects last, and whether tDCS provided at weekly intervals produces stable pain relief.

In the periphery, TENS has been studied for neuropathic pain. A recent systematic review of TENS effects in SCI-induced neuropathic pain included only randomized control trials and found good potential for beneficial effects.[281] One study appeared to be an outlier while the others all showed decline in pain scores relative to unstimulated SCI controls. A clinical based study of SCI-induced neuropathic pain with only a TENS group also found a week-over-week decline in pain scores for the 8-week treatment.[282] To gain a more clear recommendation for the use of TENS as an effective pain treatment after SCI, several clinically related factors must be considered and optimized, including electrode placement relative to the pain location, stimulation frequency with regard to pain intensity, and the dose of treatment per session, number of sessions and duration across weeks.

New approaches for SCI-related Pain: Virtual reality (VR) therapy appears to reduce neuropathic pain after SCI as shown in a recent systematic review of nine publications.[283] These studies used either immersive VR in which the headset blocks the view of the surrounding environment or non-immersive VR where vision of the real world is maintained. A suggested mechanism of action in reducing neuropathic pain after SCI is that brain processing of the virtual images reverses maladaptive plasticity. Four types of VR training proved effective at reducing pain ratings by at least 20%. However, the translation to clinical use must await more detailed studies of the impact of first-person versus third-person point of view, identification of the optimal number and length of sessions, and the length of carry-over effects days or weeks after completing VR interventions. A trend suggested that SCI characteristics like lower level or incompleteness of injury influence the magnitude of pain reduction, but larger controlled clinical trials are needed.

The Weight Bearing Shoulder

During outpatient rehabilitation and then treatment for chronic SCI, focus on the kinematics of shoulder use during WC pushing and transfers should be carefully assessed on a regular basis to avoid faulty technique and lower injury risk. The need for WC training even in people with SCI with years of WC experience has been recommended in two randomized controlled trials and a meta-analysis.[209,284,285] Higher WC skills are associated with greater independence, more social participation, and less caregiver burden.[209] Recently, a web-based, WC transfer training program designed to be direct-to-user was tested for people with chronic SCI of 10 years or more.[286] Transfer training improved and was sustained one month later. Advantages of web-based training are that it requires no extra equipment, is done in the home where the majority of transfers occur, and avoids transportation barriers.[286]

Sexual Function

A return to home and integration back into their social environment will shift priorities to resumption of sexual activities for both men and women. Sexuality is a major contributor to an individual's identity and sense of self. One of the first concerns after SCI is sexuality. As early as is feasible, an open discussion regarding sexual function should take place and continue at each stage of rehabilitation. Although this section is placed in the outpatient rehabilitation section, it is important to continually address sexuality. An open, direct, and nonjudgmental approach will be needed to allow the individual to feel comfortable communicating fears and problems. Resuming sexual function will depend on the level of SCI and completeness of the injury (Table 13-15).

Treatment to improve erectile dysfunction in men relies on phosphodiesterase type V inhibitors, like Viagra. If these are not effective, then injectable intracavernosal medications, vacuum devices, and penile implants may be used. Achieving orgasm is more likely in incomplete SCI than when the injury is complete or in the sacral region. In men, who infrequently or do not ejaculate, vibration or electrical stimulation methods can be used to obtain semen to be used in fertilization technologies like in vitro fertilization. Smoking may have a negative effect on sexual function. Erection in men and lubrication in women depend on effective circulation and blood flow; smoking is known to reduce both of these.

Limitations in sexual function, for women, often include poor arousal and impaired orgasm. For the first 4 or 5 months after SCI, women will not have a menstrual cycle, but it returns within the first year. There are no apparent impairments in

TABLE 13-15	Limitations in Sexual Function After SCI	
SEXUAL FUNCTION	**MALE**	**FEMALE**
Cauda equina Conus medullaris	• No reflex erections • Occasional ejaculation	• Absent vaginal secretions • Fertility usually intact
Thoracic/cervical	• Short-duration reflex erections • Occasional ejaculation	• Vaginal secretions present • Fertility intact • Absent sensation of labor pain

fertility or carrying a baby to term for women. However, pregnancy can worsen complications of SCI including spasticity, autonomic dysreflexia, bladder problems, and mobility.

The role of the physical therapist will be twofold – use activity-based training with potential benefits for sexual function and assist with finding safe, effective positioning for sexual activity.

Activity-based Training: There is emerging evidence that activity-based training in the form of Locomotor Training on a treadmill alone or in combination with **epidural stimulation** exoskeleton-based gait training, improves aspects of sexual dysfunction.[24,112,287] It is noteworthy that a small but well-controlled study identified that general activity like arm ergometetry or stand training did not produce improvement in sexual dysfunction.[113] Instead, gains in sexual function align specifically with locomotor training and presumptive activation of lumbosacral pathways. Unlike bowel and bladder dysfunction, sexual dysfunction is not routinely included as a health outcome in SCI rehabilitation and recovery research despite its' major impact on negative quality of life. Recent consortiums and systematic reviews have called for clinical trials to include bowel, bladder, and sexual function as routine outcomes.[117,162] Use of autonomic basic data set and reflex function warrant inclusion in clinical practice in order to ensure that treatable aspects of sexual dysfunction can be identified.[288] Greater gains in sexual function may emerge with neuromodulation itself given that sacral nerve stimulation to pelvic floor muscles improved erectile function and eliminated the need for oral medication in some men.[289]

Positioning: Sexual function will require positioning when alone and with a partner. High pressures should not occur on any body parts, during sexual activity, due to risk of fracture, dislocation, or ligament damage. Contractures may require support with pillows to reduce pressure. The therapist will also need to recommend positions, while keeping in mind the contraindications for the injury site. Avoiding positions that trigger spasticity will be critical because spasticity is a significant barrier to sexual function alone or with a partner.

Depression

Depression is a serious complication of SCI and occurs at high rates, not only in individuals with SCI but also their caregivers. It has been estimated to be as high as 42% after SCI.[290] Depression is a constellation of symptoms of such frequency and severity to negatively affect functioning of the individual. Symptoms include weight loss, insomnia, near-daily fatigue or lethargy, feelings of worthlessness, difficulty thinking or concentrating, and recurring thoughts of death. Because many of these symptoms can also be caused by pain, medications, and the injury itself (sleep, weight changes), identifying depression is difficult, making it likely that many individuals with depression go untreated. Depression may be due, at least in part, to continual challenges that the individual with SCI must face and attempt to overcome, not the least of which are environmental barriers, social difficulties, and health problems.[291] Although these represent complex issues, they are all modifiable, which suggests that depression can be limited or prevented, using holistic approaches to the well-being of the individual with SCI.

CASE A, PART XI

Ms. Roberts suffered her SCI as part of a suicide attempt, which is a definitive sign of depression. Her mental health will need to be monitored closely, during each phase of rehabilitation. Mood elevators were part of her medical care, beginning in the acute setting. Her physical rehabilitation was prioritized so that she could better participate in psychotherapy and group therapy treatments in the near future. For her to participate in group therapy, she will need to regain the ability to be upright, have good endurance, and other functions.

Physical Therapy Management

Gait Training

Perhaps the greatest divergence between training approaches occurs when considering whether to use a compensatory or plasticity-based approach for gait training. The classic gait training approach uses assistive devices and bracing to compensate for lost muscle function. In contrast, a body-weight support program minimizes bracing and allows stepping without assistive devices. There is considerable animal and human evidence that this type of training promotes greater muscle activation and restores complex firing patterns even in individuals with AIS A complete SCI.[131,292,293] Factors that promote this improvement include walking at a normal walking speed of 2.0 m/s on a treadmill, reducing the load across the legs by 50% or less, and requiring active participation by the individual rather than passively using a robot.[294] Evidence in animal studies shows remarkable cellular plasticity associated with task-specific training.[295,296] Indeed, a recent study identified greater myelin plasticity above the SCI in response to treadmill training in both animals and humans.[130] Importantly, animals also had gains in locomotor functions as measured by kinematics.[130] Therefore, implementation of a **body-weight support** program for gait training takes the approach that such training produces gains in neuroplasticity, muscle activation, and recovery of function that otherwise would be difficult or impossible to attain.

It is important that the severity, level, and completeness of SCI be considered when selecting the type of rehabilitation training for gait and overall health outcomes. Indeed, people with SCI that do not recover walking have many new options in combination with or in lieu of locomotor training to regain this function. Indeed, new neuromodulation approaches represent truly innovative options for the most severe injuries at chronic time points. However, in people that can already walk by 6 months or later after incomplete SCI, a new clinical practice guideline endorsed the use of moderate- to high-intensity gait training (i.e., 70-85% heart rate maximum) to improve gait speed. Of note, the guideline considered recovery of locomotor speed across any CNS impairment but only two SCI studies were included. Stroke studies comprised the majority of evidence used to develop the clinical practice guideline. VR for walking training was also recommended. If people with SCI are not considered chronic or have other ambulation goals besides walking faster, then other treatment options should be explored. Neither acute/subacute SCI or goals related to spasticity, pain, hyperreflexia, etc., fall within the scope of the new clinical practice guideline.

A compensatory approach takes the view that no further recovery is possible and that walking will only be restored through the use of technology, bracing, and/or assistive devices. In addition to conventional training (described below), other compensatory walking systems include implantable FES devices and new, FDA-approved exoskeletons.

Implantable FES systems supply electrical stimulation to key muscle groups for standing and walking. A computer controls the pattern of stimulation. The primary drawback of these systems is that energy costs and fatigue are quite high, while the walking speed is very slow. A **non-implantable FES system** provides stimulation over the skin and has been most widely used to perform cycle ergometry rather than walking. The surface FES system is used for strengthening, conditioning, and reducing muscle atrophy.[297]

External FES systems use stimulation electrodes applied over key muscle groups of the extremities and/or trunk and integrated computer programs for up to 40 functional tasks. The first and most familiar of these tasks was FES cycling. Now, rehabilitation training with FES stimulation includes standing, walking, trunk control, and upper extremity and hand functions. Gains in leg muscle strength, muscle metabolic markers, and quality of life occur with FES cycling.[298] In a current clinical trial, benefits of FES cycling on cardio-metabolic risk factors are being studied by establishing muscle hypertrophy beforehand.[299]

Neuromuscular electrical stimulation (NMES) is similar to FES but the NMES muscle contractions aren't specifically organized to produce functional movements like FES. Common uses of NMES after SCI are to prevent muscle atrophy, induce muscle hypertrophy, and increase muscle force/strength.[300] Recent work shows that stimulation parameters with a long pulse width produce central neuroplasticity and may improve motor relearning after SCI.[301] Evidence of central activation is easily recognized because the EMG and muscle contraction after the NMES stimulus is off.[302]

Robotic/exoskeleton devices have been designed by engineers with the hope of creating lightweight robots to perform stepping in people with SCI. The **Lokomat system** is a robotic treadmill training system, in which the patient's lower limbs are passively moved. Another form of robotic stepper is a **computer-controlled exoskeleton**, which allows the wearer to move freely in the environment. The software uses kinematic variables of the user to individualize the stepping pattern as well as movements from sit to upright and standing. There are several FDA-approved exoskeletons for personal use, but the high cost, need for high level of function, and extensive training requirements prevent wide adoption by people with SCI.[162] Instead, exoskeletons have an expanding role in gait rehabilitation within inpatient and outpatient settings both on and off the treadmill. Recent systematic reviews and clinical trials studied efficacy of a wide variety of exoskeletons including experimental and FDA-approved devices. Gait training with exoskeletons can produce significant gains in trunk control, pulmonary function, number of responders with increased gait speed, walking distance,

walking kinematics, balance, and spasticity compared to pre-training or conventional physical therapy.[162,303–307] However, these benefits may not occur broadly because most studies are very small or show modest gait effects. It is noteworthy that most people with SCI screened for exoskeleton gait training are deemed ineligible due to non-erect posture, joint contractures, pronounced spasticity, large body size (height or BMI), and/or insufficient hand function to use the controller.[308] Several complications can occur with exoskeleton training including pressure injury of the skin, fractures due to misalignment of the device or falls, joint edema especially at the ankle, dizziness, and orthostatic hypotension.[162] The risks of exoskeleton training must be carefully considered relative to the potential gains because any adverse event will compromise the rehabilitation process.

Neuromodulation for gait training epidural stimulation relies on an implantable neural stimulator that lies on the dura of the lumbar spinal cord and delivers continuous electrical pulses to the dorsal root afferents, where they enter the cord.[31] The stimulator spans several cord segments and can be individualized to optimize responses. When this stimulation is combined with task-specific training to stand or to step on a treadmill, individuals with motor complete SCI (ASIA A and B) are able to voluntarily walk overground.[309,310] Recent advances in technology and precision of stimulation resulted in clear evidence that individuals with complete SCI can be trained to walk overground, swim and stand in the community.[309,310] However, these new skills could only be performed when the stimulator was turned on. The epidural stimulator augments lumbar circuitry so that supraspinal learning, plasticity, and control can produce volitional movements like starting and stopping movements or making them larger or smaller on command.[311] Epidural stimulation does not have FDA approval for clinical use, but research has grown exponentially since groundbreaking work in 2011.[312] Remarkably, many complex functions impaired by SCI also show strong benefit from epidural stimulation, including respiration,[313] cardiovascular dysfunction,[314–316] bladder voiding,[82,317] and bowel dysfunction.[118] That a single, all-be-it invasive, intervention can benefit motor function, balance, and a range of serious secondary impairments suggests that epidural stimulation holds promise as a future SCI treatment and FDA approval.

Transcutaneous spinal cord stimulation (tSCS) is non-invasive direct or alternating electrical current over the thoracolumbar back that stimulates dorsal roots as they enter the cord.[318] There is a surge of research and clinical interest in tSCS because it is less expensive, offers the potential of self-treatment since no surgery is required, and impacts motor control after SCI.[318,319] The mechanistic theory is that motor neurons below the injury level are activated by afferent fibers or interneurons receiving stimulation with tSCS.[318] Activation of muscles with tSCS after SCI was verified using EMG, and it activated different muscles when it was moved to lower segments, meaning that tSCS can prime the spinal cord so that rehabilitation and motor learning will be even greater. It also suggests that a variety of tSCS placements will facilitate a variety of recovery opportunities. In fact, multi-segmental muscle activation from a single tSCS stimulation site at T10-T11 appears to activate locomotor CPGs after SCI. With tSCS and activity-based training, gains in gait speed, coordination, and step cycle magnitude have been reported.[318,319] Importantly, two longitudinal, cross-over studies showed the tSCS and activity-based training improved hand function after complete cervical SCI[320] and sit-to-stand transfers after primarily chronic complete SCI.[321] Stimulation with tSCS to reduce spasticity in outpatient/chronic SCI was examined in a systematic review which identified limited evidence for its use.[151] Unfortunately, no research has been done to establish that the tSCS effects outlast the intervention, and no randomized clinical trials have been conducted.[318] While promising results of tSCS are available for SCI, the absence of high-level research, clinical trials and the scope of adverse outcomes points to delayed adoption as standard of care for outpatient and chronic SCI rehabilitation.

Conventional Compensatory Gait Training

The focus of this rehabilitation will be to strengthen available arm and trunk muscles, stretch the hip to allow hip extension, and then progress to working with braces, the FES system, or exoskeletons. The physical characteristics required for conventional gait training include the following:

- Absence of hip flexion contracture. Ideally, hip ROM into hyperextension would be present because this position activates the CPG and initiates the swing phase of locomotion.
- Absence of knee flexor contractures or plantar flexor contractures. Poor limb alignment will decrease stability and prevent balance.
- Good strength in shoulder depressors and ability to support full weight through the arms without pain. This facilitates the use of crutches or a walker.
- Low levels of spasticity or well-controlled spasticity. High tone restricts movement and spasms or clonus can cause loss of balance or falls.
- Good trunk control. For people with LMN injury, the lower extremity will be advanced using momentum created by trunk and pelvic rotation. Trunk control will also be required to maintain dynamic, upright balance, during walking.
- Dynamic balance in standing. This allows assistive devices and the lower extremities to be lifted and moved.
- Low risk of fracture. Osteoporosis is highest in complete SCI and at long periods after injury.
- Non-erratic blood pressure. Standing upright will challenge the cardiovascular system more than a seated upright position. This will be compounded by high physical exertion needed to stabilize with the arms and advance the legs.
- Highly motivated. Gait training is a strenuous activity demanding significant practice in order to develop the skill.

The individual will need to be able to don, doff, and manipulate the braces. The type of brace will depend on the impairments, related to the level of SCI (Table 13-16). Braces will be needed if knee hyperextension occurs and/or if ankle dorsiflexion is weak or absent. Braces protect the joint and also prevent leg collapse, when weight is placed on the limb. The initial phase

TABLE 13-16	Types of Braces for Different Levels of SCI
BRACE TYPE	**PURPOSE**
Reciprocal gait orthosis (RGO)	SCI T5–7 Facilitates hip flexion on one side simultaneously with hip extension on the opposite side
Hip-knee-ankle-foot orthosis (HKAFO)	SCI T5–7 Stabilizes the hip
Knee-ankle-foot orthosis (KAFO)	SCI T8–12 Used if quadriceps strength is less than 3/5; stance controlled knee joints are triggered by heel contact
Ankle foot orthosis (AFO)	SCI any level Provides toe clearance and helps with knee control
FES for dorsiflexion	SCI any level A cuff placed around the upper shank that delivers electrical impulses to the tibialis anterior at the appropriate point in the step cycle to produce dorsiflexion and then shuts off
Supra-malleolar orthosis (SMO)	SCI any level To control roll-over of the ankles

will take place in the parallel bars, while wearing the braces. Activities that emphasize trunk balance with and without hand support, transfers, and walking will allow the therapist to determine the safety and feasibility of progressing to working outside the parallel bars. Once free of the parallel bars, the individual will work on mobility skills, such as transferring from the WC, walking with different assistive devices, and negotiating rough terrain, inclines, and stairs. Conventional gait training may be the best option for individuals that have failed to respond to other forms of gait training.

Task-dependent Training for Locomotion

Use of body-weight supported locomotion has been extensively used in the clinic over the last 10 years or more. Three different types have been used: (1) Lokomat robotic system, (2) manually assisted training, generally referred to as Locomotor Training, and (3) a ceiling-mounted support system for overground training. While these systems have received great scrutiny of late, a randomized clinical trial in subacute SCI (inpatient and outpatient rehabilitation) established that Locomotor Training was as effective at improving gait speed and function as an overground gait training program matched for intensity.[322] A trial comparing the Lokomat Treadmill Training system found no difference from conventional therapy.[323] In chronic individuals with SCI, there have been at least 10 studies that compared functional performance before and after a treadmill training program and 5 randomized controlled trials. Across all studies, about 70% of patients improved following treatment.[297] Some studies show that Locomotor Training increased strength, balance, gait speed, and gait distance,[23,324] while others report the greatest gains to be with body weight support, FES, and overground rather than treadmill training.[295] Importantly, Lokomat training had no benefit compared to other types of training.[295] Factors that appear to predict a good training effect and improved gait speed include shorter time since injury, lower levels of spasticity, voluntary bowel and bladder voiding, and walking speed before training.[325] In other words, individuals with greater capacity prior to training are the most likely to become fast walkers.

Locomotor Training Objectives

When using task-dependent techniques, encourage as much active movement as possible and provide as little assistance as needed. Walking is likely mediated by CPGs in the lumbar spinal cord that produce rhythmic, symmetrical stepping[326–328] (see Chapter 4 for description of CPG function). The CPG responds to afferent input from the limbs and integrates descending input from the brain to produce purposeful walking. After SCI, descending control is minimal, making the role of the afferent input more important. Training emphasizes sensory cues that induce stepping including the following:[329]

- Use normal walking speeds of 2.0 m/s or higher.
- Maximize tolerable load on the stance limb without the knee buckling, typically no greater than 50% of the body weight is unloaded.
- Maintain good upright alignment of the head and body.
- Reproduce normal movements of walking with the hip, knee, and ankle.
- Synchronize hip extension of one limb with loading of the other. Hip extension induces swing so the contralateral limb must be in or near stance when extension is reached.
- Avoid weight-bearing through the upper limbs because it inhibits EMG activity in the lower extremities.[330]
- Produce synchronized symmetrical coordination between the limbs by using equal step lengths, swing times, and arm swing.
- Reduce abnormal sensory stimulation, when assisting the movement. For stance, place the hands on extensor surfaces to increase extensor afferent cues. To assist swing, place hands on the flexor surfaces to increase flexor afferent cues.

Trainers are positioned at the pelvis, each leg, and the computer/treadmill controls. There are two components of training: (1) on the treadmill and (2) overground training. The retraining component uses manual assistance to reproduce normal stepping, as closely as possible. The trainers will adapt their assistance from step to step as they move the legs and pelvis/trunk. The second component is adaptability training, which requires the individual with SCI to reproduce the normal kinematics of stepping with as little assistance as possible. Adaptability training allows trial and error and places more emphasis on proximal trunk control, before reducing assistance at the lower joints.

Retraining and adaptability components are used for stepping and standing, while on the treadmill, and the treatment session is typically 1 hour.

Overground training translates the skills developed on the treadmill to daily activities, transfers, and mobility. During this training, it is important to avoid abnormal sensory cues. Things like braces and certain assistive devices may inhibit activity and should be avoided during treadmill and overground training sessions. Assistive devices that encourage weight-bearing through the arms and a forward-leaning trunk prevent the hip from extending and reduce the signals to initiate swing. During overground training, assistive devices should promote an upright trunk and allow higher gait speeds (e.g., a high, rolling platform walker for individuals that need greater support). For individuals with more motor control, a rolling walker that is elevated to minimize weight through the arms will better reinforce normal body position and allow faster speeds than a standard walker.

Assessment

Gait speed, assessed via the 10-m walk test or the 6-minute walk test, reflects functional performance and a return to participation in the community.[331] The minimal gait speed threshold for individuals with SCI to become community ambulators is 0.44 m/s, which is lower than has been reported for stroke. This threshold was first defined in Europe[332] and later confirmed in the United States.[331] Therapists can use this benchmark for treatment progression. Also, there is value in collecting gait speed, using both walking tests rather than the traditional 10-m walk test alone.[331] In chronic SCI, the 6-minute walk test appears to reflect endurance (the ability to sustain gait speed); whereas the 10-m walk test might translate to a short burst of speed. The **Walking Index for Spinal Cord Injury II** is a highly recommended measure of walking recovery; however, it is based on the use of braces, which task-dependent training tries to avoid.[333] The **Spinal Cord Independence Measure III** is a patient report tool that assesses activities of daily living, coordination, eating, functional mobility, respiration, and incontinence.[334] High SCIM scores are associated with better balance, upper limb control, muscle strength, and ambulation. Because the SCIM was specifically designed for SCI, it offers more detailed and appropriate assessment of functional independence than the more general Functional Independent Measure (FIM).

> ## CASE A, PART XII
>
> Because Ms. Roberts is showing continual gains in muscle activation and strength, her gait training program should start with a task-dependent neuroplasticity approach and wait to add compensatory components until recovery has plateaued. A Locomotor Training program, using a treadmill and body-weight support, would best match her current functional abilities. An overground body-weight support program might be feasible, in the future, as greater trunk control returns and her ability to manage assistive devices with her hand improves. The initial focus during adaptability

training will be to independently maintain the head and shoulders over the pelvis during standing and walking. In retraining, the focus will be to improve her endurance and tolerance of being upright. Hypotension, pain aggravation, and fatigue are likely for her because the level of her SCI is so high. Spasticity may worsen initially and then improve, due to greater time spent upright and weight-bearing. Avoid increasing spasticity medications and try to reduce them, if possible, in order to promote greater neuroplasticity from training. Progression will include reducing body-weight support and increasing treadmill speed. As the ability to take volitional steps returns and improves, stepping over obstacles, placed on the moving treadmill belt, can be added. During overground training, stepping without braces will help translate skills from the treadmill. Therapists will initially need to provide manual assistance, but as recovery occurs, Ms. Roberts should be encouraged to reproduce the stepping patterns from the treadmill.

Lifelong Considerations

Syringomyelia

Syringomyelia is the formation of a cerebrospinal fluid-filled cyst within the center of the spinal cord. It develops within months to many years after traumatic SCI and can be devastating because as the lesion expands it takes away important motor functions.[335] The symptoms of late-onset syringomyelia will be a change in sensorimotor function like radicular pain, sensory loss, segmental weakness, gait ataxia, and increased spasticity.[336] Of serious concern, is the development of syringomyelia within the cervical region because it threatens diaphragm innervation and respiration. The most typical treatments for this condition include placing a shunt to remove the CSF from the cyst to slow its progression or untethering the cord, which is a procedure that removes the scar adhesions between the cord and the dura. The role of the physical therapist, in this condition, is to differentiate the cause of any loss of function. Because the cyst is slow growing, the rate of functional loss will be slow rather than sudden, making it more difficult to recognize. A small loss of function across more than one system (e.g., sensory and motor) warrants a closer examination for syringomyelia.

Cardiovascular Deconditioning

Cardiovascular disease (CVD) is the term used to capture problems of the heart and blood vessels. It is present in 30 to 50% of individuals with SCI[337,338] and increases to 60 to 70%, when asymptomatic disease is included.[339] Unfortunately, death due to CVD is higher in people with SCI than able-bodied individuals.[337,338] Causes of CVD are a combination of loss of adrenergic control, poor diet, and physical inactivity. Adrenergic dysfunction is related to the level of SCI and directly impacts cardiac function.

- T1: No supraspinal sympathetic control
- T1–T5: Partial preservation of sympathetic control
- Below T5: Full supraspinal sympathetic control

Because SCI lesion level cannot be changed, efforts to reduce CVD must focus on modifiable factors such as physical activity. The role of the physical therapist is to promote a healthy lifestyle and create a long-term fitness program for individuals with SCI. The prevalence of CVD suggests that after SCI, daily activity using a WC and other assistance is insufficient to maintain cardiovascular health. Several physical therapy interventions have proven effective in improving cardiac function:[340]

- Treadmill training with body weight support
- FES leg cycling of moderate to high intensity several times a week
- FES leg cycling combined with arm ergometry
- Aerobic arm cycling of moderate intensity several times a week

---

CASE A, PART XIII

Following her inpatient rehabilitation, Ms. Roberts spent time in a psychiatric hospital and then lived with friends for several months, while she participated in outpatient physical therapy. She ultimately returned to living in her home, during her outpatient rehabilitation. Following 9 months of rehabilitation, Ms. Roberts was discharged with the ability to ambulate independently, using a straight cane. Right toe dragging, due to plantarflexor spasticity and weak dorsiflexors, required compensation with a Walkaide® electrical stimulator. She was able to ascend and descend stairs, using a handrail on the left. Upper limb function recovered extensively on the left, and gains in function of the right hand, as well as sensation, occurred, with somatosensory stimulation and massed practice. A home fitness program, including stationary cycling, strengthening, and stretching, was implemented. Neuropathic pain was controlled by gabapentin. Her depression was being medically managed, and she no longer attended group therapy. She was unable to return to work because of the physical demands and hand skills it required.

REFERENCES

1. Profyris C, Cheema SS, Zang D, Azari MF, Boyle K, Petratos S. Degenerative and regenerative mechanisms governing spinal cord injury. *Neurobiol Dis.* 2004;15:415-436.

2. Alizadeh A, Dyck SM, Karimi-Abdolrezaee S. Traumatic spinal cord injury: an overview of pathophysiology, models and acute injury mechanisms. *Front Neurol.* 2019;10:282.

3. Saremi J, Mahmoodi N, Rasouli M, et al. Advanced approaches to regenerate spinal cord injury: the development of cell and tissue engineering therapy and combinational treatments. *Biomed Pharmacother.* 2022;146:112529.

4. Yamazaki K, Kawabori M, Seki T, Houkin K. Clinical trials of stem cell treatment for spinal cord injury. *Int J Mol Sci.* 2020;21:3994.

5. National Spinal Cord Injury Statistical Center. Spinal Cord Injury Facts and Figures at a Glance. University of Alabama at Birmingham. nscisc.uab.edu. (2021).

6. Mahmoudi E, Meade MA, Forchheimer MB, Fyffe DC, Krause JS, Tate D. Longitudinal analysis of hospitalization after spinal cord injury: variation based on race and ethnicity. *Arch Phys Med Rehabil.* 2014;95:2158-2166.

7. McKinley WO, Tewksbury MA, Mujteba NM. Spinal stenosis vs traumatic spinal cord injury: a rehabilitation outcome comparison. *J Spinal Cord Med*. 2002;25:28-32.

8. Burns SP, Weaver F, Chin A, Svircev J, Carbone L. Cervical stenosis in spinal cord injury and disorders. *J Spinal Cord Med*. 2016;39:471-475.

9. Tatarek NE. Variation in the human cervical neural canal. *Spine J*. 2005;5:623-631.

10. West TW. Transverse myelitis: a review of the presentation, diagnosis, and initial management. *Discov Med*. 2013;16:167-177.

11. Kirshblum S, Snider B, Rupp R, Read MS. Updates of the International Standards for Neurologic Classification of Spinal Cord Injury: 2015 and 2019. *Phys Med Rehabil Clin N Am*. 2020;31:319-330.

12. Burns S, Biering-Sørensen F, Donovan W, et al. International standards for neurological classification of spinal cord injury, revised 2011. *Top Spinal Cord Inj Rehabil*. 2012;18:85-99.

13. ASIA. International Standards Training e-Learning Program (InSTeP). asia-spinalinjury.org/learning.

14. Crozier KS, Graziani V, Ditunno JF Jr., Herbison GJ. Spinal cord injury: prognosis for ambulation based on sensory examination in patients who are initially motor complete. *Arch Phys Med Rehabil*. 1991;72:119-121.

15. Waters RL, Adkins RH, Yakura JS, Sie I. Motor and sensory recovery following incomplete tetraplegia. *Arch Phys Med Rehabil*. 1994;75:306-311.

16. Spiess MR, Müller RM, Rupp R, Schuld C, van Hedel HJA. Conversion in ASIA impairment scale during the first year after traumatic spinal cord injury. *J Neurotrauma*. 2009;26:2027-2036.

17. van Middendorp JJ, Hosman AJ, Pouw MH, Van de Meent H. ASIA impairment scale conversion in traumatic SCI: is it related with the ability to walk? A descriptive comparison with functional ambulation outcome measures in 273 patients. *Spinal Cord*. 2009;47:555-560.

18. Marino RJ, Leff M, Cardenas DD, et al. Trends in rates of ASIA impairment scale conversion in traumatic complete spinal cord injury. *Neurotrauma Rep*. 2020;1:192-200.

19. Kirshblum S, Botticello A, Benedetto J, Eren F, Donovan J, Marino R. Characterizing natural recovery of people with initial motor complete tetraplegia. *Arch Phys Med Rehabil*. 2022;103:649-656.

20. Kalsi-Ryan S, Beaton D, Curt A, Popovic MR, Verrier MC, Fehlings MG. Outcome of the upper limb in cervical spinal cord injury: Profiles of recovery and insights for clinical studies. *J Spinal Cord Med*. 2014;37:503-510.

21. Dukes EM, Kirshblum S, Aimetti AA, Qin SS, Bornheimer RK, Oster G. Relationship of American Spinal Injury Association Impairment Scale grade to post-injury hospitalization and costs in thoracic spinal cord injury. *Neurosurgery*. 2018;83:445-451.

22. Kirshblum S, Millis S, McKinley W, Tulsky D. Late neurologic recovery after traumatic spinal cord injury. *Arch Phys Med Rehabil*. 2004;85:1811-1817.

23. Buehner JJ, Forrest GF, Schmidt-Read M, White S, Tansey K, Basso DM. Relationship between ASIA examination and functional outcomes in the NeuroRecovery Network locomotor training program. *Arch Phys Med Rehabil*. 2012;93:1530-1540.

24. Morrison SA, Lorenz D, Eskay CP, Forrest GF, Basso DM. Longitudinal recovery and reduced costs after 120 sessions of locomotor training for motor incomplete spinal cord injury. *Arch Phys Med Rehabil*. 2018;99:555-562.

25. Forrest GF, Lorenz DJ, Hutchinson K, et al. Ambulation and balance outcomes measure different aspects of recovery in individuals with chronic, incomplete spinal cord injury. *Arch Phys Med Rehabil*. 2012;93:1553-1564.

26. Bunge RP, Puckett WR, Becerra JL, Marcillo A, Quencer RM. Observations on the pathology of human spinal cord injury. a review and classification of 22 new cases with details from a case of chronic cord compression with extensive focal demyelination. *Adv Neurol*. 1993;59:75-89.

27. Bunge RP, Puckett WR, Hiester ED. Observations on the pathology of several types of human spinal cord injury, with emphasis on the astrocyte response to penetrating injuries. *Adv Neurol*. 1997;72:305-315.

28. Gill ML, Grahn PJ, Calvert JS, et al. Neuromodulation of lumbosacral spinal networks enables independent stepping after complete paraplegia. *Nat Med*. 2018;24:1677-1682.

29. Grahn PJ, Lavrov IA, Sayenko DG, et al. Enabling task-specific volitional motor functions via spinal cord neuromodulation in a human with paraplegia. *Mayo Clin Proc*. 2017;92:544-554.

30. Minassian K, Jilge B, Rattay F, et al. Stepping-like movements in humans with complete spinal cord injury induced by epidural stimulation of the lumbar cord: electromyographic study of compound muscle action potentials. *Spinal Cord*. 2004;42:401-416.

31. Angeli CA, Edgerton VR, Gerasimenko YP, Harkema SJ. Altering spinal cord excitability enables voluntary movements after chronic complete paralysis in humans. *Brain* 2014;137:1394-1409.

32. Basso DM, Velozo C, Lorenz D, Suter S, Behrman AL. Interrater reliability of the neuromuscular recovery scale for spinal cord injury. *Arch Phys Med Rehabil*. 2015;96:1397-1403.

33. Behrman AL, Velozo C, Suter S, Lorenz D, Basso DM. Test-retest reliability of the neuromuscular recovery scale. *Arch Phys Med Rehabil*. 2015;96:1375-1384.

34. Velozo C, Moorhouse M, Ardolino E, et al. Validity of the neuromuscular recovery scale: a measurement model approach. *Arch Phys Med Rehabil*. 2015;96:1385-1396.

35. Tester NJ, Lorenz DJ, Suter SP, et al. Responsiveness of the neuromuscular recovery scale during outpatient activity-dependent rehabilitation for spinal cord injury. *Neurorehabil Neural Repair*. 2016;30:528-538.

36. Wan IY, Angelini GD, Bryan AJ, Ryder I, Underwood MJ. Prevention of spinal cord ischaemia during descending thoracic and thoracoabdominal aortic surgery. *Eur J Cardiothorac Surg*. 2001;19:203-213.

37. Awad H, Tili E, Nuovo G, et al. Endovascular repair and open repair surgery of thoraco-abdominal aortic aneurysms cause drastically different types of spinal cord injury. *Sci Rep*. 2021;11:7834.

38. Attabib N, Kurban D, Cheng CL, et al. Factors associated with recovery in motor strength, walking ability, and bowel and bladder function after traumatic cauda equina injury. *J Neurotrauma*. 2021;38:322-329.

39. Brouwers E, van de Meent H, Curt A, Starremans B, Hosman A, Bartels R. Definitions of traumatic conus medullaris and cauda equina syndrome: a systematic literature review. *Spinal Cord*. 2017;55:886-890.

40. Mirza SK, Krengel WF 3rd, Chapman JR, et al. Early versus delayed surgery for acute cervical spinal cord injury. *Clin Orthop Relat Res*. 1999;359:104-114.

41. Gaebler C, Maier R, Kutscha-Lissberg F, Mrkonjic L, Vecsei V. Results of spinal cord decompression and thoracolumbar pedicle stabilisation in relation to the time of operation. *Spinal Cord*. 1999;37:33-39.

42. Fehlings MG, Vaccaro A, Wilson JR, et al. Early versus delayed decompression for traumatic cervical spinal cord injury: results of the surgical timing in acute spinal cord injury study (STASCIS). *PLoS One*. 2012;7:e32037.

43. Wilson JR, Witiw CD, Badhiwala J, Kwon BK, Fehlings MG, Harrop JS. Early surgery for traumatic spinal cord injury: where are we now? *Global Spine J*. 2020;10:84s-91s.

44. Bracken MB, Shepard MJ, Hellenbrand KG, et al. Methylprednisolone and neurological function 1 year after spinal cord injury. results of the national acute spinal cord injury study. *J Neurosurg*. 1985;63:704-713.

45. Bracken MB, Shepard MJ, Holford TR, et al. Administration of methylprednisolone for 24 or 48 hours or tirilazad mesylate for 48 hours in the treatment of acute spinal cord injury. Results of the Third National Acute Spinal Cord Injury Randomized Controlled Trial. National Acute Spinal Cord Injury Study. *JAMA*. 1997;277:1597-1604.

46. Anderson P. New CNS/AANS guidelines discourage steroids in spinal injury. *Medscape*. 2013. www.medscape.com/viewarticle/781669?msclkid=9616e27ab5d611ec89aa584a92126984.

47. Furlan JC, Fehlings MG. Cardiovascular complications after acute spinal cord injury: pathophysiology, diagnosis, and management. *Neurosurg Focus*. 2008;25:E13.

48. Wecht JM. Management of blood pressure disorders in individuals with spinal cord injury. *Curr Opin Pharmacol.* 2022;62:60-63.

49. Squair JW, Bélanger LM, Tsang A, et al. Spinal cord perfusion pressure predicts neurologic recovery in acute spinal cord injury. *Neurology.* 2017;89:1660-1667.

50. Hawryluk G, Whetstone W, Saigal R, et al. Mean arterial blood pressure correlates with neurological recovery after human spinal cord injury: analysis of high frequency physiologic data. *J Neurotrauma.* 2015;32:1958-1967.

51. Krassioukov A, Biering-Sørensen F, Donovan W, et al. International standards to document remaining autonomic function after spinal cord injury. *J Spinal Cord Med.* 2012;35:201-210.

52. ASIA. Autonomic Standards Training E-Program (ASTeP). asia-spinalinjury.org/learning/.

53. Katzelnick CG, Weir JP, Jones A, et al. Blood pressure instability in persons with SCI: evidence from a 30-day home monitoring observation. *Am J Hypertens.* 2019;32:938-944.

54. Wecht JM, Weir JP, Katzelnick CG, et al. Double-blinded, placebo-controlled crossover trial to determine the effects of midodrine on blood pressure during cognitive testing in persons with SCI. *Spinal Cord.* 2020;58:959-969.

55. Carlozzi NE, Fyffe D, Morin KG, et al. Impact of blood pressure dysregulation on health-related quality of life in persons with spinal cord injury: development of a conceptual model. *Arch Phys Med Rehabil.* 2013;94:1721-1730.

56. Zhu C, Galea M, Livote E, Signor D, Wecht JM. A retrospective chart review of heart rate and blood pressure abnormalities in veterans with spinal cord injury. *J Spinal Cord Med.* 2013;36:463-475.

57. Furlan JC, Fehlings MG. Role of screening tests for deep venous thrombosis in asymptomatic adults with acute spinal cord injury: an evidence-based analysis. *Spine.* 2007;32:1908-1916.

58. Vogel L, Betz R, Mulcahey MJ. Pediatric spinal cord disorders. In: Kirshblum S, Campagnolo DI, eds. *Spinal Cord Medicine.* Philadelphia: Lippincott Williams & Wilkins; 2011:533-564.

59. Weidner N, Müller OJ, Hach-Wunderle V, et al. Prevention of thromboembolism in spinal cord injury: S1 guideline. *Neurol Res Pract.* 2020;2:43.

60. Mammen EF. Pathogenesis of venous thrombosis. *Chest.* 1992;102:640s-644s.

61. Rossi EC, Green D, Rosen JS, Spies SM, Jao JS. Sequential changes in factor VIII and platelets preceding deep vein thrombosis in patients with spinal cord injury. *Br J Haematol.* 1980;45:143-151.

62. Mackiewicz-Milewska M, Jung S, Kroszczyński AC, et al. Deep venous thrombosis in patients with chronic spinal cord injury. *J Spinal Cord Med.* 2016;39:400-404.

63. Giorgi Pierfranceschi M, Donadini MP, Dentali F, et al. The short- and long-term risk of venous thromboembolism in patients with acute spinal cord injury: a prospective cohort study. *Thromb Haemost.* 2013;109:34-38.

64. Maung AA, Schuster KM, Kaplan LJ, Maerz LL, Davis KA. Risk of venous thromboembolism after spinal cord injury: not all levels are the same. *J Trauma.* 2011;71:1241-1245.

65. Matsumoto S, Suda K, Iimoto S, et al. Prospective study of deep vein thrombosis in patients with spinal cord injury not receiving anticoagulant therapy. *Spinal Cord.* 2015;53:306-309.

66. Hon B, Botticello A, Kirshblum S. Duplex ultrasound surveillance for deep vein thrombosis after acute traumatic spinal cord injury at rehabilitation admission. *J Spinal Cord Med.* 2020;43:298-305.

67. Krassioukov A, Linsenmeyer TA, Beck LA, et al. Evaluation and management of autonomic dysreflexia and other autonomic dysfunctions: preventing the highs and lows. *J Spinal Cord Med.* 2021;44:631-683.

68. Allen KJ, Leslie SW. Autonomic dysreflexia. In: *StatPearls [Internet].* Treasure Island, FL: StatPearls Publishing; 2022. www.ncbi.nlm.nih.gov/books/NBK482434/.

69. Schwab JM, Zhang Y, Kopp MA, Brommer B, Popovich PG. The paradox of chronic neuroinflammation, systemic immune suppression, autoimmunity after traumatic chronic spinal cord injury. *Exp Neurol.* 2014;258:121-129.

70. Brommer B, Engel O, Kopp MA, et al. Spinal cord injury-induced immune deficiency syndrome enhances infection susceptibility dependent on lesion level. *Brain.* 2016;139:692-707.

71. Failli V, Kopp MA, Gericke C, et al. Functional neurological recovery after spinal cord injury is impaired in patients with infections. *Brain.* 2012;135:3238-3250.

72. Kopp MA, Watzlawick R, Martus P, et al. Long-term functional outcome in patients with acquired infections after acute spinal cord injury. *Neurology.* 2017;88:892-900.

73. Welk B, Fuller A, Razvi H, Denstedt J. Renal stone disease in spinal-cord-injured patients. *J Endourol.* 2012;26:954-959.

74. Wyndaele JJ, Birch B, Borau A, et al. Surgical management of the neurogenic bladder after spinal cord injury. *World J Urol.* 2018;36:1569-1576.

75. Saadat SH, Shepherd S, Van Asseldonk B, Elterman DS. Clean intermittent catheterization: single use vs. reuse. *Can Urol Assoc J.* 2019;13:64-69.

76. Cooley LF, Kielb S. A review of botulinum toxin A for the treatment of neurogenic bladder. *PM R.* 2019;11:192-200.

77. Hu M, Lai S, Zhang Y, Liu M, Wang J. Sacral neuromodulation for lower urinary tract dysfunction in spinal cord injury: a systematic review and meta-analysis. *Urol Int.* 2019;103:337-343.

78. Garcia-Arguello LY, O'Horo JC, Farrell A, et al. Infections in the spinal cord-injured population: a systematic review. *Spinal Cord.* 2017;55:526-534.

79. Edokpolo LU, Stavris KB, Foster HE Jr. Intermittent catheterization and recurrent urinary tract infection in spinal cord injury. *Top Spinal Cord Inj Rehabil.* 2012;18:187-192.

80. Krassioukov A, Cragg JJ, West C, Voss C, Krassioukov-Enns D. The good, the bad and the ugly of catheterization practices among elite athletes with spinal cord injury: a global perspective. *Spinal Cord.* 2015;53:78-82.

81. Singh R, Rohilla RK, Sangwan K, Siwach R, Magu NK, Sangwan SS. Bladder management methods and urological complications in spinal cord injury patients. *Indian J Orthop.* 2011;45:141-147.

82. Herrity AN, Aslan SC, Ugiliweneza B, Mohamed AZ, Hubscher CH, Harkema SJ. Improvements in bladder function following activity-based recovery training with epidural stimulation after chronic spinal cord injury. *Front Syst Neurosci.* 2021;14:614691.

83. Galeiras Vazquez R, Rascado Sedes P, Mourelo Farina M., Montoto Marques A., Ferreiro Velasco ME. Respiratory management in the patient with spinal cord injury. *Biomed Res Int.* 2013;2013:168757.

84. Consortium for Spinal Cord Medicine. Respiratory management following spinal cord injury: a clinical practice guideline for health-care professionals. *J Spinal Cord Med.* 2005;28:259-293.

85. Julia PE, Sa'ari MY, Hasnan N. Benefit of triple-strap abdominal binder on voluntary cough in patients with spinal cord injury. *Spinal Cord.* 2011;49:1138-1142.

86. Edsberg LE, Black JM, Goldberg M, McNichol L, Moore L, Sieggreen M. Revised national pressure ulcer advisory panel pressure injury staging system: revised pressure injury staging system. *J Wound Ostomy Continence Nurs.* 2016;43:585-597.

87. Gelis A, Dupeyron A, Legros P, Benaïm C, Pelissier J, Fattal C. Pressure ulcer risk factors in persons with SCI: Part I: Acute and rehabilitation stages. *Spinal Cord.* 2009;47:99-107.

88. DiVita MA, Granger CV, Goldstein R, Niewczyk P, Freudenheim JL. Risk factors for development of new or worsened pressure ulcers among patients in inpatient rehabilitation facilities in the United States: data from the uniform data system for medical rehabilitation. *PM R.* 2015;7:599-612.

89. Gelis A, Dupeyron A, Legros P, Benaïm C, Pelissier J, Fattal C. Pressure ulcer risk factors in persons with spinal cord injury part 2: the chronic stage. *Spinal Cord.* 2009;47:651-661.

90. Niazi ZB, Salzberg CA, Byrne DW, Viehbeck M. Recurrence of initial pressure ulcer in persons with spinal cord injuries. *Adv Wound Care.* 1997;10:38-42.

91. Shiferaw WS, Akalu TY, Mulugeta H, Aynalem YA. The global burden of pressure ulcers among patients with spinal cord injury: a systematic review and meta-analysis. *BMC Musculoskelet Disord.* 2020;21:334.

92. Consortium for Spinal Cord Medicine. Pressure Ulcer Prevention and Treatment Following Spinal Cord Injury: A Clinical Practice Guideline for Health-Care Professionals. Second Edition. pva.org/research-resources/publications/clinical-practice-guidelines/. (2014).

93. Pickham D, Berte N, Pihulic M, Valdez A, Mayer B, Desai M. Effect of a wearable patient sensor on care delivery for preventing pressure injuries in acutely ill adults: a pragmatic randomized clinical trial (LS-HAPI study). *Int J Nurs Stud*. 2018;80:12-19.

94. Krause JS, Vines CL, Farley TL, Sniezek J, Coker J. An exploratory study of pressure ulcers after spinal cord injury: relationship to protective behaviors and risk factors. *Arch Phys Med Rehabil*. 2001;82:107-113.

95. Nino-Murcia M, Vincent ME, Vaughan C, et al. Esophagography and esophagoscopy. Comparison in the examination of patients with head and neck carcinoma. *Arch Otolaryngol Head Neck Surg*. 1990;116:917-199.

96. Krassioukov A, Eng JJ, Claxton G, Sakakibara BM, Shum S. Neurogenic bowel management after spinal cord injury: a systematic review of the evidence. *Spinal Cord*. 2010;48:718-733.

97. Glickman S, Kamm MA. Bowel dysfunction in spinal-cord-injury patients. *Lancet*. 1996;347:1651-1653.

98. Johns J, Krogh K, Rodriguez GM, et al. Management of neurogenic bowel dysfunction in adults after spinal cord injury. *J Spinal Cord Med*. 2021;44:442-510.

99. Coggrave M, Norton C, Wilson-Barnett J. Management of neurogenic bowel dysfunction in the community after spinal cord injury: a postal survey in the United Kingdom. *Spinal Cord*. 2009;47:323-330; quiz 331-3.

100. Burns AS, St-Germain D, Connolly M, et al. Phenomenological study of neurogenic bowel from the perspective of individuals living with spinal cord injury. *Arch Phys Med Rehabil*. 2015;96:49-55.

101. Rosito O, Nino-Murcia M, Wolfe VA, Kiratli BJ, Perkash I. The effects of colostomy on the quality of life in patients with spinal cord injury: a retrospective analysis. *J Spinal Cord Med*. 2002;25:174-183.

102. Coggrave M, Norton C, Cody JD. Management of faecal incontinence and constipation in adults with central neurological diseases. *Cochrane Database Syst Rev*. 2014 Jan 13;1:CD002115.

103. Del Popolo G, Mosiello G, Pilati C, et al. Treatment of neurogenic bowel dysfunction using transanal irrigation: a multicenter Italian study. *Spinal Cord*. 2008;46:517-522.

104. Hansen RB, Staun M, Kalhauge A, Langholz E, Biering-Sorensen F. Bowel function and quality of life after colostomy in individuals with spinal cord injury. *J Spinal Cord Med*. 2016;39(3):281-289.

105. Peters HP, De Vries WR, Vanberge-Henegouwen GP, Akkermans LM. Potential benefits and hazards of physical activity and exercise on the gastrointestinal tract. *Gut*. 2001;48:435-439.

106. Korsten MA, Singal AK, Monga A, et al. Anorectal stimulation causes increased colonic motor activity in subjects with spinal cord injury. *J Spinal Cord Med*. 2007;30:31-35.

107. Korsten MA, Fajardo NR, Rosman AS, Creasey GH, Spungen AM, Bauman WA. Difficulty with evacuation after spinal cord injury: colonic motility during sleep and effects of abdominal wall stimulation. *J Rehabil Res Dev*. 2004;41:95-100.

108. Hascakova-Bartova R, Dinant JF, Parent A, Ventura M. Neuromuscular electrical stimulation of completely paralyzed abdominal muscles in spinal cord-injured patients: a pilot study. *Spinal Cord*. 2008;46:445-450.

109. Mentes BB, Yüksel O, Aydin A, Tezcaner T, Leventoğlu A, Aytaç B. Posterior tibial nerve stimulation for faecal incontinence after partial spinal injury: preliminary report. *Tech Coloproctol*. 2007;11:115-119.

110. Chun A, Asselin PK, Knezevic S, et al. Changes in bowel function following exoskeletal-assisted walking in persons with spinal cord injury: an observational pilot study. *Spinal Cord*. 2020;58:459-466.

111. Gorman PH, Forrest GF, Asselin PK, et al. The effect of exoskeletal-assisted walking on spinal cord injury bowel function: results from a randomized trial and comparison to other physical interventions. *J Clin Med*. 2021;10:964.

112. Hubscher CH, Herrity AN, Williams CS, et al. Improvements in bladder, bowel and sexual outcomes following task-specific locomotor training in human spinal cord injury. *PLoS One*. 2018;13:e0190998.

113. Hubscher CH, Wyles J, Gallahar A, et al. Effect of different forms of activity-based recovery training on bladder, bowel, and sexual function after spinal cord injury. *Arch Phys Med Rehabil*. 2021;102:865-873.

114. Eng JJ, Levins SM, Townson AF, Mah-Jones D, Bremner J, Huston G. Use of prolonged standing for individuals with spinal cord injuries. *Phys Ther*. 2001;81:1392-1399.

115. Hoenig H, Murphy T, Galbraith J, Zolkewitz M. Case study to evaluate a standing table for managing constipation. *SCI Nurs*. 2001;18:74-77.

116. Baunsgaard CB, Nissen UV, Brust AK, et al. Exoskeleton gait training after spinal cord injury: an exploratory study on secondary health conditions. *J Rehabil Med*. 2018;50:806-813.

117. Pettigrew RI, Heetderks WJ, Kelley CA, et al. Epidural spinal stimulation to improve bladder, bowel, and sexual function in individuals with spinal cord injuries: a framework for clinical research. *IEEE Trans Biomed Eng*. 2017;64:253-262.

118. Walter M, Lee AHX, Kavanagh A, Phillips AA, Krassioukov AV. Epidural spinal cord stimulation acutely modulates lower urinary tract and bowel function following spinal cord injury: a case report. *Front Physiol*. 2018;9:1816.

119. Street T. Electrical stimulation of abdominal muscles for bowel management in people with spinal cord injury (BOWMAN). Identifier: NCT04307303. clinicaltrials.gov/ct2/show/NCT04307303. (2020).

120. Krassioukov A. Below the belt: non-invasive neuromodulation to treat bladder, bowel, and sexual dysfunction following spinal cord injury. Identifier: NCT04604951. clinicaltrials.gov/ct2/show/NCT04604951. (2022).

121. Grahn PJ. Epidural and dorsal root stimulation in humans with spinal cord injury. Identifier: NCT04736849. clinicaltrials.gov/ct2/show/NCT04736849. (2021).

122. Bourbeau D. High frequency SARS for neurogenic bladder and bowel emptying. Identifier: NCT05214378. clinicaltrials.gov/ct2/show/NCT05214378 (2022).

123. Herrity A. Improving bowel function and quality of life after spinal cord injury. Identifier: NCT03949660. clinicaltrials.gov/ct2/show/NCT03949660. (2019).

124. Ditunno JF, Little JW, Tessler A, Burns AS. Spinal shock revisited: a four-phase model. *Spinal Cord*. 2004;42:383-395.

125. Schwartz S, Cohen ME, Herbison GJ, Shah A. Relationship between two measures of upper extremity strength: manual muscle test compared to hand-held myometry. *Arch Phys Med Rehabil*. 1992;73:1063-1068.

126. Herbison GJ, Isaac Z, Cohen ME, Ditunno JF Jr. Strength post-spinal cord injury: myometer vs manual muscle test. *Spinal Cord*. 1996;34:543-548.

127. Harvey LA, Katalinic OM, Herbert RD, Moseley AM, Lannin NA, Schurr K. Stretch for the treatment and prevention of contractures. *Cochrane Database Syst Rev*. 2017;1:CD007455.

128. Harvey LA, Katalinic OM, Herbert RD, Moseley AM, Lannin NA, Schurr K. Stretch for the treatment and prevention of contracture: an abridged republication of a cochrane systematic review. *J Physiother*. 2017;63:67-75.

129. Hutchinson KJ, Gomez-Pinilla F, Crowe MJ, Ying Z, Basso DM. Three exercise paradigms differentially improve sensory recovery after spinal cord contusion in rats. *Brain*. 2004;127:1403-1414.

130. Faw TD, Lakhani B, Schmalbrock P, et al. Eccentric rehabilitation induces white matter plasticity and sensorimotor recovery in chronic spinal cord injury. *Exp Neurol*. 2021;346:113853.

131. Hubli M, Dietz V. The physiological basis of neurorehabilitation: locomotor training after spinal cord injury. *J Neuroeng Rehabil*. 2013;10:5.

132. Bilchak JN, Caron G, Côté MP. Exercise-induced plasticity in signaling pathways involved in motor recovery after spinal cord injury. *Int J Mol Sci*. 22(2021):4858.

133. Ziegler MD, Zhong H, Roy RR, Edgerton VR. Why variability facilitates spinal learning. *J Neurosci*. 2010;30:10720-10726.

134. Marchal-Crespo L, Schneider J, Jaeger L, Riener R. Learning a locomotor task: with or without errors? *J Neuroeng Rehabil.* 2014;11:25.

135. de Leon RD, See PA, Chow CH. Differential effects of low versus high amounts of weight supported treadmill training in spinally transected rats. *J Neurotrauma.* 2011;28:1021-1033.

136. Lance J. Spasticity: disordered motor control. In: Feldman RG, Young RR, Koella WP,eds. *Symposium Synopsis.* Chicago: Year Book Medical Publishers; 1980:485-494.

137. Adams MM, Hicks AL. Spasticity after spinal cord injury. *Spinal Cord.* 2005;43:577-586.

138. Pandyan AD, Gregoric M, Barnes MP, et al. Spasticity: clinical perceptions, neurological realities and meaningful measurement. *Disabil Rehabil.* 2005;27:2-6.

139. Billington ZJ, Henke AM, Gater DR Jr. Spasticity management after spinal cord injury: the here and now. *J Pers Med.* 2022;12:808.

140. Dietz V, Sinkjaer T. Spastic movement disorder: impaired reflex function and altered muscle mechanics. *Lancet Neurol.* 2007;6:725-733.

141. Holtz KA, Lipson R, Noonan VK, Kwon BK, Mills PB. Prevalence and effect of problematic spasticity after traumatic spinal cord injury. *Arch Phys Med Rehabil.* 2017;98:1132-1138.

142. Ertzgaard P, Nene A, Kiekens C, Burns AS. A review and evaluation of patient-reported outcome measures for spasticity in persons with spinal cord damage. Recommendations from the Ability Network: an international initiative. *J Spinal Cord Med.* 2020;43:813-823.

143. Lanig IS, New PW, Burns AS, et al. Optimizing the management of spasticity in people with spinal cord damage: a clinical care pathway for assessment and treatment decision making from the Ability Network, an international initiative. *Arch Phys Med Rehabil.* 2018;99:1681-1687.

144. Sweatman WM, Heinemann AW, Furbish CL, Field-Fote EC. Modified PRISM and SCI-SET spasticity measures for persons with traumatic spinal cord injury: results of a Rasch analyses. *Arch Phys Med Rehabil.* 2020;101:1570-1579.

145. Hsieh JTC, Connolly SJ, McIntyre A, et al. Spasticity following spinal cord injury. In: Eng JJ, Teasell RW, Miller WC, et al., eds. *Spinal Cord Injury Rehabilitation Evidence.* Version 7.0; 2019.

146. Chen XY, Chen Y, Wang Y, et al. Reflex conditioning: a new strategy for improving motor function after spinal cord injury. *Ann N Y Acad Sci.* 2010;1198(Suppl 1):E12-E21.

147. Thompson AK, Pomerantz FR, Wolpaw JR. Operant conditioning of a spinal reflex can improve locomotion after spinal cord injury in humans. *J Neurosci.* 2013;33:2365-2375.

148. Thompson AK, Wolpaw JR. H-reflex conditioning during locomotion in people with spinal cord injury. *J Physiol.* 2021;599:2453-2469.

149. Kinnear BZ, Lannin NA, Cusick A, Harvey LA, Rawicki B. Rehabilitation therapies after botulinum toxin-A injection to manage limb spasticity: a systematic review. *Phys Ther.* 2014;94:1569-1581.

150. Alashram AR, Annino G, Mercuri NB. Changes in spasticity following functional electrical stimulation cycling in patients with spinal cord injury: a systematic review. *J Spinal Cord Med.* 2022;45:10-23.

151. Alashram AR, Padua E, Raju M, Romagnoli C, Annino G. Transcutaneous spinal cord stimulation effects on spasticity in patients with spinal cord injury: a systematic review. *J Spinal Cord Med.* 2021:1-8.

152. Khan F, Amatya B, Bensmail D, Yelnik A. Non-pharmacological interventions for spasticity in adults: an overview of systematic reviews. *Ann Phys Rehabil Med.* 2019;62:265-273.

153. Oo WM. Efficacy of addition of transcutaneous electrical nerve stimulation to standardized physical therapy in subacute spinal spasticity: a randomized controlled trial. *Arch Phys Med Rehabil.* 2014;95:2013-2020.

154. Stampas A, Hook M, Korupolu R, et al. Evidence of treating spasticity before it develops: a systematic review of spasticity outcomes in acute spinal cord injury interventional trials. *Ther Adv Neurol Disord.* 2022;15:17562864211070657.

155. Bye EA, Harvey LA, Gambhir A, et al. Strength training for partially paralysed muscles in people with recent spinal cord injury: a within-participant randomised controlled trial. *Spinal Cord.* 2017;55:460-465.

156. Field-Fote E. Activating spinal circuits to improve walking, balance, strength, and reduce spasticity. Identifier: NCT05429736. clinicaltrials.gov/ct2/show/NCT05429736. (2022).

157. Afzal B. Blood flow restriction resistance exercise in lower cervical spinal cord injury patients. Identifier: NCT05425238. clinicaltrials.gov/ct2/show/NCT05425238. (2022).

158. Tolfrey V. Protein supplementation and neuromuscular electrical stimulation in persons with SCI. Identifier: NCT05249985. clinicaltrials.gov/ct2/show/NCT05249985. (2022).

159. Smith AC, Knikou M. A Review on locomotor training after spinal cord injury: reorganization of spinal neuronal circuits and recovery of motor function. *Neural Plast.* 2016;2016:1216258.

160. Stampacchia G, Rustici A, Bigazzi S, Gerini A, Tombini T, Mazzoleni S. Walking with a powered robotic exoskeleton: subjective experience, spasticity and pain in spinal cord injured persons. *NeuroRehabilitation.* 2016;39:277-283.

161. Juszczak M, Gallo E, Bushnik T. Examining the effects of a powered exoskeleton on quality of life and secondary impairments in people living with spinal cord injury. *Top Spinal Cord Inj Rehabil.* 2018;24:336-342.

162. Tamburella F, Lorusso M, Tramontano M, Fadlun S, Masciullo M, Scivoletto G. Overground robotic training effects on walking and secondary health conditions in individuals with spinal cord injury: systematic review. *J Neuroeng Rehabil.* 2022;19:27.

163. Burns AS, Lanig I, Grabljevec K, et al. Optimizing the management of disabling spasticity following spinal cord damage: the Ability Network—an international initiative. *Arch Phys Med Rehabil.* 2016;97:2222-2228.

164. Banovac K, Williams JM, Patrick LD, Haniff YM. Prevention of heterotopic ossification after spinal cord injury with indomethacin. *Spinal Cord.* 2001;39:370-374.

165. van Kuijk AA, Geurts AC, van Kuppevelt HJ. Neurogenic heterotopic ossification in spinal cord injury. *Spinal Cord.* 2002;40:313-326.

166. Citak M, Suero EM, Backhaus M, et al. Risk factors for heterotopic ossification in patients with spinal cord injury: a case-control study of 264 patients. *Spine.* 2012;37:1953-1957.

167. Pape HC, Lehmann U, van Griensven M, Gänsslen A, von Glinski S, Krettek C. Heterotopic ossifications in patients after severe blunt trauma with and without head trauma: incidence and patterns of distribution. *J Orthop Trauma.* 2001;15:229-237.

168. Garland DE, Orwin JF. Resection of heterotopic ossification in patients with spinal cord injuries. *Clin Orthop Relat Res.* 1989;242:169-176.

169. Bauman WA. Pharmacological approaches for bone health in persons with spinal cord injury. *Curr Opin Pharmacol.* 2021;60:346-359.

170. van der Scheer JW, Martin Ginis KA, Ditor DS, et al. Effects of exercise on fitness and health of adults with spinal cord injury: a systematic review. *Neurology.* 2017;89:736-745.

171. Soleyman-Jahi S, Yousefian A, Maheronnaghsh R, et al. Evidence-based prevention and treatment of osteoporosis after spinal cord injury: a systematic review. *Eur Spine J.* 2018;27:1798-1814.

172. Craven BC, Lynch C, Eng J. Bone health following spinal cord injury. In: Eng JJ, Teasell RW, Miller WC, et al., eds. *Spinal Cord Injury Rehabilitation Evidence.* Version 5.0. Vancouver; 2014:1-37.

173. Dionyssiotis Y, Kalke YB, Frotzler A, et al. S1 guidelines on bone impairment in spinal cord injury. *J Clin Densitom.* 2021;24:490-501.

174. Weaver FM, Gonzalez B, Ray C, et al. Factors influencing providers' decisions on management of bone health in people with spinal cord injury. *Spinal Cord.* 2021;59:787-795.

175. Teeter L, Gassaway J, Taylor S, et al. Relationship of physical therapy inpatient rehabilitation interventions and patient characteristics to outcomes following spinal cord injury: the SCIRehab project. *J Spinal Cord Med.* 2012;35:503-526.

176. Fyffe DC, Deutsch A, Botticello AL, Kirshblum S, Ottenbacher KJ. Racial and ethnic disparities in functioning at discharge and follow-up among patients with motor complete spinal cord injury. *Arch Phys Med Rehabil.* 2014;95:2140-2151.

177. Dru AB, Reichwage B, Neal D, et al. Race and socioeconomic disparity in treatment and outcome of traumatic cervical spinal cord injury with fracture: nationwide inpatient sample database, 1998-2009. *Spinal Cord.* 2019;57:858-865.

178. AlHuthaifi F, Krzak J, Hanke T, Vogel LC. Predictors of functional outcomes in adults with traumatic spinal cord injury following inpatient rehabilitation: a systematic review. *J Spinal Cord Med.* 2017;40:282-294.

179. Kao YH, Chen Y, Deutsch A, Wen H, Tseng TS. Rehabilitation length of stay, body mass index, and functional improvement among adults with traumatic spinal cord injury. *Arch Phys Med Rehabil.* 2022;103:657-664.

180. Kao YH, Chen Y, Deutsch A, Wen H, Tseng TS. Rehabilitation length of stay and functional improvement among patients with traumatic spinal cord injury. *Spinal Cord.* 2022;60:237-244.

181. Slocum C, Shea C, Goldstein R, Zafonte R. Early trauma indicators and rehabilitation outcomes in traumatic spinal cord injury. *Top Spinal Cord Inj Rehabil.* 2020;26:253-260.

182. Shea C, Slocum C, Goldstein R, et al. Trauma indicators in spinal cord injury rehabilitation outcomes: a retrospective cohort analysis of the National Trauma Data Bank and National Spinal Cord Injury Database. *Arch Phys Med Rehabil.* 2022;103:642-648.e2.

183. Truchon C, Fallah N, Santos A, Vachon J, Noonan VK, Cheng CL. Impact of therapy on recovery during rehabilitation in patients with traumatic spinal cord injury. *J Neurotrauma.* 2017;34:2901-2909.

184. Gedde MH, Lilleberg HS, Aßmus J, Gilhus NE, Rekand T. Traumatic vs non-traumatic spinal cord injury: a comparison of primary rehabilitation outcomes and complications during hospitalization. *J Spinal Cord Med.* 2019;42:695-701.

185. Forrest G, Reppel A, Kodsi M, Smith J. Inpatient rehabilitation facilities: the 3-hour rule. *Medicine (Baltimore).* 2019;98:e17096.

186. Natale A, Taylor S, LaBarbera J, et al. SCIRehab project series: the physical therapy taxonomy. *J Spinal Cord Med.* 2009;32:270-282.

187. Anderson KD, Field-Fote EC, Biering-Sørensen F, et al. International spinal cord injury physical therapy-occupational therapy basic data set (Version 1.2). *Spinal Cord Ser Cases.* 2020;6:74.

188. van Langeveld SA, Post MW, van Asbeck FW, Postma K, Ten Dam D, Pons K Development of a classification of physical, occupational, and sports therapy interventions to document mobility and self-care in spinal cord injury rehabilitation. *J Neurol Phys Ther.* 2008;32:2-7.

189. Zanca JM, Turkstra LS, Chen C, et al. Advancing rehabilitation practice through improved specification of interventions. *Arch Phys Med Rehabil.* 2019;100:164-171.

190. Monden KR, Hidden J, Eagye CB, Hammond FM, Kolakowsky-Hayner SA, Whiteneck GG. Relationship of patient characteristics and inpatient rehabilitation services to 5-year outcomes following spinal cord injury: a follow up of the SCIRehab project. *J Spinal Cord Med.* 2021;44:870-885.

191. Franz M, Richner L, Wirz M, et al. Physical therapy is targeted and adjusted over time for the rehabilitation of locomotor function in acute spinal cord injury interventions in physical and sports therapy. *Spinal Cord.* 2018;56:158-167.

192. Taylor-Schroeder S, LaBarbera J, McDowell S, et al. The SCIRehab project: treatment time spent in SCI rehabilitation. Physical therapy treatment time during inpatient spinal cord injury rehabilitation. *J Spinal Cord Med.* 2011;34:149-161.

193. Hachem LD, Ahuja CS, Fehlings MG. Assessment and management of acute spinal cord injury: from point of injury to rehabilitation. *J Spinal Cord Med.* 2017;40:665-675.

194. Fehlings MG, Tetreault LA, Aarabi B, et al. A clinical practice guideline for the management of patients with acute spinal cord injury: recommendations on the type and timing of rehabilitation. *Global Spine J.* 2017;7:231s-238s.

195. Badhiwala JH, Ahuja CS, Fehlings MG. Time is spine: a review of translational advances in spinal cord injury. *J Neurosurg Spine.* 2018;30:1-18.

196. Santos LV, Pereira ET, Reguera-García MM, Oliveira CEP, Moreira OC. Resistance training and muscle strength in people with spinal cord injury: a systematic review and meta-analysis. *J Bodyw Mov Ther.* 2022;29:154-160.

197. Martin Ginis KA, van der Scheer JW, Latimer-Cheung AE, et al. Evidence-based scientific exercise guidelines for adults with spinal cord injury: an update and a new guideline. *Spinal Cord.* 2018;56:308-321.

198. Grabiner MD, Owings TM. Effects of eccentrically and concentrically induced unilateral fatigue on the involved and uninvolved limbs. *J Electromyogr Kinesiol.* 1999;9:185-189.

199. Doix AM, Wachholz F, Marterer N, Immler L, Insam K, Federolf PA. Is the cross-over effect of a unilateral high-intensity leg extension influenced by the sex of the participants? *Biol Sex Differ.* 2018;9:29.

200. Eitivipart AC, de Oliveira CQ, Arora M, Middleton J, Davis GM. Overview of systematic reviews of aerobic fitness and muscle strength training after spinal cord injury. *J Neurotrauma.* 2019;36:2943-2963.

201. Alves-Rodrigues J, Torres-Pereira E, Zanúncio Araujo J, et al. Effect of functional strength training on people with spinal cord injury. *Apunts Educ Fis Deportes.* 2021;144:10-17.

202. Mulroy SJ, Thompson L, Kemp B, et al. Strengthening and optimal movements for painful shoulders (STOMPS) in chronic spinal cord injury: a randomized controlled trial. *Phys Ther.* 2011;91:305-324.

203. Yildirim A, Sürücü GD, Karamercan A, et al. Short-term effects of upper extremity circuit resistance training on muscle strength and functional independence in patients with paraplegia. *J Back Musculoskelet Rehabil.* 2016;29:817-823.

204. Harvey LA, Ristev D, Hossain MS, et al. Training unsupported sitting does not improve ability to sit in people with recently acquired paraplegia: a randomised trial. *J Physiother.* 2011;57:83-90.

205. Taylor SM, Slowinske L, Dennison M, et al. Inpatient rehabilitation wheelchair management quality improvement project: implications for patients with spinal cord injury. *J Spinal Cord Med.* 2023;46:414-423.

206. Lighthall-Haubert L, Requejo PS, Mulroy SJ, et al. Comparison of shoulder muscle electromyographic activity during standard manual wheelchair and push-rim activated power assisted wheelchair propulsion in persons with complete tetraplegia. *Arch Phys Med Rehabil.* 2009;90:1904-1915.

207. Michael E, Sytsma T, Cowan RE. A primary care provider's guide to wheelchair prescription for persons with spinal cord injury. *Top Spinal Cord Inj Rehabil.* 2020;26:100-107.

208. Tu CJ, Liu L, Wang W, et al. Effectiveness and safety of wheelchair skills training program in improving the wheelchair skills capacity: a systematic review. *Clin Rehabil.* 2017;31:1573-1582.

209. Keeler L, Kirby RL, Parker K, McLean KD, Hayden JA. Effectiveness of the wheelchair skills training program: a systematic review and meta-analysis. *Disabil Rehabil Assist Technol.* 2019;14:391-409.

210. Lemay V, Routhier F, Noreau L, Phang SH, Ginis KA. Relationships between wheelchair skills, wheelchair mobility and level of injury in individuals with spinal cord injury. *Spinal Cord.* 2012;50:37-41.

211. Giesbrecht E. Wheelchair skills test outcomes across multiple wheelchair skills training bootcamp cohorts. *Int J Environ Res Public Health.* 2021;19:21.

212. Smith EM, Best KL, Miller WC. A condensed wheelchair skills training "bootcamp" improves students' self-efficacy for assessing, training, spotting, and documenting manual and power wheelchair skills. *Disabil Rehabil Assist Technol.* 2020;15:418-420.

213. Minkel JL. Seating and mobility considerations for people with spinal cord injury. *Phys Ther.* 2000;80:701-709.

214. Anderson KD. Targeting recovery: priorities of the spinal cord-injured population. *J Neurotrauma.* 2004;21:1371-1383.

215. Hanson RW, Franklin MR. Sexual loss in relation to other functional losses for spinal cord injured males. *Arch Phys Med Rehabil.* 1976;57:291-293.

216. Snoek GJ, IJzerman MJ, Hermens HJ, Maxwell D, Biering-Sorensen F. Survey of the needs of patients with spinal cord injury: impact and

priority for improvement in hand function in tetraplegics. *Spinal Cord.* 2004;42:526-532.

217. Namrata, Mattu S. Priorities of spinal cord injured population: a survey. *Am J Appl Psychol.* 2017;6:183-187.

218. Duffell LD, Donaldson NN. A comparison of FES and SCS for neuroplastic recovery after SCI: historical perspectives and future directions. *Front Neurol.* 2020;11:607.

219. Inanici F, Brighton LN, Samejima S, Hofstetter CP, Moritz CT. Transcutaneous spinal cord stimulation restores hand and arm function after spinal cord injury. *IEEE Trans Neural Syst Rehabil Eng.* 2021;29:310-319.

220. Beekhuizen KS, Field-Fote EC. Massed practice versus massed practice with stimulation: effects on upper extremity function and cortical plasticity in individuals with incomplete cervical spinal cord injury. *Neurorehabil Neural Repair.* 2005;19:33-45.

221. Beekhuizen KS, Field-Fote EC. Sensory stimulation augments the effects of massed practice training in persons with tetraplegia. *Arch Phys Med Rehabil.* 2008;89:602-608.

222. Hoffman LR, Field-Fote EC. Cortical reorganization following bimanual training and somatosensory stimulation in cervical spinal cord injury: a case report. *Phys Ther.* 2007;87:208-223.

223. Harnett A, Rice D, McIntyre A, et al. Upper limb rehabilitation following spinal cord injury. In: *Spinal Cord Injury Rehabilitation Evidence.* Version 7.0.

224. Harvey L, de Jong I, Goehl G, Mardwedel S. Twelve weeks of nightly stretch does not reduce thumb web-space contractures in people with a neurological condition: a randomised controlled trial. *Aust J Physiother.* 2006;52:251-258.

225. Portnova AA, Mukherjee G, Peters KM, Yamane A, Steele KM. Design of a 3D-printed, open-source wrist-driven orthosis for individuals with spinal cord injury. *PLoS One.* 2018;13:e0193106.

226. Scott S, Yu T, White KT, et al. A robotic hand device safety study for people with cervical spinal cord injury. *Fed Pract.* 2018;35:S21-S25.

227. Meyers EC, Gabrieli D, Tacca N, Wengerd L, Darrow M, Friedenberg D. Decoding hand and wrist movement intention from chronic stroke survivors with hemiparesis using a user-friendly, wearable EMG-based neural interface. *medRxiv.* 2021. https://doi.org/10.1101/2021.09.07.21262896.

228. Kentar Y, Zastrow R, Bradley H, et al. Prevalence of upper extremity pain in a population of people with paraplegia. *Spinal Cord.* 2018;56:695-703.

229. Raja SN, Carr DB, Cohen M, et al. The revised international association for the study of pain definition of pain: concepts, challenges, and compromises. *Pain.* 2020;161:1976-1982.

230. Chambel SS, Tavares I, Cruz CD. Chronic pain after spinal cord injury: is there a role for neuron-immune dysregulation? *Front Physiol.* 2020;11:748.

231. Chen JT, Guo D, Campanelli D, et al. Presynaptic GABAergic inhibition regulated by BDNF contributes to neuropathic pain induction. *Nat Commun.* 2014;5:5331.

232. Chhaya SJ, Quiros-Molina D, Tamashiro-Orrego AD, Houlé JD, Detloff MR. Exercise-induced changes to the macrophage response in the dorsal root ganglia prevent neuropathic pain after spinal cord injury. *J Neurotrauma.* 2019;36:877-890.

233. Hiraga SI, Itokazu T, Hoshiko M, Takaya H, Nishibe M, Yamashita T. Microglial depletion under thalamic hemorrhage ameliorates mechanical allodynia and suppresses aberrant axonal sprouting. *JCI Insight.* 2020;5:e131801.

234. Widerström-Noga E, Cruz-Almeida Y, Felix ER, Pattany PM. Somatosensory phenotype is associated with thalamic metabolites and pain intensity after spinal cord injury. *Pain.* 2015;156:166-174.

235. Huynh V, Rosner J, Curt A, Kollias S, Hubli M, Michels L. Disentangling the effects of spinal cord injury and related neuropathic pain on supraspinal neuroplasticity: a systematic review on neuroimaging. *Front Neurol.* 2020;10:1413.

236. Widerström-Noga E, Pattany PM, Cruz-Almeida Y, et al. Metabolite concentrations in the anterior cingulate cortex predict high neuropathic pain impact after spinal cord injury. *Pain.* 2013;154:204-212.

237. Detloff MR, Fisher LC, McGaughy V, Longbrake EE, Popovich PG, Basso DM. Remote activation of microglia and pro-inflammatory cytokines predict the onset and severity of below-level neuropathic pain after spinal cord injury in rats. *Exp Neurol.* 2008;212:337-347.

238. Hansen CN, Norden DM, Faw TD, et al. Lumbar myeloid cell trafficking into locomotor networks after thoracic spinal cord injury. *Exp Neurol.* 2016;282:86-98.

239. Norden DM, Faw TD, McKim DB, et al. Bone marrow-derived monocytes drive the inflammatory microenvironment in local and remote regions after thoracic spinal cord injury. *J Neurotrauma.* 2019;36:937-949.

240. Rubinelli S, Glässel A, Brach M. From the person's perspective: perceived problems in functioning among individuals with spinal cord injury in Switzerland. *J Rehabil Med.* 2016;48:235-243.

241. Norrbrink Budh C, Hultling C, Lundeberg T. Quality of sleep in individuals with spinal cord injury: a comparison between patients with and without pain. *Spinal Cord.* 2005;43:85-95.

242. Ataoğlu E, Tiftik T, Kara M, Tunç H, Ersöz M, Akkuş S. Effects of chronic pain on quality of life and depression in patients with spinal cord injury. *Spinal Cord.* 2013;51:23-26.

243. Cardenas DD, Bryce TN, Shem K, Richards JS, Elhefni H. Gender and minority differences in the pain experience of people with spinal cord injury. *Arch Phys Med Rehabil.* 2004;85:1774-1781.

244. Burke D, Fullen BM, Stokes D, Lennon O. Neuropathic pain prevalence following spinal cord injury: a systematic review and meta-analysis. *Eur J Pain.* 2017;21:29-44.

245. Felix ER, Cardenas DD, Bryce TN, et al. Prevalence and impact of neuropathic and nonneuropathic pain in chronic spinal cord injury. *Arch Phys Med Rehabil.* 2022;103:729-737.

246. Mathur VA, Trost Z, Ezenwa MO, Sturgeon JA, Hood AM. Mechanisms of injustice: what we (do not) know about racialized disparities in pain. *Pain.* 2022;163:999-1005.

247. Hoffman KM, Trawalter S, Axt JR, Oliver MN. Racial bias in pain assessment and treatment recommendations, and false beliefs about biological differences between blacks and whites. *Proc Natl Acad Sci U S A.* 2016;113:4296-4301.

248. Widerström-Noga E, Biering-Sørensen F, Bryce TN, et al. The international spinal cord injury pain basic data set (version 2.0). *Spinal Cord.* 2014;52:282-286.

249. Jensen MP, Widerström-Noga E, Richards JS, Finnerup NB, Biering-Sørensen F, Cardenas DD. Reliability and validity of the International Spinal Cord Injury Basic Pain Data Set items as self-report measures. *Spinal Cord.* 2010;48:230-238.

250. Widerström-Noga E, Biering-Sørensen F, Bryce TN, et al. International Spinal Cord Injury Pain Basic Data Set (Version 3). 2022. asia-spinalinjury.org/international-sci-pain-basic-data-set-version-3-0.

251. Finnerup NB, Norrbrink C, Trok K, et al. Phenotypes and predictors of pain following traumatic spinal cord injury: a prospective study. *J Pain.* 2014;15:40-48.

252. Gibbs K, Beaufort A, Stein A, Leung TM, Sison C, Bloom O. Assessment of pain symptoms and quality of life using the international spinal cord injury data sets in persons with chronic spinal cord injury. *Spinal Cord Ser Cases.* 2019;5:32.

253. Widerstrom-Noga E, Anderson KD, Perez S, Martinez-Arizala A, Calle-Coule L, Fleming L. Barriers and facilitators to optimal neuropathic pain management: SCI consumer, significant other, and health care provider perspectives. *Pain Med.* 2020;21:2913-2924.

254. Nicholson Perry K, Nicholas MK, Middleton J. Spinal cord injury-related pain in rehabilitation: a cross-sectional study of relationships with cognitions, mood and physical function. *Eur J Pain.* 2009;13:511-517.

255. Interagency Pain Research Coordinating Committee. *A Comprehensive Population Health-Level Strategy for Pain: National Pain Strategy.* Washington, DC: HHS; 2015.

256. Hatch MN, Cushing TR, Carlson GD, Chang EY. Neuropathic pain and SCI: Identification and treatment strategies in the 21st century. *J Neurol Sci.* 2018;384:75-83.

257. Yu X, Liu T, Zhao D, et al. Efficacy and safety of pregabalin in neuropathic pain followed spinal cord injury: a review and meta-analysis of randomized controlled trials. *Clin J Pain.* 2019;35:272-278.

258. Cardenas DD, Jensen MP. Treatments for chronic pain in persons with spinal cord injury: a survey study. *J Spinal Cord Med.* 2006;29:109-117.

259. Polat CS, Konak HE, Akıncı MG, Onat SS, Altas EU. Misuse of gabapentinoids (pregabalin and gabapentin) in patients with neuropathic pain related to spinal cord injury. *J Spinal Cord Med.* 2022;1-6.

260. National Academies of Sciences, Engineering, and Medicine. *The Health Effects of Cannabis and Cannabinoids: The Current State of Evidence and Recommendations for Research.* Washington, DC: The National Academies Press; 2017.

261. Whiting PF, Wolff RF, Deshpande S, et al. Cannabinoids for medical use: a systematic review and meta-analysis. *JAMA.* 2015;313:2456-2473.

262. Tsai SHL, Lin CR, Shao SC, et al. Cannabinoid use for pain reduction in spinal cord injuries: a meta-analysis of randomized controlled trials. *Front Pharmacol.* 2022;13:866235.

263. Graves DE. Cannabis shenanigans: advocating for the restoration of an effective treatment of pain following spinal cord injury. *Spinal Cord Ser Cases.* 2018;4:67.

264. Acland R. The enigma of cannabis use in spinal cord injury. *Spinal Cord Ser Cases.* 2018;4:69.

265. Berliner J, Collins K, Coker J. Cannabis conundrum. *Spinal Cord Ser Cases.* 2018;4:1-3.

266. Cadel L, DeLuca C, Hitzig SL, et al. Self-management of pain and depression in adults with spinal cord injury: a scoping review. *J Spinal Cord Med.* 2020;43:280-297.

267. Heutink M, Post MWM, Bongers-Janssen HMH, et al. The CONECSI trial: results of a randomized controlled trial of a multidisciplinary cognitive behavioral program for coping with chronic neuropathic pain after spinal cord injury. *Pain.* 2012;153:120-128.

268. Detloff MR, Smith EJ, Quiros Molina D, Ganzer PD, Houle JD. Acute exercise prevents the development of neuropathic pain and the sprouting of non-peptidergic (GDNF- and artemin-responsive) c-fibers after spinal cord injury. *Exp Neurol.* 2014;255:38-48.

269. Palandi J, Bobinski F, de Oliveira GM, Ilha J. Neuropathic pain after spinal cord injury and physical exercise in animal models: a systematic review and meta-analysis. *Neurosci Biobehav Rev.* 2020;108:781-795.

270. Nees TA, Tappe-Theodor A, Sliwinski C, et al. Early-onset treadmill training reduces mechanical allodynia and modulates calcitonin gene-related peptide fiber density in lamina III/IV in a mouse model of spinal cord contusion injury. *Pain.* 2016;157:687-697.

271. Ginis KAM, Latimer A, McKechnie K, et al. Using exercise to enhance subjective well-being among people with spinal cord injury: the mediating influences of stress and pain. *Rehabil Psychol.* 2003;48:157-164.

272. Labruyere R, van Hedel HJ. Strength training versus robot-assisted gait training after incomplete spinal cord injury: a randomized pilot study in patients depending on walking assistance. *J Neuroeng Rehabil.* 2014;11:4.

273. Norrbrink C, Lindberg T, Wahman K, Bjerkefors A. Effects of an exercise programme on musculoskeletal and neuropathic pain after spinal cord injury: results from a seated double-poling ergometer study. *Spinal Cord.* 2012;50:457-461.

274. Todd KR, Van Der Scheer JW, Walsh JJ, et al. The impact of sub-maximal exercise on neuropathic pain, inflammation, and affect among adults with spinal cord injury: a pilot study. *Front Rehabil Sci.* 2021;2:700780.

275. Cruciger O, Schildhauer TA, Meindl RC, et al. Impact of locomotion training with a neurologic controlled hybrid assistive limb (HAL) exoskeleton on neuropathic pain and health related quality of life (HRQoL) in chronic SCI: a case study. *Disabil Rehabil Assist Technol.* 2016;11:529-534.

276. Yeh NC, Yang YR, Huang SF, Ku PH, Wang RY. Effects of transcranial direct current stimulation followed by exercise on neuropathic pain in chronic spinal cord injury: a double-blinded randomized controlled pilot trial. *Spinal Cord.* 2021;59:684-692.

277. Sawada T, Okawara H, Matsubayashi K, et al. Influence of body weight-supported treadmill training with voluntary-driven exoskeleton on the quality of life of persons with chronic spinal cord injury: a pilot study. *Int J Rehabil Res.* 2021;44:343-349.

278. Ditor DS, Latimer AE, Ginis KA, Arbour KP, McCartney N, Hicks AL. Maintenance of exercise participation in individuals with spinal cord injury: effects on quality of life, stress and pain. *Spinal Cord.* 2003;41:446-450.

279. Widerstrom-Noga EG, Turk DC. Types and effectiveness of treatments used by people with chronic pain associated with spinal cord injuries: influence of pain and psychosocial characteristics. *Spinal Cord.* 2003;41:600-609.

280. Shen Z, Li Z, Ke J, et al. Effect of non-invasive brain stimulation on neuropathic pain following spinal cord injury: a systematic review and meta-analysis. *Medicine (Baltimore).* 2020;99:e21507.

281. Yang Y, Tang Y, Qin H, Xu J. Efficacy of transcutaneous electrical nerve stimulation in people with pain after spinal cord injury: a meta-analysis. *Spinal Cord.* 2022;60:375-381.

282. Zeb A, Arsh A, Bahadur S, Ilyas SM. Effectiveness of transcutaneous electrical nerve stimulation in management of neuropathic pain in patients with post traumatic incomplete spinal cord injuries. *Pak J Med Sci.* 2018;34:1177-1180.

283. Chi B, Chau B, Yeo E, Ta P. Virtual reality for spinal cord injury-associated neuropathic pain: systematic review. *Ann Phys Rehabil Med.* 2019;62:49-57.

284. Worobey LA, Kirby RL, Heinemann A, et al. Effectiveness of group wheelchair skills training for people with spinal cord injury: a randomized controlled trial. *Arch Phys Med Rehabil.* 2016;97:1777-1784.e3.

285. Kirby RL, Mitchell D, Sabharwal S, McCranie M, Nelson AL. Manual wheelchair skills training for community-dwelling veterans with spinal cord injury: a randomized controlled trial. *PLoS One.* 2016;11:e0168330.

286. Rigot SK, DiGiovine KM, Boninger ML, Hibbs R, Smith I, Worobey LA. Effectiveness of a web-based direct-to-user transfer training program: a randomized controlled trial. *Arch Phys Med Rehabil.* 2022;103:807-815.e1.

287. Darrow D, Balser D, Netoff TI, et al. Epidural spinal cord stimulation facilitates immediate restoration of dormant motor and autonomic supraspinal pathways after chronic neurologically complete spinal cord injury. *J Neurotrauma.* 2019;36:2325-2336.

288. Previnaire JG, Soler JM, Alexander MS, Courtois F, Elliott S, McLain A. Prediction of sexual function following spinal cord injury: a case series. *Spinal Cord Ser Cases.* 2017;3:17096.

289. Lombardi G, Nelli F, Mencarini M, Del Popolo G. Clinical concomitant benefits on pelvic floor dysfunctions after sacral neuromodulation in patients with incomplete spinal cord injury. *Spinal Cord.* 2011;49:629-636.

290. Krause JS, Kemp B, Coker J. Depression after spinal cord injury: relation to gender, ethnicity, aging, and socioeconomic indicators. *Arch Phys Med Rehabil.* 2000;81:1099-1109.

291. Kemp B, Mosqueda L. *Aging with Disability: What the Clinician Needs to Know.* Boston: John Hopkins University Press; 2004.

292. Harkema SJ, Hurley SL, Patel UK, Requejo PS, Dobkin BH, Edgerton VR. Human lumbosacral spinal cord interprets loading during stepping. *J Neurophysiol.* 1997;77:797-811.

293. Edgerton VR, Roy RR. Activity-dependent plasticity of spinal locomotion: implications for sensory processing. *Exerc Sport Sci Rev.* 2009;37:171-178.

294. Field-Fote EC, Roach KE. Influence of a locomotor training approach on walking speed and distance in people with chronic spinal cord injury: a randomized clinical trial. *Phys Ther.* 2011;91:48-60.

295. Tillakaratne NJK, et al. Use-dependent modulation of inhibitory capacity in the feline lumbar spinal cord. *J Neurosci.* 2002;22:3130-3143.

296. Martinez M, Delivet-Mongrain H, Leblond H, Rossignol S. Recovery of hindlimb locomotion after incomplete spinal cord injury in the cat involves spontaneous compensatory changes within the spinal locomotor circuitry. *J Neurophysiol.* 2011;106:1969-1984.

297. Lam T, Wolfe D, Domingo A, Eng J, Sproule S. *Lower Limb Rehabilitation Following Spinal Cord Injury* (Vancouver, 2014).

298. Sadowsky CL, Hammond ER, Strohl AB, et al. Lower extremity functional electrical stimulation cycling promotes physical and functional recovery in chronic spinal cord injury. *J Spinal Cord Med*. 2013;36:623-631.

299. Gorgey AS, Khalil RE, Davis JC, et al. Skeletal muscle hypertrophy and attenuation of cardio-metabolic risk factors (SHARC) using functional electrical stimulation-lower extremity cycling in persons with spinal cord injury: study protocol for a randomized clinical trial. *Trials*. 2019;20:526.

300. de Freitas GR, Szpoganicz C, Ilha J. Does neuromuscular electrical stimulation therapy increase voluntary muscle strength after spinal cord injury? A systematic review. *Top Spinal Cord Inj Rehabil*. 2018;24:6-17.

301. Arpin DJ, Ugiliweneza B, Forrest G, Harkema SJ, Rejc E. Optimizing neuromuscular electrical stimulation pulse width and amplitude to promote central activation in individuals with severe spinal cord injury. *Front Physiol*. 2019;10:1310.

302. Collins DF. Central contributions to contractions evoked by tetanic neuromuscular electrical stimulation. *Exerc Sport Sci Rev*. 2007;35:102-109.

303. Xiang XN, Zong HY, Ou Y, et al. Exoskeleton-assisted walking improves pulmonary function and walking parameters among individuals with spinal cord injury: a randomized controlled pilot study. *J Neuroeng Rehabil*. 2021;18:86.

304. Alamro RA, Chisholm AE, Williams AMM, Carpenter MG, Lam T. Overground walking with a robotic exoskeleton elicits trunk muscle activity in people with high-thoracic motor-complete spinal cord injury. *J Neuroeng Rehabil*. 2018;15:109.

305. Edwards DJ, Forrest G, Cortes M, et al. Walking improvement in chronic incomplete spinal cord injury with exoskeleton robotic training (WISE): a randomized controlled trial. *Spinal Cord*. 2022;60:522-532.

306. Chang SH, Afzal T, Berliner J, Francisco GE. Exoskeleton-assisted gait training to improve gait in individuals with spinal cord injury: a pilot randomized study. *Pilot Feasibility Stud*. 2018;4:62.

307. Miller LE, Zimmermann AK, Herbert WG. Clinical effectiveness and safety of powered exoskeleton-assisted walking in patients with spinal cord injury: systematic review with meta-analysis. *Med Devices (Auckl)*. 2016;9:455-466.

308. Gorgey AS. Robotic exoskeletons: the current pros and cons. *World J Orthop*. 2018;9:112-119.

309. Hachmann JT, Yousak A, Wallner JJ, Gad PN, Edgerton VR, Gorgey AS. Epidural spinal cord stimulation as an intervention for motor recovery after motor complete spinal cord injury. *J Neurophysiol*. 2021;126:1843-1859.

310. Rowald A, Komi S, Demesmaeker R, et al. Activity-dependent spinal cord neuromodulation rapidly restores trunk and leg motor functions after complete paralysis. *Nat Med*. 2022;28:260-271.

311. Eisdorfer JT, Smit RD, Keefe KM, Lemay MA, Smith GM, Spence AJ. Epidural electrical stimulation: a review of plasticity mechanisms that are hypothesized to underlie enhanced recovery from spinal cord injury with stimulation. *Front Mol Neurosci*. 2020;13:163.

312. Harkema S, Gerasimenko Y, Hodes J, et al. Effect of epidural stimulation of the lumbosacral spinal cord on voluntary movement, standing, and assisted stepping after motor complete paraplegia: a case study. *The Lancet*. 2011;377:1938-1947.

313. Hachmann JT, Calvert JS, Grahn PJ, Drubach DI, Lee KH, Lavrov IA. Review of epidural spinal cord stimulation for augmenting cough after spinal cord injury. *Front Hum Neurosci*. 2017;11:144.

314. Aslan SC, Legg Ditterline BE, Park MC, et al. Epidural spinal cord stimulation of lumbosacral networks modulates arterial blood pressure in individuals with spinal cord injury-induced cardiovascular deficits. *Front Physiol*. 2018;9:565.

315. Harkema SJ, Legg Ditterline B, Wang S, et al. Epidural spinal cord stimulation training and sustained recovery of cardiovascular function in individuals with chronic cervical spinal cord injury. *JAMA Neurol*. 2018;75:1569-1571.

316. Harkema SJ, Wang S, Angeli CA, et al. Normalization of blood pressure with spinal cord epidural stimulation after severe spinal cord injury. *Front Hum Neurosci*. 2018;12:83.

317. Herrity AN, Williams CS, Angeli CA, Harkema SJ, Hubscher CH. Lumbosacral spinal cord epidural stimulation improves voiding function after human spinal cord injury. *Sci Rep*. 2018;8:8688.

318. Megía García A, Serrano-Muñoz D, Taylor J, Avendaño-Coy J, Gómez-Soriano J. Transcutaneous spinal cord stimulation and motor rehabilitation in spinal cord injury: a systematic review. *Neurorehabil Neural Repair*. 2020;34:3-12.

319. Laskin JJ, Waheed Z, Thorogood NP, Nightingale TE, Noonan VK. Spinal cord stimulation research in the restoration of motor, sensory, and autonomic function for individuals living with spinal cord injuries: a scoping review. *Arch Phys Med Rehabil*. 2022;103:1387-1397.

320. Freyvert Y, Yong NA, Morikawa E, et al. Engaging cervical spinal circuitry with non-invasive spinal stimulation and buspirone to restore hand function in chronic motor complete patients. *Sci Rep*. 2018;8:15546.

321. Sayenko DG, Rath M, Ferguson AR, et al. Self-assisted standing enabled by non-invasive spinal stimulation after spinal cord injury. *J Neurotrauma*. 2019;36:1435-1450.

322. Dobkin B, Apple D, Barbeau H, et al. Weight-supported treadmill vs over-ground training for walking after acute incomplete SCI. *Neurology*. 2006;66:484-493.

323. Hornby G, Campbell D, Zemon D, Kahn J. Clinical and quantitative evaluation of robotic-assisted treadmill walking to retrain ambulation after spinal cord injury. *Top Spinal Cord Inj Rehabil*. 2005;11:1-17.

324. Harkema SJ, Schmidt-Read M, Lorenz DJ, Edgerton VR, Behrman AL. Balance and ambulation improvements in individuals with chronic incomplete spinal cord injury using locomotor training based rehabilitation. *Arch Phys Med Rehabil*. 2012;93:1508-1517.

325. Winchester P, Smith P, Foreman N, et al. A prediction model for determining over ground walking speed after locomotor training in persons with motor incomplete spinal cord injury. *J Spinal Cord Med*. 2009;32:63-71.

326. Bussel B, Roby-Brami A, Neris OR, Yakovleff A. Evidence for a spinal stepping generator in man: electrophysiological study. *Acta Neurobiol Exp (Wars)*. 1996;56:465-468.

327. Bussel B, Roby-Brami A, Yakovleff A, Bennis N. Late flexion reflex in paraplegic patients: evidence for a spinal stepping generator. *Brain Res Bull*. 1989;22:53-56.

328. Calancie B, Needham-Shropshire B, Jacobs P, Willer K, Zych G, Green BA. Involuntary stepping after chronic spinal cord injury: evidence for a central rhythm generator for locomotion in man. *Brain*. 1994;117:1143-1159.

329. Behrman AL, Harkema SJ. Locomotor training after human spinal cord injury: a series of case studies. *Phys Therapy*. 2000;80:688-700.

330. Visintin M, Barbeau H. The effects of body weight support on the locomotor pattern of spastic paretic patients. *Can J Neurol Sci*. 1989;16:315-325.

331. Forrest GF, Hutchinson K, Lorenz DJ, et al. Are the 10 meter and 6 minute walk tests redundant in patients with spinal cord injury? *PLoS One*. 2014;9:e94108.

332. van Hedel HJ, Dietz V. Walking during daily life can be validly and responsively assessed in subjects with a spinal cord injury. *Neurorehabil Neural Repair*. 2009;23:117-124.

333. Dittuno PL, Ditunno JF Jr. Walking index for spinal cord injury (WISCI II): scale revision. *Spinal Cord*. 2001;39:654-656.

334. Itzkovich M, Gelernter I, Biering-Sorensen F, et al. The spinal cord independence measure (SCIM) version III: reliability and validity in a multicenter international study. *Disabil Rehabil*. 2007;29:1926-1933.

335. Ko HY, Kim W, Kim SY, et al. Factors associated with early onset posttraumatic syringomyelia. *Spinal Cord*. 2012;50:695-698.

336. Brodbelt AR, Stoodley MA. Post-traumatic syringomyelia: a review. *J Clin Neurosci*. 2003;10:401-408.

337. Myers J, Lee M, Kiratli J. Cardiovascular disease in spinal cord injury: an overview of prevalence, risk, evaluation, and management. *Am J Phys Med Rehabil*. 2007;86:142-152.

338. Myers J, Kiratli BJ, Jaramillo J. The cardiometabolic benefits of routine physical activity in persons living with spinal cord injury. *Curr Cardiovasc Risk Rep.* 2012;6:323-330.

339. Bauman WA, Raza M, Chayes Z, Machac J. Tomographic thallium-201 myocardial perfusion imaging after intravenous dipyridamole in asymptomatic subjects with quadriplegia. *Arch Phys Med Rehabil.* 1993;74:740-744.

340. Warburton DE, Eng JJ, Krassioukov A, Sproule S. Cardiovascular health and exercise rehabilitation in spinal cord injury. *Top Spinal Cord Inj Rehabil.* 2007;13:98-122.

341. Apkinar P, Atici A, Aktas I, Kulcu DG, Sari A, Durmus B. Reliability of the Modified Ashworth Scale and Modified Tardieu Scale in patients with spinal cord injuries. *Spinal Cord.* 2017;55:944-949.

Review Questions

1. **An individual with a spinal cord injury classified as AIS C will have the following functions below the level of the injury:**
   A. Complete motor paralysis only
   B. Spared motor function with complete sensory loss
   C. Complete sensory loss only
   D. Spared motor and sensory function

2. **An injury at C8 will likely produce the following impairments:**
   A. Autonomic dysreflexia
   B. Weak cough
   C. Kyphotic "C" sitting posture
   D. Weak finger abduction
   E. All of the above

3. **A central cord injury will typically have the following type of dysfunction**
   A. Loss of pain and temperature sensation only on one side of the body
   B. Severe atrophy of the hands and good motor control of the legs
   C. Paralysis of the legs and good proprioception in the legs
   D. Poor proprioception in the legs and good motor control of the legs

4. **Complete paralysis during the first week of injury means there will be no motor recovery.**
   A. True
   B. False

5. **Deep vein thrombosis is caused by which of the following:**
   A. Hypertension
   B. Spasticity
   C. Spinal shock
   D. Bed rest

6. **Which of the symptom of autonomic dysreflexia is most likely to indicate a serious life-threatening problem:**
   A. Sweating
   B. Pounding headache
   C. Piloerection
   D. Facial flushing

7. **Which of the following conditions can trigger Autonomic Dysreflexia:**
   A. Ingrown toe nail
   B. Working in an air-conditioned office
   C. Empty bladder
   D. Loose-fitting clothes

8. **A flaccid bladder causes urine retention.**
   A. True
   B. False

9. **A urinary tract infection will interfere with physical therapy treatment because it:**
   A. Increases spasticity
   B. Causes nausea
   C. Triggers autonomic dysreflexia
   D. All of the above

10. **In the acute stage of cervical SCI, loss of sympathetic drive to the lungs causes:**
    A. Spasticity
    B. Hypotension
    C. Excessive bronchial secretions
    D. Damage to the cilia

11. **A patient with C6 tetraplegia has low blood oxygenation levels when sitting in an upright body position. This is most likely due to:**
    A. Abdominal protrusion that expands the thorax
    B. Greater mucous secretions
    C. Vasomotor constriction
    D. Loss of phrenic motor drive

12. **A person with SCI at C8 that develops pneumonia during inpatient rehabilitation would be expected to:**
    A. develop a bladder infection at the same time
    B. have higher neuropathic pain intensity in the future
    C. have less motor recovery in the future
    D. develop severe spasticity in the future

13. **To prevent pressure injuries at any stage of rehabilitation after SCI, the following factors should be modified:**
    A. Eliminate nicotine
    B. Perform pressure relief every 15 minutes while sitting

C. Change positions in bed every 2 hours

D. Avoid urinary incontinence

E. All of the above

14. **An individual with a T8 SCI and upper motor neuron signs below the injury would be most at risk for which bowel dysfunction:**

A. Fecal incontinence

B. Fecal retention

C. Areflexic bowel

D. Poor motility

15. **For the patient described above with T8 SCI, the therapist will need to monitor for which of the following bowel conditions:**

A. Abdominal distention and pain

B. Autonomic dysreflexia

C. Orthostatic hypotension

D. Urinary tract infection

16. **An individual with a C5 complete SCI upon entry into inpatient rehabilitation will be expected to:**

A. Exhibit no further recovery and remain AIS A

B. Require a ventilator

C. Use a manual wheel chair

D. Have active shoulder muscles

17. **Heterotopic ossification poses a major problem for individuals with SCI because:**

A. Joint range of motion becomes severely restricted and prevents dressing

B. Of low recurrence rates

C. Stem cells prevent autonomic dysreflexia

D. Frank bone loss occurs

18. **In general, an individual with SCI would be expected to attain independent hand function if the SCI occurs below:**

A. C8

B. C6

C. C4

D. C2

19. **You are evaluating an individual with incomplete cervical SCI. What upper extremity muscle groups must have good strength in order for the individual to manually propel a wheel chair?**

A. Erector spinae

B. Deltoids

C. Elbow extensors

D. Finger extensors

20. **The upper extremity requires specific interventions as early as possible. The role of the physical therapist will be to:**

A. Deliver passive stretching only

B. Inform the occupational therapist of strength-related concerns

C. Apply somatosensory stimulation and massed practice to improve motor control

D. All of the above

21. **Neuropathic pain represents a major challenge for people with SCI because:**

A. The late onset interferes with integration into social and daily routines

B. Current treatments are ineffective

C. Normally soft stimuli are perceived as severely painful

D. All of the above

22. **The most effective treatment for neuropathic pain after SCI is anti-epilectic drugs like pregabalin and gabapentin**

A. True

B. False

23. **A return to sexual function is expected for all individuals following SCI. The role of the physical therapist will be to:**

A. Allow the nurse to discuss sexual function with the individual

B. Assume that sexual drive will be lost due to the SCI

C. Decline to treat individuals who are bisexual or homosexual due to religious beliefs

D. None of the above

24. **Which of the following complications is most likely to occur for any individual with SCI regardless of lesion severity or location?**

A. Urinary or bladder calculi

B. Pneumonia

C. Pressure ulcer

D. Depression

E. All of the above

25. **Gait training for individuals with complete SCI at T6 will most likely require:**

A. A reciprocal gait orthosis

B. A hip, knee, ankle orthosis

C. An ankle foot orthosis

D. A supra-malleolar orthosis

26. **Gait training with body weight support may benefit individuals in which of the following ways:**

A. improved bowel, bladder, and sexual function

B. reduced chronic neuropathic pain

C. higher exoskeleton-assisted walking speed

D. All of the above

E. None of the above

27. The long-term consequences of a spinal cord injury include:
    A. Osteoporosis
    B. Cardiovascular disease
    C. Shoulder pain and dysfunction
    D. Syringomyelia
    E. All of the above

28. The APTA clinical practice guideline for gait training endorses which of the following:
    A. Initiate interventions as early as possible, at acute time points
    B. Rely on treadmill training
    C. Prioritize endurance training
    D. All of the Above
    E. None of the above

29. Epidural stimulation of the spinal cord after motor complete SCI produces what effects:
    A. Overground walking
    B. Improved pulmonary function
    C. Better cardiovascular function
    D. All of the above
    E. None of the Above

30. Severe shoulder pain is typically caused by which of the following:
    A. Good body biomechanics
    B. Good muscles strength of finger flexors
    C. Sustained body weight year over year
    D. Overuse during propulsion and transfers

31. The secondary phase of SCI is deemed of:
    A. Less importance than the primary injury because motor deficits have already occurred
    B. More importance than the primary injury because it is more extensive in time and space
    C. Less importance than the primary injury because greater neuron loss doesn't occur

    D. More importance than the primary injury because it makes SCI prognosis easier

32. The most common cause of SCI is athletic activities like football.
    A. Ture
    B. False

33. To differentiate between lower motor neuron injury and upper motor neuron injury after SCI, physical therapists should:
    A. Use Beevor sign for thoracic injuries
    B. Interpret lack of deep tendon reflexes as spinal shock
    C. Understand that increased spasticity can be a result of activity-dependent training
    D. Be sure to consider antidepressants and pain medication as a cause of hyperreflexia

34. After spinal shock has resolved, muscle paralysis at the level of injury indicates:
    A. Motor neuron loss and permanent paralysis
    B. Flaccid reflexes due to loss of the final common pathway
    C. Different types of stimulation will not produce activation in these muscles
    D. All of the above
    E. None of the above

35. An SCI to the dorsal columns primarily, would present with which of the following deficits:
    A. Loss of proprioception
    B. Loss of pain and temperature sensation
    C. Loss of muscle control
    D. Loss of sweating on one side of the face

36. Which factor or factors increase AIS grades in SCI:
    A. Infection
    B. Epidural stimulation
    C. Decompression Surgery
    D. Steroid administration

Answers

1. D	2. E	3. B	4. B	5. D
6. B	7. A	8. A	9. D	10. C
11. A	12. C	13. E	14. B	15. A
16. D	17. A	18. A	19. B	20. C
21. D	22. B	23. D	24. D	25. A
26. D	27. E	28. E	29. D	30. D
31. B	32. B	33. A	34. D	35. A
36. C				

GLOSSARY

Allodynia. Intense pain to normally innocuous stimuli.

Anterior spinal cord syndrome. Lesion of the anterior two-thirds of the spinal cord due to anterior spinal artery damage, leading to bilateral impairment of motor function and pain and temperature but intact somatosensation.

ASIA Impairment Scale. SCI classification method with AIS A as a complete injury, B as sensory incomplete, C as motor incomplete, D as both motor and sensory incomplete and E normal.

Autonomic dysreflexia. A life-threatening increase in blood pressure and heart rate and vasoconstriction, associated with SCI above T6, initiated by strong sensory input.

Behavioral self-management. Strategies to manage pain through cognitive behavioral therapy, relaxation, and body awareness.

Beevor sign. Contraction of the upper rectus abdominus in the absence of lower rectus abdominus function pulls the umbilicus toward the head, when the head is raised, consistent with a lower thoracic injury.

Brown-Sequard injury. Damage to primarily one side of cord, resulting in loss of somatosensation and motor function on the side of the injury and pain and temperature on the opposite side.

Cauda equina syndrome. Lesion at L2 or below, damaging descending spinal nerve roots.

Central cord syndrome. Lesion of the center core of gray matter with greater UE loss of function than LE.

Computer-controlled exoskeleton. A robotic system that is free to roam the environment and assists the wearer to move

Condom catheter. A catheter used in men that is attached to a condom.

Conus medullaris injury. Damage at L1 where the tip of the cord is located.

Crede method. Pressing down on the lower abdomen to facilitate bladder emptying.

Detrusor muscle. Muscle forming the wall of the bladder and internal sphincter.

Digital stimulation. Circular stimulation of the rectum with a gloved finger to elicit peristalsis via the enteric nervous system.

Enteric (intrinsic) nervous system. The myenteric plexus and submucosal plexus that contribute to control of bowel function independent from brain input.

Epidural stimulation. Stimulation to the lumbar cord dorsal root afferents by an implanted electrode to provide neuromodulation of cord activity to facilitate function.

Eschar. Think hard dark tissue at the edges or bed of a pressure injury.

External anal sphincter. Under voluntary control via the pudendal nerve to maintain/allow anal closure.

External FES systems. surface electrodes apply stimulation over key muscles, integrated by a computer, to achieve multiple functional movements.

External urethral sphincter. Striated muscle at the urethral opening.

Flaccid bladder. A hyporesponsive reflex response to bladder filling, allowing the bladder to over fill.

Foley. Held in place by a partially inflated balloon.

Heterotopic ossification. Pathologic bone formation within muscle and other soft tissue.

Hyperalgesia. Exaggerated pain to a noxious stimulus.

Hypogastric nerve. Post-ganglionic sympathetic innervation (T11-L2) of bladder and bowel that inhibits detrusor contraction.

Implantable FES system. Electrical stimulation units, implanted in the muscle, to achieve movement (e.g., stimulating muscles for walking).

Indwelling catheter. Catheter that is inserted into the bladder to provide constant emptying.

Intermittent catheterization. Catheterization every 4-6 hours to empty the bladder.

Internal anal sphincter. Smooth muscle sphincter innervated by hypogastric nerve (S2-4).

Internal urethral sphincter. Functional sphincter at the bladder neck that tightens as the bladder fills to prevent leakage.

International SCI Basic Pain Data Set. Instrument for measuring pain and differentiating neuropathic pain.

International Standards for Neurological Classification of SCI. The international revision of the AIS, adopted for international use

Lokomat system. A robotic treadmill training system that provides passive LE movement.

Neurogenic Bowel Dysfunction. Disruption of the neurologic control of bowel function, leading to fecal retention and/or incontinence.

Neurogenic fever. A rise in body temperature not associated with any infection or inflammation that occurs in those with an SCI at T6 or above, caused by overheating.

Neurogenic shock. Loss of sympathetic control, affecting heart rate, vasomotor responses, and blood pressure.

Neuromuscular electrical stimulation. Electrical stimulation to achieve muscle contraction but not a functional movement; used to prevent atrophy, achieve hypertrophy, or increase strength.

Neuromuscular Recovery Scale. a 14-item measure that evaluates functional performance.

Neuropathic pain. Ongoing pain after a neural injury, resulting from damage to the somatosensory system, including allodynia and hyperalgesia.

Non-implantable FES system. Surface electrodes activate muscles for functional movement (e.g., cycling).

Paradoxical breathing. Retraction of abdomen on inspiration and protrusion on exhalation secondary to diaphragm paralysis.

Paraplegia. Involvement of legs.

Peristalsis. Reflexive contractions of smooth muscle in the wall of the colon that move stool forward.

Posterior spinal cord syndrome. damage to posterior cord, resulting in loss of somatosensation with intact motor function and pain and temperature.

Primary injury. Direct damage to spinal cord.

Puborectalis muscle. Muscle that encircles the rectum to maintain its position and fecal continence.

Pudendal nerve (S2-4). Innervates external urethral sphincter and is tonically active to keep the sphincter closed.

Reverse Trendelenburg. Elevation of the head and lowering of the feet, used to increase tolerance for sitting.

Sacral neuromodulation. An implantable stimulator is used to modulate inhibitory and excitatory bladder control.

Secondary injury. Damage to bystander neurons caused by a toxic environment.

Slough. Stringy soft moist tissue, associated with a pressure injury.

Spastic bladder. Overactive sacral reflex, resulting in bladder contraction that expels urine without allowing the bladder to fill.

Sphincter dyssynergia. Dyscoordination of bladder emptying and external sphincter relaxation.

Sphincterotomy. Surgical cutting of the external sphincter, performed on men and followed by use of a condom catheter.

Spinal Cord Independence Measure. A patient report measure of ADLS and function.

Spinal shock (diaschisis). Widespread depression of neural activity after spinal cord injury.

Spinal stenosis. Narrowing of the spinal canal that can compress the spinal cord.

Suprapubic. Surgically inserted tube through abdominal wall into bladder.

Suprapubic tapping. Intermittent pressure over the bladder to facilitate emptying.

Syringomyelia. A cyst within the spinal cord that fills with cerebrospinal fluid.

Tenodesis grip. a grip generated by tight finger flexors, achieved by wrist extension.

Tetraplegia. Involvement of arms and legs.

Transcutaneous spinal cord stimulation. Non-invasive surface stimulation to the thoracolumbar back to stimulate dorsal afferents to facilitate neural activity for functional movement.

Transverse myelitis. Bilateral inflammation of the spinal cord with a sudden onset.

Urethral stents. A mesh tube used to keep the external sphincter open, used with a condom catheter for men.

Valsalva maneuver. Bearing down or learning forward to facilitate voiding.

Walking Index for Spinal Cord Injury II. A measure of walking recovery.

ABBREVIATIONS

AIS	ASIA impairment scale
DVT	deep brain thrombosis
FES	functional electrical stimulation
HO	heterotopic ossification
ISCIPBD	International SCI Basic Pain Data Set
ISNCSCI	International Standards for Neurological Classification of SCI
LMN	lower motor neuron
NBD	neurogenic bowel dysfunction
NRS	Neuromuscular Recovery Scale
rTMS	repetitive transcranial magnetic stimulation
SCI	spinal cord injury
SCIM	Spinal Cord Independence Measure
tDCS	transcutaneous direct spinal cord stimulation
TENS	transcutaneous electrical nerve stimulation
UMN	upper motor neuron
UTI	urinary tract infection
VR	virtual reality

Multiple Sclerosis

Anne D. Kloos and Deborah A. Kegelmeyer

14

OBJECTIVES

1) Describe the demographics, risk factors, etiology, pathophysiology, common symptoms, and diagnosis of multiple sclerosis (MS)

2) Differentiate between the general progression and prognosis of the different types of MS

3) Discuss the medical management of MS

4) Design a physical therapy intervention program with appropriate goals and outcomes for the individual with MS

CASE A, PART I

Sheila Dillman is a 37-year-old white female. She came to Neurology Clinic for evaluation of her long-term neurologic complaints. Ms. Dillman relates that for the last 2 years she has noticed some strange symptoms, particularly heat intolerance which precedes the onset of difficulty with walking. She admits to several near falls and describes her gait during these episodes as a "stumbling gait." She also relates that over the last 2 years she goes through periods where her vision is blurry. Two months ago she underwent a divorce and moved to her own apartment. At this time she got sick with the flu and her condition worsened. At that time, she could not hold objects in her hands and had severe exhaustion. She also had several falls and intermittent joint pain on the left side of her body that was spread diffusely across multiple joints. More recently, her chart indicates that she abruptly developed a left hemisensory deficit. The MRI scan was performed at that time and revealed a multifocal white matter disease – areas of increased T2 signal in both cerebral hemispheres. Spinal tap was also done which revealed the presence of oligoclonal bands in CSF. Visual evoked response testing was abnormal with slowed conduction in optic nerves.

Findings on exam: She remains weak and numb on the left side; has impaired urinary bladder function, requiring multiple voids in the mornings and nocturia at times. She has become incontinent and now has to wear a pad during the day. She also has ongoing balance problems with some sensation of spinning, has continuous tinnitus with mild hearing loss, and is extremely fatigued. She complains of impaired short-term memory and irritability.

WHAT IS MULTIPLE SCLEROSIS?

MS is a chronic, progressive, inflammatory disease that affects neurons in the central nervous system. Jean-Martin Charcot is credited with the first comprehensive description of the disease in 1868.[1] He described its clinical and pathological features and outlined the symptom triad known as Charcot's triad: intention tremor, nystagmus, and scanning speech.

EPIDEMIOLOGY/RISK

The overall incidence of MS is 46.3 per 100,000 population in the United States[2]; about one million people are living with MS in the United States and an estimated 2.3 million people are living with MS globally.[3] It is one of the most common causes of neurologic disability in young adults and typically affects individuals between the ages of 20 and 50, with the mean age of onset being 32 years. Children (≤18 years) and adults over the age of 50 are rarely affected. MS is three times more common in women than men.[4] Whites of European ancestry have higher rates of MS than those of African, Asian, and Hispanic/Latino ancestry.[4] The incidence of MS increases the farther one travels from the equator, with the highest prevalence rates found in Scandinavian countries, northern Europe, northern United States, southern Canada, New Zealand, and southern Australia.[4] The estimated rate of MS is between 57 and 78 cases per 100,000 people in southern US states (below the 37th parallel), while the rate of MS is twice as high in northern states (above the 37th parallel), at about 110 to 140 cases per 100,000.[3] Migration studies indicate that individuals who move before puberty (age 15) from one geographic area to another tend to take on the risk level, either higher or lower, of the area to which they move.[4,5] However, those who move after puberty tend to retain the risk level of their birthplace. Outbreaks or "epidemics" of MS have been reported, most notably in the Faroe Islands off the coast of Scotland when they were occupied by British soldiers during World War II, but the cause and significance of these outbreaks are debated.[6]

Other modifiable environmental factors associated with increased risk of MS are smoking, low blood levels of vitamin D, and obesity. Epidemiological studies showed that smokers have a 40% increased risk of developing MS and were greater than three times more likely to develop secondary progressive MS, if they presented with relapsing-remitting MS compared to nonsmokers.[7,8] Lower vitamin D levels caused by less sunlight (ultraviolet) exposure have been proposed to explain the higher incidence of MS the further the distance from the equator. Many epidemiological studies support a protective role of vitamin D in reducing MS risk,[8] including a large prospective study of nurses in the United States that found that women who used supplemental vitamin D, largely from multivitamins, had a 40% lower risk of MS than women who did not use vitamin D supplements.[9] There is also a growing body of evidence that correcting vitamin D insufficiency in people with MS (or clinically isolated syndrome) has a beneficial effect on clinical and MRI outcomes.[8] Obesity in early life (from childhood through young adulthood) has emerged as another risk factor for MS, generally associated with a twofold increase in risk across several populations and study designs in both women and men.[8,9]

● PATHOPHYSIOLOGY/ PATHOGENESIS

The exact cause of MS is unknown, but exposure to environmental agents, particularly viruses, is believed to trigger MS in genetically susceptible individuals. Although no particular virus has been confirmed to trigger the onset of MS in humans, there is strong evidence that Epstein-Barr virus (EBV) infection is a risk factor for MS.[10,11] No genes have been directly linked to MS, but specific human leukocyte antigen (HLA) genes, particularly the *HLA-DRB1* gene, located on chromosome 6, are strongly associated with the development of the disease.[11] These genes encode proteins that are important for regulating immune cell functions. In addition, researchers have identified over 200 non-HLA genes that increase a person's risk of MS, the majority of which encode immune system-related molecules.[11] These genetic findings lend support to the idea that MS is primarily an immune-mediated disease. Twin studies have shown that the identical twin of a person with MS has about a 20 to 30% risk of developing the disease while the risk for fraternal twins is around 2 to 5%.[11,12] Siblings of an individual with MS are 10 to 15 times more likely to develop MS than the general population.[11] Second- and third-degree relatives carry a 1% increased risk of developing MS, which is modestly higher than the 0.1% risk of the general population.[13]

Tissue damage in MS results from complex interactions between the immune system, glia (oligodendrocytes and their precursors, microglia, and astrocytes), and neurons.[14] Research using autoimmune and viral animal models of MS has contributed greatly to the prevailing ideas about how environmental factors may trigger inflammation, demyelination, and neurodegeneration within the central nervous system, and to the development of treatments that target the inflammatory aspects of MS.[15] Autoimmune animal models, collectively called experimental autoimmune encephalomyelitis (EAE) models, are the best understood and most widely used in MS research. Injection of antigens (e.g., myelin-derived proteins and peptides) into the animals produces CNS inflammation and demyelination that induces progressive paralysis that follows a monophasic, relapsing-remitting, or chronic disease course depending on the antigen used and the genetic makeup of the animal.[15] Although there is debate about whether the root cause of MS originates within ("inside-out" hypothesis) or outside ("outside-in" hypothesis) of the CNS,[16] studies in animal models, along with analysis of immune cells and their products taken from cerebrospinal fluid and blood of humans, have revealed a crucial role for white blood cells (i.e., T and B cells) of the adaptive immune system.[14] The most popular "outside-in" hypothesis proposes that T cells (i.e., helper CD 4+ and cytotoxic CD8+) become activated in the peripheral circulatory system by an unknown antigen, possibly a virus such as the EBV.[17] The triggering antigen is thought to have similar sequences with myelin or other CNS antigens. For unknown reasons, the myelin-reactive T cells migrate through the blood-brain barrier into the CNS and are reactivated by intrinsic CNS immune cells (e.g., microglia, macrophages, B cells), triggering the release of inflammatory cytokines and chemokines that damage myelin and oligodendrocytes, causing demyelination as well as axonal injury (Figure 14-1A).[17] In addition, emerging evidence strongly suggests that activated B cells are involved in the pathophysiology of MS by making and releasing antibodies that attack myelin, by producing pro-inflammatory cytokines and unidentified factors that are toxic to oligodendrocytes and neurons, and by their antigen-presenting ability to activate T cells.[18]

The damage to myelin and axons slows or interrupts the conduction of nerve impulses, resulting in symptoms specific to the damaged neurons. Reduction of inflammation and its associated edema along with compensatory remyelination by oligodendrocytes and/or neural plasticity contribute to the remission of symptoms (Figure 14-1B and Box 14-1).[22-24] However, in some lesions for unknown reasons the inflammation resolves without axonal remyelination (called chronic inactive) or inflammation and slow myelin degeneration persists (called smoldering).[14] Smoldering lesions are most common in progressive multiple sclerosis (Box 14-1).[25] In general, remyelination is more robust during the early phases of MS and in younger individuals, whereas it is infrequent or absent in individuals with progressive and secondary MS.[26] Completely remyelinated lesions, called **shadow plaques**, are distinguished from **normal-appearing white matter** (NAWM) by the thinness of their myelin sheaths, possibly making them more susceptible to a second inflammatory attack.[27] NAWM refers to the areas around white matter lesions that appear normal macroscopically on conventional magnetic resonance images, yet have been shown to have abnormalities (i.e., chronically activated microglia, dysfunctional and degenerating axons, reactive astroglia, and a compromised blood-brain barrier) in people with MS. Over time, the oligodendrocytes die and remyelination is not possible. Demyelinated areas become filled with fibrous astrocytes that form scar tissue (sclerosis) or so-called sclerotic plaques that are pathologic hallmarks of the disease. The damaged axons become transected and undergo retrograde degeneration and eventually cell death.[28,29]

In addition to white matter, plaques are also found in cortical (temporal and frontal cortex, including motor areas) and subcortical (thalamus, basal ganglia, and cerebellum) grey matter and are also related to physical disability and cognitive impairments.[30,31] About half of cortical lesions are located around blood vessels, and the other half are found in cortical

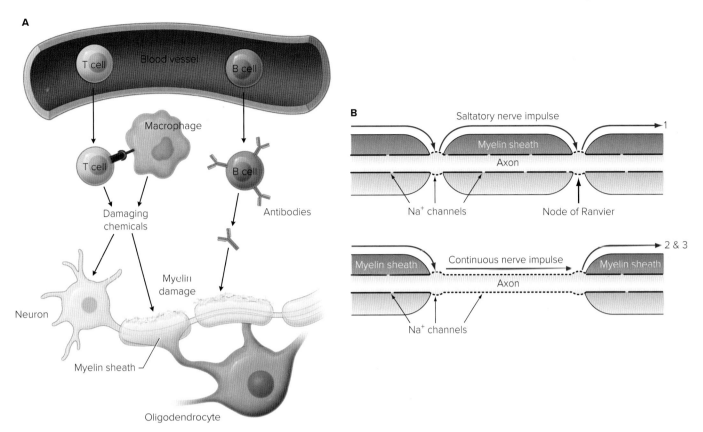

FIGURE 14-1 A. Autoimmune process of myelin damage: Activated T cells and potentially B cells, followed by macrophage activity, induce myelin inflammation that can damage the myelin. During the inflammatory phase, conduction is impaired, producing symptoms associated with the involved axons; as inflammation recedes, recovery of symptoms occurs if remyelination is achieved. **B.** Schematic representation of demyelination and axonal degeneration in MS. (1) schematic of normal neural function in a myelinated axon; (2) in acute demyelination, action potentials can't cross the open space due to low numbers of voltage-gated sodium channels in the internodal axonal regions and stop; (3) in a demyelinated axon, conduction can take place if voltage-gated sodium channels are added to the axon membrane through neuroplasticity, but is much slower; (4) with further loss of myelin, axon degeneration occurs (not shown). (B, Reproduced with permission from Hauser SL, ed. Harrison's *Neurology in Clinical Medicine,* 3rd ed., New York, NY: McGraw-Hill; 2013, Fig. 39-1, p. 475.)

sulci and deep invaginations of the brain surface that are topographically related to inflammatory infiltrates (i.e., activated macrophages, T and B cells) originating in the overlying meninges that proceed inward to affect superficial cortical layers.[14,24] Compared with white matter lesions, cortical lesions typically demonstrate less inflammation and more efficient myelin repair after demyelination, suggesting that different mechanisms underlie lesion formation in the white matter and grey matter.[24] Studies suggest that grey matter pathology is, in part, independent of white matter lesions and may precede development of the white matter pathology.[32,33] Inflammatory and neurodegenerative processes combine to eventually induce neuronal loss and brain atrophy. Axonal destruction occurs early and can be detected on MRI even before individuals are diagnosed with MS.[34]

● WHY DO SOME PEOPLE WITH MS SEEM TO GET SICKER AND THEN BETTER OVER TIME?

Question: What type of MS is Sheila most likely exhibiting?

Sheila's prior history describes a pattern of intermittent flare-ups of neurological symptoms that occurred suddenly and that resolved over time with periods of stable function between episodes, consistent with RRMS. More recently, her symptoms appear to be progressively worsening over time with evidence of multiple sclerotic lesions on the MRI, suggesting that she might be going into secondary progressive MS.

● HOW IS MS DIAGNOSED?

Early diagnosis is important as early treatment may slow or prevent worsening of disability. However, due to the heterogeneity of symptoms and the lack of a definitive diagnostic test, it may take years before the diagnosis of MS is established. The diagnosis of MS remains a clinical diagnosis based on history and neurologic examination findings of evidence of at least two episodes of neurologic symptoms referable to myelinated regions of the CNS that are separated in space (i.e., cerebral white matter, brainstem, cerebellar tracts, optic nerves, spinal cord) and time. Many physicians use the *2017 Revised McDonald Diagnostic Criteria for MS*

The clinical disease course varies widely and is unpredictable from person to person and within a particular person over time. However, there are four main subtypes that describe the most frequent clinical course for MS (Figure 14-2).[19]

Clinically Isolated Syndrome (CIS)

CIS is a monophasic clinical episode in which an individual reports symptoms and objective findings indicative of a focal or multifocal inflammatory demyelinating event in the CNS, developing acutely or subacutely, with a duration of at least 24 hours, with or without recovery, and in the absence of fever or infection. If the person with CIS is subsequently diagnosed with MS, the CIS was the person's first relapse, also called an **attack** or **exacerbation**.[19]

Relapsing-Remitting MS (RRMS)

Most individuals (about 85%) diagnosed with MS are initially diagnosed with **relapsing-remitting** MS (RRMS). People with RRMS have clearly defined relapses, defined as during which neurologic function worsens. These relapses are followed by remissions, defined as periods during which the disease does not progress, and individuals experience complete or incomplete recovery of neurologic function. RRMS can also be characterized as **active** (e.g., the person is having a relapse and/or new MRI activity), or as **not active** (e.g., no disease activity is occurring).[20] It is possible for RRMS to be **not active** but still be **worsening** (confirmed increase in disability due to symptoms persisting after a relapse), or **active** but **not worsening** (new MRI activity, but no increase in clinical symptoms). Relapse rates for untreated RRMS are about one to two relapses a year and are correlated with disability.[21]

Secondary Progressive MS (SPMS)

Following an initial period of RRMS, many people develop a **secondary progressive** (SPMS) disease course, in which the disease steadily worsens, with or without notable relapses and remissions or plateaus. As with RRMS, SPMS can be described as **active** or **not active** at different timepoints depending on whether there is evidence of disease activity. SPMS can be further characterized as **with progression**, meaning that there is sustained worsening of symptoms over time, or as **without progression**. It is possible for SPMS to be **active**, but also be described as **without progression** if there are new MRI lesions, but no observable increase in disability. Approximately 50% of people with RRMS developed SPMS within 10 years of diagnoses before the advent of disease-modifying medications.[20]

Primary Progressive MS (PPMS)

Primary progressive MS (PPMS) affects approximately 10% of people and is characterized by steadily worsening neurologic function from the time of diagnosis that is independent of relapses. The rate of progression may vary over time, with possible occurrence of symptom fluctuations, periods of stability, and superimposed relapses. As with SPMS, PPMS can be characterized as **active** or **not active**, as well as **with** or **without progression**. Individuals with PPMS tend to be older (i.e., around 40 years old) at the time of onset.[20]

(Table 14-1) to make the diagnosis.[19] All diseases that present with similar symptoms must be ruled out before the diagnosis of MS is made.

Imaging and Other Diagnostic Tests

MRI is the most important diagnostic and prognostic test in MS. It is useful for detecting **plaques** or **lesions** and cortical atrophy even before clinical symptoms are evident, identifying areas of active inflammation, and establishing **dissemination in time** (DIT, development of new CNS lesions over time) and **dissemination in space** (DIS, development of lesions in distinct anatomical areas of the CNS) (Figure 14-3).[24,34] MS lesions can be found anywhere in the CNS white matter, and 15–37% are located in the grey matter.[8] Plaques located near or around the ventricles, called periventricular lesions, and in the corpus callosum are highly suggestive of MS. In particular, lesions around small veins located perpendicular to the walls of the lateral ventricles, called **Dawson's fingers**, are common MRI findings in MS (Figure 14-3B).[35] The neurodegenerative aspect of MS is detected on T1-weighted MRI scans as dark hypointense lesions called **black holes**. Black holes, representing focal areas of complete demyelination with irreversible axonal damage, are associated with cognitive dysfunction and neurological disability in people with MS.[36] MRI findings consistent with MS are sometimes observed in seemingly healthy individuals who undergo scanning for other reasons, and are called **radiologically isolated syndrome** (RIS). Up to 50% of individuals with RIS develop MS, sometimes with a primary progressive course. Gadolinium is attracted to areas of inflammation and is used as a contrast medium in **T1-weighted MRI scans** to identify newly active lesions. **T2-weighted MRI scans** provide information about axonal loss and disease progression in terms of the total amount of lesion area and brain atrophy.[37,38]

Other important tests that support the diagnosis of MS are cerebrospinal fluid (CSF) analysis and evoked potential testing including visual, somatosensory, and brainstem auditory evoked responses. CSF-specific **oligoclonal immunoglobulin bands**, reflecting elevated secretion of immunoglobulin G (IgG) antibodies by B cells or plasma cells within the CNS, are important laboratory findings in MS due to their high prevalence in patients with MS (up to 88%) and their ability to predict a second attack in people with CIS.[24,34] Evoked potential testing showing slowed conduction of sensory signals through the CNS is thought to reflect demyelination and can identify clinically silent lesions in the CNS, that might be missed through clinical examination.[24,34]

● MS SIGNS AND SYMPTOMS: WHY ARE THE SYMPTOMS SO VARIABLE IN DIFFERENT PATIENTS WITH MS?

Signs and symptoms vary considerably, depending on the location of lesions within the CNS but can include sensory, motor, cognitive, emotional, and autonomic manifestations. A first neurologic event in which a person experiences single or multiple symptoms that last at least 24 hours is often referred to as a CIS. The most common early symptoms of MS are sensory,

2013 Subtypes of multiple sclerosis

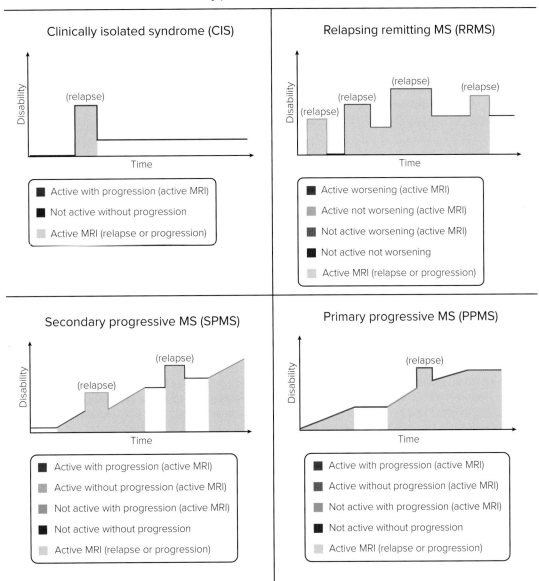

FIGURE 14-2 Schematic of clinical course associated with MS subtypes.

including **paresthesias** (e.g., numbness, tingling, pins and needles sensation, tightness, coldness, and/or swelling of the limbs or trunk), or visual disturbances (e.g., blurred vision in one or both eyes, diplopia (double vision), or diminished acuity/loss of vision).[24] Common symptoms of MS are presented in Box 14-2. Symptoms typically develop rapidly over the course of minutes or hours but can develop slowly over weeks or months. They are unpredictable and vary from person to person, and from relapse to relapse in the same person.

When primary symptoms are poorly managed, secondary symptoms develop such as infections, falls, injuries, contractures, and pressure sores that contribute to disability and decreased quality of life. As the disease progresses, individuals experience tertiary symptoms such as loss of job, loss of intimacy, role changes, family disruption, social isolation, dependency, loss of self-esteem, and all possible consequences of chronic disease.

Sensory Dysfunction

Sensory disturbances affect the majority of individuals with MS and typically include paresthesias affecting the face, body, or extremities. Numbness or tingling can be localized to a single cranial nerve or spinal nerve root distribution, a single limb (monoanesthesia), a single side of the body (hemianesthesia), as is the case for Ms. Dillman, or multiple areas (e.g., cranial nerves plus hemianesthesia). Reduced touch, pressure, pain, temperature, and proprioception sensations can interfere with performance of functional activities and in severe cases lead to injuries from secondary wounds, burns, or falls. One study involving 82 people with MS found that somatosensory impairments (proprioception, touch, and vibration) were more common in the lower extremities than upper extremities (78.2% vs 64.1%), and they were independent predictors of balance deficits as measured by the Timed Up and Go and Functional Reach tests.[39]

TABLE 14-1	The 2017 McDonald Criteria for Diagnosis of Multiple Sclerosis in Patients with an Attack at Onset	
	NUMBER OF LESIONS WITH OBJECTIVE CLINICAL EVIDENCE	**ADDITIONAL DATA NEEDED FOR A DIAGNOSIS OF MULTIPLE SCLEROSIS**
≥2 clinical attacks	≥2	None*
≥2 clinical attacks	1 (as well as clear-cut historical evidence of a previous attack involving a lesion in a distinct anatomical location[†])	None*
≥2 clinical attacks	1	Dissemination in space demonstrated by an additional clinical attack implicating a different CNS site or by MRI[‡]
1 clinical attack	≥2	Dissemination in time demonstrated by an additional clinical attack or by MRI[§] OR demonstration of CSF-specific oligoclonal bands[¶]
1 clinical attack	1	Dissemination in space demonstrated by an additional clinical attack implicating a different CNS site or by MRI[‡]
		AND
		Dissemination in time demonstrated by an additional clinical attack or by MRI[§] OR demonstration of CSF-specific oligoclonal bands[¶]

If the 2017 McDonald Criteria are fulfilled and there is no better explanation for the clinical presentation, the diagnosis is multiple sclerosis. If multiple sclerosis is suspected by virtue of a clinically isolated syndrome but the 2017 McDonald Criteria are not completely met, the diagnosis is possible multiple sclerosis. If another diagnosis arises during the evaluation that better explains the clinical presentation, the diagnosis is not multiple sclerosis. An attack is defined in panel 1. *No additional tests are required to demonstrate dissemination in space and time. However, unless MRI is not possible, brain MRI should be obtained in all patients in whom the diagnosis of multiple sclerosis is being considered. In addition, spinal cord MRI or CSF examination should be considered in patients with insufficient clinical and MRI evidence supporting multiple sclerosis, with a presentation other than a typical clinically isolated syndrome, or with atypical features. If imaging or other tests (eg, CSF) are undertaken and are negative, caution needs to be taken before making a diagnosis of multiple sclerosis, and alternative diagnoses should be considered. [†]Clinical diagnosis based on objective clinical findings for two attacks is most secure. Reasonable historical evidence for one past attack, in the absence of documented objective neurological findings, can include historical events with symptoms and evolution characteristic for a previous inflammatory demyelinating attack; at least one attack, however, must be supported by objective findings. In the absence of residual objective evidence, caution is needed. [‡]The MRI criteria for dissemination in space are described in panel 5. [§]The MRI criteria for dissemination in time are described in panel 5. [¶]The presence of CSF-specific oligoclonal bands does not demonstrate dissemination in time per se but can substitute for the requirement for demonstration of this measure.

Reproduced with permission from Thompson et al. Diagnosis of multiple sclerosis: 2017 revisions of the McDonald Criteria, Lancet Neurol. 2018;17(2):162-173.

Pain

Pain is a common disabling complaint for individuals with MS and encompasses neuropathic (i.e., pain arising directly from a lesion affecting the somatosensory system), nociceptive (i.e., musculoskeletal-related pain), or combinations of both[40] (e.g., tonic muscle spasms or spasticity). MS-related neuropathic pain is a direct or indirect result of demyelinating lesions, neuroinflammation, and/or axonal damage in the brain and spinal cord, called "central neuropathic pain" (CNP).[41,42] The most common types of neuropathic pain include dysesthesias, trigeminal neuritis, and/or Lhermitte's sign.[42] **Dysesthesias**, the most common pain in MS, are achy, tingling, or burning sensations that affect the limbs, especially the lower extremities.[41] They can be acute (sudden and spontaneous onset) or chronic and may worsen after exercise or with exposure to hot environments. Some individuals with MS experience abnormal responses to sensory stimuli including **hyperalgesia** (i.e., increased sensitivity to painful stimuli) and **allodynia** (perception of nonpainful stimuli as painful), such as a light touch or pressure stimulus to the skin from a person's clothing. **Trigeminal neuralgia** is a sudden severe, stabbing pain in the face related to damage of the trigeminal nerve. **Lhermitte's sign**, a brief electric shock-like sensation down the spine that occurs with neck flexion toward the chest, is often related to dorsal column damage in the cervical spinal cord (Figure 14-4C).[43] Musculoskeletal pain due to muscle or ligament strain can arise from mechanical stress, abnormal postures or movements, or joint immobility caused by muscle weakness, severe spasticity, and tonic muscle spasms.[40]

Visual Disturbances

Common visual disturbances in MS are decreased or blurred vision (optic neuritis), double vision (diplopia), and involuntary eye movements (nystagmus). **Optic neuritis** refers to

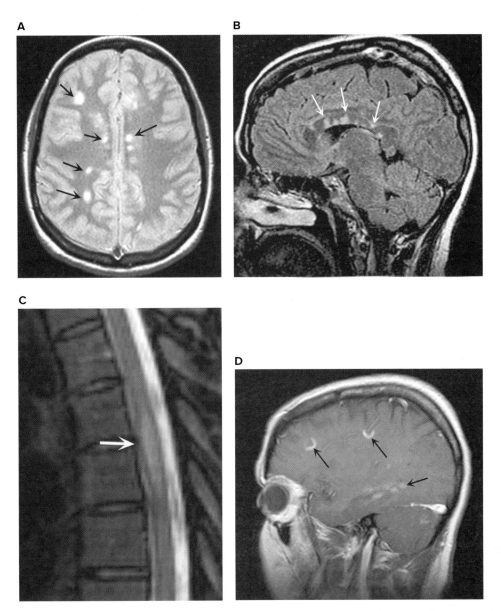

FIGURE 14-3 A–D. MRI findings in MS. Arrows point at areas of high intensity consistent with lesions. (Reproduced with permission from Hauser SL, ed. Harrison's *Neurology in Clinical Medicine*, 3rd ed., New York, NY: McGraw-Hill; 2013, Fig. 39-3, p. 481.)

inflammation of the optic nerve and causes an acute blurring or greying of vision or even blindness in one eye that is often accompanied by pain with eye movements, and alterations in the pupillary light reflex, color vision, and contrast sensitivity.[44] It is likely that Ms. Dillman was experiencing optic neuritis, during her episodes of blurred vision.

Visual symptoms following optic neuritis generally improve within three weeks, but some individuals experience long-term symptoms.[44] A **Marcus Gunn pupil** can develop after neuritis, caused by impaired optic nerve function (Figure 14-4A). Testing for the Marcus Gunn pupil is done using the swinging-flashlight test; when positive, the person's pupils dilate, instead of constricting, when a bright light is swung from the unaffected eye to the affected eye caused by poor light perception in the affected eye. Shining the light in the unaffected eye causes both pupils to constrict (normal function). Impaired contrast sensitivity

reduces the quality of vision, making it especially difficult for a person to recognize faces, read and perform activities of daily living.[44]

Diplopia occurs when eye movements are not coordinated so that the brain is getting two slightly different pictures simultaneously. This typically occurs when MS affects the brainstem, where the coordination of eye movements is controlled. **Internuclear ophthalmoplegia** (INO) is a common cause of double vision in MS (Figure 14-4B). INO can be identified by impaired horizontal eye movement with gaze away from the affected eye, characterized by weak adduction of the affected eye and abduction nystagmus of the contralateral eye. This loss of coordination of the two eyes that creates double vision results from a unilateral lesion in the **medial longitudinal fasciculus** (MLF) in the pons or the midbrain that disrupts the pathway between the abducens nucleus and the contralateral oculomotor nucleus.

Box 14-2	Common Symptoms of MS

Sensory Symptoms
Hypoesthesia, numbness
Paresthesias

Pain
Dysesthesias
Optic or trigeminal neuritis
Lhermitte's sign

Visual Symptoms
Blurred or double vision
Diminished acuity/loss of vision
Internuclear ophthalmoplegia
Nystagmus

Motor Symptoms
Weakness or paralysis
Fatigue
Spasticity
Impaired balance and coordination
Impaired gait and mobility
Impaired speech and swallowing

Cognitive Symptoms
Decreased information-processing speed
Working memory problems
Decreased attention and concentration
Executive function problems
Impaired visual spatial processing

Emotional/Behavioral Symptoms
Depression
Euphoria
Lack of insight
Adjustment disorders
Obsessive-compulsive disorders

Autonomic Dysfunction
Orthostatic hypotension
Decreased or absent sweating
Heat intolerance

Bladder and Bowel Symptoms
Urinary urgency, frequency
Constipation
Diarrhea
Incontinence

Sexual Symptoms
Erectile and ejaculatory dysfunction
Decreased vaginal lubrication
Decreased libido
Decreased ability to achieve orgasm

Individuals with MS may also develop double vision from brainstem lesions affecting cranial nerves III, IV, or VI, each of which innervate specific eye muscles. Lesions of the cerebellum or central vestibular pathways can cause saccadic dysmetria, gaze-evoked nystagmus, and saccadic intrusions during smooth pursuit eye movements (see Chapter 17).[45] When working with a person with MS, therapists should assess to see what the effects of impaired vision are on the person's balance and mobility.

Motor Dysfunction

Motor impairments, including weakness, spasticity, fatigue, and balance and coordination problems, lead to gait and mobility limitations and falls that negatively affect an individual's participation in work, school, home, and recreational activities and decrease quality of life.

Muscle Weakness

Muscle strength, rate of muscle force development, and power are impaired in people with MS compared to healthy controls. Muscle strength impairments are greatest during fast dynamic concentric contractions of lower extremity muscles,[46] as occur during sit-to-stand transfers. Weakness can be the result of central lesions, affecting motor cortical areas or projections, or secondary peripheral changes in muscle, related to denervation or diminished use.[47,48] As described in Chapter 5, force generation is associated with corticospinal projections, emanating from M1; therefore, damage to corticospinal neurons can disrupt force production within specific muscles, typically activated by the damaged neurons. Physical activity levels have been reported to be moderately reduced in people with MS compared to healthy controls, yet only about 20% of people with MS engage in sufficient amounts of moderate-to-vigorous physical activity necessary for deriving health benefits.[49,50] Inactivity can cause secondary muscle weakness from disuse, contributing to both weakness and fatigue; changes in muscle can include decreased oxidative capacity, impaired metabolic responses of muscles to exercise, and impaired excitation–contraction coupling (i.e., the process whereby action potentials cause a muscle cell to contract, followed by relaxation).[51,52] In MS, weakness can vary from mild to severe, and involve one or all extremities as well as the trunk.[46,53]

Spasticity

Spasticity occurs in approximately 80% of people with MS.[54] Those experiencing greater severity are typically males, older persons, or people with longer duration of MS.[55] Spasticity, associated with MS, results from sclerotic lesions and subsequent dysfunction or death, of **upper motor neurons** (UMN) in descending inhibitory CNS motor tracts (i.e., corticospinal, medial reticulospinal, and lateral vestibular tracts; see spasticity description in Chapter 11: Stroke), or by lesions damaging local spinal interneuron networks, that ultimately increase the excitatory inputs to alpha motor neurons.[56–58] As with other conditions that impact UMNs, this damage produces a pattern of signs and symptoms, including paresis, spasticity, hyperreflexia and clonus, involuntary flexor and extensor spasms, exaggerated cutaneous reflexes, and Babinski's sign (see Chapter 11: Stroke), also referred to as spastic paresis.[56,57] Due to the dynamic and variable disease course of MS, spasticity can present in a single limb (segmental), unilaterally (hemispasticity), or bilaterally (paraspasticity, tetraspasticity), and can fluctuate widely in severity even within a few hours.[58] Ultimately, voluntary movement is disrupted and associated with poor muscle activation, synergistic movements, and abnormal co-contraction of muscles.[56]

A Optic neuritis

1 Testing pupillary response

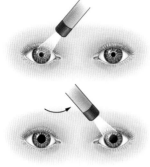

Normal eye   Affected eye

2 Fundoscopic examination of affected eye shows pallor of the optic disc

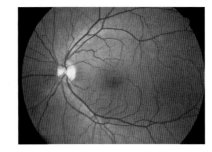

3 Localization of lesion

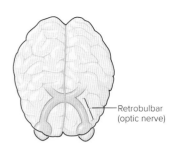

Retrobulbar (optic nerve)

B Internuclear ophthalmoplegia

1 Testing eye movement

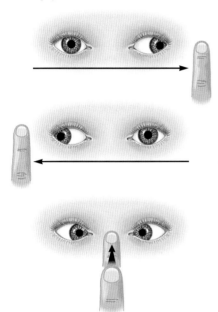

2 Localization of lesion

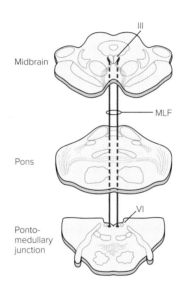

Midbrain — III

MLF

Pons

Ponto-medullary junction — VI

C Additional signs

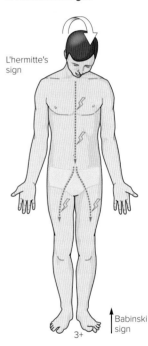

L'hermitte's sign

Babinski sign

3+

FIGURE 14-4 Common intermittent symptoms of MS. A.1: A light shown in the non-involved eye produces constriction bilaterally but a light to the involved eye produces dilation, indicating a de-afferented pupil. **A.2:** Fundoscopic exam illustrates a blurring or elevation of the optic nerve. **A.3:** In the absence of a hemianopia, the lesion can be isolated to the optic nerve. **B.1:** When following a finger across the visual field, the involved eye fails to adduct (top and middle illustrations demonstrate this for either eye). Convergence to a finger pointing at the nose illustrates normal adduction, demonstrating CN III and nucleus integrity. **B.2:** Lesion is localized to the MLF. **C.** Demonstration of testing position for L'hermitte's sign. (Reproduced with permission from Kandel ER, Schwartz JH, Jessell TM, Siegelbaum SA, Hudspeth AJ. *Principles of Neural Science*, 5th ed., New York, NY: McGraw-Hill; 2013. Fig. B-2, p. 1539.)

When severe, MS spasticity can lead to abnormal posturing and joint immobility that results in pain, contractures, and difficulty in maintaining skin integrity.[58] A cross-sectional study of 156 individuals with MS found that 56% of participants had contractures in at least one major limb joint, with the ankle being the most common contracture site (43.9%).[59] Individuals with MS with gastroc-soleus muscle spasticity demonstrated worse mobility and balance on performance (Timed 25-foot walk, Timed Up and Go, Six-Minute Walk Test, Berg Balance Scale) and self-reported (Multiple Sclerosis Walking scale-12, Activities-Specific Balance Confidence Scale) measures than those without spasticity.[60] In a survey of 10,353 participants in the North American Research Committee on Multiple Sclerosis (NARCOMS) registry, spasticity was reported to most frequently interfere with stair climbing, walking, and sleep.[54]

Fatigue

Fatigue is one of the most common symptoms of MS, occurring in approximately 80% of people.[61] It occurs in all subtypes and at all stages of the disease and is not related to the severity or to the duration of MS.[61,62] Most patients with MS describe fatigue as their worst or one of their worst symptoms.[63] Fatigue is defined by the Panel on Fatigue of the MS Council for

Clinical Practice Guidelines as "a subjective lack of physical and/or mental energy that is perceived by the individual or caregiver to interfere with usual or desirable activities."[64] Fatigue, in MS, appears to be distinctly different from fatigue seen in healthy individuals or people with other neurological diagnoses, including that it interferes with carrying out responsibilities, comes on easily and prevents sustained physical functioning, and tends to persist.[61] Fatigue is associated with poorer quality of life even when controlling for disease severity and is a major reason for people with MS leaving the workforce.[65]

The cause of fatigue is unknown but is most likely multifactorial (Figure 14-5). Four potential classes of pathophysiological mechanisms for fatigue in MS include (1) structural damage of white and grey matter resulting in reduced activity and connectivity in cortical networks that mediate motor and cognitive processes; (2) inflammatory processes within the peripheral and central nervous systems; (3) compensatory cortical reorganization and increased areas of brain recruitment during functional task performance due to lesions or inflammation; and (4) impaired metacognition (self-monitoring) of the physiological state of the body leading to feelings of helplessness or low self-efficacy (lack of control over bodily states).[48,65-69]

Fatigue may be directly related to the disease mechanisms (primary fatigue) or may be secondary to non-disease-specific factors.[48,70,71] Primary fatigue may be the result of inflammation, demyelination (i.e., slowing and desynchronization of nerve transmission or partial or complete conduction block), or axonal loss.[70] Central fatigue develops because of failing central motor drive to spinal alpha motor neurons, which also contributes to weakness. Inactivity, as described in a preceding section, leads to muscle changes that may occur independently of CNS damage and also contribute to fatigue. Other secondary contributing factors include heat intolerance, depression, pain, sleep disorders, side effects of medications (i.e., anticonvulsants, antidepressants, and analgesics), comorbid medical conditions (i.e., hypothyroidism, irritable bowel syndrome, migraine), secondary complications of MS (infections, respiratory impairment,

disability), and physical, social, and cultural aspects of the environment, in which the person lives and works.[66,71-73]

Balance and Coordination

Dizziness and problems with coordination and balance are among the most common mobility problems for people with MS.[45] Dizziness arises from demyelinating lesions affecting the cerebellum (flocculonodular lobe) or central vestibular pathways. People with MS may report feeling off balance (disequilibrium), being lightheaded, or having the sensation that they or their surroundings are spinning (vertigo). Lesions affecting the cerebellum and cerebellar tracts produce symptoms of ataxia, tremors (postural and intention), hypotonia, truncal weakness, and general asthenia (see description of cerebellar damage in Chapter 17: Vestibular/Cerebellar Disorders).[74] Postural tremors are observed as shaking, back-and-forth oscillatory movements during sitting or standing. Intention or action tremors are rhythmic shaking movements that occur with volitional movements, such as reaching for an object or moving the foot to a specific location. Severe tremors can interfere with functional activities and are associated with unemployment and poorer quality of life.[75] Numbness of the feet, secondary to damage to the dorsal column medial lemniscal pathways, can also contribute to balance and walking difficulties (sensory ataxia).

Gait and Mobility

Gait impairments are common and one of the most challenging symptoms for people with MS. Because gait patterns depend on the location and severity of CNS lesions, there is no standardized atypical gait pattern associated with MS. Coca-Tapia et al.[76] conducted a systematic review of 12 studies that used three-dimensional gait analysis systems to describe gait patterns in people with MS. They reported that decreased gait speed and stride length, and increased time spent in double stance during gait were the most consistent gait parameter changes. Kinematic and kinetic analyses revealed that people with MS had decreased

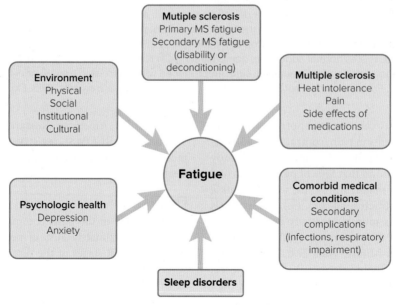

FIGURE 14-5 Multifactorial causes of fatigue.

hip extension and hip extension moment in stance, reduced knee flexion during swing, and decreased ankle dorsiflexion at initial contact and plantarflexion at the pre-swing phases of the gait cycle. A variety of impairments including weakness, fatigue, impaired sensation, vestibular symptoms, and visual deficits possibly contribute to these gait deviations.[76]

Speech and Swallowing Dysfunction

Speech and swallowing are affected by weakness, spasticity, tremor, and ataxia secondary to damage of corticobulbar tracts, cerebellar and brainstem disorders, lower cranial nerve weakness, and cognitive impairment.[77-79] Individuals may exhibit dysarthria (slurred or poorly articulated speech) and dysphonia (changes in vocal quality, such as harshness, hoarseness, breathiness, or a hypernasal sound). Scanning dysarthria, speech in which the normal "melody" or speech pattern is disrupted, with abnormally long pauses between words or individual syllables of words, is often associated with MS.[79] Swallowing problems, or dysphagia, can occur in any stage of normal swallowing within the mouth, pharynx, and esophagus. Signs of swallowing difficulties include excessive chewing duration, difficulty holding food and liquid in the mouth, inability to swallow food, and coughing during or after meals. Chronic swallowing problems can lead to poor nutrition, dehydration, airway obstruction, or aspiration pneumonia due to food particles or liquids entering the lungs while eating. Poor posture and respiratory control also contribute to speech and feeding problems.[80]

Cognitive and Emotional/Behavioral Dysfunction

Cognitive Dysfunction

An estimated 35-65% of adults with MS have cognitive dysfunction secondary to the disease.[81] Neuropathological and neuroimaging studies provide evidence that inflammation and atrophy within the grey matter, particularly within areas of the thalamus, hippocampus, and temporal cortex, play a prominent role in cognitive dysfunction in MS.[82,83] Among MRI biomarkers studied in people with MS, severe grey matter atrophy has been the most reliable for predicting future cognitive impairment.[83] The cognitive areas that are most affected in MS include information-processing speed, episodic and working memory, executive functions (abstract reasoning, problem-solving, planning, and sequencing), sustained and divided attention, and visuospatial processing.[84-87] Cognitive deficits affect people with all phenotypes of MS with the highest prevalence and fastest rate of decline found in patients with progressive phenotypes (SPMM, PPMS).[81,83] Major factors that contribute to cognitive decline in people with MS are age, fatigue, substance abuse, psychiatric and emotional disorders (depression), medications (sedatives, antidepressants), metabolic dysfunctions (diabetes, liver failure), and quality of life.[88] Cognitive dysfunction can have a negative impact on an individual's employment status, family roles, social interactions, and independence with daily activities even when motor function is adequate.[89,90] Motor learning literature has shown conflicting results regarding the impact of MS on implicit learning of motor tasks, while explicit learning of motor tasks has been shown to be impaired.[90]

Emotional/Behavioral Dysfunction

Emotional/behavioral symptoms and impairments such as depression, aggression, apathy, euphoria (exaggerated feelings of well-being and optimism that are incongruent with the person's level of disability), lack of insight, adjustment disorders (inability to adjust to or cope with a particular stressor), and obsessive-compulsive disorders (anxiety disorder characterized by intrusive thoughts that produce uneasiness, apprehension, fear, or worry) are prevalent in individuals with MS.[91] The mechanisms underlying these changes are thought to be due to white matter dysfunction within frontotemporal neuronal networks that modify a person's behavior, but maladapting coping responses that can occur in chronic illnesses with unpredictable functional decline may also contribute. Depression is the most common neuropsychiatric symptom in MS and negatively affects functioning and quality of life. Individuals with MS are at double the risk for suicide ideation and attempts compared to the general population.[92]

Autonomic Dysfunction

Autonomic dysfunction may arise in MS due to damage in CNS centers important for autonomic nervous system (ANS) function such as the insula, hypothalamus, dorsal vagal nucleus, and solitary nucleus in the brainstem and the ascending and descending autonomic tracts in the spinal cord. Dysautonomia appears more likely to occur in people with progressive types of MS and with more severe clinical disability.[93] Sweating responses have been found to be decreased or absent in some individuals with MS, and thus, measures to prevent persons with MS from overheating in a warm environment and/or while exercising are recommended.[94]

Cardiovascular Dysautonomia

Cardiovascular autonomic dysfunction has been reported to reach a prevalence between 8% and 50% in individuals with MS. Pathologic findings have been highly variable with sympathetic pathology predominating in some individuals and parasympathetic pathology in others.[95] See Box 14-3 for a discussion of autonomic heart control.

Cardiac dysautonomia typically presents as **orthostatic hypotension** (OH), with symptoms of dizziness, lightheadedness, blurred vision, and general weakness that occur with postural changes such as going from lying to sitting.[94] This is caused by inadequate sympathetic reflex vasoconstriction. Another orthostatic disorder seen in MS is **postural orthostatic tachycardia**

Box 14-3	**Autonomic Heart Control**

Heart rate (HR) is a balance of the parasympathetic and sympathetic inputs to the heart. When there is an increase in parasympathetic input, HR decreases; when there is an increase in sympathetic input, HR increases. Changing position from sitting to supine is typically associated with an increase in parasympathetic influence with an associated decrease in HR, and coming to standing, conversely, is associated with an increase in sympathetic influence and a slight increase in HR. Similarly, blood pressure (BP) is modulated by the autonomic systems with vasoconstriction increased with sympathetic activation, raising BP, and vasodilation created by parasympathetic activation, lowering BP.

syndrome (PoTS), characterized by sustained HR increase upon standing without concomitant OH.[94] Demyelinating lesions in the cerebral hemispheres and brainstem that disrupt modulation of physiological HR variability may cause PoTS in people with MS.[96] PoTS can limit a person's ability to exercise and increase feelings of fatigue, which may aggravate these already preexisting symptoms in people with MS.[94]

Bladder and Bowel Dysfunction

Bladder and/or bowel dysfunction are frequent and distressing symptoms of MS, affecting approximately 80% of individuals.[95,97] Neurogenic bladder and bowel types are either hyperreflexic spastic or hyporeflexic flaccid. Table 14-2 outlines causes and symptoms of neurogenic bladder and bowel conditions.

Progressive declines in hand function and mobility (transfers and walking) contribute to difficulties with personal hygiene and inability to toilet or manage bladder and bowel dysfunction. Large residual urine volumes increase the risk of urinary tract infections (UTIs) and kidney damage from frequent UTIs.[95] Other non-neurogenic factors that contribute to constipation are inactivity, lack of adequate fluids, poor diet and bowel habits, and medication side effects.[95] Fecal incontinence and diarrhea occur with flaccidity of the external anal sphincter and pelvic floor muscles or secondary gastrointestinal problems (gastroenteritis, inflammatory bowel disease).[98]

Sexual Dysfunction

Sexual dysfunction affects between 50 and 90% of individuals with MS and is a major cause of distress. The most frequent complaints are erectile and ejaculatory dysfunctions in men, uncomfortable sensory changes in the genitals and vaginal dryness in women, loss of sex drive, and difficulty in achieving orgasm in both genders.[94,99] These impairments may be directly related to demyelinating lesions in the CNS (see Chapter 13: Spinal Cord Injury for details),

similar to those described for bladder and bowel dysfunction. Nonsexual physical changes such as fatigue, weakness, spasticity, incoordination, difficulty with mobility, bladder and bowel problems, numbness, pain or burning in nongenital areas, side effects from MS medications, and cognitive problems can also contribute to sexual dysfunction in MS. Psychological, social, and cultural factors that may affect sexual functioning in people with MS include negative self-image or body image, performance anxiety, changes in self-esteem, feelings of dependency, communication barriers with partner, depression, and family and social role changes or role conflict.[94,99] Individuals with MS should be encouraged to talk with their neurologist or primary care physician if they are experiencing sexual problems so that they can be assessed for underlying causes and receive medical treatment or be referred to other health professionals as needed.

MS does not affect fertility or pregnancy outcomes, and pregnancy does not negatively impact the clinical course of the disease. Pregnant women with MS often experience decreased numbers of relapses, especially in the third trimester, secondary to the effects of pregnancy hormones on the immune system. Obstetric care, labor, and delivery are typically the same for women with MS as for women without MS. Disease-modifying immunomodulatory drugs are not currently approved by the US Food and Drug Administration for use during pregnancy or breastfeeding.[100]

Thermoregulatory Dysfunction

Many individuals with MS experience a transient worsening of neurological signs and symptoms in response to increases in ambient temperature (e.g., sun exposure, hot baths) or in internal body temperature (e.g., fever or vigorous exercise), or a combination of both. An increase in core body temperature of only 0.5°C may worsen symptoms, known as **Uhthoff's phenomenon**. The mechanism for this heat intolerance is thought

TABLE 14-2	Bladder and Bowel Dysfunction in Multiple Sclerosis	
NEUROGENIC BLADDER		
Types and Cause	**Description**	**Symptoms**
Hyperreflexic Spastic Bladder – UMN damage in spinal cord above sacral cord levels	Bladder is spastic; therefore, reflexively voids with minimal filling; bladder becomes smaller over time	Frequent urination; urgency with minimal bladder content
Hyporeflexive Bladder – LMN damage in sacral cord or cauda equina or pelvic nerve	Bladder becomes flaccid, loss of reflexive voiding	Hesitancy in initiating voiding; incomplete emptying (urinary retention); leakage between urination bouts
Detrusor Sphincter Dyssynergia (DSD) – UMN damage	Loss of coordination between bladder contraction and sphincter relaxation	Incomplete voiding with urinary retention, problems initiating voiding
NEUROGENIC BOWEL		
Hypperreflexic Spastic Bowel – UMN lesions above the sacral cord levels	Intact defecation reflex; spasticity in the external anal sphincter and pelvic floor muscles	Constipation
Hyporeflexic Flaccid Bowel – LMN lesions of sacral cord, cauda equina or pelvic nerve	Disrupted defecation reflex; colonic slowing and external anal sphincter dysfunction	Constipation or diarrhea; fecal incontinence

LMN, lower motor neuron; UMN, upper motor neuron.

to be temperature-induced slowing and/or blockage of conduction in demyelinated axonal segments.[101]

MEDICAL MANAGEMENT

A team approach is needed to manage MS symptoms including but not limited to physicians, nurses, social workers, mental health professionals, and rehabilitation professionals (physical therapy, occupational therapy, and speech/language pathologists).

Long-Term Medical Management

Disease-modifying therapy drugs (DMTs) are the mainstay of treatment for MS. There are many US FDA-approved DMTs (Table 14-3) for long-term use with RRMS and relapsing (i.e., active) forms of SPMS or PPMS.[102] The only FDA-approved medications for non-relapsing forms of SPMS and PPMS are mitoxantrone (Navontrone) and siponimod (Mayzent), and ocrelizumab (Ocrevus), respectively. These medications have been shown to limit relapses, progression of disease, and new inflammatory lesions seen on MRI.[103] The National Multiple Sclerosis Society's (NMSS) National Clinical Advisory Board, in recognition of the influence of DMTs on the pathogenicity of the disease, recommends that DMTs be initiated early in the disease and be continued unless there is a lack of clear benefit, intolerable side effects, or a better treatment is found. Clinicians must consider factors such as medication safety, route of administration, cost, efficacy, and adverse effects, as well as patient lifestyle and preferences when prescribing DMTs.[103] Most individuals with MS prefer to take oral medication as they experience both physical and psychological discomfort from repeated injections. Drug side effects and adverse reactions are common and may negatively affect adherence (Table 14-3).

TABLE 14-3	**Disease-Modifying Therapy Drugs**[102,103]		
DRUG/INDICATIONS	**MECHANISM OF ACTION**	**SIDE EFFECTS**	**ADMINISTRATION**
Injectable Medications			
Interferon Beta 1-a (Avonex, Plegridy, Rebif) and 1-b (Betaseron, Extavia) Indications: CIS, RRMS, and active SPMS (relapsing forms of MS)	Immune system modulator with antiviral properties	Flu-like symptoms, injection-site skin reaction	Avonex: intermuscular once weekly Plegridy: SC every 14 days Rebif: SC 3 times weekly Betaseron: SC every other day Extavia: SC every other day
Glatiramer acetate (Copaxone; Glatiramer Acetate Injection, Glatopa- generic equivalents of Copaxone) Indications: CIS, RRMS	Synthetic chain of 4 amino acids found in myelin (immune system modulator that blocks attacks on myelin)	Injection-site reactions as well as occasional systemic reaction (chest pain, palpitations, dyspnea)	SC injection daily SC 3 days per week
Ofatumumab (Kesimpta) Indications: CIS, RRMS, and active SPMS (relapsing forms of MS)	Monoclonal antibody that binds to a site on some immune B cells and depletes them	Upper respiratory tract infection, with symptoms such as sore throat and runny nose, and headache	SC injection once a month
Oral Medications			
Teriflunomide (Aubagio) Monomethyl fumarate (Bafiertam) Fingolimod (Gilenya) Cladribine (Mavenclad) Siponimod (Mayzent) Dimethyl fumarate (Tecfidera and dimethyl fumarate generic equivalent of Tecfidera) Ponesimod (Ponvory) Diroximel fumarate (Vumerity) Ozanimod (Zeposia) Indications: CIS, RRMS, and active SPMS (relapsing forms of MS)	Inhibit the function of T and B cells that have been implicated in MS	Side effects vary with the medication but may include: headache, flu, hair thinning, nausea, diarrhea, back pain, abnormal liver tests, cough, paresthesias (Aubagio), temporary slowing of the heart rate (Gilenya), flushing and gastrointestinal pain (Tecfidera)	Tablets typically taken once or twice daily

(Continued)

TABLE 14-3	Disease-Modifying Therapy Drugs[102,103] (Continued)		
DRUG/INDICATIONS	**MECHANISM OF ACTION**	**SIDE EFFECTS**	**ADMINISTRATION**
Infused Medications			
Natalizumab (Tysabri) Indications: CIS, RRMS and active SPMS (relapsing forms of MS); those with inadequate response to or inability to tolerate injectable agents	Monoclonal antibody that inhibits adhesion molecules to prevent damaging immune cells from crossing the blood-brain barrier	Headache, fatigue, depression, joint pain, abdominal discomfort, and infection; associated with rare and fatal progressive multifocal leukoencephalopathy	Intravenous infusion once every 4 weeks
Alemtuzumab (Lemtrada) Indications: CIS, RRMS, and active SPMS (relapsing forms of MS); those with inadequate response to two or more disease-modifiying therapies	Monoclonal antibody aimed at specific receptors on the surface of immune cells to modulate immune responses	Rash, HA, fever, nasal congestion, nausea, urinary tract infection, hives, itching, pain in joints, extremities, and back; infusion reactions	Intravenous infusion for 5 consecutive days, once per year
Ocrelizumab (Ocrevus) Indication: All relapsing or primary progressive forms of MS; those with inadequate response to or inability to tolerate injectable agents	Monoclonal antibody that targets CD20 positive B lymphocytes which contribute to nerve damage in MS	Infusion reactions and upper respiratory tract infections	IV infusion initially given as 2 separate infusions, 2 weeks apart. Following doses given as one infusion every 6 months
Mitoxantrone (Novantrone) Indications: worsening RRMS, SPMS, and active PPMS	Antineoplastic drug (immune system modulator and suppressor)	Nausea, thinning hair, loss of menstrual periods, bladder infections, mouth sores; urine and whites of the eyes may turn a bluish color temporarily; seldom used due to risk for cardiac disease and leukemia	Given as a short (approximately 5-15 minute) intravenous infusion every 3 months (for 2-3 years maximum)

Treatment of new symptoms depends on whether they are a **relapse** or **pseudorelapse**. A relapse refers to new neurological symptoms or worsening of already existing symptoms, reflecting one or more demyelinating lesions in the CNS, that last at least 24 hours, with or without recovery, and in the absence of fever or infection.[19] Clinicians need to differentiate a relapse from a pseudorelapse, characterized as a temporary worsening or return of previously existing neurological symptoms that is a manifestation of Uhthoff's phenomenon caused by increases in core body temperature. It is important for clinicians to consider and address possible heat-related triggers of pseudorelapse both external (ambient temperature) and internal (e.g., exercise, fever, infections, menstrual period, stress) before medications are prescribed.[104]

Medical Management of Relapses and Symptoms

Acute relapses are usually treated with high-dose corticosteroids, most commonly 1000 mg of oral or intravenous methylprednisolone given daily for 3 to 5 days. Common adverse effects of corticosteroid treatment include flushing, insomnia, gastrointestinal pain, nausea or vomiting, hypertension, hyperglycemia, hypokalemia, and psychiatric/behavioral manifestations (anxiety agitation or euphoria). Second-line therapies for MS relapses that do not respond to corticosteroids are adrenocorticotropic hormone (ACTH) gel administered by intramuscular injection and plasma exchange (plasmapheresis).[104]

Pain

Pain is managed according to its pathogenesis. Neuropathic pain from acute paroxysmal sensory symptoms (i.e., dysesthesias), trigeminal neuralgia, and Lhermitte's sign are often treated with tricyclic antidepressants (e.g., amitriptyline) or with anticonvulsant medications (gabapentin, carbamazepine; Table 14-4).[105]

Spasticity

Because spasticity varies so much from person to person, treatment must be tailored to the individual and involves a close partnership between the person with MS and health care professionals to achieve optimal dosing. First-line medications for spasticity in MS include oral baclofen and tizanidine (Table 14-4). Other oral medications used include benzodiazepines (e.g., diazepam and clonazepam), and dantrolene.[106] For severe cases of spasticity or intolerance to oral medications, a baclofen pump may be implanted to administer baclofen into the CSF of the lumbar spine. Improvements in spasticity reduction are usually greater in the lower extremities and trunk than in the upper extremities with a baclofen pump. Botulinum toxin type A

TABLE 14-4	Symptomatic Medications	
MEDICATION	**MECHANISM OF ACTION**	**SIDE EFFECTS**
Neuropathic Pain Medications[105]		
Gabapentin (Neurontin)	A gamma aminobutyric acid (GABA) analogue. *Note*: GABA is an inhibitory neurotransmitter	Dizziness, drowsiness, peripheral edema
Carbamazepine (Tegretol)	Potentiates GABA receptors	Diplopia, dizziness, hyponatremia, blood dyscrasias, lethargy; contraindicated with monoamine oxidase inhibitors (MAOIs) and bone marrow suppression
Antispasticity Oral and Injectable Medications[106]		
Baclofen (Lioresal)	GABA receptor agonist	Fatigue, somnolence, weakness, dizziness, GI symptoms, bladder dysfunction
Tizanidine (Zanaflex)	Centrally acting alpha 2 adrenergic receptor agonist	Dry mouth, sedation, dizziness, orthostatic hypotension, edema, drug-induced hepatitis
Benzodiazepines: Diazepam (Valium) and clonazepam (Klonopin)	Enhances GABA with anticonvulsant, muscle relaxant, and anxiolytic properties	Drowsiness, cognitive impairment, agitation, loss of libido
Dantrolene (Dantrium)	Muscle relaxant that abolishes excitation-contraction coupling in muscle cells	CNS effects: speech and visual disturbances, depression, confusion, hallucinations, headache, insomnia, seizures, nervousness
Botulinum toxin (Botox)	Binds to presynaptic calcium docking protein and inhibits the release of acetylcholine at the neuromuscular junction	Weakness
Fatigue Medications[107]		
Amantadine (Symmetrel)	Potentiates catecholaminergic/ dopaminergic transmission	Hallucinations, confusion, insomnia, and dizziness
Modafinil (Provigil)	Activates the hypothalamus; increases release of norepinephrine and dopamine	Cardiac contraindications and reduction of BCP efficacy. Insomnia, anxiety, irritability, nausea, diarrhea, palpitations. SAE: Stevens–Johnson syndrome
Dalfampridine (Ampyra)	Potassium channel blocker	Urinary tract infection; dizziness; headache; weakness; back pain; balance problems; burning, tingling, or itching of skin; nose and throat irritation; constipation
Ataxia and Tremor Medications[108,109]		
Levetiracetam (Keppra)	Inhibits presynaptic calcium channels	Weakness, unsteady walking, dizziness, confusion, somnolence, aggression, and irritability
Topiramate (Topamax)	Carbonic anhydrase inhibitor	Dizziness, paresthesias, somnolence, fatigue
Depression Medications[110,111]		
Paroxetine (Paxil), fluoxetine (Prozac), and sertraline (Zoloft)	Selective serotonin reuptake inhibitors (SSRIs); increases serotonin by blocking its reuptake from the synaptic junction	Anxiety, insomnia, increased appetite, tremors, GI symptoms, headaches, rash, and sexual dysfunction with decreased libido
Imipramine (Tofranil) and amitriptyline (Elavil)	Tricyclic antidepressants (TCAs); increases serotonin and norepinephrine in the brain by slowing the rate of reuptake	Dry mouth, urinary retention, constipation, BP/ HR changes

(Continued)

TABLE 14-4	Symptomatic Medications (*Continued*)	
MEDICATION	**MECHANISM OF ACTION**	**SIDE EFFECTS**
Bladder Medications[112]		
Oxybutynin (Ditropan), tolterodine (Detrol), and propantheline (Pro-Banthine)	Muscarinic acetylcholine receptor antagonists; block parasympathetic nervous system	Anticholinergic side effects: dry mouth, constipation, nausea, dysuria, abnormal vision, dizziness, somnolence
Tamsulosin (Flomax) and prazosin (Minipress)	Alpha-1 adrenergic receptor antagonist; relaxes bladder sphincter	Dizziness, unusual weakness, drowsiness, insomnia, sexual issues, orthostatic hypotension
Sexual Dysfunction Medications[112]		
Sildenafil (Viagra), vardenafil (Levitra), and tadalafil (Cialis)	Phosphodiesterase type 5 inhibitor (PDE5); prolongs phosphodiesterase (PDE) activity, causing vasodilation	Abnormal vision, diarrhea, flushing, headache, nasal congestion, urinary tract infection: contraindicated in history of cardiac disease

(Botox) can be injected into affected muscle groups to promote stretching and muscle relaxation. Effects reach their peak in 1 to 2 weeks and last up to 3 to 4 months. Injections are then repeated. Botox treatment in combination with physical therapy may improve positioning and mobility and alleviate pain.[106]

Fatigue

Pharmacological interventions to treat fatigue in MS include medications to increase energy level, such as amantadine, modafinil, and dalfampridine (Table 14-4). Less commonly used medications are antidepressants such as selective serotonin reuptake inhibitors (SSRIs).[107]

Ataxia and Tremor

Medications that have shown some limited success with treating ataxia and tremor in MS are the antiepileptic medications levetiracetam and topiramate.[108,109] Surgical interventions such as deep brain stimulation to the thalamus may be warranted for certain people.[109]

Walking

Medical management for walking involves the medication dalfampridine, a potassium channel blocker that enhances conduction in damaged nerves.[113] It is appropriate for individuals with all types of MS, who do not have a history of seizures or renal disease. Studies showed that individuals with MS taking dalfampridine had significantly increased walking speeds compared with those taking placebo.[112] Common side effects include dizziness, nervousness, and nausea.[113]

Cognitive and Emotional Problems

Cognitive and emotional management in MS focuses on medical treatment, neuropsychological rehabilitation, and lifestyle changes. Evidence suggests that disease-modifying drugs may provide some modest benefit to cognition. Antidepressant medications such as selective serotonin reuptake inhibitors (paroxetine, fluoxetine, sertraline) or tricyclic antidepressants (imipramine, amitriptyline) may be used to treat depression (Table 14-4). Cognitive rehabilitation programs that aim to improve specific cognitive skills have shown some

positive results in people with MS.[88,114] Psychotherapy and cognitive behavioral therapy (CBT) are efficacious for treatment of depression in MS.[110,111] Psychotherapy can help individuals with MS to accept and adjust to their illness; CBT can help people to improve their coping, social interaction, and problem-solving skills. Promotion of healthy behaviors such as improving sleep, engaging in regular moderate exercise, and eating a healthy diet may also be beneficial for treating cognitive and emotional symptoms in individuals with MS.[88,114]

Bladder and Bowel Problems

Management of bladder dysfunction begins with a comprehensive urodynamic work up to determine the cause of the problems. Treatment for a spastic bladder (storage problem) typically includes medications, dietary and behavioral modification, and optional surgical procedures (see Chapter 13, Spinal Cord Injury, for details about management of neurogenic bladder and bowel). Anticholinergic medications (oxybutynin, tolterodine, propantheline) or tricyclic antidepressants (imipramine, amytriptyline) are usually prescribed (Table 14-4).[95,112] Dietary modifications include increasing fluid intake to eight glasses of water per day and restricting intake of caffeine, alcohol, foods high in acid (tomato or grapefruit), and spicy foods that irritate the bladder. Behavioral modifications to prevent accidents consist of contractions of pelvic floor muscles (Kegel's exercises) to improve bladder control, using relaxation techniques to delay voiding, and going to the bathroom on a regular schedule. Some individuals may benefit from sacral nerve stimulation which involves implantation of a programmable stimulator subcutaneously at the S3 level that electrically stimulates the sacral nerve, causing contraction of the external urethral sphincter and pelvic floor muscles. **Detrusor sphincter dyssynergia** is managed with alpha-adrenergic blocking agents (tamsulosin, prazosin) and antispasticity medications (Table 14-4). A flaccid bladder (emptying problem) is managed by using techniques to facilitate voiding such as the Valsalva maneuver (squeezing the abdominal muscles to increase bladder pressure) and the Crede maneuver (applying manual pressure on the lower abdominal wall) or intermittent self-catheterization (ISC).[112]

Constipation can be treated with dietary changes including increased fluid intake, eating high-fiber foods (fruits, vegetables, whole grains), and/or adding bulking-forming supplements (Metamucil, FiberCon, Citrucel) or stool softeners such as sodium docusate (Colace). Fecal incontinence is managed with avoidance of irritating foods (caffeine, alcohol, spicy foods) or addition of anticholinergic medications (tolterodine, propantheline). Bowel programs involve regular evacuation of bowels (daily or every other day) by stimulating the defecation reflex (spastic bowel) or by manual methods (flaccid bowel).[112]

Sexual Dysfunction

Sexual dysfunction is managed with medications and counseling. Erectile dysfunction in men is treated with phosphodiesterase-5 inhibitors such as sildenafil, vardenafil, and tadalafil (Table 14-4). Hormonal therapy with estrogen and methyltestosterone may be used to treat lack of libido and vaginal dryness in women with MS.[93] Health care professionals can counsel individuals with MS regarding transferring and positioning, and managing secondary symptoms that contribute to sexual dysfunction. Referral to a psychologist for discussions about intimacy, relationships, and communication may be beneficial.

Question: What medications would most likely be prescribed for Sheila?

Sheila will most likely be prescribed a disease-modifying therapy medication, most likely one of the interferon drugs or the oral medications. In addition, she may be treated symptomatically for her bladder dysfunction (i.e., spastic bladder) with anticholinergic medications, and for her fatigue with amantadine or other fatigue medications.

● PROGNOSIS

People with MS have an approximately twofold higher mortality rate and a life expectancy that is a median of 7 years shorter than a matched healthy population.[115,116] Comorbidities such as diabetes, ischemic heart disease, and depression further elevate the risk of death in people with MS.[116] Although it is difficult to predict an individual's course with MS, one large prospective longitudinal study to determine prognostic factors for developing further attacks and disability progression in people with CIS reported that baseline demographic and topographic characteristics (i.e., male, older age, presenting symptoms in brainstem or spinal cord) were low-impact factors; the presence of oligoclonal bands was a medium-impact factor; and 10 or more lesions on T2-weighted MRI images was a high-impact factor.[117]

● PHYSICAL THERAPY MANAGEMENT

Examination

Ms. Dillman is in an acute flare-up of her MS requiring precautions to avoid overwork during physical therapy activities. As noted earlier, MS affects nearly every system in the body, including visual, auditory, autonomic, cognitive, psychological, and sensorimotor systems. Thus, a thorough systems review is performed to capture the impact on all systems and to develop a plan of care that is holistic and individualized. The neurologic assessment, outlined in Chapter 10, should be followed with adaptations made to include more detail in areas that are specifically impacted by MS. Motor control is highly dependent on sensory input, and MS affects both the motor and sensory systems; an examination of sensory function, strength, and motor control is typically performed by the physical therapist either independently or in conjunction with other team members such as an occupational therapist and/or neurologist. A thorough examination of the cranial nerves is highly recommended for individuals with MS to identify the extent of visual and auditory problems so that the therapy plan can be developed to accommodate for these losses and referrals can be made to the appropriate professionals. Assistive devices can be expensive to purchase; thus, it is appropriate to wait until remission to determine if a long-term assistive device is needed. CN assessment is also a means of identifying sensory and motor deficits in the face and neck such as Ms. Dillman's loss of sensation on the left side of her face.

CASE A, PART II

Ms. Dillman's CN assessment found no extraocular motor palsy and no difficulty with smooth pursuit (tracking of an object) or saccades (quick bilateral eye movements to orient to an object). This indicates that she will be able to utilize vision for navigation, during mobility tasks. If she were to have motor palsy in the extraocular muscles, she would have difficulties scanning for obstacles that could lead to falls and make driving difficult or even unsafe. In addition, impairments in smooth pursuit lead to difficulty tracking moving objects that can lead to mobility issues in a dynamic environment such as streets, stores, and the home. Since Ms. Dillman lives alone and has no pets, she is unlikely to experience difficulty related to smooth pursuit in the home environment. She has decreased hearing on the left, but her tongue movements are present and equal bilaterally. Ms. Dillman will be better able to hear instructions if therapy personnel stand on her right side and use visual cues that are large and stationary. Her speech has good volume and clarity, and the roof of the mouth elevates on testing; therefore, at present, there is no indication for a referral to speech therapy. Motor and sensory exams reveal intact strength in bilateral UEs except in the hands. She also has decreased finger dexterity bilaterally and *dysdiadochokinesia (difficulty with rapidly alternating movement)* on the left. There is mild strength loss in bilateral LEs. The reflex and sensory exams reveal +3 deep tendon reflexes at the ankles and knees, positive Babinski bilaterally, decreased light touch and pinprick on the left diffusely, and mild vibratory loss at bilateral halluxes and medial malleoli. Functional testing indicates increased sway with narrowed base of support (Romberg position), loss of balance with tandem gait, and slow self-selected gait speed. *Question – Involvement of which cranial nerve would lead to difficulty looking down?* Damage to Cranial Nerve IV (trochlear nerve) would lead to impairments in looking down.

The system's review provides a fairly detailed description of Ms. Dillman's major impairments and indicates that she has some difficulties with gait as noted by her decreased gait speed. The systems review has also noted deficits in strength, sensation, and balance. A more detailed examination of these systems is indicated, based on the original review's findings, which will guide the choice of assessment measures. There are many factors to consider, including the patient's and therapist's goals for therapy, expected duration of therapy episode, and natural course of the disease. Box 14-4 lists outcome measures that are commonly utilized when working with individuals with MS and are recommended by the Academy of Neurologic Physical Therapy MS EDGE task force. Given Ms. Dillman's fatigue, the examination is done with minimal position changes and using the fewest assessment measures possible. If needed some assessment measures could be collected on the second visit.

The assessment measures chosen provide an objective measure of Ms. Dillman's walking difficulties and will help guide treatment to improve safety and prevent falls. Additionally, they provide evidence that she has a slow gait and a significant impairment in dexterity. She should be educated about the benefits of occupational therapy to find ways to compensate by using assistive devices until she is out of the acute phase and then to rehabilitate her dexterity once she is in remission. Fatigue typically is one of the more common and disabling symptoms of MS and should be objectively measured. There are several measures available; however, the modified fatigue impact scale is recommended by the Academy of Neurologic Physical Therapy. Given the impact that MS has on respiratory function, respiration should be observed and measured through maximum inspiratory and expiratory pressure and VO_2 max and VO_2 peak. If deficits are found in the respiratory system, a strengthening program should be included in Ms. Dillman's treatment plan. Objective and detailed evidence of all contributing impairments, including those from systems outside the neuromuscular system, is required to design, safely implement, and measure efficacy of therapy treatments.

CASE A, PART III

Ms. Dillman's short-term goal is to stop falling, and her long-term goals are to regain finger dexterity for typing and improving walking skill for golf. A referral to occupational therapy should be made. The physical therapist decides to focus on fall prevention until Ms. Dillman has stabilized. *Assessment:* To avoid fatiguing Ms. Dillman and to get a better understanding of the problems that she is encountering in her natural environment, the 12-item MS walking scale is chosen as one of the outcome measures. This is a self-assessment and does not require any activity, but it will give a sense of areas or situations that are most dangerous for her at this time. Other assessments that would be appropriate are (1) the Dizziness Handicap Inventory to determine the impact of her dizziness on her function; (2) Timed 25-foot walk or the 10MWT – to establish gait speed; (3) the 9-hole peg test – to establish a baseline for finger dexterity. *Findings:* The MS Walking Scale indicates that Ms. Dillman is holding onto objects and is very fearful when walking outdoors. She indicated that walking is very effortful for her and she cannot walk very far. It took her 7 seconds to walk 25 feet, which means her velocity is 1.0 m/s, and she was 2 standard deviations below the age-matched norm for her performance on the 9-hole peg test.

Treatment

Therapy, for individuals with MS, is based on disease stage and areas of deficit, including fatigue, spasticity, sensory deficits, change in motor control, ataxia, and functional losses. Information in this chapter, regarding treatment of MS, is focused on the evidence for RRMS. Exceptions, for other forms of MS, are stated where appropriate. Few to no studies exist that examine the use of exercise or PT in individuals with secondary or primary progressive MS, so treatments must be based on what we know from RRMS and consideration of the underlying disease process.

Notably, treatment is very different for individuals who are experiencing an acute exacerbation. During an exacerbation, exercise is not recommended. The nerves are acutely inflamed, and exercise could aggravate the inflammatory process. Additionally, individuals with MS are often prescribed high-dose corticosteroid treatment during exacerbations, which can lead to fluid retention, high BP, osteoporosis, and aseptic necrosis.

After an acute flare-up, therapists should check for swelling in the ankles and feet and be sure to monitor BP before starting exercise. Osteoporosis and aseptic necrosis (bone death secondary to vascular changes) leave the bones vulnerable to fracture. Caution should be taken to avoid high-impact activities during and immediately after corticosteroid treatment.

Box 14-4   MS EDGE Highly Recommended Outcome Measures and G-Codes[118]

12-Item MS Walking Scale[a,b]
6-Minute Walk Test[a]
9-Hole Peg Test[c]
Berg Balance Scale[b]
Dizziness Handicap Inventory[+a,b,c,d]
MS Functional Composite[+a,c]
MS Impact Scale (MSIS-29)[a,b,c,d]
MS Quality of Life (MS QoL-54)[a,b,c,d]
Timed 25-Foot Walk[a]
Timed Up and Go (TUG) with Cognitive and Manual[a,b]

MS EDGE Recommended Measures for Acute stage
Trunk Impairment Scale[b]
Maximal Inspiratory and Expiratory Pressure
VO_2 max and VO_2 peak
Modified Fatigue Impact Scale

+, Outpatient rehabilitation setting only; G-Codes – a, mobility: walking and moving around; b, changing and maintaining body position; c, carrying, moving, and handling objects; d, self-care.

Aseptic necrosis most commonly impacts the head of the femur, so any complaint of hip pain should be taken seriously and fully investigated to rule out this condition. Individuals with MS should avoid performing exercise and daily living tasks in warm environments as they experience heat insensitivity and often become tired more easily when they are hot. Some individuals with MS experience Uhthoff's sign when they become warm. *Uhthoff's sign* is the worsening of neurologic symptoms, such as increased weakness, spasticity, or blurred vision, when the body gets overheated. These changes are temporary and indicate the need to rest and take measures to cool down.[101] Use of lightweight, layered, and loosely fitting clothing is recommended during exercise to prevent overheating. Additionally, fans can be used during exercise to help keep temperatures cooler, and individuals with MS should be encouraged to drink cold drinks and take cool showers to help refresh and reenergize. For those with severe problems, there are cooling vests that can be prescribed.

Before considering exercise programs with an individual with MS, we must first ask ourselves; "is exercise safe and beneficial for this individual?" It has been determined that exercise does not trigger exacerbations;[119] rather, it has been found to improve muscle strength, aerobic capacity, walking performance, fatigue, balance, and quality of life in individuals with MS.[120-122] High-intensity interval training or HIIT has shown promise as a modality to improve fitness and function in people with neurologic disorders. A benefit of HIIT is that it allows the individual to gain the same benefits with fewer minutes of exercise total. Exercise and rest are interspersed, typically in a 1:1 ratio. In MS a common ratio was 1 minute of exercise followed by 1 minute of rest. Studies found beneficial effects on fitness in individuals with low levels of disability.[123] Periodized exercise has also been studied in MS, showing that with substantially less training time the periodized training induced larger improvements in exercise capacity than classic endurance training at 60 to 80% of HR_{max}. Periodized training, in this study, involved cycles of high-intensity exercise for two weeks, followed by a recovery week with less exercise, and then repeated four times.[124] It is important to note that there are few studies to date of periodized exercise; plus, neither the functional benefits nor the impact on inflammatory and neurologic markers have been examined.

Although numerous studies demonstrate that exercise is safe and beneficial for individuals with MS, an additional question is whether the type of exercise matters. This question is difficult to answer currently due to the paucity of studies. There are studies to indicate that the use of robot-assisted walking may be beneficial for individuals with severe disability to improve cortical activation, gait speed, endurance, and balance.[125,126] and that whole-body vibration therapy does not yield consistent positive results for strength training.[127] Comprehensive physical therapy programs, aerobic training, and strength training all have evidence in support of their use in MS. In addition there is evidence that treadmill training improves walking speed and endurance in individuals with MS.[128] Preliminary data from early nonrandomized trials have indicated improved walking from hippotherapy,[128] aquatic therapy,[129] and the use of external focus of attention,[130] which refers to focusing on results rather than the movement details. To summarize these findings, it appears that the type of exercise or therapy does matter, so the type of exercise or therapy chosen should be based on the specific impairments and functional losses to be addressed. Some types, such as strength training, are more effective for posture, while balance improves with a combination of balance, strength, and aerobic exercise. The mechanisms underlying the benefits of exercise in MS are not yet known, but evidence to date suggests that it may impact inflammation, neurodegeneration, cytokine levels, and central nervous system structure; however, the evidence is limited.[131] Exercise guidelines have been published based on systematic reviews of the literature. They consistently recommend 2 to 3 days a week of aerobic exercise (10-30 minutes, moderate intensity) and strengthening exercise (1-3 sets with 8-15 repetitions per session).[120,131,132,135–137]

Fatigue

As stated earlier in this chapter, fatigue is a severely disabling symptom of MS and can be challenging to treat. Additionally, it is difficult to determine whether central (changes in nervous system control) or peripheral factors (changes in the muscle or neuromuscular junction) are the primary cause of fatigue. Peripheral fatigue is more easily treated through endurance activities such as riding a stationary bike or walking. Central fatigue also appears to respond to exercise but to a lesser degree. Regular exercise is strongly recommended as a means of managing fatigue.[133] In addition, clients with MS should be taught energy-conservation techniques. Energy conservation is also known as work simplification and involves performing activities in a way that minimizes muscle fatigue, joint stress, and pain so that the person's energy lasts the whole day. It includes modifying the way tasks are performed to make them as efficient as possible and emphasizes spacing activities so that periods of rest are allowed throughout the day.

Sensory Changes

Sensory changes in MS can be intermittent or chronic, leading to the need to frequently reassess sensation. Loss of sense of touch, pinprick, and localization are often in small areas and intermittent,[134] but when they become chronic or lead to numbness, they can cause safety issues such as burns and pressure sores. The primary treatment for this is to teach the individual to modify their environment to prevent exposure to hot pipes or water and to be aware of the need to check positioning and the numb area of skin at least every 2 hours.

The other common sensory loss in MS is proprioception, which results in difficulty with balance and coordination.[39] Treatment should focus on rehabilitation of the balance system and to teach safety measures when unable to rehabilitate the balance system. Therapy to improve sensory awareness of the limbs and joints focuses on weight-bearing activities that include changes in surface and base of support with or without alterations in vision. Box 14-5 has a list of exercises that can be performed to improve balance problems secondary to proprioceptive deficits. During each of these exercises, instruction should be given to focus on being aware of how the feet feel and the sensation of each weight shift. Exercises are

---

Box 14-5   Balance Exercises

Static Balance Exercises

Narrowed base of support or Romberg – stand with feet together

Sharpened Romberg stance – stand with one foot in front of the other, with the heel of the front foot touching the toes of the back foot

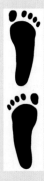

Single limb stance – stand next to a bar or solid object and stand on one leg, 60 seconds is considered normal function

Dynamic Balance

Step front and step back – first step forward then back to neutral then step backward with the same foot and back to neutral. Repeat with other leg.

Seesaw – swing arms side to side and move knees together and apart, both knees in and then both knees move out

Heel-toe walk – walk placing one foot directly in front of the other

Side stepping – step sideways using hip abduction and adduction

Braiding – lateral stepping, combined with forward and backward crossover steps

Backward walking – practice walking backward in a safe environment with a bar to grab if needed

Stairs – work on ascending and descending stairs with a reciprocal pattern

To increase difficulty also do each of these exercises with:

1. *Soft surface* – use dense foam such that the feet do not sink to the bottom of the foam
2. *Uneven surface* – walk over uneven ground outdoors
3. *Alter vision* – use dark sunglasses or place Vaseline on the lens of plastic glasses to distort vision
4. *Remove vision* – close eyes

---

progressed incrementally by narrowing the base of support, changing the surface, and altering vision. There is no difference in difficulty level between changing the surface and altering vision, but these should be added one at a time. Changes in vision and surface impact each individual differently and are dependent on the status of each individual's vestibular, somatosensory, and visual system (see Chapter 6 for a discussion of proprioception).

Sensory changes in the upper extremities are approached in the same manner with progressively more complex weight-bearing for the shoulder and elbow joints, which can be done in sitting or standing with arms on a table or in quadruped (hands and knees). Sensory loss in the hand is treated by setting up situations where the individual handles objects of different sizes, textures, and weights. To progress the activities, have the individual identify object characteristics while blocking their vision of the object. Another exercise is to place a small object in rice or something granular like rice and have them find it through the sense of touch.

Spasticity

Spasticity is difficult to treat, and the research in this area is sparse. Many pharmacological treatments have been covered in more detail earlier in this chapter. These come with the risk of side effects such as drowsiness, dizziness, confusion, nausea, and muscle weakness. Therefore, non-pharmacological treatment is still an important part of the management of spasticity. Physical activity including both daily active exercise and stretching can provide relief and is beneficial when done alone or in conjunction with pharmacological treatment. Ideally, the therapy would be initiated at the same time as the pharmacological treatment, and the person with MS is taught to perform active exercises and stretches at home at least once a day. Choose active exercises that incorporate the spastic muscle groups as primary movers. TENS as an adjunct to active exercise and stretching may also enhance the effects of those treatments in isolation.[135] **Example:** *have someone with spastic hamstrings walk backward to use the hamstrings in an eccentric activity.* Repetitive transcranial magnetic stimulation has also demonstrated positive results.[136]

Ataxia

Ataxia, common in MS, is another condition that is very disabling and refractory to treatment.[137] Physical therapy for this condition typically consists of exercises focused on relearning controlled and coordinated movements.[137,138] The individual with ataxia is placed in a position so as to easily visualize the extremity to be exercised. While focusing on the extremity, they carefully move it to a target or goal with attention directed to creating a smooth movement and then return to the starting position. Some examples are given in Box 14-6.

Exercises to improve walking in individuals with ataxia are not specific to MS. The focus is on having the individual perform balance exercises where the base of support is progressively narrowed and vision is altered such as those listed in Box 14-5. Additionally, practice with dual tasks, such as carrying a glass of water and walking while performing subtraction, are included in therapy sessions for balance and ataxia in MS.[138] Balance training should be paired with task-oriented training and where appropriate lumbar stabilization exercises to improve balance and mobility in clients with ataxia.[138] Task-oriented training should be performed in stations with

Box 14-6 Extremity Exercises for Ataxia and Coordination

Instructions: *I want you to copy the motion that I demonstrate, focusing on doing it slowly and smoothly.* Typically, these are initially done with the individual in a position to watch what they are doing so that they can use visual feedback. To work on proprioception, they can be progressed to being done without visual feedback.

Upper Extremities

Alternate Flexion and Extension – Flex the right elbow while extending the left elbow and then reverse. Also do this with the wrist and shoulder.

Supination and Pronation – Alternately supinate and pronate the forearm. Difficulty is increased by first going progressively faster, supinating and pronating in sync, and then to make it even harder do it bilaterally and out of sync (i.e., the right forearm is supinated while the left forearm is pronated). You can also do this with shoulder external and internal rotation.

Finger Dexterity – Touch the 1st digit to the thumb and then extend, touch the 2nd digit to the thumb and extend, and continue to 3rd and 4th digits. Difficulty is increased by going progressively faster.

Rock, Paper Scissors – Make a pattern using the motions of fist to palm of opposite hand, palm to palm of opposite hand, and ulnar side of hand to palm of opposite hand. Start with a combination of two motions then progress to combinations of three motions. Have the individual with MS copy the pattern that you make. You can have them practice doing the pattern repetitively.

Lower Extremities

Flexion and Extension – While in supine slide the heel toward the buttocks and then straighten the leg back out slowly, alternately flexing and then extending the hips and knees. To make this more difficult, place the heel on the shin at knee level and trace the shin bone down to the ankle, then trace it back up. Focus on making a smooth motion.

Dorsiflexion and Plantarflexion – Alternate dorsi and plantar flexion of the ankle

Bilateral Ankle Dorsi and Plantar Flexion – While seated, first dorsiflex both feet (up on heel), then plantarflex both feet (up on toes) and repeat (See A above).

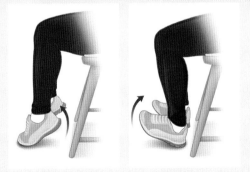

Alternate Dorsi and Plantar Flexion – While seated dorsiflex one foot (up on heel) while going into plantarflexion (up on toes) with the other foot and then reverse so that the feet are moving out of sync.

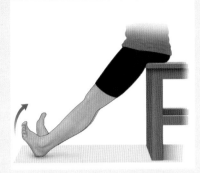

Tracing – While seated draw a circle on the floor using either the toes or heel of one foot, focus on making a smooth motion. A circle can be drawn on the floor and the individual is asked to trace the circle. Repeat with other leg.

Any pattern can be utilized and these can involve remembering and following increasingly complex patterns such as using a box diagram, created with tape on the floor (as shown below).

1	2
3	4

Instructions: "Please point your toes first to the 2 and then to the 3," followed by "please point your toes to the following numbers in the order given: 4, 1, 3, and 2." Any combination can be given and complexity and length can be progressed from simple to complex.

---

alternating exercise (~3 min.) and rest (~2 min) periods.[138,139] Tasks that have been shown to improve function in neurologic disorders including MS are described in Box 14-7. The use of stabilization exercises to improve balance has been shown to be effective across several studies, indicating these exercises should not only be utilized for strengthening but also for sensory training.[138]

It is also somewhat common for therapists to try weighting the extremities or trunk to control ataxia and improve movement quality. There is some limited case-study evidence that this technique can work. Weighting is done with light weights to avoid unduly fatiguing the individual. Weighted vests are applied to control trunk stability and are believed to help provide a stable foundation for limb movements. Distal weighting is done by either wrapping small weights on the leg or arm, at the ankle and wrist respectively, or for the upper extremity, the object being lifted can also be progressively weighted.[140] Feeding tools such as cups, forks, and spoons can be purchased that are heavier than is typical and with larger handle, which may improve coordination during

Box 14-7	Task Training to Improve Balance in Clients with Ataxia

The patient practices each of the following tasks alternating task practice and equal rest periods.

1. Move from sit to stand to sit from various chair surfaces. Begin with firm chair at least knee height and progress to lower height chairs and chairs with softer surfaces. Consider progressing to less stable surfaces such as rolling chairs and Swiss ball.

2. Step in different directions including backward and sideways. Progress to include stepping onto and over blocks or stools of different heights.

3. Reach for objects at varying distances and heights in sitting. Stand in progressively narrowed base of support, including feet together, staggered, in tandem, and single leg stance.

4. Stand up from a chair, walk a short distance, turn around, and return to sitting in the chair.

5. Walk over various surfaces, including soft, uneven, and sloped surfaces.

6. Walk up and down stairs if the individual is unable to perform step-over-step start with a step-to pattern and progress to step-over-step.

7. Walk fast and progress to running. Include practice of sudden stops and starts on the command of the therapist.

8. Hit or throw a ball to targets, and progress to throw and catch from a trampoline or wall.

feeding. Weighting should only be incorporated when rehabilitation exercises such as those described in Box 14-7 have been unsuccessful.

Functional Deficits: How Can Therapy Achieve Improved Function?

Treating functional losses in MS follows the same principles as in stroke and other neurologic diseases. Underlying impairments should be addressed, and task-oriented practice implemented to improve function. Aerobic conditioning, strengthening programs, and balance exercises are all recommended as part of a comprehensive treatment plan for the individual with MS. Given the presence of significant fatigue, it is often necessary to incorporate aerobic and strength training into functional tasks such that underlying impairments are addressed simultaneously with relearning a functional activity.

CASE A, PART IV

Ms. Dillman's short-term goal is to stop falling, and her long-term goal is to regain finger dexterity for typing and walking skill for golf. The examination revealed that she has slow walking speed (1.0 m/s) and difficulties with coordination. In addition, she has left-sided weakness with strength grades in the left leg ranging from 2/5 in the dorsiflexors to 3+/5 in the knee and hip musculature. She complains of severe

fatigue that is limiting her daily functions and causing her to be restricted to her house. During the acute stage, she is given an active range of motion program with stretching to select muscles to minimize loss of function during the exacerbation, and she is prescribed a 4-wheeled, swivel wheel walker (rollator) to improve safety during the acute phase. Once she is in remission, therapy should focus on improving strength, coordination, and independence in community ambulation. Initially, a circuit of exercises can be established with rest periods as needed. The activities should include sit to stand from a standard chair with repetitions guided by fatigue. For example, if she can do 6 before fatiguing, she should do 2 sets of 6, and as coming to standing becomes easier, the activity should be progressed by increasing the number of repetitions. Once she can do 10 repetitions, progression to a lower surface can be initiated; further progression to variable height and stability surfaces (e.g., stuffed chair, therapy ball) can also be initiated. Pulse and BP are monitored, and she should be worked to 60 to 65% of her VO_2 max as determined by the Karvonen formula: $(220 - age) \times .65$. Using this formula, she should be working at a HR of 101 to 119 bpm. During her treatment session, pulse should be monitored, and she should be encouraged to continue working until her heart rate reaches the appropriate range; then, she should continue to work, maintaining her HR in this range for aerobic training. She may initially need rest breaks every 10 minutes due to poor endurance but would slowly and progressively work up to 30 minutes of aerobic activity. See Box 14-8 for a summary of general principles of exercise progression in MS. Other activities that should be included in her therapy are the balance and coordination activities, described in Boxes 14-5 and 14-6, as well as walking. She should also perform stretching during her cool-down period. Warm-up might be done on a stationary bike, since use of the bike will not challenge her balance, as walking would. Finger dexterity should be included in her occupational therapy, and the team should also have her performing golf swings to provide active range of motion and strengthening to her shoulders.

As Ms. Dillman progresses and regains functional independence along with improvements in strength and endurance, she may initiate a strengthening program that involves weightlifting, and she may benefit from continued aerobic activity such as daily walking or use of the stationary bike to maintain fitness.

In addition to therapeutic exercise activities, Ms. Dillman, and others with MS, should be educated about energy-conservation techniques. Energy conservation and work simplification refer to completing tasks in the most energy-efficient way, in order to have enough energy for the activities enjoyed most. Box 14-9 lists principles of energy conservation and work simplification.

Box 14-8	Principles of Exercise Progression in MS[131,132,135–137]

1. Exercise should be prescribed on an intermittent basis with a pattern of a brief bout of exercise, followed by rest, and then another bout until desired exercise is completed. Training benefits using this type of exercise–rest pattern are similar to the outcomes of continuous exercise with an equal duration.

2. For resistance exercise, the rate of overload progression should be addressed with caution, and full recovery between training sessions should be allowed to prevent musculoskeletal overuse injuries.

3. Resistance can be safely increased by 2 to 5% when 15 repetitions are correctly performed in consecutive training sessions.

4. Cardiorespiratory and resistance programs should alternate training on separate days of the week, with 24 to 48 hours of recovery between training sessions.

5. Watch for Uhthoff's sign, and provide rest and cooling strategies when this occurs.

6. Given the impact of fatigue and weakness on performing activities of daily living, the exercise program progression should:
   - start by building up participation in activities of daily living;
   - progress to building in inefficiencies to normal daily tasks such as parking a little further away to increase walking distance;
   - move to participation in active recreation that the individual enjoys or typically participates in;
   - finally progress to a structured aerobic training program.

Box 14-9	Energy Conservation and Work Simplification Techniques

- Plan ahead, set priorities, and balance activities when planning a day. Keep in mind the tasks that must get done and the desired leisure activities. Plan the week ahead of time so that heavy and light tasks can be spread throughout the week.
- Make time for leisure activities.
- Pace activities by alternating rest breaks with activity. Limit each task performed so that fatigue doesn't prevent completion of the next task.
- If it is possible to sit while doing a task, it will save energy. Tasks like folding laundry and mixing up ingredients for cooking can and should be done seated. Keeping a bar stool in the kitchen provides a place to sit to work on projects at counter height.
- When possible, slide objects instead of lifting and carrying them.
- Use assistive devices to lessen the workload. Things like a rolling cart in the kitchen can save energy and enable completion of more daily activities.
- Arrange utensils, equipment, and work area to be efficient. Make sure the tools needed are in easy reach.
- Move heavy and frequently used objects to lower shelves or counter surface.
- Look for ways to make activities more efficient by sequencing activities in a more logical and efficient manner.
- Eliminate unnecessary tasks (e.g., let dishes air dry instead of towel drying them).
- Avoid doing activities in warm environments whenever possible. Do walking outdoors in the morning and evening hours, when it is coolest; use a fan during exercise; drink cold drinks; swim in pools with cooler water temperatures.
- Don't be afraid to ask for help.

Fitness

There is a growing body of evidence that aerobic fitness has a protective effect on parts of the brain that are impacted by MS,[141] including those involved with cognitive function. In addition, individuals with MS who exercise appear to have a slower rate of decline in function.[120] For individuals with MS, there are many barriers to participation in exercise programs, yet fitness is important for overall health and quality of life in these individuals. Barriers to exercise participation include fatigue and difficulty making time for exercise. Some individuals also express feeling uncomfortable working out in public due to the overt symptoms of their disease. Physical therapists can promote and assist in fitness programming by designing programs that are accessible for individuals with mobility deficits and safe to perform outside of therapy. Education is another key aspect of promoting fitness. Individuals with MS should be educated about the role exercise can play in decreasing fatigue and about energy-conservation techniques to help them deal with fatigue.

Exercise and Cognition

Emerging evidence points to possible benefits of exercise on cognitive function in the elderly and in those with neurodegenerative diseases. While this is a new field of study, exercise training to slow cognitive decline in individuals with MS is warranted based on evidence that (1) aerobic fitness, physical activity, and exercise training are associated with better cognitive function in older adults and (2) exercise training has comparable effects on mobility and quality of life outcomes in older adults and persons with MS. See Chapter 18: Aging for more information on cognition and exercise. Emerging studies in MS suggest that exercise improves cognitive function in individuals with MS who have impaired cognition.[142,143] Suggested mechanisms are improvement in remyelination and a decrease in demyelination, decrease in neuroinflammation and reduction of oxidative stress in animal models, and positive impact on cortical excitability, lesion burden, and brain volume in human trials.[132]

Treatment Strategies by Disease Stage

Early Stage

This chapter has gone through general treatment strategies, and Ms. Dillman initially presented in the early stage of her disease, allowing us to apply all of the previously discussed treatment methods to early-stage individuals.

Middle Stage

As the disease progresses, individuals with MS typically experience declines in sensory and motor function. The severity of sensory decline has been poorly documented, since sensory function is not included in the Kurtzke EDSS; however, therapists should be careful to measure sensory function and consider its impact on motor function. Individuals, in the middle stage of the disease, develop more difficulty in ambulation and may require assistive devices such as walking aids and orthotics. Canes are the most typically used walking aids, providing additional input to the balance system and improving balance during gait. Canes do not provide adequate stability to prevent falls; individuals with a history of falling usually require additional support provided by devices with a wider base of support. In choosing assistive devices, consider the impact each will have on the gait pattern and motor control. Devices such as canes and standard walkers lead to a step-to-gait pattern, which is slower and more variable than the normal reciprocal pattern. Another consideration is dual-task demands. Individuals with MS walk slower. Double support time is further increased, when walking and performing a cognitive task in those with MS, a change not seen in age-matched controls.[144] These deficits in dual tasking may also make ambulation with assistive devices that require motor planning or cognitive control more difficult. The four-wheeled, swivel wheel walker (rollator) promotes a reciprocal gait pattern and requires little motor coordination, since it is simply pushed, and thus, would be a low-level dual-task activity. Balance, gait pattern, and upper extremity function are other factors to be considered in device selection.

One of the more frequent problems associated with MS is foot drop. Common treatments for this include the use of ankle-foot orthotics (AFOs) and functional electrical stimulation (FES). Several case studies and small clinical trials have examined the benefits of AFOs in individuals with MS and produced variable findings. There is evidence that the spring-like AFO reduces the work of walking, but the impact of the AFO on spatiotemporal and kinematic aspects of gait is variable. Some studies report improvement in timed tasks with the AFO, and others report no change in time to perform the task. Another consideration in prescribing an orthotic is safety. This aspect has not been studied but is important. Some individuals with foot drop are unable to compensate through increased flexion at the hip and knee, and so, experience tripping during gait. These individuals are likely to improve safety with an AFO whether they improve speed of movement or not.[145]

FES to the peroneal nerve, triggered by a sensor in the heel of the shoe, is utilized in individuals with weak dorsiflexors and everters to produce foot clearance during gait. The FES produces an effect comparable to AFOs and can improve gait in individuals with MS. The benefits of AFOs in MS were less profound than in stroke. After a period of FES use, there are indications that some individuals are able to regain adequate dorsiflexion/eversion strength to walk without the FES.[145]

Late Stage

Ms. Dillman's MS will likely progress from RRMS to secondary progressive MS over time, and her impairments will become more disabling. It was previously believed that individuals in the later stages of neurodegenerative disease could not benefit from rehabilitative therapy. Recent studies have demonstrated that there is some ability to benefit from multidisciplinary rehabilitation, respiratory training, and cooling suits. These studies provide low-level evidence but suggest the need to further explore providing therapeutic interventions to non-ambulatory individuals with MS.

The muscles of respiration benefit from resistance training. A program of expiratory resistance training at 60% maximum expiratory pressure twice daily for 3 months can improve inspiratory and expiratory muscle strength and cough efficacy with improvements maintained after treatment is discontinued.[119,146] There are devices on the market to provide resistance training to the respiratory muscles that can be purchased at reasonable prices. Protocols typically include training five days a week and vary in duration from four to 12 weeks. Sessions typically last 15 minutes. Shorter duration studies used up to five sessions per day with longer treatment durations using only one session per day. Functional improvement was seen in individuals with MS.[119,146]

Along with disease progression, Ms. Dillman may experience difficulties in swallowing, cognitive dysfunction, and neurogenic bladder/bowel in addition to progression of her motor and sensory symptoms. Swallowing deficits can lead to aspiration that can lead to pneumonia. Ms. Dillman should be observed for any signs of swallowing deficits such as difficulty clearing food from her mouth or nonproductive cough; either warrants referral to speech therapy and/or a swallowing evaluation.

If mobility becomes severely limited, a wheelchair should be prescribed. Before purchasing a wheelchair, refer the individual with MS to a wheelchair clinic employing certified assistive technology professionals. Wheelchair prescription considers the individual's current needs and potential disease progression over time. Selection of the appropriate chair is complex. The first decision is whether the chair should be a manual or power chair. A power chair is prescribed when the individual lacks the muscle strength to self-propel a manual chair or they do not have adequate endurance to use a manual chair functionally. In addition, characteristics of the chair and the living environment need to be considered, including (1) the ability of the user or their family to place the chair in and out of a vehicle, (2) the dimensions and size of the chair in relation to the dimensions of the home or anywhere the device will be used (e.g., workplace, shops, restaurants, parks, cars, and public transportation), and (3) whether the chair is appropriate for the individual's activities.

In summary, the management of clients with MS is a complex and ongoing process that benefits from an interdisciplinary approach. Therapists should apply a holistic approach to the examination and management of impairments and functional difficulties to improve participation.

REFERENCES

1. Kumar DR, Aslinia F, Yale SH, Mazza JJ. Jean-Martin Charcot: the father of neurology. *Clin Med Res.* 2011;9(1):46-49.

2. Sharma K, Bittner F, Kamholz J. Epidemiology of multiple sclerosis in the United States. *Neurology.* 2018;90(15 Supplement):P1.140.

3. Wallin MT, Culpepper WJ, Campbell JD, et al. The prevalence of MS in the United States: a population-based estimate using health claims data. *Neurology.* 2019;92 (10):e1029-e1040.

4. Who Gets MS? (Epidemiology). National Multiple Sclerosis Society. https://www.nationalmssociety.org/What-is-MS/Who-Gets-MS#section-1. Accessed August 8, 2021.

5. Ismailova K, Poudel P, Parlesak A, Frederiksen P, Heitmann BL. Vitamin D in early life and later risk of multiple sclerosis: a systematic review, meta-analysis. *PLoS One.* 2019;27:14(8):e0221645.

6. Kurtzke JF. Epidemiology in multiple sclerosis: a pilgrim's progress. *Brain.* 2013;136(9):2904-2917.

7. Hernan MA, Jick SS, Logroscino G, Olek MJ, Ascherio A, Jick H. Cigarette smoking and the progression of multiple sclerosis. *Brain.* 2005;128:1461-1465.

8. Ascherio A, Munger KL. Epidemiology of multiple sclerosis: from risk factors to prevention – an update. *Semin Neurol.* 2016;36(2):103-114.

9. Munger KL, Zhang SM, O'Reilly E. Vitamin D intake and incidence of multiple sclerosis. *Neurology.* 2004;62:60-65.

10. Owens GP, Bennett JL. Trigger, pathogen, or bystander: the complex nexus linking Epstein-Barr virus and multiple sclerosis. *Mult Scler J.* 2012;18(9):1204-1208.

11. Canto E, Oksenberg JR. Multiple sclerosis genetics. *Mult Scler.* 2018; 24(1):75-79.

12. Hanson T, Skytthe A, Stenager E, Peterson HC, Brennum-Hanson H, Kyvik KO. Concordance for multiple sclerosis in Danish twins: an update on a nationwide study. *Mult Scler.* 2005;11:504-510.

13. Interaction of genetics and the environment. National Multiple Sclerosis Society. Available at: https://www.nationalmssociety.org/For-Professionals/Clinical-Care/About-MS/Interaction-of-Genetics-and-the-Environment/Genetics#section-1. Accessed August 8, 2021.

14. Reich DS, Lucchinetti CF, Calabresi PA. Multiple sclerosis. *N Engl J Med.* 2018;378(2):169-180.

15. Kipp M, van der Star B, Vogel DYS, et al. Experimental in vivo and in vitro models of multiple sclerosis: EAE and beyond. *Mult Scler Relat Disord.* 2012;1:15-28.

16. Milo R, Korczyn AD, Manouchehri N, Stüve O. The temporal and causal relationship between inflammation and neurodegeneration in multiple sclerosis. *Mult Scler.* 2020;26(8):876-886.

17. Yamout BI, Alroughani R. Multiple sclerosis. *Semin Neurol.* 2018; 38(2):212-225.

18. Cencioni MT, Mattoscio M, Magliozzi R, et al. B cells in multiple sclerosis: from targeted depletion to immune reconstitution therapies. *Nat Rev Neurol.* 2021;17:399-414.

19. Thompson AJ, Banwell BL, Barkhof F, et al. Diagnosis of multiple sclerosis: 2017 revisions of the McDonald criteria. *Lancet Neurol.* 2018;17(2):162-173.

20. Lublin FD, Reingold SC, Cohen JA, et al. Defining the clinical course of multiple sclerosis: the 2013 revisions. *Neurology.* 2014;83(3):278-286.

21. Maloni HW. Mutiple sclerosisa: managing patients in primary care. *Nurse Pract.* 2013;38:25-35.

22. Waxman SG. Axonal conduction and injury in multiple sclerosis: the role fo sodium channels. *Nature.* 2006;7:932-941.

23. Ksiazek-Winiarek DJ, Szpakowski P, Glabinski A. Neural plasticity in multiple sclerosis: the functional and molecular background. *Neural Plast.* 2015:Article ID 307175, 11 pages, https://doi.org/10.1155/2015/307175.

24. Filippi M, Bar-Or A, Piehl F, et al. Multiple sclerosis. *Nat Rev Dis Primers.* 2018;4(1):43.

25. Frischer JM, Weigand SD, Guo Y, et al. Clinical and pathological insights into the dynamic nature of the white matter multiple sclerosis plaque. *Ann Neurol.* 2015;78(5):710-721.

26. Goldschmidt T, Antel J, Konig FB, Bruck W, Kuhlmann T. Remyelination capacity of the MS brain decreases with disease chronicity. *Neurology.* 2009;72:1914-1921.

27. Popescu BF, Pirko I, Lucchinetti CF. Pathology of multiple sclerosis: where do we stand? *Continuum (Minneap Minn).* 2013;19(4 Multiple Sclerosis):901-921.

28. Moll NM, Rietsch AM, Thomas S, et al. Multiple sclerosis normal-appearing white matter: pathology-imaging correlations. *Ann Neurol.* 2011;70(5):764-773.

29. Gallego-Delgado P, James R, Browne E, et al. Neuroinflammation in the normal-appearing white matter (NAWM) of the multiple sclerosis brain causes abnormalities at the nodes of Ranvier. *PLoS Biol.* 2020;14:18(12):e3001008.

30. Pirko I, Lucchinetti CF, Sriram S, Bakshi R. Gray matter involvement in multiple sclerosis. *Neurology.* 2007;68:634-642.

31. Eshaghi A, Prados F, Brownlee WJ, et al. Deep gray matter volume loss drives disability worsening in multiple sclerosis. *Ann Neurol.* 2018;83(2):210-222.

32. Horkova D, Kalincik T, Dusankova JB, Dolezai O. Clinical correlates of grey matter pathology in multiple sclerosis. *BMC Neurol.* 2012;12:10-20.

33. Rocca MA, Valsasina P, Meani A, et al. On Behalf of the MAGNIMS Study Group. Association of grey matter atrophy patterns with clinical phenotype and progression in multiple sclerosis. *Neurology.* 2021;96(11):e1561-e1573.

34. Wildner P, Stasiołek M, Matysiak M. Differential diagnosis of multiple sclerosis and other inflammatory CNS diseases. *Mult Scler Relat Disord.* 2020;37:101452.

35. Lv A, Zhang Z, Fu Y, Yan Y, Yang L, Zhu W. Dawson's Fingers in cerebral small vessel disease. *Front Neurol.* 2020;11:669.

36. Nowaczyk N, Kalinowska-Łyszczarz A, Paprzycki W, Michalak S, Kaźmierski R, Pawlak MA. Spatial distribution of white matter degenerative lesions and cognitive dysfunction in relapsing-remitting multiple sclerosis patients. *Neurol Neurochir Pol.* 2019;53(1):18-25.

37. Okuda DT, Siva A, Kantarci O, et al. Radiologically isolated syndrome: 5-year risk for an initial clinical event. *PLoS One.* 2014;9(3):e90509.

38. Kantarci OH, Lebrun C, Siva A, et al. Primary progressive multiple sclerosis evolving from radiologically isolated syndrome. *Ann Neurol.* 2016;79:288-294.

39. Jamali A, Sadeghi-Demneh E, Fereshtenajad N, Hillier S. Somatosensory impairment and its association with balance limitation in people with multiple sclerosis. *Gait Posture.* 2017;57:224-229.

40. Truini A, Barbanti P, Pozzilli C, Cruccu G. A mechanism-based classification of pain in multiple sclerosis. *J Neurol.* 2013;260(2):351-367.

41. Murphy KL, Bethea JR, Fischer R. Chapter 4: Neuropathic pain in multiple sclerosis: current therapeutic intervention and future treatment perspectives. In: Zagon IS, McLaughlin PJ, eds. *Multiple Sclerosis: Perspectives in Treatment and Pathogenesis [Internet].* Brisbane, AU: Codon Publications; 2017:69-86. Available from: https://www.ncbi.nlm.nih.gov/books/NBK470151/.

42. Khan N, Smith MT. Multiple sclerosis-induced neuropathic pain: pharmacological management and pathophysiological insights from rodent EAE models. *Inflammopharmacology.* 2014;22(1):1-22.

43. Khare S, Seth D. Lhermitte's sign: the current status. *Ann Indian Acad Neurol.* 2015;18(2):154-156.

44. Hoff JM, Dhayalan M, Midelfart A, Tharaldsen AR, Bø L. Visual dysfunction in multiple sclerosis. *Tidsskr Nor Laegeforen.* 2019;139(11). English, Norwegian. doi:10.4045/tidsskr.18.0786.PMID:31429247.

45. Edwards EM, Fritz NE, Therrien AS. Cerebellar dysfunction in multiple sclerosis: considerations for research and rehabilitation therapy. *Neurorehabil Neural Repair.* 2022;36(2):103-106.

46. Jørgensen M, Dalgas U, Wens I, Hvid LG. Muscle strength and power in persons with multiple sclerosis: a systematic review and meta-analysis. *J Neurol Sci.* 2017;376:225-241.

47. Ng A, Miller R, Gelinas D, Kent-Braun J. Functional relationships of central and peripheral muscle alterations in multiple sclerosis. *Muscle Nerve.* 2004;29:843-852.

48. Manjaly ZM, Harrison NA, Critchley HD, et al. Pathophysiological and cognitive mechanisms of fatigue in multiple sclerosis. *J Neurol Neurosurg Psychiatry.* 2019;90(6):642-651.

49. Sandroff BM, Dlugonski D, Weikert M, Suh Y, Balantrapu S, Motl RW. Physical activity and multiple sclerosis: new insights regarding inactivity. *Acta Neurol Scand.* 2012;126(4):256-262.

50. Klaren RE, Motl RW, Dlugonski D, Sandroff BM, Pilutti LA. Objectively quantified physical activity in persons with multiple sclerosis. *Arch Phys Med Rehabil.* 2013;94:2342-2348.

51. Sharma KR, Kent-Braun J, Mynhier MA, Weiner MW, Miller RG. Evidence of an abnormal intramuscular component of fatigue in multiple sclerosis. *Muscle Nerve.* 1995;18(12):1403-1411.

52. Hansen D, Feys P, Wens I, Eijnde BO. Is walking capacity in subjects with multiple sclerosis primarily related to muscle oxidative capacity or maximal muscle strength? A pilot study. *Mult Scler Int.* 2014;2014:759030.

53. Yoosefinejad AK, Motealleh A, Khademi S, Hosseini SF. Lower endurance and strength of core muscles in patients with multiple sclerosis. *Int J MS Care.* 2017;19(2):100-104.

54. Bethoux F, Marrie RA. A cross-sectional study of the impact of spasticity on daily activities in multiple sclerosis. *Patient.* 2016;9(6):537-546.

55. Rizzo MA, Hadjimichael OC, Preiningerova J, Vollmer TL. Prevalence and treatment of spasticity reported by multiple sclerosis patients. *Mult Scler.* 2004;10(5):589-595.

56. Trompetto C, TMarinelli L, Mori L, et al. Pathophysiology of spasticity: implications for neurorehabilitation. *Biomed Res Int.* 2014;2014:354906.

57. Patejdl R, Zettl UK. Spasticity in multiple sclerosis: contribution of inflammation, autoimmune mediated neuronal damage and therapeutic interventions. *Autoimmun Rev.* 2017;16(9):925-936.

58. Hugos CL, Cameron MH. Assessment and measurement of spasticity in MS: state of the evidence. *Curr Neurol Neurosci Rep.* 2019;19(10):79.

59. Hoang PD, Gandevia SC, Herbert RD. Prevalence of joint contractures and muscle weakness in people with multiple sclerosis. *Disabil Rehabil.* 2014;36(19):1588-1593.

60. Sosnoff JJ, Gappmaier E, Frame A, Motl RW. Influence of spasticity on mobility and balance in persons with multiple sclerosis. *J Neurol Phys Ther.* 2011;35(3):129-132.

61. Krupp LB, Serafin DJ, Christodoulou C. Multiple sclerosis-associated fatigue. *Expert Rev Neurother.* 2010;10(9):1437-1447.

62. Garg H, Bush S, Gappmaier E. Associations between fatigue and disability, functional mobility, depression, and quality of life in people with multiple sclerosis. *Int J MS Care.* 2016;18(2):71-77.

63. Fisk JD, Pontefract A, Ritvo PG, Archibald CJ, Murray TJ. The impact of fatigue on patients with multiple sclerosis. *Can J Neurol Sci.* 1994;21(1):9-14.

64. Multiple Sclerosis Clinical Practice Guidelines. Fatigue and multiple sclerosis: evidence-based management strategies for fatigue in multiple sclerosis. Washington D.C.: Paralyzed Veterans of America; 1998.

65. Kobelt G, Langdon D,Jonsson L. The effect of self-assessed fatigue and subjective cognitive impairment on work capacity: the case of multiple sclerosis. *Mult Scler.* 2019;25(5):740-749.

66. Braley TJ, Chervin RD. Fatigue in multiple sclerosis: mechanisms, evaluation, and treatment. *Sleep.* 2010;33(8):1061-1067.

67. Tartaglia MC, Narayanan S, Arnold DL. Mental fatigue alters the pattern and increases the volume of cerebral activation required for a motor task in multiple sclerosis patients with fatigue. *Eur J Neurol.* 2008;15:413-419.

68. White AT, Lee JN, Light AR, et al. Brain activation in multiple sclerosis: a BOLD fMRI study of the effects of fatiguing hand exercise. *Mult Scler.* 2009;15:580-586.

69. Salamone PC, Esteves S, Sinay VJ, et al. Altered neural signatures of interoception in multiple sclerosis. *Hum Brain Mapp.* 2018;39:4743-4754.

70. Induruwa I, Constantinescu CS, Gran B. Fatigue in multiple sclerosis: a brief review. *J Neurol.* 2012;12:10-20.

71. Kos D, Kerckhofs E, Nagels G, D'hooghe MB, Ilsbroukx S. Origin of fatigue in multiple sclerosis: review of the literature. *Neurorehabil Neural Repair.* 2008;22:91-100.

72. Fiest KM, Fisk JD, Patten SB, et al. Fatigue and comorbidities in multiple sclerosis. *Int J MS Care.* 2016;18(2):96-104.

73. Penner I-K, Paul F. Fatigue as a symptom or comorbidity of neurological diseases. *Nat Rev Neurol.* 2017;13(11):662-675.

74. Wilkins A. Cerebellar dysfunction in multiple sclerosis. *Front Neurol.* 2017;8:312.

75. Rinker JR 2nd, Salter AR, Walker H, Amara A, Meador W, Cutter GR. Prevalence and characteristics of tremor in the NARCOMS multiple sclerosis registry: a cross-sectional survey. *BMJ Open.* 2015;5(1):e006714.

76. Coca-Tapia M, Cuesta-Gómez A. Molina-Rueda F, Carratalá-Tejada M. Gait pattern in people with multiple sclerosis: a systematic review. *Dianostics (Basel).* 2021:11(4):584.

77. Calcagno P, Ruoppolo G, Grasso MG, De Vincentiis M, Paolucci S. Dysphagia in multiple sclerosis: prevalence and prognostic factors. *Acta Neurol Scand.* 2002;105(1):40-43.

78. Feenaughty L, Guo LY, Weinstock-Guttman B, Ray M, Benedict RHB, Tjaden K. Impact of cognitive impairment and dysarthria on spoken language in multiple sclerosis. *J Int Neuropsychol Soc.* 2021;27(5):450-460.

79. Darley FL, Brown JR, Goldstein NP. Dysarthria in multiple sclerosis. *J Speech Hear Res.* 1972;15(2):229-245.

80. Ansari NN, Tarameshlu M, Ghelichi L. Dysphagia in multiple sclerosis patients: diagnostic and evaluation strategies. *Degener Neurol Neuromuscul Dis.* 2020;10:15-28.

81. Benedict RHB, Amato MP, DeLuca J, Geurts JJG. Cognitive impairment in multiple sclerosis: clinical management, MRI, and therapeutic avenues. *Lancet Neurol.* 2020;19(10):860-871.

82. Benedict R, DeLuca J, Enzinger C, Geurts J, Krupp L, Rao S. Neuropsychology of multiple sclerosis: looking back and moving forward. *J Int Neuropsychol Soc.* 2017;23(9-10):832-842.

83. Eijlers AJC, van Geest Q, Dekker I, et al. Predicting cognitive decline in multiple sclerosis: a 5-year follow-up study. *Brain.* 2018;141(9):2605-2618.

84. Rao SM, Leo GJ, Bernardin L, Unverzagt F. Cognitive dysfunction in multiple sclerosis I: frequency, patterns, and prediction *Neurology.* 1991;41(5):685-691.

85. Chiaravalloti ND, DeLuca J. Cognitive impairment in multiple sclerosis. *Lancet Neurol.* 2008;7(12):1139-1151.

86. Fritz NE, Kloos AD, Kegelmeyer DA, Kaur P, Nichols-Larsen DS. Supplementary motor area connectivity and dual-task walking variability in multiple sclerosis. *J Neurol Sci.* 2019;396:159-164.

87. Benedict R, Cookfair D, Gavett R, et al. Validity of the minimal assessment of cognitive function in multiple sclerosis (MACFIMS). *J Int Neuropsychol Soc.* 2006;12(4):549-558.

88. Miller E, Morel A, Redlicka J, Miller I, Saluk J. Pharmacological and non-pharmacological therapies of cognitive impairment in multiple sclerosis. *Curr Neuropharmacol.* 2018;16(4):475-483.

89. Benedict RH, Drake AS, Irwin LN, et al. Benchmarks of meaningful impairment on the MSFC and BICAMS. *Mult Scler.* 2016;22(14):1874-1882.

90. Goverover Y, Chiaravalloti N, DeLuca J. Brief international cognitive assessment for multiple sclerosis (BICAMS) and performance of everyday life tasks: actual reality. *Mult Scler.* 2016;22(4):544-550.

91. Rosti-Otajarvi E, Hamalainen P. Behavioural symptoms and impairments in multiple sclerosis: a systematic review and meta-analysis. *Mult Scler.* 2012;19:31-45.

92. Patten SB. Current perspectives on co-morbid depression and multiple sclerosis. *Expert Rev Neurother.* 2020;20(8):867-874.

93. Adamec I, Habek M. Autonomic dysfunction in multiple sclerosis. *Clin Neurol Neurosurg.* 2013;115(Suppl 1):S73-S78.

94. Adamec I, Krbot Skorić M, Habek M. Understanding and managing autonomic dysfunction in persons with multiple sclerosis. *Expert Rev Neurother.* 2021;21(12):1409-1417.

95. Sirbu CA, Mezei R, Falup Pecurariu C, et al. Autonomic dysfunctions in multiple sclerosis: challenges of clinical practice (Review). *Exp Ther Med.* 2020;20:196.

96. Adamec I, Lovrić M, Zaper D, et al. Postural orthostatic tachycardia syndrome associated with multiple sclerosis. *Auton Neurosci.* 2013;173(1-2):65-68.

97. Lensch E, Jost WH. Autonomic disorders in multiple sclerosis. *Autoimmune Dis.* 2011;2011:803841.

98. Wiesel PH, Norton C, Glickman S, Kamm MA. Pathophysiology and management of bowel dysfunction in multiple sclerosis. *Eur J Gastroenter Hepatol*. 2001;13(4):441-448.

99. Celik DB, Poyraz EC, Bingol A, Idlman E, Ozakbas S, Kava D. Sexual dysfunction in multiple sclerosis: gender differences. *J Neurol Sci*. 2013;324:17-20.

100. Simone IL, Tortorella C, Ghirelli A. Influence of pregnancy in multiple sclerosis and impact of disease-modifying therapies. *Front Neurol*. 2021;12:697974.

101. Davis SL, Jay O, Wilson TE. Thermoregulatory dysfunction in multiple sclerosis. *Handb Clin Neurol*. 2018;157:701-714.

102. Disease-modifying therapies for multiple sclerosis. National Multiple Sclerosis Society. Available at: https://www.nationalmssociety.org/NationalMSSociety/media/MSNationalFiles/Brochures/Brochure-The-MS-Disease-Modifying-Medications.pdf. Accessed on March 5, 2022.

103. Rae-Grant A, Day GS, Marrie RA, et al. Comprehensive systematic review summary: disease-modifying therapies for adults with multiple sclerosis: Report of the Guideline Development, Dissemination, and Implementation Subcommittee of the American Academy of Neurology. *Neurology*. 2018;90(17):789-800.

104. Repovic P. Management of multiple sclerosis relapses. *Continuum (Minneap Minn)*. 2019;25(3):655-669.

105. Solaro C, Uccelli MM. Management of pain in multiple sclerosis: a pharmacological approach. *Nat Rev Neurol*. 2011;7(9):519-527.

106. Hughes C, Howard IM. Spasticity management in multiple sclerosis. *Phys Med Rehabil Clin N Am*. 2013;24(4):593-604.

107. Tur C. Fatigue management in multiple sclerosis. *Curr Treat Options Neurol*. 2016;18(6):26.

108. Sarva H, Shanker VL. Treatment options in degenerative cerebellar ataxia: a systematic review. *Mov Disord Clin Pract*. 2014;1(4):291-298.

109. Makhoul K, Ahdab R, Riachi N, Chalah MA, Ayache SS. Tremor in multiple sclerosis: an overview and future perspectives. *Brain Sciences*. 2020;10(10):722.

110. Minden SL, Feinstein A, Kalb RC, et al. Evidence-based guideline: assessment and management of psychiatric disorders in individuals with MS: report of the Guideline Development Subcommittee of the American Academy of Neurology. *Neurology*. 2014;82:174-181.

111. Solaro C, Gamberini G, Masuccio FG. Depression in multiple sclerosis: epidemiology, aetiology, diagnosis and treatment. *CNS Drugs*. 2018; 32(2):117-133.

112. Ben-Zacharia AB. Therapeutics for multiple sclerosis symptoms. *Mt Sinai J Med*. 2011;78:176-191.

113. Jensen HB, Ravnborg M, Dalgas U, Stenager E. 4-Aminopyridine for symptomatic treatment of multiple sclerosis: a systematic review. *Ther Adv Neurol Disord*. 2014;7(2):97-113.

114. Messinis L, Kosmidis MH, Lyros E, Panathanasopoulos P. Assessment and rehabilitation of cognitive impairment in multiple sclerosis. *Int Rev Psychiatry*. 2010;22:22-34.

115. Oh J, Vidal-Jordana A, Montalban X. Multiple sclerosis: clinical aspects. *Curr Opin Neurol*. 2018;31:752-759.

116. Marrie RA, Elliott L, Marriott J, et al. Effect of comorbidity on mortality in multiple sclerosis. *Neurology*. 2015;85(3):240-247.

117. Tintore M, Rovira A, Rio J, et al. Defining high, medium and low impact prognostic factors for developing multiple sclerosis. *Brain*, 2015;138(Pt 7): 1863-1874.

118. Neurology Section. MS-EDGE Outcome Measures for In- and Out-patient Rehabilitation. Available at: https://www.neuropt.org/docs/ms-edge-documents/ms-edge_rehab_recs5417E23D4B53.pdf?sfvrsn=3a7e0ba1_2. Accessed on 4/15/2022.

119. Rietberg MB, Veerbeek JM, Gosselink R, Kwakkel G, van Wegen EE. Respiratory muscle training for multiple sclerosis. *Cochrane Database Syst Rev*. 2017;12(12):CD009424.

120. Motl RW. Exercise and multiple sclerosis. *Adv Exp Med Biol*. 2020; 1228:333-343.

121. Latimer-Cheung AE, Martin Ginis KA, Hicks AL, et al. Development of evidence-informed physical activity guidelines for adults with multiple sclerosis. *Arch Phys Med Rehabil*. 2013;94(9):1829-1836.

122. Kim Y, Lai B, Mehta T, et al. Exercise training guidelines for multiple sclerosis, stroke, and parkinson disease: rapid review and synthesis. *Am J Phys Med Rehabil*. 2019;98(7):613-621.

123. Campbell E, Coulter EH, Paul L. High intensity interval training for people with multiple sclerosis: a systematic review. *Mult Scler Relat Disord*. 2018;24:55-63.

124. Keytsman C, Van Noten P, Verboven K, Van Asch P, Eijnde BO. Periodized versus classic exercise therapy in Multiple Sclerosis: a randomized controlled trial. *Mult Scler Relat Disord*. 2021;49:102782.

125. Bowman T, Gervasoni E, Amico AP, et al. "CICERONE" Italian Consensus Group for Robotic Rehabilitation:What is the impact of robotic rehabilitation on balance and gait outcomes in people with multiple sclerosis? A systematic review of randomized control trials. *Eur J Phys Rehabil Med*. 2021;57(2):246-253.

126. Lamberti N, Manfredin F, Baroni A, et al. Motor cortical activation assessment in progressive multiple sclerosis patients enrolled in gait rehabilitation: a secondary analysis of the RAGTIME trial assisted by functional near-infrared spectroscopy. *Diagnostics (Basel)*. 2020;11(6):1068.

127. Amatya B, Khan F, Galea M. Rehabilitation for people with multiple sclerosis: an overview of Cochrane reviews. *Cochrane Database Syst Rev*. 2019;1(1):CD012732.

128. Robinson AG, Dennett AM, Snowdon DA. Treadmill training may be an effective form of task-specific training for improving mobility in people with Parkinson's disease and multiple sclerosis: a systematic review and meta-analysis. *Physiotherapy*. 2019;105(2):174-186.

129. Corvillo I, Varela E, Armijo F, Alvarez-Badillo A, Armijo O, Maraver F. Efficacy of aquatic therapy for multiple sclerosis: a systematic review. *Eur J Phys Rehabil Med*. 2017;53(6):944-952.

130. Shafizadeh M, Platt GK, Mohammadi B. Effects of different focus of attention rehabilitative training on gait performance in multiple sclerosis patients. *J Bodyw Mov Ther*. 2013;17(1):28-34.

131. Guo LY, Lozinski B , Yong VW. Exercise in multiple sclerosis and its models: focus on the central nervous system outcomes. *J Neurosci Res*. 2020;98(3):509-523.

132. Lozinski BM, Yong VW. Exercise and the brain in multiple sclerosis. *Mult Scler*. 2022;28(8):1167-1172.

133. Razazian N, Kazeminia M, Moayedi H, et al. The impact of physical exercise on the fatigue symptoms in patients with multiple sclerosis: a systematic review and meta-analysis. *BMC Neurol*. 2020;20(1):93.

134. Smith KJ, McDonald WI. The pathophysiology of multiple sclerosis: the mechanisms underlying the production of symptoms and the natural history of the disease. *Philos Trans R Soc Lond B Biol Sci*. 1999;354(1390):1649-1673.

135. Etoom M, Khraiwesh Y, Lena F, et al. Effectiveness of physiotherapy interventions on spasticity in people with multiple sclerosis: a systematic review and meta-analysis. *Am J Phys Med Rehabil*. 2018;97(11):793-807.

136. Şan AU, Yılmaz B, Kesikburun S. The effect of repetitive transcranial magnetic stimulation on spasticity in patients with multiple sclerosis. *J Clin Neurol*. 2019;15(4):461-467.

137. Mills RJ, Yap L, Young CA. Treatment for ataxia in multiple sclerosis. *Cochrane Database Syst Rev*. 2007;(1):CD005029.

138. Salcı Y, Fil A, Armutlu K, et al. Effects of different exercise modalities on ataxia in multiple sclerosis patients: a randomized controlled study. *Disabil Rehabil*. 2017;39(26):2626-2632.

139. Dean CM, Richards CL, Malouin F. Task-related circuit training improves performance of loco-motor tasks in chronic stroke: a randomized, controlled pilot trial. *Arch Phys Med Rehabil*. 2000;81:409-417.

140. Marquer A, Barbieri G, Pérennou D. The assessment and treatment of postural disorders in cerebellar ataxia: a systematic review. *Ann Phys Rehabil Med*. 2014;57(2):67-78.

141. Leavitt VM, Cirnigliaro C, Cohen A, et al. Aerobic exercise increases hippocampal volume and improves memory in multiple sclerosis: preliminary findings. *Neurocase.* 2014;20:695-697.

142. Langeskov-Christensen M, Hvid LG, Jensen HB, et al. Efficacy of high-intensity aerobic exercise on cognitive performance in people with multiple sclerosis: a randomized controlled trial. *Mult Scler.* 2021;27(10):1585-1596.

143. Rademacher A, Joisten N, Proschinger S, et al. Do baseline cognitive status, participant specific characteristics and EDSS impact changes of cognitive performance following aerobic exercise intervention in multiple sclerosis? *Mult Scler Relat Disord.* 2021;51:102905.

144. Martino Cinnera A, Bisirri A, Leone E, Morone G, Gaeta A. Effect of dual-task training on balance in patients with multiple sclerosis: a systematic review and meta-analysis. *Clin Rehabil.* 2021;35(10):1399-1412.

145. Renfrew LM, Paul L, McFadyen A, et al. The clinical- and cost-effectiveness of functional electrical stimulation and ankle-foot orthoses for foot drop in Multiple Sclerosis: a multicentre randomized trial. *Clin Rehabil.* 2019;33(7):1150-1162.

146. Martin-Sanchez C, Calvo-Arenillas JI, Barbero-Iglesias FJ, Fonseca E, Sanchez-Santos JM, Martin-Nogueras AM. Effects of 12-week inspiratory muscle training with low resistance in patients with multiple sclerosis: a non-randomised, double-blind, controlled trial. *Mult Scler Relat Disord.* 2020;46:102574.

Review Questions

1. **Which of the following statements is true regarding the epidemiology of MS?**
   A. There is an increasing prevalence of MS with increasing distance away from the equator.
   B. There is an increasing prevalence of MS with decreasing distance away from the equator.
   C. The prevalence of MS is equally distributed around the world.
   D. The incidence of MS is highest in individuals of African and Asian descent.

2. **The clear cause of MS is unknown, but which of the following factors is believed to be most important for the development of MS?**
   A. Environment, viruses, and genetics
   B. Ethnicity, diet, and antibiotic resistance
   C. Exercise, blood pressure, and sunlight
   D. Emotional health, diet, and smoking

3. **What pathophysiological process(es) in the CNS is/are involved in MS?**
   A. Inflammation and destruction of the myelin sheath
   B. Axonal degeneration
   C. Formation of amyloid plaques
   D. Both A and B
   E. Both A and C

4. **Which subtype of MS is most common?**
   A. clinically isolated syndrome
   B. secondary progressive
   C. relapsing-remitting
   D. primary progressive

5. **For an episode of neurological symptoms to be called an MS relapse or exacerbation, the duration of symptoms must be:**
   A. 6 hours duration
   B. 12 hours duration
   C. 24 hours duration
   D. 48 hours duration

6. **Which of the following baseline factors is the greatest indicator of a poor prognosis in MS?**
   A. 10 or more lesions on T2-weighted MRI images
   B. Female gender
   C. Onset at an early age
   D. Presence of oligoclonal bands

7. **What is the most common, and often the most disabling, symptom associated with MS?**
   A. Spasticity
   B. Pain
   C. Depression
   D. Fatigue

8. **What precaution in regard to exercise is specific to MS?**
   A. Exercise can cause muscle atrophy in individuals with MS.
   B. Exercise is problematic due to breathing problems in individuals with MS.
   C. Exercise-induced increases in body temperature can cause temporary worsening or return of previously existing neurological symptoms.
   D. Exercise can induce emotional stress in individuals with MS.

9. **Which of the following is currently the best medical treatment for the treatment of an acute relapse?**
   A. Plasmapheresis
   B. Interferon beta
   C. Corticosteroids
   D. Antibiotics

10. **Thomas and Sally are planning to start a family but Sally has MS. Which of the following statements is true about family planning and MS?**
    A. The risk of relapses is higher during pregnancy.

B. Certain methods of birth control are not effective for patients with MS.

C. Fertility is unaffected in women with MS.

D. Immunomodulatory drugs can be safely taken throughout pregnancy and postpartum.

11. **Sally has MS and is complaining that she cannot make it through the day due to being tired. She is worried about her job and her ability to take care of her children after work. To objectively measure her fatigue you would use which of the following measures?**

A. Berg Balance Scale

B. 6-minute walk test

C. Modified Fatigue Impact Scale

D. Timed 25-foot walk

12. **Sally who has MS has been on high-dose corticosteroid treatment immediately prior to starting therapy. During therapy she complains of hip pain that is constant and is worse with weight-bearing. Which of the following conditions should the therapist investigate and rule out before proceeding based on the history provided here?**

A. Aseptic necrosis

B. Bursitis

C. Joint instability

D. Radiculopathy

13. **Which of the following statements is true about exercise and multiple sclerosis?**

A. Exercise can trigger exacerbations.

B. Exercise does not impact quality of life.

C. Posture can be improved with strength training.

D. Robot-assisted walking is better than over-ground walking.

14. **Which of the following exercises can be done to improve static balance?**

A. Backward walking

B. Braiding

C. Sharpened Romberg stance

D. Step front and step back

15. **Sally who has MS has spasticity of the gastroc-soleus group. She should be prescribed stretching and which of the following exercises?**

A. Standing, go up on toes, and slowly lower, repeat 10 times

B. Walk backward at least 50 feet

C. Perform straight leg raises, repeat 20 times

D. Walk with toes up and weight on heels

16. **Therapy for ataxia in MS includes which of the following?**

A. Perform balance exercises that focus on weight shifting

B. Include dual-task practice such as carrying a glass of water while walking

C. Place forearm on table and concentrate on slowing spreading the fingers out and then bringing back together again

D. Perform resistance strengthening to the involved extremities with weights

17. **Individuals with MS should be worked at what percent of the Karvonen formula: (220 − age) × _____?**

A. Less than 40%

B. Greater than 80%

C. 60-65%

D. The Karvonen formula should not be used in MS

18. **Sally who has MS is married with three children and lives in a two-story home. She works full time as an elementary teacher. She has fatigue and is being taught energy conservation and work simplification. Which of the following would be an appropriate modification for Sally?**

A. Use a rolling chair or stool in the classroom so that she can roll from student to student when helping with assignments.

B. She needs to go to part-time at work.

C. Avoid attending her children's sports activities in the evening.

D. Do all strenuous activity in the morning then rest in afternoon and evening.

19. **You are educating Sally about the role of exercise for fitness in individuals with MS. Which of the following statements is true about fitness and MS? Individuals with MS who exercise regularly:**

A. Appear to have a faster rate of decline

B. Have poorer quality of life

C. Experience a protective effect on cognitive function

D. Have poorer overall health

20. **In the late stage of multiple sclerosis which therapeutic programs are beneficial?**

A. Balance training with an emphasis on narrowing the base of support

B. Resistance training to improve walking

C. Respiratory resistance training twice a day

D. Robot-assisted gait training

21. **You have your client with MS working on aerobic exercise with 30 seconds of cycling as hard as she can followed by 30 seconds of no-resistance, low-speed cycling. She repeats these intervals for 15 minutes. This exercise setup can best be described as which of the following?**

A. High-intensity interval training

B. Periodized exercise

C. High-intensity exercise

D. Ratio based training intervals.

22. **The current exercise guideline for people with MS is to perform:**
    A. 1-2 days a week of aerobic exercise and one day a week of resistance exercise
    B. High-intensity interval training four days a week
    C. 2-3 days a week of aerobic and strengthening exercise at moderate intensity
    D. Low-intensity aerobic exercise followed by stretching 3 to 4 days a week

23. **Which of the following is an evidence-based way to treat fatigue in MS?**
    A. Resistance exercise at six to eight repetitions, three sets.
    B. Educate on energy-conservation techniques
    C. High-intensity interval training
    D. Robotic walking training.

24. **Which of the following interventions is effective in improving ataxia?**
    A. Aerobic exercise
    B. Resistance exercise
    C. Task training with lumbar stabilization
    D. Treadmill training with weighting of the extremities

25. **Exercise may be able to positively impact cognitive function in which of the following clients?**
    A. Anyone with MS
    B. Newly diagnosed with MS with no signs of cognitive involvement
    C. Mild MS with cognitive impairment noted on testing of cognition
    D. Moderate to severe MS with severe cognitive impairment

26. **A positive finding for internuclear ophthalmoplegia affecting the right eye is:**
    A. Weak adduction of right eye, abduction nystagmus of left eye with gaze to the left
    B. Weak abduction of left eye, adduction nystagmus of right eye with gaze to the left
    C. Weak adduction of left eye, abduction nystagmus of right eye with gaze to the right
    D. Weak abduction of right eye, adduction nystagmus of left eye with gaze to the right

27. **Sudden, severe neuropathic pain in the face experienced by some people with MS is caused by damage of the:**
    A. Facial nerve
    B. Trigeminal nerve
    C. Optic nerve
    D. Oculomotor nerve

28. **Fatigue in MS**
    A. does not typically interfere with performance of daily life activities
    B. is related to the severity and the duration of MS
    C. only affects people with primary or secondary progressive MS subtypes
    D. is caused by many factors, both disease related and non-disease related

29. **The only FDA-approved disease-modifying therapy medication approved for primary progressive MS is:**
    A. mitoxantrone (Navontrone)
    B. glatiramer acetate (Copaxone)
    C. ocrelizumab (Ocrevus)
    D. dimethyl fumarate (Tecfidera)

30. **A medication that is specifically used to improve walking in people with MS is:**
    A. imipramine (Tofranil)
    B. dalfampridine (Ampyra)
    C. topiramate (Topamax)
    D. tizanidine (Zanaflex)

Answers

1. A	2. A	3. D	4. C	5. C
6. A	7. D	8. C	9. C	10. C
11. C	12. A	13. C	14. C	15. A
16. B	17. C	18. A	19. C	20. C
21. A	22. C	23. B	24. C	25. C
26. A	27. B	28. D	29. C	30. B

GLOSSARY

Attack. Relapse, exacerbation, and (when it is the first episode) clinically isolated syndrome are synonyms. See clinically isolated syndrome and relapse for descriptions.

Allodynia. Pain resulting from an innocuous stimulus such as light touch of the skin which would not normally cause pain.

Black holes. Dark areas representing focal axonal damage and irreversible axonal loss seen on T1-weighted MRI images.

Clinically isolated syndrome. Similar to typical multiple sclerosis relapse (also called attack and exacerbation) but in a patient not known to have multiple sclerosis. If the person is subsequently diagnosed with multiple sclerosis (by fulfilling dissemination in space and time, and ruling out other diagnoses), the clinically isolated syndrome was the person's first relapse. See relapse for description.

Dawson's fingers. A relatively specific radiographic finding of multiple sclerosis characterized by periventricular demyelinating plaques distributed along the axis of medullary veins, perpendicular to the body of the lateral ventricles.

Detrusor sphincter dyssynergia. A condition that causes bladder outlet obstruction from detrusor muscle contraction with concomitant involuntary urethral sphincter activation.

Diplopia. Double vision or seeing two images of the same object.

Dissemination in space. The development of lesions in distinct anatomical locations within the CNS, indicating a multifocal CNS process.

Dissemination in time. The development or appearance of new CNS lesions over time.

Dysesthesias. Abnormal painful sensations described by people with multiple sclerosis as burning, prickling, or aching feelings typically present in the legs and feet, or sometimes as a feeling of being squeezed around the chest or abdomen.

Exacerbation. Attack, relapse, and (when it is the first episode) clinically isolated syndrome are synonyms. See clinically isolated syndrome and relapse for descriptions.

Hyperalgesia. Abnormally increased sensitivity to or perception of a pain stimulus.

Hypoesthesia. Partial or total loss of sensation (i.e., touch, vibration, pain, temperature) in a part of the body.

Internuclear ophthalmoplegia. An eye movement disorder caused by a lesion of the medial longitudinal fasciculus resulting in symptoms of diplopia. There is a disruption in the coordination of horizontal eye movements when the person's gaze is directed away from the affected side, such that adduction of the eye on the affected side is limited, and there is nystagmus of the abducted eye on the unaffected side.

Lesions. An area of damage or scarring (sclerosis) in the CNS caused by multiple sclerosis. See plaques for a description.

Lhermitte's sign. A brief, intense sensation that feels similar to an electric shock going down the neck and spine and sometimes radiating through the trunk in response to forward flexion of the neck.

Marcus Gunn pupil. A condition caused by unilateral dysfunction of the optic nerve that results in abnormal pupillary dilation of the affected eye when a bright light is swung between the intact and the affected eye, thereby causing a size difference of the pupils between the eyes. This can occur following optic neuritis in people with multiple sclerosis.

Medial longitudinal fasciculus. A bilateral tract located near the midline within the midbrain and pons that interconnects the oculomotor nuclei (i.e., oculomotor, trochlear, and abducens) for coordination of conjugate eye movements.

Normal-appearing white matter. Normal appearing, yet mildly damaged, areas of white matter adjacent to lesions or plaques seen on MRI images.

Oligoclonal immunoglobulin bands. Immunoglobulin proteins present in the cerebrospinal fluid of people with multiple sclerosis that are considered to be an immunological biomarker of the disease.

Optic neuritis. Inflammation of the optic nerve that results in sudden partial or complete loss of vision, blurred or "foggy" vision, and pain with movement of the eye. It is a common early symptom of multiple sclerosis.

Orthostatic hypotension. An abnormal decrease in blood pressure (20 mmHg systolic, 10 mmHg diastolic) when a person stands up compared with blood pressure from the seated or supine position.

Paresthesias. Abnormal sensations described as tingling, prickling, pins and needles, or burning sensations in the absence of any stimulus. They differ from dysesthsias in that they are typically painless.

Plaques. Focal areas of demyelination within the CNS, with different amounts of inflammation, gliosis (scarring), and neurodegeneration that appear as hyperintensities on T2-weighted MRI images. They are synonymous with lesions.

Postural orthostatic tachycardia syndrome. A sympathetic dysautonomia that is characterized by orthostatic intolerance that manifests as lightheadedness or fainting accompanied by an abnormal increase in heart rate ($\geq$30 bpm or >120 bpm) upon moving from a lying down to standing-up position.

Primary progressive course. A multiple sclerosis course characterized by steadily increasing neurological disability independent of relapses from disease onset. Neurologic symptom fluctuations, periods of stability, and superimposed relapses might occur.

Pseudorelapse. Worsened neurologic symptoms not associated with active MRI lesions on MRI, but rather from increased body temperature due to overheating or other factors such as trauma, new medications, other medical conditions, and psychological stress.

Radiologically isolated syndrome. MRI findings strongly suggestive of multiple sclerosis in a person with no neurological signs or symptoms or other explanation.

Relapse. An episode of patient-reported symptoms and objective findings typical of multiple sclerosis, reflecting demyelination within the CNS, with a duration of 24 hours, with or without recovery, and in the absence of fever or infection. Attack, exacerbation, and (when it is the first episode) clinically isolated syndrome are synonyms.

Relapsing-remitting course. A multiple sclerosis course characterized by relapses with stable neurological disability between episodes.

Secondary progressive course. A multiple sclerosis course that follows an initial relapsing-remitting course, in which there is a progressive worsening of neurologic function (accumulation of disability) over time.

Shadow plaques. Plaques characterized by axons with thin myelin sheaths that are thought to represent areas of complete remyelination of previously demyelinated plaques.

T1-weighted magnetic resonance images. Used in multiple sclerosis without contrast to detect black holes where there is permanent loss of axons from neurodegeneration, and with contrast (typically gadolinium) to distinguish new active lesions with high inflammation from inactive lesions.

T2-weighted magnetic resonance image scans. Used in multiple sclerosis to identify total numbers of MS lesions as lesions appear as hyperintensities compared to the low-intensity background of white matter. To distinguish lesions from cerebrospinal fluid which also has a high signal with T2 weighting, proton density weighted (PD) or fluid attenuated inversion recovery (FLAIR) images that suppress the signal from cerebrospinal fluid can be combined with T2 weighted images.

Uhthoff's phenomenon. Worsening of neurologic symptoms in multiple sclerosis due to an increase in core body temperature by heat and exercise that blocks or slows conduction of nerve impulses in damaged axons. Once body temperature returns to normal, signs and symptoms typically reverse.

Upper motor neurons. Motor neurons that have their cell bodies above cranial nerve nuclei or the anterior horn cells of the spinal cord.

ABBREVIATIONS

ACTH	adrenocorticotrophic hormone
BP	blood pressure
CIS	clinically isolated syndrome
CSF	cerebrospinal fluid
DIS	dissemination in space
DIT	dissemination in time
DMT	disease-modifying therapy
HR	heart rate
IgG	immunoglobulin G
INO	internuclear ophthalmoplegia
ISC	intermittent self-catheterization
MLF	medial longitudinal fasciculus
MRI	magnetic resonance imaging
NAWM	normal-appearing white matter
NMSS	National Multiple Sclerosis Society
OH	orthostatic hypotension
POTS	postural orthostatic tachycardia syndrome
PPMS	primary progressive multiple sclerosis
RIS	radiologically isolated syndrome
RRMS	relapsing-remitting multiple sclerosis
SPMS	secondary progressive multiple sclerosis
UTI	urinary tract infection

Basal Ganglia Disorders: Parkinson and Huntington's Diseases

15

Anne D. Kloos and Deborah A. Kegelmeyer

OBJECTIVES

1) Discuss the demographics and etiology of idiopathic Parkinson's (PD) and Huntington's diseases (HD)

2) Compare and contrast the pathological features and pathogenesis of idiopathic PD, PD plus syndromes, and HD

3) Differentiate between the diagnosis of idiopathic PD and HD

4) Compare and contrast typical signs and symptoms of idiopathic PD and HD

5) Describe the clinical course, prognosis, and medical and surgical treatment of idiopathic PD and HD

6) Discuss evidence-based examination of the client with PD and HD

7) Discuss evidence-based management of the client with PD and HD

8) Compare and contrast examination and management of early, middle, and late-stage PD and HD

WHAT ARE PARKINSON'S AND HUNTINGTON'S DISEASES?

Parkinson's disease and Huntington's disease are progressive neurodegenerative disorders of the basal ganglia and its connections that profoundly impact motor, cognitive, and psychiatric functions of affected individuals. Parkinson's disease was named for James Parkinson, an English physician, whose work "An Essay on the Shaking Palsy" published in 1817 described six individuals with symptoms of the disease. Huntington's disease was named for George Huntington, an American physician, who published an article entitled "On Chorea" in 1872 that described the disease.

EPIDEMIOLOGY

Parkinson's disease (PD) is the second most common neurodegenerative disorder, after Alzheimer's disease, with an estimated 1 million Americans and 7 to 10 million people worldwide affected by the disease. There are approximately 60,000 new cases annually of PD in the United States.[1] The average age of onset is 60, and prevalence and incidence rates are very low in individuals under 40 years, increasing with age and peaking by age 80.[2] The disease is approximately 1.5 times more common in men than women. A large study of US Medicare beneficiaries aged 65 and older from the years 1995 and 2000-2005 found that the incidence of PD was highest among Hispanics, followed by non-Hispanic whites, Blacks, and Asians.[3] However, the prevalence of PD was highest among non-Hispanic whites, followed by Hispanics, Asians, and Blacks. Geographically, the incidence and prevalence of Parkinson's disease were 2 to 10 times greater in the Midwest and Northeast regions of the United States than Western and Southern regions.[3]

ETIOLOGY AND RISK FACTORS FOR PARKINSON'S DISEASE

Parkinsonism refers to a group of disorders with a variety of different underlying pathologies that can cause Parkinson's-like symptoms, including slowing movement (bradykinesia), tremor, rigidity or stiffness, and balance problems. PD, or idiopathic parkinsonism, is the most common disorder, affecting about 78% of individuals. **Secondary parkinsonism** results from identifiable causes such as toxins, trauma, multiple strokes, infections, metabolic disorders, and drugs. There are also conditions such as **parkinson-plus syndromes** that mimic PD in some ways but are caused by other neurodegenerative disorders.

IDIOPATHIC PARKINSON'S DISEASE

The exact cause of Parkinson's disease remains unknown,[4] but most scientists believe that it is caused by an interaction between genetic and environmental factors. Family history has been shown to be a strong risk factor for PD with a person's risk of developing PD 2.9 times greater if a first-degree relative had PD.[5] Twin studies have reported either no difference or higher concordance rates in monozygotic twins compared to dizygotic twins, when all ages were included, but among twins with PD diagnosed before age 50 the concordance rates were consistently higher in monozygotic twins.[4] These findings suggest that genetic factors play a more substantial role in early onset than late-onset PD.

Mutations in various genes named "PARK" genes have been found in familial cases of PD, accounting for about 10 to 15% of diagnosed cases.[4,5] PARK gene mutations demonstrate either autosomal dominant(e.g., PARK1, synuclein alpha [*SNCA*]; PARK8, leucine-rich repeat kinase 2 [*LRRK2*]) or autosomal recessive (e.g., PARK2, parkin RBR E3 ubiquitin protein ligase [*PRKN*]; PARK6, phosphatase and tensin homolog [*PTEN*]-induced putative kinase 1 [*PINK1*]; PARK7, Parkinsonism-associated deglycase [*DJ-1*]) inheritance. Autosomal recessive forms of PD are typically associated with an earlier age of disease onset than classical PD. Epidemiological studies have identified several environmental factors that may increase the risk of developing PD, including long-duration exposure to pesticides (e.g., rotenone), herbicides (e.g., paraquat), or heavy metals (e.g., manganese, lead, copper), which combined may account for higher rates of PD reported among some farmers, industrial workers, and miners.[4,6,7] Lifestyle factors that have been associated with a higher risk of later diagnosis of PD are previous head injury and taking beta-blocker drugs, whereas smoking, drinking coffee and tea (i.e., caffeine), physical activity, taking calcium channel blockers or nonsteroidal anti-inflammatory drugs (with exception of aspirin) are associated with a lower risk of PD.[6,7]

● SECONDARY PARKINSONISM

Toxic Parkinsonism

Carbon monoxide, mercury, and cyanide poisoning can lead to parkinsonism. MPTP (1-methyl 4-phenyl 1,2,3,6-tetrahydropyridine) is a chemical that can be produced accidentally during the manufacture of the recreational drug MPPP (1-methyl-4-phenyl-4-propionoxypiperidine), a synthetic heroin substitute. The neurotoxicity of MPTP was discovered in the early 1980s when drug addicts, who had consumed MPPP contaminated with MPTP, developed symptoms of PD within 3 days of ingestion. MPTP crosses the blood-brain barrier and is converted to a neurotoxin that selectively destroys dopamine cells in the substantia nigra.[4]

Post-Traumatic Parkinsonism

Traumatic brain injury (TBI) is a risk factor for the development of PD referred to as post-traumatic parkinsonism.[8] A study involving US veterans (n = 162,935) found that sustaining a mild TBI increased the risk of developing PD by 56% and the risk increased with the severity of injury.[9] This condition can also be associated with dementia. Boxers or other athletes, who have had multiple blows to the head or concussions, and people whose professions put them at increased risk for trauma to the head are susceptible to this condition.

Vascular Parkinsonism

Vascular (also referred to as "multi-infarct") parkinsonism is caused by one or more small strokes to the basal ganglia (BG). The onset of symptoms in a person with vascular parkinsonism can be sudden, or if strokes are very small, symptoms can progress gradually and resemble symptom progression for idiopathic PD. Symptoms of vascular parkinsonism often involve the lower extremities (e.g., gait and balance problems) more than the upper extremities. Notably, computerized tomography (CT) or magnetic resonance imaging (MRI) brain scans will show multiple minute or more extensive strokes.[4]

Infectious Diseases

Parkinsonism may occur as a result of different encephalitic conditions, most notably encephalitis lethargica, associated with a worldwide influenza epidemic between 1917 and 1926 that has not recurred. The book *Awakenings* by Oliver Sacks movingly describes the case histories of survivors of the 1917-1926 epidemic, most of whom developed parkinsonism many years after they were infected with encephalitis lethargica. Individuals with encephalitis secondary to human immunodeficiency virus (HIV), also known as HIV-associated dementia, can develop parkinsonism due to pathological changes in the BG.[4]

Metabolic Causes

In rare cases, parkinsonism can be caused by metabolic conditions that include thyroid disease (hypothyroidism, hyperthyroidism), end-stage renal disease, calcium metabolism disorders (hypoparathyroidism, hyperparathyroidism), liver failure (hepatocerebral degeneration), and inherited metabolism disorders (hereditary hemochromatosis, Gaucher's disease, phenylketonuria).[4]

Drug-Induced Parkinsonism

A variety of drugs commonly used in the treatment of other medical conditions may cause drug-induced parkinsonism by interfering with dopamine synaptic transmission (Table 15-1). The elderly are particularly susceptible to drug-induced parkinsonism; however, the parkinsonism symptoms typically resolve within a few weeks once the drug is discontinued.[10]

● PARKINSON-PLUS SYNDROMES

Parkinson-plus syndromes are a group of neurodegenerative disorders that share many of the same symptoms as idiopathic PD due to neuronal damage in the substantia nigra, along with additional neurologic symptoms that are not characteristic of PD. These syndromes include progressive supranuclear palsy (PSP), multiple system atrophy (MSA; includes striatonigral degeneration [predominant parkinsonian symptoms categorized as MSA-P], olivopontocerebellar atrophy [predominant cerebellar symptoms categorized as MSA-C], and Shy–Drager syndrome [prominent autonomic symptoms]), cortical-basal ganglionic degeneration (CBGD), and dementia with Lewy bodies (DLB) (see Table 15-2). Clinical features suggestive of parkinsonism-plus syndromes include lack of or reduced response to anti-parkinsonian drugs such as levodopa, symmetrical signs at onset, lack of or irregular resting tremor, rigidity greater in the trunk than the extremities, early onset of dementia, frequent falls, or autonomic symptoms (e.g., postural

TABLE 15-1	Drugs Associated with Drug-Induced Parkinsonism[10]	
ACTION	**DRUG TYPE**	**EXAMPLES**
Postsynaptic dopamine receptor blockers	Neuroleptics	Haloperidol (Haldol) Chlorpromazine (Thorazine) Risperidone (Risperdal)
	Antiemetics	Prochlorperazine (Compazine) Promethazine (Pherergan)
	Gastroprokinetics	Metoclopramide (Reglan)
Calcium channel blockers	Antihypertensives	Nifedipine (Procardia) Verapamil (Calan)
Presynaptic dopamine blockers		Reserpine (Serpasil) Tetrabenazine (Xenazine) Methyldopa (Aldomet)
Sodium channel blockers	Anticonvulsants	Phenytoin (Dilantin) Sodium Valproate (Depacote)
Noradrenergic uptake inhibitors	Antidepressants	Fluvoxamine (Luvox) Amitryptiline (Triavil) Trazodone (Desyrel)
Norepinephrine blocker/ Serotonin facilitator	Mood stabilizers	Lithium (Eskalith)

hypotension, incontinence), visual signs (e.g., impaired vertical gaze, nystagmus), cerebellar signs, and motor apraxia.[11]

PATHOPHYSIOLOGY

The motor symptoms of PD are caused by degeneration of nigrostriatal dopamine-containing neurons whose cell bodies are in the **substantia nigra pars compacta** (SNpc) of the midbrain and project primarily to the putamen. These neurons also produce neuromelanin, giving them a dark appearance in brain specimens. As the dopamine neurons degenerate, they develop round cytoplasmic inclusion bodies called "Lewy bodies" that consist mostly of misfolded **alpha-synuclein** protein (see Chapter 18 for Lewy body dementia). Initiation and progression of PD are mediated by several cellular mechanisms, such as alpha-synuclein misfolding and aggregation, abnormal protein degradation and clearance, mitochondrial dysfunction, oxidative stress, and neuroinflammation; a combination of these processes is believed to ultimately lead to cell death by apoptosis.[6]

Loss of nigrostriatal dopamine neurons in the substantia nigra results in **decreased dopamine levels in the striatum**, most notably in the putamen, which has important motor functions (Figure 15-1). Initially, the nervous system can compensate for this cell loss by adding axon collaterals. However, by the time symptoms are noticed, approximately 30% of the SNpc neurons have already been lost with between a 68 to 82% reduction of dopamine in the putamen. The effects of the loss of dopaminergic input from the SNpc to the striatum is a relative increased activity in the indirect motor pathway and decreased activity in the direct pathway due to the different actions of dopamine on these pathways (**refer to** Figure 5-4 **in Chapter 5**).

These changes, in combination, lead to increased activity of the BG output nuclei, namely the globus pallidus (GPi) internal segment and substantia nigra pars reticulata, and thereby, produce increased inhibition of thalamocortical neurons and the pedunculopontine nucleus (PPN) of the midbrain. The result is a state of stiffness (rigidity) with difficulty both activating and relaxing muscles for isolated movements, leading to the lack of volitional and automatic movements that are characteristic of this disorder; thus, when the person with PD attempts to move, both agonists and antagonists are activated.[13]

BG circuits are also connected to frontal and parietal lobe areas related to regulation and perception of sensation, so it is not unexpected that there would be some alterations in this system, as well. Loss of dopaminergic input to the striatum also affects associative, oculomotor, and limbic circuits, originating from dorsolateral prefrontal, frontal eye field, and anterior cingulate cortices, respectively, and contributing to cognitive, affective, and behavioral manifestations of PD (Box 15-1, Figure 15-2).[14]

A six-stage model that is widely used to explain the neuropathological progression of Parkinson's disease is the Braak hypothesis. This model suggests that the disease starts (stages 1 and 2) with the presence of abnormal alpha-synuclein inclusions in nondopaminergic neurons in the medulla of the brainstem and the olfactory bulb. This pathology is associated with non-motor symptoms such as constipation (dorsal motor nucleus of vagus nerve involvement) and hyposmia (loss of smell) that occur prior to the motor symptoms. As the disease progresses up the brainstem (stages 3 and 4), the pathology affects the substantia nigra pars compacta in the midbrain causing the classic PD motor symptoms, at which point a diagnosis is typically made.[15] In advanced PD (stages 5 and 6), the pathology affects the cerebral cortices with associated cognitive

TABLE 15-2   Parkinson-Plus Syndromes Comparison to Idiopathic PD and Evaluation and Treatment[11,12]

	EXPECTED COURSE & PROGNOSIS	GAIT/BALANCE DESCRIPTION	OTHER SYMPTOMS	EVALUATION AND TREATMENT
Vascular PD	Usually younger at onset with rapid symptom onset Shorter life expectancy than peers	Parkinsonian-ataxic gait (short shuffling steps with wider base of support and variable stride length), leading to falls; More rapid decline	UPDRS scores higher (worse) at baseline; Lower extremity pyramidal signs (i.e., Babinski sign, hyperreflexia)	Motor and sensory exam based on impairments
Dementia with Lewy bodies	Median = 8 years after diagnosis	Parkinsonian motor symptoms symmetric at onset	Progressive cognitive decline precedes parkinsonism; "fluctuations" in alertness, attention and cognition; visual hallucinations	Check cognition – MOCA Train safety as performance is highly variable
Progressive supranuclear palsy	Variable survival (median = 6.2 yrs.; range 0.5-24 yrs) Choking leads to aspiration	Axial rigidity more prominent than limb rigidity, resulting in backward lean Frequent falls early in disease, especially backward	Vertical supranuclear gaze palsy (downward > upward)	Evaluate eye movement (UPDRS) Check for ability to visually scan environment and avoid obstacles
Multiple system atrophy	Median survival 9.7 yrs	Cerebellar dysfunction (gait and limb ataxia, ataxic dysarthria, sustained gaze-evoked nystagmus); early gait impairment	Autonomic dysfunction (Severe orthostatic hypotension, urinary and erectile dysfunction)	Examine for orthostatic hypotension Teach to deal with hypotension
Corticobasal ganglionic degeneration	Severe disability; death occurs within 10 yrs	Limb apraxia, dystonia, predominantly in one extremity; bradykinesia – focal rigidity	Alien limb phenomenon (involuntary motor activity of a limb along with feeling that limb doesn't belong to person); Early cognitive dysfunction with progressive dementia	Eval coordination Look for apraxia Train coordination

Box 15-1   Four Loops of the Basal Ganglia[14]

Although Chapter 5 detailed the two circuits of the BG (direct and indirect), there are actually four loops that integrate the basal ganglia to areas throughout the brain (see Figure 15-2); each loop begins in an area or areas of the cortex, projects to different components of the BG and then to the thalamus, and back to the originating area(s). The direct and indirect circuits from Chapter 5 make up the **motor** or **skeletomotor loop**. The **oculomotor loop** receives input from the frontal and supplementary eye fields along with the posterior parietal association cortex, an area of integration of visual information, and projects back to the prefrontal eye fields. This loop helps coordinate and modulate the speed of saccadic eye movements. Also, descending projections from the substantia nigra pars compacta to the superior colliculus contribute to the BG's control of saccadic eye movements and potentially impact the initiation of these movements. Disruption of this loop can result in involuntary saccades. The **associative loop** links the BG to the dorsolateral prefrontal and premotor cortices, which are areas of convergence for projections from multiple areas of the cortex, and contribute to executive function, including goal-directed behavior, especially movement planning, as well as problem-solving, attention shifting, and dual-task performance – the ability to divide attention between two concurrent activities (e.g., talking while walking). Thus, executive dysfunction is often associated with PD; this is typically mild in early stages but presents in up to 40% of patients and can proceed to dementia in later stages. Finally, the **limbic loop** links the anterior cingulate and medial orbitofrontal cortices to the BG and back to the anterior cingulate cortex and limbic association cortex through the mediodorsal thalamic nucleus. This loop contributes to behavioral motivation and emotional regulation. Psychological disorders in PD are common and include depression, anxiety, sleep disruption, and apathy. While these might seem like common reactions to a degenerative disorder, like PD, they often predate the onset of symptoms, leading some to describe a "PD personality"; this is likely due to early disruption of this loop.

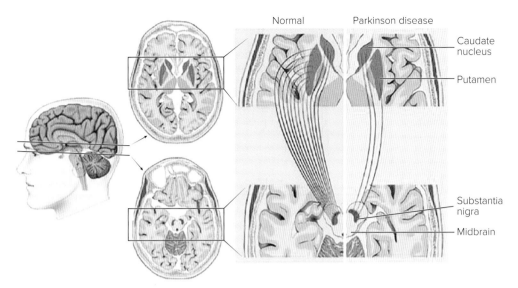

FIGURE 15-1 Pathophysiology of Parkinson's Disease. PD is associated with loss of dopaminergic neurons from the substantia nigra pars compacta (midbrain) to the striatum (putamen and caudate nucleus) with lateral fibers that project to the putamen lost early in the disease and to a greater extent than the medial fibers that project to the caudate nucleus.

impairment and hallucinations. Although this staging is widely used, there is controversy about its validity.[16] Growing evidence indicates that abnormal alpha-synuclein spreads from one brain region to another in a manner similar to the transmission of prion diseases.[17]

PARKINSON'S DISEASE SUBTYPES

Evidence suggests that Parkinson's disease has different subtypes based on motor and non-motor features that have implications for diagnosis, prognosis, and expected response to treatment.[18] One suggested subtyping consists of three groups: (1) mild motor predominant (49-53%) characterized by younger age at onset, mild motor and non-motor symptoms, slow progression, and good responses to dopaminergic medications (i.e., levodopa); (2) intermediate (35-39%) characterized by intermediate age at onset and symptomatology, moderate to good response to levodopa, and moderate disease progression; and (3) diffuse malignant (9-16%) characterized by variable age of onset, severe motor symptoms, early gait problems, rapid eye movement sleep behavior disorder (RBD), mild cognitive impairment, orthostatic hypotension, worse response to dopaminergic medications, and rapid disease progression.[18,19] An alternative but overlapping subtyping divides individuals with PD into three phenotypes based on the predominant motor symptoms, namely tremor-dominant (TD) and postural instability gait difficulty (PIGD) phenotypes.[20-22] Individuals presenting with tremor as the dominant motor symptom at onset tend to be younger in age, have a slower progression of disease, and have a good response to levodopa. In contrast, individuals with the PIGD subtype typically have an older age of onset, bradykinesia and rigidity, greater balance and gait impairments, a faster rate of cognitive decline and higher incidence of dementia, more severe non-motor symptoms, and a worse prognosis with rapid progression. Individuals with PD

that have a relatively balanced involvement of tremor and gait/balance impairments or disabilities are classified as having an indeterminate subtype.[22]

CLINICAL PRESENTATION

Primary Motor Symptoms

Tremor

Tremor is the initial symptom for approximately 70% of individuals with PD and typically presents as an involuntary slow oscillation (4-6 cycles per second) of a hand or fingers on one side of the body. The tremor is a resting tremor because it is present at rest but usually stops with voluntary use of the body part. Many people initially exhibit a tremor between the thumb and index finger, often referred to as a pill-rolling tremor, but resting tremors may be seen in other body parts such as the forearm (pronation–supination), foot, jaw, or tongue. Stress and anxiety can exacerbate tremors, while relaxation and sleep will diminish them. As the disease progresses, tremors become more severe, of longer duration, and involve both sides of the body, which can interfere with a person's ability to do daily activities. Tremors in PD may be caused by cells within the ventral intermediate (VIM) nucleus of the thalamus that receive abnormal inhibitory inputs from the GPi, as surgical lesions to the VIM nucleus abolish the resting tremors.[23]

Bradykinesia

Bradykinesia, defined as slowness of voluntary movement, manifests as difficulty with initiation of movements and changing positions, such as arising from a seated position, plus involuntary slowing during movements. **Hypokinesia**, a reduction of movement amplitude, affects all movements and is a primary cause of reduced gait speed and step length. As the disease progresses, individuals may experience freezing episodes (akinesia),

A

1. Skeletomotor loop

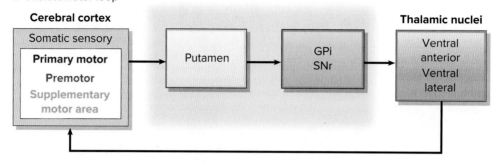

2. Oculomotor loop

3. Associative loop

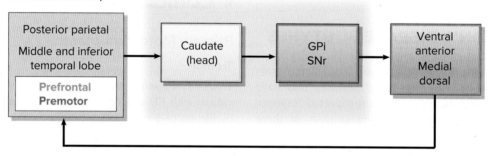

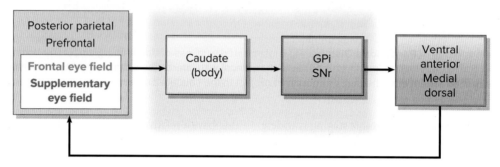

4. Limbic loop

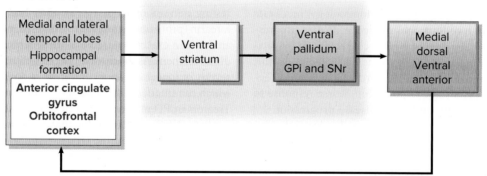

FIGURE 15-2 Four basal ganglia loops. A. Illustrations of the four loops. (1) skeletomotor; (2) oculomotor; (3) associative; and (4) limbic. **B.** Cortical areas associated with the four loops. (Reproduced with permission from Martin JH. *Neuroanatomy Text & Atlas*, 4th ed. New York, NY: McGraw-Hill; 2012.)

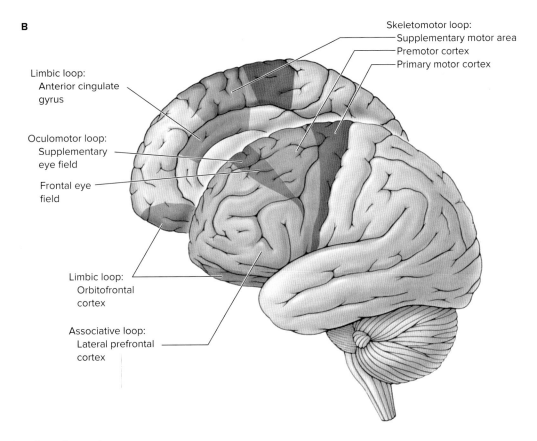

B

Limbic loop:
Anterior cingulate
gyrus

Oculomotor loop:
Supplementary
eye field

Frontal eye
field

Limbic loop:
Orbitofrontal
cortex

Associative loop:
Lateral prefrontal
cortex

Skeletomotor loop:
Supplementary motor area
Premotor cortex
Primary motor cortex

FIGURE 15-2 (*Continued*)

in which they have a sudden, temporary inability to move. To overcome the apparent inertia of the limbs, individuals with PD must concentrate intensely on doing even the simplest motor tasks. Movement initiation is particularly impaired when novel or unnatural movements are attempted or when combining several movements concurrently (e.g., flexing the elbow while simultaneously squeezing an object with the same hand).[24] A proposed mechanism for bradykinesia and hypokinesia is that motor cortical areas (i.e., supplementary and primary motor cortices), are inadequately activated by excitatory circuits that pass through the BG.[25] Motor neuron pools in the spinal cord are not provided adequate facilitation, thereby affecting recruitment and discharge rates of motor units, resulting in slow and small movements. This hypothesis is supported by observations that gait speed, step length, and arm swing are improved by administration of dopaminergic medications (i.e., levodopa),[25] and by observations of seemingly "normal" movements in otherwise akinetic individuals with PD in response to certain situations (e.g., catching a ball thrown to them or being able to suddenly run when someone calls "fire"). Excessive muscle co-contraction and rigidity may also interfere with the speed and amplitude of movements. Another contributing factor seems to be an altered perception of movement velocity and amplitude.[26] In other words, persons with parkinsonism think they are moving faster and farther than they really are.

Rigidity

Rigidity is hypertonia characterized by velocity-independent resistance to passive joint movement. In PD, it affects proximal musculature early, especially the shoulders and neck, and later spreads to muscles of the face and extremities. The rigidity can be of two types: cogwheel and leadpipe. **Cogwheel rigidity** is a jerky, ratchet-like resistance to passive movement, caused by muscles alternately tensing and relaxing, while **leadpipe rigidity** is a more sustained resistance to passive movement. Individuals with PD often complain that their limbs feel "heavy" and "stiff" making it difficult for them to move. Active movement of the contralateral limb as well as mental and emotional stress can exacerbate rigidity. Rigidity of the neck and trunk (axial rigidity) can result in a loss of arm swing, and over time, contribute to a kyphotic posture. As rigidity worsens, it can interfere with a person's ability to turn over in bed, get in and out of chairs, and turn during walking. Excessive inhibitory output from the GPi to the PPN is believed to be a primary cause of rigidity in PD, particularly axial rigidity.[25] Other proposed mechanisms that may contribute to rigidity in PD include abnormally high gain of long-latency muscle stretch reflexes, decreased inhibitory neuron activity in the spinal cord, and changes in elastic properties of muscles secondary to disuse.[23]

Postural Instability

Individuals with PD are typically not affected by postural instability in the early stages of the disease, but as the disease progresses, it becomes more prevalent and worsens. It is one of the most disabling symptoms of the disease because of its association with increased falls and loss of independence. Clinical and posturographic studies have contributed to significant advances in understanding the complex pathophysiology of postural instability in PD, but many questions still remain.

Abnormalities in balance control are a major factor contributing to postural instability in PD. These abnormalities include: (1) reduced **limits of stability** (e.g., the sway boundaries in which an individual can maintain equilibrium without changing the base of support), (2) reduced magnitude of postural responses, (3) impaired postural adaptations, and (4) altered **anticipatory postural adjustments** (APAs), which refer to activation of postural muscles in advance of performing skilled movements (see Chapter 5). When standing still, the postural sway of individuals with PD tends to be larger, particularly in the mediolateral direction, and faster with more frequent corrections than in those without PD.[27] Lateral trunk sway is also abnormally far and fast when walking in people with PD, which is worsened when stepping over objects.[28] When individuals with PD are asked to lean as far as possible in different directions while standing, they move slower and are more fearful to reach their limits of stability, particularly in the forward direction.[29] In response to balance disturbances, individuals with PD demonstrate weak and insufficient postural responses, associated with an abnormal pattern of muscle co-contraction, that delays the return of the body center of mass to within the limits of stability.[30,31] Stepping responses to correct balance loss are late and smaller than normal in PD, requiring multiple steps to stop the movement.[31] In advanced stages, individuals with PD have no postural responses to perturbations and "fall like a tree." Individuals with PD have difficulty adapting postural responses to changing conditions (e.g., switching from an ankle to a hip strategy when going from standing on a large to a narrow surface or when going from smaller to larger external perturbations) and are unable to scale the size of postural responses appropriately to the size of balance disturbances.[31-33] APAs prior to voluntary movements are also altered in PD. In early stages of the disease, the magnitude of APAs for sit-to-stand transfers (i.e., hip flexion and forward displacement of the center of mass) was larger in individuals with PD relative to controls,[34] but as the disease progresses, individuals tend to have reduced APAs.[35,36] Reduced APAs for self-initiated walking (i.e., weight shift to the opposite lower extremity in preparation for stepping) result in a longer time to initiate a step. Trembling of the knees that is observed in individuals with PD with freezing of gait (FOG) looks like multiple APAs in preparation for stepping, suggesting that there may be a problem in coupling the APA with voluntary movement (e.g., a step).[31]

Some studies have suggested that disordered sensory processing contributes to postural instability in PD. Proprioceptive deficits have been reported in individuals with PD[37] and may be related to impaired vertical body orientation in PD.[38] When individuals with PD were asked to stand upright on a tilting support platform in the absence of visual and vestibular information, they were unable to maintain a vertical trunk orientation as control subjects did.[39] Individuals with PD become increasingly dependent on visual cues for control of locomotion,[40] which may be an adaptive strategy to compensate for their proprioceptive deficits; while normal adults rely on dynamic visual information (i.e., the visual perception of motion of objects in the environment produced by a person's own movement) for ambulation only when balance is disturbed, individuals with PD are highly dependent on dynamic visual cues for the control of their gait speed, even under stable balance conditions.[40]

Over time, individuals with PD develop postural deformities. A stooped posture characterized by a forward head, rounded shoulders, and increased trunk, hip, and knee flexion commonly occurs and may contribute to postural instability by positioning the body center of mass closer to the forward limits of stability. The cause of the flexed posture is not clear but may be related to antigravity muscle weakness, increased flexor muscle tone, or an inaccurate sense of verticality.[17] Alternatively, the stooped posture may be a compensatory measure to prevent falls as individuals with PD are especially prone to become unstable with backward perturbations.[41,42] Other postural abnormalities associated with PD include **Camptocormia**, characterized by marked flexion of the trunk, and **Pisa syndrome**, which refers to a tilting of the trunk in the lateral plane, especially in sitting and standing.[39]

Falls are typically few to none in the early stages, become more prevalent in the middle stages, and then taper off in the later stages as individuals become immobile. Approximately 70% of people living in the community with PD will have fallen in the previous year, and those who have fallen two or more times in the previous year are likely to fall again in the next 3 months.[41] The incidence of limb fractures from falls is significantly higher in individuals with PD, compared with age-matched controls, with about 27% of people experiencing a hip fracture within 10 years of diagnosis.[43] The cause of falls in people with PD is multifactorial[44,45] as illustrated in Figure 15-3. Prospective studies have identified disease severity, postural instability, FOG, and cognitive impairment as strong predictors of falls in PD.[46,47] A meta-analysis found that the best predictor of falling in people with PD was a history of two or more falls in the previous year (sensitivity 68%, specificity 81%).[48] A study that compared community- versus home-based falls in individuals with mild to moderate PD (n = 196) reported that community-based falls were more likely to occur while walking and when outdoors, while home-based falls more likely occurred during FOG episodes.[44] Environmental challenges associated with community-based falls were terrain (e.g., walking on sloped or uneven ground), attention demands (i.e., distraction from postural task, dual tasking), and density (i.e., busy environment) and temporal demands (i.e., walking quickly, crossing street), while anticipated physical loads (i.e., carrying something, opening or closing door) were more often associated with home-based falls. Postural transitions (e.g., initiating or terminating walking, sitting down or standing up), unanticipated physical loads (i.e., knocked, pulled, or jolted off balance), and ambience (e.g., decreased visibility, wind) were equally associated with community- and home-based falls. "Fear of falling" in some individuals with PD with a history of falls can lead to a loss of self-confidence, activity avoidance, and increased dependence for mobility.[49]

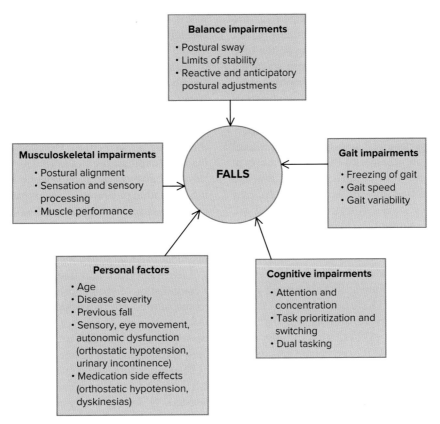

FIGURE 15-3 Fall risk factors in PD. Fall risk in PD is multifactorial, potentially stemming from musculoskeletal, balance, personal factors, gait impairments, and cognitive deficits.

CASE A, PART I

Mr. Martin was diagnosed with PD at age 60 when he noted that he had a persistent tremor in his right hand, especially when he was relaxing. He works as a vice president of a large software company. At diagnosis, the tremor is not interfering with typing or writing, but he feels it negatively impacts his image at work as it tends to be more noticeable when he is sitting in meetings. His wife and children also noticed that he was starting to slow down and walk more "like an old man." He continued to work and was started on therapy and medication at that time.

What symptoms is Mr. Martin displaying that suggest a diagnosis of PD?

Answer: His older age, resting tremor, and slowing of movements (bradykinesia) suggest a possible diagnosis of PD.

Secondary Motor Symptoms

Muscle Performance

Compared to neurologically normal adults, reduced muscle strength has been reported in individuals with PD across isometric, isokinetic, and isotonic modes of testing and across muscle groups of the upper and lower extremities.[50] Electromyography (EMG) studies of single motor units reveal multiple abnormalities, including delayed activation and relaxation of motor units, irregular and intermittent discharge patterns, a greater number of motor units recruited at low thresholds, and abnormal coactivation of antagonist muscles.[23,50] Possible explanations for the reduced ability to generate force in PD could be central imbalances in excitatory and inhibitory inputs to motor neurons, peripheral adaptations in motor neurons or muscles due to the disease or secondary disuse, or deviations in the normal aging process.[23,51] Weakness of the lower extremity musculature can compromise functional mobility and independence such as the sit-to-stand task, in which individuals with PD demonstrate reduced torques and rate of force development in the hip, knee, and ankle musculature that relate to their diminished ability to perform the task.[52] During walking, a reduction in net ankle plantarflexion torques during push-off contributes to smaller steps and slower gait speed.[25] Strength changes appear related to the disease pathology as strength is improved in individuals who are "on" dopaminergic medications (i.e., levodopa) compared to when they are in the "off" state.[51]

Gait

Gait disturbances are prevalent in middle to late stages of PD and contribute to falls, loss of independence, and institutionalization. Individuals with PD generally have slower gait velocity, shorter step length with increased forefoot loading at heel strike, increased step-to-step variability, and increased double support time.[53] Trunk rotation is reduced, resulting in decreased or absent arm swing and "**en bloc**" turning, in which individuals with PD require multiple small steps to accomplish a turn because they keep their neck and trunk rigid, rather than the usual twisting of the neck and trunk and pivoting on the toes. Heel-to-heel base of support may be widened in early stages but typically decreases as the disease progresses. **Dystonia**, involuntary sustained muscular contractions that cause abnormal movements and/or postures, often affect the foot and ankle (mainly toe flexion and foot inversion), which can interfere with gait.[54] Increased gait variability is associated with increased fall risk in the elderly and in people with PD. Other features of parkinsonian gait, specifically **festination** (i.e., acceleration and shortening of strides) and freezing (see next paragraph), may also predispose individuals to falls. A forward festinating gait (**anteropulsive**) in combination with a stooped posture leads to forward falls. Backward festinating gait (**retropulsive**) leads to backward falls.[53]

FOG is a manifestation of **akinesia**. When FOG occurs, individuals with PD describe feeling as if their feet are glued to the floor. Five subtypes of FOG have been described in PD: (1) start hesitation – as a person initiates walking, (2) turn hesitation – FOG during a turn, (3) hesitation in tight quarters, (4) destination hesitation – FOG as a person approaches a target, and (5) open space hesitation. FOG is significantly improved with levodopa therapy.[55] Not all people with PD develop FOG; known risk factors for FOG are older age, anxiety, depression, and greater severity of motor symptoms.[56] While the pathophysiology of FOG is not well understood, a shift from normal automatic control of locomotion to compensatory prefrontal executive control has been found in people with PD with FOG.[57]

Dual-tasking (e.g., walking while counting backward or talking) decreases gait speed and increases gait variability in PD and correlates with impaired executive dysfunction but not memory.[58] Healthy young adults and some older adults tend to prioritize motor over cognitive tasks, when multitasking, to avoid falls, referred to as the "posture first" strategy.[59] Studies have reported that non-demented individuals with PD have similar performance to control subjects, adopting the typical "posture first" strategy, during dual-task walking; however, when performing complex multiple motor and cognitive tasks they tend to prioritize the cognitive task and then posture, which leads to greater numbers of errors (i.e., hesitations and motor blocks) on motor tasks compared to healthy young and older adults.[59] Difficulties with multitasking also manifest as difficulties prioritizing attention in complex environments. For example, individuals with PD walked significantly slower when navigating through an obstacle course while listening to music compared to without music, while healthy older adults showed no difference in gait speed in the music and no music conditions.[60]

Other Motor Symptoms

Speech disorders and dysphagia (impaired swallowing) due to bulbar dysfunction are frequently observed in patients with PD. These symptoms are thought to result from bradykinesia and rigidity of orofacial and laryngeal muscles. Individuals with PD exhibit **hypokinetic dysarthria**, characterized by reduced speech volume, monotone speech with little inflection

in pitch, mumbled and imprecise articulation, and variable speaking rates (i.e., slow speaking rates with rushes of fast speech). Vocal quality is often described as breathy, hoarse, or harsh. Individuals with PD may have difficulties initiating speech, sometimes resulting in stuttering speech. At advanced stages, the person may only be able to whisper or may be unable to speak (**mutism**). Some individuals with PD complain of frequent word-finding difficulties, referred to as "tip-of-the-tongue phenomenon." Dysphagia is usually caused by an inability to initiate the swallowing reflex or by a prolongation of laryngeal or esophageal movement. Dysphagia leads to choking, aspiration pneumonia, and impaired nutrition with weight loss. Excessive drooling (**sialorrhea**), which may result from a decrease in spontaneous swallowing, can be particularly troubling during sleep or speech initiation, and can cause embarrassment in social situations.[61]

Loss of automatic movements in PD can result in **hypomimia**, a combination of symptoms that includes reduced facial movements, slowed eye movements, slowed blinking, and reduced facial expression. The face of a person with hypomimia is often described as "mask-like" with a static mouth and unblinking eyes. Hypomimia can be one of the most frustrating symptoms of PD, as individuals who interact with the person with PD may falsely think that the person is emotionless, depressed, or uninterested. Educating family members and close friends about hypomimia can prevent or alleviate any confusion or distress they may be feeling.[62]

Hand dexterity and finger coordination are affected in PD, even at early stages of the disease. Individuals with PD have difficulty performing rapid, repetitive, alternating movements of the hand (finger taps, hand grips, wrist pronation–supination) due to bradykinesia. Impaired fluency, coordination, and speed of fine motor movements negatively affect grasp and manipulation of objects, resulting in difficulties in performing tasks such as using a key or buttoning a shirt. **Micrographia**, a form of hypokinesia, is defined as abnormally small, cramped handwriting. Individuals with PD may demonstrate consistently small handwriting or they may start a writing segment with normal-sized handwriting and progress to continually smaller handwriting.[63]

CASE A, PART II

At age 68, Mr. Martin complains that it is becoming very difficult for him to walk on the golf course and that he has fallen three times in the 6 months, since his previous visit to the neurologist. His medications were changed and he received a prescription for therapy.

What factors could be contributing to Mr. Martin's falls?

Answer: A variety of factors could be contributing to Mr. Martin's falls (see Figure 15-3). The fact that his medications were changed raises concerns about decreased drug effectiveness or possible side effects contributing to his falls, which should be explored by the therapist.

Motor Learning

The striatum is involved in all stages of motor learning, and particularly, during consolidation of learned skills that consist of a sequence of movements. In general, studies have shown that implicit (procedural) learning of new motor skills or fine-tuning of skills is relatively preserved in early stages of PD for those without dementia, but individuals with PD generally take longer to learn motor tasks than healthy controls.[64] In contrast, explicit (declarative) learning, which involves attentional resources and cognitive strategies, is typically impaired.[65] This is supported by deficits in motor learning that have been documented for tasks that require multiple motor programs such as simultaneous movements (i.e., dual-tasks)[24,66] and sequential movements (i.e., switching from one movement to another).[67] In addition, individuals with PD have impaired speed-accuracy learning or motor skill learning that involves the ability to make fast and accurate movements such as reaching.[68] Individuals with PD also often show a decrease in retention of newly learned motor skills, even in earlier disease stages.[65] Brain imaging studies found greater neural activity in individuals with PD in the cerebellum, premotor areas, parietal cortex, precuneus, and dorsolateral prefrontal cortex bilaterally, while performing well-rehearsed sequences of finger movements compared to healthy adults, suggesting that neural circuits for learning have reduced efficiency in PD.[66,67]

Motor learning in PD has also been shown to benefit from the use of external auditory or visual cueing, particularly with respect to gait.[69] Improved retention of motor learning has been found in individuals with PD when a slightly reduced frequency (66%) of augmented feedback (i.e., knowledge of results) is used rather than continuous feedback (100%),[70] and blocked practice has been found to be better than a random practice, which is the opposite of findings for control peers.[71] Additionally, motor learning appears to be more context-specific in individuals with PD with decrements reported when retention testing was done in conditions that differed from the practice conditions.[72] Advanced disease, dementia, and visual-perceptual deficits can ultimately degrade motor learning. Despite reports of negative impacts of levodopa on upper extremity motor learning in PD, evidence to date suggests that levodopa does not worsen postural and lower extremity skill learning.[64]

CASE A, PART III

At age 75, Mr. Martin began falling again and reported that he was no longer able to enjoy golfing. His wife noted that he was rarely leaving the house, and he was falling daily. They also complained of sleep disturbances and changes in bowel and bladder.

What could be contributing to Mr. Martin's symptoms?

Answer: As the disease progresses, Mr. Martin is experiencing more frequent falls. The fact that he is rarely leaving the house raises concerns that he may have developed a fear of falling that could reduce his activity levels and opportunities to socialize with family and friends. His sleep disturbances and autonomic dysfunction (bowel and bladder changes) are common non-motor symptoms of PD that should be addressed.

● NON-MOTOR SYMPTOMS

Non-motor symptoms are common and may be more bothersome than motor symptoms for individuals with PD. These include autonomic dysfunction, cognitive/behavioral disorders, and sensory and sleep abnormalities (Table 15-3).

Autonomic Dysfunction

Autonomic dysfunction may be present in early disease stages[73] and is likely due to Lewy body pathology in the hypothalamus, intermediolateral nucleus of the spinal cord, sympathetic ganglia, dorsal motor nucleus of vagus, and the enteric nervous system.[74] Symptoms include orthostatic hypotension, thermoregulatory dysfunction (excessive sweating [**hyperhidrosis**], uncomfortable sensations of warmth and coldness), urinary symptoms (bladder urgency, frequency, and nocturia), and **sexual dysfunction** (erectile dysfunction, and problems with ejaculation in men and loss of lubrication and involuntary urination during sex in women); in rare instances, sexual dysfunction presents as **hypersexuality**, which is more common in men and in earlier onset, yet the cause is poorly understood.[75] Common skin problems that occur early in PD are **seborrhea**

TABLE 15-3	**Non-motor Symptoms of PD**		
AUTONOMIC[73–84]	**COGNITIVE/EMOTIONAL/ BEHAVIORAL**[85–93]	**SENSORY**[94–97]	**SLEEP**[98]
• Excessive sweating • Abnormal sensations of heat and cold • Seborrhea • Orthostatic hypotension • Urinary bladder dysfunction • Constipation • Sexual dysfunction • Respiratory disturbances	• Executive dysfunction • Working memory problems • Confusion/Dementia • Depression • Anxiety • Apathy • Obsessive–compulsive behavior • Fatigue	• Anosmia • Proprioceptive deficits • Visuospatial deficits • Sensory integration deficits • Paresthesias • Pain • Akathisia	• Excessive daytime somnolence • Insomnia • Rapid eye movement sleep behavior disorder • **Restless legs syndrome** • Periodic leg movement disorder • Sleep apnea • Nocturia

(increased oil secretion of the sebaceous glands) and **seborrheic dermatitis** (oily, itchy, and reddened skin). Decreased gastrointestinal motility due to Lewy body pathology in the dorsal motor nucleus of the vagus nerve and throughout the enteric nervous system, reduced appetite perhaps secondary to loss of smell, and inadequate hydration in PD result in weight loss, constipation, fecal incontinence, gastroesophageal reflux, nausea, and vomiting.[74]

Sympathetic denervation of the heart occurs early, progresses over time in most individuals with PD,[76] and may be associated with fatigue complaints.[77] Exercise capacity (maximal HR, oxygen consumption loads) in individuals with mild to moderate PD, exercising on a cycle ergometer, was not significantly different from that of age-matched controls.[78,79] However, the individuals with PD demonstrated lower peak power and higher submaximal HRs and oxygen consumption rates.[78] Similar abnormalities of increased heart rate (HR) and blood pressure (BP) and decreased maximal oxygen consumption during exercise have been reported in individuals with moderate to severe PD.[80,81]

In advanced stages, individuals with PD may present with mild to moderate edema of the feet and ankles, due to circulatory changes, causing venous pooling, related to a sedentary lifestyle and prolonged sitting. This can be relieved by increasing physical activity or with elevation of the feet.

Orthostatic hypotension (OH) is a sharp drop in BP (drop of 20 mmHg in systolic BP or 10 mmHg in diastolic BP) that happens when a person gets up from bed or from a chair and can cause fainting or falls. Symptoms of OH can include lightheadedness, dizziness, weakness, difficulty thinking, headache, and feeling faint. The two primary causes of OH in PD are (1) insufficient HR increase with position changes due to autonomic abnormalities and (2) dopaminergic medications (carbidopa/levodopa [Sinemet®], bromocriptine [Parlodel®], ropinirole [Requip®], and pramipexole [Mirapex®]).[82] Additional causes of OH include use of diuretics, dehydration, cardiac disease, fever, and anemia.

Respiratory disturbances in individuals with PD typically occur in later disease stages and can be obstructive (difficulty with exhaling all of the air in the lungs) or restrictive (difficulty fully expanding the lungs with air).[83] The obstructive pattern may be related to rigidity, cervical arthrosis, or restricted range of motion in the neck; the restrictive pattern may be related to chest wall rigidity, decreased musculoskeletal flexibility, or a kyphotic posture. Respiration may also be compromised by respiratory dyskinesia, a side effect of levodopa therapy.[84] Pulmonary dysfunction can lead to reduced daily activity and cardiopulmonary deconditioning. A serious complication of respiratory dysfunction is pneumonia, which is a leading cause of death in individuals with PD.

Cognitive and Emotional/Behavioral Abnormalities

Cognitive impairment is present in about 25% of newly diagnosed individuals with PD. Cognitive functions affected in the early stages of the disease include executive abilities (e.g., planning, decision making, concept formation, cognitive flexibility, switching between well-learned tasks), working memory (more retrieval than encoding deficits), visuospatial processing, psychomotor speed, and attention, whereas language is usually less affected.[85,86] Cognitive function may progressively decline over time, and some individuals will eventually develop dementia (called Parkinson's disease dementia [PDD]). Risk factors for early dementia in PD include older age, severe parkinsonism, and mild cognitive impairment.[87] Those with the PIGD subtype of PD are at higher risk for dementia. An estimated 50 to 80% of individuals with PD eventually develop dementia with an average onset of 10 years of diagnosis.[88] **Bradyphrenia**, slowed thinking, is present at early stages in PD and is related to striatal pathology and depression.[89] Since it may take longer to process information with bradyphrenia, it can be frustrating to both the person and caregivers.

Depression, apathy, and anxiety are also common in individuals with PD. An estimated 30 to 45% of people with PD develop major depression, characterized by symptoms of depressed mood, loss of interest or pleasure in daily activities, fatigue, poor concentration and deficits in short-term memory, insomnia, and weight loss. Apathy can occur alone or concomitant with depression in PD and is manifested by a lack of motivation or interest, reduced involvement in social aspects of life, reduced productivity, and reliance on others to structure daily activities.[90] Approximately 25 to 49% of individuals with PD have anxiety. Panic disorder (sudden and repeated attacks of fear), generalized anxiety disorder (chronic anxiety, exaggerated worry or tension, even when there is little or nothing to worry about), and social phobia (social withdrawal) are the most common anxiety disorders reported. Symptoms of anxiety can include heart palpitations, shortness of breath, sweating, and trembling. Depression, apathy, and anxiety occur at all stages of the disease, including before onset of motor symptoms. They may be related to psychological and social worries experienced by individuals with PD as well as neurochemical changes involving dopamine, norepinephrine, and serotonin.[85]

In addition to mood disorders, many individuals with PD exhibit obsessive–compulsive and impulsive behaviors, such as binge eating and cravings (especially for sweets), compulsive foraging or shopping, hypersexuality, pathological gambling, and punding (i.e., intense fascination with repetitive handling, examining, sorting, and arranging of objects).[84] These behavioral symptoms have been associated with use of dopaminergic drugs, especially dopamine agonists.[91]

Fatigue

Fatigue is a common symptom of PD and is one of the most disabling. Fatigue has been defined as an overwhelming sense of tiredness, a lack of energy, and a feeling of exhaustion. It manifests as difficulty in initiating and sustaining mental and physical tasks. Clinical studies using questionnaires have shown that fatigue is associated with motor as well as non-motor symptoms of PD.[92,93] Evidence supporting fatigue as a motor symptom of PD includes its relationship with disease severity, motor complications (i.e., motor fluctuations experienced during levodopa therapy), prominent postural instability and gait symptoms, and physical deconditioning. Non-motor symptoms that have been associated with fatigue are depression, anxiety, excessive daytime sleepiness, and cardiovascular sympathetic dysfunction. Neuroimaging studies show that fatigue is associated with involvement of non-dopaminergic (i.e., serotonergic) or extrastriatal dopaminergic pathways.[93]

Sensory Abnormalities

Sensory symptoms that are common in PD include olfactory dysfunction, pain and paresthesias, akathisia, and visual disturbances (each will be discussed in the following sections). Individuals with PD frequently report a decline or loss of smell (**anosmia**) that typically occurs a few years prior to the onset of motor symptoms, making it an important symptom for diagnosis. Loss of smell affects a person's ability to enjoy food, which may negatively impact food consumption and lead to weight loss. Olfactory dysfunction in PD has been associated with either neuronal loss in the amygdala or to decreased dopaminergic neurons in the olfactory bulb.[94]

Pain and **paresthesias** (i.e., sensations of numbness, tingling, aching, burning) are reported by approximately 50% of individuals with PD. Pain in PD typically arises from the following five causes: (1) musculoskeletal problems related to rigidity and lack of spontaneous movements, poor posture, awkward mechanical stresses, or physical wear and tear; (2) radicular or neuropathic pain, often related to neck or back arthritis; (3) dystonia-related pain; (4) discomfort due to extreme restlessness (akathisia); and (5) "central" pain, presumed to be due to alterations in central pain pathways.[95] One of the most common musculoskeletal complaints is shoulder pain or a frozen shoulder (i.e., adhesive capsulitis), which is sometimes the initial symptom of PD. Hip, back, and neck pain are all common complaints in PD. With prolonged immobility of a limb, contractures may develop, usually in the hands or feet. Radicular pain due to nerve root inflammation is often described as a burning pain that radiates in a dermatomal pattern. Dystonic spasms may cause painful foot equinovarus and toe curling, torticollis (abnormal, asymmetrical head or neck position), writer's cramp, oro-mandibular dystonia (dystonia of the face, jaw, or tongue), and blepharospasm (forced closure of the eyelids). Some individuals with PD experience discomfort from **akathisia**, a feeling of restlessness and a need to be in constant motion often manifested as rocking while standing or sitting, lifting the feet as if marching in place, and crossing and uncrossing the legs while sitting. Some people with parkinsonian akathisia are unable to sit still, lie in bed, drive a car, eat at a table, or attend social events.[96] In rare cases, individuals experience "central" pain, described as bizarre unexplained sensations of stabbing, burning, and scalding, often in unusual body distributions such as the abdomen, chest, mouth, rectum, or genitalia. Pain complaints may be greater in people experiencing depression.[95]

Visual disturbances in PD include impaired visual acuity, contrast sensitivity, color discrimination, visual fields, and motion perception. Abnormal saccadic and smooth pursuit eye movements have been reported in about 75% of people with PD. Saccadic (i.e., rapid) movements are slow and hypometric (i.e., undershoot their targets), while smooth pursuit movements have a jerky, cogwheeling appearance due to interruptions by small saccades. Convergent eye movements are associated with outward deviation of the eyes causing **diplopia** (double vision). Reduced eye blink can cause an abnormal tear film and dry, irritated eyes that itch and burn. Visual hallucinations are a chronic complication of PD, especially in people treated with levodopa and dopamine agonists. Anticholinergic drugs used in treatment of PD can cause blurred vision and sensitivity to light (photophobia). Visuospatial deficits have been identified in individuals using visual perception tasks involving spatial organization (i.e., line orientation, memory for spatial location, mental rotation [i.e., see an object and be able to rotate it mentally], object detection, and face recognition). These alterations are hypothesized to play a role in FOG and in the development of visual hallucinations.[97]

Sleep Disorders

Sleep problems may be an early sign of PD, even before motor symptoms have begun. Some of the common sleep problems for Parkinson's patients include insomnia (problems with onset and maintenance of sleep), excessive daytime somnolence (sleepiness), nightmares, sleep attacks (a sudden involuntary episode of sleep), and sleep apnea (shallow or infrequent breathing during sleep).[98] **Rapid eye movement sleep behavior disorder** (RBD) occurs in approximately one-third of individuals with PD and is a substantial risk factor for the development of PD. RBD is characterized by violent dream content that the person "acts out" with talking, yelling, swearing, grabbing, punching, kicking, jumping, and other violent and potentially injurious activities that may involve the bed partner.[99] People with PD are also at higher risk for restless legs syndrome (i.e., throbbing, pulling, creeping, or other unpleasant sensations in the legs and an uncontrollable urge to move them) and periodic leg movement disorder (i.e., periodic rhythmic movements of the limbs that last a few minutes to several hours), two conditions that may seriously disrupt sleep. **Nocturia** (frequent nighttime urination) is another cause of interrupted sleep in PD.[98]

● MEDICAL DIAGNOSIS

Parkinson's disease is primarily a clinical diagnosis based on a physician's neurological examination findings. There is no test that can clearly identify the disease. Definitive diagnosis is only made at autopsy with pathological confirmation of the hallmark Lewy bodies. Diagnosis is typically based on history and clinical examination. Diagnostic criteria have been developed by the Movement Disorder Society Clinical Diagnostic Criteria for Parkinson's disease (MDS-PD) (Table 15-4).[100]

Differentiation of PD from other forms of parkinsonism is essential. The presence of extrapyramidal signs that are bilaterally symmetrical, lack of response to levodopa, early onset of dementia or postural instability, early autonomic signs, impaired vertical gaze, and motor apraxia are suggestive of Parkinson-plus syndromes. Essential tremor is differentiated from PD by the presence of bilateral, symmetrical low amplitude, high-frequency tremors that are mostly seen during voluntary movement and affect the head and voice in addition to the limbs. Increasingly, there has been an emphasis on identifying biomarkers to help diagnose presymptomatic disease. Early prodromal signs that may indicate PD-specific pathology prior to motor symptom onset have been identified as RBD, hyposmia (reduced ability to smell), constipation, urinary dysfunction, OH, excessive

TABLE 15-4	Movement Disorder Society Diagnostic Criteria – Clinically Established Parkinson's Disease[100]		
Must have Parkinsonism – bradykinesia plus either rigidity or resting tremor			
Clinically established PD: • Absence of absolute exclusion criteria; at least two supportive criteria; no "red flags"			
Absolute exclusion criteria	**Red flags**		**Supportive criteria**
• Cerebellar signs • Supranuclear gaze palsy • Established diagnosis of Behavioral Variant Frontotemporal Dementia • Parkinsonism restricted to the lower limbs only for >3 years • Treatment with an antidopaminergic, or with dopamine-depletion agents • Absence of response to levodopa • Sensory-cortical loss • No evidence for dopaminergic deficiency on functional imaging • Other parkinsonism-inducing condition	• Rapid deterioration of gait • Absence of motor symptom progression over 5 years • Early bulbar dysfunction • Respiratory dysfunction • Early severe autonomic failure • Early recurrent falls due to misbalance • Disproportionate anterocollis • Absence of common non-motor features of disease during >5 years • Pyramidal tract signs • Bilateral symmetric presentation		• A clear and dramatic response to dopaminergic therapy • Levodopa-induced dyskinesia • Documentation of resting tremor of a limb • A positive diagnostic test of either olfactory loss or cardiac sympathetic denervation on scintigraphy

daytime sleepiness, and depression.[101] Neuroimaging (transcranial sonography, MRI [standard MRI and diffusion tensor imaging], and functional imaging using chemical markers to identify deficits in dopamine systems [positron emission imaging, PET; single photon emission computed tomography, SPECT; functional MRI]) can assist in the preclinical diagnosis of PD or in differentiating different parkinsonian syndromes.[102] In particular, the use of dopamine transporter single photon emission computed tomography imaging (DAT-SPECT) to detect presynaptic dopamine neuronal dysfunction has facilitated early and accurate diagnosis of PD, although it cannot distinguish between PD and Parkinson-plus syndromes.[103] Elevated alpha-synuclein levels in the cerebrospinal fluid, blood, or saliva are being investigated as early biomarkers of PD.[104]

CLINICAL COURSE

The expected rate of progression and survival after diagnosis is variable. In one study using the suggested subtypes, mean (SD) time from diagnosis to first milestone (regular falls, wheelchair dependence, dementia, or residential/nursing home placement) was found to be 3.5 (3.2) for the diffuse malignant group, 8.2 (5.3) for the intermediate group, and 14.3 (5.7) for the mild motor predominant group.[19] This corresponded with a mean (SD) survival of 8.1 (5.4) years for the diffuse malignant group, 13.2 (6.7) years for the intermediate group, and 20.2 (7.8) years for the mild motor predominant group. In general, individuals with young age at onset (<50 years) and those with tremor-predominant PD typically have a slower rate of progression while those with PIGD and PDD have faster rates of decline.[105] Progression is generally slower with levodopa therapy and mortality rates are improved. Death is usually due to pneumonia and cardiovascular disease.[106] The typical progression of symptoms across disease stages is shown in Table 15-5.

Two clinical measures that are widely used to measure disease progression and severity are the Unified Parkinson's Disease Rating Scale (UPDRS)[107] and the Hoehn–Yahr Classification of Disability Scale.[108] The original version of the UPDRS was modified by Goetz and colleagues in 2008 and was renamed the Movement Disorder Society-sponsored revision of the UPDRS (MDS-UPDRS).[109] It consists of the following four parts: Part I – Non-motor Aspects of Experiences of Daily Living; Part II – Motor Experiences of Daily Living; Part III – Motor Examination; and Part IV – Motor Complications. Items are rated on a five-point scale (0, normal or no problems; 1, minimal problems; 2, mild problems; 3, moderate problems; and 4, severe problems). The Hoehn–Yahr Classification of Disability Scale uses motor signs and functional status to stage the severity of the disease. Stage 1 indicates minimal disease impairment, whereas Stage 5 indicates that a person is confined to bed or a wheelchair (Table 15-6). It was modified from its original version in 2004 by Goetz and colleagues with the addition of stages 1.5 and 2.5 to help describe the intermediate course of the disease.[110]

MEDICAL MANAGEMENT

Pharmacological Management

There is no cure for PD. Medical management aims to slow down the progression of the disease through neuroprotective strategies as well as treatment of motor and non-motor symptoms. A wide range of first-line medications is available for neuroprotective and symptomatic therapy (Table 15-7). The physician's choice of medications depends on many variables, including the person's age, symptom presentation, other concurrent health issues, and lifestyle. It is important for individuals with PD to take medications on a fixed schedule to maintain adequate levels of drugs in the bloodstream. According to the National Parkinson Foundation (NPF), three out of four individuals with PD do not receive medications on time in the hospital, resulting in serious complications. The Aware in Care kit

TABLE 15-5	Progression of Symptoms Across Disease Stages in Parkinson's Disease (PD) and Huntington's Disease (HD)			
DISEASE	**PREMANIFEST**	**EARLY**	**MIDDLE**	**LATE**
PD	• Hyposmia • Constipation • Depression/Anxiety • Rapid eye movement (REM) sleep behavior disorder • Reduced arm swing • Mild motor function changes	• Unilateral tremor • Rigidity • Mild gait hypokinesia • Micrographia • Reduced speech volume	• Bilateral bradykinesia, axial and limb rigidity • Balance and gait deficits/Falls • Speech impairments • May need assistance toward end of stage	• Severe voluntary movement impairments • Pulmonary function and swallowing compromised • Dependence in mobility, self-care, and activities of daily living
HD	• Mild motor symptoms (rapid alternating movements, fine coordination, gait) • Difficulty with complex thinking tasks • Depression, aggression, irritability	• Mild chorea (mainly hands) • Mild balance problems (turns) • Abnormal extraocular movements • Mild visuospatial and cognitive deficits • Depression, irritability	• Chorea, dystonia • Voluntary movement abnormalities • Balance and gait deficits/Falls • Cognitive/Behavioral problems • Weight loss • Difficulties with self-care	• Bradykinesia, rigidity • Severe dysarthria, dysphagia • Chorea (may be less) • Global dementia • Psychosis • Dependence in mobility, self-care, and activities of daily living

TABLE 15-6	Hoehn and Yahr Staging of Parkinson's Scale[108]
STAGE (SEVERITY)	**DESCRIPTION**
1 (mild)	Ipsilateral symptoms, involving movement, facial expression, tremor, or posture but not limiting activities
1.5	Ipsilateral symptoms plus trunk impairment
2	Bilateral symptoms but no balance impairment
2.5	Mild–moderate; able to recover balance from posterior pull
Stage 3 (moderate)	Moderate disability affecting mobility and balance with bradykinesia
Stage 4 (severe)	Limited walking; requires caregiving assistance so can't live alone; diminishing tremor with increased rigidity and bradykinesia
Stage 5 (cachectic)	Unable to stand or walk; nursing care required

found on the NPF website[112] can help patients, caregivers, and health professionals to avoid these complications.

Initial Pharmacologic Treatment for PD Motor Symptoms

Levodopa is the most potent treatment for PD, since it became widely available in the late 1960s. It is a dopamine precursor that is converted into dopamine by the enzyme dopa-decarboxylase within nerve cells in the brain. Levodopa administered by itself is almost entirely (99%) metabolized in the bloodstream before it reaches the brain, requiring administration of high doses that produce unpleasant side effects (i.e., nausea and vomiting). Therefore, it is combined with carbidopa, a decarboxylase inhibitor that prevents the peripheral metabolism of levodopa, allowing therapeutic concentrations of levodopa to enter the brain without unwanted side effects. The best-known levodopa/carbidopa formulation is called Sinemet® (Table 15-7). Sinemet tablets are available in many different ratios of carbidopa to levodopa (e.g., 10/100, 25/100, 50/200, and 25/250) and formulations, including short-acting immediate-release (IR) and long-acting controlled-release (CR) forms.[113]

The primary effects of levodopa therapy are to reduce motor symptoms of bradykinesia and rigidity, allowing increased speed of movement and strength. The effect of levodopa on tremors is equivocal, with some individuals getting a reduction in tremor amplitude while others have little to no benefit. Levodopa's effects on postural instability have also been varied, with levodopa causing improvements or worsening of postural sway in quiet stance, worsening of reactive postural adjustments, and improvements in anticipator postural adjustments and dynamic balance. The greatest improvements with levodopa therapy in gait were found for gait velocity, stride length, arm swing, and turning speed. Dramatic improvements in functional status are often observed with the initiation of levodopa therapy, and for a period of time (typically between 4 and 6 years), called the "honeymoon period," the drug provides sustained symptomatic relief with minimal side effects.[114]

Levodopa is initially typically taken 3 times daily around meal times. Over time, people with PD will require more frequent and higher doses of levodopa due to decreasing short- and long-duration responses to dopaminergic medications and an

TABLE 15-7	Medications for PD[111]		
DRUG	**ACTION**	**SIDE EFFECTS**	**BRAND NAMES**
Levodopa/ Carbidopa	L-dopa converted to dopamine in brain to restore DA levels.	Orthostatic hypotension, dyskinesias, hallucinations, sleepiness.	Sinemet, immediate and sustained release; Rytary; Parcopa; Duopa; Inbrija.
Dopamine agonists	Directly stimulate postsynaptic dopamine receptors.	Nausea, sedation, dizziness, constipation, hallucinations. Linked to impulse control disorders (e.g., pathological gambling, compulsive shopping, hypersexuality).	Pramipexole (Mirapex), ropinirole (Requip), piribedil (Trivastal), rotigotine transdermal patch (Neupro), apomorphine (Uprima)
Monoamine oxidase B (MAO-B) inhibitors	Inhibits enzyme MAO-B to prevent degradation of dopamine.	Mild nausea, dry mouth, dizziness, orthostatic hypotension, confusion, hallucinations, insomnia	Selegiline hydrochloride (Eldepryl), rasagiline (Azilect)
Anticholinergics	Block acetylcholine receptors and may inhibit dopamine reuptake in striatum.	Blurred vision, dry mouth, dizziness, and urinary retention; toxicity causes impaired memory, confusion, hallucinations, and delusions.	Trihexyphenidyl HCl (Artane), benztropine mesylate (Cogentin), procyclidine hydrochloride (Kemadrin)
Catechol-o-methyl transferase (COMT) inhibitors	Inhibits enzyme COMT to prevent degradation of dopamine.	Dyskinesia, nausea, vomiting, orthostatic hypotension, sleep disorders, hallucinations, diarrhea, liver damage with tolcapone	Entacapone (Comtan), entacapone and levodopa (Stalevo), tolcapone (Tasmar)
Amantadine	Increases release of dopamine presynaptically; blocks acetylcholine receptors	Dizziness, nausea, and anorexia, livedo reticularis (i.e., purplish red blotchy spots on skin), leg edema, confusion, hallucinations	Amantadine hydrochloride (Symmetrel), Symadine; Amantadine extended release (Gocovri)

inability to store excess dopamine, resulting in a narrowing of the therapeutic window when dopaminergic medications are reducing motor symptoms ("on" time; Figure 15-4).[115] As this occurs, individuals with PD experience bothersome side effects of dyskinesia, dystonia, and motor fluctuations. **Dyskinesia** refers to uncontrolled, involuntary movements that typically present as **chorea** or **choreoathetosis** on the side most affected by PD,

usually in the legs before the arms,[116] as discussed in Chapter 20 for cerebral palsy. **Chorea** refers to involuntary, rapid, irregular, purposeless, and unsustained movements that seem to flow from one body part to another. When writhing athetoid movements are superimposed on chorea it is called **choreoathetosis**. They may start as small movements in one area of the body and progress to large amplitude movements in multiple body parts.

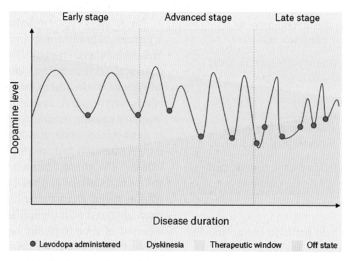

FIGURE 15-4 Interaction between medication dosing, wearing off, and dyskinesias over time. Initially levodopa is typically prescribed 3 times daily at mealtimes. With progression of the disease, the response decreases, requiring more frequent and higher dosing. When levodopa reaches maximum concentrations at these higher doses, dyskinesias can occur. The therapeutic window for diminishing motor symptoms without dyskinesias becomes narrow. (Adapted from: Armstrong MJ, Okun MS. Diagnosis and treatment of Parkinson Disease: a review. JAMA; 2020:323(6), page 553.)

Dyskinesia typically involves the trunk, neck, head, and limbs; it is commonly seen at peak dose or when levodopa levels are rising or wearing off, known as "**diphasic dyskinesia**." Individuals with young onset PD are more prone to getting dyskinesia. **Dystonia** among people on dopaminergic therapy usually occurs during "off" periods (i.e., early in morning or between doses), typically involves dystonic inversion of the foot,[54] and is present at peak dose, affecting most often the neck and face. Diphasic dystonia can also occur and usually affects the leg and ipsilateral arm. Motor fluctuations include "on–off" phenomenon and wearing-off. The **on–off phenomenon** refers to periods when the medication unpredictably starts or stops working. **Wearing-off** refers to **end-of-dose deterioration**, a worsening of symptoms near the end of the timeframe when levodopa is expected to be effective. The underlying mechanisms of levodopa-induced dyskinesia (LID) and motor fluctuations are unclear but pulsatile dopamine stimulation (fluctuation of dopamine levels) of striatal postsynaptic receptors is important in its pathogenesis.[117]

Dopamine agonists and MAO-B inhibitors give less robust motor symptom relief than levodopa but have a lower dyskinesia risk (Table 15-7). They may be administered alone or along with levodopa/carbidopa to reduce the amount of levodopa needed and thus postpone the motor complications that occur with long-term levodopa therapy.[118] In middle to late stages of the disease, they are often given, when (1) levodopa alone is not able to control symptoms and increasing the dose would cause excessive side effects or (2) the person taking levodopa is experiencing severe motor fluctuations. Treatment with dopamine agonists is associated with a higher overall risk of adverse side effects including impulse control disorders.[18,119]

Anticholinergic drugs that block the action of acetylcholine are primarily used to treat younger patients with PD, whose chief complaint is tremor, and for those individuals with dystonia that is not relieved with levodopa (Table 15-7).[18] Acetylcholine released by striatal interneurons has antagonistic effects to dopamine on medium spiny striatal neurons that are part of the BG motor pathways; acetylcholine increases the excitability of neurons in the indirect pathway and inhibits neurons in the direct pathway.[120] There are also modulatory interactions between acetylcholine and dopamine in the striatum; acetylcholine triggers release of dopamine from nigrostriatal neurons while dopamine inhibits release of acetylcholine from striatal interneurons. Depletion of striatal dopamine, due to loss of nigrostriatal neurons in PD, causes increased excitability of cholinergic interneurons, thereby, causing a reduction in movement. Anticholinergic drugs can also be helpful to reduce excessive drooling. Older individuals often experience confusion and hallucinations on anticholinergics, so these drugs are avoided in people older than 70.[118]

Middle to Late Pharmacologic Treatment for PD Motor Symptoms

In middle to late stages of PD, levodopa/carbidopa formulations that include an extended release capsule (Rytary®), a tablet that dissolves in the mouth without water (Parcopa®) for people with dysphagia, an enteral suspension (Duopa®) delivered through a surgically implanted tube, and an inhaled powder (Inbrija®)

may be prescribed to reduce "off" periods.[18,113] For individuals with severe "off" periods, apomorphine is an injectable, rapid-acting dopamine agonist that is usually effective within 10 minutes of injection and produces effects comparable to levodopa for approximately 60 to 90 minutes. Because of its rapid effects it is used as a "rescue therapy" for individuals with PD, who are experiencing freezing episodes that are not relieved with levodopa or other dopamine agonists.[121] Catechol-o-methyltransferase (COMT) inhibitors such as entacapone (Comtan®) can be taken in combination with levodopa or with other antiparkinsonian drugs, to decrease freezing episodes and motor fluctuations (Table 15-7). Amantadine, an antiviral agent, is beneficial for treating tremors and to treat dyskinesia that is unresponsive to conventional measures such as reduction of levodopa (Table 15-7).

Deep Brain Stimulation and Surgical Treatments

Deep brain stimulation (DBS) involves surgical implantation of a battery-operated medical device, called an implantable pulse generator (IPG), in the sub-clavicular area. This is connected by a thin wire that passes under the skin to electrodes that deliver high-frequency electrical stimulation to specific areas in the brain, thereby, blocking abnormal nerve signals that cause parkinsonian motor symptoms. DBS changes the brain firing pattern but does not slow the progression of the neurodegeneration. Areas that are typically stimulated in PD are the thalamus (Ventral Intermediate (VIM) nucleus), subthalamic nucleus, globus pallidus internal segment and pedunculopontine nucleus. Following surgery, the physician adjusts the amount of stimulation provided by the device to best meet the individual's needs; thereafter, the person with PD can control the IPG's "on–off" switch externally, using a controller. The IPGs typically last 3–5 years, and the replacement procedure is relatively simple. DBS is presently used only for individuals whose symptoms cannot be adequately controlled with medications but are still responsive to levodopa to some degree; DBS is not effective for those who are no longer responding to levodopa. Many individuals experience a reduction of motor symptoms (i.e., tremors, rigidity, akinesia) with DBS and can reduce their medications, thereby, reducing side effects such as dyskinesia. Some improvements in gait disturbances and FOG have been observed with DBS of the STN with better effects from bilateral stimulation. DBS has equivocal effect on balance with both improvements or worsening reported, depending on the site of stimulation. DBS does not improve cognitive symptoms in PD and may worsen them, so generally, it is not used when there are signs of dementia.[31]

MRI-guided focused ultrasound is a new non-invasive technology that reduces parkinsonian symptoms by lesioning targeted areas of the thalamus or globus pallidus. Ablation of the GPi (**pallidotomy**) reduces tremor, bradykinesia, rigidity, and LIDs, while ablation of the VIM nucleus (**thalamotomy**) relieves tremors. MRI-guided focused ultrasound is approved by the US Food and Drug Administration for the treatment of Parkinsonian tremors.[122] **Restorative surgeries** to replace striatal dopamine or improve function of dopaminergic cells, such as fetal cell transplantation, gene therapy, and stem cell therapy are promising experimental treatments for PD.

Intrastriatal transplantation of human embryonic mesencephalic dopamine rich tissue into individuals with PD has induced variable functional outcomes, with some, but not all, individuals showing significant improvements in motor symptoms.[123,124] Gene therapy for PD aims to surgically implant genetically modified cells that are incorporated into targeted cells in the striatum to produce enzymes that increase dopamine synthesis or decrease STN activity, to deliver neurotrophic factors that protect dopamine neurons, or to alleviate genetic causes of PD.[125,126] Stem cell therapy research in PD aims to create or find a renewable resource of dopamine-producing neurons for transplantation.[127]

Physical Therapy Implications of Pharmacological Management

Physical therapists need to be aware of the medications that a person with PD is taking and their potential side effects. Therapists should try to schedule their examination and treatments at a consistent time when the person is optimally dosed. If a person is experiencing motor fluctuations, the therapist should also assess the individual with PD during "off" times. Therapists need to monitor drug effectiveness on the person with PD's motor performance and functional status and communicate their observations and examination findings about any changes in functional status to the physician to assist in drug prescription.

CASE A, PART IV: PARKINSON'S DISEASE AT AGE 80

Mr. Martin requires care around the clock and is no longer ambulating. His wife reports that she has an aide that comes daily, but she has injured her back transferring her husband, when the aide is not present. She is also concerned because Mr. Martin is having difficulty eating and taking his medication. She does not feel that the medication is helping him and reports that, when they increased the dosage, he developed "jerky movements" and was complaining that he could see snakes on the walls of the bedroom at night.

What is the cause of Mr. Martin's "jerky movements" and hallucinations?

Answer: He is most likely exhibiting dyskinesia and hallucinations due to long-term levodopa therapy.

In Part I, Mr. Martin is in the early stage of PD with a typical early presentation of resting tremor in the hand and bradykinesia. He continues to work, and therapy is focused on rehabilitation of his impairments and prevention of progression of motor symptoms. He is likely taking carbidopa/levodopa (IR, CR) because of its robust effects on motor symptoms and fewer side effects. However, it is also possible that he would be taking a dopamine agonist or a MAO-B inhibitor to delay the emergence of motor fluctuations and dyskinesia.[118]

By Parts II and III of the case, he is likely to be on carbidopa/levodopa ER in combination with a dopamine agonist or a MAO-B inhibitor, and by Parts III and IV, he may also be taking a COMT inhibitor or amantadine due to on/off episodes with his medication as well as unwanted medication side effects

such as hallucinations, dyskinesia, or dystonia. If his symptoms become severe, he may be a candidate for deep brain stimulation surgery. Determining the medication schedule is particularly important for individuals who use carbidopa/levodopa because their ability to participate in therapy is best at peak dose, and some functional deficits are more likely to be evident at the end of their dose cycle. Therapists develop a plan of care to develop ways to maintain functional independence during both peak dose and end of dose times.

Nutritional Management

When foods with high protein content are ingested at the same time as levodopa, they can interfere with the absorption of levodopa. Therefore, individuals with PD may be advised to take levodopa 30–45 minutes prior to meals and may also be prescribed a low-protein diet or protein redistribution, where most protein is eaten in the evening with the advice of a dietician.[128] Individuals with PD should be encouraged to eat a healthy diet and may be advised to take food supplements for nutritional support, if they are losing weight or are underweight. Individuals with constipation are advised to drink more fluids and eat more fiber-rich foods. Occupational therapists help people with PD to improve upper extremity movements for feeding and recommend adaptive eating devices. Speech-language pathologists evaluate for dysphagia and recommend interventions to assist with swallowing dysfunction. A percutaneous endoscopic gastrostomy (PEG) may be necessary in advanced stages to maintain adequate nutrition.[129]

● EXAMINATION OF THE CLIENT WITH PARKINSON'S DISEASE

Client History

The client history involves gathering information regarding symptoms that are causing problems in daily life and elucidating the client's goals for therapy. In addition, it is important to know what medications the person with PD is taking as well as their dosing schedule. Some medications such as Sinemet® (carbidopa–levodopa) can have a significant impact on motor function, and therapy may need to be planned around the medication schedule. Falls are another issue that is common in PD and asking about fall history is an important component of the history. Typically, the fall history includes asking about a recent timeframe as well as longer timeframes such as falls in the last week and falls in the last 6 months. It is common for individuals with PD in Hoehn and Yahr stages 2.5, 3, and 4 to have frequent, even daily, falls.

Bodily Structure and Function

Neurologic System

The neurologic examination is carried out, as described in Chapter 10, with a focus on motor control and motor planning, since these are functions that are controlled by the BG. Sensation such as light touch, temperature, pinprick, and two-point discrimination are not usually altered by PD and so may be screened rather than evaluated in detail. Proprioception is typically impaired in PD with mild impairments appearing early in the course of the disease[130] therefore, vibration and proprioception should be examined in more detail (see Chapter 10) The MDS-UPDRS[110] is an assessment that enables the clinician to examine impairments that are typical to PD, such as rigidity, tremor, and bradykinesia, as well as areas of common deficits (e.g., cognition and fatigue).

Cognitive Screen: Cognitive function impacts the ability to perform motor activities such as gait and transfers and is an important consideration when assessing safety. The Montreal Cognitive Assessment is a screen for dementia that is sensitive to mild cognitive impairment,[131] with demonstrated reliability and validity in PD[132] and is recommended for use by the Parkinson Disease Evidence Database to Guide Effectiveness (PDEDGE) taskforce of the Neurology Section of the APTA. It is quick and easy to administer, but does require some training and has a fee for use. The Mini Mental Status Exam (MMSE) has also been used extensively in studies examining cognitive function in PD. It is also quick and easy to administer and requires some training and may require a fee for use; however, research suggests that the MoCA is better than the MMSE as a screening tool for cognitive decline in those with PD.[133]

Fatigue: Fatigue is difficult to assess and to treat, but it is important to identify and document its impact on the client with PD. There is a Parkinson-specific measure called the Parkinson's disease fatigue scale that is recommended for use in this population.[134]

Bradykinesia: To assess bradykinesia, the MDS-UPDRS includes finger tapping and toe tapping. It is important to assess both the UE and LE as PD can differentially affect left and right sides of the body as well as upper torso and limbs and lower torso and limbs. For finger tapping, the client is instructed to repetitively touch the index finger to the thumb, opening the hand fully each time while the therapist observes speed, amplitude, including any decrement, hesitations, and halts on each side for 10 repetitions. It is scored as 0 (no problems), 1 (mild), 2 (moderate), 3 (severe), or 4 (cannot or can only barely perform task). Further descriptors for each category are included in the test. Bradykinesia of the lower extremity is assessed in a similar fashion via toe tapping, while keeping the heel on the floor.[110]

Balance: Postural instability is assessed with the Pull Test in the MDS-UPDRS. The patient is instructed to stand with feet shoulder-width apart and to do whatever they need to do to prevent falling. The examiner stands behind the patient and without warning grabs both shoulders and pulls backward quickly. The therapist should stand behind the patient at an arm's-length away with feet spread shoulder-width apart to prevent a fall. This test is scored from 0 to 4, with 0 being a normal response of 0 to 2 steps and no loss of balance, and 4 being unable to stand unassisted.[110]

Tremor: Tremor is described in terms of location (upper extremity, lower extremity, lip/jaw), amplitude and constancy (<25% of exam period, 26–50% of exam period, 51–75% of exam period, >75% of exam period). In addition, types of tremor (resting, postural, or kinetic) should be documented.

Dyskinesia: The assessment includes information about whether dyskinesias are present and if they are bothersome to the client or interfere with the client's ability to participate in the examination process in any way. If dyskinesias are present and bothersome, timing of medications is noted and considered as they may be a side effect of medications.

Freezing: Freezing and difficulty initiating movement are debilitating problems and a major cause of falls and disability in PD, but these symptoms can be difficult to elicit in the clinic. Freezing can be assessed in the clinic using a rapid 360-degree turn in both directions[135] or by observing gait in a confined space, such as walking into a corner and turning around. Yet, this will not always elicit freezing, even in individuals with severe FOG. To assess the impact on daily life, the therapist takes a history of frequency and typical triggers of freezing episodes. This may be augmented through use of the Freezing of Gait Questionnaire (FOGQ),[136] the only validated screening tool with excellent intra-rater reliability. On this questionnaire, there are six items on how freezing impacts the ability to walk during normal daily activities. The scale ranges from 0, which denotes normal movement, to 4, which indicates an inability to walk. The maximum score is 24, indicating more severe FOG. It has also been found to be a more sensitive measure of FOG than the freezing-while-walking item on the MDS-UPDRS, which simply asks the person to rate the freezing as none, rare, occasional, frequent, or frequent falls with freezing.[137] It was also found to be the best measure available in 2021 in a COSMIN review.[136]

Movement Scale: Size or scope of movement (movement scale) is assessed for both bradykinesia and coordination by having the person perform rapid, repetitive, thumb-to-index finger movement for 30 seconds (as described for bradykinesia). The therapist observes not only speed but any change in the amplitude of the movement. The hand should open fully with each motion before closing. For an individual with PD, finger-to-finger movements will get progressively smaller the longer the individual does the movement; the movements are slow, and in mid to late-stage disease, irregular timing of the motions is noted.

Musculoskeletal System

Individuals with PD, like Mr. Martin, are often in late middle age or entering old age and commonly have musculoskeletal issues such as arthritis and disuse weakness. Declines in **strength as measured by manual muscle testing** are not typically seen early in PD. Individuals with mild PD have been shown to have deficits in both force production and power using hand-held dynamometry.[138,139] All lower extremity muscles had reduced strength when compared to controls, even when on medication. The most severely affected lower extremity muscle groups were the hip adductors and ankle plantarflexors.[138] Decreased strength and power in ankle plantarflexors would likely limit push-off during gait and negatively impact other functional activities such as stair ascent. Use of handheld dynamometry and functional strength testing is recommended to detect early, subtle strength changes. Strength, including core strength, should be monitored throughout the disease process. In addition, rigidity leads to stiffness, decreasing range of motion, and contracture; thus, assessment of **muscle length** and **joint range of motion** should also be monitored throughout the disease process. The muscle groups responsible for flexion and rotation (e.g., the pectorals, iliopsoas, hamstrings, and gastrocnemius muscles) are especially prone to shortening, so range of motion of the trunk and extremities is assessed periodically, with special attention paid to trunk extension, shoulder elevation/abduction, hip extension, knee extension, ankle dorsiflexion, and trunk and neck rotation.

Moreover, **posture** is assessed for scoliosis and kyphosis as these typically occur in later stages of the disease.

Trunk rotation is the key to many functional activities such as walking with long strides and reaching. Trunk rotation can be safely assessed by examining the individual's ability to rotate, while seated with feet on the floor and arms crossed. The therapist instructs the individual to look back over his or her shoulder, and the therapist notes any side-to-side asymmetry. If a standard seat and location are used, rotation can be measured by placing numbers on the wall at 1-inch intervals and asking the individual to indicate the last number that can be read. Rotation can also be tested in standing (see Figure 15-5).

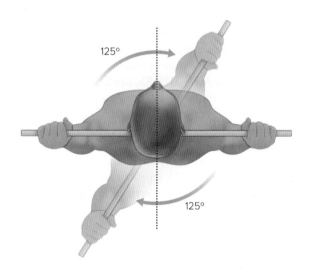

FIGURE 15-5 Overhead view of trunk rotation measurement method. A line is marked on the floor using tape, and a series of pairs of different colored points are marked on the tape, equidistant from the center mark on both the left and the right side. Clients stand (or sit) on the line with their feet shoulder-width apart, using the points as a guide to ensure that their feet are placed symmetrically on either side of the center mark. A wooden bar, approximately 4 feet long, is placed evenly across the subjects' shoulders and held in the subjects' hands, which rest as close to the shoulders as is comfortable. Clients are told to rotate as far as possible to the left or right, keeping the bar resting on their shoulders and not moving their feet. The therapist checks that the bar remains horizontal throughout the test. At the end of the rotation movement, a plumb bob or other weighted object on a string is attached to the left end of the bar for right rotation and the right end of the bar for left rotation. The bar is steadied by the rater and then the bob is allowed to drop to touch the floor. A nonpermanent marker pen is used to indicate where the plumb bob touches the floor. A long-armed goniometer is used to measure degrees of rotation. The axis of the goniometer is placed on the center of the line, and the stationary arm is placed along the line. A ruler or other lightweight long stick can be secured to the moving arm of the goniometer to reach the mark and allow for more accurate measurement. In a clinic that takes these measurements more frequently, a circle can be marked on the floor with the degrees marked along its arc at regular intervals; the therapist can simply take the measurement from the marks on the circle rather than use the goniometer every time. (Reproduced with permission from Evans KL, Refshauge KM, Adams R. Measurement of active rotation in standing: reliability of a simple test protocol. *Percept Mot Skills*. 2006:103(2):619-628.)

Functional Losses and Impact on Participation

Measurement and documentation of function provide the therapist with a means to document meaningful changes to improve the individual's ability to remain independent and active. In addition, the use of standardized measures improves communication by using a common language that allows comparison across therapists and clinics. The use of standardized measures also allows clinicians to better gauge the effectiveness of therapeutic interventions during and after therapy. Baseline measurements allow (1) quantification of any change in status throughout an episode of care, (2) documentation of disease progression, and (3) communication across different therapists and clinics.

In addition to the Academy of Neurology's core measure clinical practice guideline the PD EDGE taskforce recommends the use of a core set of nine measures across all stages of the disease and across all clinics.[140] These measures are grouped by the International Classification of Function (ICF) categories and are listed in Box 15-2. Four of the measures are part of the ANPT core measures CPG as indicated by an asterisk in Box 15-2. In addition, the ABC scale is recommended to assess fear of falling in PD. Therefore, the PD EDGE taskforce recommendation would only mean performing four additional measures in addition to the six core measures.

Function and Activity Level Measures: Measures of gait, transfers, balance, falls screening, and participation do not differ significantly from those recommended in Chapter 10

Box 15-2	PDEDGE Core Measures[140]	
Highly Recommended Measures		**Measures Recommended for Specific Constructs**
Body Structure and Function MDS-UPDRS revision* – Part III MDS-UPDRS – Part I	Montreal Cognitive Assessment	*Freezing of Gait* Freezing of Gait Questionnaire *Fatigue* Parkinson's Fatigue Scale *Fear of falling* ABC scale*
Activity 6-minute walk* 10-m walk* Mini BESTest MDS-UPDRS – Part II	Functional Gait Assessment (FGA)* Sit to stand 5 times* 9-hole peg test	*Dual-Task* Timed Up and Go cognitive
Participation PDQ-8 or PDQ-39		

*All measures in the highly recommended category are recommended for use in research and for students to learn to administer. *Part of the ANPT Core Measures CPG. (Reproduced with permission from PD EDGE Core Measures; Neurology section. 2014.)*

("Evaluation"). Specific measures for use in PD can be found in Box 15-2. The miniBESTest is recommended in PD and the Berg Balance Scale was not included in the core measures for PD as the miniBESTest was more sensitive to change over time in PD.[141] In addition, there are some unique features of PD, such as FOG, that may require the use of specific measures such as the FOGQ.[136,137] It is recommended that therapists use the ANPT core measures, and then based on the individual client's situation, choose measures from the PD EDGE to assess constructs specific to PD.

CASE A, PART V

Mr. Martin was initially evaluated (Part I) using the MDS-UPDRS revision, MoCA, 6 MWT, 10-m walk, Mini BESTest, FGA, 5 times Sit to stand, 9-hole peg test, and the PDQ-8; these are ideal for documenting baseline function and disease symptoms. At his visit at age 60 years (Part II), he reported having falls and difficulty walking outdoors. When repeating the core measures, the therapist noted that he scored in the high fall risk range on the Mini-BESTest and the FGA. Additionally, his score on the PDQ-8 had dropped, and he was walking slower and shorter distances (10-m walk test and 6 MWT). Using this data, the therapist and neurologist agreed that Mr. Martin should go through a course of individualized therapy to improve balance and walking and reassess his home exercise program. The use of the same measures allows justification for therapy and better tracking over time.

Mr. Martin moved to Florida at age 70 and at age 75 was referred for physical therapy for difficulty walking, inactivity, and falls. The therapist included the core measures in the examination, and having requested Mr. Martin's records, was able to compare his status with his last documented status, just 7 years previous. At this time, there was a marked drop in the 9-hole peg test, MoCA score, and the PDQ-8. The therapist was concerned about hand function, depression, and safety and made referrals to psychiatry and occupational therapy, based on these evaluative findings.

MANAGING THE CLIENT WITH PARKINSON'S DISEASE

Before starting an exercise program, the cardiopulmonary system must be considered. While exercise has been shown to be safe and feasible in people with mild to moderate PD,[142,143] few studies have considered the impact of PD on the **autonomic nervous system** and cardiopulmonary responses. Individuals with PD experience dysfunction in the autonomic and cardiovascular system early in the disease.[144-146] Studies show that individuals with PD exhibit a blunted cardiovascular response to exercise, specifically an attenuated **pressor response** due to disruption of the central component of autonomic reflex arches and attenuation of the muscle metaboreflex. In addition, clients with PD present with loss of sympathetic cardiac nerves, lower norepinephrine release, and lower α-adrenergic responsiveness.[146] These findings were correlated with stage of disease; with individuals in later stages of the disease exhibiting more impairment in cardiovascular response. Overall, the blunted increase in BP during exercise and accompanying lowered blood pressure and HR response, mean that general exercise guidelines are not applicable to these individuals. It is recommended that clinicians perform exercise tolerance testing whenever possible and consider using both vital signs and ratings of perceived exertion to determine appropriate exercise intensity.[147] Clinicians need to individualize treatment based on each individual's cardiovascular response. In addition, these altered responses could make participation in exercise difficult.

It is possible that appropriately prescribed exercise could moderate the effects of PD on the cardiovascular and autonomic systems. Exercise has been shown to improve **baroreflex** activation in patients with heart failure and could have the same effect in individuals with PD.[146] Overall, these studies point to the need to be vigilant in monitoring vital signs before and after exercise, especially when starting a new exercise program. In addition, therapists should use rating of perceived exertion to assess exercise intensity. Caution should be taken in prescribing and implementing higher intensity exercise for individuals who are in later stages of the disease.

Bodily Functions

Table 15-8 provides an overview of the different types of rehabilitation interventions that have been studied in PD along with a synopsis of outcomes and overall potential to provide benefit.[148-150,154,155] The following interventions are consistent with the Clinical Practice Guideline put out by the ANPT and published in 2022.[156]

Range of Motion and Stretching

Work to maintain and improve joint and tissue flexibility begins as soon as a diagnosis is made with a focus on active extension and rotation. The hamstring muscles are particularly prone to contracture and should be stretched early in the disease process to maintain length and prevent contracture. If shortening and contracture occur, stretching is done 2 to 3 times a day, using a long slow stretch (see Figure 15-6). Given the tendency for individuals with PD to develop a flexed posture and lack rotation during activities such as walking, therapy also focuses on trunk ROM into extension and rotation.

Strength

High-intensity exercise training results in myofiber hypertrophy of both type I and type II muscles, a shift to a less fatigable myofiber type profile, and increased mitochondrial complex activity.[157] In addition, strength training for greater than 8 weeks done at 60 to 70% of the single repetition max leads to significant improvements in the 6-minute walk test, stair descent time, and sit to stand.[158] There is no evidence that one type of exercise is superior to any other type, and both concentric and eccentric exercise are safe and well tolerated by individuals with PD. However, it has been suggested that eccentric exercise might minimize oxygen consumption and maximize strengthening.[159] Interestingly, a study of resistance training brought about nonsignificant improvement in isokinetic strength in the training group but still lead to significant improvements in bradykinesia

TABLE 15-8	Summary of Rehabilitation Interventions for PD[148–150]	
REHABILITATION INTERVENTION	**BODY FUNCTION AND ACTIVITIES IMPACTED**	**OVERALL CONCLUSION**
Physical Therapy	Balance – Berg Balance Scale (BBS) Gait - Timed Up and Go (TUG) and speed (comfortable and fast) Endurance (2- and 6-minute walk test) Sit to stand time Disease Burden – MDS-UPDRS	Individualized task-specific therapy leads to improvements in the tasks trained. Benefits appear to be short-term pointing to the need for an ongoing plan of care for clients with PD.
Exercise		
Aerobics	Endurance (2- and 6-minute walk test)	Moderate to high intensity aerobic exercise should be provided three times a week in 30 minute sessions to improve oxygen consumption, disease severity, and function.
Resistance Exercise	Strength – manual muscle test and isokinetics Stairs – descent time Sit to stand Endurance - 6-minute walk test	Progressive resistance exercise done for greater than eight weeks at 60-70% of the 1 rep max leads to significant improvements in function and high-intensity training leads to a shift to a less fatigable myofiber type. In addition it improves muscle activation even when force production is not improved.
Balance Exercise	Balance, - miniBESTest, Sensory Organization Test Fear of Falling – Falls Efficacy Scale, Fall rate – change in rate of falls over time.	Multimodal balance training with and without auditory stimuli improves balance in the short term for both freezers and non-freezers in people with mild to moderate disease.[151] Rhythmic auditory balance training was superior to multimodal balance training. Only RAS training had long-term effects (6 months)[151] Challenging group balance exercise improves balance and fear of falling while also reducing the rate of falls by 37%.[152]
Combination of any of the above	Balance – Berg Balance Scale, single leg stance time Falls - Fall Rate, Fall Efficacy Scale Function – 5 Times Sit to Stand Gait – Timed Up and Go, 10 meter walk test, Freezing of Gait Questionnaire	Exercise, especially when supervised by a physical therapist that applies motor learning principles such as progression from simple to difficult tasks, attentional strategies, and augmented feedback can improve gait and balance[153] and reduce fall rate by as much as 60%. It does not appear to decrease number of fallers.[149] Selection of treatment modalities should be tailored to the specific needs of each patient.[148]
Community-Based Programs		
Boxing	Potential to improve balance, gait and quality of life	Benefits have not yet been demonstrated in randomized controlled trials.
Dance	Gait speed – 10 Meter Walk Test Timed Up and Go Freezing of gait questionnaire Endurance – Six Minute Walk Test	Benefits have been demonstrated in studies but the most effective intensity, frequency, and type of music remain unclear.
Hydrotherapy	Balance – Berg Balance Scale Fear of falling – falls efficacy scale Quality of Life – Parkinson Disease Questionnaire	Aquatic exercise has been shown to provide benefits over no intervention and has also been shown to provide benefits superior to land-based exercise for balance, fear of falling and quality of life.
Tai Chi (Martial Arts)	Fall rates Balance – Berg Balance Scale and Functional Reach Gait – Timed Up and Go Test	Tai Chi improves balance and functional mobility and has a moderate effect on preventing falls. Number of studies is limited.

and functional measures of gait and transfer skills (10 MWT, TUG, 30 second chair stand).[160] This study and others support the hypothesis that strength training in PD improves connectivity of superior centers and improvement in muscle activation.[160–162] A recent review of the literature found that 10 weeks of progressive resistance training done 2-3 times per week can improve muscle strength in people with mild to moderate PD. They also suggested that resistance training should be paired with balance

A 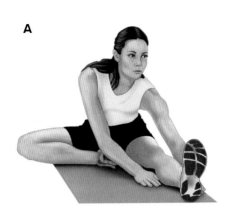   **B**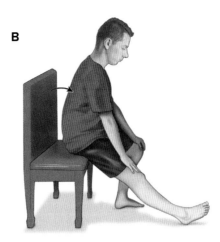

FIGURE 15-6 Illustration of hamstring stretching methods. Instruction cues the individual to keep their head up and to focus on bringing their abdomen to their thigh to ensure that the stretch is done across the hip rather than overstretching the thoracic spine, which typically occurs when individuals try to put their face to their thigh. Due to balance issues, it is best to perform stretches in sitting to better isolate the muscles to be stretched and allow the individual to perform the stretch without having to focus on maintaining their balance.

training and other types of exercise to preserve postural control, cardiorespiratory fitness, and overall function.[163] It should be noted that few studies include individuals in the later stages of the disease. Clinical judgment that factors in all aspects of each individual's case should be used to determine if resistance exercise is appropriate for clients in later stages.

Balance

Balance training is commonly recommended for individuals with PD. The balance exercises are individualized to the deficits noted in the assessment and must include exercises that are highly challenging for the individual.[149,152,164–166] Trunk exercises can improve balance in quiet stance but were not shown to improve balance confidence as measured by the ABC scale.[166] There is evidence that repetitive step training with the use of a visual cue improves reaction time, maximal excursion of the limits of stability, and movement velocity,[167] Balance training that is challenging to the individual is required to bring about meaningful improvement. Indeed, a study of challenging group balance exercise decreased fear of falling and the rate of falls by 37%.[152]

Activity

Mobility Training

Standard physical therapy typically involves task-oriented practice of gait and transfers. Practicing longer steps, turns, walking on uneven surfaces, and faster gait can lead to improved gait performance but is challenging to achieve as the individual must perform many repetitions of the correct movement pattern over a long period of time to bring about permanent changes in performance. Individualized physical therapy for 45–60 minutes, 2 to 3 times per week for at least 8 weeks, led to improvement in velocity, 2- or 6-minute walk test, step length, Timed Up and Go (TUG), BBS and disease severity scores, with effects lasting only 3-12 months.[148,150,168–171] Maintenance of improvements and prevention of decline require ongoing therapy that starts at diagnosis and continues throughout all stages of the disease.[148,170] This level of intensity is difficult to achieve in traditional therapy due to limitations on the number of visits and reimbursement.

Therapists must develop creative ways to provide ongoing care while utilizing the home program as well as community resources, during times when the client is not actively enrolled in physical therapy. Physical therapists have the expertise to prescribe individualized exercise of the correct type and dosage for each individual with PD.[172] Exercise, like medication needs to be correctly dosed, and modified over time based on individual progression of PD. We are at a place in the development of telemedicine and the use of wearables to provide lifelong, individualized care to individuals with neurodegenerative disease like PD.[172–174] Mr. Martin began therapy when diagnosed but did not receive his second round of physical therapy until two years later when he had already begun to have falls. What would be a better way for therapy to have set up Mr. Martin's plan of care?

An optimal plan of care for clients with neurodegenerative diseases is one that involves the PT at earliest symptoms, as was done with Mr. Martin. At that time the therapist should establish an ongoing relationship with the patient and plan for follow-up visits to assess Mr. Martin's status and determine if modifications are needed for his home exercise plan, as shown in Figure 15-7. Optimally, these follow-up visits occur at least once a year early in the disease and then every six months or whenever Mr. Martin notices a change in his condition, see Figure 15-7 for an example. Referral to community exercise programs and support groups are a crucial element of the plan of care. To optimize care and improve patient follow up therapists should develop relationships with community exercise program providers so that referrals between therapy and the community can be optimized.

Whole body vibration is a new technique that is not yet supported by evidence for treating balance, but may improve gait performance.[175–177]

Treadmill training improves gait speed, stride length, endurance and leads to neuroplasticity in dopaminergic signaling.[178–180] Treadmill training for individuals with PD is equally effective without body weight support, and thus, the use of a harness is only recommended when needed to ensure safety. Treadmill training is started at the individual's comfortable walking speed or slightly slower and then increased in small increments. This is known as **speed-dependent treadmill training** and is an effective means of

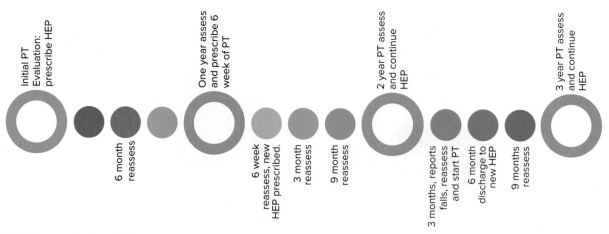

FIGURE 15-7 Example timeline. Mr. Martin Initiates PT when first diagnosed and is given an individualized home exercise program (HEP). He has been doing his home program with good success and sees PT for reassessment every 6 months. During the one-year reassessment, PT notes a decline in his 5 times sit to stand and 6-minute walk test. In addition, he is reporting significant freezing of gait on the freezing of gait questionnaire. A round of physical therapy is begun, when he meets his maximum potential, he is placed on a maintenance plan including a HEP. The PT rechecks Mr. Martin after 6 weeks, he is doing well so the PT sets the next reassessment for 3 months. Again, he is doing well and a reassessment is set for 6 months. At the two-year visit the PT assesses him and continues his HEP. Three months later he calls the neurologist due to having three falls in the last week due to freezing episodes. His medications are adjusted, and PT is again ordered. Three months after this he is discharged from PT and placed on a new HEP. He is again reassessed after three months and at the three-year annual visit. If he continues to do well, he will be regularly assessed every six months and seen whenever he notes a change in his status.

improving walking speed and stride length.[181] It is important that training utilize walking and not running, as walking and running are not the same motor skill and training in one does not fully translate to improvement in the other. Training is done for 30 to 45 minutes, 2 to 3 times per week for at least 8 weeks and followed immediately by overground training to reinforce gains made on the treadmill. Cardiovascular fitness improves with both low-intensity and high-intensity treadmill training. Therefore, if a client needs to improve gait speed and fitness, a walking program on the treadmill that encourages walking at the fastest gait speed that can be achieved safely is likely to be most effective. Treadmill training does not improve strength or range of motion. Some facilities have robotic equipment to use during treadmill training. This equipment can decrease work for therapy staff but does not add any benefit for the client with PD. Given that treadmill training is most effective for individuals with mild to moderate PD and does not typically require hands-on assistance by therapy staff, the use of robotics is not indicated in this population.[182] Combining treadmill training with music provides added benefits as compared to overground walking. The use of music with treadmill training improved quality of life, psychological well-being, motor functioning, and balance.[183] Treadmill training combined with virtual reality led to an impressive 60% decrease in fall rates in older adults a multi-center, randomized clinical trial. Inclusion of obstacles, turning, and dual tasking were important components of the virtual reality environment projected on a screen during treadmill training.[184]

Visual and auditory cueing: Individuals with PD respond well to cueing to increase movement amplitude and velocity.[185] Both visual and auditory cueing are effective and have typically been applied in an open-loop manner. **Open-loop cueing** is when the cue is fixed in its presentation while a closed-loop cue provides the cue "on-demand," using biofeedback. Typical methods for open-loop cueing include the use of visual cues on the floor to indicate appropriate step length, the use of lasers or other visual cues that move while walking, and the use of music or counting to set the step cadence. Placing tape or other visual stimuli on the floor is effective in improving step length but has the limitation of not being available in the natural environment, and it requires the individual to look down at all times, which increases the tendency to walk in a flexed posture. To alleviate these concerns, lasers are available to be attached to walkers and canes; also, there are special glasses that place a visual stimulus in front of the viewer. Both of these systems can increase step length, but the evidence on the lasers working in the natural environment is equivocal. Further, the glasses are typically bulky, and individuals are reticent to wear them in public. Auditory cueing, another form of open-loop cueing, is quite effective and has a strong body of evidence supporting its use, including improved scores on the dynamic gait index (DGI), the Tinetti mobility test (TMT), and the FOGQ. The use of external auditory cues is also difficult in community environments, so attempts have been made to use internal cueing. Unfortunately, improvements from internal cueing were not maintained.[182] **Closed-loop cueing** has been studied using wearable, visual-auditory cueing device, tactile stimulation to improve proprioceptive input and laser shoes. These methods were shown to improve both gait parameters and FOG and could be worn in the home and community. It is believed that closed-loop cueing places less cognitive attentional demands on the individual and may not lead to cue dependency.[148] These devices are new and in early stages of investigation, but they appear promising. Cueing is a strategy that can be used, but to date, has not been shown to be optimal for long-term carryover and use in community environments. It remains one of the more effective means to assist individuals who have FOG.

Assistive devices are commonly prescribed to improve safety and decrease falls. Despite their common acceptance, little research has been done looking at their effectiveness and how best to prescribe them. Individuals with PD have difficulty with transitional movements (i.e., sit ↔ stand transfers), turning, and dual-tasking.[186] Of note, the use of an assistive device is a dual-task, and thus, could be theorized to be problematic for individuals with neurologic disorders that involve the BG, such as PD. Additionally, many assistive devices (canes, standard walker, two-wheeled walkers, and walking sticks) require the user to pick them up when turning and maneuvering, which creates a destabilizing force and removes the support or assistance from the user. Given these factors, devices that can be turned without lifting them from the ground would likely be safer for use, during turning activities. In a study examining the impact of assistive devices on gait four-wheeled rollator walkers allowed people with PD to achieve the highest walking velocity, least stumbles and falls during turning, and most consistent stepping.[187] Two-wheeled walkers led to difficulty and safety issues during turning and highly variable gait. Some individuals with PD tend to walk with a forward propulsive gait, resulting in their upper body moving forward of the lower body during gait. These individuals tend to respond well to a rollator walker with reverse brakes. Reverse brakes require the user to squeeze the hand brakes to release them and let go of the brakes to apply them. This system is helpful to many individuals with PD as it appears that they maintain better control of the walker while ambulating, and during a loss of balance, they tend to let go of the brakes rather than squeeze them; thus, reverse brakes match their natural tendency. Rollator walkers are inexpensive to purchase, at many pharmacies and large retailers, and can be inexpensively converted to reverse-brake devices by personnel at bicycle and wheelchair repair shops. When prescribing an assistive device, community ambulation as well as home ambulation and the capabilities of the individual and their caregiver should be considered. Heavy devices may be difficult to place in a car, precluding use in the community, where they are most likely needed. Cost is also a consideration and may impede purchase of some devices. Insurance carriers have been reticent to provide coverage for assistive devices and may not cover devices such as the U-step walker, which has been designed for use by individuals with PD. Additionally, many devices are not useful on stairs and may even increase risk of falling on stairs. In the home, this problem can be alleviated by having a device on each level of the home so that one does not have to be carried up and down the stairs.

CASE A, PART VI

Mr. Martin benefited from the use of a cane when his balance first began to decline to improve balance and signal other people in the environment to give him more space. Once he began to experience falls, a cane wasn't sufficient to prevent the falls, and he was given an individualized therapy program and prescribed a rollator walker. It is optimal for fitness, overall health and quality of life to encourage Mr. Martin to ambulate for as long as possible. When he began to exhibit a forward propulsive gait, his walker brakes were converted to reverse brakes with good success in

decreasing his falls and improving his perceived safety. As he approached the later stages of his disease, he required assistance for ambulation, and his wife was unable to safely provide this assistance. He safely continued to walk with the Up and Go®, which is a device that partially supported his weight while walking but could also fully support his weight, during a loss of balance. It was used in the home environment to assist with ambulation while he could bear weight through his legs (Figure 15-8). The Merry Walker® is a device that provides the opportunity for upper extremity support while walking with a rolling device and additionally has a harness that provides support if the individual experiences a loss of balance. The Merry Walker is large and only feasible for use in large hallways such as are found in nursing facilities.

Fall prevention is a common goal for our clients with PD but is one that is difficult to measure and to attain. We know that appropriate therapy can reduce fall risk scores on common fall risk assessment tools,[159] and several studies have now demonstrated a reduction in fall rate but not in number of fallers.[149] Studies show that (1) there is evidence that practice of challenging balance activities, multimodal exercise, progressive strengthening, or Tai Chi reduces falls; (2) individual, facility-based exercise appears to be superior to home exercise programs;

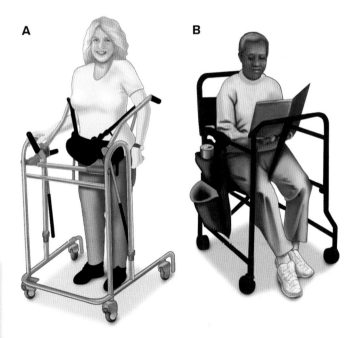

FIGURE 15-8 Walkers for assisted gait. A. Up and Go® walker partially supports body weight, via a harness and a set of gas springs, while walking but fully supports body weight, during a loss of balance. **B.** Merry Walker® provides the opportunity for upper extremity support, while walking with a rolling device that is weighted to prevent tipping and has a seat and strap, if the individual experiences a loss of balance, to prevent falls. The Merry Walker is large and only feasible for use in large hallways such as are found in nursing facilities.

(3) mobility and physical activity can be improved without increasing falls; and (4) interventions should be tailored to level of fall risk, history of falls (e.g., multiple or injurious), and presenting risk factors (e.g., cognitive impairment).[188]

Clearly, preventing falls requires individualized interventions that include balance training. Additionally, the interventions need to be based on each individual's unique impairments and situational factors. Studies that demonstrated fall reduction used an individualized and challenging balance program with or without other interventions.[149,152,189,190] Many other studies have demonstrated that increasing activity and participation in exercise do not pose an additional fall risk for this population.

Transfer training is accomplished utilizing motor learning principles of task practice on varying surfaces to optimize carryover. Individuals with PD have difficulty getting their weight forward over their feet, and thus, have increasingly more difficulty as the surface that they are transferring from is lowered. It is critical to have the patient lean forward while keeping their head up to ensure that they will get a forward weight shift with an erect spine. Bending forward with a flexed spine increases the difficulty of straightening up at the end of the transfer and can result in the person with PD becoming stuck in a flexed posture. Use of the hands on the knees can help to encourage a forward weight shift as well as providing upper extremity assist for the transfer (Figure 15-9). When going stand to sit, placing the hands on the thighs and sliding them down to the knees encourages flexion at the hips to start the transfer and helps to maintain the body mass over the feet while providing upper extremity support.

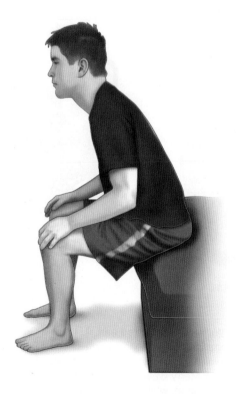

FIGURE 15-9 Sit to stand transfer with hands on knees.
Instruct the patient with PD to place their hands on their knees to encourage a forward weight shift as well as to provide upper extremity assist for coming to standing from sitting.

CASE A, PART VII

At age 80, Mr. Martin is requiring assistance with all transfers and mobility. His wife has reported a back injury from transferring him. In order to keep him at home, she is going to need assistance with transfers. She could do this by hiring round-the-clock aides, but this can be expensive. Additionally, she might be able to purchase a device to assist with transfers. There are a number of different options available. There are chairs that help lift the person up to a standing position called lift chairs (Figure 15-10A). These are good for sitting in the living room area but are not helpful in areas such as the kitchen and bathroom. For these areas, there are powered sit to stand devices or lifts that can be independently used by Mr. Martin or can assist his wife to lift him (Figure 15-10B and C). These devices are also helpful to staff in nursing facilities.

Community-Based Programs

LSVT BIG is a technique based on the Lee Silverman Voice Treatment (LSVT) that requires intensive training over 16 sessions in 1 month. The training emphasizes the use of large amplitude movements and has been shown to improve amplitude of movement, walking speed, and performance on the TUG test, and has been found to be superior to a Nordic walking program and a standard home exercise program.[191,192] The key element of the program is repetitive, task-specific practice of large amplitude movements. A shorter version of the program did not achieve equivalent results.

Nordic walking is another popular form of exercise that is often used in group exercise programs. Nordic walking is a sport-walking activity using specifically designed poles, which combines active use of the trunk and upper limbs with traditional walking. The poles are similar to those used in Nordic skiing. Several systematic reviews have been conducted with each demonstrating that Nordic walking can improve motor symptoms, balance, and gait in individuals with Parkinson's disease but it is not superior to free walking.[193–195]

Music-based movement therapy is a promising intervention that is believed to result in improved compliance due to its fun and social nature. This therapy combines cognitive, cueing, and balance strategies with a physical activity. It also uses music as an auditory cue for movement. Several forms of dance have been investigated, including partnered tango dancing and non-partnered dancing. Overall dance interventions have resulted in improved Berg balance scores, FOG, comfortable and "fast-as-you can" walking velocity.[196] Partner dancing participants expressed more enjoyment and a greater interest in continuing with the program than their non-partnered peers. A randomized controlled trial comparing tango dancing, treadmill, and stretching found no significant changes in the dance group while those in treadmill and stretching improved in gait parameters.[197]

Video games are a popular activity and have been increasingly utilized in clinical environments. When these games

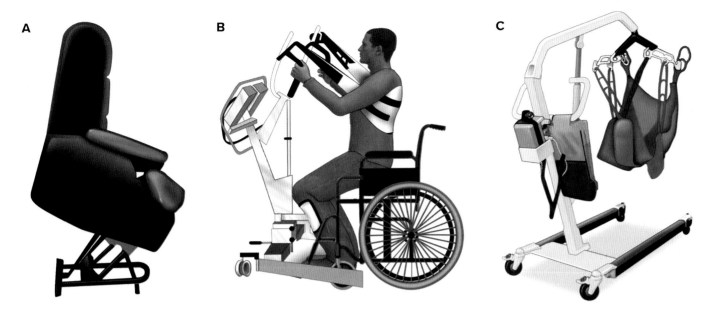

FIGURE 15-10 Devices to assist with sit–stand activities. A. Lift chair – motorized chair that slowly elevates the person to standing. **B.** Powered sit to stand device – allows person to come to standing with UE pull, harness around back to pull upward, and padded support to provide stability at calf. **C.** Full body lift device – uses a harness system for the caregiver to lift the patient to standing for transfer to bed, chair, or commode.

involve appropriate movement strategies, they can improve balance and movement in individuals with PD. Individuals with PD have poorer performance on some of the video games and have been shown to have marked learning deficits on some games but not others. The ability of individuals with PD to play video games depends on the cognitive and motor learning demands of the game, requiring the therapist to carefully analyze the game to be prescribed and each individual's ability to play each game.[198] While video games may improve compliance in some individuals due to their fun and engaging nature, they offer no additional advantages over more traditional balance training exercises.[199,200]

Writing and Hand Function

Micrographia is a common problem in individuals with PD, which has not been well studied. The standard recommendation for therapy is to practice large amplitude finger and hand movements to improve the amplitude of movement and to compensate through the use of lined paper. When using lined paper as a visual cue, individuals with PD are able to produce larger and more consistent handwriting.[201] Amplitude training improves writing size but this is at the expense of fluency.[202] Intensive motor skill learning in mild PD led to clinical improvement and altered cortical network functioning through enhancing drive to the supplementary motor area.[203]

Fitness and Wellness

Individuals with neurologic diagnoses are often more sedentary and less fit than their peers. When asked why they don't participate in community exercise programs, they report that they have low outcome expectations from exercise, lack time to exercise, and fear falling during exercise.[204] In order to improve compliance, therapists need to address these barriers. Education about the benefits of exercise and endorsements from their peers can help improve their expectations for benefit from exercise. Individualized exercise programs designed under the direction of a therapist can address the fear of falling, and if designed in partnership with the client, can address issues of time to perform exercise.

Evaluation and Treatment of Parkinson-Plus Syndromes

Vascular PD: The motor and sensory exam is based on impairments and focuses more on distal motor and sensory impairments. Treatment combines approaches for PD with those typically used for stroke rehabilitation, such as working on increasing stride length bilaterally, while also working on gait changes due to pyramidal signs such as muscular weakness or clonus (Table 11-8). Progress is typically slower than for those with either PD or CVA.

Lewy body dementia: Treatment is modified early on to accommodate for cognitive changes with a focus on teaching problem-solving and ways to manage behaviors, related to poor problem solving. Due to issues with problem-solving, there is an early focus on safety training before the cognitive issues become severe. In addition, motor learning is more severely impaired than in idiopathic PD, and therefore, therapists should employ a blocked practice schedule and avoid the use of random practice schedules. Progress will be slower than in idiopathic PD, and issues with attention will negatively impact some therapy sessions. There are very few studies examining the benefits of exercise-based interventions for Lewy body dementia but there is some evidence that exercise-based interventions lead to improvement in gait speed that exceeds the moderately important difference of 0.14 m/s.[205]

Progressive supranuclear palsy: The assessment includes an in-depth evaluation of eye movement. To assess ocular pursuit, have the client track an object up and down (vertical) and side to side (horizontal) and rate both vertical and horizontal movement using the following rating scale: (1) doesn't move to follow; (2) partial movement; or (3) complete movement. Early training should include a focus on balance activities and teaching to visually scan the environment for obstacles as well as to practice maneuvering around obstacles during gait. Gait training, balance re-education and rhythmic auditory cueing have the potential to improve balance and mobility.[206] When choosing an adaptive device, consider the need to not only provide support, during episodes of lost balance but to also provide a means to identify obstacles on the ground while also providing a means to maneuver around the obstacle. Canes are likely to allow for obstacle identification but will not prevent falls in individuals, who suffer loss of balance. Rollator walkers have been shown to provide for safe maneuvering around obstacles in both PD and HD and are, therefore, likely to work well for those with PSP.[187,207] No existing device meets all of the needs of this group of clients.

Multiple system atrophy: Since OH is prevalent and a significant problem in those with MSA, evaluation includes examination of BP during position changes. Treatment includes teaching the individual to transition slowly from supine to sit and sit to stand and to perform ankle pumps and other calf exercises before standing up. Standard physical therapy interventions should be provided based on the movement system impairments noted in each client. There is evidence from a pilot study that physical therapy followed by a home exercise program can lead to improvements in gait.[208] If coordination is impacted, include balance exercises in the treatment plan (Chapter 14, Box 14-5 and Chapter 17, Box 17-3).

Corticobasal ganglionic degeneration: Coordination is typically more severely impaired in this condition, and deficits are noted early in disease progression. A thorough evaluation of coordination is conducted, and treatment to address coordination issues is implemented immediately. Coordination treatment includes the use of balance exercises (Boxes 14-5 and 17-3) and work on coordination within function. Treatment of this disorder is challenging and requires the therapist to be flexible and creative. Table 15-2, earlier in this chapter, provides a comparison of these Parkinson-plus syndromes to idiopathic PD.

● HUNTINGTON'S DISEASE

Epidemiology

Huntington's disease (HD) affects approximately 40,000 individuals in the United States,[209] with another 200,000 at risk of developing the condition.[210] The estimated annual incidence of HD in the United States is 1.22 per 100,000 persons.[211] The onset is usually in midlife, between the ages of 30 and 50; however, about 5 to 10% of cases occur before the age of 20 (juvenile HD), and approximately 25% of cases occur after the age of 59 (late onset).[212] HD affects females and men equally and is more common in white people of Western European descent than in those of Asian or African ancestry.[213] Venezuela has the highest concentration of HD in the world, largely because of a family

that lives along the shores of Lake Maracaibo. The original progenitor of this family lived in the early 1800s and left more than 18,000 descendants.[214]

Etiology and Risk Factors

HD is caused by an autosomal dominant mutation in either of an individual's two copies of a gene called *Huntingtin*, which was mapped to chromosome 4 in 1993. The DNA nucleotide triplet of cytosine, adenine, and guanine (CAG) is repeated many more times than in the normal gene (36-125 times compared to 11-30 times in normal genes). Individuals with CAG repeats ≥40 will develop the disease, those with 36 to 39 repeats may or may not develop the disease, and those with ≤35 repeats will not develop the disease. Any child of an affected person has a 50% chance of inheriting the disease.[215]

There is a rough inverse correlation between the CAG repeat number and the age of onset of HD symptoms, such that individuals with early-onset HD tend to have longer repeat sizes. In most cases of juvenile HD the CAG repeat lengths are over 55.[216] The number of CAG repeats can expand on replication, especially in males, which accounts for the occurrence of **genetic anticipation**, in which the age of onset of HD becomes earlier in successive generations, and the likelihood of paternal inheritance is greater in children with juvenile-onset HD. New-onset cases of HD in individuals with a negative family history can arise from an expansion of the gene in the borderline or normal CAG repeat range (28-35), most often coming from the father. CAG repeat number accounts for about 60% of the variation in age of onset, with the remainder of variability due to other genes and the environment. Although CAG number does not accurately predict what symptoms an individual will have, or how severe or rapid the course of the disease will be, some data suggest that the rate of progression might be faster with longer CAG repeats, particularly for individuals with juvenile-onset disease.[217,218]

The *Huntingtin* gene produces a protein that is also called *huntingtin* (*htt*) that is normally found in all cells throughout the body. The CAG triplet repeat in the gene codes for the amino acid glutamine. An increase in the size of the CAG segment in HD leads to the production of a mutant huntingtin protein with an abnormally long polyglutamine chain. The elongated protein is cut into smaller, toxic fragments that bind together and accumulate in neurons, disrupting their normal functions and, eventually, leading to neuronal death.[217]

CASE B, PART I

WD is a 42-year-old male with HD. Onset of motor symptoms was 1 year ago, and his family notes that he has been easier to anger and clumsier for the last 3 years or so. WD's mother died of HD at age 60, after having been ill for about 20 years. WD has four siblings; his older sister has HD and an older brother has tested negative. He also has two younger brothers, one has been tested and was positive and the other has elected not to undergo genetic testing yet. WD has three children ages 16, 19, and 22. None of his children have undergone genetic testing. WD works as a pipe fitter in a local factory, and his wife works as a nurse's aide in a local nursing home. WD works day shift and his wife works 11 pm to 7 am. They live in a two-story home that they are renting with two dogs and a cat. The town they live in is small and in a very rural area.

What are the chances of WD's three children developing HD?

Answer: Because HD has an autosomal dominant inheritance pattern, each child has a 50% chance of developing the disease.

Pathophysiology

In HD, there is severe loss of neurons in the caudate and putamen nuclei of the BG. With the loss of cells, the head of the caudate becomes shrunken, and there is enlargement of the anterior horns of the lateral ventricles. Neuronal degeneration is also seen within the temporal and frontal lobes of the cerebral cortex and the Purkinje cells of the cerebellum. Early HD is characterized by loss of striatal medium spiny enkephalin/gamma-aminobutyric acid (GABA)-containing projection neurons of the indirect BG pathway. The net result is relative disinhibition of the thalamus, which in turn excites the cortex, producing **hyperkinesia**, an increase in movements. In later stages of HD, all striatal projection neurons as well as cortical neurons degenerate, resulting in a relatively **hypokinetic** state that resembles parkinsonism.[217]

Clinical Presentation

Symptoms usually evolve slowly and vary from person to person, even within the same family. Motor, cognitive, and behavioral functions can be affected. Some individuals may present with mild involuntary movements (chorea) and have more emotional/behavioral symptoms of HD while some have less emotional/behavioral symptoms with more chorea.

Motor Symptoms

Involuntary motor abnormalities in HD predominantly include **chorea** and **dystonia** (sustained muscular contractions resulting in abnormal postures or torsion movements), as described in Chapter 20 for cerebral palsy. Choreic movements initially give a person the appearance of being fidgety or restless, but as they progress, they affect the face, head, lips, tongue, and trunk, and cause flailing movements, called **ballisms**. The person with HD is often mistaken for being drunk due to the ataxic and "dancing" gait caused by chorea. Chorea in individuals with adult-onset HD initially worsens over time, but then, becomes less prominent in later stages in many with the emergence of parkinsonian symptoms (rigidity, bradykinesia). Although useful for diagnosis, chorea is a poor indicator of disease severity and typically does not interfere with functional task performance except in severe cases.[217] The most prevalent types of dystonia were reported to be internal shoulder rotation, sustained fist clenching, excessive knee flexion, and foot inversion.

Other involuntary movements that people with HD may display are **tics** (sudden, repetitive, nonrhythmic motor movement or vocalization, involving discrete muscle groups), **myoclonus** (brief, shock-like muscle contractions), and **tremors,** which may be present at rest, with posture, or with voluntary movements. Myoclonus and tremors are much more common in children and young adults with HD.[219]

Voluntary motor impairments that impede performance of daily activities include bradykinesia and akinesia, as seen in PD, as well as **apraxia** (loss or impairment of the ability to execute complex coordinated movements without muscular or sensory impairment), **motor impersistence** (inability to maintain a voluntary muscle contraction at a constant level), diminished rapid alternating movements, and difficulties performing sequences of movements. Motor impersistence manifests as frequent dropping of objects and a "milkmaid's grip" during handshakes (alternating contraction and relaxation of the grip), an inability to hold the eyes closed, incomplete chewing, and inconsistent driving speeds. Motor impersistence is independent of chorea and is linearly progressive, making it a possible marker of disease severity.[217]

Musculoskeletal impairments in muscle performance, posture, and tone also occur in HD. Overall muscle strength is not initially a problem in HD, but strength can be diminished as the disease progresses, even before a loss of functional ability is apparent.[220] It is not known whether muscle weakness is a primary impairment of the disease process or secondary to decreased mobility and disuse atrophy. Studies in symptomatic individuals with HD and asymptomatic mutation carriers found delayed recovery of ATP levels in muscles after exercise due to mitochondrial dysfunction and abnormal staining for huntingtin in skeletal muscles, which may contribute to muscle weakness in HD.[221] Muscle tightness and postural changes may develop in people with HD due to poor postural habits, dystonic posturing, and immobility. In sitting, individuals with HD tend to adopt a slouched position with excessive thoracic kyphosis and posterior pelvic tilt. In later stages, patients often assume a more massed flexion posture. Deep tendon reflexes may be increased in HD. People with chorea may exhibit "**hung-up**" reflexes, in which after the tendon is tapped and the reflex action takes place, the limb slowly, rather than quickly, returns to its neutral position.

Motor impairments can negatively impact functional task performance. Hand dexterity and fine motor skills (e.g., finger tapping skills) are often impaired early in the disease and result in problems with writing, dressing, cutting food, and handling utensils.[220,222,223] Gait and balance disturbances can lead to falls. Gait impairments begin early in HD and typically include slower gait speed, shorter and more variable stride length, a wider base of support, increased double support time, and increased trunk sway.[53,207,224] Balance deficits begin in the premanifest stage and worsen in the manifest stage.[225] Individuals with manifest HD demonstrate postural control deficits characterized by greater sway than persons without HD during eyes open in sitting and standing with a normal base of support,[226] and reduced limits of stability during multidirectional leans in standing.[227] In conditions where vision or proprioception is reduced, individuals with manifest HD demonstrated greater postural instability than controls, with greatest deficits when proprioception was attenuated such as standing on foam with the eyes open or closed. Postural deficits were detected when standing on foam with eyes closed in people with premanifest HD. Gaze fixation on a visual target improved postural stability in individuals with premanifest HD, but not in individuals with manifest HD.[228] Greater postural sway with narrowing of the base of support or with reduction or visual or proprioceptive inputs causes difficulties with tandem standing, single leg stance, and walking and standing with eyes closed.[229,230] When taking a self-initiated step, people with manifest HD demonstrated impaired APAs characterized by slower, shorter, and smaller movements of the center of mass. Use of an external auditory cue improved gait initiation in people with manifest HD.[231] Motor responses to unexpected balance disturbances are delayed, which can lead to falls.[230] Exaggerated movements, due to problems with force modulation control, may cause people with HD to lose their balance by reaching outside of their base of support or by vaulting up from a chair or out of bed. Problems with eccentric motor control can also cause falls, when people with HD sit down or descend stairs.

Speech and Swallowing Impairments

Speech disorders and dysphagia are symptoms of HD that develop over time. Individuals with HD demonstrate impaired speech performance characterized by abnormal articulation (production of speech sounds) and prosody (pitch, loudness, tempo, and rhythm in speech), a reduced speech rate with increased numbers of speech pauses, and marked difficulties with steadily repeating single syllables (e.g., /pa/, /ta/).[232] Studies of dysphagia, in individuals with HD with chorea, have shown numerous abnormalities, during all phases of ingestion: (1) oral phase – postural instability, hyperextension of the head and trunk, rapid and impulsive consumption of food, poor tongue control, uncoordinated swallow, repetitive swallow, and residual food remaining after the swallow; (2) pharyngeal phase – coughing, choking, and aspiration; and (3) esophageal phase – diaphragmatic chorea, slowed esophageal motility, and reflux.[233,234] The risk of aspiration is higher if the person engages in conversation while eating, due to exposure of the airway to food, when the vocal cords are open. Individuals with HD with rigidity and bradykinesia show mandibular rigidity, slow tongue chorea, delayed tongue transfer of food, prolonged swallow latency, and choking and coughing during meals.[234] Therapists should refer individuals with speech disorders and dysphagia to a speech-language pathologist for evaluation and treatment.

Motor Learning

Like individuals with PD, individuals with HD show deficits in motor sequence learning and speed-accuracy motor skill learning, presumably due to damage of frontostriatal circuits.[68] Some evidence suggests that explicit (conscious) motor sequence learning is impaired earlier (i.e., in premanifest stages) than implicit (unconscious) motor sequence learning, suggesting that explicit motor learning measures may be useful biomarkers of HD.[235,236] A study that examined the effects of motor imagery training on copying two Chinese letters twice in each of five sizes found that non-demented individuals with HD demonstrated

a significant improvement in movement isochrony (increased speed with greater amplitude of movement), following the motor imagery training, that was not demonstrated in non-demented individuals with PD, suggesting that motor imagery is less affected in individuals with HD than those with PD and may enhance motor skill learning in this population.[237]

Cognitive Symptoms

Cognitive problems in individuals with HD occur early in the disease and include impaired perception of time, decreased speed of processing, impaired visuospatial perception, short-term memory decline, and executive function deficits.[238] In later stages, the cognitive deficits progress to global dementia. People with HD have problems estimating time early in the disease process, with their spouses often complaining that their once-punctual spouse is frequently late and underestimates how long a task will take to complete. The speed of thinking and performance of motor skills such as finger tapping is slowed, making completion of ordinary cognitive and motor tasks tiring. Impaired visuospatial processing results in reduced awareness of body space and the environment and can lead to frequent bumping into objects. Individuals with HD have difficulties with learning new information and retrieving previously learned information, but in general, long-term memory is spared.[236] Executive functions are impaired, such as attention, planning, problem-solving, decision making, sequencing, adapting to change, and cognitive flexibility (ability to switch between two different thoughts, and to think about multiple concepts simultaneously), all of which impede the acquisition of new motor skills. Individuals with HD often report difficulty with "multitasking," and studies have reported impaired dual-task performance, especially when a cognitive load is added to a motor task, in individuals with premanifest and manifest HD.[239-241] Dual-task impairment was moderately correlated with a number of prospective falls in individuals with early-mid stage HD. Notably, individuals with HD lack awareness of their own actions and feelings, often overestimating their competency in behavioral and emotional control and performance of activities of daily living.[240,242] Speech declines more rapidly than comprehension, although individuals with HD show difficulties with initiating conversations and comprehending what's heard and said, during conversations, due to slow cognitive processing.[238]

Emotional/Behavioral Symptoms

Emotional and behavioral symptoms are very frequently present in the early stage of the disease, often prior to the onset of motor symptoms. These symptoms not only negatively impact the person with HD's daily life, but they also adversely affect the person's family. Emotional and behavioral disturbances that are common in HD include depression, anxiety, apathy, irritability, disinhibition, impulsivity, obsessions, and perseveration.[243] **Depression** is the most common symptom and is difficult to diagnose because weight loss, apathy, and inactivity are also features of HD. Depression is usually associated with feelings of low self-esteem, guilt, and **anxiety**, which often occurs in relation to uncertainty about the start and/or the course of the disease. **Apathy** manifests as loss of energy and initiative, poor perseverance and quality of work, passive behavior, impaired judgment, poor self-care, and emotional blunting; it can be difficult to discriminate from depression. Apathy is related to disease stage, whereas depression and anxiety are not. **Irritability** is often the very first sign of HD, and its expression varies from rude or hurtful comments to serious disputes and physical aggression. People with HD with **disinhibition** and **impulsivity** may develop problem behaviors such as irritability, temper outbursts, sexual promiscuity, and acting without thinking. Individuals with obsessions and **perseveration** become "stuck" on one idea or activity, making it difficult for them to change from one activity or idea to another or to deal with changes in routines. Other emotional/behavioral conditions found in individuals with HD are mania, bipolar disorders, and obsessive–compulsive disorders. Psychosis may occur in the later stages of the disease with delusions, paranoia, and hallucinations being the most frequent symptoms.[243] Sexual problems in HD are most commonly hypoactive sexual drive and inhibited orgasm, but hypersexuality can cause considerable problems in some individuals. The suicide rate for individuals with HD is estimated to be about 5 to 10 times greater than that of the general population (about 5–10%)[217] and occurs most frequently in premanifest gene carriers and early symptomatic individuals, especially around the time of gene testing or when independence diminishes.

Sleep Disturbances

Many individuals with HD experience insomnia. Electroencephalogram (EEG) studies have shown that individuals with HD show impaired initiation and maintenance of sleep, spend more time in non-rapid eye movement (NREM) sleep and less time in REM sleep, and have reduced total sleep time compared to controls. Individuals with HD also show increased awakenings, after sleep onset. The causes of insomnia may include depression and apathy, lack of daytime stimulation, disruptions of the sleep–wake cycle, medications, and involuntary movements.[244] Although choreic movements in HD tend to lessen during sleep, they may interfere with falling asleep or going back to sleep after a nighttime awakening. Poor sleep hygiene results in increased daytime somnolence. Apathetic individuals with HD often sleep excessively or spend large amounts of time in bed. Sleep studies are recommended for individuals with sleep problems.[244]

Sensory Disturbances

Individuals with HD can experience musculoskeletal pain from dystonia, muscle imbalances, immobility, and injuries from falls or uncontrolled limb movements, which can cause a person to accidentally hit objects. There are some reports of people in late stages of HD with severe "central" pain presumably due to deafferentation from the disease process. Abnormalities in skin sensations have been reported in individuals in the later stages of HD, apparently due to disturbances in cortical processing of somatosensory information (deafferentation).[245] Studies that examined proprioceptive sensory function in people with HD found some deficits, but the extent to which these deficits affect active movements is unknown.[246] Patients with HD have eye movement abnormalities including delayed initiation of movements, slowed saccadic movements, and jerky smooth pursuit movements that begin early in the disease and may affect balance and walking performance.[247] In advanced stages, individuals may use head movements to initiate eye movement.

Individuals with HD are able to detect smells, but have difficulty with identifying what smells are.[238]

Cardiovascular and Respiratory Function

Abnormalities in metabolic and physiologic responses to aerobic exercise have been reported in individuals with HD. Maximal exercise testing, using a cycle ergometer, of symptomatic individuals with HD found a normal cardiopulmonary response, with normal cardiac output and ventilation, but a reduced work capacity, lower anaerobic threshold (AT), and earlier increase in blood lactate compared to healthy controls.[248] During a submaximal aerobic exercise test, individuals with symptomatic HD did not achieve a steady-state HR, during the first phase of the cycling test with no resistance, and some individuals demonstrated a lower AT and were working anaerobically during the test.[249] Lower work capacity at a given HR may be due to reduced muscle strength or cardiorespiratory fitness levels, while the lower AT is hypothesized to be due to mitochondrial dysfunction or reduced capacity for gluconeogenesis in skeletal muscles of people with HD.[248,249]

Inactivity may lead to decreased cardiovascular endurance due to deconditioning in people with HD. Studies that investigated daytime activity levels, using activity monitors, reported significantly lower motor activity levels in people with HD compared to healthy controls[246] and significantly lower daily step counts in people with HD, who were recurrent fallers, compared to those who were non-fallers.[247] Lower daily activity levels were related to impaired voluntary movements, balance and gait disturbances, and reduced functional capacity.[250,251]

Respiratory function impairments may contribute to decreased endurance. People with HD exhibit obstructive and restrictive disorders of the respiratory system,[252] and the degree of pulmonary dysfunction is associated with motor symptom severity. However, most people do not report respiratory symptoms until later stages of the disease, presumably due to the adoption of a sedentary lifestyle. Pulmonary infections may contribute to morbidity and mortality in individuals with HD.[253]

Falls

Falls are common in people with HD and often occur while the person is performing multiple tasks simultaneously, maneuvering around obstacles on the floor, turning, or climbing stairs.[224,252] Many factors likely contribute to falls, including involuntary movements (i.e., chorea, dystonia), voluntary movement impairments (bradykinesia, impaired force modulation, and eccentric motor control), musculoskeletal impairments (decreased muscle strength and endurance, poor posture), balance problems, gait impairments (especially bradykinesia, stride variability, and excessive trunk sway), cognitive deficits (decreased attention and ability to dual-task), behavioral changes (impulsiveness, impaired judgment leading to unsafe behaviors), visual disturbances, and visuospatial deficits.[254]

Weight Loss

Many individuals with HD experience considerable weight loss throughout all stages of the disease.[255,256] While the causes of weight loss are not well understood, multiple factors including dementia, depression, chewing and swallowing difficulties, orodental problems, motor disturbances, muscle atrophy from decreased activity, inadequate access to food, and side effects of medications have been found to contribute to weight loss in this population.[257] Referral to a dietician for nutritional counseling is advised for individuals with excessive weight loss.

Juvenile HD

Individuals with juvenile HD develop the same triad of motor, cognitive, and behavioral disturbances as in adult-onset HD, but there are some distinct differences in the symptomatology. The most common presenting features of juvenile HD in the first decade of life are voluntary motor disturbances (i.e., slow, shuffling gait, rigidity of limbs or trunk, tremors, slowed speech, swallowing problems, and drooling), cognitive deficits, behavioral disturbance, and seizures. Unlike adults who typically present with involuntary motor disturbances, chorea is uncommon in children with HD. Behavioral disturbances requiring medical or legal intervention or poor school performance may be the first symptom in an adolescent. Some children develop ataxia and other cerebellar signs and severe dystonia in later stages. Slowed saccadic eye movements with compensatory jerking of the head to look to the side is common. Seizures, usually of a generalized or myoclonic type, affect up to 25% of children.[257,258]

CASE B, PART II

WD does not return to the clinic for 2 years, at which time he has marked deterioration in gait and balance; plus, his wife reports that he has been fired from his work for behavioral issues as well as difficulty performing his job. WD states that he feels he was fine at work and expresses anger at being wrongly let go. When asked what he does during the day, he says that he watches TV. His wife reports that he is up at night, while she is at work, and that he tends to get on the computer or watch TV. During the day, when he is supposed to be taking care of the dog and doing household chores, he is sleeping. She must either stay awake or frequently wake up to perform childcare duties and is experiencing high levels of fatigue. She also worries that he is going to fall and hurt himself, especially since he's beginning to have difficulty going up stairs, where he seems to catch his toe and trip.

What could be causing WD to trip on the stairs?

Answer: Factors that may be contributing to WD's tripping on stairs could include chorea, dystonia, bradykinesia, incoordination, lower extremity muscle weakness, anticipatory and dynamic balance problems, visual and visuospatial processing deficits, attention deficits and problems with dual-tasking, and going too fast due to impulsivity.

What could be causing WD's sleep to be disturbed?

Answer: WD's sleep might be disturbed by his chorea, depression and apathy, lack of daytime stimulation, and possibly disruptions of his sleep–wake cycle.

Diagnosis

Genetic testing can determine whether a person carries the HD gene. People with a positive test result risk losing health and life insurance as well as employment, which contributes to their psychological distress. For these reasons and because there is no cure for the disease, the majority of individuals "at risk" decide not to take the test. Those who undergo testing generally do so to assist in making career and family choices. Current protocols for genetic testing are designed to exclude testing for children or those with suicidal ideation, encourage genetic counseling prior to taking a blood sample for genetic analysis, inform individuals of the implications of test results for relatives, identify subsequent sources of support, and protect confidentiality.[259]

If there is a positive family history of HD, the presence of the typical motor signs and symptoms of HD are usually enough to confirm a diagnosis. A positive genetic test is cost effective and provides confirmation for individuals who have developed symptomatology consistent with HD, with or without a family history. Routine MRI and CT scans in middle to late stages of HD show a loss of striatal volume and increased size of the frontal horns of the lateral ventricles, but scans are usually unhelpful for diagnosis of HD in early stages. Functional neuroimaging (PET and functional MRI) can detect striatal atrophy in affected brains as much as 11 years before symptom onset and may be useful in diagnosing and tracking the progression of the disease.[217]

Clinical Course

The clinical course of HD can be divided into four approximate stages: premanifest, early, middle, and late. The **premanifest** stage consists of a healthy period, when the person has no detectable clinical abnormalities, and a **prodromal** phase, when individuals may show subtle changes in personality, cognition, and motor control. Once individuals with HD have symptoms that are sufficiently developed for diagnosis, they are classified into early, middle, and late stages, based on their Total Functional Capacity (TFC) score (Table 15-9).[260,261] The TFC is a 14-point scale that measures disability and participation restrictions in important life skills (work = 3 points, financial management = 3 points, family responsibilities/chores = 2 points) and activities of daily living (3 points), including where care is provided (home versus extended care facility: 3 points).[261]

The disease usually progresses slowly with an average lifespan of 10–20 years, after onset of symptoms. Progression of the disease tends to be more rapid in those diagnosed at an earlier age. Most people with HD die from complications of falls, malnourishment, infections, or pneumonia. The typical progression of symptoms across disease stages is shown in Table 15-5.

The Unified Huntington's Disease Rating Scale (UHDRS) is the standard assessment tool used to quantify disease severity and to track symptom changes over time.[264,265] It was developed as a clinical rating scale to assess four domains of clinical performance and capacity in individuals with HD: motor function, cognitive function, behavioral abnormalities, and functional capacity. The motor portion of the UHDRS includes 15 items each rated on a 0 to 4 scale (0 = normal). Scores can be calculated

TABLE 15-9	Total Functional Capacity Staging in Huntington's Disease[260]	
STAGE	**TFC SCORES**	**DESCRIPTION**
Stage I (early)	11-13	No limitations in any area
Stage II (middle)	7-10	Some problems with work and financial capacity but still able to meet responsibilities at home and complete all ADLs
Stage III (middle)	3-6	Limited work ability, needs assistance with finances and home responsibilities; some difficulty with ADLs but still living at home.
Stage IV (late)	1-2	No longer working or able to take care of finances or home chores; increased difficulty with ADLs and may no longer be living at home.
Stage V (late)	0	Requires a total care facility and is unable to care for self

CASE B, PART III

Eight years late, WD arrives at the clinic in a poorly fitted wheelchair with his wife and child. They report that they transfer him by "standing him up and turning him" and that he only walks when they walk him hand in hand with two-person assist. The patient's TFC score is 2.

Question: What stage of the disease is WD in?

Answer: WD is in Stage IV (late stage) of the disease according to his TFC score. His main mobility is a wheelchair and he is no longer able to perform ADLs without assistance.

Medical Management

Drug therapy in HD is directed toward motor, cognitive, and emotional/behavioral symptom management. Typical medications used for symptom management are summarized in Table 15-10.[216,262,263] Therapists should be aware of the medications that individuals with HD are taking and any potential side effects. Deep brain stimulation of the globus pallidus internal segment, but not the subthalamic nucleus, has shown some efficacy in treating medically refractory chorea.[216] Ribonucleic acid (RNA)-based and deoxyribonucleic (DNA)-based therapies using antisense oligonucleotides (i.e., short sequences of single stranded DNA) or RNA interference (i.e., double stranded RNA sequences) that target and interfere with the production pathway of the neurotoxic huntingtin protein are being developed and tested in clinical trials and may provide both symptomatic and disease-modifying treatment in HD.[216] Counseling can be helpful for affected individuals, their spouses, and individuals at risk for HD. Although few individuals take advantage of predictive or prenatal genetic testing, individuals with HD can benefit from frank discussions with health care professionals about family, financial, and career planning. Support groups are invaluable sources of information and insight that can help affected individuals and families deal with the difficulties of HD.

by summing questions from each section with higher scores indicating greater impairment. It has high reliability and validity[258]; however, it is intended to be performed only after training and certification to administer the different components of the test.

TABLE 15-10	Medications Used to Treat HD[216,262,263]	
SUBCLASS OF DRUG	**EXAMPLE MEDICATIONS**	**POTENTIAL SIDE EFFECTS**
Antichoreic Drugs		
Dopamine-depleting medication	Tetrabenazine (Xenazine); Deutetrabenazine (Austedo)	Depression, extrapyramidal symptoms, drowsiness, akathesia
Antidepressants (used for depression, irritability, and anxiety)		
Selective serotonin reuptake inhibitors (SSRI)	Fluoxetine (Prozac), Citalopram (Celexa), Sertraline (Zoloft), Paroxetine (Paxil)	Insomnia, gastrointestinal upset, restlessness, weight loss, dry mouth, anxiety, headache
Serotonin and norepinephrine reuptake inhibitors (SNRI)	Venlafaxine (Effexor XP), Duloxitine (Cymbalta)	Same as SSRIs
Antipsychotics (used for psychosis and sometimes for irritability or for chorea suppression)		
Atypical antipsychotics	Risperidone (Risperdal), Olanzapine (Zyprexa), Aripiprazole (Abilify), Quetiapine (Seroquel),	Extrapyramidal symptoms, drowsiness, akathesia

Physical Therapy Evaluation

Assessment of HD includes a standard neurologic assessment with the addition of chorea, eye movement, and motor testing. Eye movement and chorea are assessed using the UHDRS scale or the scale in Table 15-11. Chorea is observed while the individual sits quietly and during walking. The therapist observes all four extremities, the face, neck, and trunk.

Motor impersistence is measured on the UHDRS by having the individual stick out their tongue and document the ability to (1) fully protrude the tongue and (2) keep it out for 10 seconds. It is also important to assess for signs of motor impersistence during functional activities such as holding onto an object. This can be done by having the individual hold an object and walk; observe to see if they drop the object or change their gait pattern. Another method is to have the individual hold onto an object while talking so that they aren't looking at their hand to see whether they drop the object. Additionally, the presence of motor impersistence can negatively impact some assessment techniques. Manual muscle tests (MMT) require that the person being tested hold an isometric contraction. In anyone with HD, failure to hold the isometric muscle contraction could be due to motor impersistence rather than inability of the muscle to develop and sustain contractile force. Therapists need to be aware of the presence of motor impersistence and its severity when interpreting manual muscle test grades. It may be helpful to combine the MMT with observation of strength during function. Also, some outcome measures require that the person perform balance or coordination activities with the eyes closed, which is difficult for someone with HD to maintain due to impersistence.

TABLE 15-11	Suggested Rating Scale for Impairments Unique to HD		
Ocular Pursuit (ability of the eyes to follow an object up and down [vertical] and side to side [horizontal])			
Vertical		Horizontal	
• Doesn't move to follow • Partial movement • Completes movement		• Doesn't move to follow • Partial movement • Completes movement	
Chorea			
Upper Extremities			
Right		Left	
• Absent • Intermittent • Constant	• Mild (small movements, do not impede function) • Moderate (small- to medium-sized motions, may impede function) • Marked (medium to large size motions and impedes function)	• Absent • Intermittent • Constant	• Mild (small movements, do not impede function) • Moderate (small- to medium-sized motions, may impede function) • Marked (medium to large size motions and impedes function)
Lower Extremities			
Right		Left	
• Absent • Intermittent • Constant •	• Mild (small movements, do not impede function) • Moderate (small- to medium-sized motions, may impede function) • Marked (medium to large size motions and impedes function)	• Absent • Intermittent • Constant	• Mild (small movements, do not impede function) • Moderate (small- to medium-sized motions, may impede function) • Marked (medium to large size motions and impedes function)
Trunk			
• Absent • Intermittent • Constant	• Mild (small movements, do not impede function) • Moderate (small- to medium-sized motions, may impede function) • Marked (medium to large size motions and impedes function)		
Face			
• Absent • Intermittent • Constant	• Mild (small movements, do not impede function) • Moderate (small- to medium-sized motions, may impede function) • Marked (medium to large size motions and impedes function)		

CASE B, PART IV

When WD started to present with symptoms, as described in Part I, he is referred for physical therapy evaluation. At his first visit, a full neurologic assessment including eye movement and chorea measures is completed. He is asked to follow a pen in the examiner's hand with his eyes both in vertical and horizontal positions and has complete movement in both directions. The examiner observes all four extremities, the trunk, neck, and face, while he is sitting and when he walks, to rate his chorea. He has absent movement in the right arm and leg with constant mild movement in the face and intermittent mild movement in the trunk and the left arm and leg. The chorea remains evident during walking. On examination, using the UHDRS, WD holds out his tongue but pulls it back in, after only 8 seconds. Given the presence of early motor impersistence, the results of the MMT may be inaccurate, but WD is able to achieve normal scores in all four extremities for all major muscle groups. If he were to have any difficulty, the therapist would complete a functional examination of strength during activities that are important to WD, such as observing his ability to do sit to stand 5 times.

Individuals with HD have progressively more difficulty keeping their eyes closed on command due to motor impersistence. Verbal reminders can help them to keep their eyes closed. Testing a person with a blindfold is not the same as doing so with eyes closed and should not be substituted for the eyes closed condition. The neural system regulates according to whether or not the individual is trying to use vision, and therefore, it is important to ensure that vision is truly obscured, when testing balance without vision, and that vision is available but inaccurate when testing how well the system integrates sensory cues for balance.[266]

CASE B, PART V

For WD, at his initial PT visit, there should be some determination of how his chorea, behavior, and cognition might be impacting his work. Since lack of insight is a common early symptom of HD, it is important to be detailed in the interview and to get family input, whenever possible. WD states that work is fine, but his wife reports that he has been disciplined twice in the last 6 months, once for poor work and once for an inappropriate verbal interaction with his supervisor. WD is referred to a social worker for counseling on impulse control and issues that may arise, when he experiences stress at work. Therapy further assesses WD's fine motor control and makes a referral to occupational therapy, as the work-related issues, at this time, are related to declines in hand function. In addition, he is questioned in depth about his job requirements related to the need to walk in narrow spaces or on elevated surfaces. He does have to walk on catwalks, and this may become a safety issue in the near future. At this time, his therapy assessment shows that he can walk heel-toe without any stumbles, and his score on the Berg Balance Scale is 53, indicating that he is likely to be safe to continue with his activities at work. The therapist provides him with a home exercise program with an emphasis on balance activities, involving narrowed stances. He is also encouraged to take up an activity that would improve overall fitness and provide him with stretching and relaxation.

Chorea is measured and documented objectively using the rating scale from Table 15-11. This allows for communication with the physician and close monitoring of the progression of the chorea. When chorea interferes with function, the therapist communicates with the neurologist to assist in the initiation of pharmacological management. While chorea is quite visible and can lead to declines in function, gait and balance deficits do not decline in parallel to the progression of chorea.[267] Rather than basing decisions about ambulation safety on visualization of chorea, a thorough and standardized assessment of gait and balance should be conducted to determine fall risk and provide a basis for safety recommendations. Outcome measures for fall risk screening that are reliable and valid in HD include the TMT and BBS.[268] Box 15-3 Lists recommended and suggested outcome measures for use in Huntington's disease.[269]

Box 15-3 Outcome Measure Recommendations in Huntington's Disease[269]

Domain and Outcome Measures

Exercise capacity and/or physical capacity

    Recommended:
        *6 Minute Walk Test

    Suggested:
        International Physical Activity Questionnaire

Mobility and Function:

    Recommended:
        Tinetti Mobility Test

    Suggested:
        *10 Meter Walk Test
        Timed Up and Go

Balance and Falls Risk:

    Recommended:
        *Berg Balance Scale

    Suggested:
        Six-Condition Romberg Test
        Mini Balance Evaluation Systems Test
        *Activity-Specific Balance Scale
        Four Square Step Test

Respiratory Function

    Recommended:
        *6 Minute Walk Test

Secondary Musculoskeletal and Postural Changes

Recommended:
  Tinetti Mobility Test
  *Berg Balance Scale
  SF-36

Suggested:
  Physical Performance Test
  Timed Up and Go
  HD Quality of Life
  HD Quality of Life Caregiver
  Goal Attainment Scale

End Stage

Recommended:
  SF-36

Suggested:
  HD Quality of Life
  HD Quality of Life Caregiver
  Goal Attainment Scale

CASE B, PART VI

Two years later at WD's next clinic visit (Case Study, Part II), WD is exhibiting significant functional loss along with changes in participation and in mood. A more thorough evaluation is warranted along with focused interdisciplinary care. WD now has a TMT score of 18 and a BBS of 47 and his 10 MWT indicates a walking velocity of .7 m/s. His ability to transfer and ambulate has declined. Balance, as measured by the BBS, is impaired. Single limb stance time is now <5 seconds bilateral.

Question: Is WD at high risk of falling? And if he is, what is the basis of your conclusion?

WD is at high risk of falling based on his Tinetti score of 18, which is below the established cutoff of 21[270] but not based on his BBS score of 47. In Huntington's disease the cutoff for high fall risk is a 40 on the BBS.[271] He has impaired balance based on his BBS and single leg stance time. Given his overall impaired balance and high risk based on the Tinetti, WD is at high risk of falling.

It is quite common for individuals with HD to exhibit significant deficits in single limb stance ability early in the disease process, which has implications for their ability to ambulate on uneven surfaces and to ascend and descend curbs and steps. Individuals with HD report that the majority of their falls occur while dual-tasking, avoiding an obstacle on the floor, or when ascending and descending stairs, indicating a need to thoroughly assess these domains.[224] Stair assessment may be completed by timing how long it takes to ascend and descend a flight of stairs. This method does not provide any information about safety or biomechanics of climbing. There is a tool for stair assessment, the Step Test Evaluation of Performance on Stairs (STEPS), that has been validated in Huntington's disease and older adults.[272] It can be found here:

go.osu.edu/STEPStool. The STEPS tool allows the therapist to better identify specific areas that are problematic, and therefore, better design appropriate intervention to improve safety on stairs. One example would be that many clients with HD do not use the handrail for safety even though they repeatedly fall on stairs. In addition to working on balance training, the therapist may also train the individual with HD to use the stair rail.

MANAGING THE CLIENT WITH HUNTINGTON'S DISEASE

Based on the findings, described in Part VI, WD needs social work for assistance in dealing with his job-related issues; since he has been fired from his job, he likely needs assistance to find a new job that is more appropriate, such as stocking shelves or bagging groceries. The physical therapy assessment reveals a walking velocity of .7 m/s, BBS score of 47/56, inability to

---

Box 15-4   Summary of Clinical Recommendations to Guide Physical Therapy Practice in Huntington's Disease[207,274–279]

Action Statements

1. Physical therapists should prescribe aerobic exercise (moderate intensity, 55–90% HR maximum) paired with upper and lower body strengthening 3 times per week for a minimum of 12 weeks to improve fitness and to stabilize or improve motor function (recommendation strength: strong).

2. Physical therapists should prescribe one-on-one supervised gait training to improve spatiotemporal measures of gait (e.g., walking speed and step length) (recommendation strength: strong).

3. Physical therapists may prescribe individualized exercises, including balance exercises, delivered at a moderate frequency and intensity to improve balance and balance confidence (recommendation strength: weak).

4. Physical therapists may provide breathing exercises, including inspiratory and expiratory training, to improve respiratory muscle strength and cough effectiveness (recommendation strength: weak).

5. Physical therapists may prescribe an individually tailored program to improve postural control and may use positioning devices to optimize posture (recommendation strength: weak).

6. Physical therapists should ensure that care plans for individuals with HD with late-stage disease include appropriate positioning and seating, active movement, position, respiratory exercise, and education. Family and caregiver training to provide strategies for maintaining appropriate ongoing activity and participation for as long as possible is an important focus for the physical therapy team as part of late-stage care (recommendation strength: expert opinion).

walk heel-toe or perform single limb stance and a TMT score of 18, indicating he is at high risk of falls and walking quite slowly. At this time, he would benefit from a formal physical therapy program. Evidence for physical therapy in HD has been summarized in a clinical practice guideline based on a thorough review of the literature.[273] A summary of the recommendations is provided in Box 15-4 Interventions that have been studied include aerobic training with stationary bike, gym-based exercise program, dance using a videogame platform, multidisciplinary rehabilitation, and use of different assistive devices.[207,274–279] Areas to be addressed with therapy are determined based on identified impairments and functional losses; then, therapy is modified, based on the unique features of HD, such as chorea, cognitive changes, apathy, and dystonia. Methods of treatment are typically based on those used for PD and modified based on the unique characteristics of HD. The evidence for treatment efficacy for these methods such as strength training and treadmill walking is still evolving in HD, but given that it is also a result of damage to the BG, as is PD, similar treatment methods may be a good starting point for treatment planning.

In HD, apathy and lack of insight into their own deficits negatively impact participation in activity and exercise programs. Apathy leads individuals with HD to lead a very sedentary lifestyle and withdraw from social activities that they previously enjoyed. It also has a negative impact on participation in community and physical therapy exercising. Apathy is best overcome through individualized rewards and setting up a daily schedule with short bouts of exercise/activity.

CASE B, PART VII

By his return to therapy after 2 years (part II), WD is very inactive and is showing signs of apathy, so his care plan includes 10 minutes of exercise daily with his wife or 16-year-old child at 3:00 in the afternoon. The use of a set, daily schedule improves compliance and minimizes arguments. WD also lacks insight into his impairments and functional losses. The therapist focuses on introducing an exercise that WD has done in the past and tells WD that it is good for his "HD" rather than trying to get him to recognize that his balance is poor and his walking is unsafe. When appropriate, concrete feedback, regarding WD's impairments, may be helpful in developing some insight into his limitations. For example, if he trips during therapy, the therapist should immediately point out that he lost his footing and instruct him that his therapy/exercise program will help him walk without losing his footing. Individuals with HD may also be limited in their ability to maintain or transfer this insight into new situations, due to their cognitive losses. In this situation, safety measures need to be taken to remove WD from unsafe situations and modify his environment(s) to provide improved safety.

Bodily Functions

Range of Motion and Stretching

These interventions would be the same as outlined previously in this chapter under PD.

Transfers

Individuals with HD tend to keep their weight shifted posterior, when going sit to stand. They remain in a relatively extended posture, while shifting their weight posterior, when they go stand to sit, resulting in a fall into the seat. Additionally, they start to sit before they are aligned with the surface they plan to sit on. One method to encourage forward weight shift during transfers is to instruct the individual to place their hands on their thighs and push down through their legs, while going sit to stand and when going stand to sit, as described for PD (Figure 15-6). By doing this, the individual is forced to flex at the hips, keeping the center of mass aligned over the feet. In addition, it provides appropriate upper extremity support that facilitates, rather than hampers, proper body mechanics. Cueing with simple three-step instructions is used to encourage the individual to walk to the chair and turn, before lowering themselves onto the seat. Instruct the individual with HD to think and say "turn," "touch chair," and "now hands on legs and sit." Blocked practice of this task with many repetitions has been an effective way of teaching this transfer in our movement disorders clinic.

For those individuals who use an assistive device and cannot remember the cues, a cue card can be made and taped to the seat of their rollator walker. Caregivers are instructed to use a gait belt and to assist, by providing assistance at the hips. If chorea of the upper extremities is impeding caregivers during a transfer, the chorea can be minimized by instructing the individual with HD to "hug themselves."

Gait

Gait training is conducted, based on the impairments noted, and uses the techniques discussed in the PD section of this chapter. Research on walking devices and HD indicate that the rollator walker leads to the safest and smoothest gait.[207] As in PD, the rollator walker minimizes dual-task demands and provides a consistent source of stabilization, during turns. It is also easier to maneuver in small spaces.

Stairs

For individuals, who are still attempting curbs or stairs, the therapist should conduct a stair safety assessment. Individuals with HD report falls on stairs, while ascending and descending. They express that they have difficulty with foot placement. Observation of individuals with HD on stairs reveals a tendency to trip, while going up stairs, and to have uneven and unsafe foot placement, when going down stairs. Despite stating that they have fallen on stairs and knowing that they are not safe on stairs, individuals with HD continue to descend stairs rapidly without stopping at the top of the stairs and may not use a railing, even when it is present and needed. The stair assessment, using the STEPS tool, provides the therapist with information regarding specific deficits on stairs. Therapy at this stage focuses on teaching the individual to (1) stop, before starting the stairs and think about how to use the stairs safely; (2) grab the handrail; and (3) then, begin to ascend or descend. It is best to teach the caregiver and person with HD to use the simple cue "Stop, Think, Handrail" before ascending or descending stairs. The individual with HD may also need to be taught to go slowly when descending the stairs. In the middle and late stages of the disease, the individual with HD has impaired short-term memory and cognition, resulting in an inability to cognitively learn the rules for safe stair use. They do remain able to motor learn and to learn new habits through repetition (implicit learning). If repeated frequently and done every time stairs are used, a new pattern for stair climbing can be learned in the middle stages of the disease. In the later stages of the disease, both cognitive and motor learning are severely impaired and unlikely to occur, so stair safety training is initiated early in the disease to ensure that it is a learned habit before they enter the later stages of the disease.

Caregivers are also taught to cue the individual to stop, think, and grab the handrail and encouraged to use a gait belt, when assisting someone on the stairs.

Late-Stage Disease

In Part III of the case study, it has been 11 years since WD's diagnosis, and he is no longer ambulating. It is not unusual for clients to come to clinic having already purchased or borrowed a wheelchair. WD's wheelchair does not fit him and should be replaced with one that helps him sit upright, and if possible, maintain independent mobility. Individuals with HD often slide out of their wheelchairs due to dystonic posturing and chorea. A seatbelt positioned at the pelvis keeps the

hips back in the chair, enabling them to sit upright and remain functional. Additionally, individuals with HD are not able to use their arms to propel the wheelchair due to coordination deficits but are usually able to propel the chair using their feet. WD's wheelchair should be fitted so that he can keep his feet on the floor to propel the chair. It is recommended that the chair be fitted with elevating leg rests, as these can help to position the individual, keep them from sliding out of the chair, and will be needed as the individual becomes progressively less mobile.

WD's wife and children should be instructed on safe ways to perform transfers, including bending at the knees and using a gait belt to assist from the level of the hips. Additionally, family members are instructed that individuals with HD are slow to respond due to bradykinesia and difficulties with initiation. When the person with HD is instructed to do a task, the caregiver must allow extra time for the individual to respond. Caregivers often ask the person with HD to assist but do not give them time to respond, then, mistakenly believe that the person with HD is unwilling or unable to assist. Grab bars and other devices to assist with transfers must be firmly anchored in support beams as individuals with HD apply a great deal of shear force through objects, due to their chorea, and have been known to break furniture and grab bars, while trying to transfer.

Bathroom safety is a concern for individuals with HD, and falls are common in the bathroom and shower. Use of a tub or shower bench is highly recommended as many individuals with HD report losing their balance and falling in the shower, especially when they close their eyes. Furthermore, they fall when trying to climb over the edge of the tub. If the tub cannot be replaced with a shower, then, a bench should be placed in the tub, optimally one that extends over the edge of the tub. This facilitates having the person sit on the bench then swing the legs into or out of the tub while seated. Toileting is another time when individuals are at high risk of falling. Grab bars or an elevated bedside commode placed over the toilet are helpful. Purchasing elastic waist pants makes clothing removal safer and easier. Males may also need to be seated during all toileting as changes in balance can lead to falls.

In late-stage disease, individuals with HD typically have significant chorea and dystonic posturing, which may even lead to falls from bed. The use of padded side rails, lowering the bed close to the ground, and/or moving furniture away from the bed helps to prevent injurious falls. Positioning in chairs eventually becomes quite difficult. In the home environment, recliner chairs are the safest option, as tilting the person back helps to prevent sliding out of the chair and provides head support. In long-term care facilities, the use of reclined chairs, with padding around the head, shoulders, and hips, helps to position the client and prevent injury during choreic movements. At the time of this writing, two types of chairs are available on the market to fit the needs of the client with HD – the Broda® chair and the Carefoam® chair (Figure 15-11).

Broda Chair

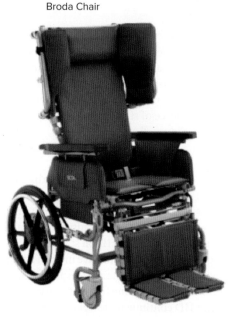

FIGURE 15-11 Specialty chairs for seating the client with HD. (Used with permission of BRODA Seating, Kitchener, Ontario.)

REFERENCES

1. Marras C, Beck JC, Bower JH, et al. Prevalence of Parkinson's disease across North America. *NPJ Parkinsons Dis.* 2018;4:21.

2. Hirsch L, Jette N, Frolkis A, Steeves TE, Pringsheim T. The incidence of Parkinson's disease: a systematic review and meta-analysis. *Neuroepidemiology.* 2016;46:292-300.

3. Wright WA, Evanoff BA, Lian M, Criswell SR, Racette BA. Geographic and ethnic variation in Parkinson disease: a population-based study of US Medicare beneficiaries. *Neuroepidemiology.* 2010;34(3):143-151.

4. Wirdefeldt K, Adami H-O, Cole P, Trichopoulos D, Mandel J. Epidemiology and etiology of Parkinson's disease: a review of the evidence. *Eur J Epidemiol.* 2011;26:S1-S58.

5. Thacker EL, Ascherio A. Familial aggregation of Parkinson's disease: a meta-analysis. *Mov Disord.* 2008;23:1174-1183.

6. Kouli A, Torsney KM, Kuan WL. Parkinson's disease: etiology, neuropathology, and pathogenesis. In: Stoker TB, Greenland JC, eds. *Parkinsons's Disease: Pathogenesis and Clinical Aspects.* Brisbane, Australia: Codon Publications; 2018.

7. Noyce AJ, Bestwick JP, Silveira-Moriyama L, et al. Meta-analysis of early non-motor features and risk factors for Parkinson disease. *Ann Neurol.* 2012;72:893-901.

8. Delic V, Beck KD, Pang KCH, Citron BA. Biological links between traumatic brain injury and Parkinson's disease. *Acta Neuropathol Commun.* 2020;8(1):45.

9. Gardner RC, Byers AL, Barnes DE, Li Y, Boscardin J, Yaffe K. Mild TBI and risk of Parkinson disease: a chronic effects of neurotrauma consortium study. *Neurology.* 2018;90:31771-31779.

10. Bondon-Guitton E, Perez-Lloret S, Bagheri H, Brefel C, Rascol O, Montastruc JL. Drug-induced parkinsonism: a review of 17 years' experience in a regional pharmacovigilance center in France. *Mov Disord.* 2011;26(12):2226-2231.

11. Poewe W, Wenning G. The differential diagnosis of Parkinson's disease. *Eur J Neurol.* 2002;9(S3):23-30.

12. Dommershuijsen LJ, Heshmatollah A, Darweesh SKL, Koudstaal PJ, Ikram MA, Ikram MK. Life expectancy of parkinsonism patients in the general population. *Parkinsonism Relat Disord.* 2020;77:94-99.

13. Cheng HC, Ulane CM, Burke RE. Clinical progression in Parkinson disease and the neurobiology of axons. *Ann Neurol.* 2010;67(6):715-725.

14. Rodriguez-Oroz MC, Jahanshahi M, Krack P, et al. Initial clinical manifestations of Parkinson's disease: features and pathophysiological mechanisms. *Lancet Neurol.* 2009;8:1128-1139.

15. Braak H, Del Tredici K, RubU, de Vos RA, Jansen Steur EN, Braak E. Staging of brain. *Neurobiol Aging.* 2003;24(2):197-211.

16. Burke RE, Dauer WT, Vonsattel JP. A critical evaluation of the Braak staging scheme for Parkinson's disease. *Ann Neurol.* 2008;65(5):485-491.

17. Ma J, Gao J, Wang J, Xie A. Prion-like mechanisms in Parkinson's disease. *Front Neurosci.* 2019;13(552):1-14.

18. Armstrong MJ, Okun MS. Diagnosis and treatment of Parkinson Disease: a review. *JAMA.* 2020:323(6):548-560.

19. De Pablo-Fernández E, Lees AJ, Holton JL, Warner TT. Prognosis and neuropathologic correlation of cinical subtypes of Parkinson disease. *JAMA Neurol.* 2019;76(4):470-479.

20. Stebbins GT, Goetz CG, Burn DJ, Jankovic J, Khoo TK, Tilley BC. How to identify tremor dominant and postural instability/gait difficulty groups with the movement disorder society unified Parkinson's disease rating scale: comparison with the unified Parkinson's disease rating scale. *Mov Disord.* 2013;28:668-670.

21. Huang X, Ng SY, Chia NS, et al. Non motor symptoms in early Parkinson's disease with different motor subtypes and their associations with quality of life. *Eur J Neurol.* 2019;26:400-406.

22. Ren J, Hua P, Li Y, et al. Comparison of three motor subtype classifications in de novo Parkinson's disease patients. *Front Neurol.* 2020;11:601225.

23. Glendinning DS, Enoka RM. Motor unit behavior in Parkinson's disease. *Phys Ther.* 1994;74(1):61-70.

24. Benecke R, Rothwell JC, Dick JP, Day BL, Marsden CD. Performance of simultaneous movements in patients with Parkinson's disease. *Brain.* 1986;109:739-757.

25. Peterson DS, Horak FB. Neural conteol of walking in people with Parinsonism. *Physiology.* 2016;31(2):95-107.

26. Demirci M, Grill S, McShane L, Hallett M. A mismatch between kinesthetic and visual perception in Parkinson's disease. *Ann Neurol.* 1997;41(6):781-788.

27. Mancini M, Carlson-Kuhta P, Zampieri C, Nutt JG, Chiari L, Horak FB. Postural sway as a marker of progression in Parkinson's disease: a pilot longitudinal study. *Gait Posture.* 2012;36(3):471-476.

28. Galna B, Murphy AT, Morris ME. Obstacle crossing in Parkinson's disease: mediolateral sway of the centre of mass during level-ground walking and obstacle crossing. *Gait Posture.* 2013;38:790-794.

29. Mancini M, Rocchi L, Horak FB, Chiari L. Effects of Parkinson's disease and levodopa on functional limits of stability. *Clin Biomech.* 2008;23(4):450-458.

30. Dimitrova D, Horak FB, Nutt JG. Postural muscle responses to multidirectional translations in patients with Parkinson's disease. *J Neurophysiol.* 2004;91(1):489-501.

31. Schoneburg B, Mancini M, Horak F, Nutt JG. Framework for understanding balance dysfunction in Parkinson's disease. *Mov Disord.* 2013;11:1474-1482.

32. Kim SD, Allen NE, Canning CG, Fung VS. Postural instability in patients with Parkinson's disease. Epidemiology, pathophysiology and management. *CNS Drugs.* 2013;27(2):97-112.

33. Smulders K, Esselink RA, De Swart BJ, Geurts AC, Bloem BR, Weerdesteyn V. Postural inflexibility in PD: does it affect compensatory stepping? *Gait Posture.* 2014;39(2):700-706.

34. Inkster LM, Eng JJ. Postural control during a sit-to-stand task in individuals with mild Parkinson's disease. *Exp Brain Res.* 2004;154(1):33-38.

35. Latash ML, Aruin AS, Neyman I, Nicholas J. Anticipatory postural adjustments during self inflicted and predictable perturbations in Parkinson's disease. *J Neurol Neurosurg Psychiatry.* 1995;58(3):326-334.

36. Bleuse S, Cassim F, Blatt JL, et al. Anticipatory postural adjustments associated with arm movements in Parkinson's disease: a biomechanical analysis. *J Neurol Neurosurg Psychiatry.* 2008;79(8):881-887.

37. Khudados E, Cody FWJ, O'Boyle DJ. Proprioceptive regulation of voluntary ankle movements, demonstrated using muscle vibration, is impaired by Parkinson's disease. *J Neurol Neurosurg Psychiatry.* 1999;67(4):504-510.

38. Vaugoyeau M, Viel S, Assaiante C, Amblard B, Azulay JP. Impaired vertical postural control and proprioceptive integration deficits in Parkinson's disease. *Neuroscience.* 2007;146(2):852-863.

39. Vaugoyeau M, Azulay JP. Sensory information in the control of postural orientation in Parkinson's disease. *J Neurol Sci.* 2010;289:66-68.

40. Azulay JP, Mesure S, Ablard B, Blin O, Sangla I, Pouget J. Visual control of locomotion in Parikinson's disease. *Brain.* 1999;122(pt 1):111-120.

41. Ashburn A, Stack E, Pickering RM, Ward CD. A community-dwelling sample of people with Parkinson's disease: characteristics of fallers and non-fallers. *Age Ageing.* 2001;30:47-52.

42. Horak FB, Dimitrova D, Nutt JG. Direction-specific postural instability in subjects with Parkinson's disease. *Exp Neurol.* 2005;193:504-521.

43. Johnell O, Melton LJ, Atkinson EJ, O'Fallon WM, Kurland LT. Fracture risk in patients with parkinsonism: a population-based study in Olmsted County, Minnesota. *Age Ageing.* 1992;21:32-38.

44. Lamont RM, Morris ME, Menz HB, McGinley JL, Brauer SG. Falls in people with Parkinson's disease: a prospective comparison of community and hombe-based falls. *Gait Posture.* 2017;55:62-67.

45. Fasano A, Canning CG, Hausdorff JM, Lord S, Rochester L. Falls in Parkinson's disease: a complex and evolving picture. *Mov Disord.* 2017;32(11):1524-1536.

46. Latt MD, Lors SR, Morris JG, Fung VS. Clinical and physiological assessments for elucidating falls risk in Parkinson's disease. *Mov Disord.* 2009;24(9):1280-1289.

47. Kerr GK, Worringham CJ, Cole MH, Lacherez PF, Wood JM, Silburn PA. Predictors of future falls in Parkinson disease. *Neurology.* 2010;75(2):116-124.

48. Pickering RM, Grimbergen YA, Rigney U, et al. A meta-analysis of six prospective studies of falling in Parkinson's disease. *Mov Disord.* 2007;22(13):1892-1900.

49. Allen NE, Schwarzel AK, Canning CG. Recurrent falls in Parkinson's disease: a systematic review. *Parkinsons Dis.* 2013;2013:906274.

50. Falvo MJ, Schilling BK, Earhart GM. Parkinson's disease and resistive exercise: rationale, review, and recommendations. *Mov Disord.* 2008;23(1):1-11.

51. Edstrom L. Selective changes in the sizes of red and white muscle fibres in upper motor lesions and parkinsonism. *J Neurol Sci.* 1970;11:537-550.

52. Inkster LM, Eng JJ, MacIntyre DL, Stoessl AJ. Leg muscle strength is reduced in Parkinson's disease and related to the ability to rise from a chair. *Mov Disord.* 2003;18:157-162.

53. Hausdorff JM, Cudkowicz ME, Firtion R, Wei JY, Goldberger AL. Gait variability and basal ganglia disorders: stride-to-stride variations of gait cycle timing in Parkinson's disease and Huntington's disease. *Mov Disord.* 1998;13(3):428-437.

54. Tolosa E, Compta Y. Dystonia in Parkinson's disease. *J Neurol.* 2006;253(suppl 7):VII7-VII13.

55. Schaafsma JD, Balash Y, Gurevich T, Bartels AL, Hausdorff JM, Giladi N. Characterization of freezing of gait subtypes and the response of each to levodopa in Parkinson's disease. *Eur J Neurol.* 2003;10(4):391-398.

56. Morris R, Smulders K, Peterson DS, et al. Cognitive function in people with and without freezing of gait in Parkinson's disease. *NPJ Parkinsons Dis.* 2020;6:9.

57. Vitorio R, Stuart S, Mancini M. Executive control of walking in people with Parkinson's disease with freezing of gait. *Neurorehabil Neural Repair.* 2020;34(12):1138-1149.

58. Ebersbach G, Moreau C, Gandor F, Defebvre L, Devos D. Clinical syndromes: parkinsonian gait. *Mov Disord.* 2013;28(11):1552-1559.

59. Amboni M, Barone P, Hausdorff JM. Cognitive contributions to gait and falls: evidence and implications. *Mov Disord.* 2013;28:1520-1533.

60. Brown LA, de Bruin N, Doan J, Suchowersky O, Hu B. Obstacle crossing among people with Parkinson disease is influenced by concurrent music. *J Rehabil Res Dev.* 2010;47:225-232.

61. Potulska A, Friedman A, Krolicki L, Spychala A. Swallowing in Parkinson's disease. *Parkinsonism Relat Disord.* 2003;9:349-353.

62. Ricciardi L, De Angelis A, Marsili L, et al. Hypomimia in Parkinson's disease: an axial sign responsive to levodopa. *Eur J Neurol.* 2020;27(12):2422-2429.

63. Proud EL, Morris ME. Skilled hand dexterity in Parkinson's disease: effects of adding a concurrent task. *Arch Phys Med Rehabil.* 2010;91(5):794-799.

64. Paul SS, Dibble LE, Peterson DS. Motor learning in people with Parkinson's disease: implications for fall prevention across the disease spectrum. *Gait Posture.* 2018;61:311-319.

65. Marinelli L, Quartarone A, Hallett M, Frazzitta G, Ghilardi MF. The many facets of motor learning and their relevance for Parkinson's disease. *Clini Neurophysiol.* 2017;128(7):1127-1141.

66. Wu T, Hallett M. A functional MRI study of automatic movements in patients with Parkinson's disease. *Brain.* 2005;128: 2250-2259.

67. Mentis MJ, Dhawan V, Feigin A, et al. Early stage Parkinson's disease patients and normal volunteers: comparative mechanisms of sequence learning. *Hum Brain Mapp.* 2003;20(4):246-258.

68. Shabbott B, Ravindran R, Schumacher JW, Wasserman PB, Marder KS, Mazzoni P. Learning fast accurate movements requires intact frontostriatal circuits. *Front Hum Neurosci.* 2013;7:752.

69. Lim I, Van Wegen E, de Goede C, et al. Effects of external rhythmical cueing on gait in patients with Parkinson's disease: a systematic review. *Clin Rehabil.* 2005;19(7):695-713.

70. Chiviacowsky S, Campos T, Domingues MR. Reduced frequency of knowledge of results enhances learning in persons with Parkinson's disease. *Front Psychol.* 2010;1:226.

71. Lin CH, Sullivan KJ, Wu AD, Kantak S, Winstein CJ. Effect of task practice order on motor skill learning in adults with Parkinson disease: a pilot study. *Phys Ther.* 2007;87(9):1120-1131.

72. Nieuwboer A, Rochester L, Muncks L, Swinnen SP. Motor learning in Parkinson's disease: limitations and potential for rehabilitation. *Parkinsonism Relat Disord.* 2009;15(suppl 3):S53-S58.

73. Magalhaes M, Wenning GK, Daniel SE, Quinn NP. Autonomic dysfunction in pathologically confirmed multiple system atrophy and idiopathic Parkinson's disease: a retrospective comparison. *Acta Neurol Scand.* 1995;91(2):98-102.

74. Pfeiffer RF. Gastrointestinal dysfunction in Parkinson's disease (review). *Parkinsonism Relat Disord.* 2011;17(1):10-15.

75. Bronner G, Vodusek DB. Management of sexual dysfunction in Parkinson's disease. *Ther Adv Neurol Disord.* 2011;4(6):375-383.

76. Shen-Ting L, Dendi R, Holmes C, Goldstein DS. Progressive loss of cardiac sympathetic innervation in Parkinson's disease. *Ann Neurol.* 2002;52:220-223.

77. Nakamura T, Hirayama M, Hara T, Hama T, Watanabe H, Sobue G. Does cardiovascular autonomic dysfunction contribute to fatigue in Parkinson's disease? *Mov Disord.* 2011;26(10):1869-1874.

78. Protas EJ, Stanley RK, Jankovic J, MacNeill B. Cardiovascular and metabolic responses to upper- and lower-extremity exercise in men with idiopathic Parkinson's disease. *Phys Ther.* 1996;76:34-40.

79. Canning CG, Alison JA, Allen NE, Groeller H. Parkinson's disease: an investigation of exercise capacity, respiratory function, and gait. *Arch Phys Med Rehabil.* 1997;78:199-207.

80. Saltin B, Landin S. Work capacity, muscle strength and SDH activity in both legs of hemiparetic patients and patients with Parkinson's disease. *Scand J Clin Lab Invest.* 1975;35(6):531-558.

81. Carter JH, Nutt JG, Woodward WR. The effect of exercise on levodopa absorption. *Neurology.* 1992;42(10):2042-2045.

82. Senard JM, Brefel-Courbon C, Rascol O, Montastruc JL. Orthostatic hypotension in patients with Parkinson's disease: pathophysiology and management. *Drugs Aging.* 2001;18(7):495-505.

83. Shill H, Stacy M. Respiratory function in Parkinson's disease. *Clin Neurosci.* 1998;5(2):131-135.

84. Jankovic J. Parkinson's disease: clinical features and diagnosis. *J Neurol Neurosurg Psychiatry.* 2008;79:368-376.

85. Kehagia AA, Barker RA, Robbins TW. Neuropsychological and clinical heterogeneity of cognitive impairment and dementia in patients with Parkinson's disease. *Lancet Neurol.* 2010;9(12):1200-1013.

86. Barone P, Aarsland D, Burn D, Emre M, Kullsevsky J, Weintraub D. Cognitive impairment in nondemented Parkinson's disease. *Mov Disord.* 2011;26(14):2483-2495.

87. Docherty MJ, Burn DJ. Parkinson's dementia. *Curr Neurol Neurosci Rep.* 2010;10(4):292-298.

88. Parkinson's disease dementia. Alzheimer's Association webpage. Accessed on July 10, 2021. https://www.alz.org/alzheimers-dementia/what-is-dementia/types-of-dementia/parkinson-s-disease-dementia.

89. Rogers D, Lees AJ, Smith E, Trimble M, Stern GM. Bradyphrenia in Parkinson's disease and psychomotor retardation in depressive illness: an experimental study. *Brain.* 1987;110:761-776.

90. Santangelo G, Barone P, Cuoco S, et al. Apathy in untreated, de novo patients with Parkinson's disease: validation study of Apathy Evaluation Scale. *J Neurol.* 2014;261(12):2319-2328.

91. Weintraub D, Koester J, Potenza MN, et al. Impulse control disorders in Parkinson disease: a cross-sectional study of 3090 patients. *Arch Neurol.* 2006;63:969-973.

92. Fabbrini G, Latorre A, Suppa A, Bloise M, Frontoni M, Berardelli A. Fatigue in Parkinson's disease: motor or non-motor symptom? *Parkinsonism Relat Disord.* 2013;19:148-152.

93. Skorvanek M, Nagyova I, Rosenberger J, et al. Clinical determinants of primary and secondary fatigue in patients with Parkinson's disease. *J Neurol.* 2013;260(6):1554-1561.

94. Haehner A, Hummel T, Reichmann H. Olfactory loss in Parkinson's disease. *Parkinsons Dis.* 2011;2011:450939.

95. Ford B. Pain in Parkinson's disease. *Movement Dis.* 2010;25(Suppl 1):S98-S103.

96. Lang AE, Johnsnon K. Akathisia in idiopathic Parkinson's disease. *Neurology.* 1987;37:477-481.

97. Caproni S, Muti M, Di Renzo A, et al. Subclinical visuospatial impairment in Parkinson's disease: the role of basal ganglia and limbic system. *Front Neurol.* 2014;5:152.

98. Stefani A, Hogi B. Sleep in Parkinson's disease. *Neuropsychopharmacology.* 2020;45:121-128.

99. Ferini-Strambi L, Fantini ML, Zucconi M, et al. REM sleep behaviour disorder. *Neurol Sci.* 2005;26(S3):s186-s192.

100. Postuma RB, Berg D, Stern M, et al. MDS clinical diagnostic criteria for Parkinson's disease. *Mov Disord.* 2015;30(12):1591-1601.

101. Berg D, Postuma RB, Adler CH, et al. MDS research criteria for prodromal Parkinson's disease. *Mov Disord.* 2015;30(12):1600-1611.

102. Tripathi M, Kumar A, Bal C. Neuroimaging in Parkinsonian disorders. *Neurol India.* 2018;66(Supplement):S68-S78.

103. Kägi G, Bhatia KP, Tolosa E. The role of DAT-SPECT in movement disorders. *J Neurol Neurosurg Psychiatry.* 2010;81(1):5-12.

104. Emamzadeh FN, Surguchov A. Parkinson's disease: biomarkers, treatment, and risk factors. *Front Neurosci.* 2018;12:612.

105. Eggers C, Pedrosa DJ, Kahraman D, et al. *PLos One.* 2012;7(10):e46813. doi:10.1371/journal.pone.0046813.

106. Moscovich M, Boschetti G, Moro A, Teive HAG, Hassan A, Munhoz RP. Death certificate data and causes of death in patients with parkinsonism. *Parkinsonism Relat Disord.* 2017;41:99-103.

107. Fahn S, Elton R. Members of the UPDRS development committee. In: Fahn S, Marsden CD, Calne DB, Goldstein M, eds. *Recent Development in Parkinson's Disease.* Vol 2. Florham Park, NJ: Macmillan Health Care Information; 1987:153-163, 293-304.

108. Hoehn MM, Yahr MD. Parkinsonism: onset, progression and mortality. *Neurology.* 1967;17(5):427-442.

109. Goetz CG, Tilley BC, Shaftman SR, et al. Movement Disorder Society UPDRS Revision Task Force. Movement Disorder Society-sponsored revision of the Unified Parkinson's Disease Rating Scale (MDS-UPDRS): scale presentation and clinimetric testing results. *Mov Disord.* 2008;23(15):2129-2170.

110. Goetz CG, Poewe W, Rascol O, et al. Movement Disorder Society Task Force Report on the Hoehn and Yahr Staging Scale: status and recommendations. The Movement disorder society task force on rating scales for Parkinson's disease. *Mov Disord.* 2004;19(9):1020-1028.

111. Pahwa R, Factor SA, Lyons KE, et al. Practice parameter: treatment of Parkinson disease with motor fluctuations and dyskinesia (an evidence-based review): report of the Quality Standards Subcommittee of the American Academy of Neurology. *Neurology.* 2006;66:983-995.

112. Aware in Care Kit. www.awareincare.org. Accessed 07/23/2021.

113. Sinemet. www.drugs.com/pro/sinemet.html. Accessed 11/7/2021.

114. Curtze C, Nutt JG, Carlson-Kuhta P, Mancini M, Horak FB. Levodopa is a double-edged sword for balance and gait in people with Parkinson's disease. *Mov Disord.* 2015;30:1361-1370.

115. Chou KL, StacyM, Simuni T, et al. The spectrum of "off" in Parkinson's disease: what have we learned over 40 years? *Parkinsonism Relat Disord.* 2018;51:9-16.

116. Thanvi B, Lo N, Robinson T. Levodopa-induced dyskinesia in Parkinson's disease: clinical features, pathogenesis, prevention and treatment. *Postgrad Med J.* 2007;83(980):384-388.

117. Stocchi F, Jenner P, Obeso JA. When do levodopa motor fluctuations first appear in Parkinson's disease? *Eur Neurol.* 2010;63(5):257-266.

118. Fox SH, Katzenschlager R, Lim SY, et al. Movement Disorder Society Evidence-Based Medicine Committee. International Parkinson and movement disorder society evidence-based medicine review: update on treatments for the motor symptoms of Parkinson's disease. *Mov Disord.* 2018;33(8):1248-1266.

119. Gray R, Ives N, Rick C, et al PD Med Collaborative Group. Long-term effectiveness of dopamine agonists and monoamine oxidase B inhibitors compared with levodopa as initial treatment for Parkinson's disease (PD MED): a large, open-label, pragmatic randomised trial. *Lancet.* 2014;384(9949):1196-1205.

120. Benarroch EE. Effects of acetylcholine in the striatum. Recent insights and therapeutic implications. *Neurology.* 2012;79(3):274-281.

121. Faulkner MA. Safety overview of FDA-approved medications for the treatment of the motor symptoms of Parkinson's disease. *Expert Opin Drug Saf.* 2014;13(8):1055-1069.

122. Schlesinger I, Sinai A, Zaaroor M. MRI-guided focused ultrasound in Parkinson's disease: a Review. *Parkinsons Dis.* 2017;2017:8124624.

123. Lindvall O, Bjorklund A. Cell therapy in Parkinson's disease. *NeuroRx.* 2004;1(4):382-393.

124. Barker R.A. Designing stem-cell-based dopamine cell replacement trials for Parkinson's disease. *Nat Med.* 2019;25:1045-1053.

125. Coune PG, Schneider BL, Aebisher P. Parkinson's disease: gene therapies. *Cold Spring Harb Perspect Med.* 2010;2(4):a009431.

126. Axelsen TM, Woldbye DPD. Gene therapy for Parkinson's disease: an update. *J Parkinsons Dis.* 2018;8(2):195-215.

127. Liu Z, Cheung HH. Stem cell-based therapies for Parkinson disease. *Int J Mol Sci.* 2020;21(21):8060.

128. Wang L, Xiong N, Huang J, et al. Protein-restricted diets for ameliorating motor fluctuations in Parkinson's disease. *Front Aging Neurosci.* 2017;9:206.

129. Burgos R, Breton I, Cereda E, Desport JC, Dziewas R, et al. ESPEN guideline clinical nutrition in neurology. *Clin Nutrition.* 2018;37:354-396.

130. José Luvizutto G, Souza Silva Brito T, de Moura Neto E, Aparecida Pascucci Sande de Souza L. Altered visual and proprioceptive spatial perception in individuals with Parkinson's disease. *Percept Mot Skills.* 2020;127(1):98-112.

131. Dalrymple-Alford J., MacAskill M, et al. The MoCA well-suited screen for cognitive impairment in Parkinson disease. *Neurology.* 2010;75(19):1717-1725.

132. Gill DJ, Freshman A, Blender JA, Ravina B. The Montreal cognitive assessment as a screening tool for cognitive impairment in Parkinson's disease. *Mov Disord.* 2008;23(7):1043-1046.

133. Hoops S, Nazem S, Siderowf AD, et al. Validity of the MoCA and MMSe in the detection of MCI and dementia in Parkinson disease. *Neurology.* 2009;73:1738-1745.

134. Brown RG, Dittner A, Findley L, Wessely SC. The Parkinson's fatigue scale. *Parkinsonism Relat Disord.* 2005;11(1):49-55.

135. Snijders AH, Haaxma CA, Hagen YJ, Munneke M, Bloem BR. Freezer or non-freezer: clinical assessment of freezing of gait. *Parkinsonism Relat Disord.* 2012;18(2):149-154.

136. Scully AE, Hill KD, Tan D, Clark R, Pua YH, de Oliveira BIR. Measurement properties of assessments of freezing of gait severity in people with Parkinson disease: a COSMIN review. *Phys Ther.* 2021;pzab009.

137. Giladi N, Azulay TJ, Rascol O, et al. Validation of the freezing of gait questionnaire in patients with Parkinson's disease. *Mov Disord.* 2009;24(5):655-661.

138. Renee S, Elisabeth P, Niruthikha M, Allyson F, Louise A. People with mild PD have impaired force produc-tion in all lower limb muscle groups: a cross-sectional study. *Physiother Res Int.* 2021;e1897.

139. Paul SS, Canning CG, Sherrington C, Fung VS. Reduced muscle strength is the major determinant of reduced leg muscle power in Parkinson's dis-ease. *Parkinsonism Relat Disord.* 2012;18(8):974-977.

140. PD EDGE Core Measures. http://www.neuropt.org. Accessed 12/11/14.

141. Duncan RP, Leddy AL, Cavanaugh JT, et al. Detecting and predicting bal-ance decline in Parkinson disease: a prospective cohort study. *J Parkinsons Dis.* 2015;5(1):131-139.

142. Landers MR, Navalta JW, Murtishaw AS, Kinney JW, Pirio Richardson S. A high-intensity exercise boot camp for persons with Parkinson disease: a phase II, pragmatic, randomized clinical trial of feasibility, safety, signal of efficacy, and disease mechanisms. *J Neurol Phys Ther.* 2019;43(1):12-25.

143. Miyasato RS, Silva-Batista C, Peçanha T, et al. Cardiovascular responses during resistance exercise in patients with Parkinson disease. *PM R.* 2018;10(11):1145-1152.

144. Pont-Sunyer C, Hotter A, Gaig C, et al. The onset of nomotor symp-toms in Parkinson's disease (the ONSET PD study). *Mov Disord.* 2015;30(2):229-237.

145. Vianna LC, Teixeira AL, Santos TS, et al. Symbolic dynamics of heart rate variability in Parkinsons's disease patients with orthostatic hypotension. *Int J Cardiol.* 2016;225:144-146.

146. Sabino-Carvalho JL, Teixeira AL, Samora M, Daher M, Vianna LC. Blunted cardiovascular responses to exercise in Parkinson's disease patients: role of the muscle metaboreflex. *J Neurophysiol.* 2018;120(4):1516-1524.

147. Werner WG, DiFrancisco-Donoghue J, Lamberg EM. Cardiovascular response to treadmill testing in Parkin-son disease. *J Neurol Phys Ther.* 2006;30(2):68-73.

148. Muller MLTM, Marusic U, van Emde Boas M, Weiss D, Bohnen NI. Treatment options for postural instability and gait difficulties in Parkinson's disease. *Expert Rev Neurother.* 2019;19(12):1229-1251.

149. Shen X, Wong-Yu IS, Mak MK. Effects of exercise on falls, balance, and gait ability in Parkinson's disease: a meta-analysis. *Neurorehabil Neural Repair.* 2016;30(6):512-527.

150. Tomlinson CL, Patel S, Meek C, et al. Physiotherapy versus placebo or no intervention in Parkinson's disease. *Cochrane Database Syst Rev.* 2012;(7):CD002817.

151. Capato TTC, de Vries NM, IntHout J, Barbosa ER, Nonnekes J, Bloem BR. Multimodal balance training supported by rhythmical auditory stim-uli in Parkinson's disease: a randomized clinical trail. *J Parkinsons Dis.* 2020;10(1):333-346.

152. Sparrow D, DeAngelis TR, Hendron K, Thomas CA, Saint-Hilaire M, Ellis T. Highly challenging balance program reduces fall rate in Parkinson dis-ease. *J Neurol Phys Ther.* 2016;40(1):24-30.

153. Olson M, Lockhart TE, Lieberman A. Motor learning deficits in Parkinson's disease (PD) and their effect on training response in gait and balance: a narrative review. *Front Neurol.* 2019;10:62.

154. Allen NE, Sherrington C, Paul SS, Canning CG. Balance and falls in Parkinson's disease: a meta-analysis of the effect of exercise and motor training. *Mov Disord.* 2011;26(9):1605-1615.

155. Olson M, Lockhart TE, Lieberman A. Motor learning deficits in Parkinson's disease (PD) and their effect on training response in gait and balance: a narrative review. *Front Neurol.* 2019;10:62.

156. Osborne JA, Botkin R, Colon-Semenza C, et al. Physical Therapist Management of Parkinson Disease: A Clinical Practice Guideline From the American Physical Therapy Association Phys Ther. 2022;102(4):pzab302.

157. Kelly NA, Ford MP, Standaert DG, et al. Novel, high-intensity exer-cise prescription improves muscle mass, mitochondrial function, and physical capacity in individuals with Parkinson's disease. *J Appl Physiol.* 2014;116(5):582-592.

158. Lima LO, Scianni A, Rodrigues-de-Paula F. Progressive resistance exercise improves strength and physical performance in people with mild to mod-erate Parkinson's disease: a systematic review. *J Physiother.* 2013;59(1):7-13.

159. Dibble LE, Hale TF, Marcus RL, Droge J, Gerber JP, LaStayo PC. High-intensity resistance training amplifies muscle hypertrophy and functional gains in persons with Parkinson's disease. *Mov Disord.* 2006;21(9):1444-1452.

160. Vieira de Moraes Filho A, Chaves SN, Martins WR, et al. Progressive resistance training improves bradykinesia, motor symptoms and func-tional performance in patients with Parkinson's disease. *Clin Interv Aging.* 2020;15:87-95.

161. David FJ, Rafferty MR, Robichaud JA, et al. Progressive resistance exercise and Parkinson's disease: a review of potential mechanisms. *Parkinsons Dis.* 2012;2012:Article ID– 124527.

162. David FJ, Robichaud JA, Vaillancourt DE, et al. Progressive resistance exer-cise restores some properties of the triphasic EMG pattern and improves bradykinesia: the PRET-PD randomized clinical trial. *J Neurophysiol.* 2016;116(5):2298-2311.

163. Paolucci T, Sbardella S, La Russa C, et al. Evidence of rehabilitative impact of progressive resistance training (PRT) programs in Parkinson disease: an umbrella review. *Parkinsons Dis.* 2020;2020:9748091.

164. Allen NE, Canning CG, Sherrington C, et al. The effects of an exercise pro-gram on fall risk factors in people with Parkinson's disease: a randomized controlled trial. *Mov Disord.* 2010;25(9):1217-1225.

165. Smania N, Corato E, Tinazzi M, et al. Effect of balance training on postural instability in patients with idiopathic Parkinson's disease. *Neurorehabil Neural Repair.* 2010;24(9):826-834.

166. Hubble RP, Silburn PA, Naughton GA, Cole MH. Trunk exercises improve balance in Parkinson disease: a phase II randomized controlled trial. *J Neurol Phys Ther.* 2019;43(2):96-105.

167. Mhatre PV, Vilares I, Stibb SM, et al. Wii fit balance board playing improves balances and gait in Parkinson's disease. *PMR.* 2013;4(9):769-777.

168. Ellis T, Motl RW. Physical activity behavior change in persons with neuro-logic disorders: overview and examples from Parkinson disease and mul-tiple sclerosis. *J Neurol Phys Ther.* 2013;37(2):85-90.

169. Cholewa J, Boczarska-Jedynak M, Opala G. Influence of physiotherapy on severity of motor symptoms and quality of life in patients with Parkinson disease. *Neurol Neurochir Pol.* 2013;47(3):256-262.

170. Ypinga JHL, de Vries NM, Bonnen LHHM, et al. Effectiveness and costs of specialized physiotherapy given via ParkinsonNet: a retrospective analysis of claims data. *Lancet Neurol.* 2018;17(2):153-161.

171. Mak MK, Wong-Yu S, Shen X, Chung CL. Long-term effects of exercise and physical therapy in people with Parkinson disease. *Nat Rev Neurol.* 2017;13:689-703.

172. Ellis T, Rochester L. Mobilizing Parkinson's disease: the future of exercise. *J Parkinsons Dis.* 2018;8:S95-S100.

173. Ellis TD, Cavanaugh JT, DeAngelis T, et al. Comparative effectiveness of mHealth-supported exercise compared with exercise alone for people with Parkinson disease: randomized controlled pilot study. *Phys Ther.* 2019;99(2):203-216.

174. Block VAJ, Pitsch E, Tahir P, Cree BAC, Allen DD, Gelfand JM. Remote physical activity monitoring in neurological disease: a systematic review. *PLoS ONE.* 11(4):e0154335.

175. Del Pozo-Cruz B, Adsuar JC, del Pozo Cruz JA, Olivares PR, Gusi N. Using whole-body vibration training in patients affected with common neuro-logical diseases: a systematic literature review. *J Altern Complement Med.* 2012;18(1):29-41.

176. Dincher A, Schwarz M, Wydra G. Analysis of the effects of whole-body vibration in Parkinson disease: systematic review and meta-analysis. *PM R.* 2019;11(6):640-653.

177. Marazzi S, Kiper P, Palmer K, Agostini M, Turolla A. Effects of vibratory stimulation on balance and gait in Parkinson's disease: a systematic review and meta-analysis. *Eur J Phys Rehabil Med.* 2021;57(2):254-264.

178. Fisher BE, Li Q, Nacca A, et al. Treadmill exercise elevates striatal dopamine D2 receptor binding potential in patients with early Parkinson's disease. *Neuroreport.* 2013;24(10):509-514.

179. Shulman LM, Katzel LI, Ivey FM, et al. Randomized clinical trial of 3 types of physical exercise for patients with Parkinson disease. *JAMA Neurol.* 2013;70(2):183-190.

180. Mehrholz J, Friis R, Kugler J, Twork S, Storch A, Pohl M. Treadmill training for patients with Parkinson's disease. *Cochrane Database Syst Rev.* 2010;(1):CD007830.

181. Mehrholz J, Kugler J, Storch A, Pohl M, Elsner B, Hirsch K. Treadmill training for patients with Parkinson's disease. *Cochrane Database Syst Rev.* 2015;(8):CD007830.

182. Picelli A, Melotti C, Origano F, Neri R, Waldner A, Smania N. Robot-assisted gait training versus equal intensity treadmill training in patients with mild to moderate Parkinson's disease: a randomized controlled trial. *Parkinsonism Relat Disord.* 2013;19(6):605-610.

183. De Luca R, Latella D, Maggio MG, et al. Do patients with PD benefit from music assisted therapy plus treadmill-based gait training? An exploratory study focused on behavioral outcomes. *Int J Neurosci.* 2020 Sep;130(9):933-940.

184. Mirelman A, Rochester L, Maidan I, et al. Addition of a non-immersive virtual reality component to treadmill training to reduce fall risk in older adults (V-TIME): a randomised controlled trial. *Lancet.* 2016;388(10050):1170-1182.

185. Kadivar Z, Corcos DM, Foto J, Hondzinski JM. Effect of step-training and rhythmic auditory stimulation on functional performance in Parkinson patients. *Neurorehabil Neural Repair.* 2011;25(7):626-635.

186. Bloem BR, Grimbergen YA, van Dijk JG, Munneke M. The "posture second" strategy: a review of wrong priorities in Parkinson's disease. *J Neurol Sci.* 2006;248(1-2):196-204.

187. Kegelmeyer DA, Parthasarathy S, Kostyk SK, White SE, Kloos AD. Assistive devices alter gait patterns in Parkinson disease: advantages of the four-wheeled walker. *Gait Posture.* 2013;38(1):20-24.

188. Canning CG, Paul SS, Nieuwboer A. Prevention of falls in Parkinson's disease: a review of fall risk factors and the role of physical interventions. *Neurodegener Dis Manag.* 2014;4(3):203-221.

189. Li F, Harmer P, Fitzgerald K et al. Tai chi and postural stability in patients with Parkinson's disease. *N Engl J Med.* 2012;366(6): 511-519.

190. Goodwin VA, Richards SH, Henley W, Ewings P, Taylor AH, Campbell JL. An exercise intervention to prevent falls in people with Parkinson's disease: a pragmatic randomised controlled trial. *J Neurol Neurosurg Psychiatry.* 2011;82(11):1232-1238.

191. Farley BG, Koshland GF. Training BIG to move faster: the application of the speed-amplitude relation as a rehabilitation strategy for people with Parkinson's disease. *Exp Brain Res.* 2005;167(3):462-467.

192. Ebersbach G, Ebersbach A, Edler D, et al. Comparing exercise in Parkinson's disease: the Berlin LSVT®BIG study. *Mov Disord.* 2010;25(12):1902-1908. doi:10.1002/mds.23212. Erratum. *Mov Disord.* 2010;25(14):2478.

193. Passos-Monteiro E, B Schuch F, T Franzoni L, et al. Nordic Walking and free walking improve the quality of life, cognitive function, and depressive symptoms in individuals with Parkinson's disease: a randomized clinical trial. *J Funct Morphol Kinesiol.* 2020;5(4):82.

194. Radder DLM, Lígia Silva de Lima A, Domingos J, et al. Physiotherapy in Parkinson's disease: a meta-analysis of present treatment modalities. *Neurorehabil Neural Repair.* 2020;34(10):871-880.

195. Granziera S, Alessandri A, Lazzaro A, Zara D, Scarpa A. Nordic walking and walking in Parkinson's disease: a randomized single-blind controlled trial. *Aging Clin Exp Res.* 2021;33(4):965-971.

196. Hackney ME, Earhart GM. Effects of dance on gait and balance in Parkinson's disease: a comparison of partnered and nonpartnered dance movement. *Neurorehabil Neural Repair.* 2010;24(4):384-392.

197. Rawson KS, McNeely ME, Duncan RP, Pickett KA, Perlmutter JS, Earhart GM. Exercise and Parkinson disease: comparing Tango, Treadmill, and Stretching. *J Neurol Phys Ther.* 2019;43(1):26-32.

198. dos Santos Mendes FA, Pompeu JE, Modenesi Lobo A, et al. Motor learning, retention and transfer after virtual-reality-based training in Parkinson's disease–effect of motor and cognitive demands of games: a longitudinal, controlled clinical study. *Physiotherapy.* 2012;98(3):217-223.

199. Pompeu JE, Mendes FA, Silva KG, et al. Effect of Nintendo Wii™-based motor and cognitive training on activities of daily living in patients with Parkinson's disease: a randomized clinical trial. *Physiotherapy.* 2012;98(3):196-204.

200. Canning CG, Allen NE, Nackaerts E, Paul SS, Nieuwboer A, Gilat M. Virtual reality in research and rehabilitation of gait and balance in Parkinson disease. *Nat Rev Neurol.* 2020;16(8):409-425.

201. Oliveira RM, Gurd JM, Nixon P, Marshall JC, Passingham, RE. Micrographia in Parkinson's disease: the effect of providing external cues. *J Neurol Neurosurg Psychiatry.* 1997;63(4):429-433.

202. Nackaerts E, Broeder S, Pereira MP, et al. Handwriting training in Parkinson's disease: a trade-off between size, speed and fluency. *PLoS One.* 2017;12(12):e0190223.

203. Nackaerts E, Michely J, Heremans E, et al. Training for micrographia alters neural connectivity in Parkinson's disease. *Front Neurosci.* 2018;12:3.

204. Ellis T, Boudreau JK, DeAngelis TR, et al. Barriers to exercise in people with Parkinson disease. *Phys Ther.* 2013;93(5):628-636.

205. Inskip M, Mavros Y, Sachdev PS, Fiatarone Singh MA. Exercise for individuals with Lewy Body dementia: a systematic review. *PLoS One.* 2016;11(6):e0156520.

206. Slade SC, Finkelstein DI, McGinley JL, Morris ME. Exercise and physical activity for people with progressive supranuclear palsy: a systematic review. *Clin Rehabil.* 2020;34(1):23-33.

207. Kloos AD, Kegelmeyer DK, White S, Kostyk S. The impact of different types of assistive devices on gait measures and safety in Huntington's disease. *PLoS One.* 2012;7(2):e30903.

208. Raccagni C, Goebel G, Gaßner H, et al. Physiotherapy improves motor function in patients with the Parkinson variant of multiple system atrophy: a prospective trial. *Parkinsonism Relat Disord.* 2019;67:60-65.

209. Yohrling G, Raimundo K, Crowell V, Lovecky D, Vetter L, Seeberger L. Prevalence of Huntington's disease in the US (954). *Neurology.* 2020;94(15 Supplement). Accessed July 31, 2021. https://n.neurology.org/content/94/15_Supplement/954.

210. National Organization for Rare Disorders. Accessed July 31, 2021. https://rarediseases.org/rare-diseases/huntington-disease/.

211. McColgan P, Tabrizi SJ. Huntington's disease: a clinical review. *Eur J Neurol.* 2018;25(1):24-34.

212. Huntington's Disease Society of America's Fast Facts. http://hdsa.org/?s=fast+facts. Accessed 07/25/2021.213.

213. Roos, R.A. Huntington's disease: a clinical review. *Orphanet J Rare Dis.* 2010;5:40.

214. Penney JB, Young AB, Shoulson I, et al. Huntington's disease in Venezuela: 7 years of follow-up on symptomatic and asymptomatic individuals. *Mov Disord.* 1990;5(2):93-99.

215. Ghosh R., Tabrizi S.J. Clinical features of Huntington's disease. In: Nóbrega C., Pereira de Almeida L., eds. *Polyglutamine Disorders. Advances in Experimental Medicine and Biology.* Vol 1049. 2018; Springer, Cham.

216. Stahl CM, Feigin A. Medical, surgical, and genetic treatment of Huntington disease. *Neurol Clin.* 2020;38(2):367-378.

217. Walker FO. Huntington's disease. *Lancet.* 2007;369:218-228.

218. Chao TK, Hu J, Pringsheim T. Risk factors for the onset and progression of Huntington disease. *Neurotoxicology.* 2017;61:79-99.

219. Louis ED, Lee P, Quinn L Marder K. Dystonia in Huntington's disease: prevalence and clinical characteristics. *Mov Disord.* 1999;14(1):95-101.

220. Busse ME, Hughes G, Wiles CM, Rosser AE. Use of hand-held dynamometry in the evaluation of lower limb muscle strength in people with Huntington's disease. *J Neurol.* 2008;255:1534-1540.

221. Saft CS, Zange J, Andrich J, et al. Mitochondrial impairment in patients and asymptomatic mutation carriers of Huntington's disease. *Mov Disord.* 2005;20:674-679.

222. Avanzino L, Pelosin E, Vicario CM, Lagravinese G, Abbruzzese G, Martino D. Time processing and motor control in movement disorders. *Front Hum Neurosci.* 2016;10:631.

223. Wiesendanger M, Serrien DJ. Neurological problems affecting hand dexterity. *Brain Res Rev.* 2001;36(2-3):161-168.

224. Grimbergen YA, Knol MJ, Bloem BR, Kremer BP, Roos RA, Munneke M. Falls and gait disturbances in Huntington's disease. *Mov Disord.* 2008;23(7):970-976.

225. Vuong K, Canning CG, Menant JC, Loy CT. Chapter 16 - Gait, balance, and falls in Huntington disease. Vol 159. In: Brian L Day, Stephen R. Lord, eds. *Handbook of Clinical Neurology.* Elsevier Amsterdam, Netherlands; 2018:251-260.

226. Kegelmeyer DA, Kostyk SK, Fritz NE, et al. Quantitative biomechanical assessment of trunk control in Huntington's disease reveals more impairment in static than dynamic tasks. *J Neurol Sci.* 2017;376:29-34.

227. Blanchet M, Prince F, Chouinard S, Messier J. Postural stability limits in manifest and premanifest Huntington's disease under different sensory conditions. *Neuroscience.* 2014;279:102-112.

228. Porciuncula F, Wasserman P, Marder KS, Rao AK. Quantifying postural control in premanifest and manifest Huntington disease using wearable sensors. *Neurorehabil Neural Repair.* 2020;34(9):771-783.

229. Rao AK, Muratori L, Louis ED, Moskowitz CB, Marder KS. Spectrum of gait impairments in presymptomatic and symptomatic Huntington's disease. *Mov Disord.* 2008;23(8):1100-1107.

230. Tian J, Herdman SJ, Zee DS, Folstein SE. Postural stability in patients with Huntington's disease. *Neurology.* 1992;42(6):1232-1238.

231. Delval A, Krystkowiak JL, Blatt E, et al. A biomechanical study of gait initiation in Huntington's dis-ease. *Gait Posture.* 2007;25(2):279-288.

232. Skodda S, Schlegel U, Hoffmann R, Saft C. Impaired motor speech performance in Huntington's disease. *J Neural Transm.* 2014;121:399-407.

233. Heemskerk AW, Roos RAC. Dysphagia in Huntington's disease: a review. *Dysphagia.* 2011;26:62-66.

234. Kagel MC, Leopold NA. Dysphagia in Huntington's disease: a 16-year retrospective. *Dysphagia.* 1992;7:106-114.

235. Feigin A, Ghilardi M-F, Huang C, et al. Preclinical Huntington's disease: compensatory brain responses during learning. *Ann Neurol.* 2006;59:53-59.

236. Schneider SA, Wilkinson L, Bhatia KP, et al. Abnormal explicit but normal implicit sequence learning in premanifest and early Huntington's disease. *Mov Disord.* 2010;25:1343-1349.

237. Yaguez L, Canavan A, Lange HW, Homberg V. Motor learning by imagery is differentially affected in Parkinson's and Huntington's diseases. *Behav Brain Res.* 1999;102:115-127.

238. Paulsen JS. Cognitive impairment in Huntington's disease: diagnosis and treatment. *Neurol Neurosci Rep.* 2011;11(5):474-483.

239. Delval A, Krystkowiak P, Delliaux M, et al. Role of attentional resources on gait performance in Huntington's disease. *Mov Disord.* 2008;23(5):684-689.

240. Fritz NE, Hamana K, Kelson M, Rosser A, Busse M, Quinn L. Motor-cognitive dual-task deficits in individuals with early-mid stage Huntington disease. *Gait Posture.* 2016;49:283-289.

241. Lo J, Reyes A, Pulverenti TS, et al. Dual tasking impairments are associated with striatal pathology in Huntington's disease. *Ann Clin Transl Neurol.* 2020;7(9):1608-1619.

242. Sitek EJ, Soltan W, Woeczorek D, et al. Unawareness of deficits in Huntington's disease. *J Int Neuropsychol Soc.* 2011;17:788-795.

243. Rosenblatt A. Neuropsychiatry of Huntington's disease. *Dialogues Clin Neurosci.* 2007;9(2):191-197.

244. Morton AJ. Circadian and sleep disorder in Huntington's disease. *Exp Neurol.* 2013;243:34-44.

245. Scherder E, Statema M. Huntington's disease. *The Lancet.* 2010;376:1464.

246. Seiss E, Praamstra P, Hesse CW, Rickards H. Proprioceptive sensory function in Parkinson's disease and Huntington's disease: evidence from proprioception-related EEG potentials. *Exp Brain Res.* 2003;148:308-319.

247. Hicks SL, Robert MP, Golding CV, Tabrizi SJ, Kennard C. Oculomotor deficits indicate the progression of Huntington's disease. *Prog Brain Res.* 2008;171:555-558.

248. Ciammola A, Sassone J, Sciacco M, et al. Low anaerobic threshold and increased skeletal muscle lactate production in subjects with Huntington's disease. *Mov Disord.* 2011;26:130-136.

249. Dawes H, Collett J, Debono K, et al. Exercise testing and training in people with Huntington's disease. *Clin Rehabil.* 2015;29(2):196-206.

250. Van Vugt JP, Siesling S, Piet KK. Quantitative assessment of daytime motor activity provides a responsive measure of functional decline in patients with Huntington's disease. *Mov Disord.* 2001;16:481-488.

251. Busse ME, Wiles CM, Rosser AE. Mobility and falls in people with Huntington's disease. *J Neurol Neurosurg Psychiatry.* 2009;80:88-90.

252. Mehanna R, Jankovic J. Respiratory problems in neurologic movement disorders. *Parkinsonism Relat Disord.* 2010;16:626-638.

253. Reyes, A., Cruickshank, T., Ziman, M. et al. Pulmonary function in patients with Huntington's Disease. *BMC Pulm Med.* 2014;14:89.

254. Quinn L, Busse M; On behalf of the members of the European Huntington's Disease Network Physiotherapy Working Group. Physiotherapy clinical guidelines for Huntington's disease. *Neurodegener Dis Manag.* 2012;2(1):21-31.

255. Djousse L, Knowlton B, Cupples LA, Marder K, Shoulson I, Myers RH. Weight loss in the early stages of Huntington's disease. *Neurology.* 2002;59:1325-1330.

256. Aziz NA, van der Marck MA, Rikkert MG, et al. Weight loss in neurodegenerative disorders. *J Neurol.* 2008;255:1872-1880.

257. Kirkwood SC, Su JL, Connealy P, Faoroud T. Progression of symptoms in the early and middle stages of Huntington's disease. *Arch Neurol.* 2001;58:273-278.

258. Nance MA, Myers RH. Juvenile onset Huntington's disease: clinical and research perspectives. *Ment Retard Dev Disabil Res Rev.* 2001;7:153-157.

259. HDSA Genetic Testing Protocol. Huntington's Disease Society of America website: http://hdsa.org/product/genetic-testing-for-huntingtons-disease-its-relevance-and-implications/. Accessed August 1, 2021.

260. Shoulson I, Fahn S. Huntington's disease: clinical care and evaluation. *Neurology.* 1979;29:1-3.

261. Total Functional Capacity Staging. http://promotingexcellence.growthhouse.org/huntingtons/monograph/pe5670.html. Accessed 12/11/14.

262. Bachoud-Lévi AC, Ferreira J, Massart R, et al. International guidelines for the treatment of Huntington's disease. *Front Neurol.* 2019;10:710.

263. Mason SL, Barker RA. Emerging drug therapies in Huntington's disease. *Expert Opin Emerg Drugs.* 2009;14(2):273-297.

264. Huntington Study Group. Unified Huntington's disease rating scale: reliability and consistency. *Mov Disord.* 1996;11:136-142.

265. Siesling S, van Vugt JP, Zwinderman KA, Kieburtz K, Roos RA. Unified Huntington's disease rating scale: a follow up. *Mov Disord.* 1998;13:915-991.

266. Asslander L, Peterka RJ. Sensory reweighting dynamics in human postural control. *J Neurophysiol.* 2014;11(9):1852-1864.

267. Rao AK, Mazzoni P, Wasserman P, Marder K. Longitudinal change in gait and motor function in pre-manifest Huntington's disease. *PLoS Curr.* 2011;3:RRN1268.

268. Quinn L, Khalil H, Dawes H, et al. Reliability and minimal detectable change of physical performance measures in individuals with pre-manifest and manifest Huntington's disease. *Phys Ther.* 2013;93(7):942-956.

269. Fritz NE, Kegelmeyer D, Rao AK, Quinn L, Kloos A. Clinical decision trees to guide physical therapy management of persons with Huntington's disease. *J Huntingtons Disease.* In Press.

270. Kloos AD, Kegelmeyer DA, Young GS, Kostyk SK. Fall risk assessment using the Tinetti mobility test in individuals with Huntington's disease. *Mov Disord.* 2010;25(16):2838-2844.

271. Rao A, Muratori L, Louis ED, Moskowitz CB, Marder KS. Clinical measurement of mobility and balance impairments in Huntinton's disease: validity and responsiveness. *Gait Posture.* 2009;29(3):433-436.

272. Kloos AD, Kegelmeyer DA, Ambrogi K, Kline D, McCormack-Mager M, et al. The step test evaluation of performance on stairs (STEPS): validation and reliability in a neurological disorder. *PLOS ONE.* 2019;14(3):e0213698.

273. Quinn L, Kegelmeyer D, Kloos A, Rao AK, Busse M, Fritz N. Clinical recommendations to guide physical therapy practice for Huntington disease. *Neurology.* 2020;94(5):217-228.

274. Quinn L, Hamana K, Kelson M, et al. A randomized, controlled trial of a multi-modal exercise intervention in Huntington's disease. *Parkinsonism Relat Disord* 2016;31:46–52.

275. Drew CJG, Quinn L, Hamana K, et al. Physical activity and exercise outcomes in Huntinton's disease (PACE_HD): protocol for a 12-month trial within cohort evaluation of physical activity intervention in people with Huntington Disease. *Phys Ther.* 2019;99(9):1201-1210.

276. Fritz NE, Rao AK, Kegelmeyer D, et al. Physical therapy and exercise interventions in Huntington's disease: a mixed methods systematic review. *J Huntingtons Dis.* 2017;6(3):217-235.

277. Kloos AD, Fritz NE, Kostyk SK, Young GS, Kegelmeyer DA. Video game play (Dance Dance Revolution) as a potential exercise therapy in Huntington's disease: a controlled clinical trial. *Clin Rehabil.* 2013;27(11):972-982.

278. Cruickshank TM, Reyes AP, Penailillo LE, et al. Effects of multidisciplinary therapy on physical function in Huntington's disease. *ACTA Neurol Scan.* 2018:138(6):500-507.

279. Zinzi P, Salmaso D, DeGrandis R, et al. Effects of an intensive rehabilitation programme on patients with Huntington's disease: a pilot study. *Clin Rehabil.* 2007;21(7):602-613.

Review Questions

1. **Parkinson's disease is caused by the loss of dopamine-containing neurons in the:**

    A. Substantia nigra pars reticulata

    B. Substantia nigra pars compacta

    C. Striatum

    D. Subthalamic nucleus

2. **A patient with Parkinson's Disease (Hoehn and Yahr Stage 3) who is taking Sinemet is receiving physical therapy for fall prevention. Which of the following impairments are most likely to contribute to the patient's balance problems?**

    A. Orthostatic hypotension, stooped posture, impaired postural reflexes

    B. Hypotonia, freezing of gait, orthostatic hypotension

    C. Chorea, stooped posture, festinating gait

    D. Stooped posture, dyskinesias, and motor impersistence

3. **A Parkinson-plus syndrome that is characterized by early postural instability and difficulty moving the eyes is:**

    A. Multiple system atrophy

    B. Corticobasal ganglionic degeneration

    C. Olivopontocerebellar atrophy

    D. Progressive supranuclear palsy

4. **A person with Parkinson's disease who is a good candidate for deep brain stimulation:**

    A. Has no response to levodopa

    B. Has never been treated with levodopa

    C. Has rigidity and dyskinesias that are no longer controlled with medications

    D. Has postural instability that is no longer controlled with medications

5. **A decarboxylase inhibitor carbidopa is given with levodopa (Levodopa) to:**

    A. Convert levodopa to dopamine in the periphery so that it can cross the blood-brain barrier

    B. Aid in the uptake of levodopa into nerve terminals

    C. Prevent the conversion of levodopa to dopamine in the periphery

    D. Aid in the active transport of levodopa across the blood-brain barrier.

6. **Which of the following neuropathological findings is characteristic of Huntington's disease?**

    A. Degeneration of olfactory bulb neurons

    B. Atrophy of the caudate nucleus

    C. Demyelinating plaques surrounding lateral ventricles

    D. Lewy bodies in striatal neurons

7. **Early symptoms of Huntington's disease include:**

    A. Balance and gait disorders

    B. Depression and irritability

    C. Swallowing and speech impairments

    D. Dementia and hallucinations

8. **If a parent has Huntington's Disease, what is the chance of one of his or her children having HD?**

    A. 10%

    B. 25%

    C. 50%

    D. 75%

9. When examining an adult with Huntington's disease, which of the following gait deviations are you MOST likely to observe?

   A. Bilaterally shortened steps and reduced arm swing

   B. Decreased hip flexion with bilateral circumduction in the swing phase

   C. Bilateral Trendelenburg limp

   D. Wide-based gait with uneven step lengths

10. In early Huntington's disease, involuntary movements like chorea are caused by damage to:

    A. Medium spiny striatal projection neurons that are part of the indirect basal ganglia pathway

    B. Dopamine-containing nigrostriatal neurons

    C. Medium spiny striatal projection neurons that are part of the direct basal ganglia pathway

    D. Glutamate-containing subthalamic nucleus neurons

11. Which of the following measures of cognitive function is validated in PD and recommended by the PD EDGE task force?

    A. Mini Mental Status Exam

    B. Montreal Cognitive Assessment

    C. St. Louis University Mental Status Exam

    D. Mini Cog

12. Which of the following is a common method for assessing bradykinesia in Parkinson's disease that is on the UPDRS?

    A. Alternating pronation and supination

    B. Finger tapping

    C. Timed Up and Go

    D. The pull test

13. Your client with PD states that freezing of gait is making it difficult for him to work and has led to 3 falls in the last 6 months. You wish to perform an assessment of his freezing that has good intra-rater reliability and is validated. Which of the following would be the best way to assess for freezing during this visit?

    A. Freezing of Gait Questionnaire

    B. Have the individual perform a rapid 360-degree turn in both directions

    C. Observe gait in a confined space

    D. Use the freezing-while-walking item on the MDS-UPDRS

14. Which of the following muscle groups is prone to shortening and contracture and has been shown to be weaker in individuals with Parkinson's disease?

    A. Ankle inverters

    B. Ankle plantarflexors

    C. Lumbar extensors

    D. Shoulder extensors

15. Limited trunk rotation can lead to which of the following functional problems?

    A. Ability to sit down on a chair

    B. Difficulty sleeping

    C. Tendency to fall posteriorly

    D. Walking with small steps

16. Which of the following is one of the core measures recommended by the Neurology section PD EDGE taskforce for use when examining an individual with Parkinson's disease?

    A. Berg balance scale

    B. Mini-mental status exam

    C. Sit to stand 5 times

    D. Timed Up and Go

17. New Q3 You receive a referral for physical therapy for a client with PD due to 2 falls in the last 3 months. This individual fractured her cheekbone on the second fall. Since that fall she reports that she no longer takes her daily walk and she is reticent to visit her son's home as she is worried she will fall. How will you best measure her functional status so that you can capture her key issues?

    A. Administer the ANPT Core Measures

    B. Administer the freezing of gait questionnaire and the Berg Balance test

    C. Adminster the ANPT Core Measures and the ABC scale

    D. Administer the Berg Balance Scale and the Mini BESTest

18. Which of the following is a true statement regarding strength training individuals with Parkinson's disease?

    A. Eccentric exercise is contraindicated

    B. High-intensity strength training is not tolerated by individuals with PD

    C. Strength training leads to improvements in gait speed and isokinetic strength

    D. Strength training improves stair descent with no improvement in isokinetic strength.

19. Balance training in individuals with PD leads to:

    A. Faster reaction time

    B. Fewer falls

    C. Minimizes the limits of stability

    D. Slower movement velocity

20. New Q4 A key element of a balance training program for individuals with PD is that it must:

    A. challenge the individual

    B. be paired with strength training

    C. be done in a group setting

    D. include reactive balance training

21. **New Q5 Which of the following is a description of an optimal physical therapy plan for a client with PD?**

    A. Initiate PT when deficits in gait and balance are first noted, discharge to continue exercise at home and with community exercise programs.

    B. Assess and teach exercises for PD at time of diagnosis. New plan of care whenever the client has declines in function.

    C. Initiate PT at time of diagnosis and then continue with maintenance therapy throughout the course of the disease.

    D. Initiate PT at time of diagnosis and provide consistent ongoing care through the use of follow up visits and home/community exercise throughout the course of the disease.

22. **Treadmill training to improve walking speed should be done using**

    A. A harness to support partial body weight

    B. An aerobic training protocol

    C. Progressive increases in speed

    D. Speeds equivalent to running

23. **Treadmill training has been shown to reduce falls in clients with PD when combined with?**

    A. Body weight support

    B. Music

    C. Virtual reality

    D. Robotics

24. **To alleviate freezing of gait the individual with PD should use**

    A. A gentle forward pull from the caregiver

    B. An assistive device

    C. Auditory cueing

    D. Rocking back and forth

25. **Which assistive device resulted in the fewest stumbles and lowest gait variability while maintaining gait speed?**

    A. A cane

    B. Front wheeled walker (2 wheels)

    C. Rollator walker (4 wheels, front two swivel)

    D. The U-Step walker

26. **Your client with PD scores as high fall risk on both the Berg Balance Scale and the Mini BESTest. The plan of care should include which of the following?**

    A. Individualized and challenging balance exercises performed at home along with progressive strengthening.

    B. Challenging balance exercises and multimodal exercise performed with the physical therapist one-on-one.

    C. A community PD exercise class that includes balance and strengthening exercises.

    D. Progressive strength training along with appropriate stretching to key muscle groups such as the hamstrings and gastrocnemius.

27. **For clients with Parkinson-Plus syndromes physical therapy interventions should:**

    A. Be based on the movement system impairments noted in the examination

    B. Include prescription of a rollator walker

    C. Include work on eye movements and visual searching strategies.

    D. Focus on coordination exercises.

28. **A common reason that individuals with PD do not participate in community exercise programs is:**

    A. It costs too much

    B. They don't think it will help them

    C. They fear being made fun of

    D. They lack transportation

29. **An individual with Huntington's disease who has motor impersistence will demonstrate which of the following on examination:**

    A. A fall when a backward pull is applied to the shoulders

    B. Dance like involuntary movements

    C. Inability to move the eye side to side to follow the examiner's finger

    D. Inability to protrude the tongue and keep it there for several seconds

30. **In individuals with HD participation in activities is negatively impacted by which of the following psychological factors?**

    A. Agoraphobia

    B. Apathy

    C. Fear of falling

    D. Mania

31. **To overcome apathy the family and therapist should use which of the following techniques?**

    A. Use low-key and low-stimulation activities

    B. A set daily schedule

    C. New activities each day

    D. A quiet and soothing environment

32. **You wish to determine if your new client with Huntington's disease is at increased risk for falling. Which of the following measures is recommended for use in this population?**

    A. Activities Specific Balance Confidence Scale

    B. Functional Reach Test

    C. Mini BESTest

    D. Tinetti Mobility Test

33. Individuals with HD often fall backward into chairs, tipping the chair over, and sometimes breaking the chair. A method to improve safety of transfers is to teach the person with HD to:

A. Keep their eyes focused on the ceiling while sitting down

B. Reach back for the chair before sitting in it

C. Place hands on hips during the transfer and do a squat motion

D. Place hands on thighs and slide the hands down while sitting

34. Which of the following interventions has strong evidence for its use with clients with Huntington's disease?

A. Balance Exercise

B. Gait training

C. Postural control exercises

D. Respiratory exercises

35. When ascending and descending stairs individuals with HD exhibit which of the following problems?

A. Buckling of the knees

B. Overuse of the railing

C. Slow descent of stairs

D. Uneven foot placement

36. Individuals with HD are slow to initiate when asked to give a verbal response or to do a task. How should the therapist instruct the family to deal with this issue?

A. Ring a bell immediately before asking the person with HD to perform a movement.

B. Ask the person with HD to perform the movement and at the same time rock them back and forth several times.

C. Pause for a minute to allow the person to make a response before giving any assistance.

D. Tap the person with HD on the leg or arm to cue them to move the limb as you ask them to move the limb.

37. Camptocormia associated with PD is characterized by excessive:

A. Extension of the trunk.

B. Flexion of the trunk.

C. Lateral tilting of the trunk.

D. Rotation of the trunk.

38. Involuntary sustained muscular contractions that cause abnormal movements and/or postures are called:

A. Ballisms

B. Myoclonus

C. Dystonia

D. Tics

39. A non-motor symptom of Parkinson's disease that typically occurs a few years prior to onset of motor symptoms and aids in diagnosis is:

A. Photophobia

B. Hallucinations

C. Depression

D. Anosmia

40. Nutritional management of individuals with Parkinson's disease includes:

A. Taking levodopa with meals

B. Eating a low-protein diet

C. Eating a high-protein diet

D. Eating a low caloric diet

41. In comparison to adult-onset Huntington's disease, individuals with juvenile Huntington's disease are more likely to have:

A. Lower numbers of CAG repeats

B. Greater severity of chorea

C. Rigidity, tremors, and seizures

D. A slower disease progression

42. A medication commonly used to treat chorea in Huntington's disease is:

A. Tetrabenazine (Xenazine)

B. Sertraline (Zoloft)

C. Duloxitine (Cymbalta)

D. Levodopa/Carbidopa (Sinemet)

Answers

1. B	2. A	3. D	4. C	5. C
6. B	7. B	8. C	9. D	10. A
11. B	12. B	13. A	14. B	15. D
16. C	17. C	18. D	19. A	20. A
21. D	22. C	23. C	24. C	25. C
26. B	27. A	28. B	29. D	30. B
31. B	32. D	33. D	34. B	35. D
36. C	37. B	38. C	39. D	40. B
41. C	42. A			

GLOSSARY

Akathisia. A feeling of inner restlessness that is reduced or relieved by movement.

Akinesia. Absence or loss of the ability to move voluntarily.

Alpha-synuclein. A neuronal protein that normally regulates synaptic vesicle trafficking and subsequent neurotransmitter release. Abnormal alpha-synuclein aggregates are found in the brains of individuals with pathological conditions characterized by Lewy bodies, such as Parkinson's disease, dementia with Lewy bodies, and multiple system atrophy.

Anticipatory postural adjustments. Unconscious muscular activities that counterbalance the perturbation caused by voluntary movements, to ensure that whole-body balance is maintained, as well as contribute to the initial displacement of the body center of mass when starting gait or when performing whole-body reaching movements.

Apathy. Lack of feeling, emotion, interest, or concern about something.

Apraxia. A neurological disorder characterized by loss of the ability to execute or perform skilled movements and gestures, despite having the intention and the physical ability to perform them.

Associative loop. A basal ganglia-thalamocortical circuit that begins and ends in the dorsolateral prefrontal and premotor cortices that is involved in cognitive functions including goal-directed behaviors, problem-solving, and dual-task performance.

Autonomic nervous system. The part of the nervous system responsible for controlling unconscious functions such as breathing, heartrate, and digestive processes.

Ballisms. Repetitive, but constantly varying, large amplitude involuntary movements of the proximal parts of the limbs.

Baroreflex. A reflex that provides a rapid response to changes in blood pressure.

Bradykinesia. Slowness in the execution of movements. It is a cardinal sign of Parkinson's disease.

Bradyphrenia. Slowed thinking.

Camptocormia. An abnormal, severe, and involuntary forward flexion of the thoracolumbar spine, which appears during standing and walking and lessens when lying flat.

Chorea. Involuntary, irregular, purposeless, nonrhythmic, abrupt, rapid, or unsustained movements that seem to flow from one body part to another, giving the appearance that a person is dancing. Chorea is a motor symptom of Huntington's disease.

Choreoathetosis. Involuntary movements in a combination of chorea (i.e., uncontrollable "dance-like" movements) and athetosis (i.e., twisting and writhing movements).

Closed-loop cueing. A signal that is provided "on-demand," such as using biofeedback to initiate an electrical stimulation to the leg muscle.

Cogwheel rigidity refers to resistance that stops and starts (i.e., rachet-like) as the limb is moved through its range of motion.

Diplopia. Double vision, such that a person sees two images of a single object.

Disinhibition. A lack of control manifested in disregard of social conventions, impulsivity, and poor risk assessment.

Dyskinesia. Abnormal involuntary movements, often choreiform in nature, that can be a complication from long-term levodopa use in people with Parkinson's disease.

Dystonia. Involuntary prolonged and repetitive muscle contractions that result in abnormal twisting body movements, and postures.

"En bloc" turning. An abnormal way of turning commonly seen in people with Parkinson's disease characterized by keeping the neck and trunk rigid, requiring multiple small steps to accomplish a turn, rather than the typical rotation of the neck and trunk and pivoting on the toes.

Festination. An abnormal gait often seen in people with Parkinson's disease characterized by short, accelerating steps, often on tiptoe, with the trunk flexed forward and the legs flexed stiffly at the hips and knees. The festination can be anteropulsive (accelerating forward) or retropulsive (accelerating backward).

Freezing of gait. Brief, episodic absence or marked reduction of forward advancement of the feet despite a person's intention to walk.

Genetic anticipation. A phenomenon in which the signs and symptoms of genetic conditions such as Huntington's disease tend to become more severe and/or appear at an earlier age as the disorder is passed from one generation to the next.

"Hung-up" reflexes. Increased relaxation time of elicited deep tendon reflexes that is observed in people with Huntington's disease.

Hyperhidrosis. Abnormally excessive sweating.

Hyperkinesia. An increase in movements, which includes abnormal involuntary movements (e.g., tremors, dystonia, chorea, tics, myoclonus) or dyskinesias.

Hypersexuality. Exhibiting unusual or excessive preoccupation with or indulgence in sexual activity.

Hypokinesia. Decreased amplitude of movements, not caused by muscular weakness or paralysis.

Hypokinetic dysarthria. A speech disorder common in people with Parkinson's disease characterized by monotony of pitch and loudness, reduced stress, and imprecise enunciation of consonants.

Hypomimia. Reduced or loss of facial expression, also referred to as "facial masking."

Irritability. Feelings of anger or frustration that often arise over even the smallest of matters.

Lead pipe rigidity A constant resistance to motion throughout the entire range of motion.

Limbic loop. A basal ganglia-thalamocortical circuit that begins and ends in the anterior cingulate area and medial orbitofrontal cortex that is involved in behavioral motivation and emotional regulation.

Limits of stability. The maximum distance that an individual is able to intentionally lean in any direction without losing his/her balance or taking a step.

Micrographia. Abnormally small handwriting or handwriting that becomes progressively smaller.

Motor (skeletomotor) loop. A basal ganglia-thalamocortical circuit, comprised of direct and indirect circuits, that begins and ends in the precentral motor areas (the premotor cortex, the supplementary motor area, and the primary motor cortex) that is involved in the preparation and execution of movements.

Motor impersistence. The inability to sustain muscle contractions for voluntary tasks such as keeping the eyes closed, protruding the tongue, or holding an object.

Mutism. Inability to speak.

Myoclonus. Sudden, brief, shock-like involuntary movements caused by muscle contractions.

Nocturia. A condition in which a person has to wake up one or more times at night for voiding.

Oculomotor loop. A basal ganglia-thalamocortical circuit that begins and ends in the frontal and supplementary eye fields that is involved in the control of saccadic eye movements.

On–off phenomenon. Sudden and unpredictable motor symptom transitions from being "on" to being "off" that are usually not related to the timing of levodopa dosing, and that typically occur in individuals with advanced Parkinson's disease.

Open-loop cueing. A signal that is fixed in its presentation such as lines painted on the floor.

Orthostatic hypotension. A sensation of lightheadedness when changing postures from lying to sitting or sitting to standing that is due to a drop in a person's blood pressure with these positional changes. Orthostatic hypotension is commonly seen in Parkinson's but can also occur as a side effect of medications commonly used to treat the disease.

Pallidotomy. A surgical procedure to ablate the globus pallidus internal segment that is used to alleviate tremor, bradykinesia, rigidity, and levodopa-induced dyskinesias.

Paresthesias. Abnormal sensations, typically tingling or pricking ("pins and needles"), caused primarily by pressure or damage to peripheral nerves.

Parkinsonism. Any condition that involves the types of movement problems (i.e., tremor, rigidity, bradykinesia/akinesia, and postural instability) seen in Parkinson's disease.

Parkinson-plus syndromes. A group of neurodegenerative diseases featuring the classical motor symptoms of Parkinson's disease (i.e., tremor, rigidity, bradykinesia/akinesia, and postural instability) with additional features that distinguish them from simple idiopathic Parkinson's disease.

Perseveration. The act of repeating something, such as words or actions, beyond an appropriate point.

Pisa syndrome. An abnormal posture characterized by lateral flexion of the trunk appearing or worsening while standing or walking and improving with passive mobilization and supine positioning.

Pressor response. A reflex response that causes vasoconstriction and thus increases blood pressure.

Rapid eye movement sleep behavior disorder. A sleep disorder in which individuals physically act out vivid, often unpleasant dreams with vocal sounds and sudden, often violent arm and leg movements during rapid eye movement sleep.

Restless legs syndrome. A disorder that causes an overwhelming urge to move the legs, usually associated with unpleasant sensations, and often occurring during sleep. Movement relieves the unpleasant sensation.

Rigidity. Non-velocity-dependent resistance to passive joint movements, typically due to lesions of the extrapyramidal pathways, such as the basal ganglia. Rigidity can be subclassified as cogwheel or lead pipe rigidity.

Seborrhea. Excessive discharge of oily secretions from the sebaceous glands.

Seborrheic dermatitis. A skin condition that affects oily areas of the body (e.g., scalp, face, sides of nose, ears, eyelids) causing scaly patches, red skin, itching, and dandruff.

Secondary parkinsonism. When symptoms similar to Parkinson's disease are caused by other diseases or disorders or caused by trauma, infection, or a medication.

Sialorrhea. Excessive salivation or drooling.

Substantia nigra pars compacta. A portion of the substantia nigra, located in the midbrain, that contains dopaminergic neurons that supply the striatum and that are damaged in Parkinson's disease.

Thalamotomy. A surgical procedure to ablate the ventral intermediate nucleus of the thalamus used to treat tremors.

Tics. Sudden, repetitive, nonrhythmic motor movement or vocalization involving discrete muscle groups.

Tremor. An involuntary, rhythmic muscle contraction that causes shaking movements in one or more parts of the body. A resting tremor is when a tremor occurs when the muscles are relaxed and supported, as when a person's hands are resting in the lap.

Wearing-off. A reemergence of parkinsonian symptoms as the effect of levodopa diminishes near the end of a dose interval, that is a common complication of long-term levodopa use.

ABBREVIATIONS

ALS/PDC	amyotrophic lateral sclerosis/parkinsonian-dementia complex
APA	anticipatory postural adjustment
AT	anaerobic threshold
BG	basal ganglia
BP	blood pressure
CAG	cytosine, adenine, and guanine
CBGD	cortical-basal ganglionic degeneration
CT	computed tomography

DAT-SPECT	dopamine transporter single positron emission computed tomography	MPTP	1-methyl 4-phenyl 1,2,3,6-tetrahydropyridine
DBS	deep brain stimulation	MRI	magnetic resonance imaging
DLB	dementia with Lewy bodies	MSA	multiple system atrophy
DNA	deoxyribonucleic acid	NPF	National Parkinson Foundation
EEG	electro-encephalogram	NREM	non-rapid eye movement
EMG	electromyography	OH	orthostatic hypotension
FOG	freezing of gait	PD	idiopathic Parkinson's disease
GABA	gamma-aminobutyric acid	PDD	Parkinson's disease dementia
Gpi	globus pallidus internal segment	PET	positron emission tomography
HD	Huntington's disease	PIGD	postural instability gait difficulty
HIV	human immunodeficiency virus	PPN	pedunculopontine nucleus
HR	heart rate	PSP	progressive supranuclear palsy
IPG	implantable pulse generator	RBD	rapid eye movement sleep behavior disorder
LID	levodopa-induced dyskinesia	RNA	ribonucleic acid
MAO-B	monoamine oxidase – B	SNpc	substantia nigra pars compacta
MDS-PD	Movement Disorder Society Clinical Diagnostic Criteria of Parkinson's Disease	SPECT	single positron emission computed tomography
		STN	subthalamic nucleus
MDS-UHDRS	Movement Disorder Society Unified Huntington's Disease Rating Scale	TBI	traumatic brain injury
		TFC	total functional capacity
MDS-UPDRS	Movement Disorder Society Unified Parkinson's Disease Rating Scale	TD	tremor-dominant
		US	United States
MPPP	1-methyl-4-phenyl-4-propionoxypiperidine	VIM	ventral intermediate nucleus

Motor Neuron Disease and Neuropathies

16

Anne D. Kloos, Deborah A. Kegelmeyer, John A. Buford, and Jill C. Heathcock

OBJECTIVES

1) Describe the general approach to and interpretation of nerve conduction studies, including motor and sensory studies of peripheral nerves, and clinical electromyography

2) Describe the demographics, risk factors, etiology, pathophysiology, diagnosis, general progression, and prognosis of Amyotrophic Lateral Sclerosis (ALS), Guillain–Barré Syndrome (GBS), Postpolio Syndrome (PPS), neuropathies, and brachial plexus injuries

3) Differentiate among signs and symptoms and impairments related to lower motor neuron pathology versus upper motor neuron pathology

4) Discuss the medical management of common symptoms found in individuals with motor neuron and neuropathy disorders

5) Design a physical therapy intervention program with appropriate goals and outcomes for the individual with motor neuron or neuropathy disorders

6) Discuss the current knowledge of degeneration and regeneration phenomena of nerve and muscle

INTRODUCTION

This chapter focuses on diseases and disorders that affect neurons. Common to each of these disorders are changes in the way muscles are activated and nerves convey information. This may involve disruption in sensory afferents, lower or upper motor neurons, or all of these. Diagnosis of these conditions typically involves electrophysiologic testing, so we will begin this chapter with an introduction to these measures.

ELECTROPHYSIOLOGIC TESTS

Electrophysiologic testing employs a variety of approaches to evaluate the function of the nervous system. This is also referred to as electrodiagnostic testing, but in a certain sense that is a misnomer. The results of these tests must always be correlated with other clinical findings and would never be diagnostic on their own. This is why the term "electrophysiologic testing" is more appropriate.

CASE A, PART I

Mr. Posner is a 40-year-old, married, father of two children, ages 7 and 9, who worked as the chief financial officer at an insurance company. He was in good health until 6 months ago when he began to have trouble using his left hand for writing, typing on a computer keyboard, cutting food, handling utensils, and buttoning his shirts. He also noticed that his walking was slower, and his legs sometimes felt "heavy and tired," after going up a flight of stairs. Mr. Posner went to a neurologist, who ordered a variety of tests, including electrophysiologic testing.

Usually, the focus of attention for electrophysiologic testing is on the peripheral nervous system, but there are approaches to measure central nervous system function as well. **Nerve Conduction Studies** (NCS) in the peripheral nervous system are most useful for detecting reduced conduction velocity due to damage to the myelination of the nerves.[1] **Clinical Electromyography** (EMG) using needle electrodes within the muscles is the most reliable way to determine whether the axons themselves are injured.[1] Needle EMG can also allow for relatively specific testing of nerve root levels to aid in the diagnosis of radiculopathy.[2-5] Overall, the clinical reasoning used to interpret results from NCS and EMG studies mimics the clinician's reasoning using a combination of sensory testing and manual muscle testing. Findings are compared with known nerve root levels and peripheral innervations to identify the pathology. Electrophysiologic testing allows a greater degree of precision in grading the severity of the injury, provides the ability to distinguish myelin from axonal damage, and can be used to determine the chronicity of the pathology.[1-5]

Nerve Conduction Studies (NCS)

Nerve conduction studies (aka Nerve Conduction Velocity Studies, NCV), are used to test the health and integrity of peripheral nerves. In general, the test is performed by using an electrical stimulator to depolarize a large number of axons in a single peripheral nerve. The response can be measured as an EMG (electromyographic) response, if the peripheral nerve innervates a muscle, or as the electrical potential created by action potentials traveling through another part of the nerve. If the nerve is damaged in some way that totally prevents transmission, the finding would be a total lack of response. Usually, however, there is partial damage. This will typically result in a response that is smaller than it should be, and conduction through the nerve that is slower than normal.

Motor versus Sensory Tests

Motor Studies

In a motor test, the objective is to test the integrity of a nerve that innervates a muscle. There are a limited number of muscles that can be studied because there is not a motor test for every muscle in the body.[6] Typically, there is reason to suspect a problem with one or more peripheral nerves when a NCS is performed. The clinician would usually pick a particular peripheral nerve, such as the median, ulnar, or radial nerve in the forearm, and study one or two muscles innervated by that nerve to check for nerve function. For example, the ulnar nerve (Figure 16-1A) is usually tested with mm. abductor digiti minimi.[3,6] This ulnar-innervated muscle is easily accessible for surface EMG recording and will typically be the first muscle in the hand to respond to ulnar nerve stimulation. For the median nerve, the mm. abductor pollicis brevis is used, and for the radial nerve, mm. extensor indicis proprius is used.[6] There will be a distal stimulation site and one or more proximal stimulation sites for most motor tests. For the median nerve, for example, the distal stimulation site is over the median nerve with a distance between the distal part of the stimulator and the proximal EMG electrode set to a standard of 8 cm.[6,7] From that point, the distance to more proximal sites must be measured, based on the individual, with a site in the antecubital fossa and another in the axilla used where the median nerve is accessible to stimulation. As an example, in the lower extremity, the muscle studied for the deep fibular (peroneal) nerve would be the extensor digitorum brevis in the foot. The stimulation sites would be a point just lateral to the tibia 8-cm proximal to the EMG electrode, and a second point over the common fibular (peroneal) nerve by the fibular head.[6,8]

The reason for having multiple stimulation sites along the length of the nerve is to be able to isolate a particular zone where nerve function is impaired.[1] In mild peripheral nerve injury, the injury mainly involves damage to the myelin sheath, with little or no actual loss of the axons themselves.[1] Because there are multiple Schwann cells that make myelin, distributed along the length of the nerve, it is possible (and indeed, common) for a particular segment of nerve to sustain a **myelin injury**, while other parts of the nerve function normally. For example, consider an ulnar nerve injury at the elbow (Figure 16-1B). The conduction through the ulnar nerve from the distal forearm to the hand would be normal. The conduction from a forearm site just a few centimeters distal to the elbow could also be normal, but conduction impairment would be evident from a site just proximal to the elbow. It is important for the clinician to locate normal segments of nerve on either side of the damaged segment, so with the ulnar nerve finding above, an additional stimulation site in the axilla would be required.[3,6] This would allow confirmation that segments of the ulnar nerve in the upper arm and in the forearm function normally, localizing the lesion to

the elbow. To complete the picture, the clinician would want to confirm that the median nerve on the same side was normal, and that both the ulnar and median nerves on the other side were also normal.[3]

An important physiologic principle that allows motor testing to be done at multiple points along the nerve is the consistency in the sizes and conduction velocities of the alpha motoneuron axons. Alpha motoneuron axons do have a slight variation in size between the fibers going to slow oxidative versus fast glycolytic motor units; however, compared to the whole range of nerve fiber sizes in a mixed peripheral nerve, the alpha motoneuron axons sizes and conduction velocities are relatively homogeneous.[1] A useful analogy is to think of an American football team running a 200-m sprint. The wide receivers and defensive backs will finish first. Running backs and linebackers will come in second. Defensive linemen will come in third, and offensive linemen will come in last. Individuals may vary, but as a rule, this would be the order of the groups. In this analogy, the very fastest group, the wide receivers and defensive backs, would be analogous to the large-diameter sensory fibers. They are the fastest fibers in the nerve. The motor axons would be like the running backs and linebackers, who are still very fast. The linemen would be like the slower sensory fibers.

If we pick out the running backs and they all run 50, 100, or 200 m, they will still be bunched in a relatively tight pack for each distance. But if the whole team runs these various distances, then the farther the race, the greater the spread will be among the packs. In NCS, this spreading out of the arrival times of the action potentials is called **temporal dispersion**. Because the motor fibers are relatively homogenous in conduction velocity (temporal dispersion is low), stimulation at a variety of distances from the muscle will still result in a relatively synchronized arrival time for action potentials from all the stimulated axons, and hence, a relatively consistent size and duration of the EMG waveform recorded. This is the underlying physiology that allows testing for motor function at relatively long distances.

Sensory Studies

Sensory studies are more technically difficult to perform.[6] First, we do not have the luxury of recording an EMG response from a muscle. We must instead record the electrical potentials associated with action potentials traveling through the axons themselves. Actually, an EMG recording is produced by the action potentials and associated ionic currents in the muscle cells themselves, not the muscle nerves. Obviously, the muscle is much larger than a nerve, and there is much more current flow involved in a muscle action potential than a nerve action potential. The voltage from a muscle recorded through the skin is about 1000 times larger than the voltage that can be recorded through the skin from a nerve. Smaller voltages are harder to measure and are more susceptible to noise and technical error in the electrode placement and equipment setup, so this makes sensory studies more difficult. Second, it is harder to be sure that the stimulating and recording electrodes are both in the proper location for a sensory study. For a motor study, we know the stimulation position is correct (if the muscle is intact) because we can see the muscle twitch, and with good knowledge of neuromuscular anatomy, it is not hard to find the muscles. In sensory studies, there is no

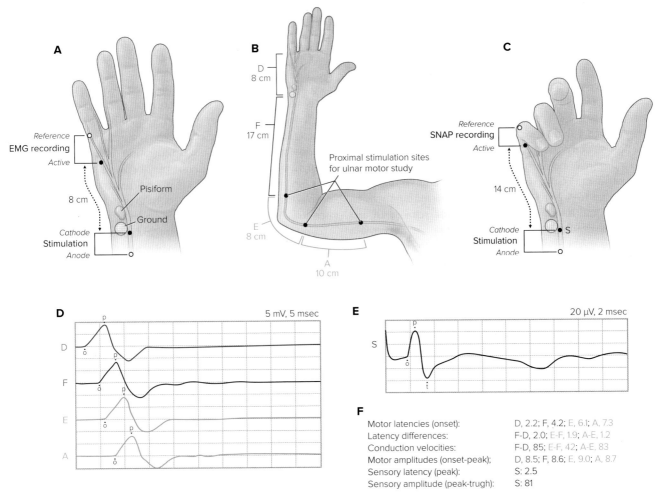

F

Motor latencies (onset):	D, 2.2; F, 4.2; E, 6.1; A, 7.3
Latency differences:	F-D, 2.0; E-F, 1.9; A-E, 1.2
Conduction velocities:	F-D, 85; E-F, 42; A-E, 83
Motor amplitudes (onset-peak);	D, 8.5; F, 8.6; E, 9.0; A, 8.7
Sensory latency (peak):	S: 2.5
Sensory amplitude (peak-trough):	S: 81

FIGURE 16-1 Examples of motor and sensory studies for the ulnar nerve. A. The setup for measuring distal motor latency for the ulnar nerve is shown. **B**. Additional proximal motor testing points are illustrated. With multiple points, the conduction velocities in the forearm, elbow, and arm segments can each be calculated. **C**. An antidromic sensory testing setup is illustrated. The stimulus is applied in a location similar to that used for the motor test. Recording electrodes around the small finger measure the SNAP as it passes antidromically through the digital nerves. **D**. Illustration of a sample ulnar nerve motor study in a case with mild slowing at the elbow. Arrows **o** and **p** indicate the onset and peak of each response. **E**. Illustration of a distal sensory antidromic study. Arrows **o**, **p**, and **t** indicate the onset, peak, and trough of each response, respectively. **F** shows the measures that would be obtained from D and E. For motor studies, the latency is based on the onset, and the amplitude is measured between the onset and peak. The segments are color coded, **D for distal**, **F for forearm**, **E for elbow**, and **A for arm**. To calculate conduction velocity for the proximal segments, the latency between responses from the two sites is divided by the distance between the sites. Normal conduction velocities should be faster than 50 m per second. Note the slowing at the elbow segment. Distal motor latency for the ulnar nerve at an 8 cm distance should be less than 4.2 msec and amplitude should exceed 2.5 mV. The values presented here should be a normal distal motor result. For a sensory study at 14 cm, the latency should be less than 3.7 msec and the amplitude should exceed 15 μV. Sensory latencies are based on the time of the first peak, and the amplitude is measured from peak to trough. Again, this is a normal sensory study. The results are consistent with a mild myelin injury at the elbow. (A–C: Adapted from Centers for Disease Control and Prevention (CDC). Performing motor and sensory neuronal conduction studies in adult humans. NIOSH Publication No. 90-113, September 1990.)

corresponding response like a muscle twitch, and we cannot see or feel the nerve. We must know the anatomy and proper electrode positions to perform the test.[6,7]

As noted above, there are also a wide variety of conduction velocities present among axons in a sensory nerve (temporal dispersion is high). As explained in the football team analogy above, this makes it hard to get accurate testing from long distances in sensory nerves. The arrivals of the action potentials are spread out, so the waveform is smaller and harder to consistently measure.

For this reason, there is usually only one distance, the most distal (shortest) segment, studied in a sensory test for a nerve conduction study. Additional distances can be tested, but this is not routine.[7]

Motor and Sensory Studies Are Both Required

A complete nerve conduction study would include at least two sensory nerves and at least two motor nerves studied in the limb where there is a concern.[1,3,8–11] In addition, the same tests would need to be performed on the other side, and at least one of the other limbs should be studied (e.g., left arm, right arm, left leg). Additional tests would be added to rule in or rule out suspected conditions. Why include sensory tests when motor tests are easier? Sensory tests are more sensitive.[1] A pebble in the shoe of the wide receiver will make more difference (and be complained about for all to hear …) than a pebble in the shoe of the offensive lineman. The largest diameter axons are most sensitive to injury – even a slight myelin injury will notably reduce their conduction velocity. Hence, in mild forms of nerve damage, motor studies may be normal, but sensory studies will reveal mild impairment.[12] Thus, sensory and motor studies must both be done. Table 16-1 provides a list of nerves commonly tested in the upper and lower limbs for motor and sensory studies, including the stimulation and recording sites.

Measurements for NCS

The two most important measurements taken for NCS are latency (and where possible, conduction velocity) and amplitude.[6,7] From the most distal stimulation site to the recording location, we measure latency (the time between the stimulus and the response). Although it might be tempting to measure the distance and divide by time to calculate conduction velocity, this is invalid for the most distal site. When electrical stimulation is applied to a nerve, there is a series of events required to initiate an action potential. The capacitance of the tissue must be charged, voltage-gated ion channels must open, and current must flow to depolarize the inside of the axon. This delay is called the **utilization time** and can take 0.5 msec or more. In a motor study, there would be an additional synaptic delay of about the same duration at the synapse for the neuromuscular junction.[1] These delays may sound brief, but conduction velocities in human nerves are fast enough that the time taken to travel from the wrist to the finger might only be 2 msec, so these delays

are substantial. Hence, for the most distal site, we measure the latency from the onset of stimulation to the response and record the number as a time without attempting to calculate velocity.

When there is more than one stimulation site on a nerve, as in a motor study, we can calculate the **conduction velocity** for the more proximal segments. Here, we take the difference in distance between the two stimulation sites and divide by the difference in latencies for the corresponding responses to calculate a conduction velocity local to the segment of nerve between the stimulation sites.[6] Whatever utilization time and synaptic delays might be present should not vary between stimulation sites, so as long as we focus on the relative times and distances, conduction velocity can be calculated. In the ulnar nerve example provided above, we would note a normal distal latency and normal conduction velocities in the forearm and upper arm segments, but a reduced conduction velocity in the segment at the elbow.[6,8]

Latency and velocity are the most reliable measures from NCS, but accurate readings require special care to use appropriate technique and to measure distances accurately.[6] Various studies have published normative values for distal latencies and segmental conduction velocities in the peripheral nervous system.[6,13] Modern testing equipment will typically have these values stored in software so that abnormal findings are automatically flagged.

Prolonged latencies or reduced conduction velocities can be interpreted as damage to the myelin.[1] In the race analogy above, we could imagine that there is a damaged section of the running track. The runners begin at normal speed, but slowdown in the damaged section. Once past the damage, they return to normal speed. Myelin injury decreases the length constant of a myelinated nerve, which reduces conduction velocity.

In addition to latency and conduction velocity, the amplitude (size) of the response must also be measured. Due to individual variations in body composition and muscle and nerve location and size, there is more variation in amplitude. Nonetheless, amplitude

TABLE 16-1	Nerves and Sites for Electrophysiologic Testing[6]		
NERVE	**TEST**	**RECORDING**	**STIMULATION SITE(S)**
Median	Motor	Abductor pollicis brevis	Wrist, elbow, and axilla
Median	Sensory (antidromic)	Index finger	Wrist
Ulnar	Motor	Abductor digiti minimi	Wrist, below elbow, above elbow, axilla
Ulnar	Sensory (antidromic)	Small finger	Wrist
Radial	Motor	Extensor indicis proprius	Forearm, upper arm, axilla
Radial	Sensory	Thumb or dorsal wrist (antidromic)	Distal forearm
Deep fibular (peroneal)	Motor	Extensor digitorum brevis	Anterior leg, fibular head, popliteal space
Posterior tibial	Motor	Abductor hallucis	Distal leg above ankle, popliteal fossa
Sural	Sensory (antidromic)	Lateral foot	Posterior lower leg
Superficial fibular (peroneal)	Sensory (antidromic)	Dorsal foot	Anterolateral leg

must always be measured. In a motor study, for example, there will be multiple stimulation points along the length of the nerve. To ensure that the nerve was stimulated with equal effectiveness at all sites, we must attempt to achieve less than 10% variation in the amplitude of the responses. Because temporal dispersion is low in motor nerves, this should be feasible if the nerve is normal.[1,6]

If NCS reveals decreased amplitude and the test is done correctly, then this indicates a failure in conduction. Imagine in the running analogy that a section of track has totally failed; there is a giant pit. The runner cannot leave his lane, so he cannot finish the race. An action potential traveling along an axon can reach a point so severely damaged (by myelin loss or axonal injury) that conduction cannot continue. Just as the runner cannot switch lanes, the action potential cannot jump to another axon, so it ends. The result is fewer action potentials reaching the recording site, which results in a smaller amplitude of the response. With NCS, there is no way to distinguish between severe myelin and axonal injury; both will result in decreased amplitude.[1] Needle EMG does allow that distinction, so both NCS and EMG should be included in electrophysiologic testing.

Finally, in reading the results of NCS, there are some abbreviations commonly used that should be understood. In a motor study, the peripheral nerve is stimulated, the action potentials reach the neuromuscular junction, the muscle depolarizes, and twitches. What is being recorded is motor action potentials from all the motor units in the muscle that responded to the stimulus. The technical name for this is a **Compound Motor Action Potential**, and this is abbreviated as **CMAP**. So, in motor studies for NCS, we record CMAPs. In sensory studies, we are also stimulating a large number of sensory axons and recording the combined voltage potential from them all as they pass under the recording site. We could call this a compound sensory nerve action potential, but the shorthand is simply **Sensory Nerve Action Potential**, and the abbreviation is **SNAP**. So, in sensory studies for NCS, we record SNAPs.[7]

Late Waves (F-Waves and H-Reflexes)

In certain locations in the body, a special kind of nerve conduction study can be performed to create a response that requires action potentials to travel from the stimulation site into the spinal cord and back out again. This can allow testing of the proximal nerve segments, including the brachial and lumbosacral plexus, when stimulation and recording sites are relatively inaccessible.

The **H-reflex** (named for the physician, Hoffmann, who described it), uses the circuits for the monosynaptic stretch reflex.[14] The peripheral nerve is stimulated to activate the Ia afferents from the muscle spindle. Action potentials travel along these fibers into the spinal cord, synapse monosynaptically on the alpha motoneurons, and cause them to make action potentials. This volley of action potentials then travels out the alpha motoneuron axons to the muscles, resulting in a muscle twitch that can be measured with EMG. Because of the long transit time required to the spinal cord and back, this is a type of late wave. The gamma motoneurons and actual muscle spindle proprioceptor organ are not involved in the H-reflex. The Ia afferent is stimulated directly, so no real muscle stretch is required.[1]

Because the Ia afferents are among the largest, most heavily myelinated fibers in the nerve, they have the longest length constant and are therefore easiest to stimulate with electrical stimulation.[14] Hence, it is possible to stimulate a nerve with minimal current and elicit an H-reflex without directly stimulating the muscle. However, this is not a reliable approach to testing. If the nerve innervates the muscle appropriately, then it should be possible to stimulate a direct motor response in the muscle without waiting for the reflex, just as if this was a regular motor study. A reliable H-reflex test creates a small M-wave (the direct motor response) to establish effective and consistent stimulation (consistent M-wave size). This M-wave should not be full sized; it should be smaller than a full-blown response. The measurement is the latency of the H-reflex that follows. The latency is the only parameter used for the H-reflex. The objective is to elicit about 10 waves and demonstrate a consistent latency. If peripheral nerve tests are normal but the H-reflex latency is delayed, this is consistent with a nerve root impingement or nerve damage of some sort proximal to the most proximal stimulation site.[1]

The **F-wave** also requires transmission through the proximal nerve to the spinal cord, but does not involve sensory fibers.[14] It was first described in the muscles of the foot, hence the abbreviation, F. Only the alpha motoneuron axons are involved in the F-wave. With stimulation of the motor axons, action potentials travel away from the stimulation site in both directions. The ones traveling toward the muscle in the normal direction (the **orthodromic volley**) produce a muscle twitch, whereas the ones traveling back toward the alpha motoneurons (the **antidromic volley**) would not be expected to do anything. However, due to special properties of motoneurons, a small subset of the motor pool will respond to the antidromic volley with depolarization sufficient to evoke an outgoing action potential. To observe this effect, maximal stimulation sufficient to produce a full-blown M-wave is required. The exact latency of the F-wave will vary across trials because the exact set of alpha motoneurons participating is not always identical. Hence, 10 to 20 tests are performed, and the best latency is taken.[1]

H-reflexes can only be elicited from certain muscles. The only H-reflex used reliably in clinical testing is the soleus.[14] F-waves can be elicited from most distal muscles. Overall, late waves can be a useful adjunct in electrophysiologic testing, but they have limited sensitivity and specificity and would always need to be combined with other tests.[1]

Clinical Electromyography

There are many uses and applications of EMG, which is the recording and measurement of electrical potentials from the muscles. As described earlier, for example, CMAPs are used to measure motor responses to peripheral nerve stimulation. For studies in biomechanics and kinesiology, EMG is often used to discern how the muscles are activated in conjunction with movements like walking. For electrophysiologic testing, a different kind of EMG recording is used. A small needle is inserted directly into the muscle to record the electrical potentials in the immediate vicinity of the muscle cells themselves.

The purpose of this form of measurement is to study the activity of a single motor unit.[13] As noted in Chapter 4, a motor unit consists of one alpha motoneuron and all the muscle fibers it innervates. When the alpha motoneuron makes an action potential, all the muscle fibers in the motor unit should respond in a consistent manner. Wherever the needle tip happens to sit in the muscle, there should be a consistent and relatively synchronized pattern of ionic current flows each time a particular motor unit fires, and the consequence is a consistent voltage record in the recording.[15] A healthy motor unit should produce a wave form with an overall shape, duration, and amplitude that falls within general boundaries for the norm. The exact shape of each motor unit's waveform in the muscle will be unique, but factors such as the number of times the voltage goes positive and negative (baseline crossings) and the expectation that at least part of the waveform, usually the largest peak, should be negative (reflecting current going into the muscle cell) are hallmarks of normal motor unit waveforms.[1,15] Waveforms that are too brief, too long, too small, too large, or too complex with multiple baseline crossings can all be signs of specific pathologies.

Technically, a needle EMG study is easy to perform. The needle is smaller than most hypodermic syringes. A physical therapist is well aware of muscle location, function, and innervation, and this is the main knowledge needed to choose and study the muscles. In rare cases, there may be cause to study challenging muscles around the face or other sensitive locations. In this case, a responsible practitioner would refer out to someone more experienced, if necessary. The majority of studies are in the limbs and paraspinal muscles, where the risk of penetrating or damaging critical structures is low, and the physical therapist has more than adequate knowledge of the neuromuscular system. With appropriate training, needle EMG studies are well within the capacity of a physical therapist.[16]

In a typical test, a muscle is selected for study based on its innervation, including the peripheral nerve and the neurological segmental level from which it is controlled. The needle EMG is connected to a loudspeaker in addition to the recording circuit. With practice, the clinician can readily learn to hear the difference between normal and pathological waveforms in EMG. Again, the clinical reasoning mimics that used in selecting muscles to test, when there is suspected neuropathy or radiculopathy. The clinician should attempt to document the waveform and firing pattern for about 12 motor units from each muscle. Studies indicate that this number provides the desired level of specificity and sensitivity. To do this, the pyramiding technique is usually employed. The needle is inserted into the muscle through the skin and recordings are made at three depths. Then the needle is withdrawn until it is not quite out of the skin, the angle is changed, and another set of three depths are studied. This is repeated two more times at differing angles, yielding 12 recording sites from one penetration of the skin.[1]

From the first depth to the second and the second to the third in each electrode track, the needle is advanced rapidly to the next depth and then held still. In a denervated muscle, this mechanical irritation will evoke involuntary electrical activity in the muscle cells that cannot be suppressed. This is called **insertional activity**. In a normal muscle, there will be a scratching sound while the electrode is advanced, but once the electrode is still, the muscle will be quiet. Therefore, significant insertional activity is abnormal and is a sign of axonal injury.[1]

When the muscle fibers of a motor unit are first disconnected from the motoneuron, they will begin to atrophy and will begin making spontaneous action potentials in individual fibers of the motor unit.[15] Because only one myofibril fires at a time, these will be brief in duration and small in amplitude. Most importantly, they occur involuntarily while the patient is attempting to keep the muscle completely relaxed. These involuntary denervation potentials, also called **spontaneous potentials**, come in two distinct forms. One is called a **positive sharp wave**. These have a V-shaped appearance (by convention, positive is downward for EMG), and hence the name. The other waveform is a **fibrillation potential**. This is both positive and negative, but is extremely brief, much too brief to be a motor unit. For clinical interpretation, positive sharp waves and fibrillation potentials both mean the same thing; these spontaneous potentials are a highly specific sign of axonal injury.[15]

Another type of spontaneous potential is called a **fasciculation**. These are not always a sign of neuromuscular pathology and can be associated with fatigue, thyroid disorders, or excessive intake of stimulants. However, they also can result from peripheral nerve injuries or in lower motor neuron injuries. On EMG examination, a fasciculation looks like a normal single motor unit action potential. However, the fasciculation is involuntary. When a person is tired and the muscles around the eye twitch involuntarily, these are fasciculations. All people experience these from time to time, and they may not have any clinical significance. However, when they are widespread and cannot be explained by other common causes, and especially with accompanying signs of a primary neuromuscular disease, they become clinically significant.[17]

In a partially denervated muscle, over time, the motor units that remain innervated will be over worked to compensate. They will hypertrophy and be used even for low levels of effort. Hence, even with minimal effort, motor units with much larger than usual amplitude will be evident. These are called **giant potentials** and are an indication of relatively recent axonal injury.[15] The next stage in recovery would be for the alpha motoneuron axons, associated with these giant potentials, to develop collaterals and find ways to innervate the denervated muscle fibers nearby. The spontaneous potentials in these denervated fibers are a signal to the axon to find them. The motor unit that is composed of a combination of hypertrophied fibers as well as some recently reinnervated fibers will have a giant potential followed by some slower, smaller potentials called **satellite potentials**.[15] As the reinnervation proceeds, the satellite potentials will become stronger and somewhat earlier, but the motor unit in this case will not be able to reproduce the synchronous activation that would be found in a normal motor unit. The result is called a **complex polyphasic potential**, a waveform with multiple baseline crossings and a bizarre shape.[1,15] This would be the endpoint of the reinnervation process. Hence, EMG can be used to detect denervation, reinnervation, and the relative chronicity of the recovery process.

Normally, an individual should be able to gradually increase the recruitment of a muscle, adding in motor units according to the size principle.[15] Hence, with low effort, relatively small motor units are recruited at frequencies of 5 to 15 Hz. As effort increases, the frequency of the motor unit firing increases and more motor units are recruited. At moderate to full effort, the EMG recorded should become what is called a **full interference pattern**. So many motor units are firing that no single waveform can be distinguished, and the waveform is a chaotic assembly of up and down voltage changes. This is normal. The person should be able to reproduce this type of normal recruitment in any muscle on command.[1,15]

In muscular dystrophy, fewer and fewer muscle fibers over time will be functioning. The result can be that even when a person puts forth a full effort, it is still possible to observe individual motor units firing. This means there are so few motor units left that their waveforms cannot interfere with each other. In general, this type of waveform is called a **myopathic potential**.[1,17,18] There is also a phenomenon called **complex repetitive discharge**. In this condition, when a person begins to initiate light effort, a particular motor unit begins firing at an extreme rate, 50 Hz or more, and continues for several seconds, gradually reducing the rate, and then abruptly shutting off. **Myotonic discharge** is a similar phenomenon with a slightly more variable amplitude and frequency. These are both considered relatively nonspecific findings that can occur in acute as well as chronic neuropathy or myopathy. A lack of complex repetitive discharges or myotonic discharge would be unexpected in myopathies, but their overall diagnostic utility is considered low.[19,20]

In sum, clinical EMG testing in any given muscle will involve the study of insertional activity, recording at rest to determine whether spontaneous potentials are present, recruitment through the range of efforts to determine whether myopathy is present, and then a systematic search to record resting activity and document motor unit waveforms from about 12 sites in the muscle.[1,15] If any abnormal findings are to be obtained, this number of sites should be sufficient to permit their observation.

RADICULOPATHY

In suspected radiculopathy, the compression is at the nerve root. In this case, peripheral nerve conduction velocities may be relatively normal, and sensory tests may also be intact, even in the presence of altered sensation from sensory testing because the lesion may be proximal to the dorsal root ganglion. The H-reflex may be helpful in S1 radiculopathy, but in general late waves are not sensitive. The most important aspect of the examination in suspected radiculopathy will be the EMG. There are published clinical guidelines that recommend selected muscles in cases of suspected radiculopathy.[2,3] The general approach is to study muscles at various segmental levels, but not all on the same peripheral nerve, to provide a contrast between the nerve roots versus the peripheral nerves to correlate with the findings.[1] In addition, it is important to include paraspinal muscles. These proximal muscles, being close to the spinal cord, may show findings different than the limb muscles, and this can aid in determining the chronicity of the lesion.[4,5] Once a particular level is suspected for the radiculopathy, additional muscles are tested for that root level. The goal is to find two or more muscles from the same nerve root level but on different peripheral nerves that both show positive findings, but muscles from other root levels on the same peripheral nerve demonstrate normal findings.[1] This is not always possible, but the logic of the clinical reasoning for confirming radiculopathy should be evident.

PLANNING THE ELECTROPHYSIOLOGIC TEST

An electrophysiologic test may be ordered when neuropathy or myopathy is suspected, or in the examination for selected neurodegenerative diseases. Typically, there is a suspicion that a particular condition is present, such as carpal tunnel syndrome, a brachial plexus injury, etc., and the test will be designed around that expectation. As mentioned above, the clinician must always test both limbs (e.g., left and right arm) when a problem is suspected in one and should also perform one test on the other extremity. For example, if a left arm problem is suspected, then the left and right arms should both be tested, and one leg should be tested, as well. This helps rule out central nervous system or systemic problems that could present as a peripheral nerve injury. The examination should include motor and sensory studies for NCS and EMG for selected muscles. In each limb, two motor tests and two sensory tests should be conducted to test different peripheral nerves. This helps differentiate nerve root levels from peripheral nerves. Finally, if radiculopathy is suspected, a set of muscles for EMG should be chosen to represent various spinal nerve root levels as well as various peripheral nerves. Late waves can be studied as well when the suspected pathology includes proximal nerve segments, as in plexus or nerve root injuries. To plan the electrophysiologic test, the clinician would review the suspected pathologies, consult the relevant clinical practice guidelines for that condition, determine which motor and sensory studies to conduct with NCS, and which muscles to study with needle EMG. In the limb with the impairment, the full set of muscles would be studied. In the limb(s) thought to be normal, EMG in key muscles would be recorded to confirm normal findings, but a full-blown study might not be indicated. During the test, as findings unfold, the clinician would be guided by the results to selected additional tests to confirm or rule out the suspected condition(s). With this approach, electrophysiologic testing is a valuable part of the examination for the diagnosis of neuromuscular disorders (Table 16-2).

AMYOTROPHIC LATERAL SCLEROSIS (ALS)

CASE A, PART II

Mr. Posner demonstrated abnormalities in both his motor NCS and the EMG studies, indicating a loss of motor axons and beginning muscle atrophy. Sensory studies in the upper and lower limbs were all normal. In the motor studies, CMAP latencies were normal (myelin intact), but amplitudes were reduced (axonal loss). EMG revealed spontaneous potentials (positive sharp waves and fibrillations) and polyphasic potentials in proximal and distal muscles of the upper and lower limbs. Recruitment was diminished, with failure to produce a full interference pattern in the muscles most affected. His neurologist diagnosed ALS.

TABLE 16-2	Common Neuropathies and the Expected Findings from Electrophysiologic Testing[21–28]
CONDITION	**TYPICAL FINDINGS**
Carpal Tunnel syndrome (median nerve mononeuropathy at the wrist)[21]	Mild: prolonged distal latency in median sensory tests. Moderate: prolonged motor latencies, reduced SNAP and CMAP amplitudes. Severe: muscle atrophy, EMG + for denervation.
Ulnar neuropathy at the elbow[21]	Reduced conduction velocity across the elbow. Motor amplitude drops for stimulation above the elbow. Ulnar SNAP reduced (sensory fibers may have axonal injury). EMG + for denervation.
Radial neuropathy at the axilla[21]	Decreased SNAP and CMAP amplitudes if axonal injury. EMG + for denervation potentials, even in Triceps.
Radiculopathy[22]	May have normal motor and sensory latencies, but reduced amplitude in the affected levels for CMAPs and SNAPs. EMG evidence of denervation in muscles at the affected level. Paraspinal muscles and limb muscles should both be examined.
Spinal stenosis[22]	Presents like a multilevel, bilateral radiculopathy.
Plexopathies[23]	NCS and EMG findings best explained by a particular part of the plexus rather than any one peripheral nerve of segmental level. CMAP and SNAP amplitudes reduced. EMG + for denervation.
Peroneal neuropathy at the fibular head[24]	Tibial and sural nerve function intact, peroneal innervated muscles show positive findings, CMAPs and SNAPs reduced for peroneal motor and sensory NCS, reduced conduction velocity located at the fibular head, H-reflex normal, but F-waves impaired or absent.
Tarsal Tunnel syndrome[24]	Prolonged distal motor latencies from tibial nerve in abductor hallucis and abductor digiti minimi pedis. Potentially prolonged latencies, reduced amplitudes, or both across the tarsal tunnel in the medial and lateral plantar nerves. Normal sural and peroneal nerve studies.
Diabetic peripheral neuropathy[25]	Gloves and socks pattern of impairment, first noted in sensory studies, with motor findings indicating more severe impairment. Multiple nerves affected by distal slowing, not attributable to any particular nerve or segmental level.
ALS[26]	Early signs would be EMG + for denervation potentials (with fasciculations considered significant) in multiple muscles at at least spinal levels and with varying degrees of chronicity (i.e., giant potentials as well as polyphasic potentials), but motor conduction velocities are normal. Reduced recruitment. Sensory testing would be normal unless there was some secondary problem (e.g., CTS).
Myopathies (limb girdle dystrophies)[20]	Reduced recruitment levels, high-frequency recruitment of motor units with minimal effort (early recruitment), small amplitude motor units, myotonic discharges.
Myasthenia gravis[27]	Sensory studies normal. CAMP amplitude decrease by 10% or more in repetitive stimulation at around 3 Hz (2-5 Hz range acceptable). The decrement should be more pronounced after a short bout of exercise with the affected muscle.
Guillain–Barré syndrome[28]	Combination of motor and sensory peripheral nerve involvement in upper and lower limbs. Motor symptoms are usually more severe than sensory in early stages. The LE sural nerve sensory test is often normal despite problems elsewhere ("sural sparing"), which is rare in other polyneuropathies. There is usually a distal onset with progression proximally. The principal signs are myelin injury (prolonged latencies with decreased amplitudes due to temporal dispersion) without axonal injury, but there can be axonal loss (EMG + for denervation) as a consequence of the myelin injury.

Epidemiology and Risk Factors

Motor neuron disease (MND) is the term given to a group of neurodegenerative diseases that selectively affect motor neurons. Amyotrophic Lateral Sclerosis (ALS) is classified as a rare disease, but it is the most common type of MND in adults. It was first described in 1869 by French neurologist Jean-Martin Charcot, but since the beloved baseball player Lou Gehrig was diagnosed with it in 1939, the disease is commonly associated with his name in the United States. The worldwide incidence of ALS is about 1 to 2.6 cases per 100,000 persons annually, and the prevalence is around 6 cases per 100,000.[29] According to the 2015 National ALS Registry, the estimated incidence of ALS in the United States was 1.6 per 100,000 persons, and the prevalence was 5.2 per 100,000 with a total of 16,583 cases identified.[30,31] ALS primarily affects adults between the ages of 40 and 70 (mean age 55 at time of diagnosis), and is 20% more common in men than women.[32] Within the United States, non-Hispanic whites are approximately twice as likely to develop ALS as African American and Hispanic populations.[33,34]

Some studies have reported links between lifestyle and environmental factors and onset of ALS. Risk factors with the strongest evidence include a history of physical trauma/injury (e.g., skeletal fractures, head trauma, severe electrical injury or burns), and previous exposure to neurotoxins in chemicals (i.e., fertilizers and pesticides), heavy metals (i.e., lead, mercury), and organic solvents (i.e., cleaning solvents and degreasers, alcohols and ketones).[29,35,36] The relationship between ALS and environmental factors is exemplified by the presence of geographical clusters with high incidence of ALS. For example, an increased incidence of ALS with parkinsonism-dementia complex (PDC) in the Pacific island of Guam (United States) and the Kii peninsula of Japan has been linked to dietary consumption of cycad plants containing the neurotoxin cycasin.[37] Similarly, an almost twofold increased incidence of ALS found among military personnel deployed to the Gulf Region during the Gulf War has been associated with their exposure to metals and chemicals during the war[29,37,38] However, current evidence is not sufficient to definitively determine the causal influence of any of these lifestyle and environmental factors on ALS.

Pathophysiology

ALS is named for its pathophysiology. The term "amyotrophy" means atrophy of muscle fibers, which are denervated as their corresponding cranial and spinal motor neurons in the brainstem and ventral horns of the spinal cord (i.e., lower motor neurons) degenerate (Figure 16-2). Lateral sclerosis refers to hardening of the ventral and lateral columns of the spinal cord as corticospinal neurons (i.e., upper motor neurons) in these areas degenerate and are replaced by fibrous astrocytes (gliosis).

Although most patients with ALS have no family history of the disease (sporadic ALS, SALS), 5 to 10% of cases inherit the disease and are considered familial (FALS) cases.[39,40] An expansion in the hexanucleotide repeat sequence (GGGGCC) in the RNA processing gene *C9ORF72* is responsible for about 40% of all familial ALS cases.[40] This gene also causes 25% of frontotemporal dementia (FTD) cases. People with this mutated gene may develop symptoms of ALS only, FTD only, or symptoms of both disorders. Mutations in the gene superoxide dismutase 1 (*SOD1*) that encodes the enzyme copper-zinc superoxide dismutase (CuZnSOD), account for about 12-20% of FALS cases.[40] The normal CuZnSOD enzyme functions to rid neurons of harmful free radicals.[41] The mutant *SOD1* enzyme's detrimental effects are thought to be mediated by a gain of one or more toxic functions.[42] Mutations in the RNA processing *TARDBP* gene that encodes the TAR DNA-binding protein 43 (TDP-43)

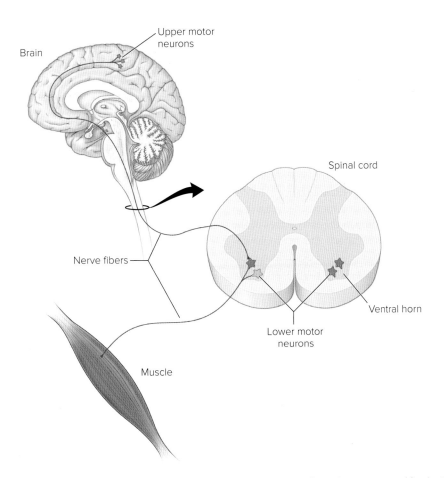

FIGURE 16-2 Pathophysiology of ALS. ALS affects upper motor neurons that arise from the cortex and brainstem as well as cranial and spinal lower motor neurons that arise from the brainstem and spinal cord.

are responsible for about 4% of FALS.[40] The protein normally functions in the cell nucleus as a gene regulator, but the mutated TDP-43 protein moves into the cytoplasm where it aggregates into abnormal clumps. Mutations in another gene, called fused in sarcoma (*FUS*), that is structurally and functionally similar to *TARDP*, is responsible for about 4% of FALS.[40] Abnormal accumulations of TDP-43 are found in almost all cases of ALS (except for *SOD1* and *FUS* cases), even if TDP-43 mutations are absent, suggesting that TDP-43 may play a pivotal role in many forms of ALS.[39] All of these gene mutations cause an autosomal dominant form of ALS. Sporadic ALS has been linked to a variety of genetic mutations, including *C9ORF72*, *SOD1*, *TARDP*, and *FUS* mutations that confer susceptibility for the disease and/or modify the age of onset and severity of the disease[39,40]

ALS is thought to develop by a complex interaction between molecular and genetic pathways.[39,43] Elevated levels of glutamate caused by increased glutamate release and reduced glutamate uptake by astrocytes leads to glutamate excitotoxicity. Glutamate overstimulation induces neurodegeneration through activation of calcium-dependent enzymatic pathways. Mutations in the *C9ORF72*, *TARDP*, and *FUS* genes impair RNA metabolism, leading to production of abnormal proteins that form damaging aggregates in the neuronal cytoplasm. Interactions between the mutated SOD1, TDP-43, and FUS proteins and the mitochondria induce (1) mitochondrial dysfunction, resulting in the increased formation of free radicals, more specifically reactive oxygen species, that are neurotoxic, and (2) defective axonal transportation. Altered axonal transportation leads to abnormal aggregation of neurofilaments in the cell body and proximal axons of motor neurons that disrupt transport of proteins and organelles from cell bodies to axon terminal endings that are critical to neuronal function and survival. In addition, activated astrocytes and microglia secrete proinflammatory molecules that are neurotoxic.[39,43]

The selective damage to motor neurons in ALS is hypothesized to be due to (1) their large size and long axonal length that require high mitochondrial activity and neurofilament content for energy and structural integrity and (2) the high content of SOD1 protein within them.[44] In addition, motor neurons appear to be especially sensitive to glutamate excitotoxicity.[44] Motor neuron loss is greater in large myelinated motor neurons than smaller ones and proceeds more rapidly in the early stages of the disease than later ones. Clinical observations and neurophysiological evidence suggest that hyperexcitability of descending corticomotoneurons, which connect monosynaptically with spinal motor neurons, mediate neurodegeneration in a "dying forward" pattern via an anterograde transsynaptic glutamate excitotoxic process[43] However, there is considerable debate about the site of ALS onset with some people proposing that lower motor neurons degenerate from the distal axon to the cell body, continuing to the upper motor neuron in a "dying back" manner, and others hypothesizing that upper and lower motor neurons degenerate independently of each other and in a random manner.[43] On biopsy, degeneration of motor axons with associated atrophy can be observed in the ventral roots in the spinal cord and within the corticospinal tracts. In advanced cases, atrophy may be present in the frontal (i.e., primary motor and premotor cortex) and temporal lobes as well. As axons degenerate in the periphery, collateral branches of surviving axons in the surrounding area will sprout and reinnervate denervated muscle fibers, thereby compensating for the motor unit loss. However, with increasing loss of motor units over time, reinnervation cannot compensate for the degeneration and motor impairments develop.[45]

Clinical Presentation and Progression

The classic presentation of ALS is slowly progressive, asymmetric muscular weakness and atrophy indicative of lower motor neuron (LMN) involvement along with upper motor neuron (UMN) signs of hyperreflexia. In 70 to 80% of patients, symptoms begin in the extremities (i.e., limb-onset ALS), while 20 to 30% of patients present with bulbar symptoms (i.e., bulbar-onset ALS) (Table 16-3).[46] Distal extremity muscles (i.e., hands and feet) are often involved before proximal extremity muscles. As in Mr. Posner's case, patients with early leg involvement often complain of tripping, stumbling, or awkwardness, when walking or running; those with arm involvement may complain of dropping things and difficulty picking up small objects or buttoning shirts. Bulbar-onset ALS occurs more frequently in middle-aged women, and initial symptoms include difficulty chewing, swallowing, and speaking. Tongue fasciculations (visible muscle twitches of the tongue) and atrophy as well as an increased jaw jerk reflex are common signs of bulbar-onset ALS. Despite the variability in symptom presentation, the course of the disease is similar in most patients with progressive spread of muscle weakness to other areas, leading eventually to total paralysis of spinal musculature and muscles innervated by the cranial nerves.[46]

Clinical features that are atypical of ALS include sensory dysfunction, bowel and bladder impairment, and abnormalities of eye movements.[46] Sensory pathways for the most part are spared

TABLE 16-3	**Motor Neuron Pathology and Associated Signs and Symptoms in ALS[46]**	
MOTOR NEURON TYPE	**AFFECTED NEURONS**	**ASSOCIATED SIGNS AND SYMPTOMS**
Upper motor neurons (UMN)	Pyramidal Betz motor neurons in the cerebral cortex, corticospinal and corticobulbar tracts	Loss of dexterity or the ability to coordinate movements; muscle paresis; spasticity; Hoffmann and Babinski reflexes; hyperreflexia; spastic dysarthria
Brainstem motor neurons (Bulbar)	Cranial nerve nuclei: V (trigeminal), VII (facial), IX (glossopharyngeal), X (vagus), and XII (hypoglossal)	Difficulty with chewing, Dysphagia; flaccid dysarthria/anarthria
Lower motor neurons (LMN)	Ventral horn cells in the spinal cord	Muscle paralysis and atrophy; fasciculations; flaccid tone; hyporeflexia; respiratory problems

in ALS, although studies have reported sensory deficits in some individuals.[47,48] Motor neurons at the second sacral level in the spinal cord (S2) that control the anal and external urethral sphincter muscles and muscles of the pelvic floor are also generally spared. However, some individuals do experience urinary urgency and constipation, suggesting that supranuclear control over sympathetic, parasympathetic, and somatic neurons may be abnormal in ALS. The oculomotor, trochlear, and abducens nerves that control external ocular muscles are also typically spared, until late stages of the disease.[49]

Longitudinal studies of the natural history of ALS have revealed that symptoms tend to progress in a contiguous manner, meaning that they spread from one focal region to an anatomically adjacent area.[46,50] For example, symptoms that start in one arm spread the fastest to the opposite arm, then to the ipsilateral leg, contralateral leg, and brainstem in that order. Thus, patients with initial unilateral arm or leg involvement often develop symptoms in spinal cord levels before they develop bulbar symptoms. To better describe clinical disease progression in ALS, two "stage" systems have been proposed by Roche et al,[51] and by Chio et al.[52] Roche et al. proposed a four-stage system with stages defined as (1) symptom onset (functional involvement including weakness, wasting, spasticity, dysarthria or dysphagia of one CNS region defined as bulbar, upper limb, lower limb or diaphragmatic), (2A) diagnosis, (2B) involvement of a second region, (3) involvement of a third region, and (4A) needing gastrostomy and (4B) noninvasive ventilation.[51] Chio et al. proposed a six-stage system in which milestones in ALS progression are defined by loss of independence in four key domains on the ALS Functional Rating Scale (ALSFRS): swallowing, walking/self-care, communicating, and breathing. Stages were defined as follows: stage 0, functional involvement but no loss of independence on any domain; stages 1 to 4, number of domains in which independence was lost; and stage 5, death.[52]

Diagnosis and Variants of ALS

Due to a lack of definitive diagnostic tests or biological markers, the diagnosis of ALS is made by clinical findings of a progressive course of weakness, with both UMN and LMN findings in four anatomically defined regions of the body: brainstem (bulbar), cervical, thoracic, and lumbar. Differential medical diagnosis includes exclusion of other musculoskeletal, neurologic, or systemic conditions. The El Escorial World Federation of Neurology criteria for the diagnosis of ALS (possible, probable, and definite)

has been widely accepted for use in clinical practice, clinical trials, and research.[44,53] The original El Escorial criteria published in 1994 has undergone two revisions, the most recent of which is called the Awaji-Shima criteria (see Table 16-4).[17]

Electrophysiological, muscle biopsy, and neuroimaging studies can be used to support the diagnosis of ALS and to rule out other diagnoses. NCS of peripheral sensory and motor neurons are usually normal or near normal in ALS in early disease stages.[26] Electromyographic studies are the most important diagnostic tests and typically reveal signs of active denervation (i.e., fibrillation and fasciculation potentials, positive sharp waves) as well as chronic denervation (i.e., large or unstable motor unit potentials, reduced motor unit recruitment) (see Electromyography section).[26] Muscle biopsy studies in ALS corroborate EMG findings, showing signs of denervation (i.e., atrophied muscle fibers) and reinnervation (i.e., fiber type grouping) (Figure 16-3).[55] Transcranial magnetic stimulation and structural and functional neuroimaging (e.g., conventional magnetic resonance imaging, diffusion tensor imaging, proton magnetic resonance spectroscopy, and functional MRI) are used to detect degeneration of corticospinal tracts and altered cortical activation, during motor tasks, thereby providing insights into the extent and effects of UMN pathology.[56,57] The combination of primary motor cortical thickness and diffusion tensor MRI measurements of corticospinal tract and corpus callosum integrity showed 94% accuracy in distinguishing persons with ALS from persons with ALS-mimicking conditions.[58] Although currently not routinely used in diagnosis, increased blood levels of neurofilament light chain, a biomarker for neurodegeneration, showed more than 90% sensitivity and specificity for distinguishing patients with ALS from healthy controls, and higher levels are associated with disease progression and shorter survival, suggesting that it may be a useful diagnostic and prognostic biomarker for ALS.[59,60]

There are several variants of ALS (primary lateral sclerosis, progressive spinal muscular atrophy, progressive bulbar palsy, and pseudobulbar palsy) that may evolve over time to become classical ALS (Table 16-5).[56] **Primary lateral sclerosis** (PLS) is a slowly progressive disorder caused by damage of the corticospinal and sometimes corticobulbar pathways resulting in purely UMN symptoms. **Progressive muscular atrophy** (PMA) is an entirely LMN disorder that affects extremity muscles initially and only later affects bulbar and respiratory muscles. Some individuals who present with subtypes of PMA called

TABLE 16-4	Revised El Escorial Criteria (Awaji-Shima) for Diagnosis of ALS[17,54]
ALS DIAGNOSTIC CATEGORY	**REQUIREMENTS**
Definite ALS*	Clinical or electrophysiological evidence of UMN and LMN signs in the bulbar region and at least two spinal regions, or UMN and LMN signs in three spinal regions
Probable ALS*	Clinical or electrophysiological evidence of UMN and LMN signs in at least two regions, with some UMN signs rostral to LMN signs
Possible ALS*	Clinical or electrophysiological evidence of UMN and LMN signs in only one region, or UMN signs alone in two or more regions, or LMN signs rostral to UMN signs

ALS, amyotrophic lateral sclerosis; LMN, lower motor neuron; UMN, upper motor neuron.
*Neuroimaging and clinical laboratory studies will have been performed and other diagnoses must have been excluded.

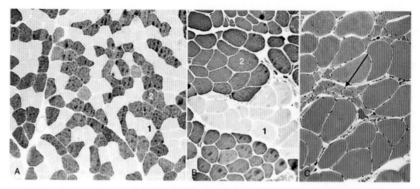

FIGURE 16-3 Muscle biopsy findings in ALS. A. Normal muscle fibers showing polygonal fiber shape and checkerboard distribution of intermingled Type I (stained light) and Type II (stained dark) fibers. B. Fiber grouping seen in ALS after reinnervation of muscle. The top and bottom fields are composed exclusively of Type II fibers (dark), while the middle field is exclusively Type I fibers (light). C. There is a cluster of atrophied muscle fibers (group atrophy) in the center (arrow) due to denervation. (Reproduced with permission from Vinay Kumar, Abul K. Abbas, Richard Mitchell M.D Ph.D., Nelson Fausto et. Al: Robbins Basic Pathology 8e,Figure 21-22.)

TABLE 16-5	Variants of Amyotrophic Lateral Sclerosis[56]	
TYPE	**UMN SIGNS AND SYMPTOMS**	**LMN SIGNS AND SYMPTOMS**
Amyotrophic lateral sclerosis (ALS)	Yes – brainstem and spinal regions	Yes – brainstem and spinal regions
Primary lateral sclerosis (PLS)	Yes – brainstem and spinal regions	No
Progressive spinal muscular atrophy (PMA)	No	Yes – spinal regions
Progressive bulbar palsy	No	Yes – brainstem region
Pseudobulbar palsy	Yes – brainstem region	No

Brainstem region refers to involvement of bulbar (mouth, face, throat) muscles; LMN, lower motor neuron; spinal regions refer to involvement of respiratory and arm, leg, and trunk muscles; UMN, upper motor neuron.

flail arm syndrome and **flail leg syndrome** have predominantly progressive atrophy, starting proximally in the arms or distally in the legs, and weakness of upper or lower extremity muscles, respectively.[61,62] **Progressive bulbar palsy** (PBP) is due to degeneration of cranial motor neurons IX, X, and XII resulting in bulbar symptoms; it is more common in older women. **Pseudobulbar palsy** (aka spastic bulbar palsy) results from corticobulbar tract degeneration and is characterized by spastic dysarthria, dysphagia, dysphonia, impairment of voluntary movements of tongue and facial muscles, and emotional lability. Patients with PLS and PMA typically have a longer survival than classical ALS, while those with bulbar variants usually have a worse prognosis.[56,61]

In addition to classical ALS, there are also variants of ALS that have additional non-pyramidal features called **ALS-Plus syndromes**.[63] Up to 50% of persons with ALS have cognitive and behavioral impairment and some develop frontotemporal dementia (ALS-FTD) or Parkinsonism-dementia complex (ALS-PDC).[64,65] ALS with cognitive impairment (ALSci) is characterized by early deficits in verbal (letter) fluency and some executive dysfunction, while ALS with behavioral impairment (ALSbi) is characterized by mild behavioral signs similar to FTD, especially apathy.[66] Some individuals with ALS have both cognitive and behavioral impairment (ALScbi). Individuals who develop ALS-FTD show progressive deterioration of behavior and/or cognition, leading to dementia.[66] Individuals with ALS-PDC show additional signs of parkinsonism (i.e., bradykinesia, rigidity, tremor),

related to neuronal degeneration in the substantia nigra.[65] Interestingly, some of the same genetic mutations can cause ALS and FTD (e.g., mutations in *C9ORF72*, *TARDBP*, *FUS*), suggesting that there may be common underlying mechanisms for these conditions.[66] Additional non-pyramidal features include oculomotor abnormalities (eye muscle weakness, impaired pursuit and saccadic eye movements, nystagmus), cerebellar symptoms (ataxia and/or limb dysmetria), autonomic dysfunction (excessive sweating), and sensory impairments (loss of taste and smell).[63,67] In general, people with ALS-Plus syndromes have a poorer survival and a higher risk of a genetic mutation than persons with ALS only.[63,68] Clinicians should monitor cognitive impairments in patients with ALS to identify potential reversible causes (e.g., medication side effects, breathing problems, depression and anxiety, sleep disturbances, or pre-existing psychiatric and neurologic diseases), to give support to patients and caregivers, and to provide personalized management of care.

Medical Prognosis

ALS is a steadily progressive disease and does not usually have periods of remission; stable plateaus are rare. The rate of progression is usually consistent for each patient but varies widely between individuals with disease durations ranging from a few months to 20 years. Death occurs on average 3 to 5 years from the time of diagnosis, primarily from respiratory failure.[69] Several factors are associated with a better or worse prognosis in patients with ALS (see Table 16-6).[70–77]

TABLE 16-6	Prognostic Factors of ALS[70–77]
POSITIVE PROGNOSTIC FACTORS	**NEGATIVE PROGNOSTIC FACTORS**
• Younger age at onset (<40 years old) • Limb versus bulbar onset • Longer interval between onset and diagnosis • Less severe involvement at the time of diagnosis • Primary lateral sclerosis or progressive muscular atrophy • Attendance at multidisciplinary ALS clinics • Use of riluzole (2-3 months) • Use of ventilator assistance	• Respiratory symptoms at onset • Cognitive abnormalities and dementia • Fast 6-month rate of decline in the ALSFRS-R • More severe corticospinal tract MRI abnormalities • Progressive bulbar palsy or pseudobulbar palsy • Malnutrition

ALSFRS-R, Amyotrophic Lateral Sclerosis Functional Rating Scale-Revised.

Medical Management

The clinical management of patients with ALS is complex and requires a comprehensive and multidisciplinary approach. Specialized centers or clinics that meet rigorous standards set by the Amyotrophic Lateral Sclerosis Association (ALSA) and the Muscular Dystrophy Association (MDA) are considered to be the most advantageous health care setting for the management of individuals with ALS.[78] Studies, comparing a cohort of patients attending a multidisciplinary clinic versus those attending a general neurology clinic, reported that the median

survival of the ALS clinic cohort was extended between 7 to 10 months longer than for patients in the general neurology cohort.[79–81] These findings suggest that more active and aggressive management, including increased use of noninvasive ventilation, attention to nutrition, and earlier referral to palliative services enhances survival.

Although there is no cure for ALS, many clinical trials to evaluate medications for reducing mortality and treating symptoms are ongoing. Riluzole[*] (Rilutec) and Edaravone (Radicava) are disease-modifying medications approved by the United States Food and Drug Administration to treat ALS.[82] Riluzole is a glutamate inhibitor and delays disease progression modestly, extending survival for about 3 months. In addition to a pill form, it is available in thickened liquid (Tiglutik) and oral film (Exservan) form for individuals with swallowing difficulties. The drug is usually well tolerated, but adverse effects include fatigue, weakness, nausea, vomiting, dizziness, and liver toxicity (requires discontinuation).[83] Edaravone is an antioxidant medication that was found to significantly decrease the rate of decline in functional abilities in individuals with ALS who met criteria of mild symptoms, normal respiratory function, and disease duration of ≤2 years.[84] It is administered via intravenous infusion, and most common side effects are bruising and gait disturbance. In addition to riluzole and edaravone, there are many medications and interventions that are used to treat symptoms (Table 16-7).[85,86] Recommendations and guidelines for the symptomatic care of patients with ALS were published by the American Academy of Neurology[87,88] and by the European Federation of Neurological Societies.[78]

Management of Respiratory Impairments

Weakness of the bulbar muscles that manage the upper airway and the spinal inspiratory and expiratory muscles leads

TABLE 16-7	Symptomatic Treatment of Amyotrophic Lateral Sclerosis[78,82]	
SYMPTOM TREATED	**MEDICAL MANAGEMENT**	**OTHER TREATMENTS**
Excessive watery saliva (sialorrhea)	Anticholinergic drugs (amitriptyline; scopolamine (transdermal patch); atropine (sublingual drops); glycopyrrolate); injections of botulinum toxin into parotid and submandibular glands; irradiation of salivary glands.	Home suction device; dark grape juice; sugar-free citrus lozenges; nebulization or steam inhalation.
Thick saliva and bronchial secretions	Mucolytics (*N-acetylcysteine*); beta-receptor antagonists (propranolol [Inderal], metoprolol [Toprol]); anticholinergic bronchodilators (ipratropium, theophylline).	Manually assisted coughing techniques; home suction device; mechanical insufflator–exsufflator cough machines; rehydration (jelly or ice); pineapple or papaya juice; reduced intake of dairy products, alcohol, and caffeine.
Dysphagia and weight loss	Enteric feeding considered if there is more than 10% loss of baseline weight; percutaneous endoscopic gastroscopy (PEG) preferably before FVC falls below 50% predicted; radiologically inserted gastrostomy (RIG) for individuals with FVC ≤50%; nasogastric tube feeding and IV hydration as temporary measure or for patients who refuse PEG.	Referrals to nutritionist or registered dietician for dietary counseling and management and SLP for swallowing evaluation; PT/OT to address proper sitting posture and adaptive eating utensils; eating and swallowing strategies such as: smaller bites of food; changes to texture and consistency of food (blending food, adding thickeners to drinks); nutritional supplements to increase caloric intake; "chin tuck" maneuver or performing a clearing cough after each swallow.

(Continued)

TABLE 16-7	Symptomatic Treatment of Amyotrophic Lateral Sclerosis[78,82] *(Continued)*	
SYMPTOM TREATED	**MEDICAL MANAGEMENT**	**OTHER TREATMENTS**
Respiratory impairments	Noninvasive positive pressure (NIPPV) ventilation (i.e., BiPAP, AVAPS) if FVC <50% predicted or there are respiratory symptoms; tracheostomy ventilation if NIPPV not tolerated or NIPPV is not able to compensate for respiratory impairment; morphine for relief from respiratory distress if ventilation is refused.	PT to provide: patient and caregiver education, breathing exercises, positioning to optimize ventilation, airway clearance techniques; prompt treatment of pneumonia and pulmonary infections, prevention by vaccination, avoidance of contact with people with colds or influenza; prevention and treatment of deep vein thromboses to avoid pulmonary emboli.
Dysarthria		Referral to SLP; speaking techniques (exaggerate articulation or decrease the rate of speech); "Low-" to "high-tech" communication devices; referral to prosthodontist for palatal lift.
Muscle cramps	Levetiracetam (Keppra), Quinine sulphate, Mexilitine	Stretching exercises; massage; hydrotherapy in heated pools; proper diet and hydration.
Spasticity	Lioresal (baclofen); tizanidine (Zanaflex); intrathecal baclofen for intractable spasticity; botulinum toxin type A.	PT/OT to provide: passive ROM, stretching exercises, postural and positioning techniques, splinting.
Muscle fasciculations	Lorazepam (Ativan)	Avoidance of caffeine and nicotine.
Depression and anxiety	Depression medications: amitriptyline (Elavil), SSRIs, mirtazapine (later stages); anxiety medications: Bupropion (Wellbutrin), benzodiazepines (diazepam)	Increased physical activity; psychological support; referral to mental health professional for counseling.
Pain	Simple analgesics; nonsteroidal anti-inflammatory drugs; narcotics for refractory pain.	PT to provide: ROM, joint mobilization, stretching exercises, pressure relief techniques (padding, seating cushions, air mattresses) and positioning, orthoses for joint support.
Urinary urgency	Oxybutynin chloride (Ditropan); tolterodine tartrate (Detrol)	Pelvic floor (Kegel) exercises; timed voiding program; biofeedback.
Constipation	Lactulose; Senna	Increased activity; hydration; increased fiber intake.
Pseudobulbar affect	Dextromethorphan and quinidine (Nuedexta); amitriptyline (Elavil); fluvoxamine (Luvox)	Educate patient and family about the nature of emotional lability and that it is part of ALS, rather than the patient being inappropriate.
Insomnia	Amitriptyline (Elavil); mirtazapine (Remeron); zolpidem (Ambien)	PT to provide pressure relief techniques and positioning; assisted ventilation (BiPAP, AVAPS).
Fatigue	Modafinil (Provigil)	PT/OT to provide: aerobic exercise program (early to middle stages), education on energy-conservation techniques (frequent rest breaks, using wheelchair for long distances, adaptive equipment use, etc.)

AVAPS, average volume-assured pressure support; BiPAP, bi-level positive airway pressure; Botox, botulinum toxin; CR, controlled release; FVC, forced vital capacity; OT, occupational therapy; PT, physical therapy; ROM, range of motion; SLP, speech language pathologist; SNP, sniff nasal pressure; SSRI, selective serotonin reuptake inhibitor.

to chronic respiratory insufficiency. Early symptoms include signs of hypercapnia such as daytime sleepiness, sleep disturbance, morning headaches, and cognitive impairment (i.e., poor concentration, confusion); **dyspnea** and **orthopnea** (difficulty breathing when lying down flat) usually develop later. Acute worsening of respiratory symptoms should immediately trigger diagnostic measures to exclude complications like atelectasis, pneumonia, or pulmonary embolism. These respiratory complications can be prevented with yearly pneumococcal and influenza vaccinations, avoidance of aspiration, and effective management of oral and pulmonary secretions. Supplemental oxygen is used very cautiously with patients with ALS because it can suppress the drive to breathe, thereby leading to worsening hypercapnia and respiratory arrest. It is recommended only for those with concomitant pulmonary disease and as a comfort measure for those who decline ventilatory support.[82]

When **forced vital capacity** (FVC) decreases to 50% of predicted normal, **noninvasive positive-pressure ventilation** (NIPPV) is recommended.[87] NIPPVV does not require placement of a tracheal tube and can be delivered by mouth, oral-nasally, or nasally. **Bi-level positive airway pressure** (BiPAP) is a positive airway pressure system that delivers different pressures, during inspiration and expiration, and is well tolerated by many individuals with ALS. Limitations of BiPAP are that pressure settings may not maintain ventilation as a person's muscle weakness progresses, and the need for a power source restricts mobility. Newer NIPPV technology called **average volume-assured pressure support** (AVAPS) overcomes these limitations by automatically adjusting the pressure support to achieve a target tidal volume and by connecting to external batteries to allow mobility. Most patients with ALS begin using NIPPV at night while asleep. As ALS progresses, the number of hours of assisted ventilation will increase and may go up to 24 hours per day. At this point, noninvasive portable ventilators (Trilogy or Astral) with internal and detachable external batteries can be easily mounted on a wheelchair to provide the person greater freedom and mobility while receiving continuous NIPPV. Several studies have reported prolonged survival times from initiation of noninvasive ventilation, ranging from 7 to 15 months, and increased quality of life in patients with respiratory compromise or moderately impaired bulbar function, who used NIPPV compared to those who did not.[89–92] Early initiation of NIPPV may increase survival, as a retrospective study of 194 patients with ALS found that initiation of NIPPV when FVC was greater than 80% of predicted normal significantly improved survival at 36 months after diagnosis, particularly in patients without bulbar symptoms, compared to patients with later-start NIPPV.[93] Eventually noninvasive ventilation will be ineffective, and a decision to either go on invasive ventilation (IV) with tracheostomy via surgical intervention or to go to hospice care must be made. Due to the emotional, social, and financial burden of IV, patients and families must be informed of the costs and benefits of this intervention. Survival rates after initiation of IV were 69% at 2 years and 33% at 5 years.[94]

Bronchial mucus plugging, exacerbated by weak cough function, is the chief precipitating factor of acute respiratory failure of individuals with ALS.[95] Manually assisted coughing techniques (e.g., abdominal thrust) applied by the clinician and/or caregiver and use of a mechanical insufflation–exsufflation (MI-E) device can facilitate clearance of respiratory and oral secretions.[87,95] The MI-E device is usually set to deliver rapid positive pressure to cause lung inflation, followed by negative pressure that mimics a cough. Three to five coughs are performed in rapid succession several times a day, which allows for the clearance of secretions.[96]

Physical Therapy Evaluation of Individuals with ALS

Due to the variety and various combinations of regions affected in ALS, therapists must conduct a careful and comprehensive examination of each patient to determine the extent of their primary, secondary, and composite impairments and determine how those impairments are related to their activity limitations and participation restrictions. Reexamination at regular intervals, using standard outcome measures, is necessary to determine the extent and rate of progression of the disease and to ensure that therapeutic interventions are administered in a timely manner (e.g., PEG placement, NIPPV, mobility aids, and equipment). The extent and timing of reexaminations may depend on whether the therapist is part of an ALS multidisciplinary team or an independent, clinic-based therapist and the severity of the patient's disease. Therapists working as team members may have a more limited role, related to assessment of gross motor function and ADLs, while clinic-based therapists may need to carry out more comprehensive assessments that also examine bulbar and respiratory function, environmental barriers to independence, and caregiver demands.

Before the patient's first visit or at the first visit, the patient or caregiver should be asked to keep an activity log for several days that records the patient's activities in 15-minute time intervals, the position the activity is performed in (i.e., lying, sitting, standing, moving), the self-reported fatigue level (no fatigue = 0, extreme fatigue = 10), and the location and intensity (0-10) of pain. The therapist should review the patient's medical record and activity logs to obtain information about the time since diagnosis, the progression of symptoms to date, other health conditions that would affect the patient's course of therapy, and the patient's current activities and his/her tolerance for them. The subjective history should include questions related to the patient's lifestyle, ability to perform ADLs, employment, hobbies or interests, chief complaints, the patient's and family members' understanding of ALS and the likely progression and prognosis, and the patient's immediate concerns and goals for physical therapy. A standard systems review and neurological examination that includes vital signs at rest, communication status and ability to follow commands, skin and sensory integrity, muscle strength, joint range of motion, and postural alignment should be performed (see Evaluation Chapter 10). The following tests and measures can be used to assess and evaluate an individual with ALS (Table 16-8). Therapists should refer to the World Federation of Neurology's *Guidelines for the Use and Performance of Quantitative Outcome Measures in ALS Clinical Trials* for a more detailed description of the standard test and measures used in clinical trials.[97] It is important to include participation tests and measures as they may be more positively impacted by physical therapy interventions than impairment and activity level measures due to the progressive nature of the disease.

Impairment Level Assessments

The therapist's examination of body structure/function impairments may include the following tests and measures:

Cognition: Two ALS-specific cognitive screening tools that can be used by physical therapists are the ALS-Cognitive Behavioural Screen (ALS-CBS) and the Edinburgh Cognitive and Behavioural ALS Screen (ECAS).[98,99] Both screens include tests of verbal fluency, which are sensitive for cognitive dysfunction in the ALS population.[100] A cutoff score of ≤10 on

TABLE 16-8 ALS Impairment, Activity, and Participation Assessments[97–99]		
IMPAIRMENT LEVEL ASSESSMENTS	**ACTIVITY LEVEL ASSESSMENTS**	**PARTICIPATION LEVEL ASSESSMENTS**
• Cognitive screen (verbal fluency, ALS-CBS, ECAS) • Psychological screen (ADI-12, BDI, HADS, STAI) • Pain (VAS, BPI) • ROM (muscle length versus joint limitations) • Muscle strength (MMT, strain gauge tensiometer, muscle dynamometer) • Hand and upper extremity function (Purdue pegboard, Nine Hole Peg Test) • Reflexes (DTRs, Babinski, Hoffmann) • Tone (Modified Ashworth Scale) • Cranial nerve screen • Respiratory Assessment (FVC, SNIP, PCEF, aerobic capacity and endurance testing) • Fatigue (FSS)	• ALSFRS, ALSFRS-R • Other functional measures (AALS, ALSS, Norris ALS Scale) • General Health (Schwab and England) • Balance (POMA, TUG, BBS, FRT) • Gait (25-foot walk test, 10MWT, 6MWT) • Functional Status (FIM)	• ALSAQ-40 (ALSAQ-5) • ALSSQOL (ALSSQOL-Revised, ALSSQOL-Short Form) • Health-related QOL (SF-36, WHOQOL-BREF, EQ-5D)

10MWT, 10 meter walk test; 6MWT, six minute walk test; AALS, Appel ALS Scale; ADI-12, ALS Depression Inventory 12; ALSAQ-40, ALS Assessment Questionnaire 40; ALS-CBS, ALS-Cognitive Behavioural Screen; ALSFRS(-R), Functional Rating Scale(-Revised); ALSSQOL, ALS-specific Quality Of Life instrument; ALSSS, ALS Severity Scale; BBS, Berg Balance Scale; BDI, Beck Depression Inventory; BPI, Brief Pain Inventory; DTR, deep tendon reflex; ECAS, Edinburgh Cognitive and Behavioural ALS Screen; EQ-5D, EuroQual-5D; FIM, Functional Independence Measure; FRT, Functional Reach Test; FSS, Fatigue Severity Scale; FVC, forced vital capacity; HADS, Hospital Anxiety and Depression Scale; MMT, manual muscle test; PCEF, peak expiratory cough flow; POMA, Performance Oriented Mobility Assessment; SNIP, sniff nasal inspiratory pressure; STAI, State-Trait Anxiety Inventory; TUG, Timed Up and Go; VAS, Visual Analogue Scale; WHOQOL-BREF, World Health Organization Quality of Life Questionnaire.

the cognitive section of the ALS-CBS had a 100% sensitivity and specificity to identify individuals with ALS with FTD, and is a quick and easily administered screening tool for cognitive and behavioral impairment in clinical settings.[66,98] If cognitive screens are abnormal, referral for a neuropsychological evaluation is indicated.

Psychosocial function: Depression and anxiety are common in patients with ALS as well as their caregivers.[101] Major depression is infrequent (around 10%), but depressive symptoms are reported by over 50% of individuals with ALS.[102,103] Some studies have shown an association between greater functional impairment and the severity of anxiety,[104] but other studies have found no correlation.[105] The ALS Depression Inventory 12 (ADI-12) is an ALS-specific screening instrument for depression that excludes statements addressing activities that depend on an intact motor system.[106] ADI-12 scores range from 12 to 48 with higher scores between 23 and 29 indicating mild depression and those >30 indicating severe depression.[107] Patients with ALS, who test positive on depression and anxiety screens, should be referred to a psychologist or psychiatrist for further evaluation. General depression and anxiety assessments used for patients with ALS in clinical trials include the Beck Depression Inventory (BDI),[108] the Hospital Anxiety and Depression Scale (HADS),[109] and the Spielberger State-Trait Anxiety Inventory (STAI).[110]

Pain: Pain is reported by many people with ALS, even in early stages of the disease.[103,111] Musculoskeletal pain develops with increased muscle weakness and abnormal muscle tone that results in immobility, contractures and joint stiffness, and/or loss of integrity. People with ALS frequently complain of pain in the low back, the neck, and the shoulder regions.[112] Some patients may develop painful adhesive capsulitis of the shoulder (i.e., "frozen shoulder").[113] Pain can also arise from muscle cramps and spasms, spasticity, skin pressure due to immobility, and constipation.[114] Pain should be assessed subjectively and objectively, either using a numerical rating scale (0 = no pain to 10 = the worst pain imaginable) or the Visual Analog Scale (VAS). The Brief Pain Inventory (BPI) is the most commonly used pain assessment in ALS studies.[115] A careful examination of the underlying causes of pain is required to determine whether it is a primary impairment of ALS (e.g., muscle sprain, ligament strains, traumatic injuries from falls) or if it arises from secondary impairments (e.g., decreased ROM, adhesive capsulitis) or composite impairments (e.g., joint malalignment secondary to spasticity or weakness).

Muscle performance: Muscle weakness is the primary deficit of ALS and leads to difficulties with performance of functional activities. Jette et al (1999).[116] found that decreases in walking ability were precipitated by small changes in lower extremity muscle force; individuals with ALS (1) dropped from being independent community ambulators to needing assistance, when their mean percentage of predicted normal maximal isometric force (%PMF) of lower extremity muscles dropped below 54%PMF; (2) became in-home ambulators when strength dropped to 37%PMF; and (3) were no longer able to walk when strength dropped to approximately 19%PMF. Assessment of maximum voluntary isometric contraction (MVIC), using a strain gauge tensiometer system, is considered the most direct technique for investigating motor unit loss and has been used extensively in clinical trials.[97,117] Advantages of this method are that it produces highly reliable and sensitive data, accurately measures muscle strength in weak as well as strong muscles, is relatively safe, and does not induce fatigue in the majority of patients. Disadvantages are that MVIC testing requires specialized equipment and extensive training. Alternative test methods are manual muscle testing (MMT) or electronic handheld dynamometer testing. One study that compared test reliability of MMT and MVIC scores in patients with ALS found that the tests had equal reproducibility, when administered by uniformly trained physical therapists.[118]

Upper extremity motor function: Hand and upper extremity function has been measured, using the Purdue pegboard and nine-hole peg test in ALS studies.[119,120] Both tests are sensitive to change over time, and normal values are published.[120–123] Initiation, modification, and control of movement patterns and voluntary postures can be assessed through observation.

Reflex integrity: Deep tendon reflexes, pathological reflexes (e.g., Babinski's and Hoffmann's signs), and muscle tone using the Modified Ashworth Scale should be assessed to discriminate UMN versus LMN involvement.[124]

Cranial nerve integrity: Dysphagia (difficulty swallowing liquids, foods, or saliva) and dysarthria (impairment in speech production) are some of the most distressing and problematic symptoms of ALS that negatively affect quality of life. With progressive weakness of the lips, tongue, palate, and mastication muscles, individuals with ALS experience swallowing problems that lead to choking, drooling, and increased risk for aspiration.[125] Among 100 individuals with ALS who underwent video fluoroscopic swallowing examination, the prevalence of unsafe and inefficient swallowing was 48% and 73%, respectively.[125] Weakness of the muscles of speech (lips, tongue, larynx, and soft palate) and respiration results in compromised speech, characterized by impaired articulation, hypernasality, slow speed and cadence, reduced volume, and reduced utterance length due to impaired breath support.[126] Evaluation of bulbar function includes testing of cranial nerves III, IV, V, VI, VII, IX, X, and XII. Oral motor function, phonation, and speech production can be assessed through the interview and observation. Referral to a nutritionist and speech language pathologist for consultation is recommended.

Respiratory system assessment: Since respiratory failure is the major cause of death in ALS, respiratory status and function should be closely monitored. Assessment of pulmonary function includes (1) the patient's reports of respiratory symptoms, (2) inspection of the patient's respiratory rate, rhythm, depth, and chest expansion, (3) auscultation of breath sounds, (4) cough effectiveness testing, and (5) measurement of FVC, **maximum inspiratory and expiratory pressures** (MIP and MEP) and/ or **sniff nasal inspiratory pressure** (SNIP) using a handheld spirometer.[127] SNIP is measured by having the person perform a short, sharp, voluntary inspiration through a pressure transducer placed in a nostril and can be used when there is bulbar involvement. In addition to a FVC of <50%, other criteria used to determine when NIPPV should be started are dyspnea at rest, abnormal nocturnal oxygen saturation (>89% for more than 5 consecutive minutes), MIP values of <60 cmH_2O, and SNIP values of <40 cmH_2O.[87,128] Supine FVC may predict diaphragm weakness better than sitting FVC because breathing is more difficult in supine because gravity is not able to assist in lowering the diaphragm.[87] **Peak cough expiratory flow** (PCEF) is a widely used measure of cough effectiveness.[87] It is measured by taking a deep breath and breathing out as fast and as hard as possible into a handheld peak flow meter. A PCEF value of <270 L/min and a MEP value of <40 cmH_2O are used to determine the need for manual or mechanical cough assistance.[129] Baseline measures

of FVC or SNIP are early predictors of survival.[129–131] Aerobic capacity and endurance may be assessed in earlier stages of ALS, using standardized exercise test protocols to evaluate and monitor responses to aerobic conditioning, and should be assessed during functional activities.[132]

Fatigue: Fatigue is a frequent and sometimes debilitating symptom in ALS that may be caused by peripheral and central mechanisms including mitochondrial dysfunction, abnormal muscle lipid metabolism, impaired muscle activation due to impaired excitation–contraction coupling, and central activation failure.[133–137] Types of fatigue often described by individuals with ALS are whole-body tiredness or muscle weakness related to muscle exertion that partially reverses with rest.[138] No ALS-specific measures exist; the Fatigue Severity Scale (FSS; scale from 9 to 63, higher scores indicate more fatigue) has been commonly used in ALS studies.[139,140]

Integumentary system assessment: Skin integrity is usually not compromised in ALS, even in the late stage, because sensation is normally preserved. Skin inspection at contact points between the body and assistive, adaptive, orthotic, protective and supportive devices, mobility devices, and the sleeping surface should be performed regularly, especially when the patient becomes immobile. Swelling of the distal limbs due to a lack of muscle pumping action from weakened limbs should also be evaluated.

Activity Level Assessments

The therapist's examination of activity limitations may include the following tests and measures.

Balance: Although muscle weakness may affect dynamic balance, such as during gait, postural sway during static stance on a firm surface with or without eyes open in ambulatory individuals with ALS was not different than control subjects despite significant weakness and spasticity, possibly due to intact sensation.[141] However, one study found that 37% of ambulatory individuals with ALS with relatively normal clinical balance and mobility test findings experienced falls during conditions 5 and 6 (i.e., altered somatosensory information with vision absent or sway-referenced) of the Sensory Organization Test (EquiTest, Neurocom), suggesting that they had decreased ability to use vestibular input and relied more on visual inputs to maintain upright balance.[142] Based on their laboratory findings they proposed that the modified Clinical Test of Sensory Interaction on Balance (mCTSIB) might be a highly sensitive test to detect balance impairments in ambulatory people with ALS in clinical settings. No ALS-specific balance test or measure exists; balance tests that have been used in ALS studies include the Tinetti Performance Oriented Mobility Assessment (POMA),[143] the Timed Up and Go (TUG) Test,[144] the Berg Balance Scale (BBS).[145] and the Functional Reach Test (FRT).[146] Low total Tinetti Balance Test scores, indicating impaired balance, have been found to be moderately to strongly related to lower extremity muscle weakness and activity limitations, in individuals with ALS,[147] and one study suggests that the Tinetti Balance Test is a reliable measure for individuals in the early or early-middle stages of ALS.[148] Another study found that TUG times increased linearly over 6 months, were negatively correlated with MMT scores and functional measures, and predicted falls using a cutoff of 14 seconds in 31 patients with ALS.[149]

Gait assessment: Gait deviations observed in the ALS population include decreased gait speed and increased mean stride time and stride time variability between one stride to the next, which have been attributed to a combination of decreased muscle strength and endurance [150,151]. Gait stability, efficiency, safety, and endurance with or without the use of orthotic and assistive devices should be assessed regularly. Timed 25-feet and 10 meter (10MWT) walk tests have been used to assess gait speed in ALS studies.[152,153] One study reported that 10MWT gait speed correlated with the ALSFRS-R score (r = 0.60), suggesting that it may serve as a measure of disability and disease severity in ALS.[152] The Six Minute Walk Test (6MWT) was found to be a valid and sensitive to change measure of walking capacity with correlations to lower extremity muscle strength and other ambulation (10MWT, TUG) measures.[153,154]

Functional status: Functional mobility skills, safety, and energy expenditure should be assessed. The Functional Independence Measure (FIM™) has been used to document functional status in clinical trials.[155] Basic and instrumental ADLs and the need for adaptive equipment may also be assessed by an occupational therapist.

Posture, body mechanics, and ergonomics: Static and dynamic postural alignment and position, ergonomics, and body mechanics, during self-care, home management, work, community, or leisure activities should be assessed. Caregivers should also be assessed in these areas, when the patient requires physical assistance from them.

Disease-specific measures: The ALS Functional Rating Scale (ALSFRS)[156] and the revised version which includes additional respiratory items (ALSFRS-R),[157] are used to measure functional status and change in patients with ALS. This instrument is available online.[158] The individual is asked to rate his/her function, for the 10 to 12 items, on a scale from 4 (normal function) to 0 (unable to attempt the task), either in person, in the clinic or via telephone interview. Both scales have been found to be valid and reliable for measuring the decline in function that results from loss of muscular strength, and to predict 9-month survival.[159] The minimal detectable change on the ALSFRS-R is 6.74.[160] Other scales that measure disease severity include: the Appel ALS Scale (AALS),[161] the ALS Severity Scale (ALSSS),[162] and the Norris Scale.[163]

Activities of daily living: The Schwab and England Scale has been used in clinical trials to evaluate ADL function in individuals with ALS.[164] It is an 11-point global measure of functioning that asks the rater to report ADL function from 100% (normal) to 0% (vegetative functions only). The ALS CNTF Treatment Study Group found the scale to have excellent test–retest reliability, to correlate well with qualitative and quantitative changes in function, and to be sensitive to changes over time.[165]

Participation Level Assessments

The therapist's examination of participation may include the following tests and measures.

Environmental barriers: Environmental assessment should focus on the patient's home and work ergonomics and energy conservation as well as safety at current and future functional levels.

Quality of life (QOL): ALS-specific QOL measures include the ALS Assessment Questionnaire 40 (ALSAQ-40)[166,167] and the ALS-specific QOL instrument (ALSSQOL).[168] The ALSAQ-40 contains 40 items that assess five distinct areas of health: mobility (10 items), ADLs (10 items), eating and drinking (3 items), communication (7 items), and emotional functioning (10 items). Patients answer each question on a five-point Likert scale, based on their condition over the past 2 weeks, and a summary score is obtained, ranging from 0 (best health status) to 100 (worst health status). The validity, reliability, and amount of change over time for each of the five domains that are meaningful to patients have been reported.[166,167] The ALSAQ-40 was shortened to five items and was also found to be valid and reliable.[168,169] The ALSSQOL contains 59 items that assess psychological, support, existential, and spiritual domains, in addition to a physical domain.[170] Patients score each item on a 0 to 10 scale, with 0 the least desirable situation and 10 the most desirable. Thus, total scores range from 0 to 590. The test was found to have concurrent, convergent, and discriminant validity for the overall instrument and convergent validity for its subscales. Shorter versions of the ALSSQOL have been validated including the 50-item ALSSQOL-Revised (ALSSQOL-R; 46 items scored for total score of 460) and the 20-item ALSSQOL-Short Form (ALSSQOL-SF).[171,172] Other generic quality-of-life measures used in clinical trials that focused on ALS rehabilitation include the Short-Form (SF-36) Health Survey, the World Health Organization Quality of Life questionnaire (WHOQOL-BREF), and the EuroQol-5D (EQ-5D).[173]

Goal Setting and Exercise Prescription

Therapists may have difficulty setting physical therapy goals for patients with ALS due to the progressive nature of the disease and a common belief that, because there is no "cure" for the disease, it is kinder to avoid additional demands on the person with ALS, who is already coping with increasing functional loss. Others believe that exercise will accelerate the disease or give people false hopes that it can delay progression. However, the literature on ALS, and other neuromuscular diseases, suggests that individuals with ALS can benefit from individually tailored exercise and activity programs throughout all stages of the disease.[112,174] Including patients in goal setting can increase their motivation to comply with exercise programs and may give them and their families a sense of control over the circumstances in which they find themselves.

The general overarching goals of physical therapy throughout all stages of ALS are to maintain optimal independence in daily living and a good quality of life. More specific physical therapy goals include (1) maintain safe and independent mobility and function; (2) maintain maximal muscle strength and endurance within the amount imposed by the disease; (3) prevent and minimize secondary impairments of the disease (e.g., contractures, disuse atrophy, decubitus ulcers, thrombophlebitis, aspiration); (4) prevent or manage pain; (5) educate on energy-conservation techniques to prevent unnecessary fatigue and respiratory discomfort; and (6) provide adaptive, assistive, and orthotic equipment to maximize functional independence.

When prescribing exercise and activity programs for individuals with ALS, therapists must carefully balance the level of activity to avoid disuse atrophy from low activity levels or, conversely, overwork damage from excessive activity. Fatigue and ambulation difficulties often lead to reduced activity levels in individuals with

ALS that can compound already low activity levels, especially if they led a sedentary lifestyle prior to diagnosis. Inadequate levels of activity, in turn, lead to cardiovascular deconditioning and muscle disuse weakness that ultimately can affect functional performance. On the other hand, excessive exercise can cause undue fatigue that limits a person's ability to perform daily activities, during recovery periods, and/or cause overuse damage to muscles and tendons that results in pain and loss of strength.

The role of therapeutic exercise in people with ALS is a controversial topic. Early studies recommended people with ALS should not exercise beyond their daily activities.[175] Some epidemiological studies demonstrated a higher incidence of ALS in people who performed intense physical work or activity before disease onset.[176,177] Other studies reported abnormal physiologic responses to exercise in people with ALS (i.e., increased lactate production, decreased anaerobic lactate threshold, decreased work capacity, increased oxygen cost of submaximal exercise, and abnormalities in plasma and muscle lipid metabolism),[178,179] which suggested that exercise might facilitate the pathogenic mechanisms of ALS (glutamate excitotoxicity, increased free radicals).[180] There is also human and animal evidence suggesting that high-intensity or highly repetitive exercise can cause prolonged or permanent loss of muscle strength in weak or partially denervated muscles.[181-185] Weak muscles may be more susceptible to overwork damage, because they are already functioning close to their maximal limits.[186] Thus, the safe range for therapeutic exercise is narrowed in people with ALS. The fear of inducing overwork damage in individuals with ALS through excessive amounts of exercise contributes to some clinicians deciding not to prescribe exercise programs for people with ALS.[187,188]

Despite these potential risks to exercise in ALS, a growing body of evidence supports the idea that exercise programs prescribed appropriately may be safe and beneficial for people with ALS.[112,174] Exercise adapted to each individual's exercise capacity that does not overload the nervous, muscular, and respiratory systems should avoid exacerbation of pathophysiologic mechanisms of ALS. Moderate intensity exercise can improve neuronal plasticity (e.g., release of neurotrophic factors, dendritic restructuring, enhanced protein synthesis, strengthening of synaptic connections to target muscles, maintaining organization and firing of muscle fibrils, improving axonal transport) and enhance cardiovascular and peripheral circulation, which may positively affect free radical balance and oxidation of muscle fibers to modify the excitotoxic environment.[131] Evidence, including several systematic reviews and meta-analyses support the safety and benefits of moderate exercise in individuals with ALS.[134,189-191] The findings of the human studies that were included in these reviews and meta-analyses are summarized in Table 16-9. In general, endurance (i.e., aerobic) and strengthening (i.e., resistance) exercises conducted at low to moderate intensities are well tolerated by individuals with ALS. There were no reported adverse effects in these human studies, related to the exercise interventions; however, some studies reported large dropout rates over time, particularly when aerobic exercise was the intervention.[193] Studies suggest that positive effects of exercise programs are greater when initiated at the early disease stage, possibly because collateral sprouting is more robust due to larger numbers of motor neurons in early stages.[194] Two

meta-analytic studies[189,191] found that studies with aerobic exercise versus resistance demonstrated the greatest improvements in functional abilities as measured by the ALSFRS or ALSFRS-R. Zucchi et al. compared the effects of a multimodal exercise program delivered high-frequency (5 times per week) versus usual intensity (2 times per week) for 5 weeks in people with ALS, and concluded that there were no benefits to high-intensity exercise over the usual intensity.[195] To avoid excessive fatigue and/or ensure safety during supervised treadmill training, researchers have successfully used body weight-support systems or NIPPV for persons with ALS.[132,196,197] While most exercise studies were conducted in clinics or research laboratories under the supervision of a physical therapist or researcher, a 6-month multimodal home-based exercise program with monthly monitoring by a physical therapist was found to be safe, feasible, and effective.[198] Tele-monitoring of vital signs during home-based endurance exercise (i.e., 15 mins walking on a treadmill or outdoors) using wireless biosensors connected to computers was found to be feasible, safe, and well accepted by persons with ALS.[132]

In animal models (i.e., transgenic mice with superoxide dismutase-1 ALS, SOD1^{G93A} mice), moderate exercise increased survival and delayed the time to reach a 50% decline in motor function (122 days exercise group versus 115 days control groups).[134,199] The few negative effects in the animal models were associated with very high-intensity exercise (e.g., progressive treadmill training at 9 to 22 m/min for 20 to 45 minutes daily) and slow rate exercise (0.1 m/min on a running wheel for 6.7 hours a day), which was less activity than usual for animals with unrestricted activity.[134,200] The beneficial motor and survival effects of exercise in the SOD1^{G93A} mice were greatest with a 6-hour duration of access to a running wheel compared to 2 or 12 hours.[201] Interestingly, swimming was found to be more beneficial in SOD1^{G93A} mice compared to running-based training.[202] Benefits of swimming-based training were related to improved skeletal muscle metabolism and reduced death of large hindlimb spinal motor neurons.[203] Thus, exercise mode, intensity, and duration appear to be critical factors influencing positive effects from endurance training in ALS mice. In contrast to animal studies, exercise studies in humans with ALS have not demonstrated prolonged survival.[200] To date, swimming has not been studied in persons with ALS, but given that it mainly incorporates concentric muscle contractions, and water minimizes stress on muscles and joints and provides resistance, it has potential to be a beneficial exercise intervention in the ALS population.[200]

Based on the evidence and current practice, general guidelines for prescribing endurance and strengthening exercises for individuals with ALS are in Box 16-1. Clinicians should monitor each person's response to exercise to determine whether the exercises are appropriate and safe and to adjust programs as the disease progresses. Possible signs and symptoms of muscle overwork include delayed onset muscle soreness, peaking between days 1 and 5 after activity; a reduction in maximum force production that gradually recovers and/or severe muscle cramping after exercise; a feeling of heaviness in the extremities; increased muscle fasciculations; or prolonged shortness of breath.[206] Patients should be advised not to carry out activities to the point of extreme fatigue (i.e., inability to perform daily activities following exercise due to exhaustion, pain, fasciculations, or muscle cramping).[207]

TABLE 16-9	Summary of Rehabilitation Interventions for Amyotrophic Lateral Sclerosis[189–192]	
REHABILITATION INTERVENTION	**BODY FUNCTION AND ACTIVITIES IMPACTED**	**OVERALL CONCLUSION**
Physical Therapy	Upper and lower extremity joint passive range of motion Hand grip strength (dynamometer) Knee extension muscle strength Norris ALS Scale Functional Ambulation Categories	Supervised group or individualized exercise programs with stretching and strengthening exercises and functional mobility training lead to improvements in range of motion, strength, and the functional tasks trained. Benefits of supervised exercise programs should be followed by long-term home exercise programs to sustain these improvements.
Exercise		
Endurance (aerobic)	ALSFRS-R total score Functional Independence Measure Norris ALS Scale (spinal subscale) Aerobic fitness-VO_2 max and anaerobic threshold Forced vital capacity ALSQ-40	Aerobic exercise using treadmill, stationary bike, cycle ergometer, or step board at a moderate intensity (e.g., 50-70% maximum heart rate, 11-13/20 rated perceived exertion, 20-30 minutes) for 2-3 days per week, for longer durations (e.g., 6-12 months) lead to improved function, and slower declines in aerobic fitness, pulmonary function, and health-related quality of life compared to controls.
Strengthening (resistance)	ALSFRS SF-36 (physical function subscale) Strength-Maximum voluntary isometric contraction (MVIC) Ashworth Spasticity Scale	Progressive resistance exercise for upper and lower extremity muscles with Medical Research Council grades of ≥3 using a moderate load (e.g., 5 reps at full 6 RM, 5 reps at 75% 6 RM, 5 reps at 50% 6 RM) for 3 days per week for 6 months lead to significantly greater function, quality of life, less decline in lower extremity strength, and less spasticity compared to controls. Most studies used submaximal isotonic exercise, but one study[192] used submaximal isometric exercise.
Combination of endurance and strengthening exercise	ALSFRS-R ALS Severity Scale Strength-Total Medical Research Council sum score Aerobic fitness-VO_2 anaerobic threshold and oxygen consumption (VO_2 submax) Mobility-Timed Up and Go Fatigue Severity Scale	Aerobic exercise using treadmill, stationary bike, or cycle ergometer (arm and legs) at a moderate intensity (e.g., 65-75% maximum heart rate, 7/10 Borg rated perceived exertion, 15-20 minutes) combined with submaximal resistance exercise for upper and lower extremity muscles with Medical Research Council grades of ≥3 using a moderate load (e.g., 65% 1 RM, 1-2 sets of 8-12 reps or 3 sets of 5 reps) for 2-3 days per week for 3 to 6 months lead to less decline in function, muscle strength, aerobic fitness, mobility and fatigue.

If a patient shows signs of prolonged muscle weakness after starting an exercise program or reports persistent morning fatigue after exercise on the previous day, the clinician should carefully adjust the exercise program intensity to eliminate any further muscle overuse. While endurance and strengthening exercises may not improve the strength of muscles already weakened by ALS or change the course of the disease, they may have positive physiological and psychological effects for individuals with ALS, especially when implemented in the early stages.

Physical Therapy Treatment

Dal Bello-Haas proposed a three-stage model for the progression of ALS as a framework for physical therapy clinical management (see Table 16-10).[208] In the early stage, individuals are independent with mobility, ADLs, and speech, despite mild to moderate weakness in

specific muscle groups. The person may experience some difficulty with mobility and ADLs toward the end of the stage. During the middle stage, the person with ALS has severe muscle weakness in some groups and mild to moderate weakness in others. There is a progressive decline in mobility and ADLs, along with increasing fatigue and pain; together these result in some compensation or dependence on others. In the late stage, the person is totally dependent with mobility and ADLs, due to severe weakness of axial and extremity muscles. Dysarthria, dysphagia, respiratory compromise, and pain are all common features of this stage.[208]

Three general approaches are used to direct physical therapy interventions across the disease stages: preventative, restorative, and compensatory. Preventative interventions aim to minimize potential impairments (e.g., loss of ROM, aerobic capacity, strength) and activity limitations. Restorative interventions

Box 16-1	General Exercise Guidelines for Individuals with ALS

- Start exercise interventions when individuals are in the early stages of the disease so that they have sufficient strength, respiratory function, and endurance to exercise without excessive fatigue.[204]
- Daily range of motion (AROM, AAROM, PROM based on abilities) and stretching exercises should be encouraged to help maintain joint mobility and prevent contractures.
- Endurance (aerobic) exercise programs should emphasize low to moderate intensity activities (50-75% peak HR, 11-13 RPE, 2-3 times per week) as tolerated without inducing excessive fatigue. Rest periods are recommended, especially if continuous activity goes beyond 15 minutes.

- Strengthening (resistance) exercise programs should emphasize concentric rather than eccentric muscle contractions, at low to moderate resistance and intensity (e.g., 1-2 sets of 8-12 reps or 3 sets of 5 reps), in muscles that have antigravity strength (i.e., ≥3 grade strength) exclusively.
- Individuals with ALS should be advised to have adequate oxygenation, ventilation, and intake of carbohydrates and fluids before exercising.[205]
- Use available technology (e.g., assistive devices, body weight-supported systems, noninvasive positive-pressure ventilation) to optimize exercise program effectiveness without causing excessive fatigue.[134,196,2027]
- Exercise compliance can be improved by integrating enjoyable physical activities along with the formal exercise program, providing opportunities for socialization, and providing rewards for accomplishment of goals.

TABLE 16-10	Amyotrophic Lateral Sclerosis Disease Stages and Common Intervention Strategies[208]	
STAGE	**COMMON IMPAIRMENTS AND ACTIVITY LIMITATIONS**	**INTERVENTIONS**
Early	• Mild to moderate weakness in specific muscle groups • Difficulty with ADLs and mobility toward the end of this stage	Restorative/Preventative: • Strengthening exercises*[128-130] • Endurance exercises[125,129] • ROM (active, active-assisted) and stretching exercises[134] Compensatory: • Assess potential need for appropriate adaptive and assistive devices • Assess potential need for ergonomic modifications of the home/workplace • Educate patient about the disease process, energy conservation, and support groups
Middle	• Severe muscle weakness in some groups; mild to moderate weakness in other groups • Progressive decrease in mobility and ADLs throughout this stage • Increasing fatigue throughout this stage • Wheelchair needed for long distances; increased wheelchair use toward end of stage • Pain (especially shoulders)	Compensatory: • Support weak muscles (assistive devices, supportive devices, adaptive equipment, slings, orthoses) • Modify the workplace/home (e.g., install ramp, move bedroom to first floor) • Prescribe wheelchair • Educate caregivers regarding functional training Preventative: • ROM (active, active-assisted, passive) and stretching exercises[134] • Strengthening exercises (early middle)[126,128] • Endurance exercises (early middle)[125,129] • Assess need for pressure-relieving devices (e.g., pressure distributing mattress)
Late	• Wheelchair dependent or restricted to bed • Complete dependence with ADLs • Severe weakness of UE, LE, neck and trunk muscles • Dysarthria, dysphagia • Respiratory compromise • Pain	Preventative: • Passive ROM • Pulmonary hygiene* • Hospital bed and pressure-relieving devices • Skin care, hygiene* • Educate caregivers on prevention of secondary complications Compensatory: • Educate caregivers regarding transfers, positioning, turning, skin care • Mechanical lift

*May be restorative.

CASE A, PART III: EARLY STAGE

Mr. Posner was referred by his neurologist to outpatient physical therapy with a diagnosis of probable ALS, laboratory supported. At his initial physical therapy session, the patient reported a previous history of an old football injury of the left knee with a chronically torn meniscus. He complained that the weakness in his hands, which was worse on the left than the right, and the stiffness in his legs were interfering with his ability to walk, go upstairs, and play golf. He stated that he could not hit the golf ball as far as in years past. Other than golfing on weekends, he stated that he did not engage in any regular exercise program. His medications included riluzole (50 mg twice daily), baclofen (10 mg twice daily), vitamin C (1000 mg once daily), vitamin E (800 units once daily), co-enzyme Q10 (600 mg once daily), and a multiple vitamin once daily. He had health care benefits through his job with 15 outpatient physical therapy visits allowed per year. The physical therapist's examination findings revealed the following impairments:

- Decreased flexibility of bilateral shoulder extensors and internal rotators, hip adductors, quadriceps, and gastrocnemius muscles on passive ROM
- Mild atrophy of the intrinsic hand muscles, left greater than right
- Decreased strength in cervical and distal extremity muscles with bilateral finger flexor and hand intrinsic muscles [Left = G (4) range; Right = G+ (4+)], ankle dorsiflexors [G (4)], neck extensors G (4), and neck flexors G+ (4+)
- Brisk reflexes (3+) at the jaw and all extremity joints; Babinski and Hoffmann's signs positive bilaterally; Modified Ashworth Scale scores were 1 in bilateral biceps and wrist flexor muscles and 1+ in bilateral hip adductors, hamstring, and gastrocnemius muscles
- Sitting FVC: 4.45 L (91% of predicted)
- Sitting posture demonstrated a forward head and rounded shoulder posture

The therapist's examination revealed the following activity limitations and participation restrictions:

- Balance (standing): Unilateral stance/eyes open, R = 25 seconds; L = 23 seconds
- Slow walking velocity (10-meter walk test = 5.2 seconds; 1.15 m/sec; no assistive device; stiff gait with bilaterally decreased hip and knee flexion during swing phase and foot flat initial contact)
- Mild ADL and mobility deficits as indicated by ALSFRS-R score: 41/48 and Schwab and England score: 90% (can do all chores but with some degree of slowness, difficulty, or impairment). See Table 16-8.
- Functional endurance deficits indicated by fatigue when going up stairs or prolonged LE activities

ALSFRS-R Assessment

Item	Score	ALSFRS-R Score Descriptor
Speech	4	Normal speech processes
Salivation	4	Normal
Swallowing	4	Normal eating habits
Handwriting (pre-ALS dominant hand)	3	Slow or sloppy; all words are legible
Cutting food and handling utensils (patients without gastrostomy)	3	Somewhat slow and clumsy, but no help needed
Dressing and hygiene	3	Independent and complete self-care with effort or decreased efficiency
Turning in bed, adjusting bed clothes	3	Somewhat slow and clumsy, but no help needed
Walking	3	Early ambulation difficulties
Climbing stairs	3	Mild unsteadiness or fatigue
Dyspnea	4	None
Orthopnea	4	None
Respiratory insufficiency	4	None, e.g., no BiPAP at present

The therapist's diagnostic impression was that the patient's hand weakness was affecting his ability to perform ADLs and the spasticity and distal weakness in his legs was affecting his gait and stair climbing. His respiratory and LE impairments were mildly affecting his endurance for LE activities.

are targeted toward remediating or improving already existing impairments and activity limitations (e.g., strengthening, balance, and endurance exercises). Compensatory interventions are directed toward modifying activities, tasks, or environments to minimize activity limitations and disablement (e.g., orthotics, assistive devices, wheelchairs).[208]

Individuals, in the early stage of ALS, such as Mr. Posner, should be encouraged to continue as many of their pre-diagnostic activities as possible. For example, Mr. Posner enjoys golfing and should be encouraged to continue playing as tolerated. If walking on the golf course is too fatiguing, the therapist can suggest that he use a golf cart, reduce the number of holes played, or hit balls at a driving range. If upper extremity weakness limits his golf swing for distance shots, he can play the greens or putting courses. He may benefit from adaptations to his club handles to prevent rotation of the club on impact through application of nonskid materials on club handles such as Dycem™[204] or a larger size grip. If Mr. Posner was leading a sedentary lifestyle before his diagnosis, he should be encouraged to increase his activity level. Walking, swimming, bicycling (three-wheeler or stationary bike, if needed), gardening, doing household chores, or working out to specific exercise routines are ways for individuals with ALS to keep active. Kamide et al.[209] reported that a combination of walking and ADL exercises significantly reduced functional decline in early-stage patients with ALS. Therapists, family members, and caregivers should support individuals with ALS to engage in activities that are safe and enjoyable for them to do for as long as possible.

Mr. Posner is likely to need physical therapy care in the future due to the progressive nature of the disease. Therefore, the therapist should not use up all of the patient's allotted yearly physical therapy visits for this episode of care. Educating the patient on a home exercise program to maintain or improve his maximum functional capacity with ongoing therapist reevaluation were priorities of the patient's plan of care. The program included the following:

1. General exercise: neck and extremity strengthening exercises (isometric or isotonic with submaximal elastic band resistance or small weights), alternating LEs on one day and the UEs on the other; AROM and stretching exercises to tight musculature; and daily walking for 10 minutes or as tolerated.

2. Energy-conservation strategies for fatigue prevention during ADLs and leisure activities (e.g., sitting down or taking a rest, when he starts to feel fatigued; doing strenuous activities during the time of day that he has the most energy; planning the week so that he doesn't have to do a lot of strenuous tasks in one day).

3. Referral to occupational therapy for evaluation of ADLs and recommendations for adaptive devices to assist with cutting food and using utensils and self-care.

4. Education on signs and symptoms of overwork fatigue and ALS resources and support groups available through the Amyotrophic Lateral Sclerosis Association (ALSA) and the MDA.

5. Follow-up appointments every 3 to 4 months for reevaluations.

CASE A, PART IV: MIDDLE STAGE

One year after his diagnosis, Mr. Posner was again referred by his neurologist for outpatient physical therapy, now diagnosed with definite ALS and adhesive capsulitis. The neurologist's orders were for gait training and reduction of shoulder pain. The patient reported that he stopped working at the insurance company about a month ago and was placed on permanent disability. He stated that he missed going to work and talking with his coworkers and had felt very depressed about it. His main social contacts were with his family and friends from church. He also contacted the local ALS Association and had been attending support group meetings with his family. The patient's baclofen had been increased to 20 mg in the morning and afternoon and 40 mg at bedtime. He was also taking Paxil 20 mg once daily for his depression. He had dropped 30 pounds, since his diagnosis. The patient's chief complaints were as follows:

- Pain throughout his shoulders bilaterally, worse on the left side than the right side, especially with overhead activities described as "a sharp ache deep in the shoulders."

- Neck pain, if he was sitting for long periods or riding in the car.

- SOB while walking, bathing, and dressing; some difficulty sleeping at night due to SOB, but not using more than two pillows; he was able to clear secretions with coughing.

He was able to do most ADLs by himself but very slowly and with much effort. He used a manual wheelchair for mobility in the community, due to fatigue when walking long distances; at home, he ambulated with the assistance of two people or a four-wheeled walker with attached forearm troughs, due to his hand grip weakness. He was no longer able to perform his home stretching program independently because of increased muscle tightness and decreased balance and muscle control. He had fallen backward on several occasions, during the past 6 months, when ambulating without assistance; one occurred in his driveway and resulted in injury to his back.

The patient had a ramp installed at his home, and his bedroom was located on the first floor. Grab bars were installed in the shower and beside the toilet, and the patient had a raised toilet seat. The patient was no longer driving. He was able to transport his manual wheelchair and walker in the trunk of his car, when going places. The patient's health coverage was currently COBRA, but he was in the process of getting Medicare with coverage to pay for his riluzole. His goals for physical therapy were to have decreased shoulder and neck pain and increased overall flexibility to move and walk better and not fall.

The physical therapist's examination findings revealed the following body/structure impairments:

- Mild edema in his feet and marked wasting of the intrinsic muscles of both hands; ankles were in a slightly plantarflexed and inverted position at rest; some fasciculations noted in the tongue and upper extremities.

- Decreased bilateral shoulder AROM: abduction (63 degrees Left; 76 degrees Right); flexion (78 degrees Left; 83 degrees Right); external rotation (25 degrees Left; 35 degrees Right) and internal rotation (40 degrees Left; 43 degrees Right) with pain (8 out of 10 on the left and 5 out of 10 on the right), during movements; PROM of shoulders limited bilaterally by muscle spasticity and guarding to 50% of NL (normal limits) in all directions; mild to moderate decreased glenohumeral mobility in all directions with mild subluxation noted bilaterally; passive ankle dorsiflexion limited bilaterally to 5 degrees.

- Decreased strength of the neck and bilateral UEs and LEs on MMT: elbow flexors F+ (3+), elbow extensors G (4), finger flexors P+ (2+), and hand intrinsics T (1), hip flexors G (4), knee extensors G (3), ankle dorsiflexors F(3), and ankle plantarflexors, evertors, invertors G− (4−), neck extensors G− (4−), neck flexors G (4)

- Brisk stretch reflexes (3+), with 2-3 beating clonus in ankles bilaterally; Modified Ashworth Scale scores were 1+ in bilateral biceps and wrist flexor muscles and 2 in bilateral hip adductors, quadriceps, hamstring, and gastrocnemius muscles.

- Sitting FVC: 3.77 L (77% of predicted).

The therapist's examination revealed the following activity limitations and participation restrictions:

- Balance (standing): Unilateral stance/eyes open, R = 10 seconds; L = 8 seconds

- Speech was slightly decreased in volume, slow, and slightly hypernasal, after the patient spoke for a while, but articulation was good; mild facial weakness as shown by difficulty holding air in his cheeks against resistance; able to swallow all foods, but sometimes choked on his saliva or when drinking water or coffee.

- Transfers sit-to-stand were slow with standby assist.

- Slow walking velocity (10 meter walk test = 7.4 seconds, 0.81 m/s), using four-wheeled walker with attached forearm troughs and standby assist; narrow base of support and forefoot contact at initial contact bilaterally)

- Moderate ADL and mobility deficits as indicated by ALSFRS-R score: 28/48 and Schwab and England score: 60% (can do most chores but very slowly and with much effort; makes errors).

Item	Score	ALSFRS-R Score Descriptor
Speech	3	Detectable speech disturbance
Salivation	3	Slight but definite excess of saliva in mouth; may have minimal drooling
Swallowing	3	Early eating problems – occasional choking
Handwriting (pre-ALS dominant hand)	2	Not all words are legible
Cutting food and handling utensils (patients without gastrostomy)	2	Intermittent assistance or substitute methods
Dressing and hygiene	2	Intermittent assistance or substitute methods
Turning in bed, adjusting bed clothes	2	Can turn alone or adjust sheets, but with great difficulty
Walking	2	Walks with assistance
Climbing stairs	0	Cannot do
Dyspnea	2	Occurs with one or more of the following: eating, bathing, dressing (ADL)
Orthopnea	3	Some difficulty sleeping at night due to SOB. Does not routinely use more than 2 pillows.
Respiratory insufficiency	4	None, e.g., no BiPAP at present

The physical therapist's diagnostic impression was that the patient was in transition from ambulation with an assistive device for short distances to dependence on a wheelchair for mobility. Pain and decreased ROM in bilateral shoulders was likely due to adhesive capsulitis secondary to immobility.

Shoulder Pain

As with Mr. Posner, shoulder pain may develop in people with ALS and can progress to significant restrictions of shoulder motions in a capsular pattern. Causative factors of pain may include (1) abnormal scapulohumeral rhythm secondary to spasticity or weakness, causing muscle imbalances that lead to impingement; (2) overuse of strong muscles; (3) prolonged immobility or reduced ROM; (4) marked shoulder weakness (in some cases "hanging arm" syndrome) and resultant glenohumeral subluxation; or (5) a fall. Depending on the cause of the pain, interventions may include modalities, ROM and passive stretching exercises, joint mobilizations, and education about proper shoulder support (e.g., using arm rests on chairs or tabletop or a shoulder support sleeve) and protection (e.g., avoid pulling the arms to assist a seated person with ALS to standing). Wearing a sling, similar to those used post-stroke, may benefit individuals with significant subluxation. Adhesive capsulitis has been managed successfully, in individuals with ALS, using intra-articular analgesic and anti-inflammatory cocktail injections, followed by a course of aggressive ROM exercises.[210]

Cervical Weakness

Mr. Posner is experiencing cervical muscle weakness that is a common problem for people with ALS.[211] Cervical extensor muscles are typically more affected than flexors. Initially, people with ALS may complain that their necks feel stiff or they feel "heavy-headed," after reading or writing, or they may notice that they have difficulty holding their heads straight with unanticipated movements, such as during sudden accelerations while sitting in a car. The weakness progresses to the point where the head begins to fall forward, and at advanced stages, the neck becomes completely flexed with the head dropped forward. The forward head position causes cervical pain and impairs ambulation and eating. For mild to moderate cervical weakness, such as Mr. Posner is experiencing, a soft collar may be worn for specific activities such as riding in the car. For people with ALS do not like to have pressure on the chin, a "baseball cap orthosis" which consists of an elastic strap that connects the back of a person's pants to the back of a baseball cap may be helpful.[212] For moderate to severe weakness, a semi-rigid or rigid collar is needed to provide adequate support. Collars such as the Philadelphia collar™,[213] Miami-J Collar™,[214] and Malibu Collar™[215] offer good support, but patients may feel confined or uncomfortably warm. The lightweight Headmaster collar™[216] has an open design that allows air circulation and is often well tolerated by individuals with ALS; it may be inadequate if rotation and lateral flexion weakness are also present.

Respiratory Weakness

Mr. Posner is experiencing shortness of breath with exertional activities and during sleep. Difficulty sleeping may be the first symptom of hypoventilation. The patient should be taught how to balance activity and rest so as not to become too fatigued. In addition, he and his family should be educated about signs and symptoms of aspiration; causes and signs of respiratory infection; management of oral secretions (oral suction device), positioning to avoid aspiration (upper cervical spine flexion ["chin tuck"

maneuver] during eating), and the Heimlich maneuver, in case of choking episodes. Respiratory muscle training appears to be feasible and safe in people with ALS.[217,218] One small double-blind, randomized study examined the effects of an inspiratory muscle training (IMT) program (10-minute sessions 3 times per day for 12 weeks) on nine individuals with ALS. Participants in the IMT group showed trends toward better FVC, VC, MIP, and SNIP values, compared to a control group that completed sham training; the gains in inspiratory muscle strength were partially reversed at an 8-week follow-up, after the training stopped.[219] Pinto et al.[220] examined the effects of IMT training (10-minute sessions twice daily for 4 months) in 26 individuals with ALS and found transient nonsignificant improvements in ASLFRS respiratory subscale scores and some respiratory function measures (SNIP, peak expiratory flow, maximal voluntary ventilation), following the intervention. Pinto and deCarvalho [221] continued to assess IMT effectiveness in surviving participants, who could perform the intervention, and found that individuals with ALS who participated in IMT longer than 8 months survived significantly longer than those in a historical control group by a mean of 12 months. Plowman et al. conducted a randomized controlled trial on the effects of expiratory muscle training (EMT, 5 sets of 5 reps of force exhalations with rests between sets, 5 days per week for 8 weeks) and reported significant improvements in MEP and swallowing function in the exercise group compared to controls.[222] Therapists should note that participants in these respiratory studies were generally in the early disease stage and had a FVC ≥ 70%. Lung volume recruitment training (LVRT, i.e., 5 breath-stacking maneuvers using a manual resuscitator with a one-way valve and mouthpiece, followed by 2 manually assisted coughs (MAC) via abdominal thrust) significantly enhanced immediate cough efficacy (FVC, PCEF) in persons with ALS; manually assisted coughs alone had less effect on PCEF.[223] Mechanical insufflation-exsufflation (assisted coughing that inflates the lungs and then stimulates a forced expiration "cough") was best at improving peak cough flow as well as the subjective evaluation of comfort and efficacy reported by persons with ALS.[224,225] One study reported that a diaphragmatic breathing exercise program was not effective in improving FVC or quality of life in 8 persons with ALS[226] In conclusion, these findings suggest that IMT, EMT, LVRT, and MAC may improve respiratory muscle strength and survival, or cough effectiveness in individuals with ALS, but rigorous studies are needed to investigate these interventions further.

LE Muscle Weakness and Gait Impairments

Mr. Posner is experiencing gait difficulties that are typical for individuals in the middle stage of the disease. Ambulatory assistive device prescription for individuals with ALS must take into account the patient's LE muscle strength or instability, UE function, extent and rate of disease progression, acceptance by the patient, and financial restrictions. At early stages, patients with ALS may benefit from use of a cane, but as the disease advances, wheeled walkers (i.e., four-wheeled walkers or front-wheeled walkers), which do not require the person to lift the device, are recommended. Mr. Posner is demonstrating bilateral ankle dorsiflexor weakness with resultant foot drop that may benefit from use of ankle-foot orthoses (AFOs). Given his good knee extensor strength with mild ankle strength deficits, light weight posterior leaf spring or carbon-fiber lateral or posterior strut dorsiflexion assist braces may be a good choice for him. For individuals with quadriceps weakness, an anterior support carbon-fiber AFO or floor reaction orthoses, such as ToeOFF® braces are commonly used.[227] If disease progression is rapid and a person will probably wear the AFO for a limited time, a commercially manufactured AFO may suffice.

Transfers and Mobility

Mr. Posner is having difficulty with sit-to-stand transfers due to LE weakness. Simple interventions include putting a firm cushion in a chair (2-3 inches) or elevating his chair with prefabricated blocks. Self-powered lifting seat cushions are portable and inexpensive, but the person needs adequate trunk control and balance for safe use. Recliner chairs with powered seat lifts may also help a person to rise from a seated position but are more expensive.

Once the individual is not able to stand, transfer boards may be used for transfers either independently, if arm strength and sitting balance are sufficient, or with caregiver assistance. Use of transfer belts can make transfers easier for the caregiver and prevent pulling on the patient's arms. Swivel cushions that swivel in both directions can make getting in and out of a car less difficult. When transfers become difficult, even with caregiver assistance, a hydraulic or mechanical lift such as the Hoyer lift™[228] is required. Use of hospital beds makes bed mobility and transfers easier for the patient and caregiver. Chair glides or stairway lifts are recommended for individuals, living in multilevel homes, that can't go up and down stairs. If insurance will not reimburse for stairway lifts, some medical supply companies may rent them, or the local ALSA or MDA chapter may have recycled lifts to loan.

Mr. Posner's muscle weakness and limited endurance necessitate that he use a wheelchair, when going long distances. Since most insurance companies will only reimburse for one wheelchair, individuals in the early to middle stages of ALS are advised to rent a manual wheelchair or obtain a loaner from a local ALSA or MDA chapter. Manual wheelchair features that were preferred by patients with ALS include lightweight frame, small wheelbase, high reclining back and supports for the head, trunk, and extremities.[229] As the disease progresses, a power wheelchair customized to the patient's needs will be required. Desirable features for powered wheelchairs are (1) tilt-in-space/recline features with a high firm back and headrest that allow the patient to shift weight and rest, while in the chair, (2) easy maneuverability (smaller wheelbase and less heavy), (3) lumbar support, (4) air or gel-filled cushion, (5) adjustable leg rests, (6) removable armrests for ease of transfer, and (7) potential mounting area for portable respirator equipment if needed.[229]

Activities of Daily Living

Mr. Posner's UE and LE weakness is impairing his ability to carry out many of his ADLs. A large variety of adaptive equipment is available to help maintain function. Foam tubing to increase the size of utensil handles, modified handles or holders on utensils and cups, long-levered jar openers, plate guards, rocker knives, universal cuffs (for holding tools and instruments) and mobile arm supports can assist a person with feeding and eating. For self-care and bathing, transfer benches (standard, slide, or swivel), shower chairs, handheld shower heads, grab bars, shower commodes, raised toilet seats, toilet frames, bidets, bath mitts, long-handled sponges, electric toothbrushes or shavers, and strap-fitted hairbrushes are recommended. Zipper pulls, Velcro clothing closures, slip-on shoes, and elastic shoelaces make dressing easier. Increasing the size of a pen/pencil with a triangular grip or cylindrical foam can make writing easier and more legible. Arm support, use of a universal cuff with a stylus, and electronic accessibility aids (e.g., Siri, Voice Control (Apple) or Access (Android/Google), Speech Recognition, Dictation, Eye gaze) help to make computer use easier. Other useful equipment includes key holders, doorknob adapters, personal alarm systems, switch-operated environmental controls for turning lights or the television on and off, and speaker phones with automatic dialing. Some of these may be too expensive for the patient and family to acquire.[227]

Psychosocial Issues

Mr. Posner is mourning the loss of his friendships at work and of his standing as a competent Chief Financial Officer. Because of the progressive nature of the disease, individuals with ALS must cope with continuous losses of physical health and abilities, body image, work and family roles, identity, and family and social networks. The physical therapist must attend to the patient's ability to cope and adapt to these changes and be able to differentiate between normal grief reactions to changes in function and symptoms of fear, anxiety, and depression. Purtilo and Haddad[230] identified four major fears of individuals with a terminal condition: fear of isolation, fear of pain, fear of dependence, and fear of death itself. Mr. Posner's fear of isolation increased when he was no longer able to go to work. Fortunately, he has maintained contacts with family members, church friends, and support group members. Mr. Posner is also experiencing increased pain and discomfort that is causing him anxiety. With aggressive management of his pain, through medications and physical therapy, these anxieties may be relieved. His increasing dependence on others for driving, walking, and ADLs are similarly causing him to feel stressed because of the increased burden that he feels he is putting on his wife and children. His wife may feel stressed and anxious about having to take over her husband's responsibilities, and his children may be frustrated with the need to provide care to their father. Referral to a psychologist for individual and family counseling may be beneficial to improve communication and resolve conflicts. Therapists must be prepared to help patients, families, and caregivers find effective ways to cope with the emotional, social, and physical stress that accompanies living with ALS.

Reduction of shoulder pain and improved shoulder ROM, family training in ROM exercises, and preparation for the patient's future mobility needs were the goals of the plan of care which included the following:

1. Therapeutic interventions for improved bilateral shoulder ROM and pain reduction;

2. Family training in passive UE and LE ROM and stretching exercises;

3. Interventions for LE edema control;

4. LE AFOs and power wheelchair prescription; and

5. Referrals to occupational therapy for ADL evaluation, to a speech and language pathologist for speech and swallowing evaluation, to a dietician for dietary counseling, and a social worker to address family or personal relationship issues, and to provide emotional support.

CASE A, PART V: LATE STAGE

Two years post-diagnosis, home physical therapy is requested to assess caregiver demands and to make recommendations. Fourteen months after Mr. Posner's diagnosis, he underwent PEG placement due to problems with dysphagia and declining respiratory status. The patient's wife quit her teaching job to be able to care full time for the patient. She stated that she is feeling exhausted and stressed by the demands of taking care of her husband. She also stated that the children, who are now ages 13 and 11, are having a difficult time dealing with their fathers' declining physical capacity, had been angry and irritable with her at times, and their grades had dropped in school. The patient does not yet have advanced directives, but the wife states that she is afraid to talk to him about it for fear that he will become depressed. The patient takes baclofen 20 mg four times daily and tizanidine 4 mg at bedtime. He also takes lithium carbonate 300 mg twice daily, per his request, following the publication of an article that suggested that it might slow the progression of the disease. The patient purchased a minivan that is equipped to transport his power wheelchair for going to church or other community events and an electric hospital bed with an anti-pressure mattress. The patient's and wife's complaints were as follows:

- Wife is unable to put the AFOs on the patient's feet due to his limited ankle ROM, making transfers very difficult because the patient stands on his toes. She almost dropped the patient several times, during transfers, and wants to be able to transfer patient with less difficulty.

- Patient is SOB even when he is sitting at rest. He has started using BiPAP every night, and states that it helps him to breathe better even during the day. He can only sleep with his head raised at night. His cough is weak, and he has some difficulty clearing his secretions.

- Patient has constant bilateral shoulder pain, left greater than right, that decreases his function and quality of life; the patient wants to have decreased shoulder pain.

- Patient needs a significant amount of help for self-care and mobility.

- Patient is able to stand with help and take a few steps with difficulty but is unable to ambulate.

- Patient enjoys socializing with family and friends at children's school and sports events and at church but is having difficulty conversing with people due to speech deficits and fatigue.

- Patient feels "useless" and wants be less of a burden on his wife and family.

The physical therapist's examination findings revealed the following impairments:

- Marked atrophy and fasciculations in the tongue and all extremities.

- Alert and oriented times 3; some psychomotor slowing as shown by a slight delay in responses to questions.

- Two finger subluxation of both shoulders.

- Shoulder pain measures 4 out of 10 on the left and 2 out of 10 on the right at rest and increases during movement.

- Minimal active movement in his UEs, and some antigravity movement in his LEs; shoulder PROM is 70% of normal limits in all directions due to spasticity, muscular tightness, and guarding; bilateral finger flexor and plantarflexor contractures.

- Decreased strength throughout neck and bilateral UEs and LEs on MMT: UE muscles in the 0 to T (1) range, LE muscles in the P+ (2+) range proximally and 0 in the ankle dorsiflexors and plantarflexors, neck extensors P (2), neck flexors F− (3−).

- Brisk stretch reflexes (3+), with continuous clonus in bilateral ankles; Modified Ashworth Scale scores are 2 in bilateral biceps and wrist flexor muscles and 3 in bilateral hip adductors, quadriceps, hamstring, and gastrocnemius muscles.

- FVC: 2.49 L (51% of predicted).

The physical therapist's examination findings revealed the following activity limitations and participation restrictions:

- Balance (standing): Unilateral stance/eyes open, unable to stand on one leg

- Speech is barely understandable with concentration; patient is on a soft mechanical diet and only uses the PEG for supplemental feedings and water; he occasionally chokes, when swallowing food and medications.

Item	Score	ALSFRS-R Score Descriptor
Speech	2	Intelligible with repeating
Salivation	2	Marked excess of saliva with some drooling
Swallowing	1	Needs supplemental tube feeding
Handwriting (pre-ALS dominant hand)	0	Unable to grip pen
Cutting food and handling utensils (patients without gastrostomy)	0	Needs to be fed
Dressing and hygiene	1	Needs attendant for self-care
Turning in bed, adjusting bed clothes	1	Can initiate, but no turn or adjust sheets alone
Walking	1	Non-ambulatory functional movement only
Climbing stairs	0	Cannot do
Dyspnea	1	Occurs at rest, difficulty breathing when either sitting or lying
Orthopnea	2	Needs extra pillow in order to sleep (more than two)
Respiratory insufficiency	3	Intermittent use of Bi PAP

- Transfers sit-to-stand and sit-to-supine with maximal assist of 1.
- Stands with his feet plantarflexed due to increased tone and muscle tightness and with his legs close together; can move his legs a couple of steps for transfers but quickly fatigues.
- Severe ADL and mobility deficits as indicated by ALSFRS-R score: 14/48 and Schwab and England score: 20% (can do nothing alone; may be able to help a little in some tasks).

The physical therapist's diagnostic impression was that the patient was quadriplegic and was dependent on his wife for ADLs. His shoulder pain and decreased ROM were likely due to a combination of instability and immobility. The patient was likely to need hospice care in the near future.

Primary goals at this stage were to maintain the patient's comfort, prevent complications, and ease caregiving burden.

1. Instruct patient's wife in basic body mechanics to use during lifting and patient care activities, PROM exercises, assisted coughing techniques, the use of a Hoyer lift™ for transfers, and use of positioning devices for the lower extremities (e.g., L-Nard boots, hip abduction splints).
2. Referrals to a speech and language pathologist for speech and swallowing evaluations and recommendations for augmentative communication devices, and to a social worker for information on respite care for the wife, family counseling, and advanced directives.

GUILLAIN–BARRÉ SYNDROME

CASE B, PART I

Mrs. Roberts is a 56-year-old registered nurse who awoke with "pins-and-needles" sensations and accompanying numbness in her hands. Upon arising, she became aware of mild incoordination and weakness of her lower extremities. The weakness progressed to involve her upper extremities, and she was hospitalized by her family physician 3 days later. She previously had been in excellent health with the exception of a 4-day hospitalization 2 weeks earlier for a flu-like syndrome, consisting of mild fever, swollen lymph nodes, general feeling of illness, and diffuse joint and muscle pains. A precise diagnosis had not been established, but her symptoms resolved. After performing an examination and ordering some tests her physician gave her a diagnosis of Guillain–Barré syndrome.

Guillain–Barré Syndrome (GBS) is a group of neuropathic conditions that affect the peripheral nervous system, causing motor neuropathy with progressive weakness and diminished or absent reflexes. Sensory and autonomic nerve involvement is also possible. In contrast to ALS, GBS has a good prognosis with most patients recovering to their prior functional status by 1 year after onset.

Incidence and Risk Factors

The annual incidence of GBS is about two per 100,000 persons, and an estimated 3000 to 6000 people develop GBS each year on average in the United States.[231] The incidence of GBS increases with age, and people over age 50 are at greatest risk for developing GBS.[231,232] The male-to-female ratio is 3:2.[232] It is more common in adults than children, and its effects do not vary with race, ethnicity, or geographic location.[231]

Etiology and Pathophysiology

Several infections are implicated in the development of GBS. About two-thirds of patients with GBS have respiratory and gastrointestinal symptoms that precede the onset of neurologic symptoms by 1 to 3 weeks. The strongest evidence implicates *Campylobacter jejuni* infection, but GBS has also been reported following infection with cytomegalovirus, varicella-zoster virus (herpes), Epstein–Barr virus (mononucleosis), Zika virus, and coronavirus 2019 (Covid-19).[28,233] Stressful events and surgeries have also been associated with the disease.[28] Despite some reports of GBS developing after vaccinations (i.e., tetanus, hepatitis, and influenza), there is not sufficient evidence to support vaccinations as a cause of GBS.

There are at least two pathologies that result in a clinical diagnosis of GBS (see Figure 16-4).[234] The demyelinating variant of GBS (**acute inflammatory demyelinating polyradiculoneuropathy [AIDP]**; see Table 16-11) is characterized by damage to the myelin sheath, surrounding axons, by white blood cells (T lymphocytes and macrophages). This process is preceded by antibodies, binding to myelin antigens that activate a group of blood proteins, known as complement, which in turn leads to the degradation of myelin. Macrophages subsequently act as scavengers to remove myelin debris (see Figure 16-4A). Axonal damage may also occur secondary to demyelination. In contrast, the axonal subtype (**acute motor axonal neuropathy [AMAN]**; see Table 16-11) is mediated by immunoglobulin G (IgG) antibodies and complement acting directly against the cell membrane covering the axon without lymphocyte involvement (see Figure 16-4B).[234] In this form of GBS, various antibodies bind to gangliosides on the cell membrane of the axons at the nodes of Ranvier. Gangliosides are groups of substances found in peripheral nerves. The key four gangliosides, against which

antibodies have been described, are GM1, GD1a, GT1a, and GQ1b, with different anti-ganglioside antibodies being associated with different subtypes of GBS (Table 16-11). After an infection, the production of these antibodies is probably the result of molecular mimicry, where the immune system reacts to the foreign infectious substance, but the resultant antibodies, in turn, attack tissues that are naturally in the body. For example, after a *Campylobacter* infection, some people will produce IgG antibodies against bacterial cell wall substances (e.g., lipooligosaccharides) that cross-react with nerve cell gangliosides. The binding of antibodies to gangliosides causes activation of complement that, in turn, leads to detachment of portions of the myelin near the nodes of Ranvier and eventually axonal degeneration of motor fibers.[234]

Clinical Presentation

AIDP typically presents as distal paresthesias or sensory loss, accompanied or followed by bilateral, and relatively symmetric, limb weakness that starts in the legs and progresses rapidly to the arms and bulbar muscles.[28] Respiratory insufficiency, due to weakness of respiratory muscles, requires mechanical ventilation for about 20% of hospitalized patients.[236] Respiratory failure is more common in patients with rapid progression of symptoms, upper limb weakness, autonomic dysfunction, or bulbar paralysis.[28] Patients typically have generalized hyporeflexia or areflexia.[237] The weakness continues to progress up to 1 to 3 weeks after the onset of symptoms, followed by a plateau of variable duration before resolution or stabilization with/without residual disability.[237] Two-thirds of patients are unable to walk

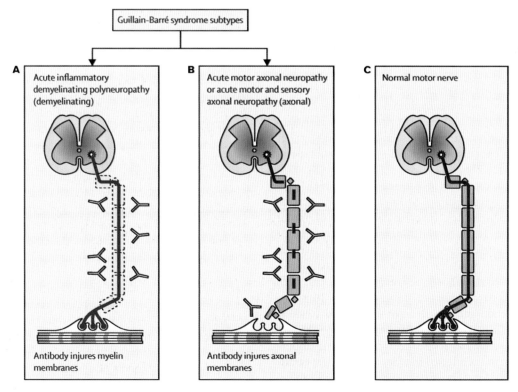

FIGURE 16-4 Major Guillain-Barre Syndrome Subtypes.[28,232,234] **A.** Antibodies bind to myelin antigens and activate blood proteins (complement) that damage myelin. **B.** Immunoglobulin G antibodies bind to gangliosides on cell membrane of axons and activate complement that damages axons. **C.** Illustration of normal motor nerve with intact axon and myelin. (Reproduced with permission from Hugh J Willison, Bart C Jacobs, Pieter A van Doorn. Guillain-Barré syndrome, Lancet 2016; 388: 717–27.)

TABLE 16-11 GBS Subtypes[235,236]

TYPE	PATHOLOGIC FEATURES	CLINICAL FEATURES	NERVE CONDUCTION STUDIES
Acute inflammatory demyelinating polyradiculo-neuropathy (AIDP)	Multifocal peripheral demyelination Slow remyelination Probably both humeral and cellular immune mechanisms	Rapidly progressive, symmetrical weakness with absent or reduced tendon reflexes; Often accompanied by sensory symptoms, cranial nerve weakness, and autonomic involvement; more common in Europe and the Americas (70%) than in Asia (30-40%).	Demyelinating polyneuropathy
Acute motor axonal neuropathy (AMAN)	Antibodies against gangliosides GM1, GD1a/b, GalNAc-GD1a in peripheral motor nerve axons; no demyelination	Strongly associated with *Campylobacter jejuni* infection; more common in the summer, younger patients, and in eastern Asia Only motor symptoms; cranial nerve involvement uncommon Deep tendon reflexes may be preserved	Axonal polyneuropathy, normal sensory action potential
Acute motor and sensory axonal neuropathy (AMSAN)	Mechanism similar to AMAN, but with sensory axonal degeneration	Similar to those of AMAN, but with predominantly sensory involvement	Axonal polyneuropathy, reduced or absent sensory action potential
Miller Fisher syndrome	Antibodies against gangliosides GQ1b, GD3, and GT1a; demyelination	Bilateral ophthalmoplegia, ataxia, areflexia Facial weakness occurs in 50% of cases Trunk, extremity weakness occurs in 50% of cases	Generally normal, sometimes discrete changes in sensory conduction or H-reflex detected
Pharyngeo-cervico-brachial variant	Antibodies against mostly gangliosides GT1a, occasionally GQ1b, rarely GD1a; no demyelination	Weakness particularly of the throat muscles, face, neck, and shoulder muscles	Generally normal, sometimes axonal neuropathy in arms

independently, when maximum weakness is reached, and among severely affected patients, 20% remain unable to walk 6 months after the onset of symptoms.[238] GBS generally follows a monophasic course and typically does not recur, but ≥2 episodes have been reported in 2 to 5% of patients[237] Recurrences occurred more frequently in patients under 30, with milder symptoms, and in patients with the Miller Fisher subtype of GBS (see Table 16-11).[238]

Other symptoms that may be present in individuals with GBS include cranial neuropathies, sensory disturbances, pain, and autonomic disturbances. Involvement of cranial motor neurons can cause facial, oropharyngeal, and oculomotor muscle weakness, associated with facial paralysis, dysarthria, dysphagia, and visual problems (i.e., diplopia, ophthalmoplegia, and pupillary disturbances). Sensory disturbances, such as distal hyperesthesias, numbness, and paresthesias (tingling, burning), are common and usually have a glove and stocking pattern. Pain, especially with movement, is common (50-89% of patients) and is described as severe, deep, aching, or cramping (similar to sciatica) in the affected muscles and back (especially lumbar, intrascapular, and cervical regions).[28] The pain is often worse at night. Autonomic symptoms occur in about two-thirds of patients and include cardiac arrhythmias, orthostasis, blood pressure instability, urinary retention, constipation, and slowing of gastrointestinal motility.[28]

Diagnosis

Two commonly used sets of diagnostic criteria for GBS were developed by the National Institute of Neurological Disorders in Stroke (NINDS)[239] and the Brighton Collaboration.[240] Both criteria include progressive, relatively symmetrical weakness with decreased or absent deep tendon reflexes as required criteria for diagnosis.[28] Symptoms must reach maximal intensity within 4 weeks of onset and other possible causes must be excluded, for a diagnosis to be made. Table 16-12 includes features necessary for the diagnosis. As described in Table 16-11, this syndrome has several distinct subtypes. AIDP is the most common subtype and accounts for up to 90% of the GBS cases in the United States.[232] Specific changes in cerebrospinal fluid (CSF) and electrodiagnostic studies are strongly supportive of the diagnosis.[28] Diagnostic lumbar puncture findings include increased protein levels (albumin) and a normal white blood cell count in the CSF (see Table 16-12). The normal CSF white blood cell count helps differentiate GBS from other infectious, inflammatory, and malignant diseases.[28] NCS may show prolonged distal motor latencies, conduction slowing, conduction block, and temporal dispersion (loss of synchrony in the nerve action potentials) of compound muscle action potentials (CMAPs) with resultant decrease in CMAP amplitude in demyelinating cases (AIDP). In addition, F-waves and H-reflexes may be prolonged or absent. In **primary**

TABLE 16-12	Diagnosis of GBS[236,239]
FEATURE	**COMMENTS**
Required for diagnosis (not applicable to all subtypes of GBS)	
Progressive weakness of more than one limb	Usually begins in bilateral legs; peaks within 4 weeks: peaks by 2 weeks in 50% of cases, and by 3 weeks in 80% of cases
Absent or decreased tendon reflexes in affected limbs	Must occur at some point in clinical course
Supportive of diagnosis	
Clinical features	
Autonomic involvement	Cardiac arrhythmias, orthostasis, blood pressure instability, urinary retention, slowing of gastrointestinal motility; absent in some subtypes
Cranial nerve involvement	Bilateral facial weakness occurs in 30-50% of cases; rarely an initial feature
Relatively symmetrical	Symptoms may not be absolutely symmetrical in affected limbs or face
Sensory involvement	Usually mild; absent in some subtypes, prominent in others (i.e., acute motor-sensory axonal neuropathy)
Symptom pattern over time	Peak by 2-4 weeks, with variable plateau, followed by recovery; permanent sequelae are possible
Cerebrospinal fluid findings	
Elevated protein levels Normal white blood cell count	Levels may be normal early, but they are elevated (>400 mg/L) by the end of the second week of symptoms in 90% of cases Less than 10 per mm³ (10×10^6 per L)
Nerve Conduction Velocity findings	
Slowing (<60% normal velocity) or blockage of nerve conduction	Slowing of nerve conduction occurs in 80% of cases, but this may take weeks to develop

axonal damage (AMAN subtype), the findings include reduced amplitude of CMAPs without conduction slowing. In the acute phase, the only needle EMG abnormality may be abnormal motor recruitment, with decreased recruitment and rapid firing motor units in weak muscles. Fibrillations may be seen after 3 to 4 weeks, if some axonal injury occurs.[241]

Other tests include blood tests and neuroimaging. Blood tests are generally performed to exclude the possibility of another cause of weakness (low potassium, Lyme disease, human immunodeficiency virus [HIV]). MRI is usually performed in GBS to rule out other potential causes of the clinical presentation, especially myelopathy.[234] A few small case series studies have looked at positive imaging findings that may be suggestive of GBS. The most often reported finding is greater gadolinium enhancement of the ventral compared to the dorsal roots of the cauda equina, especially in children.[234,242]

Prognosis

Even in developed countries, the mortality rate from GBS is about 5%, mostly due to cardiovascular and respiratory complications, which can occur in both acute and recovery phases.[237] Recovery depends on the amount of remyelination and/or axonal regrowth. The process of remyelination occurs rapidly; however, regrowth of damaged axons, after Wallerian degeneration, is a slow process, with the rate of growth being about 1 mm/day.[243] Recovery from GBS is generally good. A large literature review of outcomes in individuals with GBS, who were appropriately treated, found that 82% of individuals were able to walk unaided at 6 months, and 84.1% walked unaided at 1 year, after the onset of GBS.[244] However, only 61% of individuals had full recovery of motor strength, 38% needed to change employment due to GBS, 66% of patients reported pain, and 14% were left with severe disability at 1 year.[244,245] The most common long-term deficits are weakness of the anterior tibialis muscle and, less commonly, foot and hand intrinsics, quadriceps, and gluteal musculature. Some patients have long-term recurrences of fatigue and/or exhaustion, accompanied by pain and muscle aches, that can occur with the exertion of normal walking or working and can be alleviated by reduction of activity and rest.[246,247] Fatigue was independent of the severity of neurological deficits and was hypothesized to be due to post-infectious fatigue, dysautonomia, and psycho-sociological consequences of the disease.[246] Moderate to severe sensory deficits (impaired response to pinprick, light touch, proprioception, and vibration) were found in the arms of 38% and in the legs of 66% of 122 patients at 3 to 6 years, after recovery from acute GBS.[248] At two years after onset, individuals with GBS reported that these residual deficits negatively impacted their ability to participate in work and social activities, which affected their quality of life.[247]

The variations in the rate and extent of recovery in GBS make functional prognosis difficult. However, clinical scoring systems have been developed to aid in predicting individuals, who will need mechanical ventilation, and to predict long-term functional disability. Walgaard et al.[249] published a clinical prediction model, called the Erasmus GBS Respiratory Insufficiency Score (EGRIS), that uses the number of days between the onset of weakness and hospital admission, the presence or absence of facial or bulbar weakness, and the severity of the limb weakness (Medical Research Council [MRC] sumscore; the sum of MRC scores [0-5] on six muscles bilaterally) to predict the likelihood that respiratory insufficiency will develop. An EGRIS of 0-2 indicates a low risk of mechanical ventilation (4%), 3 to 4 indicates an intermediate risk (24%), and ≥5 indicates a high risk (65%).[236] Walgaard et al.[250] also published a clinical prediction model, called the Modified Erasmus GBS Outcome Scale, that uses the patient's age, the presence or absence of antecedent diarrhea, and severity of limb weakness (MRC sumscore) to predict whether a patient will be able to walk independently at 1, 3, or 6 months. Higher scores predict greater disability. Both scales are validated in the GBS population. Worse outcomes are associated with antecedent diarrheal illness, older age, more severe symptoms at their peak, rapid progression of symptoms, inability to walk at 14 days, and axonal involvement.[28]

Medical Management

Because of the unpredictable course and potential for death, patients with evidence of GBS should be hospitalized for intensive monitoring of cardiac, respiratory, bowel and bladder function, and provision of supportive care by a multidisciplinary team, until it has been established that there is no evidence of clinical progression. In patients with moderate to severe symptoms, respiratory compromise can develop rapidly, and mechanical ventilation may be required, if VC drops below 60% of predicted or less than 20 mL/kg.[28] Swallowing should be assessed to identify patients at risk for aspiration, necessitating the placement of a nasogastric tube. Subcutaneous heparin and compression stockings may be administered to decrease the risk of deep vein thrombosis, and patients with limited mobility should be monitored and positioned to prevent skin breakdown. If patients experience neuropathic pain, gabapentin (Neurontin) and carbamazepine (Tegretol) have been found to benefit patients with GBS, in intensive care units.[28] Increased skin sensitivity to touch may necessitate gentle handling and removal of irritating stimuli. Cardiac arrhythmia and extreme hypertension or hypotension, occurs in 20% of patients with GBS.[153] Bradycardia may be so severe that it causes asystole, necessitating the use of a temporary cardiac pacemaker.[237] Other possible complications include urinary retention and constipation, which may be addressed by bladder catheterization and the use of laxatives, respectively.

Specific treatments to speed recovery and/or eliminate symptoms of GBS include plasma exchange and intravenous immunoglobulin (IVIg).[236] Plasma exchange (removal of plasma from withdrawn blood with retransfusion of the blood cells back into the blood with a plasma subsitute) removes damaging antibodies and complement and has been shown to improve the time to recover walking ability, minimize the need for mechanical ventilation, decrease the duration of ventilation, and result in greater muscle strength after 1 year, compared with placebo, in individuals with AIDP.[251,252] IVIg treatment (intravenous infusion of immunoglobulin preparation) has been shown to hasten recovery in non-ambulatory adults and children, compared with supportive therapy alone.[251] It is thought that immunoglobulin may act by neutralizing pathogenic antibodies and inhibiting complement activation, resulting in reduced nerve injury and faster clinical improvement. In general, IVIg has replaced plasma exchange as the treatment of choice, in many medical centers, because of its greater ease of administration and availability.[237] The standard treatment regimen is a total dose of 2 g per kilogram of body weight over a period of 5 days. The combination of plasma exchange, followed by a course of IVIg, is not significantly better than plasma exchange or immunoglobulin alone.[253] Treatment with oral corticosteroids (e.g., prednisolone or methylprednisolone) showed no significant benefit to recovery.[254]

Physical Therapy Evaluation of the Individual with GBS

Physical therapy examination of the patient with GBS should start with a medical records review and history taking to obtain information about the time since diagnosis, recent illnesses or injuries, during the 4 weeks prior to GBS onset, the rate of progression and extent of symptoms, any pre-existing neuromotor or medical conditions that might impact recovery, results of electrodiagnostic testing, and the patient's goals for physical therapy. A standard systems review and neurological examination should be performed with specific consideration to the following areas.

Motor System Function

Muscle weakness is a primary impairment of GBS and should be assessed to track progression of the disease initially and later to track recovery, to predict and prevent the development of contractures, and to determine the appropriate intensity of exercise interventions to implement. Therapists should visually inspect the patient to identify muscle atrophy and the presence of muscle fasciculations. Muscle strength in the neck and extremities can be directly assessed with MMT, dynamometry, or isokinetic testing, depending on the disease stage, or indirectly through functional testing. A cranial nerve screen should be conducted. Joint ROM may be initially assessed passively and, eventually, actively, using a goniometer. Foot and wrist drop are common and may require bracing or splinting to prevent contractures.

Depending on the MMT and ROM findings, balance, mobility (e.g., transfers, wheelchair propulsion, ambulation), self-care tasks (e.g., grooming, feeding, and dressing), and other functional tasks related to the patient's work and/or leisure activities should be assessed. The BBS, TUG, and Five Times Sit-To-Stand (5TSTS) test have been used to assess balance and mobility in individuals with GBS and other neurological disorders.[255–257] Gait speed has been measured with or without use of an ambulatory assistive device using the 10MWT.[255] Gait endurance can be measured with the six-minute walk test. Finger dexterity may be measured using a nine-hole peg test.[2612] Therapists need to ensure that the patient with GBS is well rested, prior to mobility and functional testing. They should also ask the patient about and monitor for potential complications, related to weakness and immobility, such as falls and deep vein thromboses.

Three functional scales that have been used in clinical trials of individuals with GBS, include the Inflammatory Neuropathy Cause and Treatment (INCAT) group overall disability sum score (ODSS), the GBS Disability Scale (also called the modified Hughes functional scale), and the modified Rankin scale (see Table 16-13).

Respiratory failure, during the acute stage, results from progressive respiratory muscle weakness, involving both the inspiratory and expiratory muscles, and is a major complication of GBS, occurring in about 30% of patients.[262] Early signs of respiratory distress include tachypnea, tachycardia, air hunger, interrupted speech, use of accessory respiratory muscles, paradoxical breathing, and orthopnea; later signs include bradypnea, cardiac arrhythmias, loss of consciousness, and respiratory arrest.[262] Vital capacity (VC) and maximal inspiratory and

TABLE 16-13	Functional Scales Used in GBS Disability Ratings	
FUNCTIONAL SCALE	**DESCRIPTION**	**SCORING**
Overall Disability Sum Score[258,259]	Patient report with arm and leg subscales. Arm = dressing (buttons and zippers), washing and combing hair, knife and fork use, turning a key in a lock Legs = walking and use of assistive devices	Total • 0 = no signs of disability • 12 = most severe disability score Individual items: Arms • 0 = normal • 5 = severe and bilateral Individual items: Legs • 0 = walking is not affected • 7 = restricted to WC or bed with no purposeful leg movements
GBS Disability Scale[259,260]	Describes functional status along 5-point scale	1 = able to run with minor signs/symptoms 2 = able to walk 10 m but not run 3 = able to walk 10 m with help 4 = unable to walk, in bed 5 = dead
Modified Rankin Scale[261]	5-point scale	0 = no symptoms 5 = severe disability (bedridden, incontinent, requiring constant nursing care)

expiratory pressures (MIP, MEP), assessed with a handheld spirometer, are measures of respiratory muscle strength that are frequently used to monitor the breathing status of the patient with GBS. In a retrospective study of 114 patients with GBS, a VC lower than 20 mL/kg, MIP lower than 30 cm H_2O, and MEP lower than 40 cm H_2O (the so-called "20/30/40 rule"), or a greater than 30% decrease from baseline of VC, MIP, or MEP was associated with impending progression of respiratory failure and need for mechanical ventilation.[263]

Fatigue is a common complaint in individuals with GBS. Patients can rate their fatigue, using a VAS, with "no fatigue" and "worst imaginable fatigue" as opposite extremes. Other fatigue scales that have been used in individuals with GBS include the FSS, the Checklist Individual Strength (CIS) fatigue subscale, the Multidimensional Fatigue Inventory, and the Fatigue Impact Scale (FIS).[246,262] Patients should not be tested to exhaustion, since recovery from fatigue can take some time and will delay the rehabilitation process.

Sensory System Function

Sensory function, including light touch, pressure, vibration, and pinprick, should be assessed frequently in patients with GBS to track the progress of reinnervation, to monitor muscle soreness, and to avoid causing unnecessary pain during therapy. The INCAT sensory sum score is a sensory scale developed for patients with immune-mediated polyneuropathies that ranges from 0 ("normal sensation") to 20 ("most severe sensory deficit") and is the summation of pinprick and vibration grades (range 0-4) of the arms and legs and a two-point discrimination grade (range 0-4) on the index finger.[264] Pain can be reported by the patient, using a VAS, with "no pain" and "unbearable pain" as opposite extremes.[255] Therapists should use a body chart to identify both the locations and specific types of sensory loss or changes (paraesthesia, numbness, tingling, or hyperesthesia). It is also important for therapists to monitor for pressure sores

and/or teach the patient to perform skin inspections in areas where skin sensation is diminished or absent.

Autonomic System Function

Autonomic dysfunction in GBS may cause extreme fluctuations of heart rate, blood pressure, and body temperature, as well as bowel and bladder problems.[28] Therapists should monitor heart rate and blood pressure in resting and immediately after activity. If the patient reports dizziness, the therapist might consider obtaining blood pressure and heart rate while supine and then standing to identify orthostatic hypotension. Therapists should also monitor patients for signs of abnormal body temperature or bowel and bladder control.

Psychosocial Systems

GBS is often a frightening and distressful experience to patients, especially to those who progress to complete paralysis and respiratory failure.[265] Therapists should assess the patient's psychological and emotional health, coping strategies, and quality of life throughout all stages of the disease. Therapists can screen the patient for depression and anxiety using a variety of instruments (Table 16-14). Health-related quality-of-life measures that have been used in individuals with neuromuscular diseases are the Sickness Impact Profile, the SF-36, and the World Health Organization Quality of Life-Bref (WHOQOL-BREF).[266,267] It is also important to assess the caregiver and environmental support that the patient has at home and determine what their needs may be after discharge.

A summary of the tests and measures that can be used to assess and evaluate an individual with GBS is found in Table 16-14. Based on the medical records review, subjective history, and examination findings, the therapist and patient should collaborate on setting physical therapy goals. General goals for physical therapy may include the following: (1) facilitate respiratory, speech, and swallowing functions; (2) reduce pain;

TABLE 16-14	GBS Impairment, Activity, and Participation Assessments	
IMPAIRMENT LEVEL ASSESSMENTS	**ACTIVITY LEVEL ASSESSMENTS**	**PARTICIPATION LEVEL ASSESSMENTS**
• Cognitive screen (Montreal Cognitive Assessment) • Psychological screen (CES-D, HADS, HARS) • Sensation (INCAT sensory sum score) • Pain (10-point rating scale, VAS) • ROM (muscle length versus joint limitations) • Muscle strength (MMT, dynamometer, isokinetic testing, functional testing) • Hand and upper extremity function (NHPT) • Reflexes (DTRs) • Tone (Modified Ashworth Scale) • Cranial nerve screen • Respiratory Assessment (VC, MIP, MEP, aerobic capacity, and endurance testing) • Fatigue (FSS, CIS fatigue, MFI, FIS)	• Functional Status (Inflammatory Neuropathy Cause and Treatment group ODSS, modified GBS Disability Scale, modified Rankin scale, FIM) • Balance (BBS) • Gait and mobility (10 meter walk test, six minute walk test, TUG, FTSTS)	• Health-related QOL (Sickness Impact Profile, SF-36, WHOQOL-BREF)

BBS, Berg Balance Scale; CES-D, Center of Epidemiologic Study-Depression Scale; CIS, Checklist Individual Strength; DTR, deep tendon reflex; FSS, Fatigue Severity Scale; FIM, Functional Independence Measure; FIS, Fatigue Impact Scale; HADS, Hospital Anxiety and Depression Scale; HARS, Hamilton Anxiety Rating Scale; INCAT, Inflammatory Neuropathy Cause and Treatment; MEP, maximal expiratory pressure; MFI, Multidimensional Fatigue Inventory; MIP, maximal inspiratory pressure; MMT, manual muscle test; NHPT, nine-hole peg test; ODSS, overall disability sum score; TUG, Timed Up and Go; 5TSTS, Five Times Sit-To-Stand; VAS, Visual Analogue Scale; VC, vital capacity; WHOQOL-BREF World Health Organization Quality of Life-Bref.

(3) prevent secondary complications (e.g., contractures, pressure sores, DVTs, and injury to weakened or denervated muscle); (4) initiate a graduated mobility program to obtain maximal function as reinnervation occurs; and (5) facilitate return to previous life roles and improved quality of life.

Physical Therapy Interventions

The evidence, regarding exercise and rehabilitation in people with GBS, is limited with only three randomized clinical trials identified in a systematic review paper of rehabilitation interventions published in 2021.[267] One randomized controlled trial, compared high-intensity outpatient multidisciplinary rehabilitation (i.e., 3 one-hour sessions of interrupted therapy/week, involving half-hour blocks of occupational, social, psychology, speech and physical therapy sessions 2-3 times per week for up to 12 weeks) with low intensity rehabilitation (i.e., home-based program of maintenance exercises and education for self-management with a 30-minute physical program [walking, stretching] twice weekly and usual activity at home), for individuals (n = 79 enrolled, 69 completed, treatment group = 35) in the chronic phase of GBS. Physical therapy sessions consisted of strengthening and endurance exercises and gait training. Following the intervention, the individuals, in the high-intensity group, showed significantly greater improvement in function (FIM scores; $p < 0.0005$) than the low-intensity treatment group.[268] Three observational studies also support that high-intensity inpatient multidisciplinary rehabilitation, including physical therapy, minimizes disability and improves quality of life in individuals with GBS.[269] Ragupathy et al.[270] found that persons with GBS (22 enrolled, 20 completed, treatment group =10) who performed yoga (pranayama and guided medication) daily (1 hour) over 3

weeks (15 sessions total) in addition to standard inpatient rehabilitation care (i.e., pharmacotherapy, physical and occupational therapy, orthotic management) had significantly improved sleep quality (Pittsburgh Sleep Quality Index, $p < 0.05$) compared to controls that only received standard rehabilitation. Vidhyadhari et al.[271] compared the effects of proprioceptive neuromuscular facilitation (PNF) exercises/techniques (repeated stabilization and rhythmic contractions). involving respiratory muscles. in addition to diaphragmatic breathing exercises (15 minutes, 3 repetitions, 3 sets, 7 days per week for 1 week) to diaphragmatic breathing only in 30 individuals with GBS (treatment group = 15). They reported that the PNF and diaphragmatic breathing group had significant improvements in diaphragm muscle activity (surface EMG biofeedback) and pulmonary function (ratio of forced expiratory volume in the first second (FEV_1) divided by FVC) compared to the group treated without PNF techniques. Diaphragmatic breathing exercises alone also produced significant improvements in these measures, but not as great as when combined with PNF.

Several non-randomized controlled studies have investigated the effects of endurance (aerobic) exercises and physical therapy in persons with GBS with mostly positive results.[272] Four studies[273-276] that implemented endurance training (cycling, walking) showed significant improvements in physical fitness (VO_2 maximum, peak oxygen consumption, peak power output, muscular power), fatigue (FSS, FIS), isokinetic leg strength, perceived physical function (SF-36-physical, Rotterdam Handicap Scale), and pulmonary fitness (FEV_1, FVC). The exercise sessions tended to be 30 minutes, 3 times per week, at 65 to 90% of maximal HR for 12 weeks. Bulley[277] examined the effects of adding reactive balance exercises, using a podiatron (similar to a wobble board), to a physical therapy program consisting of joint and soft tissue mobilizations, stretching, strengthening, and endurance exercises (cycling, walking) in a patient 10 months post onset of GBS symptoms with toe walking due to ankle weakness resulting in tight posterior ankle muscles. After 7 days of twice daily use of the podiatron for 10 minutes, the patient had improvements in surface area of both feet contacting the ground, walking confidence, and mobility (10MWT, TUG). In another case report, a marathon runner admitted to an acute rehabilitation hospital at 10 weeks since onset of GBS symptoms underwent a daily one-hour physical therapy exercise program of progressive functional exercises (gait, transfer, and wheel-chair propulsion training and trunk and limb exercises in functional patterns for 5-10 repetitions) for 3 weeks.[278] Following the exercise program, the patient demonstrated improved function (total FIM score) and muscle strength (MMT). An important aspect of these exercise studies was that exercise tolerance was monitored and frequent rests were provided to ensure that persons with GBS did not become overly fatigued. Evidence suggests that excessive exercise, performed even when the disease has stabilized, can cause paradoxical weakening of muscle and temporary loss of function.[279,280] Therefore, it is important for physical therapists to be alert for signs of fatigue and to teach patients with GBS how to recognize the symptoms of fatigue so that they can live independently without harming themselves.

Acute/Progressive Stage

In the acute stages of GBS, patients may be in an intensive care unit (ICU) on ventilation with varying degrees of paralysis and sensory dysfunction. Physical therapy interventions in this stage typically include respiratory care, facilitation of speech and swallowing functions, pain management, bed positioning, ROM exercises, gentle stretching, massage, and initiation of functional activities in sitting and standing as tolerated. Depending on the facility, physical therapists may provide postural drainage, chest percussion, chest stretching, resistive inspiratory training, or assist with special protocols to prevent over fatigue of respiratory muscles, when weaning patients with GBS from a ventilator. Application of transcutaneous nerve stimulation (TENS) may be effective in reducing the pain of peripheral neuropathy in persons with GBS.[281,282] Therapists may manage and/or collaborate with speech pathologists and occupational therapists on dysarthria and dysphagia treatment programs. Patients with hypersensitivity to touch may benefit from a "cradle" that holds the sheets away from the body or by wrapping limbs snugly with elastic bandages. To prevent contractures and pressure sores, positioning, splinting, and ROM programs should be implemented.[283] Turning patients, who are immobile, at least every 2 hours, and protecting bony prominences, such as elbows and heels, using foam or sheepskin pads prevents pressure sores. Prolonged positioning with ankle-foot and resting wrist and hand splints or a rolled cloth in the hand helps to maintain good alignment of the feet and hands. Passive ROM that includes accessory and physiological motions to the ends of normal range for all extremity joints, neck, and trunk should be performed at least twice daily. With proper instruction from the therapist, caregivers may be able to safely perform passive ROM exercises. If patients can move actively without pain or excessive fatigue, they can be instructed to perform the ROM themselves. If the patient can't complete a movement, the

therapist or a well-trained caregiver can assist them to get the full range. To increase compliance, therapists should post the positioning, splinting, and ROM recommendations with diagrams as needed in a prominent location near the patients' beds. If tightness of muscles that span two joints (i.e., hamstrings, gastrocnemius) develops, gentle stretching at endpoint range for 10 to 30 seconds may alleviate the problem.[284] Swelling of limbs, due to prolonged immobility or concomitant cardiac conditions, may be treated with limb elevation and edema-specific massage. Upright activities can be started in the ICU, using a circle electric or standing bed or by initiating a sitting program as soon as tolerated. Patients who experience orthostatic hypotension may benefit from wearing an abdominal binder, foot-to-thigh compression stockings, and getting good hydration.

CASE B, PART II

Mrs. Robert's weakness progressed to flaccid quadriplegia with complete cranial nerve involvement that required mechanical ventilation. While in the ICU, she received physical therapy interventions of chest stretching exercises, bed positioning, a passive ROM program, and application of ankle splints to maintain 90 degrees of dorsiflexion with neutral eversion–inversion. A positioning and ROM schedule with pictures of the positions and ROM movements was posted at her bedside. Due to her complaints of extreme hypersensitivity to touch, a cradle was placed on the bed to prevent sheets from touching her, and she was fitted with above-knee light pressure stockings. OT fabricated bilateral wrist and finger splints, a speech therapist helped her to relearn safe swallowing patterns, and a dietician ensured that she got proper nutrition by adjusting the texture of her food.

Progression of her symptoms appeared to plateau at approximately 14 days after onset, followed by gradual return of respiratory functions. She was weaned from the ventilator after 25 days, which was a difficult process. Her PT provided instruction in breathing exercises, which she performed every 1 or 2 hours, that were vital to her ability to wean off of the ventilator. After weaning, she was transferred to a general floor and was brought to the PT department for her therapy. As her strength returned, she progressed to doing active assistive, active, and finally resistive trunk and extremity exercises. A mat program of rolling and supine to sit activities was implemented. Her therapist carefully monitored all of her activities to make sure that she was not over-working weak muscle groups.

Chronic/Recovery Stage

Once the weakness stops progressing, the plateau period may last only a few days to a few weeks, depending on whether only myelin or the axons themselves were affected. Strength will return over weeks to months and usually occurs in a descending pattern with arm function returning sooner than leg function. As strength begins to return, the therapist can slowly add active exercise, with frequent breaks, and monitoring for signs of fatigue.[279,284] Therapists should avoid putting any antigravity strain on muscles until strength reaches at least a 3/5 (Fair) MMT grade. Slings or adaptive devices (e.g., powder boards) that support the weight of the limb in a gravity-eliminated position will allow patients to perform active movements in muscles that lack antigravity strength. Exercises should be stopped at the first signs of fatigue or muscle ache. Any progression of resistance or repetitions of strengthening exercises should be monitored for 3 to 7 days for increased weakness, muscle spasm, or soreness, before progressing further.[280] If weakness or soreness follows exercise, it is best to not repeat the activity for several days and, then, reinitiate it at a lower level of resistance or number of repetitions and increase gradually. Low numbers of repetitions and high frequency of short periods of exercise are recommended initially.[243] Once reinnervation occurs and motor units are responsive, muscle re-education can begin. To help patients to contract a muscle, the therapist must first demonstrate a movement and, then, teach the patient which muscle to contract to make the movement. As strength and exercise tolerance increases, resistive exercises that incorporate multijoint and across-plane movements such as PNF patterns have been recommended.[243] Individuals with GBS have problems with fast-twitch muscle fiber recruitment for unknown reasons, which may benefit from practice of activities that push speed or rapid rises and falls in muscle force production (e.g., fast walking, jumping, quick changes in direction during walking and lunges).[243]

Most patients require a wheelchair for mobility, for several months, until their strength and endurance improve. Initially, they may need a wheelchair with a high, reclining back, but as strength improves, they may switch to a more lightweight and easily maneuverable chair. Deciding whether a patient with GBS should rent or purchase a wheelchair can be a difficult decision for a therapist to make, since it may be hard to predict how long the wheelchair will be necessary. When transitioning from wheelchair mobility to independent ambulation, patients may start in the parallel bars and progress to walking with a rollator walker with a seat to allow frequent rests. Eventually, they may progress to using Lofstrand crutches or a cane. Since wheelchairs and ambulatory assistive devices are not always covered by insurance, therapists need to carefully consider the cost to the patient. Some individuals with GBS have residual weakness of the anterior compartment musculature that requires the use of an AFO.

Even when strength has returned, rehabilitation and exercise may need to continue to address fatigue. Cardiopulmonary fitness may be decreased in patients recovering from GBS, due to altered muscle function or sedentary lifestyle.[243,285] An individualized physical therapy plan that includes interventions such as aerobic and strengthening exercises and functional task training, as described above, may be implemented to address the patient's specific impairments and activity limitations. Modifications to interventions should be used to prevent excessive fatigue. For example, Tuckey and Greenwood[286] reported positive effects of partial body-weight support treadmill exercise for a 44-year-old male 6 months post-onset of severe GBS, who was unable to stand independently. Ultimately, if fatigue symptoms persist,

the therapist may recommend work simplification and energy-conservation strategies.

Patients with GBS, who had prolonged ICU experiences, especially those who had respiratory failure and were on a ventilator, can have posttraumatic stress disorder (PTSD) and are likely to have increased incidence of anxiety, depression, and panic disorders years after discharge.[287] Although many people recover well from GBS, some patients report that they have had to make job changes, alter their leisure activities, and have had psychosocial changes due to their GBS.[288] Therapists must assess the patient's levels of fears and try to alleviate anxieties by talking with the patient and family members about their concerns. Therapists should refer patients to local GBS support groups, if they are available. If overwhelming anxiety and depression persist, a referral to a psychologist or psychiatrist is warranted.

CASE B, PART III

After 2 months of hospitalization, Mrs. Roberts was discharged home to return for daily outpatient rehabilitation. Her PT recommended an ultralight rental wheelchair, and she was fitted with prefabricated adjustable AFOs, for her bilateral foot drop, with the plan to order custom molded AFOs, after 4 to 6 months, if her dorsiflexor weakness persisted. Both the PT and OT visited her home with a social worker to determine what home adaptations and support services she and her husband needed. She continued to show gradual recovery over the next 1.5 years and progressed to a walker, then to Lofstrand crutches, and eventually to independent ambulation. She used her AFOs at all times for the first 12 months and then was able to cut back to only wearing them for walking long distances or when prolonged eccentric activity was required (e.g., hiking downhill). She was able to do all of her previous activities but needed to pace her activities, during the day, to prevent excessive fatigue.

● POSTPOLIO SYNDROME (PPS)

CASE C, PART I

Megan is a 57-year-old female, who had polio at age 11 months, resulting in weakness of the left leg and right arm. She is a human resources manager in a large accounting firm. Six months ago, she began to have pain in her shoulders and left leg and states that she felt fatigued all day and began having trouble keeping up with work and other daily activities. Prior to this, she relates that she has always been able to walk independently but did have a "limp." Physician records indicate that her strength 2 years ago was F (3) in her left hip flexors and abductors, F+ (3+) in her left dorsiflexors and the rest of her left LE musculature was G (4). Her right UE strength was grossly F-G (3-4) with scapular winging on shoulder elevation. Her right grip strength was G− (4−). On examination at this time, she has P (2) strength in her left dorsiflexors and hip musculature and F+ (3+) strength in her right dorsiflexors. Right UE shoulder elevators are F− (3−), external and internal rotators are P (2), and grip strength is F (3). She has taken a family medical leave of absence from work, as she is too fatigued to put in a 40-hour work week, and states that once home, she mostly rests and no longer participates in social activities. Her shoulder pain is achy in nature and generalized across her shoulders and upper back. It is constant and keeps her awake at night at times.

CASE C, PART II

Megan has residual involvement of the calf muscles in her left leg but was able to ambulate with only a mild limp.

If innervation of her tibialis anterior was severely compromised, how did she manage to dorsiflex her foot during gait?

The tibialis anterior may have continued to work through reinnervation by surviving motor neurons. Also, she may have been using other muscles of the foot and ankle, such as the toe extensors, to substitute.

Acute anterior poliomyelitis is a viral disease in which the *poliovirus* enters the body by oral ingestion and multiplies in the intestine. The majority of infected individuals (95-99%) remain asymptomatic, but 1 to 5% of persons develop a fever, fatigue, headache, vomiting, stiffness in the neck, and pain in the limbs, similar to viral meningitis. It can strike at any age but affects mainly children under 3 (over 50% of all cases). It has largely been eradicated through vaccination programs, but cases still occur in Pakistan and Afghanistan.[289]

Polio leads to asymmetric, flaccid paralysis, with the legs more commonly involved than the arms. In 10 to 15% of all paralytic cases, severe bulbar weakness occurs. After the initial infection, the virus is shed in feces for several weeks and can spread rapidly through a community.

Pathology of the Polio Virus

The pathological findings consist of inflammation of meninges and anterior horn cells, with loss of spinal and bulbar motor neurons. Less common findings include abnormalities in the cerebellar nuclei, basal ganglia, reticular formation, hypothalamus, thalamus, cortical neurons, and dorsal horn.[290] Recovery begins in weeks and reaches a plateau in 6 to 8 months. The extent of neurological and functional recovery is determined by three major factors:

1. The number of motor neurons that recover and resume their normal function;
2. The number of motor neurons that sprout axons to reinnervate muscle fibers left denervated by death of motor neurons (i.e., collateral sprouting); and
3. The degree of muscle hypertrophy wherein muscle fibers may increase in size from 2 to 3 times normal size.

Due to collateral sprouting, a single motor neuron that normally innervates 100 muscle fibers might eventually innervate 700 to 2000 fibers. As a result, survivors of acute polio have a few, significantly enlarged motor units, doing the work previously performed by many units. Fiber type grouping occurs in the reinnervated muscle, and the normal mosaic interspersion of Type I and Type II fibers will be diminished or absent (see Figure 16-3). Compensation by collateral sprouting and muscle hypertrophy may result in normal manual muscle tests even though more than half the original anterior horn cells are destroyed in some patients.[291]

Post-polio Syndrome Presentation

Post-polio syndrome (PPS) is a condition that affects people who have had polio, followed by a period of neurological stability, and then develop new or exacerbated symptoms several years after the acute poliomyelitis infection.[292] During the 1940s and 1950s, before polio vaccines were available, polio outbreaks in the United States caused more than 15,000 cases of paralysis each year.[293] Researchers estimate that PPS affects 25 to 40% of every 100 polio survivors who had paralysis.[293,294] Factors associated with PPS development and typical signs of PPS are listed in Table 16-15.

Fatigue has been identified as the most common and most debilitating symptom of PPS[290,292] Fatigue can have physical, cognitive, and psychological components.[292] Patients with PPS may experience and can differentiate between generalized or focal muscle fatigue, associated with new muscle weakness, and "central fatigue" that causes attention and cognitive problems, suggesting that fatigue in PPS may be caused by impaired brain

TABLE 16-15	Factors Associated with PPS Development and Signs of PPS	
FACTORS ASSOCIATED WITH PPS DEVELOPMENT[295]	**SIGNS OF PPS**[296]	
Age greater than 10	New muscular weakness	
Prior hospitalization for the acute illness	Fatigue	
Ventilator dependency	Pain	
Paralytic involvement of all four extremities	Onset or aggravation of muscle atrophy	
Rapid return of functional strength following extensive initial involvement	Onset or aggravation of pre-existing difficulties in accomplishing daily life activities	
	Cold intolerance	
	Sleep disorders	
	Dysphonia or dysphagia	
	Respiratory deficiency	

function as well as degenerated motor units.[290] Fatigue in PPS may not appear at the time of the activity, and recovery may not occur with typical rest periods.[297]

Muscle weakness, in PPS, is most prominent in muscles that were severely affected in the initial infection, but it may also occur in clinically unaffected muscles.[298] The pattern of weakness is typically asymmetric but may be proximal, distal, or patchy[299]; it is primarily observed with repetitive and stabilizing contractions, rather than with single maximum contractions, possibly due to a decreased ability of muscles to recover rapidly after contracting.[300] New muscle involvement may also cause signs and symptoms such as muscle fasciculations, cramps, atrophy, and elevation of muscle enzymes in the blood.[301] Individuals with previous poliomyelitis may have been able to maintain a high functional level for years, despite having only a few strong muscle groups, due to compensatory mechanisms, but late-onset muscle weakness of a significant muscle group can lead to disproportionately large functional losses, including reduced balance, increased falling, and the need to use assistive devices for walking or a wheelchair.[302,303]

Pain is a common complaint with PPS.[303,304] The pain intensity is high and is more often located in parts of the body that were previously affected by polio than in parts that were not.[304] Patients with PPS frequently report cramping pain in the legs (most often the upper leg musculature) and aching pain in the neck and shoulders.[303,304] Although the pain can have multiple causes, it is mostly associated with mechanical stress on muscles, tendons, and joints, from altered biomechanics, and is related to the amount of physical activity.[303] An EMG study of walking in people with PPS found overuse and substitution activity of the vastus lateralis, biceps femoris, and gluteus maximus muscles, when the soleus muscle is not functioning.[305] Over the long term, this substitution and overcompensation may lead to microtrauma of ligaments and joints and over-exhaustion of motor units that results in pain. Similarly, pain may arise from overuse of muscles with use of assistive devices or propelling manual wheelchairs. The incidence of pain in 114 patients with PPS increased from 84%, in those who ambulated without orthoses, to 100% in those who used crutches or wheelchairs for locomotion.[304]

Diagnosis of PPS

The March of Dimes diagnostic criteria for PPS are shown in Box 16-2. Diagnostic workup will be performed to exclude other conditions that might cause the health problems listed above. In addition, the physician will do blood tests to see if creatine kinase is elevated which is consistent with PPS. Electromyographic testing will show abnormalities of chronic denervation. Muscle biopsy is done to see if there is evidence of fiber type grouping due to chronic denervation/reinnervation or active denervation as shown by the presence of small angulated fibers that arise with terminal sprouting.

Does Megan show signs and symptoms of postpolio syndrome?

Yes, she has muscle weakness, excessive fatigue, muscle atrophy, and joint and muscle pain. She previously had polio and had a stable period of recovery for >20 years. She now has new onset of symptoms that fit PPS.

Box 16-2	March of Dimes Criteria for Post-Polio Syndrome[306]

- Prior paralytic poliomyelitis with evidence of motor neuron loss, as confirmed by history of the acute paralytic illness, signs of residual weakness and atrophy of muscles on neurologic examination, and signs of denervation on electromyography;
- A period of partial or complete functional recovery after acute paralytic poliomyelitis, followed by an interval (usually 15 years or more) of stable neurologic function;
- Gradual or sudden onset of progressive and persistent new muscle weakness or abnormal muscle fatigability (decreased endurance), with or without generalized fatigue, muscle atrophy, or muscle joint pain; sudden onset may follow a period of inactivity, or trauma or surgery; less commonly, symptoms attributed to PPS include new problems with breathing or swallowing;
- Symptoms persist for at least one year;
- Exclusion of other neurologic, medical, and orthopedic problems as causes of symptoms.

Etiology of PPS

The cause of PPS is unknown, but experts have offered several theories. As in ALS, loss of motor units leads to collateral sprouting of intact axons to innervate "orphaned" (i.e., denervated) muscle fibers, which results in a larger number of muscle fibers being innervated by a smaller pool of motor neurons. For motor units to supply high numbers of denervated muscle fibers, they must establish a dynamic equilibrium of adding and losing muscle fibers over time. The most common theory of PPS pathogenesis is that this equilibrium becomes unstable such that the enlarged motor units can't maintain their terminal axon sprouts, thereby resulting in new weakness.[292] This distal motor unit degeneration/dysfunction process seems to be aggravated by muscle overwork. Anecdotal evidence from therapists and physicians, working with individuals during the poliomyelitis epidemics in the 1940s and 1950s, reported that patients, who exercised muscles with below fair grades either repeatedly or against heavy loads, often lost the ability to contract the muscle.[181] Testing of this observation, in rats, found similar findings; vigorous exercise caused muscle damage in denervated muscles (i.e., less than one-third of the motor units were functional), whereas it caused hypertrophy in muscles that had more than one-third of motor units functional.[182] Studies have demonstrated this effect in the tibialis anterior but not the biceps brachii muscle, leading to the hypothesis that muscles with intense, regular activity demands are subject to a more intense denervation-reinnervation process.[307] While the cause of the disturbance in the denervation-reinnervation equilibrium remains unclear, one hypothesis is that the giant motor units that are formed, during the initial recovery process, may not be able to sustain indefinitely the metabolic demands of all their sprouts; therefore, more pruning than sprouting occurs. In addition, the denervation process leads to changes in muscle fiber type, typically from Type II to Type I – slow twitch; this change may lead to difficulty in adapting to the constraints, placed on a muscle, and eventually to overwork. The energy production capacity of Type I muscle fibers in polio survivors is decreased, leading to greater fatigability.[308] Other theories about PPS pathogenesis include that the virus triggers an inflammatory or immune system response, or the virus persists or reactivates to cause progressive motor neuron degeneration.[292,308]

Medical Management and Prognosis of PPS

There is no specific pharmaceutical treatment for the syndrome itself, but studies indicate that intravenous human immunoglobulin may reduce pain, increase quality of life, and improve strength.[308,309] Lamotrigine, a glutamate release blocker, was shown to have a positive effect on activity limitations as measured by the Nottingham Health Profile-Physical Mobility and pain after 4 weeks of treatment.[310,311] Joint deformities, arthrosis, and limb-length inequality may require surgery. Increased function can be achieved by arthrodesis, tendon transfers, and muscle transplantation.[303]

PPS is typically a very slowly progressing condition, with muscle strength declining at a rate of 1 to 3% per year. The decline in muscle strength usually follows a linear progression, without steep declines, but some individual with PPS have periods of symptom stability that last for years.[309] Notably, men have been shown to have a greater progressive decline in muscle strength than women.[312]

Physical Therapy Examination

Clients who have had poliomyelitis should undergo careful MMT of individual muscles to determine which muscles are weak. It is important to focus on individual muscles rather than muscle groups, in order to implement a focused treatment plan that is safe and avoids overworking affected muscles. In addition, endurance and fatigue are evaluated as they are two of the areas that negatively impact function, in individuals with PPS. Outcome measures that are reliable for assessing gait and mobility in PPS are the TUG, 6-minute walk test, 10MWT, and the five times sit-to-stand test.[313] Disease-specific scales that can be used as outcome measures are the Neurological Fatigue Index for PPS (NFI-PP) and Post-Polio Quality of Life Scale (PP-QoL).[314,315]

CASE C, PART III

Megan underwent strength testing, which demonstrated progressive weakness in previously affected muscles (left dorsiflexors, hip flexors, and abductors; right shoulder elevators and grip strength) as well as some new muscles (left hip extension and adduction, right dorsiflexion). Additionally, her 6-minute walk test was 400 feet, which is well below age-matched norms and her comfortable walking speed was 1.0 m/sec, considered slow for her age. She filled out a fatigue questionnaire that indicated significant decline in function and participation due to fatigue. These examination findings indicated a need to work on endurance, strength in unaffected muscle groups, and fatigue to assist in improving function. She may also benefit from use of assistive devices.

Physical Therapy Management of PPS

Because fatigue is a major complaint in individuals with PPS, it should be a focus of physical therapy. Low to moderate intensity exercise programs, including aerobic (i.e., treadmill, bicycle, fast walking, swimming) and resistive exercises, have been shown to reduce fatigue in individuals with PPS.[296,316] Individuals should use the Borg rating of perceived exertion to determine appropriate exercise intensity for aerobic exercise[317] Graded exercise programs that are slowly progressed and include supervision, by a physical therapist, are recommended. Oncu et al.[316] showed that individuals with PPS, who performed an exercise program under the supervision of a physical therapist in a rehabilitation clinic, demonstrated greater improvements in functional capacity, while the group doing the program as a home exercise program did not improve functional capacity. In addition, clients should be taught energy-conservation measures, including the use of handicap license plates to allow parking closer to establishment doors, balancing activity and rest throughout the day, sitting instead of standing, rearranging their home so that frequently used objects are in easy reach, and use of a scooter or similar motorized vehicle, when traveling a distance.

The key factor in prescribing exercise for individuals with PPS is to avoid overwork of weakened muscles, which can present as muscle aches or tenderness to touch. Some authors have recommended that strengthening exercises in PPS should only be done on muscles with at least antigravity strength or muscles with more strength in reserve than is required for minimum function.[295] To objectively measure if a muscle has enough reserve, the therapist can measure a person's muscle strength before and after walking for 1 to 2 minutes.[295] Strengthening programs should focus on (1) unaffected muscle groups that can take over some functions of the overworked muscles and (2) submaximal exercise to maintain strength and function in affected muscle groups. Halstead and colleagues established a limb classification system based on EMG evidence of anterior horn cell disease, remote and recent history, and formal physical examination to help guide exercise prescription in people with PPS.[318] The limb is classified into one of five classes, according to the most affected muscle in that extremity. Exercise guidelines have been recommended for each of the five classes.[295,318] See Box 16-3 for general principles for designing exercise programs. If muscle weakness is severe and/or overwork signs and symptoms persist, it may be necessary to prescribe assistive devices including orthoses, wheelchairs, and/or adaptive equipment. In individuals with quadriceps weakness, carbon-fiber knee-ankle-foot orthoses (KAFOs) may improve gait efficiency and reduce overuse.[319] A stance control knee joint, that locks only during the stance phase improved gait mechanics and efficiency compared with a fully locked knee. Modalities are also helpful for pain relief including heat, TENS, and massage.[320,321]

Psychosocial Considerations in PPS

Psychological symptoms such as chronic stress, depression, anxiety, compulsiveness, and type A behavior have been described in polio survivors.[322] These symptoms may not only be distressful but may interfere with the individual's ability to make lifestyle changes to manage late-onset symptoms.

Box 16-3	General Principles for Designing Exercise Programs

- Use a low to moderate exercise intensity.
- Slowly progress exercise, especially if muscles have not been exercised for a while and/or have obvious chronic weakness from acute poliomyelitis.
- Strengthening exercises should only be attempted with muscles that can move against gravity.[193]
- Pace exercise to avoid fatigue (intermittent periods of rest and exercise).
- Rotate exercise types, such as stretching, general (aerobic) conditioning, strengthening, endurance or joint range of motion exercises.
- Exercise should not cause muscle soreness or pain.
- Exercise should not lead to fatigue that prevents participation in other activities that day or the days following.

Understanding the background and the social milieu that influenced their lives is beneficial to their care. During the polio epidemics in the 1940s and 1950s, fear of contracting polio was rampant. A coping strategy, at that time, was to encourage children to achieve high levels of physical performance. If a child contracted polio, the recommended treatment at that time was to hospitalize the person for months away from their families and friends, causing many children to feel abandoned and anxious. Polio patients were expected to be a "good patient," by working hard, and were not encouraged to talk about their disabilities. These acute experiences may have pushed survivors into lifelong patterns of type A behavior, making it difficult for them to cope with new post-polio symptoms, emerging years later.[322] Patients may have difficulty shifting from a philosophy of "no pain, no gain" to one of energy conservation and rest. Fear of loss of independence and prospects of role changing may cause the breakdown of the coping strategies that they have used for years. The therapist's sensitivity, support, and respect will play a major role in the patient's compliance with treatment. Conservative management that does not involve major lifestyle changes should be tried first. Therapists should also provide information about support groups in the community.

CASE C, PART IV

Megan is prescribed a submaximal, progressive aerobic program of pedometer walking to improve fatigue and endurance. She is also given strengthening for all muscles not previously affected by polio that have a strength grade of 3+ or greater. Additionally, she is prescribed ankle orthotics to assist with dorsiflexion and improve her gait pattern to be safer and more energy efficient. She performs her exercise program under the supervision of a therapist and is closely monitored before and after exercise for muscle pain or tenderness to ensure that she is not pushed to the point of overworking any muscle groups.

PERIPHERAL NEUROPATHIES

Peripheral neuropathy is damage to nerves, leading to impaired sensation, movement, gland, or organ function. If the damage is isolated to one nerve, it is known as **mononeuropathy**, and if it involves more than one nerve it is **polyneuropathy**. When multiple nerves are affected but the pattern is not symmetrical, it is referred to as **multifocal mononeuropathy** or **multiple mononeuropathy**. Neuropathies are common, affecting 3 to 4% of those over the age of 55 with damage secondary to diabetes, being the most common cause of peripheral neuropathies.[323,324] It is estimated that 50% of individuals, diagnosed with diabetes (Type I and II), have peripheral neuropathy.[324] Other causes of neuropathy are trauma, infection, autoimmune disorders, and inherited disorders (Table 16-16). When there is damage to nerves through any of these mechanisms, it is the large-diameter fibers that are more vulnerable than small-diameter fibers, meaning that light touch is the first sensation to be impaired followed by pain and temperature.

Classifications of Traumatic Nerve Injuries

Nerve injuries can be classified by the extent of injury and the chance of spontaneous recovery. The two most widely accepted nerve injury classification systems were developed by Seddon and Sunderland (see Table 16-17).[328,329] Seddon classifies injuries as follows: Class I (neurapraxias) – segmental demyelination due to focal compression but the axon remains intact; Class II (axonotmesis) – the axon is damaged but the **endoneurium** (the connective tissue around the myelin sheath of each myelinated nerve fiber) remains intact; and Class III (neurotmesis) – a complete severance of nerve fibers and the supporting endoneurium. With Class II and III injuries, there is degeneration of the fiber distal to the cell body that is called Wallerian degeneration.[330]

In **neurapraxia** (Seddon's Class I Injury), there is a reversible blockade of nerve conduction due to mild or moderate focal compression. This may result in decreased strength, absence of DTRs, and loss of sensation (confined to large-diameter fibers). There is usually no loss of autonomic nerve function and no permanent damage to the axon. Recovery is usually spontaneous and occurs within 3 months. **Axonotmesis** (Class II) is usually caused by crush injuries and results in a variable loss of sensory, motor, and autonomic nerve function. There is a complete disruption of the nerve axon and surrounding myelin but the epineurium and **perineurium** (connective tissues that surround bundles of axons called nerve **fascicles**) remain intact. Prognosis for effective regeneration is good because the integrity of the endoneurium is maintained but may be slow (several months to a year) as regeneration occurs at rate of 1 mm/day. **Neurotmesis** (Class III) is typically caused by stab wounds, high-velocity projectiles, or nerve traction that completely transects the nerve. Axonal regeneration may occur, but generally occurs with low fidelity (i.e., axon may not regrow to reconnect to the same end target) because the connective tissue layers are disrupted. Deficits may involve sensory, motor, and autonomic nerves and may be permanent.[328,329] This type of injury has a high incidence of neuroma formation. A **neuroma** is a growth or tumor of nerve tissue that is most often benign.

TABLE 16-16	Causes of Peripheral Neuropathies[325–327]	
CATEGORY	**MECHANISM OF NERVE DAMAGE**	**EXAMPLES**
Trauma		
Stretch injury	Severance or tearing of the nerve due to a traction force	• Brachial plexus damage at birth (Erb's Palsy) • Radial nerve injury secondary to a humeral fracture
Lacerations, stab wounds, and penetrating trauma	Partial or complete severing of the nerve	• May be a clean cut (surgical incision, glass) or • Irregular (blunt instruments, knife stabbings)
Compression	Mechanical deformation and ischemia	• "Saturday night palsy" in which the radial nerve is compressed while sleeping either from a partner laying on the arm or from placement of the arm under the body. It is known as "Saturday night palsy" because it is thought to be more common when the person is impaired by alcohol. • Bone displacement from fracture • Hematoma • Compartment syndrome – swelling within the facial sheath following severe trauma
Repetitive stress injury	Repetitive flexing of a joint leads to irritation and swelling. When swelling is in a constricted area through which a nerve passes the nerve becomes compressed.	• Carpal tunnel is a well-known condition that is thought to be caused by repetitive stress such as typing or working with a jack hammer.
Systemic Disease		
Diabetes I and II	Most common form in the United States; mechanism is usually loss of peripheral blood flow leading to ischemia of the distal nerve endings.	• Usually a symmetrical distal polyneuropathy. • Sensorimotor neuropathy found in up to 50% of patients involves paresthesia, hyperesthesia, sensory loss of vibration, pressure, pain and temperature; presence of a foot ulcer may clue physician into diagnosis.[210] • Acute diabetic mononeuropathy (carpal tunnel, cranial nerves): common nerves compressed are the median at the wrist (carpal tunnel), ulnar at the elbow, peroneal at the fibular head, lateral cutaneous nerve of the thigh at the inguinal ligament. • Diabetic autonomic neuropathy is a widespread disorder of the cholinergic, adrenergic and peptidergic autonomic fibers that leads to dysregulation of one or more of the following systems: cardiac, sexual, gastrointestinal, sudomotor (sweating), pupillomotor (blurred vision), and bladder dysfunction.
Kidney disorders	Leads to high levels of ammonia in the blood	• Caused by uremic toxicity
Autoimmune diseases	Sjogren's syndrome Lupus Rheumatoid arthritis and other connective tissue disorders Guillain–Barré syndrome Chronic inflammatory demyelinating polyradiculopathy (CIDP) Multifocal motor neuropathy	• Immune system attacks the body's own tissues, leading to nerve damage. • Inflammation in tissues around nerves can spread directly into nerve fibers. • Chronic autoimmune conditions can destroy joints, organs, and connective tissues, making nerves vulnerable to compression injuries and entrapment. • Guillain–Barré can damage motor, sensory, and autonomic nerve fibers. • CIDP usually damages sensory and motor nerves, leaving autonomic nerves intact. • Multifocal motor neuropathy affects motor nerves exclusively; it may be chronic or acute.

(Continued)

TABLE 16-16 Causes of Peripheral Neuropathies[325–327] (*Continued*)

CATEGORY	MECHANISM OF NERVE DAMAGE	EXAMPLES
Vitamin deficiencies and alcoholism	Deficiencies of vitamins E, B1, B6, B12, niacin, thiamine Alcohol abuse	• Damage to the nerves associated with long-term alcohol abuse may not be reversible when a person stops drinking alcohol. • Chronic alcohol abuse also frequently leads to nutritional deficiencies (including B12, thiamine, and folate) that contribute to the development of peripheral neuropathy.
Vascular disease	Lack of blood to the nerves, most commonly the terminal nerve endings leads to ischemia	• Vasculitis leads to loss of distal blood supply and anoxic damage to distal nerve fibers
Cancers	Neuroblastomas, tumors, paraneoplastic syndromes	• Cancer can infiltrate nerve fibers or exert damaging compression forces on nerve fibers. • Tumors also can arise directly from nerve tissue cells. • Paraneoplastic syndromes can indirectly cause widespread nerve damage. • Toxicity from the chemotherapeutic agents and radiation used to treat cancer also can cause peripheral neuropathy.
Infections	Herpes varicella zoster (shingles), Epstein–Barr virus, West Nile virus, cytomegalovirus, and herpes simplex members of the large family of human herpes viruses. Lyme disease, diphtheria, and leprosy are bacterial diseases HIV, human immunodeficiency virus leading to AIDs Lyme disease, diphtheria, and leprosy	• The viruses can severely damage sensory nerves, causing attacks of sharp, lightning-like pain. Post-herpetic neuralgia is long-lasting, particularly intense pain that often occurs after an attack of shingles. • The bacterial infections are characterized by extensive peripheral nerve damage. • A rapidly progressive, painful polyneuropathy affecting the feet and hands is often the first clinically apparent sign of HIV infection. • Bacterial diseases characterized by extensive peripheral nerve damage.
Inherited neuropathies	Charcot–Marie–Tooth disease Mutations in genes that produce proteins involved in the structure/function of the peripheral nerve axon or the myelin sheath.	Symptoms include: • Extreme weakening and wasting of muscles in the lower legs and feet • Foot deformities, such as high arches and hammertoes • Gait abnormalities: foot drop and a high-stepped gait • Loss of tendon reflexes and numbness in the lower limbs • Decreased or increased sensation • Autonomic changes: decreased sweating; edema; uncontrolled BP, HR; bowel and bladder problems • Motor changes: weakness or paralysis; muscle atrophy • Trophic changes: shiny skin, brittle nails, neurogenic joint damage
Toxins		
Heavy metals and environmental toxins	Lead, mercury, arsenic, insecticides, and solvents	• Symptoms vary according to the metal but can include sensory and/or motor involvement.
Drugs	Anticonvulsants Antiviral agents Antibiotics Some heart and blood pressure medications Chemotherapy drugs	• In most cases, the neuropathy resolves when these medications are discontinued, or dosages are adjusted. • About 30-40% of people who undergo chemotherapy develop peripheral neuropathy and it is a leading reason why people with cancer stop chemotherapy early. • The severity of chemotherapy-induced peripheral neuropathy (CIPN) varies from person to person.

TABLE 16-17	Classification of Traumatic Nerve Injuries[328,329]				
SEVERITY	**DESCRIPTION**	**RECOVERY PATTERN**	**RATE OF RECOVERY**	**SURGERY**	
First: Neurapraxia	Local ion-induced conduction block or demyelination with restoration in weeks	Complete	Fast (days –12 weeks)	None	
Second: Axonotmesis	Disruption of axon with regeneration and full recovery	Complete	Slow (3 cm/month)	None	
Third: Axonotmesis	Disruption of axon and endoneurium causing disorganized regeneration	Varies	Slow (3 cm/month)	Varies	
Fourth: Axonotmesis	Disruption of axon, endoneurium, perineurium, with intact epineurium and no regeneration	None	None	Yes	
Fifth: Neurotmesis	Transection of the nerve	None	None	Yes	

Sunderland further refined Seddon's categories based on the realization that injuries had widely variable prognoses. **Neurapraxia** corresponds to a Sunderland type 1 injury, axonotmesis corresponds to Sunderland type 2, 3, and 4 injuries, and neurotmesis corresponds to Sunderland type 5 injury (Table 16-17). In a Sunderland type 2 injury, the endoneurium, perineurium, and **epineurium** (the outermost layer of connective tissue surrounding a peripheral nerve) are still intact, but the axons are physiologically disrupted. Because the endoneurium is intact, the regenerating axons are directed along their original course, and complete functional recovery can be expected. The time for recovery depends on the level of injury, as the axon must regenerate distal to the end-organ. It can usually be measured in months, as opposed to weeks, for a Sunderland type 1 injury.[329,330]

Sunderland's third-degree injury involves disruption of the axon and endoneurium, but the perineurium and epineurium are intact. This injury can result in axon misdirection and potential debilitating consequences as recovery is incomplete in this grade of injury for a number of reasons. There is more severe retrograde injury to cell bodies, which either destroys neurons or slows their recovery, and without an intact endoneurium, fibrosis occurs, which hinders axonal regeneration. Finally, end-organs may undergo changes that impede full recovery.[329,330]

Sunderland's fourth-degree injury involves disruption of all structures except the epineurium. Axon regeneration is disorganized, and surgical intervention is required to restore function. Sunderland's fifth-degree injury involves complete loss of continuity of the nerve.[329,330]

In both Seddon's Class II (Sunderland's 2, 3, 4) and III (Sunderland's 5) injuries, there is Wallerian degeneration, meaning a degeneration of the axon distal to the site of injury. The axon shrinks, fragments, and becomes irregular in shape. Schwann cells and macrophages that migrate to the area break down axonal fragments and myelin. Schwann cells also proliferate and form columns of cells, called bands of Bungner, that guide regenerating axons toward their original target tissue.[329,331]

There are also changes in the nerve proximal to the site of injury, including retraction of the proximal stump, clot formation at the severed end, increased numbers of ribosomes around the nucleus (chromatolysis), and an enlarged and decentralized cell body. Axonal degeneration occurs in the proximal stump for a minimum of two to three nodes of Ranvier. The proximal stump sprouts many axons that grow toward the distal Schwann cell tube initially, but eventually only one axon will remain. The Schwann cells at the end of the proximal stump also proliferate and attempt to form a bridge between the proximal and distal stumps. As regeneration continues distally, axons may become re-myelinated and eventually connect with the target tissue (Figure 16-5).[332]

Effects of Muscle Denervation

When muscles become denervated, they undergo several changes in structure, including atrophy of both Type I and II fiber types and proliferation of extra-junctional acetylcholine receptors, which are normally found only at the neuromuscular junction. When complete denervation of a muscle lasts longer than 21 days, the muscle becomes fibrotic, leading to a substantial decrease in the recovery of muscle mass and force production.[333]

Surgical Repair

Direct nerve repair in which the entire nerve is sutured as a unit, using sutures placed in the epineurium, is the gold standard surgical treatment for severe axonotmesis and neurotmesis injuries. Alternatively, grouped fascicular repair involving suturing of fascicular groups (bundles of nerve fibers) within the nerve trunk can be performed.[334]

Signs of Recovery Following Neurotmesis

When neurotmesis occurs, healing can occur if the proximal and distal stumps are sutured; axons in the proximal stumps will sprout and may regenerate connections to the target tissue. The axon regrowth typically proceeds at rate of 1 mm/day. Sensory recovery occurs before return of voluntary movement and is assessed by looking for the presence of deep pressure pain sensation, as this is the first sign of recovery. Deep pressure pain

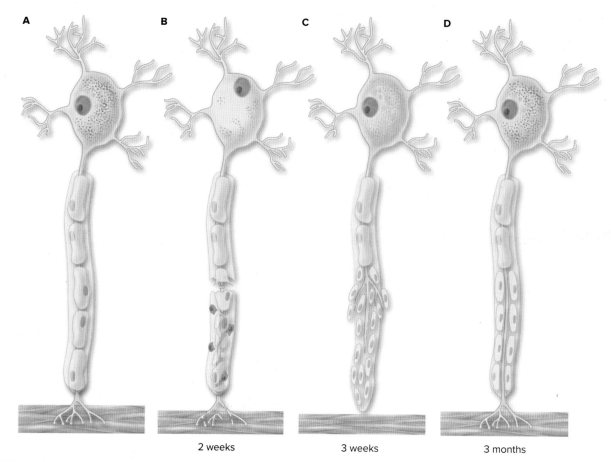

FIGURE 16-5 Class II peripheral nerve injury and recovery. (Reproduced with permission from Mescher AL, ed. *Junqueira's Basic Histology*, 13ed. New York, NY: McGraw-Hill; 2013. Fig. 9-30, p. 185-186.)

sensation is followed by superficial pain, then heat and cold, and finally, light touch and tactile discrimination. When motor nerves are affected, recovery is based on strength of contraction. For both sensory and motor recovery the Medical Research Council Grading System for Nerve Recovery is commonly used to assess and document recovery[335] (Table 16-18).

Nerve Grafts

When primary repair cannot be performed without putting undue tension on the remaining nerve, nerve grafting is required.[334] **Autografts** (donor and recipient are the same biologic organism) remain the standard for nerve grafting material. **Allografts** (graft from a different species) have not shown

TABLE 16-18	Medical Research Council Grading System for Nerve Recovery[335]		
MOTOR RECOVERY		**SENSORY RECOVERY**	
M0	No contraction	S0	None
M1	Return of palpable contraction in the proximal muscles	S1	Deep cutaneous pain only
M2	Poor muscle grade activity in proximal muscles; palpable (trace) intrinsics	S1+	Deep and superficial pain
M3	Fair strength in proximal and distil muscles	S2	Superficial pain and some touch
M4	Good muscle strength, still weak intrinsics	S2+	As in S2, but with an exaggerated response
M5	Recovered strength in all muscles	S3	Disappearance of exaggerated response with >15 mm 2-point discrimination
		S3+	Better localization of stimulation with 7-15 mm of 2-point discrimination
		S4	Complete recovery

recovery equivalent to that obtained with autogenous nerve. The most common source of autograft is the sural nerve, which is easy to obtain, the appropriate diameter for most surgical needs, and loss of this nerve, from its primary site, has minimal impact on function. Other graft sources include the anterior branch of the medial antebrachial cutaneous nerve, the lateral femoral cutaneous nerve, and the superficial radial sensory nerve.[332] If an autograft is not feasible, then a **nerve conduit** (artificial nerve graft) is often used to provide a pathway for nerve regeneration to occur. Potential advantages of nerve conduits, over allografts, include absorbability, lack of donor-site morbidity, and lack of axonal escape.[336]

CASE D, PART I

Tina, a 50-year-old woman, was injured 2 days ago, when a load of lumber fell from a shelf, pinning her left forearm. The following signs and symptoms are noted on her left side:

- She does not feel pinprick, touch, temperature, or vibration on the medial hand, little finger, and medial half of the ring finger.

- Sweating is absent in the same distribution as the sensory loss.

- Radial wrist extension and flexion and finger extension strength are normal on manual muscle tests.

- She is unable to flex the middle and distal phalanges of the fourth and fifth digits, abduct or adduct her fingers, or adduct the hand.

What nerve is injured in this patient? Ulnar nerve

What is the most likely classification of this injury (i.e., Class I, II, or III)? Class II axonotmesis

Suppose that the nerve was crushed near the elbow, about 20 cm from her fingers. Approximately how long will it be before she regains the ability to abduct and adduct her fingers? 200 days

---

Diabetic and Related Neuropathies

Diabetic neuropathy is a frequent sequela of both Type I and II diabetes, occurring in up to 75% of those with diabetes and involves either motor or sensory nerves, or both (see Table 16-19).[338] Individuals who smoke, are of older age, and have uncontrolled blood glucose levels are at higher risk of developing neuropathy as are those with a longer duration of diabetes. There are many types of diabetic neuropathy, including (1) distal symmetric polyneuropathy, (2) autonomic neuropathy, (3) diabetic radiculoplexus neuropathy (DRPN; aka diabetic proximal motor neuropathy or diabetic amyotrophy), and (4) diabetic focal peripheral neuropathies (cranial mononeuropathy; aka diabetic ophthalmoplegia).[339]

Diabetic distal symmetric polyneuropathy (DSP) is the most common type of diabetic neuropathy, presenting with foot pain and paresthesias that occur bilaterally and symmetrically in a stocking distribution in the distal legs. Large-fiber sensory nerve involvement results in tingling paresthesias and a perception that the feet feel "numb or asleep" along with distally impaired vibration, joint position, and touch-pressure sensation, and diminished or absent ankle reflexes.[337] If small sensory fibers are involved, the patient reports pricking, stabbing, and burning sensations. DSP may also be associated with motor weakness that leads to foot drop and reduced ankle reflexes. **Diabetic autonomic neuropathy** usually accompanies diabetic DSP, but in rare cases, it occurs alone. Autonomic symptoms and deficits are usually mild until late stages of disease. It potentially involves all organs that receive autonomic innervation. The pathogenesis of diabetic DSP is multifactorial and involves complex interactions between the degree of blood glucose level control, diabetes duration, age-related nerve loss, and other factors such as blood pressure, lipid levels, and weight. These risk factors act together to activate biochemical pathways that damage nerves and small blood vessels.[337]

Severe diabetic DSP may cause loss of sensation, extreme sensitivity to touch, including light touch (allodynia), loss of balance and coordination, and loss of reflexes and muscle weakness. These impairments lead to widening of the foot, foot ulcers, and gait changes. When the foot widens and structures shift, weight bearing occurs through structures that don't commonly bear weight, and this leads to foot ulcers that can lead to amputation. Foot care and proper footwear should be initiated early in the disease to prevent these secondary complications. Wearing well-fitted shoes with good support and padding for the metatarsal heads and examining the feet daily can help prevent amputations.[337]

Diabetic radiculoplexus neuropathy (DRPN) can affect cervical, thoracic, and/or lumbosacral regions but the most common is lumbosacral DRPN.[337] Lumbosacral DRPN typically affects middle-aged or older individuals with Type II diabetes. It presents with severe unilateral or asymmetric proximal pain, involving the back, hip, or anterior thigh, followed by asymmetric proximal leg weakness and profound atrophy. The pain and weakness spread in a progressive or stepwise manner, over weeks to months, to nearby and contralateral segments with some people becoming wheelchair-dependent or developing asymmetric quadriparesis. Weight loss and dysautonomia are common with about half of patients experiencing orthostatic hypotension and changes in sexual, bladder, and bowel function. The pathogenesis of DRPN is an ischemic injury caused by an immune-mediated microvasculitis, involving motor, sensory, and autonomic fibers. Recovery usually begins within 9 to 12 months, although recovery can be incomplete and last for many years.[337]

Some **focal peripheral mononeuropathies** (DMN), involving cranial, thoracic, or extremity nerves, are associated with diabetes.[338] Cranial mononeuropathy presents as isolated lesions of cranial nerves III, IV, or VI. Symptoms include unilateral headache, ptosis, and impaired extraocular movements, resulting in diplopia that develops over a few hours. Another common focal neuropathy of diabetes is a **unilateral truncal** (thoracic) **radiculopathy**, which presents as acute abdominal pain suggestive of an intra-abdominal process, herpes zoster, or a spinal process.[337] In addition, nerves that are susceptible

TABLE 16-19 Comparison of Diabetic Polyneuropathy and Subtypes[337]

FEATURES/SYMPTOMS/SIGNS	DSP	DRPN	CIDP	DMN
Symptoms				
Acute/subacute onset	No	Yes	Yes	At times
Progression rate	Years	Weeks/months	Weeks/months	Variable
Pain/allodynia	<20% (feet)	Yes	No	Yes (focal)
Numbness/tingling	Yes	At times	Yes	Yes (focal)
Weakness	Late	Yes	Yes	Motor nerve
Dysautonomia	Yes	Yes (about 50%)	No	No
Signs				
Decreased vibration, joint position	Yes	Variable	Yes	No
Decreased pain, temperature	Yes	Variable	At times	Yes (focal)
Weakness/atrophy	Late distal	Proximal, at times distal	Proximal and distal	Proximal and distal (at times)
Orthostatic hypotension	Mild	Yes	No	No
Anatomical pattern				
Symmetric	Yes	No	Yes	No
Proximal predominant	No	Yes	When severe	Variable
Stocking-glove	Yes	No	Yes	No
Prognosis				
Chronic/progressive	Yes	No	About 33%	Yes
Monophasic/resolution	No	Yes (partial)	Often	No
Pathophysiology	Metabolic/microvascular	Immune-mediated	Immune-mediated	Compressive/ischemic

CIDP, chronic inflammatory demyelinating polyradiculopathy; DMN, diabetic mononeuropathy; DRPN, diabetic radiculoplexus neuropathy; DSP, distal symmetric polyneuropathy.

to compression or cumulative trauma, including the median, ulnar, radial, lateral femoral cutaneous, fibular, and plantar nerves, are frequently injured in patients with diabetes.[337]

Chronic inflammatory demyelinating polyradiculopathy (CIDP), sometimes called chronic relapsing polyneuropathy, is an immune-mediated neuropathy that may be associated with diabetes. One study reported that patients with diabetes were 11 times more likely to have CIDP, compared with those without diabetes, but other studies have failed to confirm an increased risk.[337,340] The disorder causes demyelination of peripheral nerves, resulting in progressive weakness and impaired sensory function in the extremities. Young adults and men are more commonly affected. It often presents with symptoms of tingling or numbness (beginning in the toes and fingers), weakness of the arms and legs, areflexia, and fatigue. The course of CIDP varies widely among individuals. Some individuals may have a bout of CIDP, followed by spontaneous recovery, while others may have many bouts with partial recovery in between relapses. CIDP is closely related to GBS and is considered the chronic counterpart of that acute disease. Medical treatment for

CIDP includes corticosteroids, such as prednisone, which may be prescribed alone or in combination with immunosuppressant drugs. Plasmapheresis (plasma exchange) and intravenous immunoglobulin (IVIg) therapy are also effective. IVIg may be used even as a first-line therapy.[340]

Physical Therapy Assessment of Neuropathies

When assessing for neuropathy, the sensory, motor, and autonomic systems should be thoroughly examined. It is important to identify the cause of neuropathy so that appropriate treatment and prevention can be implemented. For instance, diabetic neuropathy tends to primarily involve the sensory system, and it is important to prevent further progression through tight control of blood glucose levels. In Guillain–Barré, the motor system is more involved. Sensory and motor findings are usually in a symmetrical glove and stocking distribution. Sensory and motor assessment are covered in Chapter 10 (Evaluation). When sensory neuropathy is suspected, a thorough examination, using monofilaments and other tests for all sensory modalities, is necessary to implement the most effective treatment plan.

In addition to these standard evaluation techniques, it is also helpful to obtain NCV and electromyography (EMG) testing (see the discussion at the beginning of this chapter). Another specialized test is Tinel's sign, in which you tap over the nerve; a positive sign is pain or tingling, in the distribution of the nerve, and indicates that the nerve is irritated. Assessment should be done systematically, noting the distribution of sensory and motor loss. Use of **dermatomes** and **myotomes** allows clinicians to identify the nerve(s) involved (see Figure 3-5 in Chapter 3 of this text for a dermatome map). Finally proprioceptive, kinesthetic, and vibratory testing are used to assess the dorsal column-medial lemniscus pathway. Of these tests, vibratory testing is the most sensitive and valid.

Many diseases, including diabetes, autoimmune disease, and degenerative neurologic disorders, impact the autonomic nervous system and can lead to autonomic neuropathy (AN), including cardiovascular, gastrointestinal, and genitourinary autonomic neuropathy. Dysautonomia, including cardiovascular autonomic neuropathy (CAN) is present in the prodromal stages of Parkinson disease[341] and in about 20% of individuals with diabetes, increasing to 60% in long-standing diabetics.[342] Physical therapists must be acutely aware of the potential for autonomic neuropathies when prescribing exercise for their patients with diabetes or other disorders that affect the autonomic system. CAN contributes to myocardial infarction, arrhythmia, and sudden death. It also impacts response to exercise. Symptoms include exercise intolerance, early fatigue and weakness with exercise, resting tachycardia, abnormal blood pressure regulation, postural hypotension, dizziness, and syncope. **Subclinical** CAN has been detected in individuals with Type II diabetes 1 year after diagnosis and in those with Type I diabetes 2 years after diagnosis. Gastrointestinal neuropathy can lead to gastroparesis (abnormal gastric emptying), and genitourinary neuropathy can cause neurogenic bladder and sexual dysfunction.[343]

Tests for Autonomic Neuropathy

Physical therapists can screen for autonomic neuropathies by testing for orthostatic hypotension, taking pulse and noting any resting tachycardia; and administering a screening questionnaire developed to assess for symptoms of AN. The **Survey of Autonomic Symptoms** (see Table 16-20) is a validated questionnaire that can be administered in about 15 minutes.[344] A score of >3 on the SAS symptom total score indicates a high probability of autonomic dysfunction and the need to refer for further testing. This survey also asks patients to rate the degree to which each symptom bothers them in column B which is their Total Symptom Impact Score (TIS).[344]

Measuring blood pressure in supine and standing is a long-recognized method of testing for orthostatic hypotension. Have the patient lay down for 5 minutes, and then, blood pressure and heart rate (HR) are taken. Then, have the patient stand up and take the pressure and HR after 1 minute and 3 minutes. A drop of systolic pressure ≥20 mmHg or ≥10 mmHg in diastolic pressure or if the patient experiences dizziness or lightheadedness indicates an abnormal test and the probability of orthostatic hypotension.[345] In addition, the **NASA 10 Minute Lean Test** may also be administered to detect orthostatic intolerance (Table 16-21).[346] This test assesses for orthostatic intolerance,

which is the development of symptoms when standing upright that are relieved by reclining. This includes orthostatic hypotension, neurally mediated hypotension and postural orthostatic tachycardia syndrome (POTS). You can also use this test as an outcome measure following treatment for orthostatic intolerance. The patient should not wear compression garments during this test and if possible, should limit fluid and salt intake for 24 hours prior to the test. The test is done by first having the patient rest in supine for 15 minutes and then record the blood pressure (BP) and HR. Repeat one minute later and every minute until two consecutive readings are relatively close. Next have the patient stand up and assume a standing position leaning against a wall with heels about six inches from the wall (Table 16-21). They will remain in this position for 10 minutes. Take BP and HR after one minute and repeat every minute until 10 minutes have elapsed. The patient should not move or shift their weight during the test. Observe for signs of pre-syncope such as lightheadedness and alterations in the color and temperature of the extremities.[346]

In at-risk patients even with minimal evidence of CAN, altered cardiac autonomic balance has been found to be present and can be detected through an exercise-based assessment for CAN. The early post-exercise recovery period in those with altered autonomic function is characterized by enhanced sympatho-excitation, diminished parasympathetic reactivation, and delay in heart rate recovery.[347-349] In addition, the squatting test is an active posture maneuver that imposes significant orthostatic stresses. In normal subjects, this maneuver does not lead to any symptoms, but in those with CAN, both the increase in BP, during squatting, and the decrease in BP, during standing, may be exaggerated and sustained, potentially leading to complaints and adverse events.[350] To do this screen, monitor pulse and BP carefully, during the transition from standing to squatting, from squatting to standing, and for several minutes after the individual returns to standing. If the screen is positive with these abnormal changes, the client should be referred for cardiovascular autonomic reflex tests, prior to instituting any significant aerobic exercise program.

Treatment of CAN involves cardiovascular risk reduction and lifestyle intervention. Exercise should be graded, with a slow progression, and should be supervised.[343] Low-level, slowly progressive aerobic exercise is beneficial for improving orthostatic tolerance for those with diabetes and CAN.[351,352] If the individual has resting tachycardia, beta-blocker medications may be used. Compression garments have been shown to be effective.[353] Physical therapists can teach the individual with orthostatic hypotension to use physical counter-maneuvers when experiencing symptoms of orthostatic hypotension. Squatting as a physical counter-maneuver, produced the most dramatic change in BP while leg crossing also increased BP.[353] Physical therapists can also teach clients to rise from supine and sitting, in increments, resting after each position change to allow time for the body to make adjustments to the position change. In addition, isometric contraction of the plantarflexors along with ankle pumps can help to improve blood flow from the lower extremities.[353] Resistance exercise has mixed results as a study demonstrated that low-intensity resistance training improved left ventricular function in

TABLE 16-20	Autonomic Screening: Survey of Autonomic Symptoms (SAS) Questionnaire[344]						
Symptom/health problem	A. Symptom Score		B. Total Symptom Impact Score (TIS)				
	Have you had any of the following health symptoms during the past 6 months?		If you answered yes to any question in column A, how much would you say the symptom bothers you?				
	0 = No	1 = Yes	Not at all	A little	Some	A moderate amount	A lot
1. Do you have lightheadedness?	0	1	1	2	3	4	5
2. Do you have a dry mouth or dry eyes?	0	1	1	2	3	4	5
3. Are your feet pale or blue?	0	1	1	2	3	4	5
4. Are your feet colder than the rest of your body?	0	1	1	2	3	4	5
5. Is sweating in your feet decreased compared to the rest of your body?	0	1	1	2	3	4	5
6. Is sweating in your feet decreased or absent (for example, after exercise or during hot weather)?	0	1	1	2	3	4	5
7. Is sweating in your hands increased compared to the rest of your body?	0	1	1	2	3	4	5
8. Do you have nausea, vomiting, or bloating after eating a small meal?	0	1	1	2	3	4	5
9. Do you have persistent diarrhea (more than 3 loose bowel movements per day)?	0	1	1	2	3	4	5
10. Do you have persistent constipation (less than 1 bowel movement every other day)?	0	1	1	2	3	4	5
11. Do you have leaking of urine?	0	1	1	2	3	4	5
12. Do you have difficulty obtaining an erection (men)?	0	1	1	2	3	4	5
	Symptom Total =		TIS =				

Scores on the SAS symptoms column A >3 indicate possible autonomic neuropathy. (Reproduced with permission from Zilliox L, Peltier AC, Wren PA, et al. Assessing autonomic dysfunction in early diabetic neuropathy: the Survey of Autonomic Symptoms. Neurology. 2011;76(12):1099-1105.)

CASE E, PART I

RT is a 68-year-old obese male with history of hypertension, who retired from an office job with the government and presently teaches part-time at a local business college. Approximately 3 months ago, he noticed some burning and tingling in his feet and was evaluated by his physician. Laboratory studies taken at that time revealed a fasting blood glucose of 146 mg/dL and his HbA$_{1c}$ was 7.2% (normal 4.0-6.0%). His physician referred him to physical therapy for difficulty walking, per the patient's self-report. RT's HbA$_{1c}$ indicates that he has not had good glycemic control over the last few months and is at increased risk for peripheral and AN.

What type of neuropathy is RT at highest risk for developing? A symmetrical distal polyneuropathy

What tests and measures specific to neuropathy should be done with RT? Monofilament testing of the foot, for protective sensation, proprioceptive and vibratory testing to determine if his gait problems stem from issues in the dorsal medial lemniscal pathway.

Should he be tested for CAN? If so what tests should the PT administer? Tests for AN should also be completed. A squatting test and an assessment of orthostatic hypotension during supine to stand should be administered.

If the screen for CAN is positive can RT begin an exercise program? If so what type? Yes, he can begin exercise if it is supervised and progressed slowly. He might benefit from both resistance exercise to improve left ventricular function and aerobic exercise to improve overall health, glycemic control, and cardiopulmonary function.

TABLE 16-21   MLT 10 Minute Lean Test[346]

		Blood Pressure		Heart Rate	Symptom report (lightheadedness, dizzy, change in color in hands, feet, etc...
		Systolic	Diastolic		
Supine	1 minute				
	2 minute				
Standing	1 minute				
	2 minute				
	3 minute				
	4 minute				
	5 minute				
	6 minute				
	7 minute				
	8 minute				
	9 minute				
	10 minute				

rats with diabetes but studies in humans have had nonsignificant results on meta-analysis.[353,354] It may also be helpful for patients to drink more fluids, sleep with the head of the bed elevated, take extra precautions after eating due to postprandial hypotension, and possibly switch to eating more frequent, small meals.[353]

Physical Therapy Management of Individuals with Peripheral Neuropathies

Pain Management

The best treatment for peripheral neuropathies is prevention. In those with prediabetes and diabetes, long-term control of blood glucose levels through appropriate diet, oral drugs, or insulin injections is key to preventing tissue damage. Exercise can be an effective modality for prevention and treatment. In a mouse model of Type I diabetes, exercise delayed the onset of mechanical hypersensitivity (independent of glucose control), reduced changes in calcium ion function to improve electrophysiological deficits,[355] and reduced myelin loss.[356] Peripheral

neuropathies are also present in neurodegenerative and autoimmune diseases.[357,358] While the research was performed in diabetes, it demonstrates that exercise is an effective means of reducing oxidative stress, which is the underlying mechanism of nerve damage in many disorders. Research in chemotherapy-induced neuropathy and other disorders demonstrates benefit of exercise to reduce pain and improve function as well as to stimulate nerve regeneration.[359-361] Another non-pharmaceutical treatment that is effective is TENS, which activates central mechanisms to provide analgesia[360,362] Low-frequency TENS activates K-opioid receptors in the spinal cord and the brainstem, whereas high-frequency TENS produces its effect via C-opioid receptors. Deep heat can make pain worse, and massage has not been shown to be effective.[363] Medications that are used to decrease neuropathic pain include tricyclic antidepressants (Elavil, Pamelor), anti-epileptics (Gabapentin or Pre-gabalin), serotonin and norepinephrine reuptake inhibitors (venlafaxine or duloxetine) and analgesics (Vicodin, topical lidocaine or capsaicin cream).[364] These each have side effects and variable effectiveness.

Functional Training

In those with diabetic and chemotherapy-induced peripheral neuropathy, exercise decreases pain,[365] improves balance,[366] trunk proprioception, and strength,[366–368] and improves 6-minute walk (6MW) distance[369] and habitual physical activity.[370] In a controlled clinical trial, individuals with CIDP, who performed an exercise program, had improved strength and quality of life (SF-36) as compared to no improvements in control subjects who did not exercise.[371] The exercise program was a relatively mild one, including body weight resistance exercises, active range of motion, some elastic band exercises, and stretching (10 repetitions of each per day). In addition, they did a progressive walking and cycling program, 10 to 20 minutes daily, at 60 to 70% of maximum heart rate, or the "somewhat hard" Borg rating of perceived exertion.[371] Similarly, long-term aerobic brisk walking, 4 hours per week over 4 years, in individuals with diabetes prevented the onset of or slowed the progression of motor and sensory neuropathies,[372] while aerobic exercise at a moderate intensity improved NCV in individuals with diabetic peripheral neuropathy.[373] Exercise has also been shown to improve function in older adults with diabetic neuropathies as measured by the BBS, FRT, TUG, and the 10-m walk.[367] There is emerging evidence that exercise may slow the progression of disease in diabetic peripheral neuropathy. Research to date is limited but supports the use of moderate-intensity aerobic exercise, balance exercises, functional activity, and resistance exercise as having beneficial effects in peripheral neuropathy.[374] Type, dose, duration, and intensity of exercise have not been adequately explored to make specific recommendations. Glycemic control remains the gold standard for preventing diabetic neuropathy but there is evidence that moderate-intensity aerobic exercise can also play a positive role in preventing the development of and slowing the progression of diabetic neuropathy.[375]

CASE E, PART II

RT already has sensory changes and would benefit from a walking program. If he complains of pain, the most effective treatment would be TENS. He has been referred to therapy due to complaints of difficulty walking. The evidence shows that a multifactorial program of strengthening, balance training, and range of motion is likely to improve his balance and walking function.

Denervated Muscle

The effectiveness of electrical stimulation after axonotmesis is still under investigation. For the patient who is expected to have nerve regrowth after complete denervation, electrical stimulation, using galvanic current to the denervated muscle, has been used to maintain the connective tissue mobility within the denervated muscle, with the goal of minimizing fibrosis and having a mobile end-organ, when reinnervation takes place. However, there is controversy in the literature about the use of electrical stimulation in denervated muscle, as it has been found to slow but not prevent muscle atrophy. In an animal model of a crush injury, the addition

of electrical stimulation slowed recovery compared to animals that did not receive electrical stimulation.[376] In addition, the longer pulse duration needed to cause a contraction in denervated muscle may be too painful for some people to tolerate. For partially denervated muscle, the recommended treatment is muscle re-education. Available evidence does not support the use of electrical stimulation in partially denervated muscles.[376,377] Ohtake et al.[377] recommended deferring the use of electrical stimulation in individuals with Bell's palsy for 3 months because 64% of patients with Bell's palsy will have regained normal function within this time period. **In Case D, Tina has a recent compression injury of her ulnar nerve. Based on the evidence, she would not benefit from electrical stimulation but, instead, should be treated initially with rest, followed by muscle re-education.**

Sensory Impairment

Treatment for sensory impairment is focused on teaching the client that they are at risk of injuring the limb, since they cannot feel it nor painful stimuli that might harm the limb. The therapist should teach the client to frequently check the position of the limb, observe the skin for any signs of irritation, and avoid tight or restrictive clothing and shoes. They will also need to learn to check water temperature and use extra caution around extremely hot or cold objects. **RT has sensory impairment of the feet and will need to select supportive shoes with good padding. He should also be educated to check his feet daily for redness or sores and to use caution, when initially wearing a new pair of shoes.**

● BRACHIAL PLEXUS INJURIES

CASE F, PART I

Jonathon was a full-term, 9 lb, 10 oz, 22½ inch baby boy, born via vaginal delivery at his rural home, delivered by a midwife with a minor complication at delivery due to his shoulder width, which required some minor manipulation of the shoulder. His mother contacted her pediatrician on day 5 post-delivery because he did not seem to move his left arm as much as his right.

The brachial plexus, made up of spinal nerves from C5 to T1, makes up a large complex network of nerves (plexus) that run through the cervical-axillary canal. This plexus provides motor and sensory innervation to the upper extremity. The brachial plexus is at risk for some types of injury, typically accidental trauma, from traction to the arm or head that results in sheer, stretch, compression, or tear of the peripheral nerve. As seen in Figure 16-6, the brachial plexus is described, using the designations of roots, trunks, divisions, cords, and branches (nerves). As such, injury to a certain area of the plexus will present with common characteristics as the innervation path to the arm and hand can be traced. For example, if there is injury to the upper plexus, at the superior trunk, motor and sensory damage from C5 and C6 are expected, as is innervation through the lateral and posterior cords, and radial and ulnar nerves.[378]

A

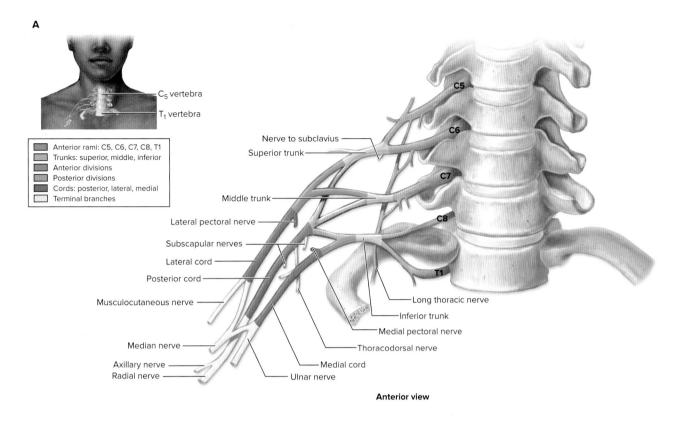

C₅ vertebra
T₁ vertebra

▨	Anterior rami: C5, C6, C7, C8, T1
▨	Trunks: superior, middle, inferior
▨	Anterior divisions
▨	Posterior divisions
▨	Cords: posterior, lateral, medial
▢	Terminal branches

Nerve to subclavius
Superior trunk

Middle trunk

Lateral pectoral nerve
Subscapular nerves
Lateral cord
Posterior cord
Musculocutaneous nerve

Median nerve
Axillary nerve
Radial nerve

C5
C6
C7
C8
T1

Long thoracic nerve
Inferior trunk
Medial pectoral nerve
Thoracodorsal nerve
Medial cord
Ulnar nerve

Anterior view

B

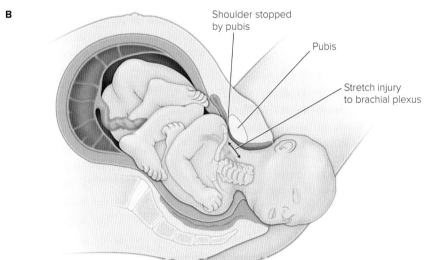

Shoulder stopped
by pubis

Pubis

Stretch injury
to brachial plexus

FIGURE 16-6 A. Brachial plexus with divisions, branches, and nerves detailed. **B.** Common injury mechanism when neck is stretched laterally to expel shoulder(s). (Part A: Reproduced with permission from McKinley M, O'Laughlin VD. *Human Anatomy.* 3rd ed. New York, NY: McGraw-Hill; 2012. Fig. 16.9A, p. 498.)

Brachial Plexus Palsy

Peripheral nerve injuries at the brachial plexus from a trauma are relatively common in pediatrics. The most common mechanism of injury is during birth, when the head of the infant is pulled into lateral flexion as the baby is delivered or before the shoulders are delivered, causing stress on the brachial plexus; this is more likely with a larger baby, like Jonathon. During a breech birth (feet or bottom first) the arm(s) of the infant can be raised overhead, which can also result in stress on the brachial plexus during delivery; however, typically babies with breech presentation are now delivered by C-section, so this is less likely a cause of BPP in the United States. Risk factors for brachial plexus injury include shoulder dystocia (where the head has been delivered but the shoulder is stuck), prolonged delivery, difficult delivery, needing assistance such as forceps, and an infant greater than 4000 g (8.8 pounds). More than half of the cases of brachial plexus injury do not

TABLE 16-22	Brachial Plexus Injury[378]		
CLASSIFICATION	NERVE ROOTS INVOLVED	SYMPTOMS	LIKELIHOOD OF SPONTANEOUS RECOVERY
Grade I Erb-Duchenne palsy Waiter's tip	C5 & C6	Shoulder adduction and internal rotation; elbow extended	90%
Grade II Extended Erb palsy	C5-C7	Grade I plus wrist weakness	65%
Grade III	C5-T1	Weakness of all arm muscles; minimal movement	
Grade IV	C5-T1 plus ipsilateral Horner's syndrome due to damage of the sympathetic chain	Grade III plus miosis, ptosis, anhidrosis	Unlikely
Klumpke's palsy (rare)	C8 & T1 with or without Horner's syndrome	Wrist and hand paresis with normal proximal muscle movement.	Uncertain due to rarity

have these risk factors. Accidental traction of the arm, during play, is also a common mechanism of injury to the brachial plexus in childhood.[379,380] The incidence of BPP is about 1.5 per 1,000 live births in the United States but is higher in other countries and in the United States where obstetric care is not as good.[381] Resulting injuries are categorized by the nerve roots damaged and the degree of injury (see Table 16-22 for nerve root classification). Degree of injury is classified as with other neuropathies (defined earlier in this chapter): neuropraxia, axonotmesis, neurotmesis. Neurotmesis involves tearing in the central portion of the nerve with grades that refer to the layers of the axon damaged; avulsion refers to detachment at the nerve root. Causes of brachial plexus injury are categorized as traumatic or non-traumatic. Obstetrical trauma is the most common cause in infants; however, motorcycle accidents and gunshot wounds are common causes in adults. Non-traumatic injury is associated with nerve inflammation (neuritis) caused by infection, radiation or a metabolic condition, compression or entrapment of the nerve, and benign or malignant tumors.[379] Symptoms are consistent with other nerve injuries, including motor and sensory dysfunction (see Box 16-4).

Recovery

Spontaneous recovery happens in the majority of birth injuries to the brachial plexus. By 2 months of age, 60% of infants with brachial plexus injuries show no residual weakness, and at 4 months the percentage rises to 75% that spontaneously recover. The nerves may regrow or heal at 1 mm per day or 1 inch per month. Isolated elbow flexion, using the biceps, and spontaneous finger movement is a predictor of recovery at 3 months. After 4 months of age, only 4% of infants show any spontaneous recovery. The site of injury (preganglionic or postganglionic) also influences the likelihood of spontaneous recovery with postganglionic lesions much more likely to recover than preganglionic (avulsion) injuries.[382] Permanent damage remains in 10 to 18% of obstetric brachial plexus injuries, typically when

---

CASE F, PART II

Jonathan demonstrates weakness of the left arm, especially at the shoulder and elbow (deltoids and biceps); when he's happy and kicking with arm movement, he moves the left much less than the right, but he does open and close his hand. While he responds to tickling and pressure on his right arm and his left hand (except for the thumb), he does not respond to either on most of his left arm. At rest, his arm is held in adduction and internal rotation.

What would be the appropriate classification of this injury? Grade I Erb-Duchenne palsy

---

Box 16-4   Symptoms on the Injured Side[380,381]

- *Hypotonia of the arm and hand*
- *Muscle weakness; absence of antigravity movements*
- *Muscle atrophy*
- *Abnormal positioning of the shoulder, elbow (and especially) wrist, and hand*
- *Lack of sensation or referred sensation*
- *Less perspiration*
- *Lack of awareness of arm or hand*
- *Neglect*
- *Drooping eyelid*
- *Contractures of joints*
- *Pain*
- *Numbness or tingling*
- *Decreased girth*
- *Decreased grip strength*
- *Absent/weak Moro reflex*
- *Absent/weak protective reflexes*

there is more severe damage to the nerve. These children will have residual weakness and permanent disability of the arm and hand.[379,382]

Physical Therapy Intervention

Physical therapy for infants with a brachial plexus injury may begin immediately after the injury is identified, likely in the nursery/NICU, and continues when the infant goes home. First, a complete neurological examination should be completed to rule out central nervous system involvement and identify specific locations in the brachial plexus that are likely damaged. Recommended assessments are as follows: (1) Active Movement Score (AMS) – evaluates 15 spontaneous movements against or without gravity and (2) Toronto Test – evaluates 5 movements at elbow, wrist, and fingers. MRI or CT may be recommended for infants with suspected avulsion or severe injury. In older children and adults with BPI, EMG and NCV studies may be done to identify lesion levels; these are not typically preformed in infants. SNAPs are reduced or absent in postganglionic lesions but normal in preganglionic lesions. EMG is most useful as recovery occurs (3-6 weeks after injury) to document the degree of reinnervation as polyphasic motor potentials begin to appear.[381] Early treatment focuses on maintaining range of motion, including positioning and teaching the parents stretching and passive range of motion exercises to be completed multiple times per day as well as for handling, bathing and dressing and positioning to prevent skin breakdown.[383] Passive and active ROM exercises will be prescribed after an initial period of rest and recovery. Treatment over the first few months will include use of towels, rolls, and props for positioning; using gravity-eliminated positions to encourage some UE movement; promoting midline behaviors and avoiding neglect; encouraging tummy time and looking at both arms; and avoiding stretch on the arm and neck. As the infant develops, facilitation of symmetry in fine and gross motor skills is necessary as there is some indication that infants with brachial plexus palsy are delayed in crawling, walking, and other motor skill development. Joint mobilization, common strengthening and ROM exercises, taping, and electrical stimulation have all been used successfully in older children and patients with brachial plexus injuries. Splints, casts, and Botox may be indicated for prevention of contractures. Weight-bearing postures are good ways to increase muscle strength. Sensory stimulation may facilitate awareness of the arm and encourage the infant to incorporate it into activities.[383] Recently, modified constraint-induced movement therapy (CIMT) was provided to children 17 to 48 months with residual BPP impairment; the non-impaired arm was casted in a soft cast and treatment included 1 hour/day of active clinic-based treatment plus 2 hours/day of home-programming, 5 days per week for 3 weeks. This was followed by a 5-week home program to encourage arm use in play activities (transition training). this was superior to standard care in improving arm use in bimanual activities; however, it didn't increase the use of the arm in activities of daily living beyond that of assisting.[384] Its use with younger infants has not been evaluated yet. (See discussion in Chapter 11 – Stroke – and Chapter 20 – Cerebral Palsy – for details of CIMT therapy.) A recent pilot study reported that mirror therapy, using a virtual reality program, improved spontaneous use and quality of life, as measured by the Pediatric Quality of Life Inventory Generic Core Scales.[385]

Surgical intervention is considered if infants have not made spontaneous recovery in the first few months or for a known avulsion. For avulsion injuries and serious scarring, surgical interventions may be the only option. Surgical options include (1) direct nerve repair where the nerve ends are stitched together; (2) nerve graft where either an autograft or allograft is used to bridge the gap between the nerve components; or (3) nerve transfer, where another peripheral nerve is resected and connected to appropriate muscles to restore function. Tendon transfers may also be done to improve function. Surgical goals for avulsion injuries are directed primarily to achieve shoulder abduction and elbow flexion to provide some functional use of the arm.[379]

CASE F, PART III

Jonathon's parents were instructed in a program of positioning and passive range of motion to prevent loss of motion of the left arm. They were encouraged to stimulate reaching activities by (1) placing mobiles and toys on the left side of the crib; (2) placing a Velcro-strapped rattle in Jonathon's left hand to reinforce arm movement for short periods of time; (3) encouraging midline movements and bilateral reaching and grasping by placing toys in midline on and above his chest; and (4) teaching cause and effect to link the movement of his left arm and hand to the movement of a toy (e.g., under direct supervision with a parent, attach a tether from his arm to an overhead mobile, for brief periods of time, so that arm movement makes the mobile move). By age 4 months, Jonathon's palsy had resolved, and he demonstrated full range of motion, typical antigravity movement, and equal use of his left arm in activities.

REFERENCES

1. Weiss L, Silver J, Weiss J. Easy EMG: a guide to performing nerve conduction studies and electromyography. 1st ed. Waltham, MA: Butterworth-Heinemann; 2004. ISBN 0750674318.

2. Cho SC, Ferrante MA, Levin KH, Harmon RL, So Y T. Utility of electrodiagnostic testing in evaluating patients with lumbosacral radiculopathy: an evidence-based review. *Muscle Nerve.* 2010;42:276-282.

3. American Association of Electrodiagnostic Medicine (So YT, Weber CF, and Campbell WW). Practice parameter for needle electromyographic evaluation of patients with suspected cervical radiculopathy: summary statement. *Muscle Nerve.* 1999;22(suppl 8):S209-S211.

4. Dillingham TR, Lauder TD, Andary M, et al. Identifying lumbosacral radiculopathies: an optimal electromyographic screen. *Am J Phys Med Rehabil.* 2000;79(6):496-503.

5. Dillingham TR, Lauder TD, Andary M, et al. Identification of cervical radiculopathies: optimizing the electromyographic screen. *Am J Phys Med Rehabil.* 2001;80(2):84-91.

6. NIOSH. Performing motor and sensory neuronal conduction studies in humans: a NIOSH technical manual (NIOSH) Publication No. 90-113. Washington, DC: National Institute for Occupational Safety and Health; 1990. Available at: https://www.cdc.gov/niosh/docs/90-113/.

7. Tavee J. Nerve conduction studies: basic concepts. *Handb Clin Neurol.* 2019;160:217-224.

8. Practice parameter: electrodiagnostic studies in ulnar neuropathy at the elbow. American Association of Electrodiagnostic Medicine, American Academy of Neurology, and American Academy of Physical Medicine and Rehabilitation. *Neurology.* 1999;52(4):688-690.

9. Jablecki CK, Andary MT, Ball RD, et al. American Association of Electrodiagnostic Medicine. Practice parameter for electrodiagnostic studies in carpal tunnel syndrome: summary statement. *Muscle Nerve.* 2002;25:918-922.

10. Marciniak C, Armon C, Wilson J, Miller R. Practice parameter: utility of electrodiagnostic techniques in evaluating patients with suspected peroneal neuropathy: an evidence based review. *Muscle Nerve.* 2005;31:520-527.

11. Patel AT, Gaines K, Malamut R, Park TA, Del Toro DR, Holland N. Usefulness of electrodiagnostic techniques in the evaluation of suspected tarsal tunnel syndrome: an evidence based review. *Muscle Nerve.* 2006;32:236-240.

12. Oh SJ, Hatanaka Y, Ohir M, Kurokawa K, Claussen GC. Clinical utility of sensory nerve conduction of medial femoral cutaneous nerve. *Muscle Nerve.* 2012;45:195-199.

13. AANEM. American Association of Neuromuscular and Diagnostic Medicine Reference Values. Available at: https://www.aanem.org/getmedia/6a8afa49-cb56-40ad-a83b-4d25c120bbc8/NDTF-Chart-Final.pdf. Accessed August 26, 2022.

14. Barboi AC, Barkhaus PE. Electrodiagnostic testing in neuromuscular disorders. *Neurol Clin.* 2004;22(3):619-641.

15. Kraft GH. The electromyographer's guide to the motor unit. *Phys Med Rehabil Clin N Am.* 2007;8(4):711-732.

16. APTA (American Physical Therapy Association). Electrophysiologic Examination and Evaluation HOD P06-96-20-04. Available at: http://www.apta.org/uploadedFiles/APTAorg/About_Us/Policies/Practice/ElectrophysiologicExaminationEvaluation.pdf. Updated August 7, 2012. Accessed August 26, 2022.

17. De Carvalho M, Dengler R, Eisen A, et al. Electrodiagnostic criteria for diagnosis of ALS. *Clin Neurophysiol.* 2008;119:497-503.

18. Narayanaswami P, Weiss M, Selcen D, et al. Evidence-based guideline summary: diagnosis and treatment of limb-girdle and distal dystrophies. *Neurology.* 2014;83(16):1453-1463.

19. Fellows LK, Foster BJ, Chalk CH. Clinical significance of complex repetitive discharges: a case-control study. *Muscle Nerve.* 2003;28(4):504-507.

20. Fournier E, Tabti N. Clinical electrophysiology of muscle diseases and episodic muscle disorders. *Handb Clin Neurol.* 2019;161:269-280.

21. Dimberg EL. Electrodiagnostic evaluation of ulnar neuropathy and other upper extremity mononeuropathies. *Neurol Clin.* 2012;30:479-503.

22. Plastaras CT. Electrodiagnostic challenges in the evaluation of lumbar spinal stenosis. *Phys Med Rehabil Clin N Am.* 2003;14:57-69.

23. Dhawan PS. Electrodiagnostic assessment of plexopathies. *Neurol Clin.* 2021;39:997-1014.

24. Bowley MP, Doughty C. Entrapment neuropathies of the lower extremity. *Med Clin North Am.* 2019;103:371-382.

25. Feldman EL, Callaghan BC, Pop-Busui R, et al. Diabetic neuropathy. *Nat Rev Dis Primers.* 2019;5(1):42.

26. Joyce NC, Carter GT. Electrodiagnosis in persons with amyotrophic lateral sclerosis. *PM R.* 2013;5(5 Suppl):S89-S95.

27. Pasnoor M, Dimachkie MM, Farmakidis C, Barohn RJ. Diagnosis of myasthenia gravis. *Neurol Clin.* 2018;36:261-274.

28. Walling AD, Dickson G. Guillain-Barré syndrome. *Am Fam Physician.* 2013;87(3):191-197.

29. Talbott EO, Malek AM, Lacomis D. The epidemiology of amyotrophic lateral sclerosis. *Handb Clin Neurol.* 2016;138:225-238.

30. Mehta P, Raymond J, Punjani R, et al. Incidence of amyotrophic lateral sclerosis in the United States, 2014-2016. *Amyotroph Lateral Scler Frontotemporal Degener.* 2022;23(5-6):378-382.

31. Mehta P, Kaye W, Raymond J, et al. Prevalence of amyotrophic lateral sclerosis: United States, 2015. *MMWR Morb Mortal Wkly Rep.* 2018;67(46):1285-1289.

32. The ALS Association. Available at: http://www.alsa.org/about-als/facts-you-should-know.html. Accessed April 1, 2022.

33. Cronin S, Hardiman O, Traynor BJ. Ethnic variation in the incidence of ALS. *Neurology.* 2007;68:1002-1007.

34. Roberts AL, Johnson NJ, Chen JT, Cudkowicz ME, Weisskopf MG. Race/ethnicity, socioeconomic status, and ALS mortality in the United States. *Neurology.* 2016;87(22):2300-2308.

35. Wang MD, Little J, Gomes J, Cashman NR, Krewski D. Identification of risk factors associated with onset and progression of amyotrophic lateral sclerosis using systematic review and meta-analysis. *Neurotoxicology.* 2017;61:101-130.

36. Andrew AS, Bradley WG, Peipert D, et al. Risk factors for amyotrophic lateral sclerosis: a regional United States case-control study. *Muscle Nerve.* 2021;63(1):52-59.

37. Spencer PS, Lagrange E, Camu W. ALS and environment: clues from spatial clustering? *Rev Neurol (Paris).* 2019 Dec;175(10):652-663.

38. Horner RD, Kamins KG, Feussner JR, Grambow SC, Hoff-Lindquist J, Harati Y. Occurrence of amyotrophic lateral sclerosis among Gulf War veterans. *Neurology.* 2003;61:742-749.

39. Mejzini R, Flynn LL, Pitout IL, Fletcher S, Wilton SD, Akkari PA. ALS genetics, mechanisms, and therapeutics: where are we now? *Front Neurosci.* 2019;13:1310.

40. Amado DA, Davidson BL. Gene therapy for ALS: a review. *Mol Ther.* 2021;29(12):3345-3358.

41. Shaw PJ. Molecular and cellular pathways of neurodegeneration in motor neuron disease. *J Neurol Neurosurg Psychiatry.* 2005;76:1046-1057.

42. Rossi FH, Franco MC, Estevez AG. Pathophysiology of amyotrophic lateral sclerosis. In: Estévez AG, ed. *Current Advances in Amyotrophic Lateral Sclerosis.* 2013. doi:10.5772/56562.

43. van den Bos M, Geevasinga N, Higashihara M, Menon P, Vucic S. Pathophysiology and diagnosis of ALS: insights from advances in neurophysiological techniques. *Int J Mol Sci.* 2019;20(11):2818.

44. Shaw PJ, Eggett CJ. Molecular factors underlying selective vulnerability of motor neurons to neurodegeneration in amyotrophic lateral sclerosis. *J Neurol.* 2000;247(suppl 1):117-127.

45. Martineau É, Di Polo A, Vande Velde C, Robitaille R. Dynamic neuromuscular remodeling precedes motor-unit loss in a mouse model of ALS. *Elife.* 2018;7:e41973.

46. Salameh JS, Brown RH Jr, Berry JD. Amyotrophic lateral sclerosis: review. *Semin Neurol.* 2015;35(4):469-476.

47. Pugdahl K, Fuglsang-Frederiksen A, de Carvalho M, et al. Generalised sensory system abnormalities in amyotrophic lateral sclerosis: a European multicentre study. *J Neurol Neurosurg Psychiatry.* 2007;78(7):746-749.

48. Lulé D, Diekmann V, Müller HP, Kassubek J, Ludolph AC, Birbaumer N. Neuroimaging of multimodal sensory stimulation in amyotrophic lateral sclerosis. *J Neurol Neurosurg Psychiatry.* 2010;81(8):899-906.

49. Piccione EA, Sletten DM, Staff NP, Low PA. Autonomic system and amyotrophic lateral sclerosis. *Muscle Nerve.* 2015;51(5):676-679.

50. Brooks BR. Natural history of ALS: symptoms, strength, pulmonary function, and disability. *Neurology.* 1996;47(suppl 2):S71-S81.

51. Roche JC, Rojas-Garcia R, Scott KM, et al. A proposed staging system for amyotrophic lateral sclerosis. *Brain.* 2012;135(Pt 3):847-852.

52. Chiò A, Hammond ER, Mora G, Bonito V, Filippini G. Development and evaluation of a clinical staging system for amyotrophic lateral sclerosis. *J Neurol Neurosurg Psychiatry.* 2015;86(1):38-44.

53. Al-Chalabi A, Hardiman O, Kiernan MC, Chiò A, Rix-Brooks B, van den Berg LH. Amyotrophic lateral sclerosis: moving towards a new classification system. *Lancet Neurol.* 2016;15(11):1182-1194.

54. Brooks BR, Miller RG, Swash M, Munsat TL. El Escorial revisited: revised criteria for the diagnosis of amyotrophic lateral sclerosis. *Amyotroph Lateral Scler Other Motor Neuron Disord.* 2000;1:292-299.

55. Jensen L, Jørgensen LH, Bech RD, Frandsen U, Schrøder HD. Skeletal muscle remodelling as a function of disease progression in amyotrophic lateral sclerosis. *Biomed Res Int.* 2016;2016:5930621. doi:10.1155/2016/593062.

56. Van Es MA, Hardiman O, Chio A, et al. Amyotrophic lateral sclerosis. *Lancet.* 2017;390(10107):2084-2098.

57. Agosta F, Spinelli EG, Filippi M. Neuroimaging in amyotrophic lateral sclerosis: current and emerging uses. *Expert Rev Neurother.* 2018 May;18(5):395-406.

58. Ferraro PM, Agosta F, Riva N, et al. Multimodal structural MRI in the diagnosis of motor neuron diseases. *Neuroimage: Clin.* 2017;16:240-247.

59. Gaiottino J, Norgren N, Dobson R, Topping J, Nissim A, Malaspina A. Increased neurofilament light chain blood levels in neurodegenerative neurological diseases. *PLoS One.* 2013;8(9):e75091.

60. Verde F, Steinacker P, Weishaupt JH, et al. Neurofilament light chain in serum for the diagnosis of amyotrophic lateral sclerosis. *J Neurol Neurosurg Psychiatry.* 2019;90:157-164.

61. Wijesekera LC, Mathers S, Talman P, et al. Natural history and clinical features of the flail arm and flail leg ALS variants. *Neurology.* 2009;72(12):1087-1094.

62. Hübers A, Hildebrandt V, Petri S, et al. Clinical features and differential diagnosis of flail arm syndrome. *J Neurol.* 2016;263:390-395.

63. McCluskey L, Vandriel S, Elman L, et al. ALS-Plus syndrome: non-pyramidal features in a large ALS cohort. *J Neurol Sci.* 2014;345(1-2):118-124.

64. Rascovsky K, Grossman M. Clinical diagnostic criteria and classification controversies in frontotemporal lobar degeneration. *Int Rev Psychiatry.* 2013;25(2):145-158.

65. Kaji R, Izumi Y, Adachi Y, Kuzuhara S. ALS-parkinsonism-dementia complex of Kii and other related diseases in Japan. *Parkinsonism Relat Disord.* 2012;18(suppl 1):S190-S191.

66. Rusina R, Vandenberghe R, Bruffaerts R. Cognitive and behavioral manifestations in ALS: beyond motor system involvement. *Diagnostics (Basel).* 2021;11(4):624.

67. Sharma R, Hicks S, Berna CM, Kennard C, Talbot K, Turner MR. Oculomotor dysfunction in amyotrophic lateral sclerosis: a comprehensive review. *Arch Neurol.* 2011;68(7):857-861.

68. Ye S, Jin P, Chen L, Zhang N, Fan D. Prognosis of amyotrophic lateral sclerosis with cognitive and behavioural changes based on a sixty-month longitudinal follow-up. *PLoS One.* 2021;16(8):e0253279.

69. Brown RH, Al-Chalabi A. Amyotrophic lateral sclerosis. *N Engl J Med.* 2017;377:162-172.

70. Czaplinski A, Yen AA, Appel SH. Forced vital capacity (FVC) as an indicator of survival and disease progression in an ALS clinic population. *J Neurol Neurosurg Psychiatry.* 2006a;77:390-392.

71. Magnus T, Beck M, Giess R, Puls I, Naumann M, Toyka KV. Disease progression in amyotrophic lateral sclerosis: predictors of survival. *Muscle Nerve.* 2002;25:709-714.

72. Mandioli J, Faglioni P, Nichelli P, Sola P. Amyotrophic lateral sclerosis: prognostic indicators of survival. *Amyotroph Lateral Scler.* 2006;7:217-220.

73. Agosta F, Pagani E, Petrolini M, et al. MRI predictors of long-term evolution in amyotrophic lateral sclerosis. *Eur J Neurosci.* 2010;32:1490-1496.

74. Bock M, Duong YN, Kim A, Allen I, Murphy J, Lomen-Hoerth C. Progression and effect of cognitive-behavioral changes in patients with amyotrophic lateral sclerosis. *Neurol Clin Pract.* 2017;7:488-498.

75. Tramacere I, Dalla Bella E, Chiò A, Mora G, Filippini G, Lauria G. EPOS Trial Study Group. The MITOS system predicts long-term survival in amyotrophic lateral sclerosis. *J Neurol Neurosurg Psychiatry.* 2015;86(11):1180-1185.

76. Westeneng HJ, Debray TPA, Visser AE, et al. Prognosis for patients with amyotrophic lateral sclerosis: development and validation of a personalised prediction model. *Lancet Neurol.* 2018;17(5):423-433.

77. Xu L, He B, Zhang Y, et al. Prognostic models for amyotrophic lateral sclerosis: a systematic review. *J Neurol.* 2021;268(9):3361-3370.

78. EFNS Task Force on Diagnosis and Management of Amyotrophic Lateral Sclerosis. Andersen PM, Abrahams S, Borasio GD, et al. EFNS guidelines on the clinical management of amyotrophic lateral sclerosis (MALS): revised report of an EFNS task force. *Eur J Neurol.* 2012;19(3):360-375.

79. Chiò A, Bottacchi E, Buffa C, Mutani R, Mora G. The PARALS. Positive effects of tertiary centres for amyotrophic lateral sclerosis on outcome and use of hospital facilities. *J Neurol Neurosurg Psychiatry.* 2006;77:948-950.

80. Miller RG, Mitchell JD, Lyon M, Moore DH. Riluzole for amyotrophic lateral sclerosis (ALS)/motor neuron disease (MND). *Cochrane Database Syst Rev.* 2007;1:CD001447.

81. Paipa AJ, Povedano M, Barcelo A, et al. Survival benefit of multidisciplinary care in amyotrophic lateral sclerosis in Spain: association with non-invasive mechanical ventilation. *J Multidiscip Healthc.* 2019;12:465-470.

82. Dorst J, Ludolph AC, Huebers A. Disease-modifying and symptomatic treatment of amyotrophic lateral sclerosis. *Ther Adv Neurol Disord.* 2017;11:1756285617734734. doi:10.1177/1756285617734734.

83. Miller RG, Mitchell JD, Moore DH. Riluzole for amyotrophic lateral sclerosis (ALS)/motor neuron disease (MND). *Cochrane Database Syst Rev* 2012;3:CD001447.

84. Edavarone Study Group. Safety and efficacy of edaravone in well defined patients with amyotrophic lateral sclerosis: a randomised, double-blind, placebo-controlled trial. *Lancet Neurol.* 2017;16: 505-512.

85. Leigh PN, Abrahams S, Al-Chalabi A, et al. King's MND Care and Research Team. The management of motor neuron disease. *J Neurol Neurosurg Psychiatry.* 2003;74(suppl IV):iv32-iv47.

86. Radunovic A, Mitsumoto H, Leigh PN. Clinical care of patients with amyotrophic lateral sclerosis. *Lancet Neurol.* 2007;6:913-925.

87. Miller RG, Jackson CE, Kasarskis EJ, et al., Quality Standards Subcommittee of the American Academy of Neurology. Practice parameter update: the care of the patient with amyotrophic lateral sclerosis: drug, nutritional, and respiratory therapies (an evidence-based review): report of the Quality Standards Subcommittee of the American Academy of Neurology. *Neurology.* 2009;73(15):1218-1226.

88. Miller RG, Jackson CE, Kasarskis EJ, et al., Quality Standards Subcommittee of the American Academy of Neurology. Practice parameter update: the care of the patient with amyotrophic lateral sclerosis: multidisciplinary care, symptom management, and cognitive/behavioral impairment (an evidence-based review): report of the Quality Standards Subcommittee of the American Academy of Neurology. *Neurology.* 2009b;73(15):1227-1233.

89. Kleopa KA, Sherman M, Neal B, Romano GJ, Heiman-Patterson T. BiPAP improves survival and rate of pulmonary function decline in patients with ALS. *J Neurol Sci.* 1999;164:82-88.

90. Bourke SC, Tomlinson M, Williams TL, Bullock RE, Shaw PJ, Gibson GJ. Effects of non-invasive ventilation on survival and quality of life in patients with amyotrophic lateral sclerosis: a randomised controlled trial. *Lancet Neurol.* 2006;5:140-147.

91. Lechtzin N, Scott Y, Busse AM, Clawson LL, Kimball R, Wiener CM. Early use of non-invasive ventilation prolongs survival in subjects with ALS. *Amyotroph Lateral Scler.* 2007;8:185-188.

92. Radunovic A, Annane D, Rafiq MK, Brassington R, Mustfa N. Mechanical ventilation for amyotrophic lateral sclerosis/motor neuron disease. *Cochrane Database Syst Rev.* 2017;10(10):CD004427.

93. Vitacca M, Montini A, Lunetta C, et al. ALS RESPILOM Study Group. Impact of an early respiratory care programme with non-invasive ventilation adaptation in patients with amyotrophic lateral sclerosis. *Eur J Neurol.* 2018;25(3):556-e33.

94. Laub M, Midgren B. Survival of patients on home mechanical ventilation: a nationwide prospective study. *Respir Med.* 2007;101:1074-1078.

95. Hanayama K, Ishikawa Y, Bach JR. Amyotrophic lateral sclerosis: successful treatment of mucous plugging by mechanical insufflation-exsufflation. *Am J Phys Med Rehabil.* 1997;76(4):338-339.

96. Bach JR. Amyotrophic lateral sclerosis: prolongation of life by noninvasive respiratory aids. *Chest.* 2002;122(1):92-98.

97. Brinkmann JR, Andres P, Mendoza M, Sanjak M. Guidelines for the use and performance of quantitative outcome measures in ALS clinical trials. *J Neurol Sci.* 1997;147:97-111.

98. Woolley SC, York MK, Moore DH, et al. Detecting frontotemporal dysfunction in ALS: utility of the ALS cognitive behavioral screen (ALS-CBS). *Amyotroph Lateral Scler.* 2010;11(3):303-311.

99. Beeldman E, Govaarts R, de Visser M, et al. Screening for cognition in amyotrophic lateral sclerosis: test characteristics of a new screen. *J Neurol.* 2021;268(7):2533-2540.

100. Abrahams S, Leigh PN, Goldstein LH. Cognitive change in ALS: a prospective study. *Neurology.* 2005;64:1222-1226.

101. Chen D, Guo X, Zheng Z, et al. Depression and anxiety in amyotrophic lateral sclerosis: correlations between the distress of patients and caregivers. *Muscle Nerve.* 2015;51(3):353-357.

102. Mitchell JD, Borasio GD. Amyotrophic lateral sclerosis. *Lancet.* 2007; 369:2031-2041.

103. Nicholson K, Murphy A, McDonnell E, et al. Improving symptom management for people with amyotrophic lateral sclerosis. *Muscle Nerve.* 2018;57(1):20-24.

104. Oh H, Sin MK, Schepp KG, Choi-Kwon S. Depressive symptoms and functional impairment among amyotrophic lateral sclerosis patients in South Korea. *Rehabil Nurs.* 2012;37:136-144.

105. McElhiney MC, Rabkin JG, Gordon PH, Goetz R, Mitsumoto H. Prevalence of fatigue and depression in ALS patients and change over time. *J Neurol Neurosurg Psychiatry.* 2009;80:1146-1149.

106. Kubler A, Winter S, Kaiser J, Birbaumer N, Hautzinger M. The ALS Depression Inventory (ADI): a questionnaire to measure depression in degenerative neurological diseases. *Z Klin Psychol Psychother.* 2005;31:19-26.

107. Atassi N, Cook A, Pineda CM, Yerramilli-Rao P, Pulley D, Cudkowicz M. Depression in amyotrophic lateral sclerosis. *Amyotroph Lateral Scler.* 2011;12(2):109-112.

108. Beck AT, Ward CH, Mendelson M, Mock J, Erbaugh J. An inventory for measuring depression. *Arch Gen Psychiatry.* 1961;4:561-571.

109. Zigmond AS, Snaith RP. The hospital anxiety and depression scale. *Acta Psychiatr Scand.* 1983;67:361-370.

110. Spielberger CS, Gorsuch RL, Lushene RE. *Manual for the state trait anxiety inventory.* Palo Alto, CA: Consulting Psychologists Press; 1970:1-36.

111. Rivera I, Ajroud-Driss S, Casey P, et al. Prevalence and characteristics of pain in early and late stages of ALS. *Amyotroph Lateral Scler Frontotemporal Degener.* 2013;14(5-6):369-372.

112. Paganoni S, Karam C, Joyce N, Bedlack R, Carter GT. Comprehensive rehabilitative care across the spectrum of amyotrophic lateral sclerosis. *NeuroRehabilitation.* 2015;37(1):53-68.

113. Ho DT, Ruthazer R, Russell JA. Shoulder pain in amyotrophic lateral sclerosis. *J Clin Neuromuscul Dis.* 2011;13(1):53-55.

114. The UK Motor Neurone Disease Networking Group. A pathway for the management of pain in motor neurone disease. 2001. Available from: https://parkinsonsacademy.co/resources/care-pathways/. Accessed April 26, 2022.

115. Chiò A, Mora G, Lauria G. Pain in amyotrophic lateral sclerosis. *Lancet Neurol.* 2017;16(2):144-157.

116. Jette DU, Slavin MD, Andres PL, Munsat TL. The relationship of lower-limb muscle force to walking ability in patients with amyotrophic lateral sclerosis. *Phys Ther.* 1999;79:672-681.

117. Munsat TL, Andres P, Skerry L. Therapeutic trials in amyotrophic lateral sclerosis: measurement of clinical deficit. In: Rose C, ed. *Amyotrophic Lateral Sclerosis.* New York, NY: Demos Publications; 1990:65-76.

118. Great Lakes ALS Study Group. A comparison of muscle strength testing techniques in amyotrophic lateral sclerosis. *Neurology.* 2003;61:1503-1507.

119. Purdue Pegboard Test: User Intructions. Lafayette Instrument. 2015. Lafayette IN. Available at: http://www.limef.com/downloads/MAN-32020A-forpdf-rev0.pdf.

120. Czell D, Neuwirth C, Weber M, Sartoretti-Schefer S, Gutzeit A, Reischauer C. Nine Hole Peg Test and transcranial magnetic stimulation: useful to evaluate dexterity of the hand and disease progression in amyotrophic lateral sclerosis. *Neurol Res Int.* 2019;2019:7397491.

121. Desrosiers J, Hebert R, Bravo G, Dutil E. The Purdue Pegboard Test: normative data for people aged 60 and over. *Disabil Rehabil.* 1995;17:217-224.

122. Buddenberg LA, Davis C. Test-retest reliability of the Purdue Pegboard Test. *Am J Occup Ther.* 2000;54:555-558.

123. Oxford Grice K, Vogel KA, Le V, Mitchell A, Muniz S, Vollmer MA. Adult norms for a commercially available Nine Hole Peg Test for finger dexterity. *Am J Occup Ther.* 2003;57(5):570-573.

124. Bohannon RW, Smith MB. Interrater reliability of a modified Ashworth scale of muscle spasticity. *Phys Ther.* 1987;67:206-207.

125. Robison R, DiBiase L, Ashley A. et al. Swallowing safety and efficiency impairment profiles in individuals with amyotrophic lateral sclerosis. *Dysphagia.* 2022;37(3):644-654.

126. Fried-Oken M, Mooney A, Peters B. Supporting communication for patients with neurodegenerative disease. *NeuroRehabilitation.* 2015;37(1):69-87.

127. Tilanus TBM, Groothuis JT, TenBroek-Pastoor JMC, et al. The predictive value of respiratory function tests for non-invasive ventilation in amyotrophic lateral sclerosis. *Respir Res.* 2017;18(1):144.

128. Sferrazza Papa GF, Pellegrino GM, Shaikh H, Lax A, Lorini L, Corbo M. Respiratory muscle testing in amyotrophic lateral sclerosis: a practical approach. *Minerva Med.* 2018;109(6 Suppl 1):11-19.

129. Morgan RK, McNally S, Alexander M, Conroy R, Hardiman O, Costello RW. Use of sniff nasal-inspiratory force to predict survival in amyotrophic lateral sclerosis. *Am J Respir Crit Care Med.* 2005;171:269-274.

130. Czaplinski A, Yen AA, Appel SH. Amyotrophic lateral sclerosis: early predictors of prolonged survival. *J Neurol.* 2006b;253:1428-1436.

131. Schmidt EP, Drachman DB, Wiener CM, Clawson L, Kimball R, Lechtzin N. Pulmonary predictors of survival in amyotrophic lateral sclerosis: use in clinical trial design. *Muscle Nerve.* 2006;33:127-132.

132. Braga ACM, Pinto A, Pinto S, de Carvalho M. The role of moderate aerobic exercise as determined by cardiopulmonary exercise testing in ALS. *Neurol Res Int.* 2018;2018:8218697. doi:10.1155/2018/8218697.

133. Lou JS. Fatigue in amyotrophic lateral sclerosis. *Phys Med Rehabil N Am.* 2008;19(3):533-543.

134. Lui AJ, Byl NN. A systematic review of the effect of moderate intensity exercise on function and disease progression in amyotrophic lateral sclerosis. *J Neurol Phys Ther.* 2009;33(2):68-87.

135. Sharma KR, Kent-Braun JA, Majundars S, et al. Physiology of fatigue in amyotrophic lateral sclerosis. *Neurology.* 1995;45:733-740.

136. Aboussouan LS. Mechanisms of exercise limitation and pulmonary rehabilitation for patients with neuromuscular disease. *Chron Respir Dis.* 2009; 6:231-249.

137. Kent-Braun J, Miller RG. Central fatigue during isometric exercise in amyotrophic lateral sclerosis. *Muscle Nerve.* 2000;23:909-914.

138. Gibbons CJ, Thornton EW, Young CA. The patient experience of fatigue in motor neurone disease. *Fron Psychol.* 2013;4(788):1-9.

139. Gibbons C, Pagnini F, Friede T, Young CA. Treatment of fatigue in amyotrophic lateral sclerosis/motor neuron disease. *Cochrane Database Syst Rev.* 2018;1(1):CD011005. doi:10.1002/14651858.CD011005.pub2.

140. Lou JS. Techniques in assessing fatigue in neuromuscular diseases. *Phys Med Rehabil Clin N Am.* 2012;23(1):11-22.

141. Nardone A, Galante M, Lucas B, Schieppati M. Stance control is not affected by paresis and reflex hyperexcitability: the case of spastic patients. *J Neurol Neurosurg Psychiatry.* 2001;70(5):635-643.

142. Sanjak M, Hirsch MA, Bravver EK, Bockenek WL, Norton HJ, Brooks BR. Vestibular deficits leading to disequilibrium and falls in

ambulatory amyotrophic lateral sclerosis. *Arch Phys Med Rehabil.* 2014;95(10):1933-1939.

143. Tinetti ME. Performance-oriented assessment of mobility problems in elderly patients. *J Am Geriatr Soc.* 1986;34:119-126.

144. Podsiadlo D, Richardson S. The timed "Up & Go": a test of basic functional mobility for frail elderly persons. *J Am Geriatr Soc.* 1991;9:142-148.

145. Berg KO, Wood-Dauphinee SL, Williams JI, Maki B. Measuring balance in the elderly: validation of an instrument. *Can J Pub Health.* 1992;83(suppl 2):S7-S11.

146. Duncan PW, Weiner DK, Chandler J, Studenski S. Functional reach: a new clinical measure of balance. *J Gerontol.* 1990;45:M192-M197.

147. Kloos AD, Dal Bello-Haas V, Proch C, Mitsomoto H. Validity of the Tinetti Assessment Tool in individuals with ALS. In: Proceedings of the 9th International Symposium on Amyotrophic Lateral Sclerosis/Motor Neuron Disease Conference. Munich, Germany; 1998:149.

148. Kloos AD, Dal Bello-Haas V, Thome R. et al. Interrater and intrarater reliability of the Tinetti Balance Test for individuals with amyotrophic lateral sclerosis. *J Neurol Phys Ther.* 2004;28(1):12-19.

149. Montes J, Cheng B, Diamond B, Doorish C, Mitsumoto H, Gordon PH. The timed up and go test: predicting falls in ALS. *Amyotroph Lateral Scler.* 2007;8:292-295.

150. Goldfarb BJ, Simon SR. Gait patterns in patients with amyotrophic lateral sclerosis. *Arch Phys Med Rehabil.* 1984;65(2):61-65.

151. Hausdorff JM, Lertratanakul A, Cudkowicz ME, Peterson AL, Kaliton D, Goldberger AL. Dynamic markers of altered gait rhythm in amyotrophic lateral sclerosis. *J Appl Physiol.* 2000;88(6):2045-2053.

152. Inam S, Vucic S, Brodaty NE, Zoing MC, Kiernan MC. The 10-metre gait speed as a functional biomarker in amyotrophic lateral sclerosis. *Amyotroph Lateral Scler.* 2010;11(6):558-561.

153. Sanjak M, Langford V, Holsten S, et al. Six-minute walk test as a measure of walking capacity in ambulatory individuals with amyotrophic lateral sclerosis. *Arch Phys Med Rehabil.* 2017;98(11):2301-2307.

154. Russo M, Lunetta C, Zuccarino R, et al. The 6-min walk test as a new outcome measure in Amyotrophic lateral sclerosis. *Sci Rep.* 2020;10(1):15580.

155. Guide for the Uniform Data System for Medical Rehabilitation (Adult FIM™), version 4.0. Buffalo, NY: State UNIPPVersity of New York at Buffalo; 1993.

156. Cedarbaum JM, Stambler N. Performance of the ALS functional rating scale (ALSFRS) in multicenter clinical trials. *J Neurol Sci.* 1997;152(suppl 1):S1-S9.

157. Cedarbaum JM, Stambler N, Malta E, et al. The ALSFRS-R: a revised ALS Functional Rating Scale that incorporates assessments of respiratory function. BDNF ALS Study Group (Phase III). *J Neurol Sci.* 1999;169:13-21.

158. ALS Functional Rating Scale. Available at: http://www.outcomes-umassmed.org/ALS/alsscale.aspx. Accessed on April 30, 2022.

159. Kaufmann P, Levy G, Montes J, et al., QALS study group. Excellent interrater, intra-rater, and telephone-administered reliability of the ALSFRS-R in a multicenter clinical trial. *Amyotroph Lateral Scler.* 2007;8:42-46.

160. Miano B, Stoddard GJ, Davis S, Bromberg MB. Inter-evaluator reliability of the ALS functional rating scale. *Amyotroph Lateral Scler Other Motor Neuron Disord.* 2004 Dec;5(4):235-239.

161. Appel V, Stewart SS, Smith G, Appel SH. A rating scale for amyotrophic lateral sclerosis: description and preliminary experience. *Ann Neurol.* 1987;22:328-333.

162. Hillel AD, Miller RM, Yorkston K, McDonald E, Norris FH, Konikow N. Amyotrophic Lateral Sclerosis Severity Scale. *Neuroepidemiology.* 1989;8:142-150.

163. Norris FH Jr, Calanchini PR, Fallat RJ, Panchari S, Jewett B. The administration of guanidine in amyotrophic lateral sclerosis. *Neurology.* 1974; 24:721-728.

164. Schwab RS, England AC Jr. Projection techniques for evaluating surgery in Parkinson's disease. In: Gillingham J, Donaldson I, eds. *Third Symposium on Parkinson's Disease.* Edinburgh: Livingstone Ltd.; 1969:152-157.

165. The ALS CNTF Treatment Study (ACTS) Phase I-II Study Group. The amyotrophic lateral sclerosis functional rating scale: assessment of activities of daily living in patients with amyotrophic lateral sclerosis. *Arch Neurol.* 1996;53:141-147.

166. Jenkinson C, Fitzpatrick R, Brennan C, Bromberg M. Development and validation of a short measure of health status for individuals with amyotrophic lateral sclerosis/motor neuron disease: the ALSAQ-40. *J Neurol.* 1999a;246:16-21.

167. Jenkinson C, Fitzpatrick R, Brennan C, Swash M. Evidence for the validity and reliability of the ALS assessment questionnaire: the ALSAQ-40. *Amyotroph Lateral Scler Other Motor Neuron Disord.* 1999b;1:33-40.

168. Gołąb-Janowska M, Honczarenko K, Stankiewicz J. Usefulness of the ALSAQ-5 scale in evaluation of quality of life in amyotrophic lateral sclerosis. *Neurol Neurochir Pol.* 2010;44(6):560-566.

169. Jenkinson C, Fitzpatrick R. Reduced item set for the amyotrophic lateral sclerosis assessment questionnaire: development and validation of the ALSAQ-5. *J Neurol Neurosurg Psychiatry.* 2001;70:70-73.

170. Simmons Z, Felgoise SH, Bremer BA, et al. The ALSSQOL: balancing physical and nonphysical factors in assessing quality of life in ALS. *Neurology.* 2006;67(9):1659-1664.

171. Simmons Z, Felgoise SH, Rodriguez JL, Walsh SM, Bremer BA, Stephens HE. Validation of a shorter ALS-specific quality of life instrument: the ALSSQOL-R. *Neurology.* 2010;74(suppl 2):A177-A178.

172. Felgoise SH, Feinberg R, Stephens HE, et al. Amyotrophic lateral sclerosis-specific quality of life-short form (ALSSQOL-SF): a brief, reliable, and valid version of the ALSSQOL-R. *Muscle Nerve.* 2018;58(5):646-654.

173. Rosa Silva JP, Santiago Júnior JB, Dos Santos EL, de Carvalho FO, de França Costa IMP, Mendonça DMF. Quality of life and functional independence in amyotrophic lateral sclerosis: a systematic review. *Neurosci Biobehav Rev.* 2020;111:1-11.

174. Bello-Haas VD. Physical therapy for individuals with amyotrophic lateral sclerosis: current insights. *Degener Neurol Neuromuscul Dis.* 2018;8:45-54.

175. Sinaki M, Mulder DW. Rehabilitation techniques for patients with amyotrophic lateral sclerosis. *Mayo Clin Proc.* 1978;53:173-178.

176. Chiò A, Benzi G, Dossena M, Mutani R, Mora G. Severely increased risk of amyotrophic lateral sclerosis among Italian professional football players. *Brain.* 2005;128:472-476.

177. Feddermann-Demont N, Junge A, Weber KP, Weller M, Dvorak J, Tarnutzer AA. Prevalence of potential sports-associated risk factors in Swiss amyotrophic lateral sclerosis patients. *Brain Behav.* 2017;7:e00630.

178. Siciliano G, Pastorini E, Pasquali L, Manca ML, Iudice A, Murri L. Impaired oxidative metabolism in exercising muscle from ALS patients. *J Neurol Sci.* 2001;191(1-2):61-65.

179. Sanjak M, Paulson D, Sufit R, et al. Physiologic and metabolic response to progressive and prolonged exercise in amyotrophic lateral sclerosis. *Neurology.* 1987;37(7):1217-1220.

180. Longstreth WT, Nelson LM, Koepsell TD, van Belle G. Hypotheses to explain the association between vigorous physical activity and amyotrophic lateral sclerosis. *Med Hypotheses.* 1991;34(2):144-148.

181. Bennett RL, Knowlton GC. Overwork weakness in partially denervated skeletal muscle. *Clin Orthop.* 1958;12:22-29.

182. Reitsma W. Skeletal muscle hypertrophy after heavy exercise in rats with surgically reduced muscle function. *Am J Phys Med.* 1969;48:237-258.

183. Johnson EW, Braddom R. Overwork weakness in facioscapulohumeral muscular dystrophy. *Arch Phys Med Rehabil.* 1971;52(7):333-336.

184. Tam SL, Archibald V, Jassar B, Tyreman N, Gordon T. Increased neuromuscular activity reduces sprouting in partially denervated muscles. *J Neurosci.* 2001;21:654-667.

185. Tam SL, Archibald V, Tyreman N, Gordon T. Effect of exercise on stability of chronically enlarged motor units. *Muscle Nerve.* 2002;25:359-369.

186. Coble NO, Maloney FP. Interdisciplinary rehabilitation of multiple sclerosis and neuromuscular disorders. In: Maloney FP, Burks JS, Ringel SP,

eds. *Effects of Exercise in Neuromuscular Disease*. New York: JB Lippincott; 1985:228-238.

187. Kurtzke JF. Risk factors in amyotrophic lateral sclerosis. *Adv Neurol.* 1991;56:245-270

188. Strickland D, Smith SA, Dolliff G, Goldman L, Roelofs R. Physical activity, trauma, and ALS: a case-control study. *Acta Neurol Scan.* 1996;94(1):45-50.

189. Meng L, Li X, Li C, et al. Effects of exercise in patients with amyotrophic lateral sclerosis: a systematic review and meta-analysis. *Am J Phys Med Rehabil.* 2020;99(9):801-810.

190. Ortega-Hombrados L, Molina-Torres G, Galán-Mercant A, Sánchez-Guerrero E, González-Sánchez M, Ruiz-Muñoz M. Systematic review of therapeutic physical exercise in patients with amyotrophic lateral sclerosis over time. *Int J Environ Res Pub Health.* 2021;18(3):1074.

191. Park D, Kwak SG, Park JS, Choo YJ, Chang MC. Can therapeutic exercise slow down progressive functional decline in patients with amyotrophic lateral sclerosis? a meta-analysis. *Front Neurol.* 2020;11:853.

192. Merico A, Cavinato M, Gregorio C, et al. Effects of combined endurance and resistance training in Amyotrophic Lateral Sclerosis: a pilot, randomized, controlled study. *Eur J Transl Myol.* 2018;28(1):7278.

193. Clawson LL, Cudkowicz M, Krivickas L, et al. Neals consortium. A randomized controlled trial of resistance and endurance exercise in amyotrophic lateral sclerosis. *Amyotroph Lateral Scler Frontotemporal Degener.* 2018 19(3-4):250-258.

194. Kato, Naoki et al. Effect of muscle strengthening exercise and time since onset in patients with amyotrophic lateral sclerosis: a 2-patient case series study. *Medicine (Baltimore).* 2018;97(25): e11145.

195. Zucchi E, Vinceti M, Malagoli C, et al. High-frequency motor rehabilitation in amyotrophic lateral sclerosis: a randomized clinical trial. *Ann Clin Transl Neurol.* 2019;6(5):893-901.

196. Sanjak M, Bravver E, Bockenek WL, Norton J, Brooks BR. Supported treadmill ambulation for amyotrophic lateral sclerosis: a pilot study. *Arch Phys Med Rehabil.* 2010;91:1920-1929.

197. Pinto AC, Alves M, Nogueira A, et al. Can amyotrophic lateral sclerosis patients with respiratory insufficiency exercise? *J Neurol Sci.* 1999;169: 69-75.

198. Kitano K, Asakawa T, Kamide N, et al. Effectiveness of home-based exercises without supervision by physical therapists for patients with early-stage amyotrophic lateral sclerosis: a pilot study. *Arch Phys Med Rehabil.* 2018;99(10):2114-2117.

199. Carreras I, Yuruker S, Aytan N, et al. Moderate exercise delays the motor performance decline in a transgenic model of ALS. *Brain Res.* 2010;1313: 192-201.

200. Tsitkanou S, Della Gatta P, Foletta V, Russell A. The role of exercise as a non-pharmacological therapeutic approach for amyotrophic lateral sclerosis: beneficial or detrimental? *Front Neurol.* 2019;10:783.

201. Kaspar BK, Frost LM, Christian L, Umapathi P, Gage FH. Synergy of insulin-like growth factor-1 and exercise in amyotrophic lateral sclerosis. *Ann Neurol.* 2005;57:649-655.

202. Deforges S, Branchu J, Biondi O, et al. Motoneuron survival is promoted by specific exercise in a mouse model of amyotrophic lateral sclerosis. *J Physiol.* 2009;587(Pt 14):3561-3572.

203. Desseille C, Deforges S, Biondi O, et al. Specific physical exercise improves energetic metabolism in the skeletal muscle of amyotrophic-lateral-sclerosis mice. *Front Mol Neurosci.* 2017;10:332.

204. Dycem Non-slip products. Available at: www.dycem.com.

205. Chen A, Montes J, Mitsumoto H. The role of exercise in amyotrophic lateral sclerosis. *Phys Med Rehabil Clin N Am.* 2008;19:545-557.

206. Mayadev AS, Weiss MD, Distad BJ, Krivickas LS, Carter GT. The amyotrophic lateral sclerosis center: a model of multidisciplinary management. *Phys Med Rehabil Clin N Am.* 2008;19:619-631.

207. Dal Bello-Haas V, Kloos AD, Mitsumoto H. Physical therapy for a patient through six stages of amyotrophic lateral sclerosis. *Phys Ther.* 1998;78:1312-1324.

208. Dal Bello-Haas V. A framework for rehabilitation in degenerative diseases: planning care and maximizing quality of life. *Neurol Rep.* 2002;26(3): 115-129.

209. Kamide N, Asakawa T, Shibasaki N, et al. Identification of the type of exercise therapy that affects functioning in patients with early-stage amyotrophic lateral sclerosis: a multicenter, collaborative study. *Neurol Clin Neurosci.* 2014;2:135-139.

210. Ingels PL, Rosenfeld J, Frick SL, Bryan WJ. Adhesive capsulitis: a common occurrence in patients with ALS. *Amyotroph Lateral Scler Other Motor Neuron Disord.* 2001;2(S2):60.

211. Gourie-Devi M, Nalini A, Sandhya S. Early or late appearance of "dropped head syndrome" in amyotrophic lateral sclerosis. *J Neurol Neurosurg Psychiatry.* 2003;74(5):683-686.

212. Hansen A, Bedore B, Nickel E, Hanowski K, Tangen S, Goldish G. Elastic head support for persons with amyotrophic lateral sclerosis. *J Rehabil Res Dev.* 2014;51(2):297-303.

213. Philadelphia Cervical Collar Co., Thorofare, NJ 08086. https://www.calabresegroup.com/phillycollar/.

214. Ossur Americas, Irvine, CA 92618 https://www.ossur.com/.

215. Trulife Group Limited Company, Jackson, MI 49203 https://trulife.com/.

216. Headmaster Collar. Available at symmetric Designs LTD, Salt Spring Island, BC, Canada ViK 1C9. https://www.symmetric-designs.com/our-products.

217. Su CL, Tam KW, Fang TP, Chiang LL, Chen HC. Effects of pulmonary rehabilitation program on amyotrophic lateral sclerosis: a meta-analysis of randomized controlled trials. *NeuroRehabilitation.* 2021;48(3):255-265.

218. Macpherson CE, Bassile CC. Pulmonary physical therapy techniques to enhance survival in amyotrophic lateral sclerosis: a systematic review. *J Neurol Phys Ther.* 2016;40(3):165-175.

219. Cheah BC, Boland RA, Brodaty NE, et al. INSPIRATIonAL-INSPIRAtory muscle training in amyotrophic lateral sclerosis. *Amyotroph Lateral Scler.* 2009;10:384-392.

220. Pinto S, Swash M, de Carvalho M. Respiratory exercise in amyotrophic lateral sclerosis. *Amyotroph Lateral Scler.* 2012;13(1):33-43.

221. Pinto S, deCarvalho M. Can inspiratory muscle training increase survival in early-affected amyotrophic lateral sclerosis patients? *Amyotroph Lateral Scler Frontotemporal Degener.* 2013;14:124-126.

222. Plowman EK, Tabor-Gray L, Rosado KM, et al. Impact of expiratory strength training in amyotrophic lateral sclerosis: results of a randomized, sham-controlled trial. *Muscle Nerve.* 2019 Jan;59(1):40-46.

223. Cleary S, Misiaszek JE, Karla S, Wheeler S, Johnston W. The effects of lung volume recruitment on coughing and pulmonary function in patients with ALS. *Amyotroph Lateral Scler Frontotemporal Degener.* 2013;14: 111-115.

224. Mustfa N, Aiello M, Lyall RA, et al. Cough augmentation in amyotrophic lateral sclerosis. *Neurology.* 2003;61(9):1285-1287.

225. Senent C, Golmard JL, Salachas F, Chiner E, Morelot-Panzini C, et al. A comparison of assisted cough techniques in stable patients with severe respiratory insufficiency due to amyotrophic lateral sclerosis. *Amyotroph Lateral Scler.* 2011;12(1):26-32.

226. Nardin R, O'Donnell C, Loring SH, et al. Diaphragm training in amyotrophic lateral sclerosis. *Clin Neuromuscul Dis.* 2008;10(2):56-60.

227. Majmudar S, Wu J, Paganoni S. Rehabilitation in amyotrophic lateral sclerosis: why it matters. *Muscle Nerve.* 2014;50(1):4-13.

228. Hoyer Lift. Available from Sunrise Medical, Longmont, CO 80503. https://www.sunrisemedical.com/.

229. Trail M, Nelson N, Van JN, Appel SH, Lai EC. Wheelchair use by patients with amyotrophic lateral sclerosis: a survey of user characteristics and selection preferences. *Arch Phys Med Rehabil.* 2001;82(1):98-102.

230. Purtilo R, Haddad A. *Health professional and patient interaction.* 7th ed. Philadelphia, PA: WB Saunders; 2007.

231. Centers for Disease Control and Prevention. Available at: https://www.cdc.gov/campylobacter/guillain-barre.html. Accessed May 22, 2022.

232. Sejvar JJ, Baughman AL, Wise M, Morgan OW. Population incidence of Guillain-Barré syndrome: a systematic review and meta-analysis. *Neuroepidemiology*. 2011;36:123-133.

233. Toscano G, Palmerini F, Ravaglia S, et al. Guillain-Barré syndrome associated with SARS-CoV-2. *N Engl J Med*. 2020 Jun 25;382(26):2574-2576.

234. Rinaldi S. Update on Guillain-Barré syndrome. *J Peripher Nerv Syst*. 2013;18(2):99-112.

235. van den Berg B, Walgaard C, Drenthen J, Fokke C, Jacobs BC, van Doorn PA. Guillain-Barré syndrome: pathogenesis, diagnosis, treatment and prognosis. *Nat Rev Neurol*. 2014;10(8):469-482.

236. Leonhard SE, Mandarakas MR, Gondim FAA, Bateman K, Ferreira MLB, et al. Diagnosis and management of Guillain-Barre syndrome in ten steps. *Nat Rev Neurol*. 2019;15(11):671-683.

237. Yuki N, Hartung H-P. Guillain-Barré syndrome. *N Engl J Med*. 2012; 366(24):2294-2304.

238. Kuitwaard K, van Koningsveld R, Ruts L, Jacobs BC, van Doorn PA. Recurrent Guillain-Barré syndrome. *J Neurol Neurosurg Psychiatry*. 2009;80:56-59.

239. Asbury AK, Cornblath DR. Assessment of current diagnostic criteria for Guillain-Barré syndrome. *Ann Neurol*. 1990;27(Suppl):S21-S24.

240. The Brighton Collaboration GBS Working Group. Guillain-Barré syndrome and Fisher syndrome: case definitions and guidelines for collection, analysis, and presentation of immunization safety data. *Vaccine*. 2011;29(3):599-612.

241. Willison HJ, Jacobs BC, van Doorn PA. Guillain-barré syndrome. *Lancet*. 2016;388:717-727.

242. Yikilmaz A, Doganay S, Gumus H, Per H, Kumandas S, Coskun A. Magnetic resonance imaging of childhood Guillain-Barre syndrome. *Childs Nerv Syst*. 2010;26(8):1103-1108.

243. Bassile CC. Guillain-Barré syndrome and exercise guidelines. *Neurol Rep*. 1996;20(2):198-203.

244. Rajabally YA, Uncini A. Outcome and its predictors in Guillain-Barré syndrome. *J Neurol Neurosurg Psychiatry*. 2012;83:711-718.

245. Ruts L, Drenthen J, Jongen JL, et al., Dutch GBS Study Group. Pain in Guillain-Barré syndrome: a long-term follow-up study. *Neurology*. 2010;75: 1439-1447.

246. de Vries JM, Hagemanns MLC, Bussmann JBJ, van der Ploeg AT, van Doorn PA. Fatigue in neuromuscular disorders: focus on Guillain-Barré and Pompe disease. *Cell Mol Life Sci*. 2010;67(5):701-713.

247. Forsberg A, Press R, Holmqvist LW. Residual disability 10 years after falling ill in Guillain-Barré syndrome: a prospective follow-up study. *J Neurol Sci*. 2012;317(1-2):74-79.

248. Bernsen RA, Jager AE, Schmitz PI, van der Meché FG. Long-term sensory deficit after Guillain-Barré syndrome. *J Neurol*. 2001;248:483-486.

249. Walgaard C, Lingsma HF, Ruts L, et al. Prediction of respiratory insufficiency in Guillain-Barré syndrome. *Ann Neurol*. 2010;67:781-787.

250. Walgaard C, Lingsma HF, Ruts L, van Doorn PA, Steyerberg EW, Jacobs BC. Early recognition of poor prognosis in Guillain-Barré syndrome. *Neurology*. 2011;76:968-975.

251. Hughes RA, Wijdicks EF, Barohn R, et al. Practice parameter: immunotherapy for Guillain-Barré syndrome: report of the Quality Standards Subcommittee of the American Academy of Neurology. *Neurology*. 2003; 61(6):736-740.

252. Raphaël JC, Chevret S, Hughes RA, Annane D. Plasma exchange for Guillain-Barré syndrome. *Cochrane Database Syst Rev*. 2012;7:CD001798.

253. Plasma Exchange/Sandoglobulin Guillain-Barré Syndrome Trial Group. Randomised trial of plasma exchange, intravenous immunoglobulin, and combined treatments in Guillain-Barré syndrome. *Lancet*. 1997;349: 225-230.

254. Hughes RA, Swan AV, van Doorn PA. Intravenous immunoglobulin for Guillain-Barré syndrome. *Cochrane Database Syst Rev*. 2014;19(9): CD002063.

255. Forsberg A, Press R, Einarsson U, de Pedro-Cuesta J, Widén Holmqvist L, Swedish Epidemiological Study Group. Impairment in Guillain-Barré syndrome during the first 2 years after onset: a prospective study. *J Neurol Sci*. 2004;227:131-138.

256. Whitney S L, Wrisley DM., Marchetti GF, Gee MA, Redfern MS, Furman JM. Clinical measurement of sit-to-stand performance in people with balance disorders: validity of data for the Five-Times-Sit-to-Stand Test. *Phys Ther*. 2005;85(10):1034-1045.

257. Nordon-Craft A, Moss M, Quan D, Schenkman M. Intensive care unit-acquired weakness: implications for physical therapist management. *Phys Ther*. 2012;92(12):1494-1506.

258. Merkies IS, Schmitz PI, van der Meché FG, Samijn JP, van Doorn PA, Inflammatory Neuropathy Cause and Treatment (INCAT) group. Clinimetric evaluation of a new overall disability scale in immune mediated polyneuropathies. *J Neurol Neurosurg Psychiatry*. 2002;72(5):596-601.

259. Fokke C, van den Berg B, Drenthen J, Walgaard C, van Doorn PA, Jacobs BC. Diagnosis of Guillain-Barré syndrome and validation of Brighton criteria. *Brain*. 2014;137:33-43.

260. Hughes RA, Newsom-Davis JM, Perkin GD, Pierce JM. Controlled trial prednisolone in acute polyneuropathy. *Lancet*. 1978;2:750-753.

261. van Swieten JC, Koudstaal PJ, Visser MC, Schouten HJ, van Gijn J. Interobserver agreement for the assessment of handicap in stroke patients. *Stroke*. 1988;19:604-607.

262. Orlikowski D, Prigent H, Sharshar T, Lofaso F, Raphael JC. Respiratory dysfunction in Guillain-Barré Syndrome. *Neurocrit Care*. 2004;1(4):415-422.

263. Lawn ND, Fletcher DD, Henderson RD, Wolter TD, Wijdicks EF. Anticipating mechanical ventilation in Guillain-Barré syndrome. *Arch Neurol*. 2001;58:893-898.

264. Merkies IS, Schmitz PI, Van Der Meché FG, Van Doorn PA. Psychometric evaluation of a new sensory scale in immune-mediated polyneuropathies. Inflammatory Neuropathy Cause and Treatment (INCAT) Group. *Neurology*. 2000;54(4):943-949. doi:10.1212/wnl.54.4.943

265. Bernsen RA, de Jager AE, Kuijer W, van der Meché FG, Suurmeijer TP. Psychosocial dysfunction in the first year after Guillain-Barré syndrome. *Muscle Nerve*. 2010;41(4):533-539.

266. Féasson L, Camdessanché JP, El Mandhi L, Calmels P, Millet GY. Fatigue and neuromuscular diseases. *Ann Readapt Med Phys*. 2006;49:375-384.

267. Sulli S, Scala L, Berardi A, et al. The efficacy of rehabilitation in people with Guillain-Barrè syndrome: a systematic review of randomized controlled trials. *Expert Rev Neurother*. 2021;21(4):455-461.

268. Khan F, Pallant JF, Amatya B, Ng L, Gorelik A, Brand C. Outcomes of high- and low-intensity rehabilitation programme for persons in chronic phase after Guillain-Barré syndrome: a randomized controlled trial. *J Rehabil Med*. 2011;43(7):638-646.

269. Khan F, Ng L, Amatya B, Brand C, Turner-Stokes L. Multidisciplinary care for Guillain-Barré syndrome. *Cochrane Database Syst Rev*. 2010; 10:CD008505.

270. Ragupathy S, Anupam G, Raghuram N, et al. Effect of pranayama and meditation as an add-on therapy in rehabilitation of patients with Guillain-Barré syndrome: a randomized control pilot study. *Disabil Rehabil*. 2013;35(1):57-62.

271. Vidhyadhari BSL, Madavi K. Influence of proprioceptive neuromuscular facilitation techniques on diaphragm muscle activity and pulmonary function in subjects with Guillain-barre syndrome. *Indian J Physiother Occup Ther*. 2015;9(2): 24-28.

272. Arsenault NS, Vincent PO, Yu BH, Bastien R, Sweeney A. Influence of exercise on patients with Guillain-Barré syndrome: a systematic review. *Physiother Can*. 2016;68(4):367-376.

273. Karper WB. Effects of low-intensity aerobic exercise on one subject with chronic-relapsing Guillain-Barré syndrome. *Rehabil Nurs*. 1991; 16(2):96-98.

274. Pitetti KH, Barrett PJ, Abbas D. Endurance exercise training in Guillain-Barre syndrome. *Arch Phys Med Rehabil*. 1993;74(7):761-765.

275. Garssen MP, Bussmann JB, Schmitz PI, et al. Physical training and fatigue, fitness, and quality of life in Guillain-Barré syndrome and CIDP. *Neurology*. 2004;63(12):2393-2395.

276. Bussmann JB, Garssen MP, van Doorn PA, Stam HJ. Analysing the favourable effects of physical exercise: relationships between physical fitness, fatigue and functioning in Guillain-Barré syndrome and chronic inflammatory demyelinating polyneuropathy. *J Rehabil Med.* 2007;39(2):121-125.

277. Bulley P. The podiatron: an adjunct to physiotherapy treatment for Guillain-Barré syndrome? *Physiother Res Int.* 2003;8(4):210-215.

278. Fisher TB, Stevens JE. Rehabilitation of a marathon runner with Guillain-Barré syndrome. *J Neurol Phys Ther.* 2008;32(4):203-209.

279. Herbison GJ, Jaweed MM, Ditunno JF Jr. Exercise therapies in peripheral neuropathies. *Arch Phys Med Rehabil.* 1983;64(5):201-205.

280. Bensman A. Strenuous exercise may impair muscle function in Guillain-Barré patients. *JAMA.* 1970;214:468-469.

281. McCarthy JA, Zigenfus RW. Transcutaneous electrical nerve stimulation: an adjunct in the pain management of Guillain-Barré syndrome. *Phys Ther.* 1978;58(1):23-24.

282. Gersh MR, Wolf SL, Rao VR. Evaluation of transcutaneous electrical nerve stimulation for pain relief in peripheral neuropathy. *Phys Ther.* 1980;60(1):48-52.

283. Mullings KR, Alleva JT, Hudgins TH. Rehabilitation of Guillain-Barré syndrome. *Dis Mon.* 2010;56(5):288-292.

284. Khan F, Amatya B. Rehabilitation interventions in patients with acute demyelinating inflammatory polyneuropathy: a systematic review. *Eur J Phys Rehabil Med.* 2012;48(3):507-522.

285. Vajsar J, Fehlings D, Stephens D. Long-term outcome in children with Guillain-Barré syndrome. *J Pediatr.* 2003;142(3):305-309.

286. Tuckey J, Greenwood R. Rehabilitation after severe Guillain-Barré syndrome: the use of partial body weight support. *Physiother Res Int.* 2004;9(2):96-103.

287. Simmons S. Guillain-Barré syndrome: a nursing nightmare that usually ends well. *Nursing.* 2010;40:24-29.

288. Bernsen RA, de Jager AE, Schmitz PI, van der Meché FG. Long-term impact on work and private life after Guillain-Barré syndrome. *J Neurol Sci.* 2002;201:13-17.

289. World Health Organization. Poliomyelitis (polio). https://www.who.int/health-topics/poliomyelitis#tab=tab_1. Accessed May 30, 2022.

290. Bruno RL, Sapolsky R, Zimmerman JR, Frick NM. Pathophysiology of a central cause of post-polio fatigue. *Ann N Y Acad Sci.* 1995;753:257-275.

291. Grimby G, Einarsson G, Hedberg M, Aiansson A. Muscle adaptive changes in post-polio subjects. *Scan J Rehabil Med.* 1989;21(1):19-26.

292. Lo JK, Robinson LR. Postpolio syndrome and the late effects of poliomyelitis. Part 1: pathogenesis, biomechanical considerations, diagnosis, and investigations. *Muscle Nerve.* 2018 Dec;58(6):751-759.

293. Centers for Disease Control and Prevention. Polio. Available at: https://www.cdc.gov/polio/index.htm. Accessed May 30, 2022.

294. Ramlow J, Alexander M, LaPorte R, Kaufmann C, Kuller L. Epidemiology of the post-polio syndrome. *Am J Epidemiol.* 1992;136(7):769-786.

295. McDonald-Williams MF. Exercise and postpolio. *Neurol Rep.* 1996;20(2):31-36.

296. Tiffreau V, Rapin A, Serafi R, et al. Post-polio syndrome and rehabilitation. *Ann Phys Rehabil Med.* 2010;53(1):42-50.

297. Berlly MH, Strauser WW, Hall KM. Fatigue in postpolio syndrome. *Arch Phys Med Rehabil.* 1991;72:115-118.

298. Halstead L. Assessment and differential diagnosis for post-polio syndrome. *Orthopedics.* 1991;14:1209-1217.

299. Jubelt B, Agre JC. Characteristics and management of postpolio syndrome. *JAMA.* 2000;284:412-414.

300. Rodriquez AA, Agre JC. Electrophysiological study of the quadriceps muscles during fatiguing exercise and recovery: a comparison of symptomatic and asymptomatic postpolio patients and controls. *Arch Phys Med Rehabil.* 1991;72:993-997.

301. Peach PE. Overwork weakness with evidence of muscle damage in a patient with residual paralysis from polio. *Arch Phys Med Rehabil.* 1990;71:248-250.

302. Lord S, Allen G, Williams P, Gandevia S. Risk of falling: predictors based on reduced strength in persons previously affected by polio. *Arch Phys Med Rehabil.* 2002;83:757-763.

303. Gonzalez H, Olsson T, Borg K. Management of postpolio syndrome. *Lancet Neurol.* 2010;9:634-642.

304. Smith L, McDermott K. Pain in post-poliomyelitis: addressing causes versus effects. In: Halstead L, Wiechers D, eds. *Research and Clinical Aspects of the Late Effects of Poliomyelitis.* White Plains, NY: March of Dimes Birth Defect Foundation. Birth Defects Orig Artic Ser. 1987;23(4):121-134.

305. Perry J, Burnfield JM. *Gait Analysis: Normal and Abnormal Function.* 2nd ed. Thorofare, NJ: Slack; 2010.

306. March of Dimes. Identifying best practices in diagnosis and care. From: International Conference on Post-Polio Syndrome; May 19–20, 2000; Warm Springs, GA. http://www.polioplace.org/sites/default/files/files/MOD-Identifying.pdf. Accessed May 18, 2018.

307. Sandberg A, Stalberg E. Changes in macro electromyography over time in patients with a history of polio: a comparison of two muscles. *Arch Phys Med Rehabil.* 2004;85:1174-1182.

308. Boyer FC, Tiffreau V, Rapin A, et al. Post-polio syndrome: pathophysiological hypotheses, diagnosis criteria, medication therapeutics. *Annal Phys Rehabil Med.* 2010;53:34-41.

309. Lo JK, Robinson LR. Post-polio syndrome and the late effects of poliomyelitis: Part 2: treatment, management, and prognosis. *Muscle Nerve.* 2018;58(6):760-769.

310. On AY, Oncu J, Uludag B, Ertekin C. Effects of lamotrigine on the symptoms and life qualities of patients with post polio syndrome: a randomized, controlled study. *NeuroRehabilitation* 2005;20:245-251.

311. Koopman FS, Beelen A, Gilhus NE, de Visser M, Nollet F. Treatment for post-polio syndrome. *Cochrane Database Syst Rev.* 2015(Issue 5):CD007818.

312. Flansbjer UB, Brogårdh C, Horstmann V, Lexell J. Men with late effects of polio decline more than women in lower limb muscle strength: a 4-year longitudinal study. *PM R.* 2015;7(11):1127-1136.

313. Li Hi Shing S, Chipika RH, Finegan E, Murray D, Hardiman O, Bede P. Post-polio syndrome: more than just a lower motor neuron disease. *Front Neurol.* 2019;10:773.

314. Young CA, Wong SM, Quincey AC, Tennant A. Measuring physical and cognitive fatigue in people with post-polio syndrome: development of the neurological fatigue index for post-polio syndrome (NFI-PP). *PM R.* 2018;10(2):129-136.

315. Young CA, Quincey AC, Wong SM, Tennant A. Quality of life for post-polio syndrome: a patient derived, Rasch standard scale. *Disabil Rehabil.* 2018;40(5):597-602.

316. Oncu J, Durmaz B, Karapolat H. Short-term effects of aerobic exercise on functional capacity, fatigue, and quality of life in patients with post-polio syndrome. *Clin Rehabil.* 2009;23(2):155-163.

317. Voorn EL, Gerrits KH, Koopman FS, Nollet F, Beelen A. Determining the anaerobic threshold in postpolio syndrome: comparison with current guidelines for training intensity prescription. *Arch Phys Med Rehabil.* 2014;95(5):935-940.

318. Halstead LS, Gawne AC, Pham BT. National rehabilitation hospital limb classification for exercise, research, and clinical trials in post-polio patients. *Ann N Y Acad Sci.* 1995;753:343-353.

319. Brehm MA, Beelen A, Doorenbosch CA, Harlaar J, Nollet F. Effect of carbon-composite knee-ankle-foot orthoses on walking efficiency and gait in former polio patients. *J Rehabil Med.* 2007;39(8):651-657.

320. Hebert JS, Liggins AB. Gait evaluation of an automatic stance-control knee orthosis in a patient with postpoliomyelitis. *Arch Phys Med Rehabil.* 2005;86(8):1676-1680.

321. Kim JH, Ji SG, Jung KJ, Kim JH. Therapeutic experience on stance control knee-ankle-foot orthosis with electromagnetically controlled knee joint system in poliomyelitis. *Ann Rehabil Med.* 2016;40(2):356-361.

322. Bruno RL, Frick NM. The psychology of polio as prelude to post polio syndrome: behavior modification and psychotherapy. *Orthopedics.* 1991;14:1185-1193.

323. Said G. Diabetic neuropathy. *Handb Clin Neurol.* 2013;115:579-589.

324. Hicks CW, Selvin E. Epidemiology of peripheral neuropathy and lower extremity disease in diabetes. *Curr Diab Rep.* 2019;19(10):86.

325. Tagliafico A, Altafini L, garello I, Marchetti A, Gennaro S, Martinoli C. Traumatic neuropathies: spectrum of imaging findings and postoperative assessment. *Semin Musculoskelet Radiol.* 2010;14(5):512-522.

326. Siao P, Kaku M. A clinician's approach to peripheral neuropathy. *Semin Neurol.* 2019;39(5):519-530.

327. Hughes R. Peripheral nerve diseases. *Prac Neurol.* 2008;8:396-405.

328. Campbell WW. Evaluation and management of peripheral nerve injury. *Clin Neurophysiol.* 2008;119:1951-1965.

329. Bhandari PS. Management of peripheral nerve injury. *J Clin Orthop Trauma.* 2019;10(5):862-866.

330. Seddon HJ. A classification of nerve injuries. *Br Med J.* 1942;27(12):237-239.

331. Menorca RM, Fussell TS, Elfar JC. Nerve physiology: mechanisms of injury and recovery. *Hand Clin.* 2013;29(3):317-330.

332. Lee SK, Wolfe SW. Peripheral nerve injury and repair. *J Am Acad Orthop Surg.* 2000;8(4):243-252.

333. Carlson BM. The biology of long-term denervated skeletal muscle. *Eur J Transl Myol.* 2014;24(1):3293.

334. Houschyar KS, Momeni A, Pyles MN, et al. The role of current techniques and concepts in peripheral nerve repair. *Plast Surg Int.* 2016;2016:4175293.

335. Medical Research Council. *Aids to the Investigation of Peripheral Nerve Injuries.* London: Her Majesty's Stationary Office; 1943, revised, 1976.

336. Griffin JW, Hogan MV, Chhabra AB, Deal DN. Peripheral nerve repair and reconstruction. *J Bone Joint Surg Am.* 2013;95(23):2144-2151.

337. Albers JW, Pop-Busui R. Diabetic neuropathy: mechanisms, emerging treatments, and subtypes. *Curr Neuro Neurosci Rep.* 2014;14(8):473.

338. Harris-Hayes M, Schootman M, Schootman JC, Hastings MK. The role of physical therapists in fighting the Type 2 diabetes epidemic. *J Orthop Sports Phys Ther.* 2020;50(1):5-16.

339. Sasaki H, Kawamura N, Dyck PJ, Dyck PJB, Kihara M, Low PA. Spectrum of diabetic neuropathies. *Diabetol Int.* 2020;11(2):87-96.

340. Sharma KR, Cross J, Farronay O, Ayyar DR, Shebert RT, Bradley WG. Demyelinating neuropathy in diabetes mellitus. *Arch Neurol.* 2002;59(5):758-765.

341. Chen Z, Li G, Liu J. Autonomic dysfunction in Parkinson's disease: implications for pathophysiology, diagnosis, and treatment. *Neurobiol Dis.* 2020;134:104700.

342. Duque A, Mediano MFF, De Lorenzo A, Rodrigues LF Jr. Cardiovascular autonomic neuropathy in diabetes: pathophysiology, clinical assessment and implications. *World J Diabetes.* 2021;12(6):855-867.

343. Deli G, Bosnyak E, Pusch G, Komoly S, Feher G. Diabetic neuropathies: diagnosis and management. *Neuroendocrinology.* 2013;98(4):267-280.

344. Zilliox L, Peltier AC, Wren PA, et al. Assessing autonomic dysfunction in early diabetic neuropathy: the survey of autonomic symptoms. *Neurology.* 2011;76(12):1099-1105.

345. Phipps D, Butler E, Mounsey A, et al. PURL: best timing for measuring orthostatic vital signs? *J Fam Pract.* 2019;68(9):512-514.

346. Hyatt KH, Jacobson LB, Schneider VS. Comparison of 70 degrees tilt, LBNP, and passive standing as measures of orthostatic tolerance. *Aviat Space Environ Med.* 1975;46(6):801-808.

347. Banthia S, Bergner DW, Chicos AB, et al. Detection of cardiovascular autonomic neuropathy using exercise testing in patients with type 2 diabetes mellitus. *J Diabetes Complications.* 2013;27(1):64-69.

348. Goldberger JJ, Arora R, Buckley U, Shivkumar K. Autonomic nervous system dysfunction: JACC focus seminar. *J Am Coll Cardiol.* 2019;73(10):1189-1206.

349. Pierpont GL, Adabag S, Yannopoulos D. Pathophysiology of exercise heart rate recovery: a comprehensive analysis. *Ann Noninvasive Electrocardiol.* 2013;18(2):107-117.

350. Fornasiero A, Zignoli A, Rakobowchuk M, et al. Post-exercise cardiac autonomic and cardiovascular responses to heart rate-matched and work rate-matched hypoxic exercise. *Eur J Appl Physiol.* 2021;121(7):2061-2076.

351. Takahagi VCM, Costa DC, Crescencio JC, Gallo Junior L. Physical training as non-pharmacological treatment of neurocardiogenic syncope. *Arq Bras Cardiol.* 2014;102(3):288-294.

352. Voulgari C, Pagoni S, Vinik A, Poirier P. Exercise improves cardiac autonomic function in obesity and diabetes. *Metabolism.* 2013;62(5):609-621.

353. Logan A, Freeman J, Pooler J, et al. Effectiveness of non-pharmacological interventions to treat orthostatic hypotension in elderly people and people with a neurological condition: a systematic review. *JBI Evid Synth.* 2020;12:2556-2617.

354. Mostarda CT, Rodrigues B, de Moraes OA, et al. Low intensity resistance training improves systolic function and cardiovascular autonomic control in diabetic rats. *J Diabetes Complications.* 2014;28(3):273-278.

355. Shankarappa SA, Piedras-Rentería ES, Stubbs EB Jr. Forced-exercise delays neuropathic pain in experimental diabetes: effects on voltage-activated calcium channels. *J Neurochem.* 2011;118(2):224-236.

356. Selagzi H, Buyukakilli B, Cimen B, Yilmaz N, Erdogan S. Protective and therapeutic effects of swimming exercise training on diabetic peripheral neuropathy of streptozotocin-induced diabetic rats. *J Endocrinol Invest.* 2008;31(11):971-978.

357. Roth B, Schiro DB, Ohlsson B. Diseases which cause generalized peripheral neuropathy: a systematic review. *Scand J Gastroenterol.* 2021;56(9):1000-1010.

358. Pavlakis PP. Rheumatologic disorders and the nervous system. *Continuum (Minneap Minn).* 2020;26(3):591-610.

359. Lin WL, Wang RH, Chou FH, Feng IJ, Fang CJ, Wang HH. The effects of exercise on chemotherapy-induced peripheral neuropathy symptoms in cancer patients: a systematic review and meta-analysis. *Support Care Cancer.* 2021;29(9):5303-5311.

360. Gordon T, English AW. Strategies to promote peripheral nerve regeneration: electrical stimulation and/or exercise. *Eur J Neurosci.* 2016;43(3):336-350.

361. Kleckner IR, Kamen C, Gewandter JS, et al. Effects of exercise during chemotherapy on chemotherapy-induced peripheral neuropathy: a multicenter, randomized controlled trial. *Support Care Cancer.* 2018;26(4):1019-1028.

362. Makhtari T, Ren Q, Li N, Wang F, Bi Y, Hu L. Transcutaneous electrical nerve stimulation in relieving neuropathic pain: basic mechanisms and clinical applications. *Curr Pain Headache Rep.* 2020;24(4):14.

363. Akyuz G, Kenis O. Physical therapy modalities and rehabilitation techniques in the management of neuropathic pain. *Am J Phys Med Rehabil.* 2014;93:253-259.

364. Murnion BP. Neuropathic pain: current definition and review of drug treatment. *Aust Prescr.* 2018;41(3):60-63.

365. Bland KA, Kirkham AA, Bovard J, et al. Effect of exercise on taxane chemotherapy-induced peripheral neuropathy in women with breast cancer: a randomized controlled trial. *Clin Breast Cancer.* 2019;19(6):411-422.

366. Ahmad I, Noohu MM, Verma S, Singla D, Hussain ME. Effect of sensorimotor training on balance measures and proprioception among middle and older age adults with diabetic peripheral neuropathy. *Gait Posture.* 2019;74:114-120.

367. Song CH, Petrofsky JS, Lee SW, Lee KJ, Yim JE. Effects of an exercise program on balance and trunk proprioception in older adults with diabetic neuropathies. *Diabetes Technol Ther.* 2011;13:803-811.

368. Nardone A, Godi M, Artuso A, Schieppati M. Balance rehabilitation by moving platform and exercises in patients with neuropathy or vestibular deficit. *Arch Phys Med Rehabil.* 2010;91(12):1869-1877.

369. Melese H, Alamer A, Hailu Temesgen M, Kahsay G. Effectiveness of exercise therapy on gait function in diabetic peripheral neuropathy patients: a systematic review of randomized controlled trials. *Diabetes Metab Syndr Obes.* 2020;13:2753-2764.

370. Mueller MJ, Tuttle LJ, LeMaster JW, Strube MJ. Weight-bearing versus nonweight-bearing exercise for persons with diabetes and peripheral neuropathy: a randomized controlled trial. *Arch Phys Med Rehabil.* 2013;94(5):829-838.

371. Ruhland JL, Shields RK. The effects of a home exercise program on impairment and health-related quality of life in persons with chronic peripheral neuropathies. *Phys Ther.* 1997;77:1026-1039.

372. Balducci S, Iacobellis G, Parisi L, et al. Exercise training can modify the natural history of diabetic peripheral neuropathy. *J Diabetes Complications.* 2006;20:216-223.

373. Gholami F, Nikookheslat S, Salekzamani Y, Boule N, Jafari A. Effect of aerobic training on nerve conduction in men with type 2 diabetes and peripheral neuropathy: a randomized control trial. *Neurophysiol Clin.* 2018;48(4):195-202.

374. Streckmann F, Balke M, Cavaletti G, et al. Exercise and neuropathy: systematic review with meta-analysis. *Sports Med.* 2022;52(5):1043-1065.

375. Carvajal-Moreno L, Coheña-Jiménez M, García-Ventura I, Pabón-Carrasco M, Pérez-Belloso AJ. Prevention of peripheral distal polyneuropathy in patients with diabetes: a systematic review. *J Clin Med.* 2022;11(6):1723.

376. Gigo-Benato D, Russo TL, Geuna S, Domingues NR, Salvini TF, Parizotto NA. Electrical stimulation impairs early functional recovery and accentuates skeletal muscle atrophy after sciatic nerve crush injury in rats. *Muscle Nerve.* 2010;41(5):685-693.

377. Ohtake PJ, Zafron ML, Poranki LG, Fish DR. Does electrical stimulation improve motor recovery in patients with idiopathic facial (Bell) palsy? *Phys Ther.* 2006;86(11):1558-1564.

378. Govidan M, burrows HL. Neonatal brachial plexus injury. *Pediatr Rev.* 2019;40(9):494-496.

379. Gilcrease-Garcia BM, Deshmukh SD, Parsons MS. Anatomy, imaging, and pathologic conditions of the brachial plexus. *Radiographics.* 2020;40:1686-1714.

380. Chauhan SP, Blackwell SB, Ananth CV. Neonatal brachial plexus palsy: incidence, prevalence, and temporal trends. *Semin Perinatol.* 2014;38(4):210-218.

381. Smania N, Berto G, La Marchina E, Melotti C, Midiri A, et al. Rehabilitation of brachial plexus injuries in adults and children. *Eur J Phys Rehabil Med.* 2012;48:483-506.

382. Yang LJ. Neonatal brachial plexus palsy: management and prognostic factors. *Semin Perinatol.* 2014;38:222-234, 243.

383. Schmieg S, Nguyen JC, Pehnke M, Yum SW, Shah AS. Team approach: management of brachial plexus birth injury. *J Bone Joint Surg.* 2020;8(7):e19.00200.

384. Werner JM, Berggren J, Loiselle J, Lee GK. Constraint-induced movement therapy for children with neonatal brachial plexus palsy: a randomized crossover trial. *Dev Med Child Neurol.* 2021;63:545-551.

385. Yeves-Lite A, Zuil-Escobar JC, Martinez-Cepa C, romay-Barrero H, Ferri-Morales A, Palomo-Carrion R. Conventional and virtual reality mirror therapies in upper obstetric brachial palsy: a randomized pilot study. *J Clin Med.* 2020;9:3021.

Review Questions

1. **If a sensory study shows prolonged latencies but a motor study on the same peripheral nerve is normal, what does this typically indicate?**
   A. Mild axonal injury
   B. Mild myelin injury
   C. Moderate axonal injury
   D. Moderate myelin injury

2. **In a needle EMG study, why is it important to study insertional activity?**
   A. To find evidence of axonal injury
   B. To find evidence of myopathy
   C. To study the neuromuscular junction
   D. To study the nociceptors

3. **What is the difference between H-reflex testing and F-wave testing?**
   A. Only F-wave testing requires normal motor neuron and motor axon function
   B. Only H-reflex testing is useful for detecting radiculopathy
   C. Only F-wave testing requires an intact nerve plexus
   D. Only H-reflex testing requires normal sensory axons

4. **Death from amyotrophic lateral sclerosis (ALS) from the time of diagnosis occurs on average in:**
   A. 6-12 months
   B. 1-3 years
   C. 3-5 years
   D. 5-7 years

5. **A variant of sporadic ALS that features spasticity with only slight weakness of the extremities due to dysfunction of the corticospinal tract without lower motor neuron involvement is:**
   A. Primary lateral sclerosis
   B. Progressive bulbar palsy
   C. Pseudobulbar palsy
   D. Progressive muscular atrophy

6. **Which of the following impairments is relatively rare in people with ALS?**
   A. Sensory deficits
   B. Dysphagia
   C. Weakness/paralysis of spinal muscles
   D. Fatigue

Questions 7 and 8 refer to the following scenario:

Mary Thomas is a 40-year-old female with familial ALS. She reports she has always been active prior to her diagnosis, playing tennis on the weekends and walking a mile every day with her dog.

Mary complains that her left (L) toes have been catching on the floor when she walks quickly and that she has occasional mild cramping in her calf muscles, L greater than R. Otherwise, she has no other complaints and is independent with all mobility and ADLs. On physical examination, you note L DF strength is 3/5. Bilateral quads and hamstring strength = 4/5; bilateral plantarflexor strength = 4+/5.

7. **Your best exercise prescription for Mary would be:**
   A. Passive ROM exercises for the L foot and ankle
   B. High-intensity walking program
   C. Instructing Mary to take frequent rests when walking longer distances
   D. A lower extremity strengthening program for the proximal muscles
   E. All of the above

8. **Which of the following findings would indicate a need to modify Mary's exercise plan?**
   A. A Grade of 2 when you reevaluate the muscle strength of her lower extremities
   B. Increased incidences of calf cramping after exercise
   C. Reports of increased fatigue the day after exercise
   D. Increased fasciculations in the lower extremities with exercise
   E. All of the above

9. **The tests that are most commonly used to diagnose Guillain–Barré syndrome (GBS) are:**
   A. Lumbar puncture, somatosensory evoked potentials, magnetic resonance imaging (MRI)
   B. Blood tests, electromyography (EMG), magnetic resonance imaging (MRI)
   C. Lumbar puncture, electromyography (EMG), magnetic resonance imaging (MRI)
   D. Lumbar puncture, electromyography (EMG), positron emission tomography (PET)

10. **In relation to the various subtypes of GBS, the most frequent subtype occurring in North America and Europe, which accounts for 90% of all GBS cases in these regions is:**
    A. Acute motor and sensory axonal neuropathy (AMSAN)
    B. Acute motor axonal neuropathy (AMAN)
    C. Acute inflammatory demyelinating polyradiculoneuropathy (AIDP)
    D. Miller Fisher syndrome

11. **Which of the following types of GBS has the worst prognosis?**
    A. Acute motor and sensory axonal neuropathy (AMSAN)

B. Acute inflammatory demyelinating polyradiculoneuropathy (AIDP)
    C. Chronic inflammatory demyelinating polyradiculopathy (CIDP)
    D. Miller Fisher syndrome

12. **Acute inflammatory demyelinating polyradiculoneuropathy (AIDP) attacks what part of the peripheral nerve?**
    A. Basement membranes surrounding Schwann cells
    B. Schwann cells
    C. Nodes of Ranvier
    D. Myelin sheath

13. **Which of the following immunotherapies has not demonstrated efficacy in the treatment of GBS?**
    A. Corticosteroids
    B. Plasma exchange
    C. Intravenous immunoglobulin
    D. All of the above have demonstrated efficacy in treating GBS

14. **Which of the following prognostic factors are associated with the WORST prognosis with GBS?**
    A. Progression of symptoms ≥7 days; did not require assisted ventilation; poor upper extremity muscle strength
    B. Progression of symptoms ≥7 days; respiratory muscle involvement requiring assisted ventilation; decreased amplitude findings on nerve conduction studies
    C. Progression of symptoms <7 days; did not require assisted ventilation; poor upper extremity muscle strength
    D. Progression of symptoms in <7 days; respiratory muscle involvement requiring assisted ventilation; decreased amplitude findings on nerve conduction studies

15. **The most appropriate initial exercise progression for a patient recovering from GBS with limb muscle strength ranging between P+ (2+) to F− (3−/5) strength is:**
    A. Functional based exercise → light progressive resistive exercise → active range of motion
    B. Passive range of motion → active range of motion gravity-eliminated → active range of motion against gravity
    C. Active range of motion against gravity → light progressive resistive exercise → functional-based exercise
    D. Active range of motion gravity-eliminated → active range of motion against gravity → light progressive resistive exercise

16. **Which form of neuropathy affects motor and sensory and leaves autonomic nerves intact?**
    A. Chronic inflammatory demyelinating polyradiculopathy
    B. Diabetic peripheral neuropathy
    C. Guillain–Barré
    D. Multifocal motor neuropathy

17. **Which classification of nerve injury by Sunderland involves disruption of the axon and endoneurium with the perineurium and epineurium being left intact?**
    A. 1st degree
    B. 2nd degree
    C. 3rd degree
    D. 4th degree

18. **Which nerve is the most common source for autografts?**
    A. Brachial
    B. Femoral
    C. Radial
    D. Sural

19. **Tinel's sign is when you:**
    A. Put the nerve on a stretch and the distal limb goes numb
    B. Tap over the nerve and there is tingling in its distribution
    C. Compress the nerve and there is tingling in its distribution
    D. Tap over the nerve and the limb forcefully flexes

20. **A therapy client who is using the stationary bike as part of his therapy completes 20 minutes of pedaling and his heart rate is elevated to 110 bpm. After 5 minutes his heart rate is still 110 bpm. This response indicates:**
    A. A possible myocardial infarction (MI)
    B. Enhanced parasympathetic activation
    C. Possible cardiac autonomic neuropathy
    D. Orthostatic hypotension

21. **An appropriate intervention for diabetic clients to prevent or slow neuropathy is:**
    A. Brisk walking for at least 8 hours a week for 8 weeks
    B. Brisk walking for at least 4 hours a week as a lifelong activity
    C. Resistance training of major muscle groups at least 3 times a week
    D. Daily electrical stimulation to involved muscles

22. **In individuals who have recovered from polio which of the following is a true statement regarding the neuromuscular unit?**
    A. Type I fibers are disproportionately impacted
    B. Remaining muscle fibers are unable to hypertrophy
    C. Single motor neurons may innervate up to 2000 muscle fibers
    D. Anterior horn cells may recover and regenerate to reinnervate the muscle

23. **Postpolio syndrome is diagnosed based on which of the following criteria?**
    A. There is a new onset of problems within 10 years of original infection

B. There is onset of weakness in previously unaffected muscles years after the original infection
    C. Blood tests show low levels of creatine kinase
    D. Muscle biopsy indicates long-term denervation with no signs of reinnervation

24. **True or False: It is believed that overwork plays a role in postpolio syndrome.**
    A. True
    B. False

25. **A client with postpolio syndrome comes to therapy with foot drop. She wishes to regain walking without the use of an AFO or with the least intrusive AFO possible. On testing the tibialis anterior is graded 1/5 or trace strength. A recommended therapy would be to:**
    A. Prescribe resistance strengthening for the tibialis anterior
    B. Prescribe a rigid AFO and discourage active dorsiflexion
    C. Implement strengthening of the extensor hallicus longus and extensor digitorum longus muscles to perform dorsiflexion
    D. Use a maximal exercise protocol working muscles to failure

26. **Principles for designing exercise programs for individuals who have postpolio syndrome include:**
    A. Working to the point of fatigue and mild muscle soreness
    B. Strengthening exercises for muscles with fair or lower strength grades
    C. High intensity, brief exercise
    D. Rotating exercise types such as aerobic and strengthening

27. **The name of brachial plexus injury with only C5 and C6 involvement is:**
    A. Erb's-Duchenne Palsy
    B. Klumpke's Palsy
    C. Smith's Palsy
    D. Class II Palsy

28. **Spontaneous recovery for obstetric brachial plexus injury occurs:**
    A. Rarely
    B. After surgery
    C. In a majority of cases
    D. With hypotonia

29. **Which of the following diagnoses should the therapist consider the risk for autonomic neuropathy in assessing and treating the patient?**
    A. Brachial Plexus Injury
    B. Brain tumor
    C. Parkinson disease
    D. Sciatica

30. Which of the following tests for autonomic neuropathy provides an indication of the impact of symptoms on daily life?
    A. Symptoms of autonomia survey
    B. Supine to stand test
    C. 10 minute lean test
    D. Survey of autonomic symptoms

31. Doing this is an effective means of raising blood pressure
    A. lying with feet elevated
    B. squatting
    C. sitting with legs externally rotated
    D. pursed lip breathing

32. Your client with autoimmune disease has peripheral neuropathies and is referred for physical therapy to improve function and mobility. Which of the following treatments has been shown to be beneficial for treating peripheral neuropathies?
    A. Long-term moderate or high-intensity aerobic exercise
    B. Stretching
    C. Yoga
    D. Aquatic therapy

33. A mutation in which of the following genes is responsible for about 40% of familial amyotrophic lateral sclerosis cases?
    A. SOD1
    B. FUS
    C. C9ORF72
    D. TARDBP

34. Pseudobulbar palsy in amyotrophic lateral sclerosis is caused by damage to:
    A. cranial motor neurons III, IV, and VI
    B. corticobulbar tract motor neurons
    C. corticospinal tract motor neurons
    D. cranial motor neurons IX, X, and XII

35. A type of dementia that some individuals with amyotrophic lateral sclerosis develop is:
    A. frontotemporal dementia
    B. Alzheimer's dementia
    C. Vascular dementia
    D. Lewy body dementia

36. The forced vital capacity (FVC) percent predicted criteria used to determine when noninvasive positive-pressure ventilation should be started in a person with amyotrophic lateral sclerosis is:
    A. <70%
    B. <60%
    C. <50%
    D. <40%

37. The most common long-term deficit of individuals with Guillain–Barré syndrome is weakness of the:
    A. quadriceps muscle
    B. tibialis anterior muscle
    C. gluteus maximus muscle
    D. peroneal muscle

38. Which of the following interventions significantly improved sleep quality in people with Guillain–Barré syndrome?
    A. Treadmill walking
    B. Cycling on a recumbent bike
    C. Proprioceptive neuromuscular facilitation exercises to extremities
    D. Yoga

39. A patient with type II diabetes presents to your physical therapy clinic with severe left-sided back pain with progressive proximal weakness and atrophy of muscles in the left leg. Based, on the history, you suspect that the patient might have:
    A. Cardiovascular diabetic neuropathy
    B. Lumbosacral diabetic radiculoplexus neuropathy
    C. Unilateral truncal radiculopathy
    D. Chronic inflammatory demyelinating polyradiculopathy

40. Which of the following is associated with EMG/NCS in infants with postganglionic brachial plexus injury?
    A. Absent or reduced SNAP
    B. Normal SNAP
    C. Exaggerated CMAPs
    D. Normal CMAP

41. Early physical therapy treatment prior to discharge from the nursery for a neonatal brachial plexus injury focuses on what?
    A. Instruction on how to stimulate motor milestones
    B. Muscle re-education, using electrical stimulation
    C. Parental instruction of positioning and passive stretching
    D. Splinting the hand to prevent contractures.

Answers

1. B	2. A	3. D	4. C	5. A
6. A	7. D	8. E	9. C	10. C
11. A	12. D	13. A	14. D	15. D
16. A	17. C	18. D	19. B	20. C
21. B	22. C	23. B	24. A	25. C
26. D	27. A	28. C	29. C	30. D
31. B	32. A	33. C	34. B	35. A
36. C	37. B	38. D	39. B	40. A
41. C				

GLOSSARY

Allograft. A donor graph from a cadaver.

Antidromic volley. Conduction of a nerve stimulus back toward the nerve cell body.

Autograft. A nerve graph from another site on the individual.

Complex polyphasic potential. An abnormal waveform with multiple baseline crossings, associated with partial reinnervation of a damaged axon.

Complex repetitive discharge. Motor unit firing at an extreme rate for several seconds, followed by a gradual reduction and abrupt shutoff, associated with neuropathy or myopathy.

Conduction velocity. The difference in the distance between 2 stimulation sites, divided by the latency difference.

Dermatome. An area of the skin that is supplied by a single spinal nerve.

Dyspnea. Difficult, painful breathing, or shortness of breath.

Fasciculation. A spontaneous potential of an entire motor unit.

Fibrillation. An abnormal spontaneous potential that has both a positive and negative wave form but involves a single muscle fiber.

Forced vital capacity. The amount of air that a person can forcibly exhale from the lungs after taking the deepest breath possible.

Full interference pattern. A chaotic waveform caused by a moderate to full muscle contraction.

F-wave. Stimulation of alpha motor axons, leading to an antidromic response.

Giant potential. An abnormally large action potential associated with a partially denervated muscle.

H-reflex. Peripheral stimulation of the monosynaptic stretch reflex.

Maximum expiratory pressure. A measure of the strength of respiratory muscles, obtained by having a person exhale as strongly as possible against an occluded airway.

Maximum inspiratory pressure. The maximum inspiratory pressure that a person can generate against a completely occluded airway; used to evaluate inspiratory muscle strength and a person's readiness for weaning from mechanical ventilation. A maximum inspiratory pressure above −25 cm H_2O is associated with successful weaning.

Myopathic potential. Waveform associated with loss of muscle fibers.

Myotome. Set of muscles that are innervated by a single spinal nerve.

Myotonic discharge. An abnormal waveform with a variable pattern of increased and decreased activity within the muscle, typically associated with myopathy.

Nerve conduction studies. Test health and integrity of peripheral nerves.

Noninvasive positive-pressure ventilation. Delivery of mechanical ventilation to patients with respiratory failure through a face mask, nasal mask, or helmet.

Orthodromic volley. An action potential conducted from the cell body to the axon terminal.

Orthopnea. A feeling of breathlessness when lying down, relieved by sitting or standing.

Peak cough expiratory flow. Peak expiratory flow measured during a cough used to determine cough effectiveness.

Positive sharp wave. A spontaneous potential that is brief and only in a positive (downward direction).

Primary lateral sclerosis. A rare motor neuron disease that affects the upper motor neurons causing progressive spasticity affecting the lower extremities, trunk, upper extremities, and bulbar muscles, usually in that order.

Progressive bulbar palsy. A motor neuron disease that causes degeneration of cranial motor neurons in the lower brainstem resulting in dysarthria, dysphagia, facial weakness, tongue weakness, and fasciculations of the tongue and facial muscles.

Progressive muscular atrophy. A rare motor neuron disease that causes degeneration of lower motor neurons, resulting in generalized, progressive loss of muscle function mostly limited to the upper and lower extremities.

Pseudobulbar palsy. A neurologic condition due to bilateral damage of upper motor neurons in the corticobulbar tracts, causing spasticity and weakness in bulbar muscles, and resultant dysarthria, dysphagia, facial and tongue weakness, and emotional lability.

Satellite potentials. A small slower potential that follows a giant potential.

Sniff nasal inspiratory pressure. A measure of inspiratory muscle strength, obtained by measuring peak nasal pressure in one occluded nostril during a maximal sniff performed from relaxed end-expiration through the contralateral patent nostril.

Spontaneous potentials. Involuntary denervation potentials.

Subclinical. A disease or symptoms that are not severe enough to present easily observable symptoms.

Temporal dispersion. The spreading of the arrival of action potentials.

Utilization time. The delay in the onset of an action potential from the time of stimulation to the onset of the action potential.

ABBREVIATIONS

6MWT	six minute walk test
10MWT	10 meter walk test
ADL	activities of daily living
AIDP	acute inflammatory demyelinating polyneuropathy
ALS	amyotrophic lateral sclerosis
ALSAQ-40	ALS-Specific Quality of Life-40
ALS-CBS-ALS	Cognitive Behavioral Screen
ALSbi	ALS with behavioral impairment
ALSci	ALS with cognitive impairment

ALScbi	ALS with cognitive and behavioral impairment		FVC	forced vital capacity
ALSFRS-R	ALS Functional Rating Scale-Revised		GBS	Guillian-Barre syndrome
ALS-FTD	ALS-frontotemporal dementia		HADS	Hospital Anxiety and Depression Scale
ALS-PDC	ALS-parkinsonism dementia complex		HR	heart rate
AMAN	acute motor axonal neuropathy		HIV	human immunodeficiency virus
AMS	active movement score		INT	inspiratory muscle training
AVAPS	average volume-assured pressure support		IV	intravenous
BBS	Berg Balance Scale		IVIg	intravenous immunoglobulin
BDI	Beck Depression Inventory		LMN	lower motor neuron
BiPAP	bi-level positive airway pressure		LVRT	lung volume recruitment training
BP	blood pressure		MAC	manually assisted coughs
BPI	Brief Pain Inventory		MEP	maximum expiratory pressure
BPI	Brachial Plexus Injury		MI-E	mechanical insufflation-exsufflation
BPP	Brachial Plexus Palsy		MIP	maximum inspiratory pressure
CAN	cardiovascular autonomic neuropathy		MMT	manual muscle test
CIDP	chronic inflammatory demyelinating polyneuropathy		MND	motor neuron disease
			MRI	magnetic resonance imaging
CIMT	constraint-induced movement therapy		MVIC	maximum voluntary isometric contraction
CMAPS	compound muscle action potentials		NCS	nerve conduction study
ECAS	Edinburgh Cognitive and Behavioral ALS Screen		NFI-PP	Neurological Fatigue Index for Post-Polio
			NINDS	National Institute of Neurological Disorders
EMG	clinical electromyography		NIPPV	noninvasive positive-pressure ventilation
EMT	expiratory muscle training		PCEF	peak cough expiratory flow
EQ-5D	EuroQuol-5D		PEG	percutaneous endoscopic gastrostomy
FEV1	forced expiratory volume in 1 second		POMA	Tinetti Performance Oriented Mobility Assessment
FIM	Functional Independence Measure			
FRT	Functional Reach Test		SNAP	sensory nerve action potential
FSS	Fatigue Severity Scale			

Vestibular/Cerebellar Disorders

17

Anne D. Kloos

OBJECTIVES

1) Compare and contrast the pathophysiology of common disorders of the vestibular system

2) Describe the medical and surgical management of common vestibular disorders

3) Differentiate between signs and symptoms caused by peripheral versus central vestibular pathology

4) Describe the physical therapist management of individuals with vestibular dysfunction

5) Discuss the physical therapy goals and expected outcomes of vestibular rehabilitation

6) Discuss the common causes of cerebellar pathology

7) Describe the physical therapist management of individuals with movement dysfunction secondary to cerebellar damage

8) Discuss the physical therapy goals and expected outcomes of rehabilitation for individuals with movement dysfunction secondary to cerebellar damage

CASE A, PART I

Mrs. O'Hara, a 55-year-old woman, is experiencing episodes of "dizziness," beginning 2 weeks ago. She reports that her initial episode of "dizziness" occurred while she was rolling over in bed from her right to left side, and she describes feeling as if "the room was spinning." The episode lasted for a few seconds and went away by keeping her head completely still. She had mild nausea but no vomiting. The "dizziness" returned when she attempted to get out of bed to go the bathroom, lessened once she was upright, and worsened when she went to lie back down in bed. Mrs. O'Hara also noted that, over the past 2 weeks, the spinning sensations occurred when she looked up to reach for something in a cupboard in her kitchen or when she looked down to put on her shoes. While sitting, she has no symptoms. She notes that her symptoms started after she slipped on a patch of ice that caused her to fall and hit her head.

● ANATOMY AND PHYSIOLOGY OF THE VESTIBULAR SYSTEM

The anatomy and physiology of the vestibular system and its role in the control of eye movements (via the vestibulo-ocular reflex) and postural stability (via the vestibulospinal reflex) are discussed in Chapter 6.

● DISORDERS OF THE VESTIBULAR SYSTEM

Disorders of the vestibular system are common, especially among the elderly. One large epidemiological study estimated that as many as 35% of adults aged 40 years or older in the United States (approximately 69 million Americans) have experienced some form of vestibular dysfunction,[1] which increases to 50% of community-dwelling adults older than 80 years reporting dizziness.[2] Elderly individuals with dizziness also report memory problems and anxiety more frequently than non-dizzy elderly, which negatively impacts their quality of life.[3]

Vestibular disorders can be categorized by their location into peripheral and central vestibular disorders. Peripheral vestibular disorders involve the inner ear vestibular structures and/or the vestibular nerve. Central vestibular disorders primarily result from damage to the vestibular nuclei, the cerebellum, and the brainstem, including vestibular pathways within the brainstem that mediate vestibular reflexes (i.e., vestibulo-ocular reflex [VOR] and the vestibulospinal reflex [VSR]).

Peripheral Vestibular Disorders

Based on the anatomy, pathophysiology, and signs and symptoms, peripheral vestibular disorders can be further divided into the following three types: (1) acute unilateral vestibular hypofunction with the main symptom of acute onset rotatory vertigo; (2) bilateral vestibular hypofunction with the main symptom of postural imbalance; and (3) recurrent pathological excitation or inhibition of the peripheral vestibular system with the main symptom of recurrent attacks of vertigo.[4]

Unilateral Vestibular Hypofunction

Unilateral vestibular hypofunction (UVH) is characterized by a reduction or loss of peripheral vestibular function and can be caused by viral or bacterial infections (e.g., **vestibular neuritis** or neuronitis, **labyrinthitis**), head trauma, vascular occlusion, and unilateral vestibulopathy, following surgical procedures (e.g., labyrinthectomy and acoustic neuroma resections). Individuals with UVH experience (1) acute onset of severe rotational **vertigo** (a sensation of spinning), (2) **spontaneous horizontal-rotatory nystagmus**, beating toward the unaffected ear, (3) slight **oscillopsia** (perception that visualized objects are oscillating), when turning the head quickly to the affected side, (4) postural instability with a tendency to fall toward the affected side, and (5) nausea and vomiting. The symptoms of vertigo and nystagmus are produced by an imbalance of the tonic firing rates of the left and right sides of the vestibular system. At rest, vestibular afferents and their corresponding vestibular nuclei typically have a tonic firing rate of approximately 70 to 100 spikes per second. Damage to the vestibular system that decreases function unilaterally creates an imbalance between the two sides that results in the brain's misperception that movement of the head has occurred (in the direction of the more neutrally active healthy ear) and triggers the VOR in a corrective response.[5] Vision may become blurred with quick head movements to the affected side due to an impaired VOR. Imbalance, especially with head turns, results from decreased activation of the VSR on the affected side. Thus, a person with left UVH may experience sensations of spinning in a clockwise direction (i.e., toward the healthy right ear), spontaneous horizontal right-beating nystagmus (slow-phase VOR eye movement to the left followed by fast saccades to the right), and blurred vision and loss of balance to the left side with head rotations to the left. With acute vertigo, excessive autonomic nervous system activity causes nausea, vomiting, pallor, and perspiration. Hearing loss occurs with labyrinthitis or following labyrinthectomy. Resolution of vertigo and spontaneous nystagmus usually occurs within 3 to 7 days in lit environments, as the patient can suppress the nystagmus with visual fixation, but spontaneous nystagmus may always be present in the dark. The dynamic VOR and postural instability resolution is usually slower and may take up to a year.[6] Initial treatment includes administration of vestibular suppressants (e.g., dimenhydrinate, scopolamine), antiemetic, and antinausea medications, and the patient may be put on bed rest. However, once the symptoms diminish, the patient should start to ambulate, and vestibular suppressants are stopped to promote CNS compensation. Individuals with residual gaze instability and balance impairments may benefit from physical therapy.

Vestibular Schwannoma (Acoustic Neuroma)

Vestibular schwannomas (VSs), historically called **acoustic neuromas**, are the most common intracranial tumors producing vestibular symptoms (Figure 17-1).[7] They are usually slow-growing, benign tumors that originate from the Schwann cells, lining the vestibular portion of the eighth cranial nerve, often within the internal auditory canal (IAC). The IAC also contains the facial nerve (cranial nerve VII). Early in the disease, when the tumor is small, patients may complain of vertigo, disequilibrium, tinnitus, and asymmetric hearing loss due to compression of the vestibulocochlear nerve. The slow growth of the tumor often allows for the brain to compensate, thereby, alleviating symptoms (see Figure 17-1B). With continued growth, the tumor can

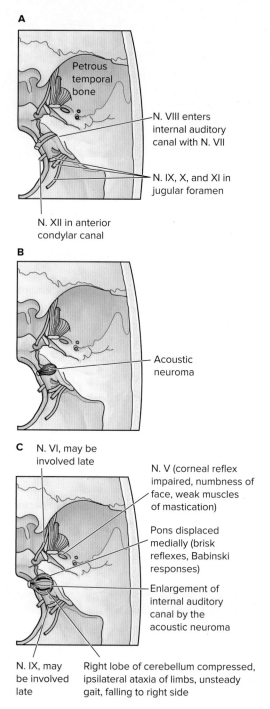

FIGURE 17-1 Vestibular schwannoma (acoustic neuroma). A. View of CN VII and VIII as they enter the internal auditory canal in proximity to CN IX, X, and XI. **B.** Early stage acoustic neuroma impinging on CN VII and VIII. **C.** Late stage acoustic neuroma impinging on pons. (Reproduced with permission from Martin JH (Ed). *Neuroanatomy Text and Atlas*, 4th Ed. New York, NY: McGraw-Hill; 2012.)

compress the facial nerve within the IAC or the trigeminal nerve (cranial nerve V) at its root or ganglion, causing facial weakness and numbness, respectively. Eventually, the tumor grows to a size where it compresses the brainstem and cerebellum, causing difficulty in swallowing, impaired eye movements, gait ataxia, and possibly death (see Figure-1C). VS may be treated with observation, microsurgical resection, stereotactic radiotherapy (e.g., gamma knife), or a combination of these, with the goal of maximal control of tumor growth with functional deficits.[8] With tumor removal, there is loss of vestibular nerve function, resulting in asymmetrical vestibular inputs. Ideally, physical therapy is started in the postoperative period to help relieve disequilibrium and oscillopsia symptoms, followed by outpatient treatment similar to treatment for UVH as needed.

Bilateral Vestibular Hypofunction

Bilateral vestibular hypofunction (BVH) or loss is most commonly caused by ototoxicity from taking certain classes of antibiotics (e.g., aminoglycosides gentamicin and streptomycin). Other possible causes include infections (meningitis, bilateral sequential vestibular neuritis), inner-ear autoimmune disorders, (e.g., Cogan's syndrome, ulcerative colitis, rheumatoid arthritis), bilateral Ménière's disease, bilateral tumors (VSs in neurofibromatosis), and bilateral vestibulopathy due to aging. The prominent symptoms of BVH are disequilibrium, severe postural instability with resultant gait ataxia, and oscillopsia with head movement due to bilaterally impaired or absent VSR and VOR, respectively.[9] Unless BVH is asymmetrical, individuals will not complain of nausea, vertigo, or nystagmus, because there is no asymmetry of tonic resting firing rates of vestibular afferents. BVH symptoms are likely permanent, but people can return to high functional levels.

Recurrent Vestibular Disorders

Vestibular disorders that produce recurrent disruptions in vestibular function include benign paroxysmal positional vertigo, Ménière's disease (endolymphatic hydrops), and perilymphatic fistula. These disorders are characterized by intermittent periods of normal vestibular function with periods of abnormal function.[10]

Benign Paroxysmal Positional Vertigo (BPPV)

Benign paroxysmal positional vertigo (BPPV) is the most common peripheral vestibular disorder and is the cause of approximately 40% of dizziness in older people.[11] It typically affects women more than men, in their fourth and fifth decades of life.[12] This condition occurs as a result of otoconia detaching from the otolithic membrane in the utricle and migrating into one of the semicircular canals (SCCs). BPPV can be categorized by the particular SCC involved and whether the detached otoconia are free-floating within the affected canal (**canalithiasis**) or attached to the cupula (**cupulolithiasis**). The most common form, accounting for 81 to 90% of all cases, is canalithiasis in the posterior SCC.[13] Because the otoconia have more than twice the density of the endolymph within the SCCs, the involved canal becomes gravity-sensitive. The shifting of otoconia with head movements causes deflection of the cupula, thereby sending abnormal input to the brain, resulting in the person's complaints of vertigo as well as observable nystagmus. Other symptoms of BPPV may include disequilibrium, mild postural instability, and nausea. BPPV is typically unilateral; bilateral involvement is rare but can occur in association with head trauma. Activities that provoke symptoms vary across individuals, but they all involve rapidly changing the head's position with respect to gravity.

With posterior SCC involvement, common problematic head movements include looking up, or rolling over and getting out of bed. In most people, the cause of BPPV is unknown, but conditions associated with higher incidence of BPPV are traumatic head injury, vestibular neuritis, labyrinthine ischemia, and age-related degeneration of the otolithic membrane.[14] Physical therapy, consisting of head maneuvers and vestibular rehabilitation exercises, is the first choice of treatment for BPPV (see Physical Therapy Treatment section of this chapter). If the maneuvers and exercises are ineffective in controlling symptoms, surgical plugging to stop the movement of particles within the affected posterior SCC or sectioning of the nerve to the posterior SCC has >96% success rate.[12]

Ménière's Disease

Ménière's disease is a recurrent disorder of the inner ear that typically affects women more than men in their fourth and fifth decades of life.[7] The pathophysiology involves increased endolymphatic pressure within the inner ear possibly caused by malabsorption of endolymph in the endolymphatic duct and sac, leading to inappropriate nerve excitation.[15] Magnetic resonance imaging of the inner ear of patients with Meniere's disease shows enlargement of the endolympathic space into areas that are normally occupied by perilymphatic space, a condition called **endolymphatic hydrops**.[16] This finding in addition to the three cardinal symptoms of Meniere's disease, namely vertigo, hearing loss, and tinnitus, aid in making the diagnosis.[15,16] Attacks typically start as aural fullness (e.g., pressure, discomfort, fullness sensation in the ears), a reduction in hearing, and tinnitus (usually low-tone roaring), followed by rotational vertigo, postural imbalance, nystagmus, and nausea and vomiting after a few minutes.[17] The severe vertigo and disequilibrium typically last from 20 minutes to up to 24 hours and can be debilitating.[16] Within 72 hours, these symptoms usually subside and the person can walk. Hearing and tinnitus will also recover, but there may be residual permanent sensorineural hearing loss, particularly in the lower frequencies. With advanced disease, hearing does not return after the attack, and the symptoms of vertigo lessen in frequency and severity.

Medical treatment aims to prevent or reduce the severity and frequency of vertigo attacks, and relieve and prevent hearing loss, tinnitus, and aural fullness. Patients with Ménière's disease should be educated on lifestyle changes that may reduce symptoms such as dietary restrictions of salt and caffeine, and stress and allergy management.[18] Pharmacologic treatments include vestibular suppressant, antiemetic, and antinausea medications during acute episodes. Long-term use of betahistine (SERC; not currently FDA-approved but can be obtained by prescription at many compounding pharmacies in the United States) to prevent vertigo attacks and diuretics to decrease endolymph volume may be prescribed, but their effectiveness is unclear.[18,19] In patients with disabling vertigo that does not respond to medications, surgical interventions to stop abnormal vestibular inputs, completed via chemical ablation with transtympanic gentamicin injection, vestibular neurectomy, or labyrinthectomy may be indicated.[20,21] Vestibular exercises are not recommended during acute attacks, but physical therapy may be beneficial for patients in treating the effects of chronic UVH or BVH, in the later stages of the disease or in treating disequilibrium after destructive surgical procedures.[18]

Perilymphatic Fistula (PLF)

A perilymphatic fistula (PLF) is commonly caused by a tear or defect in the oval and/or round windows that separate the air-filled middle ear and the fluid-filled perilymphatic space of the inner ear. This small opening allows perilymph to leak into the middle ear. PLF is usually caused by head trauma (often minor), excessive intracranial or atmospheric pressure changes as in rapid airplane descent or scuba diving, extremely loud noises, objects perforating the tympanic membrane, ear surgery (stapedectomy), or vigorous straining as in lifting a heavy object. Patients report a "pop" in the ear, followed by the onset of sudden vertigo, hearing loss, and loud tinnitus.[18] Other symptoms may include postural imbalance, nystagmus, nausea, and vomiting. Some people experience pressure sensitivity, meaning that their symptoms may get worse with coughing, sneezing, or blowing their nose, as well as with exertion and activity. Conservative treatment focuses on avoidance of anything that could increase inner ear or intracranial pressure such as sneezing, coughing, or straining to allow spontaneous healing of the membrane. If the cause of the PLF is known or conservative treatment fails, surgery to seal the fistulas, using tissue grafts, is performed.[21] Physical therapy is usually not needed for PLF, unless disequilibrium continues or UVH develops following surgery.

A particular variant of PLF, called **superior semicircular canal dehiscence**, occurs when a portion of the temporal bone that normally covers the superior (i.e., anterior) SCC is thin or missing, exposing the membranous SCC to stimuli that it normally does not receive (e.g., sound, changes in intracranial pressure, vibrations). Individuals with this condition often experience an unusual symptom called **Tullio's phenomenon** in which vestibular symptoms (i.e., vertigo, oscillopsia, nystagmus, ocular tilt reaction, and postural imbalance) are induced by auditory stimuli (e.g., loud noises, their own voice, or a musical instrument).[22]

Table 17-1 summarizes the hallmark symptoms of the peripheral vestibular disorders.

Central Vestibular Disorders

Causes of central vestibular disorders occurring with dizziness are vertebrobasilar ischemic disease (including vertebrobasilar insufficiency [VBI] and stroke), traumatic head injury, migraine-associated dizziness, and conditions that affect the brainstem and cerebellum (e.g., cerebellar degeneration, multiple sclerosis [MS], and tumors).

Vertebrobasilar Ischemic Stroke/Insufficiency

The blood supply to the brainstem, cerebellum, and inner ear is derived from the vertebrobasilar system (see Chapter 11). Occlusion of the subclavian, vertebral, or basilar arteries or their major branches, including the posterior inferior cerebellar

TABLE 17-1	Symptomatology of Peripheral Vestibular Disorders				
	UVH	**BVH**	**BPPV**	**MÉNIÈRE'S DISEASE**	**PERILYMPHATIC FISTULA**
Vertigo	+	−	+	+	+
Nystagmus	+	−	+	+	−/+
Duration of vertigo	Days to weeks	Not applicable	30 seconds–2 minutes	30 minutes–24 hours	Seconds to minutes
Nausea	+	−	−/+	+	−/+
Postural imbalance	+	++	+	+	+
Specific symptoms	Acute onset, tinnitus, hearing loss with labyrinthitis	Gait ataxia	Onset latency, adaptation	Fullness of ear, tinnitus, hearing loss	Loud tinnitus, Tullio's phenomenon
Precipitating event	Upper respiratory or gastrointestinal infection	Treatment with antibiotics (gentamicin, streptomycin)	Looking up, turning in bed	Not applicable	Head trauma, ear surgery, coughing, sneezing, straining
Outcome	Resolution of most symptoms by 1 year; vertigo in dark may be permanent	Symptoms are typically permanent	Resolved with PT or surgery in most people	Vertigo severity diminishes but hearing loss is often permanent	Usually resolves in 4 weeks

Abbreviations: BPPV, benign paroxysmal positional vertigo; BVH, bilateral vestibular hypofunction; UVH, unilateral vestibular hypofunction; Key: −, Absent; +, present; ++, very strong.

artery, anterior inferior cerebellar artery, or superior cerebellar artery may result in vertigo. Posterior inferior cerebellar artery occlusion to the dorsolateral aspect of the medulla will result in Wallenberg's syndrome (lateral medullary syndrome). Lateral pontomedullary infarction secondary to occlusion of the anterior inferior cerebellar artery will result in lateral inferior pontine syndrome. Lateral superior pontine syndrome occurs when the superior cerebellar artery is occluded. For description of these syndromes, refer to Chapter 11.

Vertebrobasilar insufficiency is synonymous with a transient ischemic attack (TIA) of the vertebrobasilar system and is a common cause of vertigo in the elderly. Other associated symptoms of VBI include blurred vision or diplopia, drop attacks (sudden fall without loss of consciousness), syncope (fainting) or weakness, ataxia, and headaches. If left untreated, the disease process can progress to a stroke with long-lasting or permanent sequela. In fact, 29% of 84 patients with vertebrobasilar ischemic strokes had at least one episode of vertigo prior to their strokes.[23] Thus, it is important for clinicians to consider stroke in any person with acute vertigo and other concomitant neurologic signs and symptoms.

Traumatic Head Injury

Central vestibular disturbances are common, following head trauma secondary to diffuse damage to long white fiber tracts.[24] About 50 to 75% of individuals with mild traumatic brain injury (TBI) may complain of vertigo that can persist for years, while almost all individuals with moderate brain injury complain of vertigo at some time.[25] Central vestibular lesions from head trauma often result in vestibular symptoms of vertigo, nystagmus, and balance dysfunction that are accompanied by other neurologic signs such as hemisensory loss, hemiparesis, or ataxia depending on the CNS area involved.[26] BPPV is a common cause of vertigo after TBI.[26] The evaluation of individuals with head trauma is complicated because the peripheral vestibular system and the neck may also be injured. Peripheral vestibular injuries are often associated with temporal and/or facial bone fractures. Flexion–extension (i.e., "whiplash") injuries to the neck can also result in dizziness (see Cervicogenic Dizziness section).

Vestibular Migraine (VM)

Migraine-associated dizziness, referred to as vestibular migraine (VM), affects an estimated 6.1 million individuals in the United States, or 2.7% of the population.[27] People with a history of migraine headaches may experience episodic symptoms of vertigo, dizziness, imbalance, and motion sickness that can last minutes to hours.[28,29] About 50% of patients also experience cochlear symptoms (tinnitus, aural fullness, and hearing loss) with vertigo.[29] In most patients, these symptoms are associated with a migraine headache and/or photophobia (intolerance to light) or phonophobia (intolerance to loud sounds), but some patients may experience these symptoms without a headache.[4] The diagnosis of VM is complicated because it presents very similar to UVH, BPPV, or Ménière's disease.[30] Diagnostic criteria for definite VM include vestibular symptoms lasting 5 minutes to 72 hours with concurrent or previous history of migraine headaches, and at least half of the episodes of vestibular symptoms occur simultaneously with migraine symptoms.[30]

Risk factors associated with VM are age less than 40, female sex, a self-reported history of anxiety or depression, and prior head trauma.[27] Migraine headaches can be controlled with medications and lifestyle changes to avoid triggers for migraines (e.g., stress, diet, fluorescent lights). Vestibular rehabilitation may be beneficial for individuals with migraines that are controlled,[31,32] but exercises that stimulate the vestibular system can trigger migraines, if they are not controlled.[33]

Conditions Affecting the Brainstem and Cerebellum

Individuals with conditions that cause cerebellar degeneration (e.g., spinocerebellar ataxias, episodic ataxias, Friedreich's ataxia, cerebellar cortical atrophy, multiple system atrophy) may present with oculomotor deficits (abnormal ocular pursuit and improperly sized saccades), nystagmus (especially with downward and lateral gaze), incoordination of the extremities, a wide-based ataxic gait with uneven stride lengths, and inability to tandem walk.[31] Patients with disorders affecting the vestibulocerebellum may have difficulty with sensory integration, particularly visual-vestibular interaction, which may manifest as difficulty performing rapid head movements and maintaining balance while walking.[31] Demyelinating diseases such as MS may affect the vestibular nuclei, medial longitudinal fasciculus, and/or cerebellum, causing central vestibular dysfunction. Symptoms of vertigo, nystagmus (gaze-evoked and pendular), and disequilibrium are common in patients with MS.[26] Tumors in the brainstem and cerebellum may affect vestibular nuclei, central vestibular pathways, and the vestibulocerebellum.

OTHER DIAGNOSES INVOLVING THE VESTIBULAR SYSTEM

Motion Sickness/Persistent Postural-Perceptual Dizziness (PPPD)

Many individuals with or without vestibular disorders experience dizziness and imbalance with self-movement (e.g., passively riding in a car or airplane), or when they are in stimulating visual environments, such as walking in supermarket aisles, driving in traffic, or watching car-chase scenes in films. These different types of motions also provoke symptoms of nausea and vomiting, that are often preceded by pallor, malaise, drowsiness, and irritability.[34] This so-called motion sickness is thought to be caused by conflict between the vestibular, visual, and other proprioceptive systems.[35] For example, consider the situation when you read in the car. Your eyes, fixed on the page, say that your head and body are not moving. However, as the car goes over bumps and accelerates/decelerates, your ears (i.e., vestibular system) say that you are moving. This mismatch between what the visual and vestibular systems may explain why motion sickness is common in this scenario. Individuals who have a current or prior vestibular disorder are particularly susceptible to developing dizziness in visually stimulating environments, called visual vertigo, thought to be due to an overreliance on visual cues for balance control, leading to "visual dependency."[36,37]

Motion sickness is a component of a chronic functional disorder called PPPD. Primary symptoms of PPPD are dizziness, unsteadiness, or non-spinning vertigo present on most days for at least 3 months. These symptoms are exacerbated by upright posture, moving about actively or being moved passively (e.g., standing, walking, or riding in a vehicle), or exposure to moving visual stimuli or complex visual patterns (i.e., visual vertigo). Secondary effects of PPPD include fear of falling, anxiety or depressive disorders, and agoraphobia. Individuals with PPPD often demonstrate significant stiffening in their postural strategies leading to reduced horizontal and increased vertical body sway in quiet stance and gait disorders described as a slow or hesitant gait and/or a "walking on ice" gait pattern.[38,39]

Treatment for motion sickness and PPPD generally consists of vestibular rehabilitation, cognitive-behavioral interventions, and medications. Vestibular rehabilitation programs for patients with motion sickness and PPPD include education about the condition, integrated relaxation/mindfulness practice, habituation exercises that gradually increase the amount of body/visual motion to promote desensitization and increase tolerance to the provoking stimuli, and balance training.[36,40,41] Cognitive-behavioral interventions include psychotherapeutic counseling and education on strategies to reduce symptoms that focus on synchronizing the visual system with the motion by looking at the visual horizon, and mentally rehearsing a trip route in advance.[39,42] Medications such as scopolamine, antihistamines (dimenhydrinate [Dramamine] and cyclizine [Marezine]), and selective serotonin reuptake inhibitors are prescribed for relief of dizziness and unsteadiness.[34,39,42]

Cervicogenic Dizziness

Cervicogenic dizziness (also called cervical vertigo) is defined as symptoms of dizziness (including vertigo, disequilibrium, and light-headedness) arising from the cervical spine.[43] The main causes of cervicogenic dizziness are believed to be altered proprioceptive signals from the upper cervical spine, caused by disorders in vertebral segments C1–C3 and VBI (see Vertebrobasilar Ischemic Stroke/Insufficiency section). Similar to motion sickness, conflict between the vestibular, visual, and cervical inputs has been proposed to explain how cervical pain can lead to dizziness.[43] Inaccurate afferent inputs from inflamed or irritated cervical roots, proprioceptors of the facet joints, or the cervical musculature conflict with vestibular and visual inputs converging on brainstem nuclei (i.e., vestibular nuclei and reticular formation), resulting in altered oculomotor function and VOR, altered balance function, and perceptions of dizziness. Dizziness associated with neck pain is most common in patients with whiplash injuries, but also occurs in patients with cervical spondylosis and those treated with cervical traction.[27] Physical therapy for cervical dysfunction and/or vestibular rehabilitation may be beneficial for these individuals.[44,45]

● MEDICAL ASSESSMENT AND MANAGEMENT

Physicians use information from a person's medical history and findings from a physical examination as a basis for ordering diagnostic tests to assess the vestibular system function and to rule out alternative causes of symptoms.

Vestibular Function Tests

Electronystagmography/Videonystagmography

Electronystagmography (ENG) is a battery of eye movement tests that look for signs of vestibular dysfunction or neurological problems. During ENG, eye movements are recorded and analyzed, using small surface electrodes placed on the skin around the eyes. Alternatively, eye movements may be recorded using videonystagmography (VNG), using an infrared video camera mounted inside **Frenzel goggles** that the patient wears. Frenzel goggles consist of magnifying glasses and a lighting system that, when worn in a darkened room, allow the illuminated and magnified patient's eyes to be easily seen and prevent the patient from being able to suppress nystagmus by focusing the eyes. ENG/VNG tests include measures of (1) oculomotor function (including gaze stability and velocity, latency, and gain of smooth pursuit and saccadic eye movements) to identify pathology within the central oculomotor and vestibular systems, (2) positional testing (various head and whole body positions including the Dix–Hallpike maneuver) to determine positions that cause nystagmus, and (3) the caloric test (warm or cold water or air is circulated in the ear canal) to test horizontal SCC function (see Chapter 6 – Special Senses for Specifics on this test).[46] Eye movements for warm and cold irrigations in each ear are recorded, specifically, the peak slow component eye velocity (SCEV) is measured (i.e., slow phase of nystagmus); from this, and a unilateral weakness percent (UW%), also referred to as the percent reduced vestibular response (%RVR), is calculated between the two ears. A difference of ≥26% is usually indicative of a clinically significant unilateral weakness in the ear producing lesser responses.[46] The caloric test is considered the "gold standard" for identifying peripheral UVH and is particularly useful for determining the side of the deficit because each labyrinth is tested separately.[47]

Rotational Chair Testing

Rotational chair testing allows evaluation of both horizontal SCCs at head movement frequencies that are more physiologically natural (1-20 Hz) in contrast to caloric test (0.025 Hz). In individuals with normal vestibular function, rotational chair testing should induce nystagmus. Common rotational chair tests are the **sinusoidal harmonic acceleration test** (SHA) and the **velocity step test.** In the SHA, the patient is rotated in a pendular pattern (left/right) at various frequencies (0.01-0.64 Hz) while the peak chair velocity is typically fixed at 50 to 60 degrees per second.[46] VOR parameters that are measured by this test include **gain** (ratio of slow phase eye velocity to head velocity [measured as chair velocity]), **phase** (the timing relationship between the eye and head movement), and **symmetry** (comparison of the VOR measures from rotations toward one ear with those from rotations to the opposite ear). The SHA test is the "gold standard" for identifying a bilateral vestibular weakness.[47] In the **velocity step test**, a stationary patient accelerates quickly to a predetermined peak velocity, continues to rotate in one direction at that velocity, and then is quickly stopped. The decay rate of nystagmus following both the abrupt angular acceleration and deceleration is measured and is called the **time constant**. The time constant is defined as the amount of time it takes for the slow phase velocity of the nystagmus to decline by 37% of its peak velocity, which typically takes 10 to 25 seconds (normal).[46] VOR phase and VOR time constant are measures of the same processes, namely transduction and velocity storage. Stimulation of hair cells by movement of the cupula generates a brief signal that lasts as long as the cupula is deflected. However, this response is sustained in the medial vestibular nucleus for longer than 10 seconds in individuals with normal vestibular function, supposedly as a means for the brain to detect low-frequency head rotation.[46] Lower velocity step rotations (about 60 degrees/sec) are used to determine the time constant and whether functional recovery of VOR gain has occurred from a chronic UVH, while higher velocity step rotations (>100 degrees/sec) are useful for detecting pathologically low VOR gains. Reduced gain, abnormal phase lead (i.e., eye movement is shifted slightly ahead of head movement), and shorter time constants are typically associated with peripheral vestibular pathology, while abnormally high gain, phase lag (eye movement is shifted slightly behind head movement), and longer time constants may indicate central (i.e., cerebellar) pathology. Symmetry measures are used to determine whether weakness is present on one side.[46]

Vestibular-Evoked Myogenic Potential

Otolith function (saccule and utricle) is tested with vestibular-evoked myogenic potential (VEMP). The two types of VEMP tests are **cervical VEMP** (cVEMP) and **ocular VEMP** (oVEMP). Both types measure the latency, amplitude, and threshold of a muscle contraction, recorded using electromyography (EMG), to locate vestibular pathology.[48] The cVEMP is used to evaluate whether the saccule and the inferior vestibular nerve are intact and functioning normally. During cVEMP testing, headphones are placed over the ears and electrodes are placed over the contracted sternocleidomastoid (SCM) muscle. When sounds (i.e., loud clicks) are delivered to the ipsilateral ear in individuals with normal vestibular function, the electrodes record a transient inhibition of the ipsilateral contracted SCM muscle that occurs about 13 msec after the click.[46] This reflex is activated by sound stimulation of the saccular afferents that have ipsilateral disynaptic connections with the SCM muscle.[46,48] The oVEMP is used to evaluate the function of the utricle and the superior vestibular nerve. In healthy individuals, loud clicks to the ear or bone vibrations to the forehead result in transient excitation of the contralateral inferior oblique (IO) eye muscle at a latency of 10 msec as recorded by electrodes placed under the eye.[46]

Gaze Stabilization Test

The gaze stabilization test (GST) assesses the most rapid head movement velocity at which a person can correctly maintain visual acuity of a computer-based target (e.g., letter E), thereby providing an estimate of VOR function. Patients with UVH had reduced scores on the GST compared to healthy controls, and the GST demonstrated 64% sensitivity and 93% specificity, and a high-reliability index of 0.91 to detect UVH with ipsilesional head movements.[49]

Computerized Dynamic Posturography (CDP)

Computerized dynamic posturography (CDP) provides information about motor control or balance function under varying environmental conditions. It utilizes force plates to measure a person's center of pressure (COP) under challenging conditions. CDP is divided into sensory and motor components. The sensory portion, called the Sensory Organization Test (SOT), assesses an individual's ability to integrate visual, proprioceptive, and vestibular inputs to maintain balance. Patients are asked to stand still for 30 seconds for three trials under six increasingly difficult conditions with variations in reliable information provided by the visual and somatosensory systems (Figure 17-2).

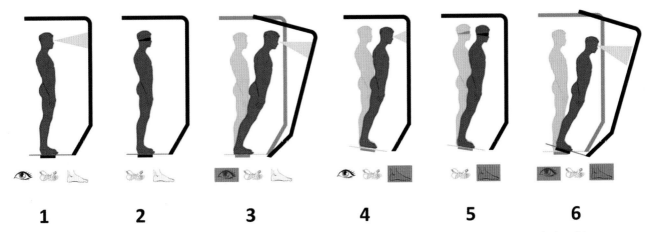

Conditions of SOT in which controlled perturbation to visual and somatosensory inputs could be applied. Red boxes denote perturbation of the corresponding sensory input. Participant's eyes were closed in conditions 2 and 5.

FIGURE 17-2 Six testing conditions for the Sensory Organization Test (Reprinted, with permission, from *NeuroCom International*). Vision is absent in Conditions 2 and 5. In Conditions 3 and 6, the surrounding wall sways with the person's body in the anterior/posterior (AP) direction, thereby reducing the accuracy of visual inputs for the perception of the body's motion relative to the visual field. In Conditions 4 to 6, the support surface sways along with the person's body, thereby, reducing the accuracy of somatosensory inputs for the perception of the body's AP motion relative to the support surface. (Reproduced with permission from Charkhkar H, Christie BP, Triolo RJ. Sensory neuroprosthesis improves postural stability during Sensory Organization Test in lower-limb amputees. Sci Rep. 2020;10(1):6984.)

TABLE 17-2	Interpretation of Patterns of Responses for the Sensory Organization Test	
PATTERN	**ABNORMAL TEST CONDITION**	**INTERPRETATION**
Vestibular dysfunction or loss	5, 6	Suggests difficulty using vestibular input for stance; early falls seen with bilateral loss of vestibular function; falls late in the trial seen with reduced bilateral peripheral vestibular function and uncompensated loss of unilateral function.
Support surface dependence	4, 5, 6	Suggests abnormal reliance on foot support surface inputs for stance; person has difficulty using both visual and vestibular or vestibular inputs alone.
Visual preference	3, 6	Suggests that central adaptive mechanisms for suppression of conflicting visual input may be impaired.
Visual dependence	2, 3, 5, 6	Suggests abnormal reliance on vision for stance; person has difficulty using foot support surface and/or vestibular inputs for stance.
General sensory selection	3, 4, 5, 6	Suggests difficulty with balance control in conditions with any sensory conflict.

The SOT is not diagnostic, but it is useful in patients with postural instability to determine patterns of dysfunction produced by six SOT test conditions (Table 17-2). The motor portion includes the Motor Control Test (MCT) that assesses the latency, weight distribution, and amplitude of a person's postural responses to sudden displacements of the support surface, and an Adaptation Test (ADT) that assesses a person's ability to adapt to repeated perturbing stimuli (i.e., support surface tilts up or down at the same amplitude).[48]

Visual Perception Tests

The **subjective visual vertical** (SVV) and **subjective visual horizontal** (SVH) tests are used to assess otolith function and the central pathways that convey gravitational information. The tests do not distinguish between saccular or utricular pathology. During these tests, patients are asked to align a dimly lit luminous bar (in a completely dark room) with what they perceive as being vertical (SVV) or horizontal (SVH). Individuals with normal vestibular function align the bar within ±2.0 degrees of true vertical or horizontal, while patients with either central or peripheral pathology align the bar with larger angular deviations. The direction of pathological SVV tilt is usually on the same side as the lesion (ipsiversive) in patients with unilateral peripheral vestibular neuritis and those with unilateral brainstem lesions that are lower than the upper pons.[50,51] With pathology of the cerebellum or unilateral brainstem lesions above the upper pons (i.e., midbrain, thalamus), the direction of SVV tilt is usually opposite to the side of the lesion (contraversive).[50,52]

Hearing Tests

Audiometry measures hearing function. Hearing evaluations are an important part of vestibular diagnostics. Several different audiometry tests, performed by an audiologist, may be completed. Individuals with vestibular disorders may have their hearing monitored at intervals over time, especially when there is evidence of tinnitus, hearing loss, or a sensation of fullness in the ears.

Neuroimaging

Magnetic resonance imaging (MRI) of the brain can reveal the presence of tumors, damage from strokes, and other soft-tissue abnormalities that might cause dizziness or vertigo. MRIs of structures in and around the inner ear may show problems such as an acoustic neuroma. Computerized axial tomography (CT) scans of the temporal bone (within which the inner ear resides) are often used to locate fractures.

Pharmacological Treatment

Treatment of Vertigo

Vestibular suppressant medications that are used for symptomatic treatment of acute vertigo, nausea, and vomiting are listed in Table 17-3. These drugs are not recommended for long-term use as they may inhibit central compensation and recovery of symptoms.

Treatment of Nystagmus

Several medications are used to suppress different forms of nystagmus. Pendular nystagmus, often associated with MS and brainstem strokes, can be suppressed with the anticonvulsant drug, gabapentin (Neurontin), or with memantine, a drug that blocks glutamate *N*-methyl-D-aspartate (NMDA) receptors.[53] Downbeat nystagmus, associated with cerebellar pathology, is effectively treated with potassium channel-blocking agents 4-aminopyridine (fampridine or dalfampridine), which is available as a sustained-release preparation (Ampyra). Other drugs that may be used to treat nystagmus are baclofen (Lioresal) and clonazepam (Klonopin).[54]

● PHYSICAL THERAPY EXAMINATION

Medical and Subjective Histories

Physical therapists, treating individuals with complaints of dizziness and imbalance, must first take thorough medical

TABLE 17-3	Common Drugs Used to Treat Acute Vertigo and Associated Nausea and Emesis[53,54]				
MEDICATION	**CLASS**	**SEDATION**	**ANTIEMESIS**	**SIDE EFFECTS**	
Dimenhydrinate (Dramamine)	Antihistamine; phosphodiesterase inhibitor	+	++	Dry mouth, tinnitus, blurred vision, coordination problems	
Diphenhydramine (Benadryl)	Antihistamine	+	++	Tachycardia, urinary retention	
Promethazine (Phenergan)	Antihistamine; anticholinergic; phenothiazine	++	++	Dry mouth, constipation, blurred vision	
Meclizine (Antivert, Bonine)	Antihistamine; anticholinergic	++	+	Dry mouth, tiredness	
Prochlorperazine (Compazine)	Antihistamine; anticholinergic; phenothiazine	+	+++	Dry mouth, blurred vision, constipation	
Scopalamine (Transderm Scop)	Anticholinergic (nonselective muscarinic)	+	++	Dry mouth, dilated pupils, blurred vision	
Ondansetron (Zofran)	Serotonin 5-hydroxytryp-tamine$_3$ (5-HT$_3$) receptor antagonist		+++	Headache, constipation, blurred vision	
Lorazepam (Ativan)	Benzodiazepine	++	+	Addiction, effects increased with other sedative drugs	

+, Mild; ++, moderate; +++, prominent.

and subjective histories and perform a systems review to sort out potential causes. The patients' current symptoms and past medical histories may assist the therapist to identify potential problems such as diabetes, heart disease, or neurological dysfunction that could negatively impact the patient's recovery. Patients should be asked about any medications that they are currently taking to determine if they are taking vestibular suppressant drugs (e.g., meclizine, scopolamine) that could delay recovery or might worsen their dizziness. For individuals taking vestibular suppressant drugs, the therapist should consult with the physician to see if they can be reduced or stopped. Therapists should also ask the patient or obtain from the medical record any diagnostic test reports, such as ENG/VNG, caloric, rotational chair, or VEMP tests.

Physical therapists must distinguish exactly what the patient is experiencing when feeling "dizzy" to be able to make appropriate clinical management decisions. Common types of dizziness symptoms and their possible causes are listed in Table 17-4. Notably, some patients, particularly patients with migraine, are chronically sensitive to motion, either of themselves or of the environment. Patient descriptions of their dizziness as an out-of-body experience, floating, or a spinning sensation inside of their head without accompanying nystagmus suggest a psychophysiological disorder (i.e., a combination of psychiatric factors and physiologic responses, such as hyperventilation).

Information about the onset, frequency, duration, and intensity of symptoms, and what circumstances exacerbate and relieve the symptoms should be obtained. Examples of questions to ask patients with vestibular disorders are given in Box 17-1. Intensity of symptoms like vertigo, lightheadedness, disequilibrium, and oscillopsia can be quantified using visual analogue scale (VAS). Patients are asked to answer a question (e.g., how intense is your vertigo right now?) by making a mark on a 10-cm line on a continuum from "none" at one end to "worst possible intensity" at the other to indicate

Box 17-1	Questions to Ask People with Vestibular Disorders[55]

1. Do you have spells of vertigo (sensation of spinning)? If yes, how long do they last?
2. When was the last time the vertigo occurred?
3. Is the vertigo spontaneous (present at rest), caused by motion, or caused by position changes?
4. Do you feel like you are going to lose your balance? If yes, is the feeling of being off balance constant, spontaneous, caused by motion, caused by position changes, worse with fatigue, worse in the dark, worse outside, worse on uneven surfaces?
5. Do you feel off balance when you are lying down, sitting, standing, or walking?
6. Do you stumble, stagger, or side-step while walking?
7. Do you veer to one side while you walk? If yes, to which side do you veer?
8. At what time of the day do you feel best? worst?
9. How many times per day do you have symptoms?
10. Do you have hearing problems?
11. Do you have visual problems?
12. Have you been in an accident (e.g., motor vehicle)?
13. Do you live alone?
14. Do you have stairs in your home?
15. Do you smoke? If yes, how much per day?
16. Do you drink alcohol? If yes, how much per day/week?

TABLE 17-4	Common Dizziness Symptoms and Possible Causes	
SYMPTOM	**DESCRIPTION**	**POSSIBLE CAUSES**
Vertigo (e.g., visualized spinning, tilting, dropping of the environment)	Illusion of movement, most commonly described as a feeling that they are spinning or that the room (environment) is spinning, often with nystagmus	Imbalance in tonic firing rates of left and right divisions of the vestibular system caused by unilateral peripheral (UVH, BPPV) or central lesions of vestibular nuclei.
Presyncope (near-faint)	Perception that he/she is about to faint; often associated with a buzzing sensation in the head, rubbery legs, constriction of the visual field, pallor, diaphoresis, and nausea.[5]	Diffuse decreased cerebral blood flow (i.e., cardiac arrhythmia, orthostatic hypotension)
Lightheadedness ("woozy")	Nonspecific type of dizziness that may be described as feeling "woozy" or disoriented	Decreased blood pressure (if accompanied by presyncope), hypoglycemia, drug intoxication, anxiety or panic disorders (associated with hyperventilation)
Disequilibrium (e.g., unsteadiness in standing and walking)	Feeling that a person is off balance. Patients typically do not experience disequilibrium while sitting or lying down but report unsteadiness upon standing or walking	Vestibular (BVH, chronic UVH), loss of lower extremity somatosensation, brainstem/vestibular cortex lesions, cerebellar and motor pathway lesions.
Motion intolerance	Sensitivity to riding in a car or other moving vehicle	Sensory conflict (e.g., motion sickness), migraine headaches
Oscillopsia	Visual instability with head movement in which objects in the environment appear to move or bounce, often resulting in blurring or diplopia	Peripheral vestibular disorders (BVH, UVH, BPPV) and brainstem and cerebellar lesions
Out of body feeling, floating, spinning inside of head		Psychophysiological disorder (e.g., anxiety, functional neurologic disorder, depression)

Abbreviations: BPPV, benign paroxysmal positional vertigo; BVH, bilateral vestibular hypofunction; UVH, unilateral vestibular hypofunction.

the intensity of their symptoms at a particular moment. Other vertigo assessments are the **Vertigo Symptom Scale**[56] **(VSS)** and the **UCLA Dizziness Questionnaire (UCLA-DQ)**.[57] The VSS evaluates symptoms related to vestibular disorders using a 6-point scale from 0 (never) to 5 (very often, more than once a week).[56] The UCLA-DQ uses a 5-point scale to describe a patient's vertigo and may be useful as a quick screening before a comprehensive evaluation.[57] Visual vertigo symptoms can be assessed using the **Visual Vertigo Analogue Scale** (VVAS), which asks a person to rate the intensity of visual vertigo provoked in nine challenging situations of visual motions using analogue scales.[58]

A fall history, including number of falls in the past 6 months, conditions under which falls occurred, whether the patient sought medical intervention as a result of a fall, and any lifestyle modifications made to prevent recurrent falls, should be obtained. The **Activities-Specific Balance Confidence Scale** (ABC Scale) is useful for determining the patient's perceptions of his/her ability to balance.[59] The patient should be asked about previous and current functional status and activity level. Some patients will stay in their homes to avoid highly textured visual stimulation (e.g., light flickering through trees, walking down aisles in stores) or develop phobias such as fears of elevators and heights.[55] The **Vestibular Activities of Daily Living Scale** (VD-ADL) can assist therapists to identify current limitations in activity and participation. Patients rate the effects of vertigo and balance disorders on their independence in performing 28 activities of daily living on a scale of 1 to 10 with 1 being "independent" and 10 being "too difficult, no longer perform."[60]

The **Dizziness Handicap Inventory** (DHI) assesses a person's perception of the effects of a balance problem and the emotional, physical, or functional adjustments that he or she makes.[61] The questionnaire consists of 25 items that are divided into functional (9 items), emotional (9 items), and physical (7 items) subscales. Each item is assigned a value of four points for a "yes," two points for a "sometimes," and zero points for a "no." The inventory is reliable and DHI scores are highly correlated with scores on the impairment-based SOT.[62] Clinicians can administer the DHI (1) before a patient's initial examination to help determine the physical tests that should be performed and to establish a baseline and (2) after treatment to determine treatment efficacy.[63]

Therapists should ask patients about their functional goals for physical therapy and discuss with them whether they are realistic and attainable.[55] The **Vestibular Rehabilitation Benefit Questionnaire** is utilized clinically to assess the effectiveness of physical therapy interventions on an individual's symptoms and the impact of those symptoms on quality of life. The 22-item questionnaire consists of items falling into three subscales: dizziness and anxiety (6 items), motion-provoked dizziness (5 items), and quality of life (11 items). The score for the entire tool ranges from 0 to 100%; 0% indicates no deficit, and 100% indicates significant deficit as compared to the normal state.[64]

Tests and Measures

Examination of the patient with dizziness includes assessment of eye movements (i.e., nystagmus, oculomotor, and vestibulo-ocular testing), positional testing, balance and gait. These tests should be performed along with a systems review and standard neurological assessment that includes evaluation of somatosensation, pain, coordination, range of motion, muscle strength, and posture to identify concurrent impairments that might affect the patient's prognosis and treatment (see Chapter 10 – Neurologic Evaluation). To assess the contribution of vertebral artery occlusion to the patient's symptoms, a **seated vertebral artery test** can be performed, in which the patient performs in consecutive order: (1) rotation of the head opposite to the tested side as far as possible, (2) extension of the head, and then (3) a combination of head rotation and extension opposite to the tested side.[65] If the patient experiences symptoms such as dizziness, diplopia, dysarthria, dysphagia, drop attacks, nausea, vomiting, or sensory changes at any time, the test is positive and testing is stopped. A positive test may indicate VBI, but a negative test cannot rule it out.[66] If cervicogenic dizziness is suspected, a more detailed examination of the upper quarter, including cervical-thoracic mobility, tests for instability of the upper cervical spine, palpation of cervical spine musculature and facet joints, and segmental mobility testing of the cervical spine should be performed.[65] A clinical test that can be performed to differentiate whether the patient's dizziness originates from cervical or vestibular dysfunction is the **head–neck differentiation test**. In the head–neck differentiation test, the patient sits on a swivel chair and the therapist rotates the chair left and right while simultaneously stabilizing the patient's head and the patient reports the presence of any dizziness. The therapist then rotates the chair without stabilizing the patient's head and the patient again reports the presence of any dizziness. Complaints of dizziness with trunk rotation under a stabilized head implicates cervical spine dysfunction, whereas dizziness with head and trunk rotation together (en bloc rotation) indicates a vestibular component to the patient's symptoms. If symptoms are provoked in both conditions, it is likely that cervicogenic dizziness and vestibular dysfunction are both present.[67] Other testing procedures and interpretation of findings are as follows.

Spontaneous Nystagmus

Procedure: Ask the patient to fixate on a stationary target in neutral gaze position and observe for nystagmus or rhythmic refixation eye movements. Repeat with the patient wearing Frenzel goggles so that the person cannot suppress the nystagmus by fixating on an object.

Interpretation: If nystagmus is observed, the amplitude, direction, and effect of target fixation should be noted. Lesions of the labyrinth, vestibular nerve, and rarely the vestibular nuclei produce intense, horizontal-rotatory nystagmus that is enhanced under Frenzel goggles. In contrast, central lesions (e.g., brainstem, cerebellum, and cerebrum) cause less-intense horizontal, vertical, torsional, or pendular (i.e., eyes oscillate at equal speeds) nystagmus that is usually reduced under Frenzel goggles.[68]

Gaze-Holding Nystagmus

Procedure: Ask the patient to gaze at a target placed 20 to 30 degrees to the left of center for 20 seconds. Observe for gaze-evoked nystagmus or change in direction, appearance, or intensity in spontaneous nystagmus. Repeat the procedure to the right.

Interpretation: The ability to maintain eccentric gaze is controlled by neural pathways in the brainstem and cerebellum, particularly the vestibulocerebellum. When these mechanisms fail to hold the eye in the eccentric position, the eye drifts toward the midline, followed by corrective saccades toward the target. Thus, central lesions produce direction-changing gaze-evoked nystagmus (i.e., the fast component of the nystagmus always beats in the direction of intended gaze). In contrast, acute peripheral UVH produces direction-fixed gaze holding nystagmus (the direction of the nystagmus is the same regardless of the eye-in-orbit position) and the nystagmus intensifies (i.e., the slow-phase velocity of the nystagmus increases) when gazing in the direction of the fast phase.[55,69]

Smooth Pursuit

Procedure: Ask the patient to keep the head stationary, while following your finger with the eyes, as you slowly move it left and right, up and down.

Interpretation: Normal eye tracking of a slowly moving object generates a smooth eye movement that involves central pathways and cranial nerves III, IV, and VI. Smooth pursuit is abnormal if, during tracking, the patient repeatedly loses the target and then catches up with a small saccade. Abnormal smooth pursuit is consistent with a central lesion and is never a sign of peripheral vestibular impairment.[70]

Saccades

Procedure: Ask the patient to look back and forth between two outstretched fingers held about 12 inches apart in the horizontal and vertical planes. Observe for latency of onset, speed, accuracy, and conjugate movement.

Interpretation: Saccadic eye movements are rapid eye movements that involve the frontal lobes, brainstem reticular formation, and cranial nerves III, IV, and VI. Healthy individuals can reach the targets with one eye movement or with one small corrective saccade. Abnormal saccadic eye movements are consistent with a central lesion and are never a sign of peripheral vestibular impairment.[71]

Vestibulo-Ocular Reflex Cancellation (VORc)

Procedure: Ask the patient to voluntarily fixate on a moving target, while the patient's head is moved in the same direction.

Interpretation: The normal smooth pursuit system is able to override or "cancel" the VOR at slow head velocities, as a patient focuses his or her gaze on a target that moves simultaneously and in the same direction as the head moves. An abnormal response is observed when a patient's fixation on a target, moving synchronously with his or her head, is interrupted by saccades. An impaired VORc is consistent with a central nervous system disorder.[55]

Ocular Alignment

Procedure: Observe the seated patient for head tilt (associated with abnormal SVV), skew deviation (one eye being superiorly displaced in comparison with the other eye), ocular torsion (the superior pole of the eyes are rotated together in the frontal plane), or a combination of the three symptoms called the **ocular tilt reaction** (OTR).

Interpretation: In a healthy individual, the SVV is aligned with the gravitational vertical, and the axes of eyes and the head are horizontal and directed straight ahead. The OTR indicates either a unilateral peripheral vestibular deficit (labyrinth or vestibular nerve) or a unilateral lesion of brainstem pathways. OTR from vestibular loss on the right-side manifests as head tilts to the right, right eye drops down in the orbit, and both eyes statically rotate to the right.[72]

Head Impulse Test (HIT, also called Head Thrust Test [HTT])

Procedure: Ask the patient to fixate on a near target (e.g., the clinician's nose), grasp the patient's head, and apply a brief, small-amplitude (5-10 degrees), and high-acceleration (3000-4000 degrees/sec^2) head turn, first to one side and then to the other. When the head stops moving, the clinician looks to see if the eyes are still directed toward the target and watches for corrective saccades toward the target.

Interpretation: When the VOR is functioning normally, the eyes move in the direction opposite to the head movement and gaze remains fixated on the target during the head thrust. Observations of "catch-up" saccades, after a head thrust to one side, is a sign of decreased neural input from the ipsilateral horizontal SCC afferents or central vestibular neurons to the VOR because the contralateral vestibular afferents and central vestibular neurons are inhibited and cannot supply enough neural activity to stabilize gaze. Patients with unilateral peripheral or central vestibular pathology will not be able to maintain gaze on the target, when the head is moved quickly toward the side of the lesion; individuals with bilateral loss of vestibular function will make corrective saccades after high-velocity head movements to both sides. Schubert et al.[73] reported that the HTT had a sensitivity of 71% for identifying UVH and 84% for BVH, and a specificity of 82% when the test was performed with the patient's head flexed forward 30 degrees and the head was moved unpredictably.[47]

Head-Shaking Induced Nystagmus Test (HSN)

Procedure: The patient is instructed to close the eyes. Tilt the head of the patient forward 30 degrees and oscillate the head in the horizontal plane at 2 Hz for 20 seconds. On stopping the oscillation, the patient opens the eyes and the clinician looks for nystagmus. The maneuver may be repeated in the vertical direction.

Interpretation: In individuals with normal vestibular function, nystagmus will not be present after the head shaking stops. An imbalance in the peripheral vestibular inputs to central vestibular nuclei can result in HSN. In cases of UVH, the patient may display nystagmus with the fast phase directed toward the healthy ear. Patients with complete bilateral vestibular function loss will not show HSN because there is no asymmetry between the vestibular inputs. Vertical nystagmus, following horizontal or vertical head shaking, indicates central pathology.[74]

Dynamic Visual Acuity (DVA)

Procedure: Ask the patient to read the lowest (smallest) line possible on a wall-mounted acuity chart (Snellen eye chart or Lighthouse distance visual acuity test) with best corrected vision (glasses, contact lenses). Repeat the maneuver while passively oscillating the patient's head at 2 Hz and record the number of lines of acuity "lost" during the headshake.

Interpretation: In normal individuals, visual acuity changes by one line in younger individuals and by two lines in older individuals. If the person can only read lines more than 3 lines above the initial static visual acuity, he or she likely has vestibular dysfunction. Patients with bilateral vestibular loss, especially acutely, often lose 6 to 8 lines of visual acuity. A computerized version of the DVA has the benefit of being able to determine DVA for right and left head movements separately.[55]

Positional Testing

Static and dynamic position tests are performed to determine which head positions or movements provoke the patient's symptoms of vertigo, dizziness, nausea, and nystagmus. Static positions that are tested typically include the following: (1) sitting with the head upright, (2) supine with head flexed forward approximately 30 degrees, (3) supine with the head turned right, and (4) supine with the head turned left. The Motion Sensitivity Test (MST) measures motion-provoked dizziness in patients using a series of 16 movements from least to most provocative (Table 17-5).[75,76] The severity and duration of the dizziness are recorded for each position and a cumulative score, the MST quotient, is calculated. A final score of 0 to 10 indicates mild motion sensitivity, with scores of 11 to 30 indicating moderate motion sensitivity, and scores of 31 to 100 indicating severe motion sensitivity.[55] The MST has been found to be reliable and valid.[77] Clinicians can use the results of static and dynamic position tests to develop exercise programs for patients and to provide evidence of intervention efficacy.

Positional testing is used to identify whether a person has BPPV. Vestibular tests that identify BPPV, affecting the vertical SCCs (i.e., posterior and anterior SCCs), include the Dix–Hallpike Test (see Figure 17-3) and the Sidelying Test (Figure 17-4). The Dix–Hallpike Test has been considered the gold standard for diagnosing BPPV.[78] Starting from a long-sitting position with the head rotated 45 degrees to one side, the patient is moved to a supine position with the head extended 30 degrees below the horizontal and still rotated 45 degrees.

The clinician, then, observes the patient's eyes for nystagmus and asks if vertigo is felt. The patient is then slowly brought back to the starting position, and the other side is tested. When the Dix–Hallpike Test is contraindicated, such as in individuals

TABLE 17-5	Motion Sensitivity Test		
BASELINE SYMPTOMS	**INTENSITY (A)**	**DURATION (B)**	**SCORE (A+B)**
1. Sitting to supine			
2. Supine to left side			
3. Supine to right side			
4. Supine to sitting			
5. Left Dix–Hallpike test			
6. Return from left Dix–Hallpike test			
7. Right Dix–Hallpike test			
8. Return from right Dix–Hallpike test			
9. Sitting: nose toward left knee			
10. Return to sitting			
11. Sitting: nose toward right knee			
12. Return to sitting			
13. Sitting: head rotation (5 times)			
14. Sitting: head flexion and extension (5 times)			
15. Standing: 180-degree turn to right			
16. Standing: 180-degree turn to left			

Duration of dizziness: rated 0–3 (5–10 seconds = 1 point; 11–30 seconds = 2 points; ≥30 seconds = 3 points).
Intensity of dizziness: rated 0–5 (0 = no symptoms; 5 = severe dizziness).
Duration score + Intensity score = MST score (Maximum score for each position is 8 points; the total possible raw score is 128 [8 points × 16 positions]).
Motion sensitivity quotient: Number of symptom-provoking positions × MST score × 100 divided by 2048 (16 [total number of positions] × 128 [total possible MST score]).
Note: An MST quotient of 0 indicates no symptoms, whereas an MST quotient of 100 indicates severe unrelenting symptoms in all positions.
(Reproduced with permission from Smith-Wheelock M, Shepard NT, Telian SA. Physical therapy program for vestibular rehabilitation. Am J Otol. 1991;12(3):218-225.)

with neck and back problems or those with a positive vertebral artery test, the Sidelying Test may be used as an alternative. The patient is quickly moved from a seated position on the side of a plinth to sidelying with the head rotated 45 degrees in the opposite direction (Figure 17-4). Horizontal SCC BPPV is diagnosed by the Roll Test (also called the Pagnini–McClure maneuver), in which the head is turned by about 90 degrees to each side while supine (Figure 17-5).[78]

A positive test for BPPV from canalithiasis is characterized by (1) delayed onset of vertigo by 1 to 40 seconds after the person is placed in the provoking position; (2) presence of nystagmus with the same latency as the complaints of vertigo; and (3) increasing followed by decreasing intensity of vertigo and nystagmus that disappears within 60 seconds.[79] BPPV from cupulolithiasis is much less common than canalithiasis and is characterized by (1) immediate onset of vertigo when the person is moved into the provoking position; (2) nystagmus that appears with the same latency as the complaints of vertigo, and (3) persistence of the vertigo and nystagmus as long as the person's head is maintained in the provoking position.[79] The problematic SCC can be identified based on the characteristics of the observed nystagmus (Table 17-6). For the Dix–Hallpike and Sidelying tests, the involved side in posterior SCC BPPV is always the side that

reproduces nystagmus and vertigo (i.e., the downside ear in a dependent position). Therapists should use the direction of the torsional component of the nystagmus to identify the involved side in anterior SCC BPPV with the Dix–Hallpike and Sidelying tests rather than which ear is dependent because it could be in either ear. Determination of the affected horizontal SCC side with the roll test is more difficult because vertigo and nystagmus will be elicited in both the head left and head right positions. The clinician must carefully observe the nystagmus to determine whether the patient has the canalithiasis or the cupulolithiasis form of horizontal SCC BPPV. In the canalithiasis form of horizontal SCC BPPV, the nystagmus is **geotropic**, meaning that the fast phase beats toward the Earth and lasts <60 seconds. In the cupulolithiasis form of horizontal SCC BPPV, the nystagmus is **apogeotropic**, meaning that the fast phase beats away from the Earth, and lasts >60 seconds. The affected side is typically considered to be the more symptomatic side in canalithiasis and the less symptomatic side in cupulolithiasis.[79]

Balance and Gait Assessment

Examination of balance and gait problems is important to determine the patient's functional status and fall risk. **Balance**, also referred to as **postural stability,** is the dynamic process by

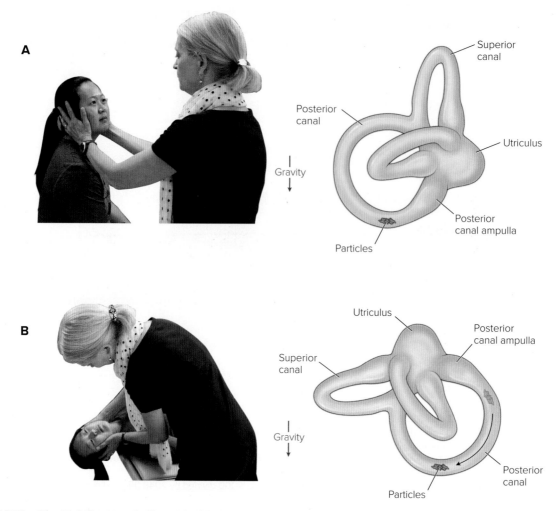

FIGURE 17-3 The Dix–Hallpike test. A. The patient long-sits on the examination table and the clinician turns the head horizontally 45 degrees. **B.** the clinician maintains the 45-degree head rotation while bringing the patient quickly to a supine position with the neck extended 30 degrees beyond the horizontal. This figure shows testing for right posterior or right anterior semicircular canal BPPV. The corresponding illustrations demonstrate the orientation of the semicircular canals and location of the otolithic debris in the posterior canal (viewed from the patient's right side).

which the body is in equilibrium either at rest (static equilibrium) or in steady-state motion (dynamic equilibrium). In general, balance is greatest when the body's center of mass (COM), a point that corresponds to the center of the total body mass, is

TABLE 17-6	Nystagmus Features by Canal Affected in BPPV
CANAL AFFECTED	**INITIAL RESPONSE IN DIX–HALLPIKE TEST**
Posterior	Upbeating and torsional (torsional toward affected ear)
Anterior	Downbeating and torsional (torsional toward affected ear)
Horizontal: canalithiasis	Geotropic (right-beating in head right position, left-beating in head left position)
Horizontal: cupulolithiasis	Apogeotropic (left-beating in right head position, right-beating in head left position)

maintained over its base of support (BOS). The term "limits of stability" refers to the sway boundaries in which an individual can maintain equilibrium without changing his or her BOS. Testing should address static and dynamic steady-state balance, anticipatory postural control, reactive balance control, sensory and movement strategies, and balance during functional activities. Table 17-7 includes common static and dynamic steady-state balance tests and expected results in patients with specific vestibular disorders.

As a sensor of gravity and head acceleration, the vestibular system contributes important information for both static (i.e., maintaining stability in different postures) and dynamic (maintaining stability as the support surface moves or the body moves on a stable surface) balance control. However, vestibular information has to be integrated with visual and somatosensory inputs for people to perceive body position and movement necessary for balance control, since the vestibular system only provides information about head movements and not the position or movement of any other parts of the body or of the head on the trunk.[80] For example, vestibular information alone cannot be used to distinguish a simple head nod (head movement on a

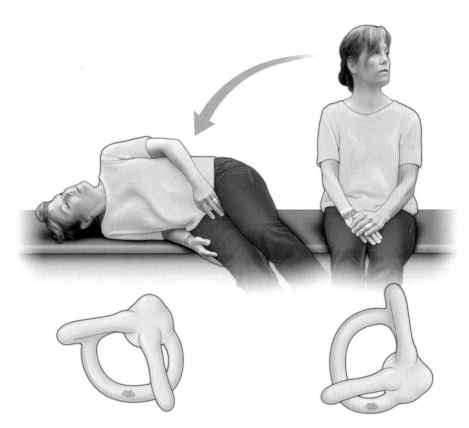

FIGURE 17-4 Sidelying test. After seating the patient on the examination table, the clinician turns the head horizontally 45 degrees away from the involved ear. The clinician maintains the 45-degree head rotation while bringing the patient quickly to the side opposite to the head rotation. The corresponding illustrations demonstrate the orientation of the semicircular canals and location of the otolithic debris in the posterior canal (viewed from the front).

stable trunk) from a forward tilt over the feet (head movement in conjunction with a moving trunk). The visual system provides information regarding (1) the position of the head relative to the environment, (2) the direction of vertical (e.g., walls and doorframes aligned vertically) for orientation of the head to maintain level gaze, and (3) the direction and speed of head movements because as a person's head moves, surrounding objects move in the opposite direction. The addition of visual information helps the CNS to determine whether sensory signals coming from the otoliths are due to a head tilt with respect to gravity or linear movement of the head. The somatosensory system provides information about the position and motion of the body and body parts relative to each other and the support surface. The addition of somatosensory information allows the CNS to discern whether information about head rotation coming from the vertical (anterior and posterior) SCCs is due to head motion on the neck or because of a whole-body movement like falling. Thus, information from vestibular, visual, and somatosensory systems about body position and self-motion must be integrated and interpreted by the CNS before it can be used to maintain body orientation and equilibrium.

Normally, the coordination of sensory information from vestibular, visual, and somatosensory systems for body orientation and movement sensation is a seamless process. CNS areas involved in integration and processing of sensory inputs are the cerebellum, basal ganglia, and supplementary motor area.[81]

Somatosensory information has the fastest processing time for rapid responses, followed by visual and vestibular inputs.[81] However, when sensory inputs from one system change due to environmental conditions or injuries that decrease the information-processing rate, individuals may need to re-weight their relative dependence on each of the senses. For example, in a well-lit environment with a firm BOS, healthy individuals will rely primarily on surface somatosensory information for balance.[82] However, if they stood on an unstable surface (sand, boat) or incline (ramp) with good lighting for vision, they would increase their reliance on visual and vestibular information and decrease their dependence on the unreliable somatosensory inputs. This adaptive re-weighting process is called **sensory organization**. Most individuals can compensate well if one of the three systems is impaired.

Static steady-state balance can be assessed by observing the patient's ability to maintain different postures. The **Clinical Test of Sensory Integration on Balance Test** (CTSIB), formerly called the "Foam and Dome" Test,[83] measures the patient's ability to balance under six different sensory conditions: (1) eyes open, stable surface (floor); (2) eyes closed, stable surface; (3) visual conflict (dome), stable surface; (4) eyes open, unstable surface (foam); (5) eyes closed, unstable surface; and (6) visual conflict, unstable surface. The SOT is the computerized version of this test (see preceding section on posturography).[84] A modified version (mCTSIB), also referred to as the modified

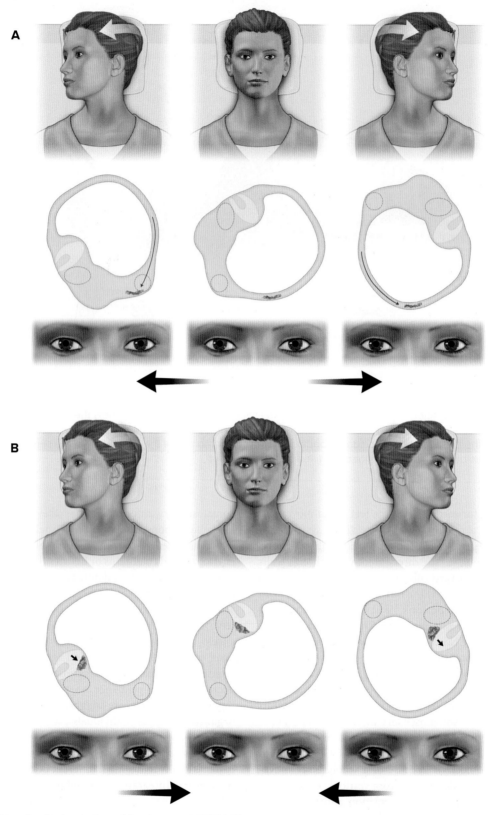

FIGURE 17-5 Roll test for horizontal semicircular canal BPPV. The patient is positioned in supine with the head placed in 20-degree cervical flexion. The head is quickly turned about 90 degrees to each side. **A.** Canalithiasis. **B.** Cupulolithiasis. The corresponding illustrations demonstrate the location of the otolithic debris in the horizontal canal during each maneuver, and the direction of the induced nystagmus (arrows).

TABLE 17-7	Common Balance Test Results for Vestibular Conditions			
TEST	**BPPV**	**UVH**	**BVH**	**CENTRAL LESION**
Tandem Romberg	Normal	Acute: cannot perform Chronic: abnormal, eyes closed	Abnormal; cannot perform with eyes closed	Abnormal
Single-legged stance	Normal	Acute: cannot perform Chronic: normal	Difficult to perform even during compensated stage, with EO	May be unable to perform
Gait	Acute: Normal or wide-based, slow, decreased trunk rotation Compensated: Normal	Acute: wide-based, slow, decreased trunk rotation; may need help initially Compensated: normal	Acute: wide-based, slow, decreased trunk rotation; cannot tandem walk EC Compensated: mild deviations	May be slow or shuffling, or marked ataxia
Turn head while walking	May cause slight unsteadiness	Acute: cannot keep balance Compensated: normal; some may slow cadence	Gait slows, BOS widens, step length decreases; may lose balance	May lose balance, increased ataxia

Abbreviations: BPPV, benign paroxysmal postural vertigo; UVH, unilateral vestibular hypofunction; BVH, bilateral vestibular hypofunction; EO, eyes open; EC, eyes closed; BOS, base of support.

Romberg test of Standing Balance on Firm and Compliant Support Surfaces (modified Romberg), has the dome portion removed, using only four conditions of eyes open and closed while standing on the floor and then a dense piece of foam.[85,86] Each condition is tested three times for 30 seconds. A failure is defined as opening the eyes, moving the feet or arms to maintain stability, or needing support to prevent a fall before 30 seconds. Interpretation of the results of the CTSIB and mCTSIB is the same as for the SOT (see Table 17-2). Patients lacking labyrinthine inputs become more dependent on accurate ankle proprioceptive and visual inputs to correctly organize their postural responses.[87] Inaccurate or distorted proprioceptive or visual inputs, or conditions in which they are forced to use only vestibular inputs will often produce increased sway and/or falls in these individuals.[87] Giray et al.[88] demonstrated significant differences on the instrumented mCTSIB (NeuroCom Balance Master) between subjects with unilateral vestibular dysfunction who participated in a 4-week vestibular rehabilitation program and those who did not ($p < 0.05$) for all conditions and for the composite score.[88]

If the patient demonstrates no difficulty performing the CTSIB or mCTSIB test, the patient can be further challenged with the **sharpened Romberg** and **Single-Leg Stance (SLS)** tests. The **sharpened Romberg**, also known as the tandem Romberg, requires the patient to stand with the feet in a heel-to-toe position with arms folded across the chest and eyes closed for 1 minute.[89] The SLS test asks the patient to stand on one leg without shoes with arms placed across the chest without letting the legs touch each other. Five 30-second trials are performed for each leg with a maximum possible score of 150 seconds per leg. Normal adults should be able to balance for 20 to 30 seconds on each leg.[90]

Dynamic steady-state balance control can be assessed by therapist observation of the patient's self-initiated movements and performance on standardized tests. Observations of weight shifts performed in standing to the limits of stability in all directions, reaching tasks such as picking up objects off the floor or putting an object on a high shelf, or transitions from one position to another (e.g., supine-to-sit or sit-to-stand transfers) can be used to determine whether the patient moves efficiently, symmetrically, and safely. The **Five Times Sit-to-Stand Test** (FTSST) assesses the patient's ability to balance while standing up and sitting down five times as quickly as possible from a standard armless chair. The FTSST has been shown to be a reliable and valid measure in individuals with balance disorders.[91] The **Fukuda Stepping Test** (FST) is a dynamic test that was originally developed as a test of vestibular function. The test is performed by having the patient stand with eyes closed and arms extended to shoulder height. The patient marches in place for 50 steps at the pace of a brisk walk. Progressive turning toward one side of 45 degrees or more is considered a positive test and suggests a unilateral peripheral or central vestibular deficit.[92] Honaker and Shepard[93] measured FST as a function of the patient's degree of caloric weakness on ENG and found that the FST was only sensitive in detecting individuals with severe weakness on ENG (>75% weakness).[93] A screening test of walking balance that is commonly used is **tandem walking**, in which the person walks heel to toe with either eyes open or closed. Using a cutoff of ≤5 correct steps out of 10 performed with eyes closed identified individuals with vestibular disorders with a sensitivity of 67% and a specificity of 71%.[94]

Anticipatory postural control helps a person to maintain balance by compensating for destabilization associated with voluntary movements, such as postural transitions and walking. Anticipatory control involves activation of postural muscles in advance of performing skilled movements, such as activation of posterior leg and back extensor muscles prior to a person pulling on a handle when standing,[95] or weight shifts toward the stance foot prior to unloading the stepping leg during walking.[96] These proactive postural changes that occur before and at the onset of a movement to reduce destabilization caused by the movement are called **anticipatory postural adjustments (APAs)**.

Anticipatory postural control is evaluated by having the patient perform voluntary movements that require the development of a postural set to counteract a predicted postural disturbance. The patient's ability to catch or kick a ball, open doors, lift objects of different weights, step over obstacles, and reach without losing balance is indicative of adequate anticipatory control. The **Functional Reach Test**[97] and the **Multi-Directional Reach Test**[98] require the patient to reach in different directions as far as possible without changing the BOS. Normative data are available, and the tests are reliable and valid.[97,98]

Reactive balance control is used to recover balance in response to unexpected losses of balance that either displace a person's BOS (e.g., tripping on an object on the ground), or move the COM beyond the limits of stability (e.g., a strong wind striking the body). After an unexpected external perturbation, **automatic postural reactions** are the first responses that effectively prevent falls. They produce quick, relatively stereotyped movements among individuals (similar to reflexes), but they require coordination of responses among body regions and are modifiable depending on the demands of the task. Automatic postural reactions may be followed by a variety of motor outputs dependent on task parameters (e.g., reach for a nearby stable support surface or step away from a destabilizing condition). Together, these automatic reactions and motor outputs ensure that the response is proportionate to the postural challenge.[84]

Horak and Nashner[99] described four movement strategies called ankle, hip, stepping, and suspensory that healthy adults use to recover balance, when standing on a surface that suddenly moves under them. In quiet stance and during small perturbations (i.e., slow-speed perturbations usually occurring on a large, firm surface), the **ankle strategy** acts to restore a person's center of mass (COM) to a stable position. The muscle activation sequence associated with the ankle strategy is a distal-to-proximal firing pattern of the ankle, hip, and trunk musculature. For rapid and/or large external perturbations or for movements executed with the COM near the limits of stability, a **hip strategy** is employed. The hip strategy uses rapid hip flexion or extension to move the COM within the BOS. The muscle activation sequence associated with the hip strategy occurs in a proximal-to-distal pattern. If a large force displaces the COM beyond the limits of stability, a forward or backward **stepping strategy** is used to take a step, enlarging the BOS to regain balance control. The **suspension strategy** is observed during balance tasks when a person quickly lowers his or her body COM by flexing the knees, causing associated flexion of the ankles and hips or a slight squatting motion.[99]

Automatic postural responses or reactive control can be assessed by the patient's response to external perturbations. Pushes (small or large, slow or rapid, anticipated and unanticipated) applied to the sternum, posterior trunk, or pelvis in different directions are widely used, but they are not quantifiable or reliable. The clinician subjectively rates the responses as normal, good, fair, poor, or unable. The **Pull Test**,[100] **Backwards Push and Release Test**,[101,102] and the **Postural Stress Test**[103] are more objective and reliable measures of reactive postural control. The pull test (item #30 of the Unified Parkinson's Disease Rating Scale) is administered by delivering a strong posterior pull to the shoulders of the patient and rating the response on a 5-point scale from 0 (normal) to 4 (unable to stand without assistance). The Backwards Push and Release Test is administered by standing in the back and to the side of the patient with one hand on each scapula and asking them to lean backward into the hands. Once the patient is in place, the examiner releases the hold, requiring the patient to take a step. The examiner rates the patient's performance using a 5-point scale from 0 (recovers independently with 1 step of normal length and width) to 4 (falls without attempting a step or unable to stand without assistance). The Postural Stress Test measures an individual's ability to withstand a series of destabilizing forces applied at the level of the waist using a pulley weight system. Scoring of the postural responses is based on a 10-point scale, where a score of 0 represents a complete failure to remain upright and a score of 9 represents the most efficient postural response.[104]

During the functional evaluation of individuals with vestibular deficits, the clinician should observe and document the patient's movement strategies in response to postural disturbances.[55] Horak et al. found that patients with bilateral vestibular loss displayed normal ankle strategies in response to surface translations, but they did not use a hip strategy even when it was necessary to maintain balance while standing on a narrow balance beam.[105] Clinicians should observe the patient's individual movement strategies to determine if they are sufficient and safe to achieve task goals.

Clinicians should assess the patient's gait through clinical observation, videotape analysis, or computerized gait or motion analysis systems. Observe patients walk at different speeds and directions, in crowded versus uncrowded settings, while moving the head, with interruptions of sudden stops, in obstacle courses, and with secondary motor or cognitive tasks to simulate activities that patients perform in their daily lives. Record whether specific activities increase their symptoms. Refer to Table 17-7 for common gait deviations found in patients with vestibular disorders. Individuals with peripheral vestibular disorders may adopt a stiff or robot-like gait pattern that limits movement of the head and trunk with excessive use of visual fixation.[55] A variety of gait disorders are seen with central pathology, but gait ataxia is usually associated with cerebellar dysfunction.

Functional tests are used to determine activity limitations and to identify tasks that a patient needs to practice. Three mobility scales Four Square Step Test,[106] Timed Up and Go Test (TUG),[107] Berg Balance Scale (BBS),[108] and two gait scales (i.e., Dynamic Gait Index,[109] Functional Gait Assessment[110]) can be easily used to assess balance performance during functional activities. Most of these tests were designed to assess fall risk in the elderly, with the exception of the Functional Gait Assessment which was developed specifically for use with patients with vestibular disorders.[110] A complete list of the Vestibular Evidence Database to Guide Effectiveness (VEDGE) task force recommended vestibular outcome measures are available online.[111]

Clinicians should be alert to "red flags" that may appear during patient examinations. For example, undiagnosed CNS signs and symptoms such as spontaneous nystagmus in room light after 2 weeks or vertical nystagmus without a torsional component [not BPPV] in room light, or a positive vertebral artery test should be reported to the referring physician or appropriate health care professional.

DIFFERENTIATING PERIPHERAL VESTIBULAR PATHOLOGY FROM CENTRAL VESTIBULAR PATHOLOGY

Table 17-8 delineates some of the characteristic features that can help distinguish patients with central vestibular pathology from those with peripheral vestibular pathology. Patients with central vestibular lesions more often complain of disequilibrium and ataxia rather than true vertigo. Often their inability to stand or walk distinguishes them from patients with peripheral lesions, who more commonly are able to stand or ambulate with assistance. Unlike peripheral lesions, nystagmus of central pathology changes direction with gaze, may be pendular, or purely vertical or torsional. Individuals with central vestibular lesions may have neurologic symptoms such as diplopia, altered consciousness, hemisensory loss, hemiparesis, and lateropulsion (tendency to fall to one side) that are not present with peripheral lesions. Peripheral vestibular lesions are more often associated with auditory symptoms.[111]

A three-step test, called the Head Impulse–Nystagmus–Test of Skew (HINTS) test, is helpful for differentiating an acute central vestibular lesion, possibly due to stroke, from a peripheral lesion with a sensitivity of more than 90%.[112,113] The examiner first administers the HIT to test the VOR, followed by observation of the eyes for spontaneous nystagmus using Frenzel's glasses, and skew deviation using the cover test. The cover test for skew deviation is performed by asking the patient to maintain his/her gaze on your nose, while alternately covering each of the patient's eyes. A positive result is the deviation of one eye while it is being covered, followed by an upward or downward corrective movement of the eye observed by the examiner when the eye is uncovered. Findings of a negative HIT test, a change in direction of the fast-phase of horizontal nystagmus (i.e., opposite in direction of spontaneous nystagmus) with gaze shifts, and a positive test of skew points to a central lesion. An acronym mnemonic to remember this is INFARCT—IN: Impulse Negative, FA: Fast phase Alternating, and RCT: Refixation during Cover Test.[112]

PHYSICAL THERAPY TREATMENT

CASE A, PART II

Based on Mrs. O'Hara's complaints of episodic vertigo that was provoked by rolling in bed and commenced following a head injury, the therapist suspected a possible diagnosis of BPPV. A Dix–Hallpike test was performed with the patient wearing Frenzel goggles and identified a robust up-beating torsional nystagmus accompanied by worsening vertigo and nausea that occurred about 20 seconds after the patient was put in the test position (supine with her head extended over the examination table 30 degrees and rotated to the right 45 degrees) and disappeared 30 seconds later. Dix–Hallpike testing on the left side was negative. The clinician determined that the patient had canalithiasis BPPV involving the right posterior SCC.

TABLE 17-8	Common Symptoms Differentiating Central versus Peripheral Vestibular Pathology[106,107]
CENTRAL VESTIBULAR PATHOLOGY	**PERIPHERAL VESTIBULAR PATHOLOGY**
Uncommon to have hearing loss	Symptoms may include hearing loss, fullness in ears, tinnitus
Nystagmus direction is purely vertical or torsional.	Nystagmus is horizontal and torsional.
Pendular nystagmus (eyes oscillate at equal speeds)	Jerk nystagmus (nystagmus has slow and fast phases)
Nystagmus either does not change or reverses direction with gaze.	Nystagmus increases with gaze toward the direction of the fast phase (i.e., away from the side of the lesion).
Nystagmus either does not change or it increases with visual fixation.	Nystagmus is decreased with visual fixation.
Symptoms of acute vertigo not usually suppressed by visual fixation.	Symptoms of acute vertigo usually suppressed by visual fixation.
Nausea/vomiting more mild.	Nausea/vomiting usually severe.
Oscillopsia is severe.	Oscillopsia is mild unless lesion is bilateral.
Abnormal performance on smooth pursuit and/or saccades	Smooth pursuit tracking and saccade performance normal
If sudden onset, likely not able to stand and walk even with assistance (severe ataxia).	If sudden onset, can stand and walk with assistance (mild ataxia).
Other neurologic symptoms are present.	Other neurologic symptoms are rare.
Symptoms may recover slowly or never resolve.	Symptoms usually resolve within 7 days in people with UVH.

Benign Paroxysmal Positional Vertigo

General physical therapy goals and expected outcomes for patients with BPPV are (1) removal of otoconia from the SCCs, (2) remission of vertigo with head movement, (3) improved balance, and (4) independence in all functional activities, involving head motions. Recommended treatment for BPPV utilizes particle repositioning head maneuvers that move the displaced otoconia out of the affected SCC. The three main maneuvers used to treat posterior and anterior SCC BPPV are the (1) Epley maneuver, (2) Liberatory maneuver, and (3) Brandt–Daroff habituation exercises. Evidence for the efficacy of these treatments to achieve remission of symptoms is strongest for the use of the Epley maneuver for posterior SCC BPPV.[79] However, even with successful treatment with such maneuvers, BPPV recurs in about one-third of individuals after 1 year and in roughly 50% of all individuals treated by 5 years.[114,115]

The **Epley maneuver** is based on the canalithiasis theory of free-floating debris in the SCC and is used to treat the canalithiasis form of posterior and anterior SCC BPPV.[116] The maneuver involves sequential movement of the head into five positions that will move the debris out of the SCC and into the vestibule (Figure 17-6).

The **Liberatory maneuver** (also called the Semont maneuver) is based on the cupulolithiasis theory of debris, adhering to the cupula in the SCC, and is used to treat cupulolithiasis of the posterior and anterior SCC BPPV. It can also be used as an alternative treatment for patients who do not tolerate or respond to the Epley maneuver. The Liberatory maneuver involves rapidly moving an individual from lying on one side to lying on the other (Figure 17-7). The rapid acceleration and deceleration of the movement from the initial sidelying position to the second (opposite side) sidelying position is presumed to dislodge debris adhering to the cupula of the SCC.[79] Elderly patients and those with back problems may not tolerate the quickness of movement required in this procedure.

Brandt–Daroff exercises consist of repeated movements into and out of positions that cause vertigo (Figure 17-8).[116] The mechanism by which they work is not entirely understood, but proposed mechanisms are: (1) habituation of the CNS to the provoking positions, (2) dislodging debris from the cupula, or (3) causing debris to float out of the SCC.[79] These exercises are typically prescribed for patients who continue to have persistent or mild vertigo even after the Epley and/or Liberatory maneuvers or do not tolerate those maneuvers. The exercises should be performed for 5 to

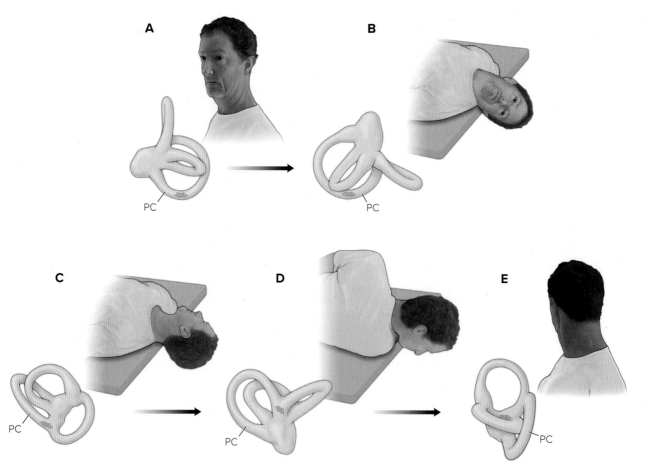

FIGURE 17-6 Epley maneuver. The patient is taken through five positions to move the debris through the canal: (**A**) long-sitting with the head rotated 45 degrees toward the affected side; (**B**) quickly moved to supine with head extended 30 degrees while maintaining the 45 degree rotation to the affected side, then maintained for 1–2 minutes; (**C**) turn head to the opposite side while maintaining extension over the end of the table; (**D**) roll to side without moving the head, again maintained for 1–2 minutes; (**E**) return to sitting on the side of the plinth.

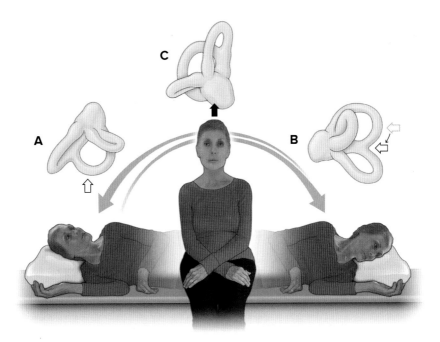

FIGURE 17-7 Liberatory maneuver. The Liberatory maneuver is used to dislodge the debris within the cupula. To treat posterior SCC cupulolithiasis the (**A**) patient sits with head rotated 45 degrees towards the unaffected ear; (**B**) the patient is quickly brought to sidelying on the side of the affected ear keeping the head rotated and the position is held one minute; (**C**) patient is rapidly brought to sidelying on the opposite side without changing the position of the head; and the patient slowly returns to sitting. For treatment of anterior SCC cupulolithiasis, the head is rotated initially 45 degrees toward the affected ear.

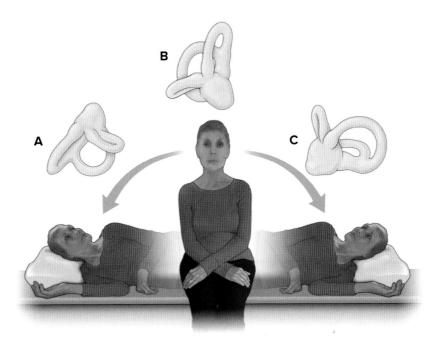

FIGURE 17-8 Brandt–Daroff exercises. (**A**) The patient begins by sitting sideways on the bed; then, (**B**) quickly lies down on her side with her head turned 45 degrees toward the ceiling. She returns to upright and then (**C**) quickly lies down on the other side, again with the head turned 45 degrees toward the ceiling.

10 repetitions, three times per day until the patient has no vertigo for 2 consecutive days. Patients should be instructed that movements must be performed rapidly, which will probably provoke the symptoms. If vertigo is too severe, the number of repetitions can be reduced to three, performed three times per day. It is normal for patients to experience residual symptoms (i.e., disequilibrium and nausea) after doing the exercises, but these are usually temporary and should not prevent the patient from continuing the exercises.[116]

Because of the relative rarity of horizontal SCC BPPV, there are no best practices established for treatment maneuvers.

The canalithiasis form of horizontal canal BPPV can be effectively treated with either the Bar-B-Que Roll or the Casani (also known as the Gufoni) maneuvers.[117,118] The Bar-B-Que Roll maneuver entails moving the head through a series of 90-degree angles and

pausing between each turn for 10 to 30 seconds (Figure 17-9). The Casani (or Gufoni) maneuver (Figure 17-10) is the primary treatment for the cupulolithiasis form of horizontal SCC BPPV.[119] For horizontal SCC canalithiasis BPPV that does not

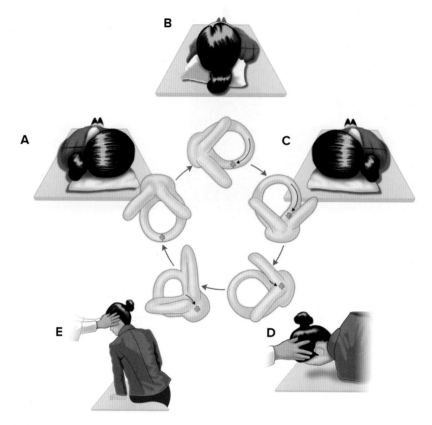

FIGURE 17-9 Bar-B-Que Roll maneuver for the treatment of geotropic right horizontal SCC-BPPV. Turn head toward the involved ear while lying supine (**A**), then turn head 270 degrees toward the unaffected side through a series of stepwise 90-degree turns (**B–D**); then resume the sitting position (**E**). Each position should be maintained for at least 1 or 2 minutes, or until the induced nystagmus and vertigo are resolved. The corresponding illustrations demonstrate the orientation of the semicircular canals and the location of the otolithic debris in the horizontal canal.

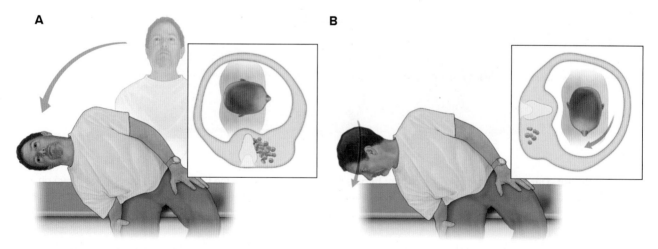

FIGURE 17-10 Casani maneuver – for the treatment of horizontal SCC cupulolithiasis BPPV. In the Casani maneuver, the patient moves quickly from sitting position to sidelying on the affected side (**A**). The patient then quickly turns the head so that the nose points down 45 degrees (**B**) and remains in that position for 2 to 3 minutes before coming back to sitting. (Reproduced, with permission, from Casani AP, Vannucci G, Fattori B, et al. The treatment of horizontal canal positional vertigo: our experience in 66 cases, *Laryngoscope.* 2002 Jan;112(1):172–178.)

respond to head maneuvers, a home treatment called forced prolonged positioning may be recommended. The patient goes to bed and lies in sidelying on the affected side (more symptomatic side) for 30 to 60 seconds and then slowly rolls over to sidelying with the unaffected ear down. The patient remains in this position all night, permitting the otoconia to gradually move out of the canal.[120]

Originally, posttreatment instructions, following particle repositioning maneuvers, asked patients to keep their heads upright for 48 hours, including sleeping with the head elevated 45 degrees. The evidence does not support that sleeping upright after the Epley and Liberatory maneuvers is necessary.[121–123] After successful treatment with particle repositioning maneuvers, some patients may continue to experience residual disequilibrium and balance problems that may require further physical therapy interventions. Before discharging the patient, the physical therapist should teach the patient how to perform the appropriate techniques at home in case of recurrence.

CASE A, PART III

Based on Mrs. O'Hara's diagnosis of right posterior SCC canalithiasis BPPV, the patient was treated with the Epley maneuver. Following treatment, the Dix–Hallpike test was performed again in the same position that had exacerbated her symptoms previously. The nystagmus had resolved and the patient reported marked improvement of her symptoms. The patient was given a BPPV education sheet, scheduled a follow-up in 2 weeks, and instructed to return to physical therapy as soon as possible if she experienced worsening symptoms. At the patient's follow-up, she reported complete resolution of symptoms and was able to lie flat in bed, roll over, and pitch her head up and down without causing vertigo.

CASE B, PART I

Mr. Huffman is a 65-year-old accountant who experienced a sudden onset of vertigo, nausea, vomiting, and imbalance 2 weeks after he had a flu-like illness. Ten days after the onset of his vertigo, he was referred to physical therapy for vestibular rehabilitation with a diagnosis of right UVH secondary to vestibular neuritis. Previous caloric testing reported a 35% weakness in the right ear. Oculomotor testing revealed a left-beating spontaneous vestibular nystagmus, which was suppressed in light. Gaze stability testing revealed an impaired VOR with a positive right head impulse test, and there was a change of visual acuity from 20/20 to 20/40 (i.e., 3-line decrement) on the DVA test. Mr. Huffman scored 15/24 on the DGI (score of <19 indicates increased risk of falls).[104] His mCTSIB results showed an impaired ability to maintain balance in condition 6 (eyes closed and standing

on foam). His DHI of 40% indicated a moderate perception of handicap due to dizziness. The patient exhibited imbalance during the FGA, stepping outside a 12-inch wide path six times over a 20-feet long walkway. Mr. Huffman reported functional problems on the VD-ADL with scores of 4 (slower, cautious, more careful) on most activities. At the beginning of his evaluation, he rated his dizziness as 3/10 using a VAS. His self-rated dizziness increased to 7/10 during the evaluation, particularly with head turns.

Unilateral Vestibular Hypofunction

General physical therapy goals for individuals with UVH and expected outcomes are to (1) improve the patient's gaze stability to see clearly, during head movements, (2) decrease the patient's sensations of disequilibrium and oscillopsia with head motions, (3) improve static and dynamic postural stability, during functional tasks, and (4) return the patient to his or her previous level of activity and participation in society. Mechanisms that are involved in the recovery of function after unilateral vestibular loss include functional recovery of hair cells or vestibular nerves, spontaneous rebalancing of the tonic firing rate centrally, adaptive changes in the residual vestibular system, the substitution of alternative strategies, and habituation of unpleasant sensations.[124] A Cochrane review in 2015 on vestibular rehabilitation concluded that there is moderate to strong evidence that vestibular rehabilitation is a safe and effective treatment for patients with UVH or loss, and moderate evidence exists that vestibular rehabilitation is an effective treatment of patients during the acute onset of vestibular neuritis or after resection of VS.[125] Clinical practice guidelines for vestibular rehabilitation for patients with peripheral vestibular hypofunction were published in 2016 by the American Physical Therapy Association, based on evidence supporting the effectiveness of vestibular rehabilitation in improving balance function, functional recovery, quality of life, and reducing fall risk in patients with acute (first 2 weeks after symptom onset), subacute (2 weeks to 3 months), and chronic (>3 months) unilateral and bilateral peripheral vestibular hypofunction.[126] Patients should expect improved function within 6 weeks, if they are compliant with vestibular rehabilitation exercises.[124]

Gaze Stability Exercises

Individuals with visual blurring and dizziness, when performing tasks that require visual tracking or gaze stabilization, can benefit from specific exercises. In patients with some vestibular function, adaptation of the VOR can be facilitated by exposing the patient to small amounts of **retinal slip**, which occurs when the image of an object moves off the fovea. The error signal that is generated by retinal slip stimulates vestibular adaptation within the brain. Exercises that are used to induce adaptation via retinal slip include having the patient maintain visual fixation of an object (i.e., thumb or business card) while the head is moving under the following two paradigms: (1) with the visual target stationary, the patient moves the head back and forth while maintaining visual fixation (X1 paradigm) and (2) the persons'

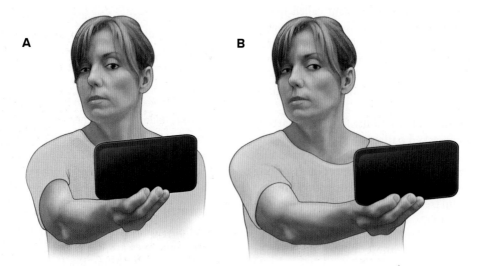

FIGURE 17-11 Gaze stability exercise. A. X1 Paradigm – Patient moves head back and forth while maintaining gaze on stable target. **B.** X2 Paradigm – Patient moves head back and forth while moving target in the opposite direction.

head and the visual target move in opposite directions while the person keeps the target in focus (X2 paradigm) (Figure 17-11). These exercises can be progressed by (1) increasing the directions of head movements, (2) the duration and frequency of exercise bouts (e.g., start with 3 to 5 times daily for a total of 12 minutes as tolerated and progress to 20 minutes a day), (3) the speed of head movements, (4) the distance of the target (start with near target [3 feet] and progress to far target [8–10 feet]), (5) the size of the target (e.g., checkerboard, outdoors), or (6) changing body position (e.g., start sitting or standing, progressing to walking forward or backward, stepping up or down).[126,127]

In individuals with poor or no VOR, substitution exercises that promote the use of saccadic and pursuit eye movements and central preprogramming are prescribed.[119] These exercises include (1) active eye movements followed by head movements between two horizontal targets and (2) visualization of remembered targets. In the eye followed by head movement exercise, two letters (e.g., X and Z) are placed on a wall about 2-feet apart (i.e., close enough that the patient can look at one of the targets and see the other target out of the corner of the eye). The patient is asked to look directly at the X, with the head rotated so that the nose is aligned with the X. Without moving the head, the patient shifts gaze to the other target. Then, the patient turns his/her head toward the second target, while maintaining fixation on the target during the head movement. The exercise is repeated to both sides multiple times. In the remembered target exercise, the patient starts by looking directly ahead at a target. Then the patient closes the eyes and turns the head, while attempting to maintain the eyes on the remembered target location. The patient opens the eyes and sees if he is looking at the target. This exercise may enhance use of cervical inputs to generate eye movements that keep the eye on target or cortical co-activation, producing the head and eye movement.[124]

Habituation Exercises (Motion Sensitivity)

Habituation exercises can be used to treat continual complaints of movement- or visual-provoked dizziness. These exercises are based on the concept that repeated exposure to provoking body or visual motion stimuli causes a reduction in symptoms over time. The original habituation exercises were developed and studied by Cawthorne[128] and Cooksey[129] (see Box 17-2), Norre and De Weerdt,[130] and Dix.[131] Many clinicians use the Motion

---

Box 17-2 Cawthorne and Cooksey Habituation Exercises

The patient completes 4 to 5 repetitions of each exercise first slowly and then faster; many can be done initially with eyes open and then progressed to eyes closed.[124,128,129]

Eye movements (sitting and standing):

- Holding the head still, looks up and down, to each side
- Looks at their finger as it moves closer to their eyes and further away

Head movement (sitting and standing):

- Alternately rotates head to the right and left
- Alternately moves head up and down

Body movement (sitting)

- Bends to the floor to pick up an object, returns to upright and lifts above head
- Circular shoulder movements
- Bends forward to retrieve object through their knees, returns to upright and then places back through knees
- Coming to standing
- Rises to stand from sitting and returns (eyes open, eyes closed)
- Comes to standing and turns to right or left, returns to sitting (eyes open or closed)

Standing: can be done on firm surface and progress to soft surface

- Tosses a ball back and forth from one hand to another at waist level

- Tosses ball back and forth through knees while bent forward
- Single limb stance

Walking: can be done initially on a firm surface and progressed to a soft surface; can also progress to eyes closed

- Alternately turns head to right and left
- Tip toe walking
- Moves in a circle while therapist unexpectedly tosses a ball to them

Sensitivity Quotient (MSQ) results (see Tests and Measures section) to determine provoking movements and to develop an individualized exercise program.[65,132] In this approach, up to four movements are chosen from the MSQ as the basis of the patient's exercise program. The patient repeats the movements three to five times, two to three times a day, with rests between movements to allow the symptoms to stop. To address visual motion sensitivity (i.e., visual vertigo), optokinetic stimuli (i.e., repetitive moving patterns) or immersion in virtual reality environments that simulate realistic, visually challenging environments are used for habituation exercises.[133,134] The visual stimuli can be delivered via high-tech equipment (optokinetic discs, moving rooms or virtual reality simulations), or low-tech equipment (busy computer screen savers or videos of busy environments). The effectiveness of habituation exercises is improved if the stimuli are of sufficient intensity to produce mild to moderate symptoms.[124] Whenever possible, the habituation exercises should be incorporated into the person's daily activities, and a home exercise program (HEP) based on the provoking movements should be provided. Table 17-9 provides a progression of habituation exercises used to reduce dizziness in patients with UVH. It may take 4 weeks for symptoms to decrease.[124]

Postural Stability Exercises

Postural stability exercises aim to improve the patient's balance control and prevent falls. When developing an intervention program for balance impairments, clinicians need to consider their patients' impairments across all systems and decide which impairments can be rehabilitated and which require compensation or substitution. For example, individuals with vestibular deficits often experience postural instability, when performing activities with reduced visual and/or somatosensory inputs. Therefore, they may benefit from performing exercises and tasks that remove or alter visual and somatosensory cues to force them to utilize the remaining sensory inputs. Head movements should be included in exercises as many people with vestibular loss will decrease their head movement. Motor learning concepts (i.e., practice parameters, feedback, stages of learning, task analysis, environmental conditions) should be incorporated into balance training. Box 17-3 provides examples of balance exercises and progressions to address identified deficits in static, dynamic, anticipatory, and reactive balance control as well as problems involving sensory organization, functional performance, and safety. Physical therapists must properly supervise and/or guard patients when they are performing balance exercises to ensure their safety.

TABLE 17-9	Progression of Habituation Exercises to Treat Patients with Unilateral Vestibular Hypofunction[119]
WEEK	**HABITUATION EXERCISE**
1	Large amplitude, rapid cervical movements (horizontal or vertical), consisting of 5 complete movements (cycles) performed 3 times in sitting
2	Large amplitude, rapid horizontal cervical rotation (seated) and standing pivots, or large amplitude, rapid vertical cervical movement (seated) and seated trunk flexion-extension, 3 sets of 5 cycles
3	Large amplitude, rapid horizontal and vertical cervical movements (seated) and standing pivots, or large amplitude, rapid horizontal and vertical cervical movements (seated) and seated trunk flexion-extension, 3 sets of 5 cycles
4	Large amplitude, rapid horizontal and vertical cervical movements (seated), standing pivots, and seated trunk flexion-extension, 3 sets of 5 cycles
5	Large amplitude, rapid horizontal and vertical cervical movements (standing), standing pivots, and seated trunk flexion-extension, 3 sets of 5 cycles
6	Large amplitude, rapid horizontal and vertical cervical movements (standing), standing pivots (180 degrees), seated trunk flexion-extension, Brandt–Daroff exercises (Figure 16-8), 3 sets of 5 cycles

Box 17-3 Postural Stability Exercises and Interventions

Static balance control

To promote static balance control, the patient can start by maintaining a standing posture on a firm surface. More challenging activities include practice in the tandem and single-leg stance, lunge, and squat positions. Progress these activities by standing on soft surfaces (e.g., foam, sand, and grass), narrowing the BOS, moving the head, or closing the eyes. Add a secondary task (i.e., catching ball or mental calculations) to further increase the level of difficulty.

Dynamic balance control

To promote dynamic balance control, interventions may involve the following:

- Maintain equal weight distribution and upright trunk postural alignment while standing on a soft surface (e.g., carpeting, foam, wobble boards). Progress the activities by superimposing movements such as shifting the body weight, rotating the trunk, rotating the head side-to-side or up and down.
- Perform standing bends and squats on firm surface. Progress to narrow BOS, eyes closed, soft surface, reaching to touch floor.

- Transitions into and out of chair or on and off floor. Progress to without arm support, eyes closed.
- March in place with eyes open on a firm surface. Progress to marching with eyes closed, on soft surfaces, and with head turns.
- Walk and turn suddenly or walk in a circle while gradually decreasing the circumference of the circle, first in one direction and then in another.

Anticipatory balance control

To practice anticipatory balance control, the patient can perform the following:

- Reach in all directions to touch or grasp objects, catch a ball, or kick a ball.
- Bend and pick up objects off of lower surfaces.
- Perform step-up and down exercises or lunges in multiple directions.
- Maneuver through an obstacle course.

Reactive balance control

To train reactive balance control, the patient can perform the following activities:

- Work to gradually increase the amount of sway in standing in different directions while on a firm stable surface.
- Practice forward walking with abrupt stops. Progress to backward walking.
- To emphasize training of the *ankle strategy*, practice swaying while standing on one leg with the trunk erect.
- To emphasize training of the *hip strategy*, walk on lines drawn on the floor, perform tandem stance, perform single-leg stance with trunk bending, or stand on a rocker balance board.
- To emphasize the *stepping strategy*, practice stepping up onto a stool or curb or over progressively larger obstacles (i.e., electric cord, shoe, phone book) or practice stepping with legs crossed in front or behind the other leg (e.g., weaving or braiding).
- To increase the challenge during these activities, add anticipated and unanticipated external forces. For example, have the patient lift boxes that are identical in appearance but of different weights, throw and catch balls of different weights and sizes.

Sensory organization

Many of the activities previously described can be utilized while varying the reliance on specific sensory systems.

- To reduce or destabilize the *visual inputs*, have the patient close the eyes or practice in low lighting or darkness, or move the eyes and head together during the balance activity.
- To decrease reliance on *somatosensory cues*, patients can narrow the BOS, stand on a soft surface, or stand on an unstable surface (i.e., rocker or incline board).

Examples of these types of activities might include the following:

- Walking backward, side-stepping, and braiding performed with the eyes closed.
- Walking while watching a ball being tossed from one hand to the other.
- Standing or marching in place on foam performed first with eyes open and later with eyes closed.

Balance during functional activities

Clinicians should focus on activities like the activity limitations identified in the evaluation. For example, if reaching is limited, then the patient should work on activities such as reaching for a glass in the cupboard, reaching behind (as putting arm in a sleeve), or catching a ball off center. Having the patient perform two or more tasks simultaneously increases the level of task complexity. Practicing recreational activities that the patient enjoys, such as golf, increases motivation for practice while challenging balance control.

Safety during gait, locomotion, or balance

To emphasize safety, clinicians should have the patient practice postural sway activities within the person's actual stability limits and progress dynamic activities with emphasis on promoting function. If balance deficits cannot be changed, environmental modifications (e.g., better lighting, installation of grab bars, removal of throw rugs), assistive devices, and increased family or external support may be required to ensure safety.

CASE B, PART II

Based on Mr. Huffman's diagnosis of right UVH and the results of his physical therapy examination, the therapist developed an individualized vestibular rehabilitation program for Mr. Huffman that included progressive gaze stabilization exercises and static and dynamic balance exercises. Gaze stability exercises included horizontal and vertical head movements, performed while the patient moved his head as quickly as possible, while keeping a stationary target in focus. These exercises were performed with near and far targets four to five times a day. Static and dynamic balance exercises were performed on compliant surfaces (carpeting, foam) with varied foot positions. Visual input was altered by having Mr. Huffman close his eyes or wear blurry glasses to obscure his vision. He rated his dizziness at the beginning and end of each session, using a VAS to determine correct exercise intensity. The physical therapist periodically provided education about his diagnosis, the course of treatment, and prognosis. After completing seven 1-hour treatments, spaced 1-week apart, Mr. Huffman reported 0/10 dizziness and scored a 5% on the DHI, indicating minimal perception of handicap from dizziness. Since the MCID value for the DHI is 18 points, Mr. Huffman's change of 35 points may be considered clinically important.[61] He had a normal score on the mCTSIB and a score of 24/24 on the DGI. Over a long walkway, he easily stayed inside a 12-inch-wide path. Mr. Huffman's gaze stability was within normal limits, with a change in visual acuity from 20/20 to 20/30 on the DVA test. He scored "independent" on the VD-ADL and was able to resume his previous activities and roles and responsibilities without symptoms.

Bilateral Vestibular Hypofunction

General physical therapy goals for individuals with BVH and expected outcomes are to (1) improve the patient's gaze stability, (2) decrease the patient's complaints of disequilibrium and oscillopsia with head motions, (3) improve static and dynamic postural stability, during functional tasks, and (4) prevent physical deconditioning by engaging in a walking program. Mechanisms of recovery of gaze stability in BVH are central pre-programming of eye movements and modifications in saccadic and smooth pursuit eye movements.[135] A study that examined recovery of postural stability in patients with bilateral vestibular deficits over a 2-year period found that patients initially rely on visual inputs as a substitute for loss of vestibular inputs, but over time, they become more dependent on somatosensory inputs to maintain balance.[135] Several studies support the use of a vestibular rehabilitation exercise program to decrease subjective complaints, improve visual acuity during head movement, and improve postural stability during functional activities.[126,136–140] Recovery for individuals with bilateral vestibular deficits is slower than for unilateral lesions and may take up to 2 years.[136] Certain activities will always be limited, such as walking in low-vision conditions or over uneven surfaces, night driving, and sports that involve quick movements of the head.[135,141]

For patients with BVH, who have some remaining function, gaze stability exercises can be similar to the X1 paradigm exercises used for people with UVH. Some individuals with BVH do not tolerate the X2 paradigm exercises due to excessive retinal slip, but those with asymmetrical BVH may tolerate and benefit from the exercise. Patients with very low or no peripheral vestibular function will benefit from the sequenced eye and head movement and imaginary target exercises (see Physical Therapy Treatment section) that substitute smooth pursuit and saccadic eye movements to stabilize gaze. Additional substitution strategies to improve eye stabilization include performing eye movements without head motion (i.e., stop and stand still while reading signs) and with head movement while focusing on a distant object (i.e., walk in open spaces while focusing the eyes on a distant object).

Balance exercises for individuals with BVH should enhance the substitution of visual and somatosensory information to improve postural stability and develop compensatory strategies that can be used in situations where balance is highly stressed.[135] People with BVH are at high risk of falls, and therefore, clinicians must be careful that balance exercises are performed safely. Balance exercises that vary the reliance on specific sensory systems similar to those for individuals with UVH may be beneficial. Compensatory strategies that can be taught to prevent falls are (1) using night lights, if they get out of bed at night, (2) using lights that come on automatically, (3) having emergency lighting inside and outside of the house in case of power failure, and (4) learning how to safely move around places with busy visual environments such as shopping malls and grocery stores.[135] Some individuals with BVH may require the use of an assistive device when walking at night, on uneven surfaces, and in busy environments.

Patients with BVH may become physically deconditioned due to decreased activity levels, resulting from a fear of falling or increased dizziness from movement.[135] Therefore, it is very important to get individuals with BVH on a walking program, preferably daily. This program should be progressed to challenge patients by having them walk over different surfaces (e.g., carpeting, foam, grass, sand) and in different environments (e.g., mall, grocery store). Exercises in a pool may be advantageous, as the buoyancy of the water may allow the person with BVH to move without fear of falling to the ground. Patient should be educated on the importance of maintaining daily activity after vestibular rehabilitation ends.

Central Vestibular Disorders

General physical therapy goals and expected outcomes for patients with central vestibular disorders include (1) demonstration of appropriate fall prevention strategies and precautions for safe functioning in daily life, (2) demonstration of appropriate selection of compensatory strategies for gaze stability, and (3) prevention of physical deconditioning by engaging in a walking program. Recovery from central lesions is often prolonged (≥6 months) and may be incomplete because areas of the central nervous system that are likely responsible for adaptive mechanisms may be damaged by the initial lesion.

Physical therapy interventions for individuals with central vestibular lesions will depend on the location of the lesion and the patient's signs and symptoms. Treatment of people with lesions of the vestibular nuclei will probably be similar to treatment for a person with UVH. Treatment of patients with complaints of dizziness may respond to gaze stability and/or habituation exercises. Gait and balance exercises that promote integration of somatosensory, visual, and vestibular inputs are often effective with these patients. While the literature in the efficacy of vestibular rehabilitation in central disorders has been mostly small, uncontrolled studies, there is supportive evidence from a few randomized controlled trials that vestibular rehabilitation is effective in the management of individuals with MS.[142,143]

● CEREBELLAR DISORDERS

CASE C, PART I

Mrs. Falstaff is a 52-year-old homemaker, who has experienced progressive balance problems, for the last 3 years, and several episodes of spontaneous vertigo, lasting for a few seconds while walking. She was referred to physical therapy for balance and gait training and fall prevention with a genetically confirmed diagnosis of spinocerebellar atrophy type 6 (SCA 6). Her subjective history reveals that she has fallen five times in the past 6 months, all of which occurred in her home while walking, and she once sustained an ankle sprain, while descending stairs, that required medical care. She uses a cane, when walking in the community, but at home, prefers to use walls and furniture to navigate in her house. Her father, sister, and two brothers all have the same condition. The result of a recent head MRI indicates cerebellar atrophy.

Anatomy and Physiology of the Cerebellum

For a discussion of the anatomy and physiology of the normal cerebellum and its role in control of movements, refer Chapter 5.

Disorders of the Cerebellum

Due to the cerebellum's critical role in coordinating and adapting movements, damage to the cerebellum often results in disabling **ataxia**, defined as the loss of muscle coordination without apparent weakness. Cerebellar ataxia results from a variety of acquired and hereditary causes as described in Table 17-10. Strokes that involve any of the three arteries that supply blood to the cerebellum (e.g., superior, anterior inferior, and posterior inferior cerebellar arteries; refer Chapter 10) can result in cerebellar damage. The cerebellum is also sensitive to toxins, including heavy metals, solvents, and alcohol. Chronic alcoholism causes cerebellar atrophy primarily in the anterior superior vermis.[144] Medications that can cause cerebellar ataxia are certain antiepileptic drugs (e.g., carbamazepine [Tegretol], phenytoin [Dilantin]), lithium salts (Eskalith, Lithobid), certain cancer chemotherapeutic drugs, cyclosporine (Gengraf, Neoral, Sandimmune), and the antibiotic metronidazole (Flagyl). Tumors in the posterior fossa, in or near the cerebellum, occur more frequently in children than in adults.[145] Multiple sclerosis is the most common nonhereditary cause of cerebellar damage.[146] Chiari and other congenital malformations cause damaging pressure and mechanical deformation of the cerebellum (see Chapter 19). Studies in animals and individuals with TBI demonstrate that the cerebellum is often damaged in traumatic brain injuries, even when the initial mechanical forces are directed at the cerebral cortex (see Chapter 11).[147,148]

Of the hereditary causes of cerebellar damage, the highest prevalence is Friedreich's ataxia, followed by the spinocerebellar ataxias.[146] **Friedreich's ataxia** (also called FA or FRDA) is an autosomal recessive inherited disease that causes progressive damage to the spinal cord (dorsal columns, corticospinal, and spinocerebellar tracts), dorsal root ganglia, cerebellum, and cranial nerves VII, X, and XII, causing progressive limb and gait ataxia, dysarthria, loss of proprioception and vibration sensations, absent tendon reflexes, abnormal eye movements, and upper motor neuron signs. Other symptoms that often accompany FA are hypertrophic cardiomyopathy, diabetes, scoliosis, pes cavus, and restless leg syndrome. Symptoms typically begin between the ages of 5 and 15 years, and generally patients lose the ability to transfer and walk without assistance between 10 and 15 years after disease onset.[145] **Spinocerebellar ataxias** (SCAs) are a group of over 35 distinct autosomal dominant hereditary diseases, which are named by numbers (e.g., SCA1, SCA2).[145] Depending on the genetic abnormality, cerebellar damage may occur alone or may be combined with extracerebellar damage. Onset is usually during the third or fourth decade of life, and progression is usually slow, which means that children of affected parents will likely not know until they are adults whether they are affected. Related autosomal dominant inherited diseases that are more rare are the **episodic ataxias** (EAs), characterized by recurrent, discrete episodes of vertigo, ataxia, and often migraine headaches and nausea, lasting minutes to hours that are provoked by stress, excitement, or exercise.[145]

Clinical Manifestations of Cerebellar Damage

Ataxia is the primary sign of cerebellar damage, which can be used to describe uncoordinated gait (**gait ataxia**) or uncoordinated arm and leg movements (**limb ataxia**). Cerebellar ataxia worsens with movements of multiple joints and with quick movements. Table 17-11 shows the common signs and symptoms of cerebellar dysfunction.

Limb Movements

Limb movements, in cerebellar disease, are characterized by dysmetria, dyssynergia, dysdiadochokinesia, movement decomposition, and rebound. **Dysmetria** is an inaccuracy of movement in which the desired target is either under-reached (hypometria) or over-reached (hypermetria). Dysmetria is generally worse with multi-joint compared to single-joint limb movements, and slow movements tend to produce hypometria

TABLE 17-10	Selected Causes of Cerebellar Damage[140,141]
ACQUIRED CAUSES	**HEREDITARY CAUSES**

• Stroke (ischemic, hemorrhagic)
• Toxicity (alcohol, heavy metals [mercury, lead, thallium], medications, organic solvents [toluene, benzene], phencyclidine [PCP])
• Tumor (primary cerebellar tumor, metastatic disease)
• Immune-mediated (multiple sclerosis, celiac disease, vasculitis [Behcet's disease, lupus], paraneoplastic cerebellar degeneration)
• Congenital and developmental (Chiari malformation, agenesis, hypoplasias [Joubert syndrome, Dandy–Walker cyst], dysplasias)
• Infection (cerebellitis, abscess)
• Metabolic (hypothyroidism, acute thiamine [B1] deficiency, chronic vitamin B_{12} and E deficiencies)
• Trauma
• Degenerative nonhereditary diseases (multiple system atrophy [MSA], idiopathic late-onset cerebellar ataxia [ILOCA])
	Autosomal recessive:
	  • Friedreich's ataxia (FA)
	  • Early onset cerebellar ataxia (EOCA)
	  • Ataxia telangiectasia
	Autosomal dominant:
	  • Spinocerebellar ataxias (SCAs)
	  • Episodic ataxias (EAs)
	  • Dentato-rubral-pallidoluysian atrophy (DRPLA)
	  • Gerstmann–Straussler–Scheinker (GSS) disease
	X-linked disorders:
	  • Mitochondrial disease
	  • Fragile X-associated tremor/ataxia syndrome

TABLE 17-11	Signs and Symptoms of Cerebellar Damage		
SYMPTOM/SIGN	AREA OF CEREBELLAR DAMAGE	FUNCTIONAL MANIFESTATION	EXAMINATION FINDINGS
Limb ataxia • Dysmetria • Dyssynergia • Dysdiadochokinesia • Decomposition • Rebound	Lateral cerebellum, deep cerebellar nuclei (globose, emboliform, part of dentate nuclei)	Uncoordinated movement of ipsilateral arm and/or leg	• Impaired FTN* and HTS** • Impaired rapid alternating movements • Slow, effortful fine finger movements • Impaired limb rebound
Tremor	Cerebellar efferent pathways to the red nucleus and inferior olivary nucleus, deep cerebellar nuclei	• Postural tremor • Kinetic tremor • Intention tremor (<5 Hz)	• Side-to-side tremor of out-stretched arms or tremor when standing still • End-point tremor on FTN or HTS test
Hypotonia	Vermis, flocculonodular lobe	Decreased ability to maintain a steady force	• Ipsilateral hypotonia of limbs • Pendular deep tendon reflexes
Balance and gait dysfunction	Anterior lobe, vermis, fastigial nucleus	• Wide-based stance • Uncoordinated gait • Difficulty with stopping or turning • Frequent falls	• Impaired sharpened Romberg test • Impaired spatiotemporal/ kinematic gait parameters • Unsteady tandem gait • Impaired stopping and turning
Oculomotor dysfunction	Flocculonodular lobe, vermis, fastigial nucleus	• Oscillopsia • Blurred or double vision	• Nystagmus • Impaired slow pursuit • Impaired shift of gaze/saccades • Impaired VOR cancellation
Speech impairments	Rostral paravermal region of the anterior lobes	• Dysarthria • Slurred speech	• Impaired articulation and prosody • May be slow, hesitant, or accentuate some syllables
Cognitive and psychiatric impairments	Bilateral posterior lobes (cognitive), vermis (emotional)	• Memory problems, difficulty functioning at work or in home • Impaired communication skills • Personality changes	• Impaired executive functions • Impaired visuospatial function • Agrammatism, dysprosodia • Blunted affect or disinhibited, inappropriate behavior

*FTN, finger-to-nose.
**HTS, heel-to-shin.

while fast movements produce hypermetria.[149] **Dyssynergia** describes uncoordinated multi-joint movements, where movements of specific segments are not properly sequenced or of the appropriate amplitude or direction. Dysmetria and dyssynergia appear to be related and are thought to be due to a deficit in predicting and accounting for the dynamics of the limbs.[149] **Dysdiadochokinesia** refers to an impaired ability to perform rapid alternating movements (e.g. supination-pronation). Patients with cerebellar dysfunction typically demonstrate excessive slowness with inconsistency in the rate and range of alternating movements, which worsen as the movement continues.[150] **Movement decomposition** refers to the breakdown of a movement sequence or multi-joint movement into separate movements that are simpler to perform than the combined movement. A well-known example of this is that patients with cerebellar damage, when asked to reach for an object in front and above the resting arm, will often flex the shoulder first and then, while holding the shoulder fixed, extend the elbow.[149] This produces a slower and more curved path of the finger to the target, compared to the faster and straight-line path of healthy individuals. Movement decomposition may be a compensatory strategy for dealing with impaired multi-joint movements.[149] **Rebound** refers to an inability to rapidly and sufficiently stop movement of a body part after strong isometric resistance of the body part is suddenly removed. Healthy individuals are able to quickly halt the movement, while patients with cerebellar damage show considerable movement in the direction opposite to the applied resistance. This phenomenon is thought to be caused by delayed cessation of the agonist muscles and/or delayed activation of the antagonist muscles.

Tremor

Tremors caused by cerebellar damage are called **action tremors**, meaning that they are elicited during muscle activation and not when the person is at rest. Action tremors are further classified as **kinetic or postural tremors**. Kinetic tremors are observed in muscles that are producing an active voluntary movement, while postural tremors are seen in muscles that are maintaining a static position against gravity. Kinetic tremors typically occur at low frequencies below 5 Hz.[151] **Intention tremor** is a specific type of kinetic tremor that is observed as an increase in tremor amplitude that occurs in the terminal portion of visually guided movements toward a target. It occurs because the person is using visual feedback to make corrective movements to reach the target; an intention tremor is diminished or absent, if vision is removed.[146] **Titubation** is a specific type of postural tremor characterized by slow-frequency oscillations (about 3 Hz) of the head or trunk.[152] The cause of cerebellar tremors is not well understood but proposed mechanisms are (1) an inability to anticipate movements with excessive reliance on sensory feedback (i.e., vision, proprioception) and (2) central influences involving pathways connecting the dentate nucleus, red nucleus, and inferior olivary nucleus.[146,151]

Hypotonia and Muscle Force Generation

Hypotonia, in individuals with cerebellar damage, usually manifests as a decrease in extensor tone necessary to keep the body upright against gravity. Pendular deep tendon reflexes (e.g., leg swings more than four times in response to briskly tapping the quadriceps tendon) and inability to check forearm movement in the rebound test have been attributed to hypotonia but may have other explanations.[151] Hypotonia may be due to decreased excitatory inputs to the vestibulospinal and reticulospinal tracts from the cerebellar vermis and flocculonodular lobe, as individuals with severe cerebellar hypoplasias, affecting the vermis, such as Joubert syndrome, have greater degrees of hypotonia.[153] Notably, hypotonia usually does not interfere with physical function in individuals with cerebellar damage.[154]

Although cerebellar damage does not typically cause loss of functional motor strength, many patients experience problems with sustaining a steady force with their hands, which they may refer to as weakness. A reduced rate of force generation (power) as well as variability in maintaining a constant level of force have been reported in individuals with cerebellar damage.[155,156] These deficits in force generation may affect performance of precision manipulative hand tasks.

Balance and Gait Dysfunction

Individuals with cerebellar damage demonstrate impaired static, dynamic, reactive, and anticipatory balance control. Increased postural sway is typically observed in quiet stance, with some variations in sway frequency, amplitude, and direction depending on the site of the lesion.[157,158] Individuals with cerebellar damage, isolated to the anterior lobe, show increased postural sway, which is high-frequency, low amplitude, and mainly in the anterior–posterior direction. They also exhibit postural tremor and increased movements of the head, trunk, and legs and tend to improve their stability with visual feedback. In contrast, individuals with isolated damage to the flocculonodular lobe tend to exhibit low-frequency, high-amplitude sway without a preferred direction and without associated head, trunk, and leg movements. These individuals do not improve performance with visual feedback. Individuals with lateral cerebellar lesions tend to have slight or even no postural instability.[156,158]

In response to an unexpected perturbation of the support surface, individuals with cerebellar damage show hypermetric responses, characterized by abnormally large and prolonged muscle activity and greater surface-reactive torque responses that cause them to overshoot the initial posture during the balance recovery phase.[159] This seems to indicate an inability to set the correct size (or gain) of the response.[146] However, similar to healthy individuals, people with cerebellar damage are able to decrease the size of their postural responses with repeated trials of a predictable perturbation and can change their response magnitude appropriately to an expected change in the size of a perturbation, although the overall size of the responses remain increased compared to normal. Lack of APAs results in imbalance during self-generated movements, as for example not leaning forward prior to standing on the toes, resulting in the person falling backwards.[160,161]

Gait ataxia in individuals with cerebellar dysfunction is characterized by reduced speed, prolonged time in double stance, abnormal interlimb coordination, and increased variability in stride lengths and kinematics of the hip, knee, and ankle joints, although their BOS may not be increased as commonly presumed.[162–164] Balance deficits have a direct and marked impact on walking, as individuals with cerebellar damage and significant imbalance typically demonstrate the classic features of gait ataxia, while those with cerebellar damage and significant leg coordination deficits, but slight to no balance deficits, typically have few gait abnormalities.[165] Gait variability (i.e., coefficient of variation in stride time), during slow walking, is associated with a history of falls in individuals with cerebellar ataxia.[166] During walking, individuals with cerebellar ataxia have great difficulty in stopping abruptly and adopt a multistep stopping strategy to compensate for their inability to control the upper body and to generate appropriate braking forces in the lower extremities to stop the progression of the body in the forward direction.[167] Some patients with cerebellar ataxia occasionally stop abruptly with feet parallel instead of one foot forward in relation to the other, which is never seen in control subjects.[167] They also have difficulty performing large turns and adopt compensatory strategies such as enlarging the BOS, shortening step length, increasing the number of steps, and using multiple steps to turn rather than a "spin-turn" strategy.[168,169] Deficits in balance and walking may contribute to the reported high incidence of falls in cerebellar ataxia.[170]

Oculomotor Dysfunction

Since normal oculomotor function relies heavily on the cerebellum for adaptive control, it is not surprising that cerebellar damage can significantly affect eye movements.[146] Smooth pursuit eye movements are slowed, requiring catch-up saccades to keep the eyes fixated on the moving target.[151] The speed of saccadic eye movements is normal in cerebellar disease, but the accuracy is impaired so that both hypometric or hypermetric saccades are seen.[166] VOR cancellation may be diminished or absent.[151,171] There is also reduced velocity of divergent eye movements, which affects the ability to shift gaze from targets close and far away.[146] Numerous types of nystagmus can be seen with cerebellar damage, but the most common form is gaze-evoked nystagmus, elicited near the end ranges of lateral and/or vertical gaze.[151,171] Gaze-evoked nystagmus results in the inability to maintain an eccentric position of gaze. Individuals with significant oculomotor dysfunction should be referred to a vestibular specialist.

Speech Impairments

The speech deficit of individuals with cerebellar dysfunction is **ataxic dysarthria**. The most consistent impairments are found for articulation (pronunciation of speech sounds) and prosody (patterns of stress and intonation of speech). The speech is described as scanning in nature, consisting of hesitations, accentuations of some syllables, the addition of pauses or omission of appropriate pauses, and, in some cases, slurring of syllables.[172] Speech intelligibility may be decreased with problems in distinguishing the difference between plosives (e.g., [p], [t], [k]) at the end of words.[173]

Impaired Motor Learning

Motor learning may be impaired in individuals with cerebellar damage. The cerebellum is very important for motor skill learning through repeated practice of a motor behavior and using error information from one trial to improve performance on the next trial. It is also important for **motor adaptation**, a form of motor learning that involves modification of an already well learned motor skill in response to altered conditions (e.g., adaptation to prism glasses or walking on a split-belt treadmill), which is also an error-driven process. Studies suggest that the type of error that drives cerebellar-dependent learning of reaching is a sensory prediction error (i.e., "How far am I from where I initially predicted that I would be?") rather than a target-referenced error (i.e., "How far am I from the desired target?").[174,175] Similarly, studies have shown that individuals with cerebellar damage have difficulty learning both simple and complex motor behaviors, including recovery from a balance disturbance,[176] walking in a new pattern,[177] or adjusting arm movements for reaching.[178] Thus, clinicians should be aware that individuals with cerebellar damage may take longer to acquire motor skills and adapt motor behaviors and may not ever attain full recovery.

Cognitive and Psychiatric Impairments

Evidence suggests that cerebellar damage can result in a cerebellar–cognitive–affective syndrome that consists of executive dysfunctions (i.e., impairments in planning, set-shifting, verbal fluency, abstract reasoning, and working memory), impaired visuospatial functions (organization and memory), mild language difficulties (i.e., agrammatism [inability to construct a grammatical sentence] and dysprosodia [impaired speech intonation patterns]), and personality changes (i.e., blunting of affect, disinhibition, and inappropriate behavior).[179] Certain cerebellar ataxias are associated with neuropsychiatric symptoms such as distractibility, hyperactivity, compulsive obsessive behavior, anxiety, depression, aggression, hallucinations, lack of empathy, and avoidant behavior.[180]

MEDICAL MANAGEMENT OF CEREBELLAR DAMAGE

There are no curative interventions for people with cerebellar damage. Pharmacological interventions to date have had limited success in reducing symptoms or slowing or stopping disease progression. Medications with some evidence to improve ataxia are 4-aminopyridine (Ampyra) for patients with episodic ataxia type 2, riluzole for patients with ataxia of mixed etiology, Friedreich ataxia or SCA, valproic acid for patients with SCA type 3, and thyrotropin-releasing hormone for patients with spinocerebellar degeneration.[181] The mainstays of treatment for people with degenerative cerebellar ataxias are physical therapy, occupational therapy, and speech therapy.[139,145]

PHYSICAL THERAPY EXAMINATION

Examination of the patient with cerebellar damage includes assessment of limb movement coordination, tremor, balance and gait. These tests would be performed in addition to a systems review and standard neurological assessment that includes evaluation of somatosensation (including cutaneous sensation and proprioception), pain, passive muscle tone, range of motion, muscle strength, muscle endurance, and posture to identify concurrent impairments that might affect the patient's prognosis and treatment (refer Chapter 10 – Neurologic Evaluation).

Limb Movements

Dysmetria, dyssynergia, and movement decomposition are typically tested with the finger-to-nose (FTN) and heel-to shin (HTS) tests. The FTN test asks the patient to repeatedly touch the tip of his/her nose and then the tip of the clinician's nose or finger. The HTS test is performed by having the patient bring the heel of the tested leg to the opposite knee and sliding it in a straight line down the anterior aspect of the tibia to the ankle, while keeping the foot nearly vertical. The clinician assesses for movement decomposition, movement speed, variability in the spatial path, and over/undershooting of the target.[146] Dysdiadochokinesia is typically tested by asking the patient to (1) supinate and pronate the forearm or (2) tap the hand or foot. The clinician assesses the rate and amplitude of movement on these tests, which should be performed (1) on both sides to make comparisons, (2) at slow and fast speeds to determine severity of ataxia, (3) with and without vision to determine if vision improves movement quality, and (4) multiple times on the same limb to observe variability in movements (i.e., hypometric on some, hypermetric on others). It is also important to give the patient the proper amount of head and trunk support so that balance deficits do not affect limb movements and to ensure that the patient does not have visual or other oculomotor impairments that would prevent accurate location of a target. Rebound is tested by asking the patient to flex the elbow against the clinician's hand and then the clinician abruptly removes the resistance and assesses the patient's ability to stop the sudden flexion.[151]

Tremor

Postural tremor is tested by asking the patient to stand in place or with the arms out in front of the body with palms facing down. Kinetic tremor can be tested during non-target directed movements (forearm pronation/supination, hand and foot tapping) or during targeted movements such as the FTN or HTS tests. Intention tremor can be tested by repeating targeted movements with eyes closed; a decrease or disappearance of the tremor with eyes closed compared to eyes open indicates an intention tremor. The clinician assesses tremor amplitude and frequency during these tasks. Tremor may also be observed by asking the patient to write something.[146]

Balance and Gait

Examination of balance and gait for individuals with cerebellar damage is performed in the same manner as for individuals with other neurological diagnoses and so is not described in detail here (see Chapter 10 – Neurologic Evaluation). Documentation of level of assistance needed, movement quality, including severity and frequency of specific features of ataxia (e.g., postural tremor or titubation, movement decomposition, rebound), and time taken to perform functional tasks is useful for treatment planning and tracking patient progress.

Standardized Clinical Scales

The best studied and validated standardized rating scales for quantifying the severity of cerebellar ataxia are the International Cooperative Ataxia Rating Scale (ICARS) and the Scale for the Assessment and Rating of Ataxia (SARA).[182] The ICARS is a semi-quantitative 100-point scale that measures a person's ability to perform 19 specific activities and movements, divided into four categories: posture and gait, limb movements, speech, and oculomotor function.[183] The higher the score, the worse is the patient's performance. The SARA has eight items, yielding a total score of 0 (no ataxia) to 40 (most severe ataxia) and rates quality of movement during gait, stance, sitting, speech, finger movement, and limb coordination functions.[184] Although the SARA was initially developed and tested for the quantification of ataxia due to SCA, it has proven validity in the evaluation of ataxia with other diagnoses.[178] The Brief Ataxia Rating Scale (BARS) is a shorter modified version of ICARS that consists of five items that evaluate walking capacity, decomposition, using the HTS and FTN tests, and dysmetria, dysarthria, and abnormalities of ocular pursuit.[179] Higher scores, on the 30-point scale, indicate worse performance. Use of these scales provides the therapist with an objective and quantifiable measure to demonstrate severity of ataxia and to track progress of therapy. Using a Delphi survey, a panel of experts recommended the SARA, BBS, and TUG tests for the assessment of balance in people with cerebellar ataxia.[185] A systematic review of the psychometric properties of balance measures of cerebellar ataxia found that the posture and gait subcomponent of ICARS demonstrates strong psychometric properties with acceptable clinical utility.[186]

● PHYSICAL THERAPY TREATMENT

Recovery of motor function in individuals with cerebellar damage depends on the cause, extent, and site of the damage as well as numerous other factors such as damage to other brain regions, coexisting medical conditions, and age. Prognosis for recovery may be better for individuals with ataxia, following stroke, neurosurgery, trauma, or MS because only specific areas of the cerebellum are affected, leaving intact regions that might be able to compensate for the damaged parts. In contrast, the prognosis for individuals with degenerative cerebellar diseases may be worse due to the progressive nature and widespread effects of these diseases on all areas of the cerebellum. One study showed that people with damage to the deep cerebellar nuclei did not recover as completely as those with damage isolated to the cerebellar cortex and white matter.[187]

General physical therapy goals and expected outcomes for individuals with cerebellar ataxia include to: (1) improve static and dynamic postural stability during functional tasks, (2) develop appropriate fall prevention strategies and precautions for safe functioning in daily life, and (3) prevent physical deconditioning by engaging in aerobic exercise and/or resistance training.[188] Several systematic reviews have been published that examined the efficacy of rehabilitation in treating cerebellar ataxia.[188–191] The fact that the studies in these reviews contained relatively few randomized controlled trials, featured a multitude of different patient populations (e.g., MS, stroke, TBI, cerebellar degeneration), and implemented interventions with varying types, intensities, and durations, makes it difficult for clinicians to make evidence-based decisions about the most effective interventions for their patients. However, some preliminary evidence suggests that rehabilitation interventions may be more effective if they are (1) multifaceted interventions targeting more than one impairment (e.g., balance and coordination, multidisciplinary inpatient programs); (2) intensive (e.g., ≥60 minutes for 3 days or more per week) and individualized to provide the greatest challenge according to the patient's needs and abilities; (3) durations of a minimum of 4 weeks for improvements in ataxia; and (4) delivered earlier in disease progression, especially interventions targeted to improve ambulation.[189–193] A summary of only the major findings is provided to assist clinicians with their decision-making.

Treatment of Body Structure/Function Impairments

Depending on the patient's individual body structure or function impairments, interventions such as stretching of tight hip flexors, hamstrings, quadriceps, and ankle plantarflexors or strengthening of pelvic and lower extremity musculature may be needed.[194] If the patient is experiencing vertigo, nystagmus, or oculomotor symptoms, he/she may benefit from gaze stability exercises for the VOR and habituation exercises (see Physical Therapy Treatment section).[194] Individuals with cerebellar ataxia expend more energy and require greater concentration levels to perform their daily activities than nondisabled individuals, which may result in excessive fatigue. Integration of aerobic exercise (i.e., walking, stationary cycling, swimming and aquatic exercise, arm ergometry) and submaximal resistance exercise to improve cardiovascular endurance and reduce muscle fatigue is recommended for the majority of individuals with cerebellar ataxia.

Gait and Balance Interventions

Most of the intervention studies for cerebellar ataxia to date emphasize intensive static and dynamic balance exercises and coordination exercises to improve stability, particularly during gait.[188] For specific exercises to improve coordination and motor control of the extremities, see Chapter 14 – Multiple Sclerosis. Initially, the exercises are performed using vision to assist in controlling the movement and progressed to working on movement without the aid of vision. Examples of static and dynamic balance exercises that are commonly prescribed can be found in Box 17-3 and Table 17-12. According to a systematic review conducted by Barbuto et al.[191], most studies that examined the effects of balance training in individuals with degenerative cerebellar disease reported improvements in ataxia severity, gait (only if walking was part of the balance training), and balance measures, with more robust responses associated with therapist supervision, increased balance challenge and frequency of training. Among studies which implemented home-based balance training programs, those conducted with video game-based training[195,196] demonstrated reductions in ataxia severity that were not seen with traditional balance training, possibly due to greater adherence.[191] Gait training overground as well as on treadmills (with or without body weight support) has had some success.[192,197–199]

Two clinical studies with relatively large sample sizes provide some of the best evidence that motor rehabilitation can be beneficial to individuals with degenerative cerebellar disease. Miyai et al. (2012) examined the effects of a combination of physical and occupational therapy delivered 12 hours per week for 4 weeks in patients (n=42) with pure cerebellar degeneration. Following the intervention, the patients demonstrated improvements in ataxia severity, gait speed, fall frequency, and activities of daily living. Improvements were greater in trunk ataxia than in limb ataxia. Despite a trend for functional status to decline to the baseline level within 24 weeks, gains were maintained in more than half of the participants.[192] Ilg et al. (2009) reported that individuals with progressive ataxia due to cerebellar degeneration (n=10) or degeneration of afferent pathways (n=6), who participated in a 4-week physical therapist-directed intensive coordinative training program, focused on static and dynamic balance exercises and walking, followed by performance of an HEP of similar exercises for one hour each day for an additional 4 weeks, had significant improvements in ICARS, SARA, and BBS scores and in gait speed, step length, and lateral trunk sway measures that were sustained 8 weeks after the intervention (see Table 17-12).[193] Individuals with cerebellar ataxia benefitted substantially more from the intervention than individuals with sensory ataxia, likely because sensory inputs are necessary for adequate cerebellar processing.[200] Assessments after one year revealed that individuals who continued to perform the HEP retained the training benefits for executing activities of daily living, despite gradual declines in motor performance and increases of ataxia symptoms due to disease progression.[201] Thus, patients with cerebellar degeneration may benefit the most when physical therapist-directed in person supervised exercise programs are augmented by continuous unsupervised in home exercise training.

TABLE 17-12	Exercises for Cerebellar Ataxia[188]
EXERCISE TYPE	**VARIATIONS**
Static balance activities	Single limb stance Quadruped weight shift – lift one arm, lift one leg, lift one arm and the opposite leg
Dynamic balance 　Kneeling	• Alternately put one foot in front and then the other (1/2 kneeling position) • Alternately put one foot to the side and then the other • Alternately come to standing, using a ½ kneel position and return to kneeling
Standing	• Swing arms • Step in each direction – front, side, back • Braiding stepping • Stair climbing • Overground walking on different surfaces
Whole body movements 　Quadruped	• Raise one arm and the opposite leg; flex them to touch elbow and knee under the trunk and then extend (repeat multiple times then complete with opposite arm and leg)
Kneeling	• Crouch to floor, bending knees, arms and trunk; then extend back up into a kneeling position • Move into side-sitting to one side, return to kneeling and then to side-sitting on the opposite side
Fall prevention activities 　Standing	• Therapist disturbs balance in forward, backward, and lateral positions • Toe touches – bends to touch toes and returns to upright; therapist may introduce a balance displacement • Repeatedly move to quadruped from standing and return to upright; therapist may introduce a balance displacement • When pushed in upright, patient practices flexing forward to the floor
Walking	• Therapist provides balance displacement while the patient is walking
Trunk and shoulder mobility	• From prone lying, push up into extended arms position to stretch upper back • Spine rotation: supine lying – bend knees and alternately rotate the knees to the right and left side • Flexion of the shoulder: supine lying – lift the arms in the direction of the head

Compensatory Strategies

Ataxia can be difficult to treat and individuals with cerebellar lesions often rely on compensatory techniques, including (1) replacing rapid multi-joint movements with slower sequential single joint movements, (2) the use of vision to guide movement, (3) balance-based torso weighting, (4) the use of ambulatory assistive devices, such as a rollator walker, to maximize function and minimize fall risk, and (5) training on safe fall strategies and how to get up from the floor if falls occur.[202-204] Canes and standard walkers may be difficult to use, if ataxia is present in the upper extremities, as the individual may not be able to coordinate the use of the assistive device.

CASE C, PART II

The physical therapist's examination findings of Mrs. Falstaff included dysarthric speech and cerebellar ataxia in the lower extremities. Her SARA score was 28/40 and her performance on the TUG was 25 seconds with use of a cane. Her mCTSIB results showed an impaired ability to maintain balance when her vision was removed or standing on foam (i.e., Conditions 2–4). She rated herself as 30% on the ABC Scale. Based on Mrs. Falstaff's diagnosis of SCA 6 and her physical therapy examination findings, the physical therapist instructed Mrs. Falstaff in exercises for balance and gait that were updated weekly. Balance retraining was performed with varying sensory conditions (i.e., standing with eyes open and then closed, on firm surface and then on foam). The patient practiced standing in a modified single-leg stance position (i.e., patient placed her foot on an egg carton and maintained her balance without crushing the egg carton) with eyes open and then closed, with and without a handhold, and eventually stepping, while alternating foot placement on the egg carton. Gait training initially included walking forward, backward, and sideways on level surfaces with a cane. Later, walking under a variety of challenges was progressed, including (1) while making head turns slowly side-to-side, (2) through an obstacle course that required stepping over small objects, (3) walking over uneven surfaces (foam mat, grass), and (4) walking up and down slight inclines. She was instructed in a HEP that included lower extremity coordination and balance exercises, including tandem stance, marching in place, sit-to-stand, sideways and backward walking with stand-by assistance from her husband. After completing nine 1-hour sessions spaced 1-week apart, Mrs. Falstaff scored a 10/40 on the SARA and completed the TUG in 12.5 seconds. She was able to maintain her balance on the mCTSIB in all conditions except for Condition 4 (standing on the foam with eyes closed). Her ABC Scale score was 75%. The patient was instructed to continue a home program that included a walking program and balance exercises. At a 2-week follow-up appointment, the patient reported that she was able to perform all of her daily activities with no episodes of dizziness and did not need further therapy.

REFERENCES

1. Agrawal Y, Carey JP, Della Santina CC, Schubert MC, Minor LB. Disorders of balance and vestibular function in US adults. *Arch Intern Med.* 2009; 169(10):938-944.

2. Alyono JC. Vertigo and dizziness: understanding and managing fall risk. *Otolaryngol Clin North Am.* 2018 Aug;51(4):725-740.

3. Grimby A, Rosenhall U. Health-related quality of life and dizziness in old age. *Gerontology.* 1995;41(5):286-298.

4. Strupp M, Brandt T. Diagnosis and treatment of vertigo and dizziness. *Dtsch Arztebl Int.* 2008;105(10):173-180.

5. Megna J. The differential diagnosis of dizziness in the older adult. In: Hardage J, ed. *Topics in Geriatrics.* Vol 6, Issue 3. *An Independent Study Course Designed for Individual Continuing Education.* Alexandria, VA: Geriatric Section, American Physical Therapy Association; 2010.

6. Curthoys IA, Halmagyi GM. Vestibular compensation-recovery after unilateral vestibular loss. In: Herdman SJ, Clendaniel RA, eds. *Vestibular Rehabilitation.* 4th ed. Philadelphia, PA: F.A. Davis Company; 2014:121-150.

7. Thompson TL, Amadee R. Vertigo: a review of common peripheral and central vestibular disorders. *Ochsner J.* 2009;9(1):20-26.

8. Kaul V, Cosetti MK. Management of vestibular schwannoma (including NF2): facial nerve considerations. *Otolaryngol Clin North Am.* 2018 Dec;51(6): 1193-1212.

9. Strupp M, Kim JS, Murofushi T, et al. Bilateral vestibulopathy: diagnostic criteria consensus document of the classification committee of the bárány society. *J Vestib Res.* 2017;27(4):177-189.

10. Strupp M, Iugaiczyk J, Erti-Wagner BB, Rujescu D, Westhofen M, Dieterich M. Vestibular disorders: diagnosis, new classification and treatment. *Desch Arztebl Int.* 2020;117(17):300-310.

11. von Brevern M, Bertholon P, Brandt T, et al. Benign paroxysmal positional vertigo: diagnostic criteria. *J Vestib Res.* 2015;25(3-4):105-117.

12. Bhattacharyya N, Gubbels SP, Schwartz SR, et al. Clinical practice guideline: Benign paroxysmal positional vertigo (update). *Otolaryngol Head Neck Surg.* 2017;156(3_suppl):S1-S47.

13. Fife TD, Iverson DJ, Lempert T, et al. Practice parameter: therapies for benign paroxysmal positional vertigo (an evidence-based review): report of the quality standards subcommittee of the American Academy of Neurology. *Neurology.* 2008;70:2067-2074.

14. Nuti D, Masini M, Mandalà M. Benign paroxysmal positional vertigo and its variants. *Handb Clin Neurol.* 2016;137:241-256.

15. Gürkov R, Pyykö I, Zou J, Kentala E. What is Menière's disease? A contemporary re-evaluation of endo-lymphatic hydrops. *J Neurol.* 2016;263(Suppl 1):S71-S81.

16. Lopez-Escamez JA. et al. Diagnostic criteria for menière's disease. *J Vestib Res.* 2015 Jan;25(1): 1-7.

17. Fetter M. Vestibular system disorders. In: Herdman SJ, Clendaniel RA, eds. *Vestibular Rehabilitation.* 4th ed. Philadelphia, PA: F.A. Davis Company; 2014:50-58.

18. Basura GJ, Adams ME, Monfared A, et al. Clinical practice guideline: Ménière's disease. *Otolaryngol Head Neck Surg.* 2020 Apr;162(2_suppl):S1-S55.

19. Lacour M, van de Heyning PH, Novotny M, Tighilet B. Betahistine in the treatment of Meniere's disease. *Neuropsychiatr Dis Treat.* 2007;3(4) 429-440.

20. Magnan J, Özgirgin ON, Trabalzini F, et al. European position statement on diagnosis, and treatment of Meniere's disease. *J Int Adv Otol.* 2018;14(2): 317-321.

21. Sarna B, Abouzari M, Merna C, Jamshidi S, Saber T, Djalilian HR. Perilymphatic fistula: a review of classification, etiology, diagnosis, and treatment. *Front Neurol.* 2020 Sep 15;11:1046.

22. Basura GJ, Cronin SJ, Heidenreich KD. Tullio phenomenon in superior semi-circular canal deshiscence syndrome. *Neurology.* 2014 Mar;82(11):1010.

23. Grad A, Baloh RW. Vertigo of vascular origin. Clinical and electronystagmographic features in 84 cases. *Arch Neurol.* 1989;46:281-284.

24. Cooke DL. Central vestibular disorders. *Neurol Rep.* 1996;20:22-29.

25. Berman JM, Fredrickson JM. Vertigo after head injury – a five year follow-up. *J Otolaryngol.* 1978;7(3):237-245.

26. Haripriya GR, Mary P, Dominic M, Goyal R, Sahadevan A. Incidence and treatment outcomes of post traumatic BPPV in traumatic brain injury patients. *Indian J Otolaryngol Head Neck Surg.* 2018;70(3):337-341.

27. Formeister EJ, Rizk HG, Kohn MA, Sharon JD. The epidemiology of vestibular migraine: a population-based survey study, *Otol Neurotol.* Sep 2018;39(8):1037-1044.

28. Dieterich M. Central vestibular disorders. *J Neurol.* 2007;254:559-568.

29. Radtke A, von Brevern M, Neuhauser H, Hottenrott T, Lempert T. Vestibular migraine: long-term follow-up of clinical symptoms and vestibulo-cochlear findings. *Neurology.* 2012;79(15):1607-1614.

30. Lempert T, Olesen J, furman J, et al. Vestibular migraine: diagnostic criteria. *J Vestib Res.* 2012;22(4): 167-172.

31. Furman JM, Whitney SL. Central causes of dizziness. *Phys Ther.* 2000;80(2):179-187.

32. Wrisley DM, Whitney SL, Furman JM. Vestibular rehabilitation outcomes in patients with a history of migraine. *Otol Neurotol.* 2002;23(4):483-487.

33. Murdin L, Davies RA, Bronstein AM. Vertigo as a migraine trigger. *Neurology.* 2009;73(8):638-642.

34. Brainard A, Gresham C. Prevention and treatment of motion sickness. *Am Fam Physician.* 2014;90(1):41-46.

35. Shupak A, Gordon CR. Motion sickness: advances in pathogenesis, prediction, prevention, and treatment. *Aviat Space Environ Med.* 2006;77(12):1213-1223.

36. Bronstein AM, Golding JF, Gresty MA. Visual vertigo, motion sickness, and disorientation in vehicles. *Semin Neurol.* 2020 Feb;40(1):116-129.

37. Hebert JR, Subramanian PS. Perceptual postural imbalance and visual vertigo. *Curr Neurol Neurosci Rep.* 2019 Mar 16;19(5):19.

38. Staab JP, Eckhardt-Henn A, Horii A, et al. Diagnostic criteria for persistent postural-perceptual dizziness (PPPD): consensus document of the committee for the classification of vestibular disorders of the Bárány Society. *J Vestib Res.* 2017;27(4):191-208.

39. Popkirov S, Staab JP, Stone J. Persistent postural-perceptual dizziness (PPPD): a common, characteristic and treatable cause of chronic dizziness. *Pract Neurol.* 2018 Feb;18(1):5-13.

40. Rine RM, Schubert MC, Balkany TJ. Visual-vestibular habituation and balance training for motion sickness. *Phys Ther.* 1999;79:949-957.

41. Dunlap PM, Holmberg JM, Whitney SL. Vestibular rehabilitation: advances in peripheral and central vestibu-lar disorders. *Curr Opin Neurol.* 2019 Feb;32(1):137-144.

42. Schmäl F. Neuronal mechanisms and the treatment of motion sickness. *Pharmacology.* 2013;91(3-4):229-241.

43. Clendaniel RA, Landel R. Physical therapy management of cervicogenic dizziness. In: Herdman SJ, Clendaniel RA, eds. *Vestibular Rehabilitation.* 4th ed. Philadelphia, PA: F.A. Davis Company; 2014:590-609.

44. Wrisley DM, Sparto PJ, Whitney SL, Furman JM. Cervicogenic dizziness: a review of diagnosis and treatment. *J Orthop Sports Phys Ther.* 2000;30(12):755-766.

45. Reid SA, Rivett DA, Katekar MG, Callister R. Comparison of mulligan sustained natural apophyseal glides and maitland mobilizations for treatment of cervicogenic dizziness: a randomized controlled trial. *Phys Ther.* 2014 Apr;94(4):466-476.

46. Schubert MC. Vestibular function tests. In: Herdman SJ, Clendaniel RA, eds. *Vestibular Rehabilitation.* 4th ed. Philadelphia, PA: F.A. Davis Company; 2014:178-194.

47. Fife TD, Tusa RJ, Furman JM. Assessment: vestibular testing techniques in adults and children: report of the therapeutics and technology assessment subcommittee of the American Academy of Neurology. *Neurology.* 2000;55:1431-1441.

48. Slattery EL, Sinks BC, Goebel JA. Vestibular tests for rehabilitation: applications and interpretation. *Neurorehabilitation.* 2011;29:143-151.

49. Goebel JA, Tungsiripat N, Sinks B, Carmody J. Gaze stabilization test: a new clinical test of unilateral vestibular dysfunction. *Otol Neurotol.* 2007;28(1):68-73.

50. Dieterich M, Brandt T. Ocular torsion and tilt of subjective visual vertical are sensitive brainstem signs. *Ann Neurol.* 1993;33(3):292-299.

51. Min KK, Jong S, Kim MJ, Cho CH, Cha HE, Lee JH. Clinical use of subjective visual horizontal and vertical in patients of unilateral vestibular neuritis. *Otol Neurotol.* 2007;28(4):520-525.

52. Baier B, Dieterich M. Ocular tilt reaction: a clinical sign of cerebellar infarctions? *Neurology.* 2009;72(6):572-573.

53. Pfieffer ML, Anthamatten A; Glassford M. Assessment and treatment of dizziness and vertigo. *Nurse Pract.* 2019;44: 29-36.

54. Schneider R, Leigh RJ. Pharmacological and optical methods to treat vestibular disorders and nystagmus. In: Herdman SJ, Clendaniel RA, eds. *Vestibular Rehabilitation.* 4th ed. Philadelphia, PA: F.A. Davis Company; 2014:250-265.

55. Whitney SL, Herdman SJ. Physical therapy assessment of vestibular hypofunction. In: Herdman SJ, Clendaniel RA, eds. *Vestibular Rehabilitation.*4th ed. Philadelphia, PA: F.A. Davis Company; 2014:359-393.

56. Yardley L, Masson E, Verschuur C, Haacke N, Lux L. Symptoms, anxiety and handicap in dizzy patients: development of the vertigo symptom scale. *J Psychosom Res.* 1992;36:1-11.

57. Honrubia V, Bell TS, Harris MR, Baloh RW, Fisher LM. Quantitative evaluation of dizziness characteristics and impact on quality of life, *Amer J Otol.* 1996;17:595-602.

58. Dannenbaum E, Chilingarian G, Fung J. Validity and responsiveness of the visual vertigo analogue scale. *J Neurol Phys Ther.* 2019 Apr;43(2):117-121.

59. Powell LE, Myers AM. The activities-specific balance confidence (ABC) scale. *J Gerontol A Biol Sci Med Sci.* 1995;50:28-34.

60. Cohen HS, Kimball KT. Development of the vestibular disorders activities of daily living scale. *Arch Otolaryngol Head Neck Surg.* 2000;126:881-887.

61. Jacobson GP, Newman CW. The development of the dizziness handicap inventory. *Arch Otolaryngol Head Neck Surg.* 1990;116(4):424-427.

62. Jacobson GP, Newman CW, Hunter L, Balzer GK. Balance function test correlates of the dizziness handicap inventory. *J Am Acad Audiol.* 1991;2(4):253-260.

63. Coward JL, Wrisley DM, Walker M, Strasnick B, Jacobson JT. Efficacy of vestibular rehabilitation. *Otolaryngol Head Neck Surg.* 1998;118(1):49-54.

64. Morris AE, Lutman ME, Yardley L. Measuring outcome from vestibular rehabilitation, part II: refinement and validation of a new self-report measure. *Int J Audiol.* 2009;48(1):24-37.

65. Clendaniel R. The effects of habituation and gaze-stability exercises in the treatment of unilateral vestibular hypofunction - preliminary results. *J Neurol Phys Ther.* 2010;34(2):111-116.

66. Côté P, Kreitz BG, Cassidy JD, Thiel H. The validity of the extension-rotation test as a clinical screening procedure before neck manipulation: a secondary analysis. *J Manipulative Physiol Ther.* 1996;19(3):159-164.

67. Reiley AS, Vickory FM, Funderburg SE, Cesario RA, Clendaniel RA. How to diagnose cervicogenic dizziness. *Arch Physiother.* 2017;7:12.

68. Serra A, Leigh RJ. Diagnostic value of nystagmus: spontaneous and induced ocular oscillations. *J Neurol Neurosurg Psych.* 2002;73:615-618.

69. Jeffcoat B, Shelukhin A, Fong A, Mustain W, Zhou W. Alexander's law revisited. *J Neurophysiol.* 2008;100(1):154-159.

70. Sharpe JA. Neurophysiology and neuroanatomy of smooth pursuit: lesion studies. *Brain Cogn.* 2008;68(3):241-254.

71. Ramat S, Leigh RJ, Zee DS, Optican LM. What clinical disorders tell us about the neural control of saccadic eye movements. *Brain.* 2007;130:10-35.

72. Dieterich M, Brandt T. Vestibular lesions of the central vestibular pathways. In: Herdman SJ, Clendaniel RA, eds. *Vestibular Rehabilitation*. 4th ed. Philadelphia, PA: F.A. Davis Company; 2014:59-84.

73. Schubert MC, Tusa RJ, Grine LE, Herdman SJ. Optimizing the sensitivity of the head thrust test for identifying vestibular hypofunction. *Phys Ther*. 2004;84(2):151-158.

74. Kim MB, Huh SH, Ban JH. Diversity of head shaking nystagmus in peripheral vestibular disease. *Otology Neurotol*. 2012;33(4):634-639.

75. Smith-Wheelock M, Shepard NT, Telian SA. Physical therapy program for vestibular rehabilitation. *Am J Otol*. 1991;12:218-225.

76. Telian SA, Shepard NT. Update on vestibular rehabilitation therapy. *Otolaryngol Clin North Am*. 1996;29(2):359-371.

77. Akin FW, Davenport MJ. Validity and reliability of the motion sensitivity test. *J Rehabil Res Dev*. 2003;40(5):415-421.

78. Seung-Han L, Kim JS. Benign paroxysmal positional vertigo. *J Clin Neurol*. 2010;6:51-63.

79. Herdman SJ, Hoder JM. Physical therapy management of benign paroxysmal positional vertigo. In: Herdman SJ, Clendaniel RA, eds. *Vestibular Rehabilitation*. 4th ed. Philadelphia, PA: F.A. Davis Company; 2014: 324-354.

80. King LA, Horak FB. The role of the vestibular system in postural control. In: Herdman SJ, Clendaniel RA, eds. *Vestibular Rehabilitation*. 4th ed. Philadelphia, PA: F.A. Davis Company; 2014.

81. Winstein CJ, Mitz, AR. The motor system. II Higher centers. In: Cohen, H, ed. *Neuroscience for Rehabilitation*. Philadelphia: JB Lippincott; 1993.

82. Horak FB. Postural orientation and equilibrium: what do we need to know about neural control of balance to prevent falls? *Age Ageing*. 2006;35 (Suppl 2): ii7–ii11.

83. Shumway-Cook A, Horak FB. Assessing the influence of sensory interaction of balance. Suggestion from the field. *Phys Ther*. 1986;66(10):1548-1550.

84. Nashner LM. Sensory neuromuscular and biomechanical contributions to human balance. In: Duncan PW, ed. *Balance Proceedings of the APTA Forum*. Alexandria, VA: American Physical Therapy Association; 1990.

85. Bermúdez Rey MC, Clark TK, Merfeld DM. Balance screening of vestibular function in subjects aged 4 years and older: a living laboratory experience. *Front Neurol*. 2017 Nov 28;8:631.

86. Horn LB, Rice T, Stoskus JL, Lambert KH, Dannenbaum E, Scherer MR. Measurement characteristics and clinical utility of the clinical test of sensory interaction on balance (CTSIB) and modified CTSIB in individuals with vestibular dys-function. *Arch Phys Med Rehabil*. 2015;96: 1747-1748.

87. Keshner EA, Galgon AK. Postural abnormalities in vestibular disorders. In: Herdman SJ, Clendaniel RA, eds. *Vestibular Rehabilitation*. 4th ed. Philadelphia, PA: F.A. Davis Company; 2014:85-109.

88. Giray M, Kirazli Y, Karapolat H, Celebisoy N, Bilgen C, Kirazli T. Short-term effects of vestibular rehabilitation in patients with chronic unilateral vestibular dysfunction: a randomized controlled study. *Arch Phys Med Rehabil*. 2009;90(8):1325-1331.

89. Newton RA. Review of tests of standing balance abilities. *Brain Inj*. 1989; 3:335-343.

90. Vellas BJ, Wayne SJ, Romero L, Baumgartner RN, Rubenstein LZ, Garry PJ. One-leg balance is an important predictor of injurious falls in older persons. *J Am Geriatr Soc*. 1997;45(6):735-738.

91. Whitney SL, Wrisley DM, Marchetti GF, Gee MA, Redfern MS, Furman JM. Clinical measurement of sit-to-stand performance in people with balance disorders: validity of data for the five-times-sit-to-stand test. *Phys Ther*. 2005(10):1034-1045.

92. Fukuda T. The stepping test: two phases of the labyrinthine reflex. *Acta Otolaryngol*. 1959;50(2):95-108.

93. Honaker JA, Shepard NT. Performance of Fukuda Stepping Test as a function of the severity of caloric weakness in chronic dizzy patients. *J Am Acad Audiol*. 2012;23(8):616-622.

94. Cohen HS, Stitz J, Sangi-Haghpeykar H, et al. Tandem walking as a quick screening test for vestibular disorders. *Laryngoscope*. 2018;128: 1687-1691.

95. Cordo PJ, Nashner LM. Properties of postural adjustments associated with rapid arm movements. *J Neurophysiol*. 1982;47(2):287-302.

96. Mouchnino L, Blouin J. When standing on a moving support, cutaneous inputs provide sufficient information to plan the anticipatory postural adjustments for gait initiation. *PLOS ONE*. 2013;8(2):e55081.

97. Duncan PW, Weiner DK, Chandler J, Studenski S. Functional reach: a new clinical measure of balance. *J Gerontol*. 1990;45(6):M192-M197.

98. Newton RA. Validity of the multi-directional reach test: a practical measure for limits of stability in older adults. *J Gerontol A Biol Sci Med Sci*. 2001;56(4):M248-M252.

99. Horak FB, Nashner LM. Central programming of postural movements: adaption to altered support surface configurations. *J Neurophysiol*. 1986; 55:1369-1381.

100. Munhoz RP, Li JY, Kurtinecz M, et al. Evaluation of the pull test technique in assessing postural instability in Parkinson's disease. *Neurology*. 2004;62(1):125-127.

101. Jacobs JV, Horak FB, Van Tran K, Nutt JG. An alternative clinical postural stability test for patients with Parkinson's disease. *J Neurol*. 2006 Nov;253(11):1404-1413.

102. Smith BA, Carlson-Kuhta P, Horak FB. Consistency in administration and response for the backward push and release test: a clinical assessment of postural responses. *Physiother Res Int*. 2016;21(1):36-46.

103. Wolfson LI, Whipple R, Amerman P, Kleinberg A. Stressing the postural response. A quantitative method for testing balance. *J Am Geriatr Soc*. 1986;34(12):845-850.

104. Chandler JM, Duncan PW, Studenski SA. Balance performance on the postural stress test: comparison of young adults, healthy elderly, and fallers. *Phys Ther*. 1990 Jul;70(7):410-415.

105. Horak FB, Nashner LM, Diener HC. Postural strategies associated with somatosensory and vestibular loss. *Exp Brain Res*. 1990;82(1):167-177.

106. Dite W, Temple VA. A clinical test of stepping and change of direction to identify multiple falling older adults. *Arch Phys Med Rehabil*. 2002; 83:1566

107. Podsiadlo D, Richardson S. The timed "Up & Go": a test of basic functional mobility for frail elderly persons. *J Am Geriatr Soc*. 1991;39(2): 142-148.

108. Berg KO, Wood-Dauphinee SL, Williams JI, Maki B. Measuring balance in the elderly: validation of an instrument. *Can J Public Health*. 1992;83(suppl 2): S7-S11.

109. Whitney SL, Hudak MT, Marchetti GF. The dynamic gait index relates to self-reported fall history in individuals with vestibular dysfunction. *J Vestib Res*. 2000;10(2):99-105.

110. Wrisley DM, Marchetti GF, Kuharsky DK, Whitney SL. Reliability, internal consistency, and validity of data obtained with the functional gait assessment. *Phys Ther*. 2004;84(10):906-918.

111. Vestibular Evidence Database to Guide Effectiveness (VEDGE). Available at: http://www.neuropt.org/professional-resources/neurology-section-outcome-measures-recommendations/vestibular-disorders.

112. Kattah JC. Update on HINTS Plus, with discussion of pitfalls and pearls. *J Neurol Phys Ther*. 2019 Apr;43(Suppl 2):S42-S45.

113. Brandt T, Dieterich M. The dizzy patient: don't forget disorders of the central vestibular system. *Nat Rev Neurol*. 2017 Jun;13(6):352-362.

114. Nunez RA, Cass SP, Furman JM. Short and long-term outcomes of canalith repositioning for benign paroxysmal positional vertigo. *Arch Otolaryngol Head Neck Surg*. 2000;122:647-652.

115. Sakaida M, Takeuchi K, Ishinaga H, Adachi M, Majima Y. Long-term outcome of benign paroxysmal positional vertigo. *Neurology*. 2003;60(9): 1532-1534.

116. Brandt T, Daroff RB. Physical therapy for benign paroxysmal positional vertigo. *Arch Otolaryngol.* 1980;106:484-485.

117. Kim JS, Oh SY, Lee SH, et al. Randomized clinical trial for geotropic horizontal canal benign paroxysmal positional vertigo. *Neurology.* 2012;79(7):700-707.

118. Mandalà M, Pepponi E, Santoro GP, et al. Double-blind randomized trial on the efficacy of the Gufoni maneuver for treatment of lateral canal BPPV. *Laryngoscope.* 2013;123(7):1782-1786.

119. Casani AP, Vannucci G, Fattori B, Berrettinin S. The treatment of horizontal canal positional vertigo: our experience in 66 cases. *Laryngoscope.* 2002;112:172-178.

120. Vannucchi P, Giannoni B, Pagnini P. Treatment of horizontal semicircular canal benign paroxysmal positional vertigo. *J Vestib Res.* 1997;7:1-6.

121. Bhattacharyya N, Gubbels SP, Schwartz SR, et al. Clinical practice guideline: Benign paroxysmal positional vertigo (Update) executive summary. *Otolaryngol Head Neck Surg.* 2017 Mar;156(3):403-416.

122. Massoud EAS, Ireland DJ. Post-treatment instructions in the nonsurgical management of benign paroxysmal positional vertigo. *J Otolaryngol.* 1996;25:121-125.

123. Nuti D, Nati C, Passali D. Treatment of benign paroxysmal positional vertigo: no need for postmaneuver restrictions. *Otol Heal Neck Surg.* 2000;122:440-444.

124. Herdman SJ, Whitney SL. Physical therapy treatment of vestibular hypofunction. In: Herdman SJ, Clendaniel RA, eds. *Vestibular Rehabilitation.* 4th ed. Philadelphia, PA: F.A. Davis Company; 2014:394-431.

125. McDonnell MN, Hillier SL. Vestibular rehabilitation for unilateral peripheral vestibular dysfunction. *Cochrane Database Syst Rev.* 2015;1: CD005397.

126. Hall CD, Herdman SJ, Whitney SL, et al. Vestibular rehabilitation for peripheral vestibular hypofunction: an evidence-based clinical practice guideline: from the American Physical Therapy Association Neurology Section. *J Neurol Phys Ther.* 2016;40(2):124-155.

127. Tee LH, Chee NWC. Vestibular rehabilitation therapy for the dizzy patient. *Ann Acad Med Singapore.* 2005;34:289-294.

128. Cawthorne T. The physiological basis for head exercises. *J Chart Soc Physiother.* 1944;30:106.

129. Cooksey FS. Rehabilitation in vestibular injuries. *Proc Royal Soc Med.* 1946;39:273-278.

130. Norre ME, De Weerdt W. Treatment of vertigo based on habituation. 1. Physiopathological basis. *J Laryngol Otol.* 1980;94:689-696.

131. Dix MR. The rationale and technique of head exercises in the treatment of vertigo. *Acta Otorhinolaryngol Belg.* 1979;33:370-384.

132. Shepard NT, Telian SA, Smith-Wheelock M. Habituation and balance retraining therapy. *Neurol Clin.* 1990;5:459-475.

133. Pavlou M, Kanegaonkar R, Swapp D, Bamiou D, Slater M, Luxon L. The effect of virtual reality on visual vertigo symptoms in patients with peripheral vestibular dysfunction: a pilot study. *J Vestib Res: Equilibrium & orientation.* 2012;22(5-6):273-281.

134. Pavlou M. The use of optokinetic stimulation in vestibular rehabilitation. *J Neurol Phys Ther,* June 2010;34(2):105-110.

135. Herdman SJ, Clendaniel RA. Physical therapy management of bilateral vestibular hypofunction and loss. In: Herdman SJ, Clendaniel RA, eds. *Vestibular Rehabilitation.* 4th ed. Philadelphia, PA: F.A. Davis Company; 2014:432-456.

136. Krebs DE, Gill-Body KM, Riley PO, Parker SW. Double-blind, placebo-controlled trial of rehabilitation for bilateral vestibular hypofunction: preliminary report. *Otolaryngol Head Neck Surg.* 1993;109(4):735-741.

137. Brown KE, Whitney SL, Wrisley DM, Furman JM. Physical therapy outcomes for persons with bilateral vestibular loss. *Laryngoscope.* 2001;111:1812-1817.

138. Krebs DE, Gill-Body KM, Parker SW, Ramirez JV, Wernick-Robinson M. Vestibular rehabilitation: useful but not universally so. *Otolaryngol Head Neck Surg.* 2003;128(2):240-250.

139. Patten C, Horak FB, Krebs DE. Head and body center of gravity control strategies: adaptations following vestibular rehabilitation. *Acta Otolaryngol.* 2003;123(1):32-40.

140. Herdman SJ, Hall CD, Schubert MC, Das VE, Tusa RJ. Recovery of dynamic visual acuity in bilateral vestibular hypofunction. *Arch Otolaryngol Head Neck Surg.* 2007;133(4):383-389.

141. Cohen HS, Wells J, Kimball KT, Owsley C. Driving disability and dizziness. *J Safety Res.* 2003;34(4):361-369.

142. Hebert JR, Corboy JR, Vollmer T, et al. Efficacy of balance and eye-movement exercises for persons with multiple sclerosis (BEEMS). *Neurology.* 2018; 90:e797-e807.

143. Ozgen G, Karapolat H, Akkoc Y, Yuceyar N. Is customized vestibular rehabilitation effective in patients with multiple sclerosis? A randomized controlled trial. *Eur J Phys Rehabil Med.* 2016;52:466-478.

144. Sullivan EV, Rose J, Pfefferbaum A. Effect of vision, touch and stance on cerebellar vermian-related sway and tremor: a quantitative physiological and MRI study. *Cereb Cortex.* 2006;16:1077-1086.

145. Mancuso M, Orsucci D, Siciliano G, Bonuccelli U. The genetics of ataxia: through the labyrinth of the Minotaur, looking for Aridne's thread. *J Neurol.* 2014;261(suppl 2):S528-S541.

146. Marsden J, Harris C. Cerebellar ataxia: pathophysiology and rehabilitation. *Clin Rehabil.* 2011;25:195-216.

147. Park E, Ai J, Baker AJ. Cerebellar injury: clinical relevance and potential in traumatic brain injury research. *Prog Brain Res.* 2007;161:327-338.

148. Potts MB, Adwanikar H, Noble-Haeusslein LJ. Models of traumatic cerebellar injury. *Cerebellum.* 2009;8(3):211-221.

149. Bastian AJ, Martin TA, Keating JG, Thach WT. Cerebellar ataxia: abnormal control of interaction torques across multiple joints. *J Neurophysiol.* 1996;76:492-509.

150. Holmes G. The cerebellum of man. *Brain.* 1939;62:1-30.

151. Javalkar V, Khan M, Davis DE. Clinical manifestations of cerebellar disease. *Neurol Clin.* 2014;32:871-879.

152. Deuschl G, Bain P, Brin M. Consensus statement of the movement disorder society on tremor. Ad Hoc Scientific Committee. *Mov Disord.* 1998; 13(suppl 3):2-23.

153. Chance PF, Cavalier L, Satran D, et al. Clinical nosologic and genetic aspects of Joubert and related syndromes. *J Child Neurol.* 1999;14: 660-666.

154. Diener HC, Dichgans J. Pathophysiology of cerebellar ataxia. *Mov Disord.* 1992;7:95-109.

155. Boose A, Dichgans J, Topka H. Deficits in phasic muscle force generation explain insufficient compensation for interaction torque in cerebellar patients. *Neurosci Lett.* 1999;261:53-56.

156. Mai N, Diener H-C, Dichgans J. On the role of feedback in maintaining constant grip force in patients with cerebellar disease. *Neurosci Lett.* 1989;99:340-344.

157. Mauritz KH, Dichgans J, Hufschmidt A. Quantitative analysis of stance in late cortical cerebellar atrophy of the anterior lobe and other forms of cerebellar ataxia. *Brain.* 1979;102:461-482.

158. Diener HC, Dichgans J, Bacher M, Gompf B. Quantification of postural sway in normals and patients with cerebellar diseases. *Electroencephalogr Clin Neurophysiol.* 1984;57:134-142.

159. Horak FB, Diener HC. Cerebellar control of postural scaling and central set in stance. *J Neurophysiol.* 1994;72:479-493.

160. Mummel P, Timmann D, Krause UW, et al. Postural responses to changing task conditions in patients with cerebellar lesions. *J Neurol Neurosurg Psychiatry.* 1998;65:734-742.

161. Schwabe A, Drepper J, Maschke M, Diener H-C, Timmann D. The role of the human cerebellum in short- and long-term habituation of postural responses. *Gait Posture.* 2004;19:16-23.

162. Palliyath S, Hallett M, Thomas SL, Lebiedowska MK. Gait in patients with cerebellar ataxia. *Mov Disord.* 1998;13:958-964.

163. Earhart GM, Bastian AJ. Selection and coordination of human locomotor forms following cerebellar damage. *J Neurophysiol.* 2001;85:759-769.

164. Seidel B, Krebs DE. Base of support is not wider in chronic ataxic and unsteady patients. *J Rehabil Med.* 2002;34:288-292.

165. Morton SM, Bastian AJ. Relative contributions of balance and voluntary leg-coordination deficits to cerebellar gait ataxia. *J Neurophysiol.* 2003;89:1844-1856.

166. Schniepp R, Wuehr M, Schlick C, et al. Increased gait variability is associated with the history of falls in patients with cerebellar ataxia. *J Neurol.* 2014;261(1):213-223.

167. Serrao M, Conte C, Casali C, et al. Sudden stopping in patients with cerebellar ataxia. *Cerebellum.* 2013;12(5):607-616.

168. Mari S, Serrao M, Casali C, et al. Turning strategies in patients with cerebellar ataxia. *Exp Brain Res.* 2012;222(1-2):65-75.

169. Serrao M, Mari S, Conte C, et al. Strategies adopted by cerebellar ataxia patients to perform U-turns. *Cerebellum.* 2013;12(4):460-468.

170. van der Warrenberg BP, Steijens JA, Muneke M, Kremer PB, Bloem BR. Falls in degenerative cerebellar ataxias. *Mov Disord.* 2005;20:497-500.

171. Lewis RF, Zee DS. Ocular motor disorders associated with cerebellar lesions: pathophysiology and topical localization. *Rev Neurol (Paris).* 1993;149(11):665-677.

172. Urban PP. Speech motor deficits in cerebellar infarctions. *Brain Lang.* 2013;127(3):323-326.

173. Blaney B, Hewlett N. Dysarthria and Friedreich's ataxia: what can intelligibility assessment tell us? *Int J Lang Commun Disord.* 2007;42:19-37.

174. Tseng YW, Diedrichsen J, Krakauer JW, et al. Sensory prediction errors drive cerebellum-dependent adaptation of reaching. *J Neurophysiol.* 2007;98:54-62.

175. Shadmehr R, Smith MA, Krakauer JW. Error correction, sensory prediction, and adaptation in motor control. *Ann Rev Neurosci.* 2010;33:89-108.

176. Timmann D, Horak FB. Perturbed step initiation in cerebellar subjects. 1. Modifications of postural responses. *Exp Brain Res.* 1998;119:73-84.

177. Earhart GM, Fletcher WA, Horak FB, et al. Does the cerebellum play a role in podokinetic adaptation? *Exp Brain Res.* 2002;146:538-542.

178. Smith MA, Shadmehr R. Intact ability to learn internal models of arm dynamics in Huntington's disease but not cerebellar degeneration. *J Neurophysiol.* 2005;93:2809-2821.

179. Schmahmann JD, Sherman JC. The cerebellar cognitive affective syndrome. *Brain.* 1998;121(pt 4):561-579.

180. Marmolino D, Manto M. Past, present, and future therapeutics for cerebellar ataxias. *Curr Neuropharmacol.* 2010;8:41-61.

181. Zesiewicz TA, Wilmot G, Kuo SH, et al. Comprehensive systematic review summary: treatment of cerebellar motor dysfunction and ataxia: report of the guideline development, dissemination, and implementation subcommittee of the American Academy of Neurology. *Neurology.* 2018 Mar 6;90(10):464-471.

182. Saute JA, Donis KC, Serrano-Munuera C, et al.; Iberoamerican multidisciplinary network for the study of movement disorders (RIBERMOV) study group. Ataxia rating scales – psychometric profiles, natural history and their application in clinical trials. *Cerebellum.* 2012;11(2):488-504.

183. Trouillas P, Takayanagi T, Hallett M, et al. International cooperative Ataxia rating scale for pharmacological assessment of the cerebellar syndrome. The Ataxia neuropharmacology committee of the world federation of neurology. *J Neurol Sci.* 1997;145:205-211.

184. Schmitz-Hübsch T, du Montcel ST, Baliko L, et al. Scale for the assessment and rating of ataxia: development of a new clinical scale. *Neurology.* 2006;66:1717-1720.

185. Winser SJ, Smith C, Hale LA, Claydon LS, Whitney SL. Balance outcome measures in cerebellar ataxia: a Delphi survey. *Disabil Rehabil.* 2015;37(2):165-170.

186. Winser SJ, Smith C, Hale LA, Claydon LS, Whitney SL, Mehta P. Systematic review of the psychometric properties of balance measures for cerebellar ataxia. *Clin Rehabil.* 2015;29(1):69-79.

187. Schoch B, Dimitrova A, Gizewski ER, Timmann D. Functional localization in the human cerebellum based on voxelwise statistical analysis: a study of 90 patients. *Neuroimage.* 2006;30(1):36-51.

188. Marquer A, Barbieri G, Perennou D. The assessment and treatment of postural disorders in cerebellar ataxia: a systematic review. *Ann Phys Rehabil Med.* 2014;57:67-78.

189. Fonteyn EMR, Keus SHJ, Verstappen CCP, Schöls L, De Groot IJM, Van De Warrenburg BPC. The effectiveness of allied health care in patients with ataxia: a systematic review. *J Neurol.* 2014;261:251-258.

190. Milne SC, Corben LA, Georgiou-Karistianis N, Delatycki MB, Yiu EM. Rehabilitation for individuals with genetic degenerative ataxia: a systematic review. *Neurorehabil Neural Repair.* 2017 Jul;31(7):609-622.

191. Barbuto S, Kuo SH, Stein J. Investigating the clinical significance and research discrepancies of balance training in degenerative cerebellar disease. *Am J Phys Med Rehabil.* Nov 2020;99(11):989-998.

192. Miyai I, Ito M, Hattori N, et al. Cerebellar ataxia rehabilitation trial in degenerative cerebellar diseases. *Neurorehabil Neural Repair.* 2012;(5):515-522.

193. Ilg W, Synofzik M, Brötz D, et al. Intensive coordinative training improves motor performance in degenerative cerebellar disease. *Neurology.* 2009;73:1823-1830.

194. Gill-Body KM, Popat RA, Parker SW, Krebs DE. Rehabilitation of balance in two patients with cerebellar dysfunction. *Phys Ther.* 1997;77:534-552.

195. Ilg W, Schatton C, Schicks J, et al. Video game-based coordinative training improves ataxia in children with degenerative ataxia. *Neurology.* 2012;79:2056-2060.

196. Wang RY, Huang FY, Soong BW, et al.: A randomized controlled pilot trial of game-based training in individuals with spinocerebellar ataxia type 3. *Sci Rep.* 2018;8:7816.

197. Cernak K, Stevens V, Price R, Shumway-Cook A. Locomotor training using body-weight support on a treadmill in conjunction with ongoing physical therapy in a child with severe cerebellar ataxia. *Phys Ther.* 2008;88:88-97.

198. Vaz DV, Schettino Rde C, Rolla de Castro TR, et al. Treadmill training for ataxic patients: a single-subject experimental design. *Clin Rehabil.* 2008;22:234-241.

199. Freund JE, Stetts DM. Use of trunk stabilization and locomotor training in an adult with cerebellar ataxia: a single system design. *Physiother Theory Pract.* 2010;26:447-458.

200. Ilg W, Bastian AJ, Boesch S, et al. Consensus paper: management of degenerative cerebellar disorders. *Cerebellum.* 2014;13(2):248-268.

201. Ilg W, Brötz D, Burkard S, Giese MA, Schöls L, Synofzik M. Long-term effects of coordinative training in de-generative cerebellar disease. *Mov Disord.* 2010 Oct 15;25(13):2239-2246.

202. Bateni H, Maki BE. Assistive devices for balance and mobility: benefits, demands, and adverse consequences. *Arch Phys Med Rehabil.* 2005;86:134-145.

203. Gibson-Horn C. Balance-based torso-weighting in a patient with ataxia and multiple sclerosis: a case report. *JNPT.* 2008;32:139-146.

204. Widener GL, Allen DD, Gibson-Horn C. Randomized clinical trial of balance-based torso weighting for improving upright mobility in people with multiple sclerosis. *Neurorehabil Neural Repair.* 2009;23:784-791.

Review Questions

1. A sensation of motion which is associated with various vestibular disorders in which the person experiences a feeling that he/she is spinning or the person's surroundings are spinning is called:
   A. Lightheadedness
   B. Oscillopsia
   C. Disequilibrium
   D. Vertigo

2. Benign paroxysmal positional vertigo is most commonly caused by particles in the:
   A. Utricle
   B. Saccule
   C. Posterior semicircular canal
   D. Anterior semicircular canal

3. Horizontal semicircular canal BPPV can be identified with the:
   A. Dix–Hallpike test
   B. Roll test
   C. Rotational chair test
   D. Sidelying test

4. Dysdiadochokinesia refers to the inability to:
   A. Perform coordinated multi-joint movements
   B. Perform rapid alternating movements
   C. Perform tandem gait
   D. Control the distance or speed of a movement

5. An early symptom of a vestibular schwannoma (acoustic neuroma) is:
   A. Gait ataxia
   B. Impaired eye movements
   C. Hearing loss
   D. Facial numbness

6. The most prominent symptom of bilateral vestibular loss is:
   A. Nystagmus
   B. Vertigo
   C. Nausea
   D. Postural imbalance

7. Ménière's disease is caused by:
   A. Increased endolymphatic pressure within the ear
   B. An inflammation of the membranous labyrinth
   C. Leakage of perilymph into the middle ear
   D. An inflammation of the vestibular nerve

8. The ocular vestibular-evoked myogenic potential (VEMP) test is used to evaluate the function of the:
   A. Horizontal semicircular canals
   B. Saccule
   C. Utricle
   D. Saccule and utricle

9. The best exercise to improve gaze stability in an individual with bilateral vestibular loss with no peripheral vestibular function is the:
   A. X1 paradigm exercise
   B. X2 paradigm exercise
   C. Sequenced eye and head movement exercise
   D. Brandt–Daroff exercise

10. When evaluating a patient with residual balance deficits from vestibular neuritis, you observe that the patient bends her hips and trunk when she experiences a small perturbation or weight shifts while standing on a firm surface. The exercise intervention that would retrain the patient to use a more normal balance strategy under these conditions is:
    A. Tandem standing or walking
    B. Balancing on a narrow beam or line
    C. Standing on one leg
    D. Small forward and backward sways

11. A person with an acute right unilateral vestibular nerve function loss will likely experience:
    A. Spontaneous right-beating nystagmus and loss of balance to the left side with head rotations to the right
    B. Spontaneous right-beating nystagmus and loss of balance to the right side with head rotations to the right
    C. Spontaneous left-beating nystagmus and loss of balance to the left side with head rotations to the left.
    D. Spontaneous left-beating nystagmus and loss of balance to the right side with head rotations to the right.

12. The treatment of choice for a patient with posterior semicircular canal canalithiasis BPPV is the:
    A. Liberatory (Semont) maneuver
    B. Brandt–Daroff exercises
    C. Canal repositioning (Epley) maneuver
    D. Bar-B-Que roll maneuver

13. A patient who presents with spontaneous down-beating nystagmus that does not change with visual fixation most likely has:
    A. Ménière's disease
    B. Bilateral vestibular nerve function loss
    C. Unilateral vestibular nerve hypofunction
    D. Central vestibular dysfunction

14. **The most common hereditary cerebellar disease is:**
    A. Spinocerebellar atrophy
    B. Friedreich's ataxia
    C. Episodic ataxia
    D. Ataxia telangiectasia

15. **A patient with cerebellar damage who has difficulty performing rapid forearm supination and pronation is demonstrating:**
    A. Dyssynergia
    B. Dysmetria
    C. Dysdiadochokinesia
    D. Rebound

16. **When performing the finger-to-nose test you note that a patient with cerebellar damage exhibits a tremor as his finger approaches a target. When the patient repeats the test with the eyes closed, the tremor is no longer present. This tremor is called:**
    A. Intention tremor
    B. Postural tremor
    C. Essential tremor
    D. Resting tremor

17. **Spinocerebellar ataxias:**
    A. Typically have their onset in childhood
    B. Typically have a rapid progression
    C. Are a group of over 35 diseases
    D. Are autosomal recessive inherited diseases

18. **Individuals with vestibular dysfunction or loss are likely to have difficulty maintaining their balance in which of the following Sensory Organization Test conditions:**
    A. Conditions 3, 4, 5
    B. Conditions 3,6
    C. Conditions 3, 4, 5, 6
    D. Conditions 5, 6

19. **A subjective complaint that objects appear to be constantly jumping or vibrating is called:**
    A. Dizziness
    B. Lightheadedness
    C. Vertigo
    D. Oscillopsia

20. **Common signs and symptoms of Friedreich's ataxia include:**
    A. Pes cavus, gait ataxia, loss of proprioception, and vibration
    B. Scoliosis, absent tendon reflexes, loss of pain, and temperature
    C. Pes planus, gait ataxia, dysarthria
    D. Limb ataxia, migraine headaches, diabetes

21. **The areas of cerebellar damage most associated with balance and gait dysfunction are:**
    A. Lateral cerebellar hemispheres, interposed, and dentate nuclei
    B. Anterior lobe, vermis, and fastigial nucleus
    C. Bilateral posterior lobes, vermis
    D. Flocculonodular lobe, vermis

22. **Nystagmus caused by central vestibular pathology can be distinguished from nystagmus caused by peripheral pathology by which of the following characteristics:**
    A. Direction is horizontal and torsional, has slow and fast phases, and it does not change direction with gaze
    B. Direction is horizontal and torsional, eyes oscillate at equal speeds, and it does not change direction with gaze
    C. Direction is purely vertical or torsional, has slow and fast phases, and it reverses direction with with gaze
    D. Direction is purely vertical or torsional, eyes oscillate at equal speeds, and it reverses direction with gaze

23. **Balance assessments recommended for use in people with cerebellar ataxia by a panel of experts are the:**
    A. Scale for the Assessment and Rating of Ataxia, Berg Balance Scale, Timed Up and Go
    B. Scale for the Assessment and Rating of Ataxia, Berg Balance Scale, Single-Leg Stance Test
    C. International Cooperative Ataxia Rating Scale, Berg Balance Scale, Functional Gait Assessment
    D. International Cooperative Ataxia Rating Scale, Timed Up and Go, Sharpened Romberg

Answers

1. D	2. C	3. B	4. B	5. C
6. D	7. A	8. C	9. C	10. D
11. D	12. C	13. D	14. B	15. C
16. A	17. C	18. D	19. D	20. A
21. B	22. D	23. A		

GLOSSARY

Acoustic neuroma. A slow-growing benign tumor that develops on the vestibulocochlear nerve, causing loss of hearing, dizziness, and imbalance.

Action tremor. Any tremor that is produced by voluntary muscle contraction, including postural and kinetic tremors.

Ankle strategy. Movements of the whole body at the ankle like an inverted pendulum often used to maintain balance during quiet stance and during small perturbations (i.e., slow-speed perturbations usually occurring on a large firm surface).

Apogeotropic nystagmus. Nystagmus beating toward the ceiling in supine with the head rotated to the left or right that is associated with horizontal semicircular canal cupulolithiasis.

Ataxia. The presence of abnormal uncoordinated movements.

Ataxic dysarthria. A speech disorder associated with damage to the cerebellum that is characterized by impaired articulation and prosody.

Benign paroxysmal positional vertigo (BPPV). A disorder of the inner ear characterized by repeated episodes of positional vertigo.

Canalithiasis. A theory for the pathogenesis of BPPV that proposes that there are free-floating particles (otoconia) that have moved from the utricle and collect near the cupula of the affected canal, causing forces in the canal leading to abnormal stimulation of the vestibular apparatus.

Cervical vestibular-evoked myogenic potential. A potential measured from the sternocleidomastoid muscle in response to repetitive sounds in the ipsilateral ear that is used to evaluate function of the saccule and the inferior vestibular nerve.

Cupulolithiasis. A theory for the pathogenesis of BPPV that proposes that otoconial debris attached to the cupula of the affected semicircular canal cause abnormal stimulation of the vestibular apparatus.

Dysdiadochokinesia. Impaired ability to perform rapid alternating movements.

Dysmetria. A condition in which there is inaccuracy of the distance in movements to a target, which manifests as hypermetria (i.e., over-reaching or over-stepping) or hypometria (under-reaching or under-stepping).

Dyssynergia. Uncoordinated, multi-joint movements, where movements of specific segments are abnormally sequenced, or have inappropriate amplitude or direction.

Endolymphatic hydrops. A disorder of the vestibular system caused by abnormal fluctuations in endolymph within the inner ear, resulting in a distended endolymphatic space.

Frenzel goggles. The combination of magnifying glasses and a lighting system, that when worn by a person, allow examiners to observe the person's eye movements without the person being able to fixate the eyes.

Gait ataxia. A staggering gait, with variability of the step timing and distance between the steps, often due to cerebellar dysfunction.

Geotropic nystagmus. Nystagmus beating toward the ground in supine with the head rotated to the left or right that is associated with horizontal semicircular canal canalithiasis.

Hip strategy. Rapid hip flexion or extension movements often used to maintain balance in response to rapid and/or large external perturbations or for movements executed with the center of gravity near the limits of stability.

Intention tremor. A tremor that occurs during target directed movement. It is a type of kinetic tremor.

Kinetic tremor. A tremor that occurs during any voluntary movement, including both visually or non-visually guided movements.

Labyrinthitis. An inflammatory disorder of the membranous labyrinth, typically caused by viral and bacterial infections. In adults it usually occurs in the fourth to seventh decades of life. The inflammation damages the vestibular and cochlear end organs, causing vestibular and hearing impairments.

Limb ataxia. Inability to make smooth, coordinated movements of arms or legs as when touching an examiner's finger with an index finger (finger to finger test) or running the heel straight down the opposite shin (heel-to shin test).

Motor adaptation. The ability to modify a learned motor skill to compensate for changes in our body and in the environment.

Movement decomposition. The breakdown of a movement sequence or multi-joint movements into separate more simple movements instead of being executed smoothly.

Nystagmus. A rapid, involuntary oscillatory movement of the eyeball.

Ocular tilt reaction. A combination of head tilt, ocular torsion (i.e., bilateral eye rotation), and skew deviation (i.e., vertical misalignment of the eyes) that can be caused by peripheral or central vestibular damage.

Ocular vestibular-evoked myogenic potential. A potential measured from the contralateral inferior oblique eye muscle in response to repetitive sounds in an ear that is used to evaluate function of the utricle and the superior vestibular nerve.

Oscillopsia. Visual disturbance in which objects appear to jump, jiggle, or vibrate when they are actually not moving.

Persistent postural-perceptual dizziness. A functional vestibular disorder that manifests with increasing and decreasing symptoms of dizziness, unsteadiness, or nonspinning vertigo lasting $\geq$ 3 months that are exacerbated by upright posture, active or passive self motion, and exposure to environments with complex or moving visual stimuli.

Positional vertigo. Vertigo produced by changes in the head position relative to gravity.

Postural tremor. Tremor that is present while voluntarily maintaining a position against gravity (i.e., holding arms outstretched at shoulder height).

Rebound. An inability to rapidly and sufficiently stop movement of a body part after strong isometric resistance of the body part is suddenly removed.

Sinusoidal harmonic acceleration test. A test used to assess the vestibulo-ocular reflex (i.e., gain, phase, and symmetry) by rotating a person in a pendular pattern at frequencies ranging from 0.01 Hz to 0.64 Hz with vision denied.

Spontaneous horizontal-rotatory nystagmus. Abnormal nystagmus that occurs due to unilateral peripheral vestibular system damage.

Stepping strategy. A step made in response to a large force that displaces a person's center of mass beyond the limits of stability.

Superior semicircular canal dehiscence. A vestibular disorder caused by a hole in the bone overlying the superior (aka anterior) semicircular canal of the inner ear causing symptoms of vertigo, oscillopsia, autophony (hearing one's voice or sounds like breathing and blinking louder than normal), and sensitivity to loud sounds.

Suspension strategy. A quick lowering of a person's body center of mass by flexing the knees, used to enhance the effectiveness of balance strategies.

Titubation. A postural tremor of the head and/or trunk in an anterior–posterior plane at 3 to 4 Hz.

Tullio's phenomenon. Sound-induced disequilibrium, oscillopsia, or nystagmus often associated with superior semicircular canal dehiscence.

Velocity step test. A test used to assess the vestibulo-ocular reflex by measuring the decay rate of nystagmus (i.e., time constant) following an abrupt angular acceleration or deceleration with rotation of a person to the right or the left with vision denied.

Vertigo. An illusory sensation of motion of either the self or the surroundings in the absence of true motion.

Vestibular neuritis/neuronitis. An inflammatory disorder that selectively affects the vestibular portion of the vestibulocochlear nerve and causes severe vertigo. It mainly affects individuals between 30 and 60 years and is thought to be due to a viral infection.

Vestibular schwannoma. See acoustic neuroma.

Vestibular system/apparatus. The sensory system within the inner ear that, with the vestibular nerve and its connections in the brain, provides the fundamental input to the brain regarding balance and spatial orientation.

Visual vertigo. A condition in which symptoms of dizziness, vertigo, and imbalance are provoked by situations involving visual conflict or intense visual stimulation, such as walking in supermarket aisles or being in environments with moving objects.

ABBREVIATIONS

ABC Scale	Activities-specific Balance Confidence Scale
ADT	Adaptation Test
APA	anticipatory postural adjustments
BARS	Brief Ataxia Rating Scale
BBS	Berg Balance Scale
BPPV	benign paroxysmal positional vertigo
BVH	bilateral vestibular hypofunction
CDP	computerized dynamic posturography
COM	center of mass
CRM	canalith repositioning maneuver
CT	computerized axial tomography
CTSIB	Clinical Test of Sensory Integration on Balance Test
cVEMP	cervical vestibular-evoked myogenic potential
DGI	Dynamic Gait Index
DHI	Dizziness Handicap Inventory
DVA	Dynamic Visual Acuity
ENG	electronystagmography
FTN	finger-to-nose test
FST	Fukuda Stepping Test
FTSST	Five Times Sit-to-Stand Test
HEP	home exercise program
HINTS	Head Impulse-Nystagmus-Test of Skew
HIT	head impulse test
HTS	heel-to-shin test
HTT	head-thrust test
HSN	head-shaking induced nystagmus test
ICARS	International Cooperative Ataxia Rating Scale
MAD	migraine-associated dizziness
MCID	minimal clinically important difference
MCT	Motor Control Test
mCTSIB	Modified Clinical Test of Sensory Integration on Balance Test
MRI	magnetic resonance imaging
MST	Motion Sensitivity Test
NMDA	N-methyl-D-aspartate
OTR	ocular tilt reaction
oVEMP	ocular vestibular-evoked myogenic potential
PLF	perilymphatic fistula
PPPD	persistent postural-perceptual dizziness
SARA	Scale for the Assessment and Rating of Ataxia
SCC	semicircular canal
SCM	sternocleidomastoid
SLS	Single-Leg Stance Test
SOT	Sensory Organization Test
SVH	subjective visual horizontal
SVV	subjective visual vertical
TIA	transient ischemic attack
TUG	Timed Up and Go
UCLA-DQ	UCLA Dizziness Questionnaire
UVH	unilateral vestibular hypofunction
VD-ADL	Vestibular Activities of Daily Living Scale
VAS	visual analogue scale

VEDGE	Vestibular Evidence Database to Guide Effectiveness
VBI	vertebrobasilar insufficiency
VEMP	vestibular-evoked myogenic potential
VM	vestibular migraine
VNG	videonystagmography

VOR	vestibulo-ocular reflex
VORc	vestibulo-ocular reflex cancellation
VS	vestibular schwannoma
VSR	vestibulospinal reflex
VSS	Vestibular Symptom Scale
VVAS	Visual Vertigo Analogue Scale

Age-Related Neurologic Changes

Deborah A. Kegelmeyer and Deborah S. Nichols-Larsen

18

OBJECTIVES

1) Distinguish the aging process from pathologic conditions of aging

2) Differentiate the epidemiology and pathophysiology of conditions that produce dementia

3) Identify and discuss optimal treatment options for older adults and those with dementia to maximize function

The nervous system, including the autonomic, central, and peripheral components, along with our muscles and special senses experiences changes with aging. Combined, these changes lead to declines in executive function and memory, sensory transmission and processing, motor performance such as slowing of movement, impaired coordination, balance, and gait as compared to young adults. Coordination is most impaired in bimanual and multi-joint movements. Balance impairment can be noted in increased postural sway and diminished dynamic balance, and gait is slower and affected by cognitive, motor, and sensory system changes.[1] The special senses (vision, hearing, taste, and smell) all experience changes, associated with aging, as early as ages 40 to 50, and each has been linked to declines in cognitive function, overall health, and/or quality of life.[2–5] Low visual acuity is present in approximately 20% of adults over 80 with another 7% experiencing blindness[2,5]; similarly, there is bilateral hearing loss in nearly 30% of adults over 65 with 2 to 3% severe.[6] Deficits in both vision and hearing (dual loss) occur in 4.6 to 9.7% of older adults, resulting in greatly reduced odds of successful aging.[5] Nearly 50% of those aged 65 to 80 have a detectable loss in olfaction, and this increases to 75% in those over 80. While taste is also diminished with aging, the complexity of taste perception and its integration with olfaction have made it difficult to determine the extent of loss associated with aging.[7] However, in combination changes in olfaction and taste affect eating in older adults.

The nervous system experiences declines at a rate of 5% per decade, after age 40.[8] Not all changes in function can be attributed to aging, and it is important for therapists to have an understanding of normal age-related changes versus pathologies, as behaviors that fall outside of what is considered to be the range of normal function should be assessed and treated. An understanding of the aging brain is necessary for successful examination and treatment of individuals with age-related decline in function.

CASE A, PART I

Carol Schmidt is a 70-year-old female who has begun to experience some slowing of movement and difficulty with her tennis game. She has noted that she is slower to get to the ball and cannot make some of the trickier shots that she was able to make just a few years ago. Mrs. Schmidt's mother, Adele Weiss, is 94 years old and moves quite slowly with a stooped posture, tends to hold onto furniture when walking around her apartment, and is no longer able to safely ambulate in low light conditions. She has fallen twice in the last year and no longer leaves her home other than to shop and go to religious services with her daughter. In addition, both women complain of being forgetful and needing to make shopping lists. Adele recently told Carol that she is having more difficulty bathing and cooking.

CASE A, PART II

Mrs. Schmidt (Carol) would be expected to have changes in motor control, as compared to when she was younger, but is expected to continue to be able to function in normal daily activities. She would also be expected to function better than her 94-year-old mother. Adele is in the "old–old" age group and is expected to move slower than her daughter and to have difficulty with high-level balance activities.

• TYPICAL NEUROMUSCULAR CHANGE WITH AGING

Changes in the Brain with Aging

There is a progressive loss in brain weight, beginning in the fifth decade (ages of 45–50) with nearly an 11% loss in those over 85. Similarly, brain volume declines linearly over adulthood with a nearly 14% loss by age 90, averaging 0.5% per year after age 60.[9] This change in brain weight and volume is associated with decreases in gray matter, subcortical structures (caudate, cerebellum, and hippocampus), and white matter as well as the expansion of the ventricles with advancing age. Brain volume loss was originally thought to be the result of progressive neuron death, but more recent studies have found only a 10% loss of neurons by age 90. Rather, gray matter thinning seems to result from a decrease in neuron size and dendritic density.[10] Nonetheless, the gray matter cortical mantle is thinner in older adults with the greatest age-related differences in gray matter volume occurring in the prefrontal and orbitofrontal cortices, areas critical for executive function and memory.[1,11] Other areas with significant volume loss are the supramarginal gyrus and inferior parietal cortex, associated with higher level sensory processing, yet the primary sensory cortex and superior parietal cortex have little loss.[12] While the primary motor cortex seems largely spared, motor control is dependent on sensory processing areas and even more so in the elderly than in young adults. Subcortical structures, including the cerebellum and caudate nucleus of the basal ganglia, also exhibit reduced volume with aging. The cerebellum is important for movement timing and coordination, while the caudate nucleus is involved in skill acquisition, specifically motor planning.[1]

Decreased white matter contributes even more to brain volume loss than changes in gray matter, beginning at age 50 with nearly a 20 to 30% loss reported in those over 70 years of age. This loss appears greatest in the precentral gyrus and corpus collosum.[10] Declines in white matter volume begin later but continue at a more accelerated rate than gray matter changes. Specifically, the corpus callosum, the largest white matter bundle, exhibits changes that may, in part, be due to deterioration of the myelin in multiple fiber bundles.[10,13] Changes in the corpus callosum significantly impact the efficiency of interhemispheric communication that is critical for bimanual coordination (Table 18-1). Similarly, there is a decrease in myelin in the gracilis fasciculus and an associated decrement in vibration threshold in the feet, indicating that fibers conveying proprioception are most affected by aging, which may contribute to balance deficits due to the loss of long latency postural reactions.[14] Fortunately, some brain areas seem to have fewer age-related changes, including the medial parts of the temporal lobe (declarative memory), the anterior cingulate gyrus (motivational learning), and the occipital cortex (vision).[15]

TABLE 18-1	Age-Related Changes in the Brain[10–15]
AREAS OF DECLINE	**FUNCTIONAL IMPACT**
Gray matter	
Cortical mantle	Deficits in memory, attention, perceptual awareness, thought, language, and consciousness
Prefrontal cortex	Disrupted learning, memory, problem-solving, and planning
Orbitofrontal cortices	Decreased taste and smell, reward value of taste and smell; impaired learning and reversal of stimulus-reinforcement associations
Parietal cortex	Poorer body scheme, attention, and perception
Hippocampus	Declining memory, especially for recent memories
Thalamus	Impaired sensory perception and regulation of motor functions
Basal ganglia	Disrupted motor planning, limb movement, and skill acquisition
Cerebellum	Poorer coordination and movement timing
White matter	
Myelin	Slower or impaired stimulus conduction
Corpus callosum	Disrupted interhemispheric communication and decline in bimanual skills

CASE A, PART III

Tennis requires fast coordinated movements that are highly dependent on sensory feedback and integration. Based on a rate of loss of 5% per decade after age 40, Carol has likely lost 15+% of her brain volume in the frontal and parietal lobes as well as the cerebellum and basal ganglia, which would be expected to slow her tennis game and lead to more missed shots.[8] In addition, she may be having more difficulty with tennis due to changes in the corpus callosum that are affecting her bimanual skills. Her mother, Adele, has experienced up to 25% decline in some areas, explaining her slower walking speed and making it impossible for her to run or play tennis as her daughter can.

Neurotransmitters

Aging is associated with decreased levels of critical neurotransmitters, including acetylcholine, serotonin, norepinephrine, and dopamine.[1] Acetylcholine declines are noted in the hippocampus and surrounding temporal lobe (basal forebrain); the cholinergic hypothesis proposes that this decline in acetylcholine is responsible for declines in memory, associated with aging, as well as the significant cognitive decline in Alzheimer's disease.[16] Age-related decreases in dopamine are associated with slowing of movement, increased postural instability, and loss of fine motor dexterity. The dopaminergic system has the broadest impact on motor function and is the most widely studied system. When compared to young adults, older adults exhibit a decrease in the absolute level of dopamine, the number of receptors, and transporter proteins responsible for moving the neurotransmitter across the cell membrane.[1] Ultimately, loss of dopamine is closely linked to impairments in gait, balance, and fine motor control. Additionally, dopaminergic symptoms contribute to executive function, especially working memory, so loss of dopamine activity may also contribute to age-related executive function and memory deficits. Based on these findings, the aging brain is on "the preclinical continuum of Parkinson's disease."[1] Similarly, the serotonin system of the midbrain projects widely throughout the brain, including other areas of the brainstem, the cerebellum, hypothalamus and thalamus, as well as the hippocampus and frontal lobes. Alterations in serotonin in aging have been correlated with declines in activity level, diminished balance, sleep regulation, and mood, contributing to increased rates of sleep disorders, anxiety, and depression. Further, serotonin contributes to gastrointestinal secretions and motility as well as bone formation, and therefore, diminished levels may contribute to age-related weight and bone loss.[17] Norepinephrine serves a modulatory function in arousal, attention, and memory (working and episodic). Aging is associated with decreased levels of norepinephrine, which correlates with the degree of cognitive decline, including memory, visuospatial capacity, and processing speed. Notably, secondary changes in norepinephrine levels are also associated with Alzheimer's and Parkinson's Diseases.[18]

CASE A, PART IV

Adele is exhibiting changes in her gait that are likely due to the loss of dopamine and changes in her basal ganglia and cerebellum.

Peripheral Nervous System

With aging, there is also degeneration of components of the peripheral nervous system. These changes lead to slowing of neural conduction of both motor and sensory fibers. Components of the peripheral nervous system known to degenerate are the anterior horn cells (alpha motor neurons), neuromuscular junctions, and dorsal root ganglia along with a reduction in the density of myelinated fibers in the spinal nerve roots. Further, there is a reduction in myelinated fibers in the fasciculus gracilis that is more apparent at rostral levels, indicating that, with increasing age, there is distal degeneration of afferent fibers. This likely contributes to diminished sensation in the feet and the potential for falling in older adults. There is also an average 8% loss of the sympathetic preganglionic cell bodies in the thoracic ventral horn, which project to the sympathetic ganglia.[14] These fibers contribute to autonomic regulation of blood vessel dilation/constriction, heart rate, and ultimately blood pressure; a decrease in these fibers likely contributes to a diminished cardiovagal response in older adults.[19] However, an overall hyperexcitability of the sympathetic nervous system also occurs with aging, which may contribute to hypertension (HTN) and cardiovascular disease; this is particularly evident in those who increase their body mass as they age.[20]

Distally, there is axonal degeneration and greater internodal length variability with shorter internodes more prevalent, suggesting a process of denervation and then regeneration.[14] The capacity for axonal regeneration and reinnervation is maintained throughout life but tends to be slower and less effective with aging.[21] This pattern of degeneration and reinnervation also leads to changes in the muscle (see Box 18-1). Interestingly, there is also a decrease in the number of neurons per muscle fiber, leading to **fiber grouping**, where like muscle fiber types (e.g., Type 1) cluster together rather than being distributed

Box 18-1 | Muscle Changes with Aging[22]

There are many changes in muscle, associated with aging, including a loss of muscle mass and fiber number (**sarcopenia**), loss of strength and elasticity, and an increase in adipose tissue between muscle fibers. The loss in muscle mass seems to particularly result from a decrease in Type II muscle fiber mass, while Type I fibers seem to maintain their size better with only a mild decline in size in older adults; thus, **strength** may only marginally decline while **power** (quick maximal contraction) declines to a much greater degree. Changes in fiber type ratio and innervation may contribute to this decrement in power by slowing the velocity of the muscle contraction. Old–old adults have fewer Type II fibers (fast twitch) with a secondary increase in the relative proportion of slow twitch to fast twitch fibers. More Type I fibers may result from the reinnervation of denervated Type II fibers by neurons that typically control Type I fibers. Of interest is the accumulation of adipose tissue between muscle fibers (not within them), which may contribute to the changing power of muscle contractions. Additionally, the elasticity of muscle is diminished with aging, resulting in increased muscle stiffness that actually may contribute to maintained strength. Another contributor to muscle loss with aging may be the subclinical occurrence of inflammation, noted in the elderly, which may result in the metabolic breakdown of muscle (**muscle catabolism**).

throughout the muscle as in younger muscle, which is thought to be a consequence of denervation and subsequent reinnervation by motor neurons. The result of this pattern of changes is likely an increased recruitment of motor units for a given task in older adults with the increased effort required for any given functional task.[22] Yet, neural changes do not entirely account for changes in muscle function with aging.

CASE A, PART V

Both Carol and Adele are likely to say that it takes more effort to do their daily activities than it did when they were in their 30s and 40s; both are probably using more muscle tissue to do the same amount of work due to fiber grouping. However, Adele has likely lost significant muscle mass and has limited muscle elasticity. Notably, continued tennis playing may delay muscle changes for Carol, and strength training could help Adele recapture some of the strength loss that she's experiencing.

In general, normal age-related changes in the nervous system lead to small declines in the sensory and motor systems, including all three systems related to balance: the visual, vestibular, and somatosensory systems. These age-related declines result in slowing of movement and difficulty in situations that require faster responses or a higher level of sensory–motor integration. Overall, individuals experiencing healthy aging remain able to engage in typical daily activities such as transferring on and off of furniture, walking in their home, walking outside and in crowded environments, and balancing during functional activities. In the old–old, such as Adele, we would expect to see slowing of function and an inability to engage in high-level motor activities such as balancing on a moving surface or negotiating an unfamiliar area in low light. Any loss of function beyond this would potentially be beyond normal age-related changes and may be due to a treatable pathology. Adele's restriction of movement to her home and difficulty with bathing and cooking indicate a need for her to undergo an evaluation for problems beyond normal age-related changes.

Motor Function

Healthy aging leads to slowing of movement, declines in bimanual and multi-joint coordination, and declines in balance as compared to young adults. Changes in muscles and joints also contribute to these changes. Gait becomes slower with smaller steps, a wider base of support, decrease in the swing-to-stance ratio (more time in double stance), initial contact in a flat-footed posture and decreased rotation leading to a stiff, one-dimensional gait. These factors lead to an increase in the work of walking. Fine motor movements of the upper extremities are also impacted by the aging process, specifically fine motor movements of the fingers for tasks like writing. Activities that require multi-joint movements, such as dressing, and those that require the simultaneous use of both upper extremities in a coordinated fashion (bimanual movement), such as stirring food in a held bowl, are also impacted by changes in the aging nervous system.[1]

Negative (Maladaptive) Plasticity of Aging

The **negative plasticity model of aging** states that, during normal aging, individuals undergo physical, behavioral, and environmental changes that promote negative plastic changes. In aging, sensory inputs become degraded, and thus, the sensation transmitted to the central nervous system is diminished, inaccurate, or not transmitted at all. Ultimately, this leads to a decline in CNS processing and inaccurate output from the cognitive and motor systems. Over time, neural systems change, based on these erroneous inputs, inducing negative plasticity changes in the brain and resulting in even greater impairments of function. Once this cycle of events begins, it induces a cascade of negative interactions, resulting in worsening cognitive and motor function. Four interrelated and mutually reinforcing factors have been identified as central to this process: (1) reduced schedules of activity, (2) noisy processing, (3) weakened neuromodulatory control, and (4) negative learning[23] (see Table 18-2).

CASE A, PART VI

Adele's withdrawal into her home and diminished involvement in activities outside of the home are an example of *reduced levels of activity*. It is likely that she is experiencing **noisy processing** due to declines in vision (see Box 18-2), somatosensation, and cerebellar and vestibular function. Noisy inputs from blurry vision and poor somatosensory feedback make it difficult for her to maintain a safe balance in situations where the surface is soft or uneven with even greater difficulty in low lighting, bright lighting with a glare, or darkness. Adele experiences fewer situations in which these systems have to interact in a complex manner (*leading to weakened neuromodulatory control*), and due to neural plasticity, the system remodels in response to this situation (**negative learning**). This remodeling leads to degradation of movement that is labeled negative plasticity.

TABLE 18-2	Factors of Negative Plasticity[24]
FACTORS	**DESCRIPTION**
Reduced schedules of activity	The level of engagement in cognitively demanding activities is lessened.
Noisy processing	Sensory input from all systems is degraded as a result of deterioration of peripheral sensory organs. Degraded sensory inputs lead to difficulty in accurately responding to relevant stimuli with an increased likelihood of responding to irrelevant stimuli. These adaptive changes slow the speed of information processing.
Weakened neuromodulation	The metabolism, connectivity, and eventually, the structure of neuromodulatory control systems, which regulate learning and plasticity in adults, become degraded. In aggregate, this degradation weakens the brain's control over its own plasticity, lowering learning rates and trapping the brain in potentially inappropriate or unhelpful patterns of activation.
Negative learning	As reduced schedules of activity, noisy processing, and weakened neuromodulatory control interact to make novel or demanding activities more challenging to perform, individuals naturally adapt their behaviors in ways that can reinforce negative aspects of the sensory input and motor output. For example, as it becomes harder to hear in a crowded environment, an older adult might ask the speaker to talk louder (increasing signal distortion along with loudness), find it more frustrating to have such conversations (decreasing neuromodulatory responses required to maintain high brain function), or simply choose to have fewer of such interactions (further reducing involvement in higher level brain activity).

Vision: Changes in visual function with aging may be noted as early as age 40 but include a variety of changes within the visual system; some are natural consequences of aging while others are pathologic changes. (1) **Presbyopia:** To accommodate to close vision, the ciliary muscles of the eye contract and pull the lens into a more rounded shape; the ability of the lens to be stretched in this way diminishes in the fifth and sixth decades, resulting in the loss of accommodation ability, and thereby, the development of presbyopia (poor near vision) that requires reading glasses for correction in almost all older adults. For some near-sighted individuals, this is associated with improved distance vision.[24] (2) **Cataracts:** The lens of the eye is made up of proteins that over time can be destabilized by decades of ultraviolet light and chemical exposure; other pathologic conditions, especially diabetes, can further destabilize these proteins, leading to aggregation within the lens such that there are areas of protein aggregates and areas of sparse proteins. This disrupts refraction and creates poor visual acuity and light sensitivity.[25] (3) **Degeneration of the Vitreous Body:** The vitreous body fills the interior of the eye, providing architectural support for the shape of the eye; however, with aging, there can be some level of degradation of this gelatinous structure. Such loss places the aging adult at risk for **retinal detachment**.[24] (4) **Retinal Ganglion Cell Loss:** With aging, there can be up to a 30% loss of rods in the retina, yet there is almost no loss of cones; this loss of rods is related to the diminished "night" vision that older adults display. In addition to the loss of rods, there is also a slowing of rhodopsin regeneration, which prolongs the adaptation that normally takes place when one enters a darkened room that allows for enhanced rod activity and "night" vision; this delay can take up to 10 minutes longer for older adults than for 20-year-olds.[24,25] (5) **Glaucoma:** Although some loss of retinal ganglion cells is part of aging, glaucoma is a pathological loss of these cells and their axonal projections that can ultimately result in blindness in about 13% of those diagnosed. While a small percent of individuals inherit glaucoma through an autosomal dominant inheritance (5%), most acquire it, but the exact causes remain elusive. Diminished blood flow to the retina, associated with hypotension or atherosclerosis, increased ocular pressure that creates mechanical stress on optic neurons, or a primary neurodegenerative process in retinal cells have been hypothesized as potential causes. Signs of glaucoma include increased intraocular pressure and changes in vision (blurriness) or visual field (tunnel vision or black patches), but many individuals have no symptoms in the early stages of the disorder.[26] (6) **Macular Degeneration (MD):** The macula is the central part of the retina, and a combination of genetic, environmental, and health conditions (smoking, hypertension, hyperlipidemia. diabetes) can result in its degeneration in greater than 25% of older adults. In some (10%), this degeneration is also accompanied by abnormal blood vessel proliferation (**wet MD**) while in others, there is no change in blood vessels (**dry**). Dry MD is more common and less severe than wet MD.[27]

Hearing: Hearing loss associated with aging is known as **presbycusis** and typically involves a progressive, symmetrical, and bilateral loss of hearing with 50 to 80% of adults over 80 impaired, and up to 30% have significant loss.[6] There are at least four causes of this disorder: (1) **Sensory** (5% of presbycusis) – damage to hair cells in the organ of Corti disrupts high frequency hearing but hearing for speech remains intact; (2) **Neural** – loss of cochlear neurons impedes hearing in the speech frequencies and thereby, impairs speech discrimination; (3) **Strial/metabolic** – the vascular support to the endolymph in the stria vascularis is disrupted with atrophy of the stria resulting in a general loss of hearing (all frequencies); (4) **Conductive** – increased stiffness of the basal cochlea results in loss of low frequencies but also does not impede speech discrimination.

In addition, some presbycusis seems to result from a mix of these four types, and yet changes in other structures not encompassed by these four types may result from vascular changes or metabolic disorders such as diabetes with secondary hearing loss. Central processing of hearing may also be affected by aging, including slowing of neuronal conduction, loss of axons within the cochlear nerves, and cellular changes in the cochlear and olivary nuclei.[28]

Taste and Smell: Similar to the loss of brain tissue with aging, there is a concomitant loss of olfactory receptors of 10% each decade; thus by age 80, 75% of adults have an impaired sense of smell. Similarly, there seems to be a loss of taste buds with aging, most specifically in the epiglottis. However, there is wide variability in the number of taste buds between individuals, so the loss of these receptors may differentially affect taste ability in older adults, depending on their density at younger ages.[29] Nonetheless, loss of taste and smell receptors contributes to the decrease in appetite (**aging anorexia**) experienced by many older adults; some decrease in appetite is expected due to a decrease in activity level plus there are other changes in GI function that contribute to the noted weight loss. However, for 20 to 40% of older adults, this decrease in appetite can result in dangerous weight loss, malnutrition, poorer overall health, and a diminished ability to combat illness.[30]

Theoretically, age-related changes due to negative plasticity should be somewhat reversible with skilled training that promotes positive plasticity. Amelioration of negative plasticity has been reported, using training methods that ensure optimization of sensory inputs and intense cognitive task practice, characterized by many repetitions over 8 to 10 weeks, and resulting in improved memory.[23]

CHANGE IN COGNITIVE FUNCTION

Teaching and Learning with Aging

CASE B, PART I

Mr. Thomas retired at age 65 and spent the next decade traveling and actively involved on several community-based committees. He is now 75 years old and feels like his "mind is slipping." He received a flyer in the mail offering free college courses to seniors and is considering signing up for a course on astronomy and one on using tablet computers. *What are the benefits of these classes for Mr. Thomas?* Coursework will provide mental stimulation and novel inputs that will help to keep him engaged and lead to the maintenance of his cognitive functions.

Aging adults undergo changes that lead to slowing of processing speed and deficient reasoning skills (*fluid intelligence*). Overall intelligence does not decline and *crystallized intelligence (acquired factual knowledge)* improves or remains unchanged (see Box 18-3).[31] To accommodate for changes in fluid intelligence and maximize maintained crystallized intelligence, a class for older adults should provide examples and relate new concepts to previously well-learned information.

CASE B, PART II

For example, the instructor in the tablet computer course could relate functions of the computer to that of a typewriter. It is likely that individuals in Mr. Thomas' generation spent many years using a typewriter and are familiar with how one works; therefore, they could use this crystallized knowledge as a building block for new learning. Yet, novel concepts such as Wi-Fi and the internet that do not easily connect with any prior crystallized concepts will be more challenging for the older adult to learn.

Changes in cognitive function vary across individuals, differentially impacting the spectrum of cognitive functions, including attention, working memory, memory, perception, and higher level cognitive functions; however, changes may be interrelated or additive.[10] Further, some areas of function are more likely to decline than others; for example, older adults may have difficulty with divided attention or attention switching but do well on sustained attention[32] (Table 18-3). Working memory is like computer RAM; it relates to the amount of information that the brain can process at any given time, and it decreases with age. Older adults also have increasing difficulty processing multiple information elements at the same time and exhibit slowing of processing speed. Interestingly, while most older adults have good long-term memory, they typically remember the essence of the event but not all of the context or details of it.[10]

CASE B, PART III

To accommodate for these age-related changes in working memory and processing speed, information within classes for older adults should be presented in smaller units; the instructor should speak more slowly than usual and pause after each group of facts to allow increased time for processing. In addition, the room should be quiet and set up with a microphone and speaker to ensure that everyone can hear; also, materials should be presented in a large print of at least 14 fonts. Repeating information allows the older learner a second chance to process the information and improves retention and learning. Box 18-4 presents strategies to use when teaching older adults. Despite all of these challenges, the elderly are typically very motivated learners, and new learning may be effective in preventing or ameliorating the negative plasticity of aging.

Box 18-3	Fluid versus Crystallized Intelligence[31]	
FACTORS OF GENERAL INTELLIGENCE	**DEFINITION**	**AGE-RELATED CHANGE**
Crystallized	The ability to use skills, knowledge, and experience. It does not equate to memory, but relies on accessing information from long-term memory. It is demonstrated largely through one's vocabulary and general knowledge.	This improves somewhat with age, as experiences tend to expand one's knowledge
Fluid	The ability to analyze novel problems, identify patterns and relationships that underpin these problems, and the extrapolation of these using logic.	Peaks in adolescence and begins to decline progressively beginning around age 30 or 40

Box 18-4	Strategies to Use When Teaching Older Adults

- Connect new information to prior knowledge
- Utilize collaborative learning
- Allow learning to be self-paced
- Slow down
- Encourage elderly to use anticipation and self-cueing
- Use aids to compensate for sensory changes (decreased vision and hearing)

● DEMENTIA

While some changes in executive function and cognition occur with aging, some older adults have a greater degree of change beyond that described as "normal" yet continue to manage their self-care and function fairly independently; the best term for this is **mild cognitive impairment (MCI)**. MCI is diagnosed when an individual has a greater than expected deficit for their age in one of five areas of cognitive function (executive function [abstraction, judgment, calculation], learning and memory, language, visuospatial ability, or psychomotor skills). Often those with MCI are aware of their cognitive change. Mild cognitive impairment can remain stable, progressively worsen into true dementia, or improve and even go back to baseline.

TABLE 18-3	Areas of Cognitive Function and the Impact of Aging[10,32]	
AREA OF COGNITIVE FUNCTION	**DESCRIPTION**	**IMPACT OF AGING**
Basic cognitive function		
Perception	The process of becoming aware of something through the senses such as vision, hearing, and somatosensation. Highly integrated with cognition.	Reduced in older adults. Has a large impact on other cognitive functions and so should be thoroughly assessed. Frequently when declines in vision and hearing are accounted for, there are no longer age-related differences in cognitive functioning
Attention: Some form of attention is involved in all other cognitive domains except when the task has become automatic.		
Selective	Ability to attend to a stimuli while disregarding irrelevant stimuli	Maintained ability to concentrate and select relevant stimuli
Divided/Switching	Processing two or more sources of information at the same time requires dividing attention and the ability to switch smoothly between the information sources. It is assessed through dual task performance outcome measures.	Significant impairments on tasks that require dividing or switching attention among multiple tasks.
Working memory: The system that involves the manipulation of information that is currently being maintained in focal attention.		
Attentional resources	There is a limitation in the resources available for attention-related tasks	Older adults demonstrate significant deficits in tasks that involve the use of working memory such as active manipulation, reorganization, or integration of the contents of working memory. Attentional resources are reduced and the speed of processing is significantly slower. Research results are mixed on whether inhibitory control is lacking.
Processing Speed	The speed with which information is manipulated, stored, or retrieved (processed)	
Inhibitory control	The ability to suppress irrelevant information in working memory	
Long-term memory: Stored information that is no longer present in or being manipulated in an active state.		
Episodic	Memory for personally experienced events that occurred in a particular place and time	Aging has the largest impact on episodic memory. Older adults believe that their long-term memory is better than their short-term memory but they have difficulty remembering the context or source of information like where or when they saw or did something or whether they actually did something or just thought about it. **Semantic memory is largely preserved.** Older adults have normal acquisition and retention of skills. Implicit memory remains intact. Prospective memory can be successfully augmented through the use of calendars and lists. When no such tool is available, deficits become noticeable.
Semantic	General knowledge about the world (factual information)	
Autobiographical	Memory for one's personal past	
Procedural	Knowledge of skills and procedures like driving a car	
Implicit	Refers to a change in behavior that occurs as a result of prior experience without conscious memory or recollection of that experience (the method for learning skills)	
Prospective	Remembering to do things in the future like a doctor's appointment.	
Higher level cognitive functions		
Speech and language	Ability to produce and understand speech and language, including written language.	Largely intact in older adults; may even improve with aging

(Continued)

TABLE 18-3	Areas of Cognitive Function and the Impact of Aging[10,32] (*Continued*)	
AREA OF COGNITIVE FUNCTION	**DESCRIPTION**	**IMPACT OF AGING**
Decision making	The thought process of selecting a logical choice from the available options.	There is little research but studies to date show that older adults come to the same decisions as young adults but reach them in a different way. Older adults tend to rely on prior knowledge and less on new information while younger adults consider more alternatives in coming to a conclusion. Older adults also rely more heavily on expert opinion.
Executive control	A multicomponent construct consisting of a range of different processes that are involved in the planning, organization, coordination, implementation, and evaluation of nonroutine activities. Depends heavily on the prefrontal cortex.	Declines in executive control are noted in aging and correlate with findings of neuroimaging studies showing volume and function decline in the prefrontal brain regions.

Those diagnosed with MCI in their 70s, have an approximate 7% chance of progressing to dementia.[33]

Dementia is a general term that refers to a decline in cognitive ability in comparison to the person's previous level that progressively interferes with activities of daily living and cannot be explained by delirium or other psychiatric disorder. Mild dementia is diagnosed when there is a deficit in at least two of the cognitive domains listed for MCI but also impairment in occupation, self-care, or social interactions.[33,34] Individuals with mild dementia invariably worsen with time. Dementia is a common disorder involving 14% of those over age 70 with increasing incidence at older ages[34]. The annual cost of managing dementia is more than $355 billion in the United States alone.[35]

Some forms of cognitive impairment are amenable to treatment and can be slowed or even reversed; for this reason, it is very important that patients get a diagnostic workup to identify any reversible causes of cognitive impairment (Box 18-5) so that individualized treatment specific to the cause can be initiated. Note that the most common cause of treatable cognitive impairment is depression, which can be screened by the therapist and is amenable to treatment. The Patient Health Questionnaire or **PHQ-2** (Box 18-6), a two-question depression screen, is a simple, fast, and easy tool to screen for depression and should be used in physical therapy practice.[37]

Box 18-5	Potentially Reversible Causes of Cognitive Impairment[36]

Depression (most common) – depression and dementia often occur together; however, depression in older adults may be misdiagnosed as dementia, since it is associated with social withdrawal, poor concentration, and apathy; treatment of depression in older adults may be confounded by their responses to medications (see Polypharmacy).

Polypharmacy – aging is associated with physiological changes that affect pharmacokinetics (drug absorption, metabolism, and excretion) and pharmacodynamics (tissue sensitivity/responsiveness); plus, many older adults are prescribed multiple medications. Thus, drug interactions and these physiological changes may combine to create dementia-like symptoms.

Normal pressure hydrocephalus – described later in this chapter.

Vision and hearing – loss of hearing creates social isolation, deceased participation, and excessive cognitive effort to interact with others; similarly significant visual loss can also contribute to social isolation. Deficits in both hearing and vision can mirror symptoms of dementia. However, cognitive decline to dementia can be accelerated by the presence of significant visual and/or hearing loss.

Vitamin deficiencies – deficits in vitamin B_{12} and B_6 (niacin) as well as folate can contribute to cognitive decline. Replenishing B_6 can result in a return of mentation, yet the effect of replenishing B_{12} or folate is equivocal.

Sodium levels – substantial changes in sodium levels (hyponatremia or hypernatremia) can present with cognitive changes; correction of levels, including changing medications that may contribute to these changes, can result in improved mentation.

Hyperparathyroidism and hypoparathyroidism result in changes in calcium levels and resultant cognitive deficits, which can be ameliorated with normalization of calcium levels.

Diabetes – hypoglycemia and hyperglycemia present with cognitive impairment, so diabetes needs to be carefully managed.

Neoplasms or hematomas can induce progressive cognitive deficits that can be potentially reversed with appropriate treatment.

Infections – many infections (Lyme disease, syphilis, HIV) are associated with neural damage and changes in cognition. Appropriate treatment can improve cognitive function before significant damage occurs.

Box 18-6   PHQ-2 Depression Screen[37]

OVER THE LAST 2 WEEKS, HOW OFTEN HAVE YOU BEEN BOTHERED BY ANY OF THE FOLLOWING PROBLEMS?	NOT AT ALL	SEVERAL DAYS	MORE THAN HALF THE DAYS	Nearly Every Day
	0	1	2	3
1. Little interest or pleasure in doing things?	☐	☐	☐	☐
2. Feeling down, depressed, or hopeless?	☐	☐	☐	☐
A score of 3 or more indicates a positive screen for depressive symptoms.				

Dementia versus Delirium

Dementia can be confused with delirium, which is a transient condition with a rapid onset and fluctuating symptoms that include poor maintained and shifting attention to external stimuli and disorganized thinking, manifested by rambling and incoherent speech. Two significant differences between dementia and delirium are as follows: (1) the acute onset of delirium and (2) consciousness is affected in delirium and not in dementia (Table 18-4).[38,39] Delirium is typically caused by a severe stressor to the system such as surgery, anesthesia, infection, or disease with *post-anesthetic* delirium most common. When working with an elderly individual who has undergone a recent trauma or significant change in health status, therapists should assess for cognitive impairment but remember that the impairment may be delirium. If cognitive impairment is due to delirium, then the individual's prognosis will be significantly better due to its temporary and time-limited status. In older individuals, delirium can last up to 12 months. Notably, individuals with dementia are likely to have delirium in times of stress, and so, health care professionals need to be aware that both conditions may be present during illness and after injury or surgery. In those with dementia, a larger percentage of individuals developed post-operative delirium, than those without dementia.[40] Individuals who develop delirium following a stressor are at increased risk of going on to develop dementia.[38] Early interventions to prevent or minimize delirium are key to improving outcomes in hospitalized older adults. These interventions include early and frequent mobilization, appropriate sensory stimulation and allowing for normal sleep-wake cycles. Promoting early mobility is the only intervention that has been shown to decrease the duration of delirium.[41] The physical therapist can be a key team member in promoting safe mobility. Ways to improve safety are to provide appropriate assistive devices and encourage the use of gait belts. If the patient is very hypoactive, have them sit up in a chair and participate in activities such as chair exercises, as appropriate.

CASE C, PART I

Mrs. Ludwig is 72 years old with an uncomplicated medical history. She recently lost her husband and moved from the home in which they had lived for 40 years to a condominium on a single level, where she lives alone. She was seen by her family physician for complaints of back pain and referred for therapy. On initial evaluation, she is quiet and answers questions with single-word responses. She presents with unkempt hair and her shoes do not match. She states that she has to get up at night to go to the bathroom and feels that her gait is unsteady. On her second visit, the therapist asks her to demonstrate the three home exercises she was prescribed, but Mrs. Ludwig does not remember two of the three exercises. The therapist is concerned that Mrs. Ludwig may have dementia due to her unkempt hair, mismatched shoes, single-word answers, and poor memory for her exercise program.

Causes of Dementia

The most common form of dementia is Alzheimer's disease, accounting for 50 to 60% of all cases of dementia. The next most common cause is vascular dementia, 20% of all cases.[34,42] Yet, there are many causes of dementia, associated with different diseases that damage the nervous system through different pathologic processes (Table 18-5). In this section, we will discuss the most common causes.

CASE C, PART II

Which conditions may be the cause of Mrs. Ludwig's poor cognitive functioning?

Based on Mrs. Ludwig's presentation and uncomplicated medical history, the most likely causes would be depression, Alzheimer's, normal pressure hydrocephalus, thyroid disease, or Parkinson's disease.

How should the therapist assess Mrs. Ludwig in light of these concerns?

Mrs. Ludwig is at risk for depression due to the major life changes she has experienced in the recent past. The PHQ-2 would be a simple tool that the therapist could use to screen for depression, and if positive, refer Mrs. Ludwig to her physician to follow up on this finding.

TABLE 18-4	Differentiating Dementia from Delirium and Depression[36]		
	DEMENTIA	**DELIRIUM**	**DEPRESSION**
Onset	Insidious	Acute	Acute
Conscious state	Impaired very late	Variable consciousness	Unusual
Mood	Stable	Highly variable	Depressed with diurnal variation
Duration	Long term	Short (days)	Short (weeks)
Cognitive features	Reduced short > long-term memory	Short attention span	Reduced short- and long-term memory
Sleep/Wake cycle	Day/Night reversible	Hour-to-hour variation	Hypersomnia or insomnia
Psychomotor changes	Late	Marked	–
Associated features	–	Medical conditions – medications	Past history

Neurodegenerative Causes of Dementia

Alzheimer's disease (AD) accounts for about half of all dementia cases.[34,42] It is more common in women[44] and in those who have first-degree relatives with the disease or a history of head

TABLE 18-5	Causes of Dementia[34,36,42,43]
Neurodegenerative disorders	AD Parkinson's disease Lewy body dementia Frontotemporal dementia (Pick's disease) Huntington's disease
Cerebrovascular disorders	Vascular dementia (20%) Vasculitis Subarachnoid hemorrhage
Toxic/Metabolic encephalopathies	Endocrine gland disorders Drugs (e.g., anesthetics, antibiotics, antidepressants, antivirals, chemotherapeutic) Alcohol Carbon monoxide poisoning Industrial agent Heavy metals
Prion associated disorders	Creutzfeldt–Jakob disease
Neurogenetic disorders	Down syndrome Myotonic dystrophy Spinocerebellar ataxias Wilson disease
Infectious disorders	Meningitis Encephalitis Neurosyphilis
Miscellaneous	Depression Posttraumatic dementia Demyelinating MS Neoplasm Normal pressure hydrocephalus

trauma.[35] Memory and cognitive problems associated with AD have a very slow, insidious onset between 40 and 90 years of age, most commonly after age 65. The intellectual decline eventually results in lasting changes in personality and the inability to perform activities of daily living due to memory loss and other features of AD such as apraxia, expressive aphasia, and visuospatial impairment (Box 18-7); this decline can be characterized by three descriptive stages (Box 18-8). It is important to note that pathological changes associated with AD precede clinical symptoms and the progression of the disease is along a continuum in which there is no clear distinction between stages.[46] Changes in cognition and function progress in a continuous manner with cognitive impairment preceding functional impairment (Figure 18-1).

Alzheimer's disease is associated with multiple changes in the central nervous system, including a decrease in the overall number of synapses, the formation of amyloid plaques and neurofibrillary tangles, angiopathy, and ultimately brain atrophy that is symmetric and widespread, including loss of cortex and white matter with secondary ventricular enlargement. **Amyloid plaques**, also called **senile plaques**, are composed of abnormally folded proteins that aggregate together with some neuritic components. Notably, many older adults without AD exhibit amyloid plaques, those with AD have a much higher number of plaques. Similarly, **neurofibrillary tangles** are aggregates of

Box 18-7	Clinical Features of AD[45]

- Apraxia – impaired ability to do previously learned motor activities despite intact motor function
- Agnosia – failure to recognize or identify objects despite intact sensory function
- Memory loss – initially short-term memory with progression to include long-term memory
- Visuospatial impairment – diminished ability to identify stimuli and their location
- Concreteness – recognize concrete concepts but not abstract concepts or words
- Motor function – preserved motor function except in later stages

Box 18-8	Disease Progression of Alzheimer's Disease[46]

Prodromal AD – The individual appears normal but pathological changes have begun in the brain. The individual may be aware of mild cognitive changes that cannot be detected with testing. Also known as MCI due to AD. In this phase, the individual remains functionally independent.

Early – Problems retaining new information and forgetfulness, social withdrawal, and may stop participating in activities and hobbies they formerly loved. Moody, time disoriented and exhibiting poor judgment.

Intermediate – Behavioral and personality changes, parkinsonism, and psychotic symptoms are most evident. They begin to exhibit changes in gait, wandering starts, and confusion of day and night appears. Late in this stage, there may be excessive wandering behavior, and they forget how to eat. Weight loss is a problem. The individual requires care in this stage.

Late – Loss of most functional abilities. Incontinence, loss of ability to walk, and the individual is at risk for contracture and development of decubiti, anorexia, and illogical thinking.

a protein, called tau, that are found in the cytoplasm of neurons (cell body and axons) and the extracellular space; tau is an elongated structure, and in neurofibrillary tangles, as the name suggests, they wind around each other to produce a tangled bundle. Neurofibrillary tangles are also present in other neurologic conditions so are not unique to AD. The angiopathy of AD is referred to as **cerebral amyloid angiopathy** and is characterized by amyloid material replacing the smooth muscle cells of the capillaries, arterioles, and sometimes larger arteries within the cerebral cortex but may also occur in the subarachnoid space and cerebellum. This change in the wall of these small vessels places them at risk for hemorrhage. Of note, AD and cerebrovascular disease are often found together; when this occurs, it is called mixed dementia. Interestingly, it has been shown that effective, early treatment of hypertension can protect against cognitive decline.[47]

Lewy body dementia (LBD) is the presence of dementia with relative *sparing of memory*; other symptoms include gait and balance dysfunction, prominent *hallucinations and delusions* with *sensitivity to antipsychotics*, and *fluctuations in attention* and *cognition*. Individuals with LBD are more impaired than those with AD on attention tests but continue to have fluctuations in cognition even in late stages. Yet, cognitive tests by themselves do not differentiate AD and LBD. Neuropsychiatric problems or symptoms are more common in LBD, often leading to entry into health care within psychiatric centers. In one-third of cases, **visual hallucinations** are a presenting symptom. Depressive symptoms are also more common in LBD than AD. The hallmark **sensitivity to antipsychotic medications**, found in LBD, is due to the extrapyramidal syndrome features that are present in LBD. Gait and balance disorders are clinically the same as those seen in Parkinson's disease (PD); therefore individuals with LBD may also be initially diagnosed as having PD. In addition, individuals with LBD show more rapid motor deterioration than those with AD.[43] Recent studies have shown that individuals with LBD have worse gait, balance, and finger dexterity than those with PD and AD at the same stage of their disease.[48]

Lewy body dementia is part of a group of disorders, including PD, associated with an abnormal accumulation of a protein

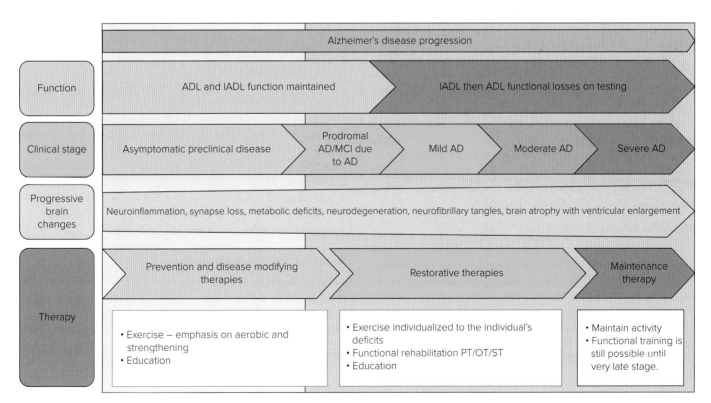

FIGURE 18-1 Continuum of Alzheimer's disease and management.

(**alpha-synuclein** or **α-Syn**) in the presynaptic terminals of neurons. This protein's normal function is to regulate neurotransmitter release and modulate synaptic function. However, in LBD, α-Syn aggregates into clusters, called Lewy bodies, in the axon terminals, becoming toxic and damaging the synaptic membrane and axonal mitochondria, thereby disrupting neuronal function, especially in dopaminergic and cholinergic neurons. Ultimately, there is a loss of synapses and neuronal death. The motor deficits mirror those of PD; yet, there are also some similarities to AD, including the presence of amyloid plaques (common) and neurofibrillary tangles (less common). However, unlike AD, there is little brain atrophy with LBD.[49]

Frontotemporal dementias (FTD) are a group of disorders with a basic degenerative pattern within the frontal and temporal lobes with three presentations: (1) behavioral variant frontotemporal dementia (bvFTD or Pick disease); (2) nonfluent-agrammatic progressive aphasia with speech characterized by short phrases with word omissions; and (3) semantic progressive aphasia, characterized by maintained speech fluency but loss of vocabulary. The latter two are also referred to as primary progressive aphasias. The most common form of FTD is Pick disease, which is characterized by mild to moderate frontal lobe atrophy with temporal lobe sparing early and degeneration later, often localized to the right hemisphere, a mean age of onset of 45 to 70 years and duration of 3 to 17 years. Compared to AD, these patients are less disoriented but have more difficulty with problem-solving. Short-term memory and the ability to negotiate in the environment (visuospatial ability) are relatively spared until later in the disease course. Speech is involved early, as it is in AD, as well as changes in personality and behavior, including disinhibition. Hypochondriasis, schizophrenia, obsessive-compulsive disorder, depression, and anxiety can be so severe that these individuals may end up in a psychiatric emergency room or being treated for these psychiatric problems long before the diagnosis of dementia is made.[50]

Similar to the other dementias already discussed (AD, LBD), FTDs result from protein anomalies of tau protein, transactive response DNA binding protein 43 (TDP-43), or sarcoma protein. The psychiatric symptoms, in FTD, stem from early degeneration of the paralimbic cortex in the ventromedial prefrontal cortex along with the anterior cingulate and insular cortex. About 15% of FTD cases will also present with motor neuron diseases and 20% with parkinsonism that can be distinguished from PD by the lack of rigidity in the arms, absence of a resting tremor, and presence of supranuclear palsy.[50]

Vascular Dementia (VaD)

The second most common form of dementia is VaD. Like many of the dementias, VaD encompasses a group of disorders, including multi-infarct, strategic infarct, and subcortical ischemic vascular dementia. VaD is associated with three common blood vessel disorders: atherosclerosis (ATS), small vessel disease (SVD), or cerebral amyloid angiopathy (CAA), which are described in Box 18-9. VaD is common in those with a history of diabetes and/or HTN; interestingly, HTN has been associated with hypoperfusion of the brain and diminished cortex thickness that may also contribute to the development of dementia. **Multi-infarct dementia**, consistent with its name, results from

---

Box 18-9	Vessel Disorders Associated with VaD[51]

Atherosclerosis (ATS) is the buildup of lipids, typically cholesterol, and proteins into plaques within the walls of larger arteries, weakening the arterial wall and creating the potential for rupture and hemorrhage, manifested as a stroke. However, pieces of these plaques can also break off and cause downstream blockage and ischemia within smaller vessels (smaller often subclinical infarcts).

Small vessel disease (SVD), as the name implies, is a disorder of smaller vessels that can be similar to that of ATS in larger vessels, characterized by a hardening of the arterial wall and hypoperfusion of the surrounding tissue. Alternatively, arteriosclerosis is associated with a thickening of small vessel walls that impedes blood flow and can result in **lacunar** (small) or even smaller **micro** infarcts. SVD is typically localized to the basal ganglia early but expands into the white matter, thalamus, and cerebellum over time.

Cerebral amyloid angiopathy (CAA) results from amyloid β-protein deposits within the smooth muscle of blood vessels that eventually lead to blockage or rupture of the vessel. This occurs first in the small vessels within the pial and arachnoid maters that provide collateral circulation to the brain's surface but eventually occurs in vessels to deeper structures (hippocampus, amygdala) and finally within the basal ganglia, thalamus, and brainstem.

---

a number of small infarcts (lacunar or micro) in concert with or without larger infarcts that can result from ATS, SVD, or CAA, although ATS seems to play a greater role. **Strategic infarct dementia** is induced by ischemia of vessels within regions that are critical for cognitive and memory function (e.g., hippocampus, thalamic paramedian nuclei, subiculum). Vascular damage, primarily from ATS, within the smaller penetrating blood vessels of the cortical white matter, can result in axonal demyelination and destruction of critical projecting neurons; this is known as **subcortical ischemic vascular dementia**.[51]

Because the lesions in VaD are typically small and functional deficits begin to appear when the burden of lesions is high enough to create significant tissue loss, progression is usually in a step-wise fashion rather than linear. Unlike AD, vascular dementia may be accompanied by early gait disturbances, frequent falls, and personality changes. Because subcortical areas are more at risk for perfusion problems, individuals with VaD may be apathetic and depressed but are less likely to be agitated or psychotic as compared to those with AD.[51] See Table 18-6 for a comparison of the most common dementias.

Normal Pressure Hydrocephalus

Normal pressure hydrocephalus (NPH) is associated with enlargement of the ventricles without an increase in intracranial pressure or interstitial edema; this enlargement creates ischemia of the deep white matter such that the myelinated fibers appear pale. Ultimately, there is tissue atrophy and dementia. NPH seems to result from a disturbance in the outflow of cerebrospinal fluid into the subarachnoid space (see Chapter 19 for a review of CSF flow). There is some indication that NPH occurs in individuals who may have had infantile external hydrocephalus, a condition of poor

TABLE 18-6	Distinguishing Features of the Common Dementias[43,46,48-51]					
	MEMORY	**LANGUAGE**	**EXECUTIVE FUNCTION**	**VISUOSPATIAL**	**BEHAVIOR**	**MOTOR SYMPTOMS**
AD	Early, short-term loss > long term	Poor word list generation	Preceded by memory loss	Early topographic disorientation	Socially inappropriate, late agitation	Apraxia, agnosia, mid-stage develop shuffling gait
VaD	Variable	Aphasia if cortex involved	Variable	Variable	Apathy or depression	Focal findings: mild bradykinesia if basal ganglia involved
LBD	Fluctuating alertness, memory spared	Slower	Impaired	Impaired	Hallucinations, bizarre delusions	Rigidity, bradykinesia, hypokinesia (parkinsonian gait)
FTD	Decreased concentration > short-term memory loss	Unrestrained but empty. Aphasia may precede dementia	Early decline	Spared	Early disinhibition, hypochondriasis, affective disorders, mania	Lack of coordination, rigidity and may feel weak

CSF absorption in young infants secondary to immature arachnoid granulations that resolve. One hypothesis is that this condition triggers an alternate CSF flow pathway that transfers the fluid into the interstitial space and then via small channels (aquaporin-4 channels) within the linings of veins into the venous system. However, with aging, this secondary system is disrupted, resulting in NPH.[52] Other causes can include previous trauma, brain surgery or subarachnoid hemorrhage, or infection (meningitis).[36]

Normal pressure hydrocephalus creates motor disturbances and dementia; however, it is one of the reversible causes of dementia. With therapists' roles in assessing gait and mobility, they are often the first to pick up on the pattern of symptoms associated with normal pressure hydrocephalus. NPH usually presents with progressive mental impairment, a broad-based shuffling gait, and impaired bladder control, especially at night. Gait changes and reported dizziness leaves these individuals at high risk for falling, and they often first present to the health care system after suffering an injury from a fall. NPH has symptoms much like Alzheimer's and Parkinson's diseases so is often misdiagnosed or unrecognized. Magnetic resonance imaging (MRI) can elucidate subtle changes to distinguish NPH from AD. When NPH is caught early, at the point of gait disruption without significant mental deterioration, shunting (as described here) can be effective in improving function (memory and gait) in the early stages; however, many patients with NPH eventually progress to dementia of another type (AD, FTD, VaD) for unknown reasons.[36]

CASE C, PART III

Mrs. Ludwig is exhibiting symptoms that are consistent with both AD and NPH. For this reason, a cognitive screen such as the Folstein Mini-Mental Status Examination (MMSE) or the Montreal Cognitive Assessment (MoCA) should be administered with a referral to the physician if she scores in the at-risk range on the screening assessment.

Additionally, Mrs. Ludwig could have thyroid disease or PD. The therapist would be able to screen for these disorders through a complete systems review including skin, hair, and weight changes, as changes in these systems are consistent with thyroid disorders. A thorough assessment of tone, gait, and motor skills would identify if the motor symptoms of PD such as rigidity, hypokinesia, and bradykinesia are present.

Medical Management of Dementia

Evaluation and Diagnosis of Dementia

The physician will screen for depression and do blood tests to identify signs of reversible causes of dementia (e.g., medication issues, infection, hypothyroidism, B12 deficiency), including testing serum electrolytes, serum glucose, urea, nitrogen, and creatinine, B12 level, liver function tests, and thyroid function tests. For reversible cases of cognitive impairment (**reversible dementia**), the specific remedy should be administered as soon as possible in order to reverse damage, if possible, and stop progression of damage.[53] Imaging remains somewhat controversial; however, for NPH, imaging is critical for diagnosis to look for enlargement of the ventricles and changes in white matter and the caudate nucleus.[36] In individuals with AD, imaging changes are typically not evident early in the disease, do not dictate the care provided or affect the outcome of that care. Patients with non-AD dementias are likely to have findings on CT or MRI; therefore, the use of imaging is recommended in patients with less common dementia presentations such as onset before age 60, focal signs or symptoms, or the presence of early gait disturbance.[34,53]

Intervention

Anyone diagnosed with dementia should receive family, caregiver, and patient education at the time of diagnosis. Treatment for AD includes the use of cholinesterase inhibitors and *N*-methyl-D-asparate receptor agonists, which may slow the disease progression, improving cognition and behavior, but do not alter the ultimate course of the disease. There is evidence that a healthy lifestyle, including regular aerobic exercise, a healthy diet, and ongoing mental and social activity that stimulate the brain can help prevent AD. Vascular dementia is managed through aggressive treatment of cardiovascular risk factors. Treatment of LBD can be challenging. Anti-parkinsonian agents may reduce extrapyramidal symptoms but, in general, are not as efficacious as they are in those with PD.[54] NPH, as mentioned earlier, is treated with shunting.

Individuals with dementia may exhibit behaviors such as agitation, wandering, pacing, and aggressive behaviors. These are often made worse or triggered by the environment or physical problems. If a client with dementia is exhibiting one or more of these behaviors, check for potential triggers that can be addressed. See Box 18-10 for a list of potential triggers. Once the potential trigger is identified, the therapist should attempt to remove or address the problem. If the problem is physical such as pain, is there a way that you can help alleviate the pain? Often a change in position or stopping a particular activity or exercise will alleviate pain. Rest is the most appropriate intervention for fatigue and may require moving the individual to a quiet room with low lighting. It is important to collaborate with nursing so that problems such as urinary tract infections can be investigated and treated. Environmental triggers are best handled by either making changes, such as dimming lights, eliminating background noise, and minimizing the number of people in the environment or moving the individual to a quiet, familiar environment where sensory stimulation is minimal.

Box 18-10	Trig Common Triggers for Behavioral Changes

Physical
- Pain
- Fatigue
- Cognitive overload – may be due to having to process too many sensory inputs, especially if in a new environment.
- Illness such as urinary tract infection may first present in worsening of behavior.

Environmental (often due to sensory overload)
- bright lights
- loud noise (music and/or talking at a party or restaurant)
- movement in the environment
- even itchy or tight clothing
- new or unfamiliar environment

or a combination of any of these things.

Box 18-11	Behavioral Management Techniques

- Identify and address potential triggers for worsening behavior (Box 18-10)
- Stay calm and exemplify calm behavior
- Reassure and acknowledge their feelings
- Listen to what they are saying
- Maintain eye contact
- Simplify your instructions and if possible the environment
- Try to distract them
- Explain what you are about to do
- Reorient without arguing or demanding that they understand
- Slow down
- Avoid change in caregivers and the environment in which they live
- Encourage familiarity with consistent caregivers
- Use touch to connect with the person but do not use it to restrain or control them
- Educate and support the family
- Respect individuals' integrity and encourage independence

Aggressive behaviors can be a common symptom in individuals with dementia and lead to challenges in caregiving. The use of restraints should be avoided as they increase agitation and can lead to injuries and even death. Behavioral management techniques are quite effective if implemented correctly and consistently (Box 18-11) and should help therapists deal with individuals with aggressive behavior as well. If behavioral and nonpharmacological management fail, physicians may use antipsychotic medications. These medications are only used if the patient is a danger to himself or others.[55]

Physical Therapy Management of the Patient with Dementia

Screening

Signs or symptoms that would suggest dementia in a client include superficial answers to probing questions, inappropriate dress or hygiene, and inability to remember therapy from previous sessions. In at-risk individuals or someone who demonstrates signs or symptoms of dementia, the therapist should administer a cognitive screening exam such as the MMSE or the MoCA. Prior to assessing for cognitive function, first ensure that the individual has adequate vision and hearing to understand instructions. The MMSE is the most common neurocognitive test. This is a screening tool that allows the clinician to identify potential cognitive issues but does not diagnose dementia or the type of dementia. The MMSE measures concentration, memory, visuospatial ability, and basic language. The MMSE is influenced by the person's culture and educational background but is the most commonly utilized test in the United States. It does not include any assessment of executive function. An individual scoring <24 on the MMSE should be referred to a physician as having a positive screen for cognitive impairment. The Clock Task is a means of assessing executive function and is commonly administered in conjunction with the MMSE; this is a simple test where the individual is asked to (1) draw the face of a clock with the numbers on it and (2) place the hands of the clock at a specified time (11:10 or 1:45). Patients with impaired executive function have difficulty performing complex tasks such as the clock task. They can perform the elements of the task but cannot put it all together to accomplish the entire task. Problems with executive function are found in the old–old, those with dementia, and individuals with diabetes, AIDS, or uncontrolled HTN. The MoCA is a 30-point test that can be administered in 10 minutes with a cut-off score for cognitive impairment of 26. The sensitivity and specificity of the MoCA for detecting early cognitive impairment were 100% and 87%, respectively, compared with 78% and 100% for the MMSE. Since the MoCA assesses multiple cognitive domains, it may be a useful cognitive screening tool for several neurological diseases that affect younger populations, such as PD, vascular cognitive impairment, Huntington's disease, brain metastasis, primary brain tumors (including high- and low-grade gliomas), multiple sclerosis, and other conditions, such as traumatic brain injury, depression, schizophrenia, and heart failure.[56] Another popular cognitive screen is the St. Louis University Mental Status Exam (SLUMS). It also assesses multiple cognitive domains and has comparable sensitivity and specificity as the MMSE and the MoCA.[57,58]

CASE C, PART IV

Mrs. Ludwig undergoes a thorough assessment and the therapist communicates with the physician regarding the new concerns related to cognition. Therapy can move forward with treatment for Mrs. Ludwig's back pain. Treatment for the back pain is modified to account for cognitive issues such as ensuring Mrs. Ludwig has written directions, maintaining a consistent structure and exercise program, and keeping all instructions simple.

Motor Learning in Dementia

Individuals with dementia have deficits in areas related to memory, mood, and executive function but do not necessarily have damage in the areas related to motor learning. In fact, individuals with dementia can learn motor skills. **Remember, procedural learning uses different areas of the brain than semantic learning and does not require explicit knowledge of how a task is done** (see Chapter 7). Indeed, implicit learning remains intact in individuals with dementia. However, in individuals with dementia, random and variable practice offers no benefit and may impede learning, while constant and blocked practice results in learning even when the individual has no explicit recall of the practice or learning. Blocked-variable practice has also been investigated in individuals with AD but resulted in no appreciable learning. It appears that patients with AD can acquire a motor skill and demonstrate intact implicit memory and learning, but no explicit memory or learning. Therefore, they are able to learn motor skills even though they do not remember having practiced the skill and could not describe what they are about to do. Motor learning is possible because the subcortical

structures (e.g., cerebellum and basal ganglia), involved in skill acquisition, are not as affected by AD as the cortex and hippocampus. There is a supposition that individuals with AD fail to develop a motor schema, which is associated with the storage of the sensation of the movement, the context in which it occurred, the movement parameters, and the knowledge of the results; the inability to form a motor schema is likely due to involvement of the cortex and hippocampus such that some aspects of the schema are not encoded, limiting the transfer of newly learned skills to novel situations. Thus, physical therapy should be effective if the motor skill is practiced in the environment in which the skill will be performed.[59] Feedback can be given in summary or constant, and the mode of feedback can vary.[60] Constant feedback improves performance but is unlikely to result in learning. Intrinsic feedback relies on information generated by the movement and appears to remain intact in clients with AD. The majority of studies examining motor learning in people with AD utilized visual feedback. When vision was excluded, performance degraded. It appears that constant visual feedback is important for AD clients learning motor skills. Extrinsic feedback can be given as either knowledge of results or knowledge of performance. Both rely heavily on cognitive abilities and are unlikely to be helpful in motor learning in clients with cognitive disorders. In summary, implicit motor learning is preserved in people with AD and occurs through repeated exposure to the movement. Performance is unlikely to reach normal levels. Training should take place in the environment in which the movement will be performed as individuals with dementia have difficulty generalizing motor skills and therefore carryover is limited.[60]

Physical Therapy Interventions for Individuals with Dementia

Individuals with dementia should receive therapy for any musculoskeletal disorders such as sprains, fractures, or joint replacements just as a nonimpaired patient would. Therapy will be managed according to the guiding principles of implicit learning, using a high number of repetitions and low variability, and allowing few errors during learning.[61] The goals and timing of therapy should also be modified to fit the abilities of the client with dementia. In some situations, the most appropriate therapy may be training the individual to use a Rollator walker to improve safety. This can be initiated by the physical therapist and then continued by caregivers. Therefore, an appropriate care plan would be for therapy to see the client two to three times to determine the appropriate assistive device and then train caregivers to continue with the plan. Alternatively, an individual with dementia who is falling when walking and transferring, while using a Rollator, may require more therapy sessions than the individual without dementia in order to provide an adequate quantity of massed practice of each skill in which falls are occurring.

One method of training that has been found to be effective for individuals with dementia is **errorless learning**. Errorless learning refers to teaching procedures that are designed in such a way that the learner does not have to resort to trial and error and is not allowed to make mistakes during acquisition of learning. Errors are prevented by providing prompts that guide the patient to the correct response. The goal is not that the patient is 100% accurate but that the patient be successful in completing the skill. This technique will not work with every patient in every situation but has been shown to improve learning of specific tasks. Errorless learning has been shown to work with discrete tasks that have an invariant sequence of steps such as performing a sit-to-stand transfer from the patient's favorite chair. It should be noted that it has not been studied with continuous tasks like gait and is not likely to be as effective with this type of task. To use errorless learning, choose a specific task to train such as a sit-to-stand transfer with a walker in front of a patient. Use cues based on the mode of communication that works best for that patient. Some may respond better to hand over hand assist while others may respond best to verbal cueing. Cueing can also be demonstrative or environmental. Cues should be provided as needed to ensure the patient recalls the information needed to complete the task, such as providing hand-over-hand cueing to ensure the patient grabs the walker on standing up. If the patient is performing the task correctly do not provide cues. Step in with a cue when the patient exhibits signs that they do not know the next step or are about to do something unsafe. Over time, cueing should fade. It is helpful to document specifically how many times the patient needed a corrective cue to better track fading of cueing. It is vital that caregivers carry over the errorless learning. If the patient continues to need frequent cueing, another approach to improving safety and function should be considered.[62]

Functioning in the home and external environment typically requires the person to perform dual tasks. Performing a dual task such as carrying a full coffee cup to the kitchen table requires that the individual be able to sustain attention on the task when required, be selective as to which element of the task requires attention at any moment, be able to alternate attention between the task of carrying the coffee cup and walking without falling, and divide attention such that the person simultaneously attends to walking and carrying. The more automatic a skill is the less likely the patient will need to focus on that task as it has become automatic. Well-learned, familiar skills are pulled from long-term memory, which is intact in Alzheimer's disease. Dual tasking requires cognitive resources to determine how to perform the task in a safe manner. When cognitive function declines the ability to dual task declines and this can lead to difficulty in functioning in the home and external environments.[63]

There are several screening tools that assess dual task function including the Timed up and Go Cognitive (TUGcog), TUG manual, and Walking While Talking Test (WWTT).[64,65] Each of these tests has the individual walk while performing a concurrent task. It is recommended that the assessor calculate dual task costs when performing any of these assessments. **Dual task cost** is a way to demonstrate the interference that is caused by performing the second task (dual tasking). An example of how to calculate dual task cost for the TUGcog is given in Box 18-12.

Box 18-12	Caclulating Dual Task Cost

$$\frac{TUGcog\,(time) - TUG\,(time)}{TUG\,(time)} \times 100 = Dual\,Task\,Cost$$

Before beginning an intervention to improve dual task function in patients with dementia, the therapist must consider the patient's relative experience with the task (e.g., Is it familiar and automatic or a new skill?), the severity of the patient's dementia, and is the training likely to transfer to the patient's home environment? If the patient is falling when walking and talking, then an intervention that focuses on practicing walking while talking may be attempted. It should be noted that it may not be possible to train dual tasking in those with later stages of dementia. When a patient is not responding to dual task training then the therapist should consider other interventions such as assistive devices (e.g., Rollator), environmental modification, and caregiver education to limit dual tasking such as not conversing while walking.[66]

Therapists need to monitor for signs of both physical and cognitive fatigue when working with clients with dementia. Patients who are having to work hard at a task may be using a great deal of their cognitive reserve and can become cognitively overloaded (fatigued) before developing physical fatigue. It is important to recognize and respond to cognitive fatigue as well as physical fatigue. The goal is to rest or stop the session before the client becomes so fatigued that they develop behavioral outbursts such as agitation. Signs that a patient is becoming overloaded include agitation, increased confusion, pacing, and increased aphasia and apraxia. It is important to note that these behaviors may also be triggered by pain. If rest and a quiet environment do not improve the behavior, an assessment for potential sources of pain or illness such as urinary tract infection should be conducted.

Impact of Exercise on Cognitive Function

Interestingly, there have been a number of studies that have evaluated the impact of exercise on cognitive function and self-care in individuals with dementia, most frequently those with AD. Exercise programs can improve cognitive function and ADLs in those with dementia. Aerobic exercise appears to be a key component in successful programs and either aerobic or aerobic + nonaerobic exercise was effective. Interventions given for <150 min/week were equally as effective as interventions given for >150 min/week (Figure 18-2).[67,68]

Fitness and the Role of Exercise in Preventing Dementia

Aerobic exercise has a focused benefit on both neurogenesis and angiogenesis in the hippocampus with increased synaptic plasticity, facilitating the integration of hippocampal neurons into existing brain networks. In one study of individuals at high risk for developing AD, those who were more physically active exhibited less hippocampal atrophy over an 18-month period than those who were inactive. However, the protective effects of physical activity were not observed in individuals who were at low risk for developing AD, indicating that the benefits of exercise may be dependent on the individual's genetic or physiologic makeup. The type of exercise is important as benefits vary by type of exercise. **Brain-derived neurotrophic factor** (BDNF) is important as it supports the survival of existing neurons and the growth of new neurons, while insulin-like growth factor 1 (IGF-1) supports neurogenesis, angiogenesis, and neural plasticity,

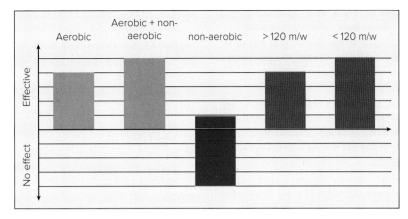

FIGURE 18-2 Effect of different types of exercise on cognitive function in people with AD[Jia].

especially after brain injury. Aerobic exercise upregulates BDNF while resistance exercise upregulates both BDNF and IGF-1. There is overwhelming evidence that BDNF is an important factor in exercise-induced improvement in brain function and cognition, yet the impact of age is not yet known.[69]

The evidence suggests that aerobic exercise benefits cognitive performance, brain function, and brain structure. Aerobic training in late life preferentially benefits executive functions, including multitasking, planning, and inhibition of extraneous information. All of these functions are performed in the prefrontal cortex. Animal models indicate that exercise brings about structural integrity improvement (neurogenesis and angiogenesis) and increased production of neurochemicals that promote growth, differentiation, survival, and repair of brain cells. Since improvement in function is often seen without apparent neurogenesis, it may not play an important role in improvement of functional performance. Thus, **angiogenesis** may underlie the improvement in function found in these studies.[70]

Epidemiologic and prospective studies support the role of aerobic fitness in healthy cognitive brain function and in delaying the onset of dementia. Studies in humans, to date, have primarily been observational, and so, their conclusions are limited. They indicate that individuals who are more active in middle age have a lower likelihood of cognitive decline or dementia in old age. In addition, these studies do not tell us specifically what led to the protection from cognitive decline.

Resistance exercise has also been investigated as a means to protect cognitive function, but the findings to date have been equivocal. Protocols with positive benefits used 50 to 80% of a single repetition maximum lift and led to improvements in memory, when training was progressive and lasted more than 6 months. Another study showed improved selective attention and conflict resolution after 1 year of one or two times weekly resistance training. Given the differences across studies, it is possible that aerobic training will be more effective for some individuals, resistance training for others, and a combination of both for yet others.[70,71]

In addition, there is a wide inter-individual variation in response to exercise across studies, with some responding well to exercise interventions and others having little response. This inter-individual variability points to the need to prescribe exercise on an individual basis rather than "one size fits all".[71] In addition, evidence points to the benefits of multi-modal exercise over purely aerobic or purely strengthening. Overall the limited evidence to date supports starting younger and maintaining an active lifestyle to reduce the risk of developing dementia.[72]

Despite positive findings related to exercise and cognition, there are no definitive guidelines describing the best exercise parameters to improve cognitive function in older adults.[73] Based on the evidence to date, recommendations for exercise parameters such as type, frequency, intensity, and duration can be made[72] (see Table 18-7).

REFERENCES

1. Seidler RD, Bernard JA, Burutolu TB, et al. Motor control and aging: links to age-related brain structural, functional, and biochemical effects. *Neurosci Biobehav Rev*. 2010;34(5):721-733.

2. Schott JM. The neurology of ageing: what is normal? *Pract Neurol*. 2017;17:172-182.

3. Brai E, Hummel T, Albert L. Smell, an underrated early biomarker for brain aging. *Front Neurosci*. 2020;14(792):1-6.

4. Mick PT, Hamalaien A, Kolisang L, et al. The prevalence of hearing, vision, and dual sensory loss in older Canadians: an analysis of data from the Canadian longitudinal study on aging. *Canadian J Aging*. 2021;40(1):1-22.

5. Gopinath B, Liew G, Burlutsky G, McMahom CM, Mitchell P. Association between vision and hearing impairment and successful aging over five years. *Maturitas*. 2021;143:203-208.

TABLE 18-7	Exercise Parameters for Improved Cognitive Health in Older Adults			
TYPE	**FREQUENCY**	**INTENSITY**	**SESSION DURATION**	**PROGRAM DURATION**
Multimodal combining aerobic and resistance	Increases over time to 3–5 times/week	Light, moderate or high	45–60 minutes	Key is at least 52 hours total.

6. Davis A, McMahon CM, Pichora-Fuller KM, et al. Aging and hearing health: the life-course approach. *Gerontologist.* 2016;56(S2):S256-S267.

7. Sergi G, Bano G, Pizzato S, Veronese N, Manzato E. Taste loss in the elderly: possible implications for dietary habits. *Crit Rev Food Sci Nutrition.* 2017;57:384-3689.

8. Peters R. Aging and the brain. *Postgrad Med J.* 2006;82(964):84-88.

9. Hedman AM, van Haren NEM, Schnack HG, Kahn RS, Hulshof HE. Human brain changes across the life span: a review of 56 longitudinal magnetic resonance imaging studies. *Hum Brain Mapp.* 2012;33:1987-2002.

10. Harada CN, Natelson Love MC, Triebel KL. Normal cognitive aging. *Clin Geriatr Med.* 2013 Nov;29(4):737-752.

11. Yuan P, Raz N. Prefrontal cortex and executive functions in healthy adults: a meta-analysis of structural neuroimaging studies. *Neurosci Biobehav Rev.* 2014;42:180-192.

12. Fjell AM, Walhovd KB, Fennema-Notstine C, et al. One-year brain atrophy evident in healthy aging. *J Neurosci.* 2009;29(48):15223-15231.

13. Liu H, Yang Y, Xia Y, et al. Aging of cerebral white matter. *Ageing Res Rev.* 2017;34:64-76.

14. Wickremaratchi MM, Llewelyn JG. Effects of ageing on touch. *Postgrad Med J.* 2006;82:301-304.

15. Fjell AM, Westlye LT, Amlie I, et al. High consistency of regional cortical thinning in aging across multiple samples. *Cereb Cortex.* 2009;19:2001-2012.

16. Terry AV Jr, Buccafusco JJ. The cholinergic hypothesis of age and Alzheimer's disease-related cognitive deficits: recent challenges and their implications for novel drug development. *J Pharmacol Exp Ther.* 2003;306:821-827.

17. Fidalgo S, Ivanov DK, Wood SH. Serotonin: from top to bottom. *Biogerontology.* 2013;14:21-45.

18. Mather M. Harley CW. The locus coeruleus: essential for maintaining cognitive function and the aging brain. *Trends Cogn Sci.* 2016;20(3):214-226.

19. Idiaquez J, Guiloff RJ. Cardiovagal and somatic sensory nerve functions in healthy subjects. *Clin Auton Res.* 2015;25:193-197.

20. Balasubramanian P, Hall D, Subramanian M. Sympathetic nervous system as a target for aging and obesity-related cardiovascular diseases. *Geroscience.* 2019;41(1):13-24.

21. Neumann B, Segel M, Chalut KJ, Franklin RJ. Remyelination and ageing: reversing the ravages of time. *Mult Scler.* 2019 Dec;25(14):1835-1841.

22. Larsson L, Degens H, Li M, et al. Sarcopenia: aging-related loss of muscle mass and function. *Physiol Rev.* 2019;99:427-511.

23. Mahncke HW, Bronstone A, Merzenich MM. Brain plasticity and functional losses in the aged: scientific bases for a novel intervention. *Prog Brain Res.* 2006;157:81-109.

24. Petrash JM. Aging and age-related diseases of the ocular lens and vitreous body. *Invest Ophthalmol Vis Sci.* 2013;54:ORSF54-ORSF59.

25. Owsley C. Vision and aging. *Annu Rev Vis Sci.* 2016 Oct 14;2:255-271.

26. Stein JD, Khawaja AP, Weizer JS. Glaucoma in adults-screening, diagnosis, and management a review. *JAMA.* 2021;325(2):164-174.

27. Al-Zamil WM, Yassin SA. Recent developments in age-related macular degeneration: a review. *Clin Interv Aging.* 2017;12:1313-1330.

28. Lee KY. Pathophysiology of age-related hearing loss. *Korean J Audiol.* 2013;17:45-49.

29. Doty RL. Age-related deficits in taste and smell. *Otolaryngol Clin N Am.* 2018;51:815-825.

30. Cox NJ, Morrison L, Ibrahim K, Robinson SM, Sayer AA, Roberts HC. New horizons in appetite and the anorexia of ageing. *Age Ageing.* 2020 Jul 1;49(4):526-534.

31. Beier ME, Ackerman PL. Age, ability, and the role of prior knowledge on the acquisition of new domain knowledge: promising results in a real-world learning environment. *Psychol Aging.* 2005;20(2):341-355.

32. Mioni G, Capizzi M, Stablum F. Age-related changes in time production and reproduction tasks: involvement of attention and working memory processes. *Neuropsychol Dev Cogn B Aging Neuropsychol Cogn.* 2020 May;27(3):412-429.

33. Knopman DS, Petersen RC. Mild cognitive impairment and mild dementia: a clinical perspective. *Mayo Clin Proc.* 2014;89(10):1452-1459.

34. Gale SA, Acar D, Daffne KR. Dementia. *Am J Med.* 2018;131:1161-1169.

35. 2021 Alzheimer's disease facts and figures. *Alzheimers Dement.* 2021 Mar; 17(3):327-406.

36. Little MO. Reversible dementias. *Clin Geriatr Med.* 2018;34:537-562.

37. Kroenke K, Spitzer RL, Williams JBW. The patient health questionnaire-2: validity of a two-item depression screener. *Med Care.* 2003;41: 1284-1292.

38. Pereira JV, Thein MZA, Nitchingham A, Caplan GA. Delirium in older adults is associated with development of new dementia: a systematic review and meta-analysis. *Int J Geriatr Psychiatry.* 2021;36:993-1003.

39. Dening KH. Differentiating between dementia, delirium and depression in older people. *Nurs Stand.* 2019 Aug 31;35(1):43-50.

40. Chaiwat O, Chanidnuan M, Pancharoen W, et al. Postoperative delirium in critically ill surgical patients: incidence, risk factors, and predictive scores. *BMC Anesthesiol.* 2019;19(39):1-10

41. Ghaeli P, Shahhatami F, Mojtahed Zade M, Mohammadi M, Arbabi M. Preventive intervention to prevent delirium in patients hospitalized in intensive care unit. *Iran J Psychiatry.* 2018;13(2):142-147.

42. Kuo CY, Stachiv I, Nikolai T. Association of late life depression, (non-) modifiable risk and protective factors with dementia and Alzheimer's disease: literature review on evidence, preventive interventions and possible future trends in prevention and treatment of dementia. *Int J Environ Res Public Health.* 2020;17(7475):1-24.

43. Vicioso BA. Dementia: when is it not Alzheimer's disease? *Am J Med Sci.* 2002;324(2):84-95.

44. Scheyer O, Rahman A, Hristov H, et al. Female sex and Alzheimer's disease. *J Prev Alzheimers Dis.* 2018;5(4):225-230.

45. Jacobs DH, Adair JC, Williamson DJ, Na DL, Gold M, et al. Apraxia and motor-skill acquisition in Alzheimer's disease are dissociable. *Neuropsychologia.* 1999;37:875-880.

46. Aisen PS, Cummings J, Jack CR Jr, et al. On the path to 2025: understanding the Alzheimer's disease continuum. *Alzheimers Res Ther.* 2017 Aug 9; 9(1):60:1-10.

47. Vinters HV. Emerging concepts in Alzheimer's disease. *Ann Rev Pathol: Mech Dis.* 2014;16(57):291-319.

48. Fritz NE, Kegelmeyer DA, Kloos AD, et al. Motor performance differentiates individuals with lew body dementia, Parkinson's and Alzheimer's disease. *Gait Posture.* 2016;50:1-7.

49. Overk CR, Masliah E. Pathogenesis of synaptic degeneration in Alzheimer's disease and lewy body disease. *Biochem Pharmacol.* 2014;88:508-516.

50. Karageorglou E, Miller BL. Frontotemporal lobar degeneration: a clinical approach. *Semin Neurol.* 2014;34:189-201.

51. Thal DR, Grinberg LT, Attems J. Vascular dementia: different forms of vessel disorders contribute to the development of dementia in the elderly brain. *Exp Gerontol.* 2012;47(11):816-824.

52. Bradley WG. CSF flow in the brain in the context of normal pressure hydrocephalus. *Am J Neuroradiol.* 2015;36:831-838.

53. Day GS. Reversible dementias. *Continuum (Minneap Minn).* 2019;25(1): 234-253.

54. Taylor JP, McKeith IG, Burn DJ, et al. New evidence on the management of Lewy body dementia. *Lancet Neurol.* 2020;19(2):157-169.

55. Kales HC, Gitlin LN, Lyketsos CG; for the Detroit Expert Panel on the Assessment and Management of the Neuropsychiatric Symptoms of Dementia. Management of neuropsychiatric symptoms of dementia in clinical settings: recommendations from a multidisciplinary expert panel. *J Am Geriatr Soc.* 2014;62(42):762-769.

56. Vásquez KA, Valverde EM, Aguilar DV, Gabarain HH. Montreal cognitive assessment scale in patients with Parkinson disease with normal scores in the mini-mental state examination. *Dement Neuropsychol.* 2019;13(1):78-81.

57. Tariq SH, Tumosa N, Chibnall JT, Perry MH, Morley JE. Comparison of the Saint Louis University mental status examination and the mini-mental state examination for detecting dementia and mild neurocognitive disorder – a pilot study. *Am J Geriatr Psychiatry*. 2006;14:900-910.

58. Patnode CD, Perdue LA, Rossom RC, et al. Screening for cognitive impairment in older adults: an evidence update for the US preventive services task force. 2020;Reports NO:19-05257-EF-1.

59. Dick MB, Hsieh S, Dick-Muehlke C, Davis DS, Cotman CW. The variability of practice hypothesis in motor learning: Does it apply to Alzheimer's disease? *Brain Cogn*. 2000;44:470-489.

60. van Halteren-van Tilborg IADA, Sherder EJA, Hulstijn W. Motor skill learning in Alzheimer's disease: a review with an eye to the clinical practice. *Neuropsychol Rev*. 2007;17(3):203-212.

61. White L, Ford MP, Brown CJ, Peel C, Triebel KL. Facilitating the use of implicit memory and learning in the physical therapy management of individuals with Alzheimer disease: a case series. *J Geriatr Phys Ther*. 2014;37:35-44.

62. Kessels RPC, Olde Hensken LMG. Effects of errorless skill learning in people with mild-to-moderate or severe dementia: a randomized controlled pilot study. *Neurorehabil*. 2009;25:307-312.

63. Ahman HB, Giedraitis V, Cedervall Y, et al. Dual-task performance and neurodegeneration: correlations between timed up-and-go dual task test outcomes and Alzheimer's disease cerebrospinal fluid biomarkers. *J Alzheimer's Dis*. 2019;71:S75-S83.

64. Cedervall Y, Stenberg AM, Åhman HB, et al. Timed up-and-go dual-task testing in the assessment of cognitive function: a mixed methods observational study for development of the UDDGait protocol. *Int J Environ Res Public Health*. 2020;17(5):1715.

65. Ceide ME, Ayers EI, Lipton R, Verghese J. Walking while talking and risk of incident dementia. *Am J Geriatr Psych*. 2018;26(5):580-588.

66. Lemke NC, Werner C, Wiloth S, Oster P, Bauer J, Hauer K. Transferabiity and sustainability of motor-cognitive dual-task training in patients with dementia: a randomized controlled trial. *Gerontology*. 2019;65:68-83.

67. Groot C, Hooghiemstra AM, Raijmakers PG, et al. The effect of physical activity on cognitive function in patients with dementia: A meta-analysis of randomized control trials. *Ageing Res Rev*. 2016 Jan;25:13-23.

68. Jia RX, Liang JH, Xu Y, et al. Effects of physical activity and exercise on the cognitive function of patients with Alzheimer disease: a meta-analysis. *BMC Geriatr*. 2019;19:181.

69. Smith JC, Nielson KA, Woodard JL, et al. Physical activity reduces hippocampal atrophy in elders at genetic risk for Alzheimer's disease. *Front Aging Neurosci*. 2014;6:61.

70. Stimpson NJ, Davison G, Javadi AH. Joggin' the Noggin: towards a physiological understanding of exercise-induced cognitive benefits. *Neurosci Biobehav Rev*. 2018 May;88:177-186.

71. Müllers P, Taubert M, Müller NG. Physical exercise as personalized medicine for dementia prevention? *Front Physiol*. 2019 May 29;10:672.

72. Brasure M, Desal P, Davila H, et al. Physical activity in preventing cognitive decline and Alzheimer-type dementia: a systematic review. *Ann Inter Med*. 2018;168:30-38.

73. Quigley A, MacKay-Lyons M, Eskes G. Effects of exercise on cognitive performance in older adults: a narrative review of the evidence, possible biological mechanisms, and recommendations for exercise prescription. *J Aging Res*. 2020 May 14;2020:1407896.

Review Questions

1. **The greatest age-related differences in gray matter occur in which area of the brain?**
   A. Prefrontal cortex
   B. Motor cortex
   C. Occipital cortex
   D. Sensory cortex

2. **Juggling is a bimanual task and these bimanual skills would be expected to decline with aging due to changes in which area of the brain?**
   A. Cingulate gyrus
   B. Corpus callosum
   C. Hippocampus
   D. Occipital cortex

3. **Decreased levels of which of the following neurotransmitters have been correlated with declines in activity levels in an animal model?**
   A. Acetylcholine
   B. Dopamine
   C. Norepinephrine
   D. Serotonin

4. **In aging it is noted that muscle fiber conversion to a slow twitch type occurs. This is proposed to be at least in part due to:**
   A. Degeneration of the dorsal root ganglion
   B. Denervation followed by regeneration of distal axons
   C. Loss of preganglionic cell bodies in the sympathetic outflow tract
   D. Reduction in myelinated fibers in the fasciculus gracilis

5. **Mrs. Smith who is 90 years old is unable to leave her home without assistance due to difficulty ambulating on uneven surfaces and an inability to step up or down from curbs. These functional losses would be considered normal age-related declines associated with aging. True or False.**
   A. True
   B. False

6. **Mr. Thomas who is 70 years old goes to his local gym and lifts weights four times a week. He does not participate in any aerobic exercises. This exercise program could provide which of the following benefits to Mr. Thomas:**
   A. Upregulation of BDNF
   B. Less atrophy of the cerebellum
   C. Reversal of fiber type conversion in exercised muscles
   D. None of the above, only aerobic exercise improves neurologic function

7. According to the negative plasticity model, typical age-related changes in somatosensation can lead to which of the following?

A. Reduction in motor output

B. Impaired or wrong sensory input

C. Increasing complexity of sensory input

D. An inability of the nervous system to remodel with age

8. Therapy for impaired balance can limit or reverse negative plasticity in aging individuals by?

A. Reducing sensory inputs during activity such as limiting feedback

B. Providing a balance program with progressively more difficult activities

C. Instructing the person to avoid walking on uneven surfaces

D. Providing an assistive device for use during all mobility

9. Typical age-related changes in gait include which of the following?

A. Increased cadence

B. Decreased swing-to-stance ratio

C. Increased rotation of the trunk

D. Landing on the toes at initial contact

10. Which of the following is an example of crystallized intelligence? Mr. Smith

A. Relates a story to his grandchild about battle strategies he used in WWII and how they are similar to ones being used currently

B. Announces he knows how a recent battle could have been won and describes a strategy that is a modification of one he used in WWII

C. Announces that he has come up with a novel battle strategy that should be used in a current war zone

D. Calculates the number of bombs dropped in a recent battle based on his knowledge of the number of bombs per plane and his count of planes from newsreel footage.

11. Aging impacts attention in which of the following ways?

A. Reduces ability to select relevant stimuli to focus on

B. Decreases concentration

C. Impairs ability to divide attention

D. Impairs ability to reorganize information

12. Aging has the largest impact on which type of memory?

A. Episodic

B. Implicit

C. Procedural

D. Semantic

13. Which of the following is considered a higher-level cognitive function?

A. Attention

B. Memory

C. Speech and language

D. Speed of processing

14. The most common cause of treatable or reversible dementia is?

A. Alzheimer's disease

B. Depression

C. Normal pressure hydrocephalus

D. Alcoholism

15. Delirium is different from dementia in that delirium

A. Consciousness is not affected

B. Onset is acute

C. There is impairment in attention

D. The person has insomnia

16. Changes in gait first occur in which stage of Alzheimer's disease?

A. Early

B. Intermediate

C. Late

17. Mr. Thomas has decreased concentration, impaired memory, and his wife complains that he has become very flirtatious and has begun to approach young women and tell them they are beautiful. She states that he has always been a shy and reserved person. Based on this description which form of dementia does Mr. Thomas most likely have?

A. Alzheimer's

B. Frontotemporal dementia

C. Lewy body dementia

D. Vascular dementia

18. True or False. The Mini-Mental Status Exam includes an assessment of executive function

A. True

B. False

19. Mrs. Ludwig is taught to scoot to the edge of the chair and lean forward when transferring sit to stand. She is able to perform this skill when in the dining room with no cueing. When asked to tell her daughter about her therapy she does not remember the therapist or ever being in therapy. Which of the following statements is true about Mrs. Ludwig's learning?

A. She has not learned how to transfer

B. She has explicitly learned transfer skills

C. She exhibits implicit learning of the transfer skills

D. She has impaired motor learning and should not receive therapy

20. **When working with Mrs. Ludwig who has Alzheimer's disease Mrs. Ludwig becomes agitated and starts yelling "get off of the boat." The therapist should respond in what manner?**

    A. Ask the PT assistant to take over as a change in caregiver may help calm her down

    B. Avoid eye contact while explaining that everything is okay

    C. Place both hands on Mrs. Ludwig's shoulders and apply firm downward pressure

    D. Say "I understand you are upset, do you need to get up?" based on what Mrs. Ludwig is shouting

21. **Your client with cognitive impairment has been working with you in therapy for 35 minutes and you note that they have become more confused than when you started and are exhibiting increased aphasia. What is the likely cause of this?**

    A. These are common signs/symptoms of cognitive impairment and are not significant

    B. The patient is fatigued and needs to rest

    C. This may be indicative of a medical emergency such as increased pressure on the brain or a stroke

    D. These are symptoms of delirium

22. **You have been asked to design an exercise program to improve both cognitive and daily function in individuals with Alzheimer's disease. Which of the following is a critical component to include?**

    A. Aerobic exercise

    B. Resistance exercise

    C. Sessions must be at least 45 minutes long

    D. Must be done for over 150 minutes a week

23. **If you want to reduce your risk of developing dementia when you are older the best evidence-based recommendation at this time is to do which of the following?**

    A. High intensity aerobic exercise, starting before age 65

    B. Exercise 5-7 times a week, must include some resistance training

    C. Any type of exercise for at least 52 hours total

    D. Individualized, multi-modal exercise that progresses in frequency over time

24. **A patient with a diagnosis of Alzheimer's disease has had three falls in the last 2 months. His partner reports that he fell while returning from getting their mail from the mailbox at the end of their driveway. You suspect that the added task of carrying the mail is increasing his fall risk. Which of the following assessments would best help you confirm or reject this hypothesis?**

    A. Timed Up and Go Cognitive

    B. Calculate dual task cost when doing the Timed Up and Go Cognitive

    C. Timed Up and Go Manual

    D. Walking While Talking Test

25. **Which of the following is an example of a correct use of errorless learning?**

    A. Provide a verbal cue to scoot to the edge of the chair prior to going sit to stand whenever the patient does not initiate scooting at the start of the transfer.

    B. Provide hand-over-hand assistance in steering the rollator walker during walking.

    C. Demonstrate leaning forward at the start of the sit-to-stand movement prior to the individual attempting the transfer.

    D. If the patient does not bend forward on initiating sit to stand provide a verbal cue on the next attempt.

Answers

1. A	2. B	3. D	4. B	5. B
6. A	7. B	8. B	9. B	10. A
11. C	12. A	13. C	14. B	15. B
16. B	17. B	18. B	19. C	20. D
21. B	22. A	23. D	24. C	25. A

GLOSSARY

Aging anorexia. Loss of appetite, resulting in extreme weight loss, malnutrition, and poor health.

Amyloid plaques (senile plaques). Aggregations of abnormally folded proteins, containing neural material, associated with aging and Alzheimer's disease.

Atherosclerosis. A buildup of lipids within the walls of the large arteries.

Cataracts. An aggregation of proteins within the lens of the eye that disrupts refraction.

Cerebral amyloid angiopathy. Replacement of the smooth muscle of blood vessels with amyloid material.

Delirium. A transient condition of rapid onset impaired cognition and consciousness caused by a severe stressor.

Dementia. A decline in cognitive ability that is associated with a diminished ability to complete activities of daily living.

Dry. Occurs without blood vessel proliferation.

Dual task cost. A measure of the interference a second task (e.g., talking) imposes on the performance of the primary task (e.g., walking).

Errorless learning. Providing ongoing prompts during procedural learning so that the learner does not make mistakes.

Fiber grouping. The clustering of like muscle fiber type in aging muscle.

Glaucoma. A pathological loss of retinal ganglion cells.

Lewy body. Alpha-synuclein aggregates that cluster in axon terminals and disrupt neural function.

Macular degeneration. Degeneration of the central part of the retina.

Mild cognitive impairment. Greater than expected loss of cognitive function than is expected without a deficit in independent function.

Muscle catabolism. Metabolic breakdown of muscle associated with subclinical inflammation.

Negative learning. Adaptation of behavior instigated by aging in sensory and motor function that reduces brain activity and further impedes function.

Negative plasticity of aging Decreased environmental, sensory, and behavioral stimulation results in decreased neural activity and subsequent brain deterioration.

Neurofibrillary tangles. Aggregates of tau protein found in the cytoplasm of neurons in a bundled configuration.

Noisy processing. Aging of sensory systems, leading to degraded sensory processing.

Presbycusis. Progressive, bilateral hearing loss of aging.

Presbyopia. Impaired visual accommodation due to aging of the lens.

Reversible dementia. Conditions that present as dementia (loss of cognition & impaired activities of daily living) but may be treated with a return to better function, if caught early.

Sarcopenia. The loss of muscle mass and strength associated with aging.

Wet. Occurs with blood vessel proliferation.

ABBREVIATIONS

AD	alzheimer's disease
AT	Atherosclerosis
CAA	Cerebral amyloid angiopathy
FTD	Frontotemporal dementia
LBD	Lewy body dementia
MCI	Mild Cognitive Impairment
MD	Macular degeneration
MMSE	Mini Mental State Examination
MoCA	Montreal Cognitive Assessment
NPH	Normal pressure hydrocephalus
VaD	Vascular dementia

Neural Tube Disorders and Hydrocephalus

19

Jill C. Heathcock and Deborah S. Nichols-Larsen

OBJECTIVES

1) Distinguish the epidemiology and pathophysiology of neural tube defects

2) Identify the common sensorimotor deficits and associated comorbidities of myelomeningocele

3) Identify and help physical therapists choose optimal treatment interventions for children with myelomeningocele

CASE A, PART I

Dylan is a 15-year-old male with myelomeningocele. His birth history includes myelomeningocele (see Figure 19-1) identification from an ultrasound at 20 weeks of gestation. He was born via scheduled C-section at 38 weeks gestational age. He had postnatal surgery to close the lesion 24 hours later, and during surgery, the highest lesion level identified was L1/L2; he had a second surgery to implant a ventriculoperitoneal shunt at 3 weeks of age. He wore a Pavlik harness for his first 6 months of life for bilateral hip dysplasia. He has had multiple episodes of physical therapy care throughout his lifetime. Dylan does not ambulate but wore braces up to the age of six to facilitate standing and home ambulation with a walker. Currently, he is s/p spinal fusion for scoliosis and has restrictions, including no flexion of his trunk and no pushing or pulling with his arms; he has been fitted with a thoracolumbosacral orthosis (TLSO) to prevent trunk flexion during recovery. Dylan is unable to push or pull with his legs. His ankle ROM is lacking 5 degrees bilaterally, and 20+ degrees of hip flexion contractures were corrected as part of his scoliosis surgery. In the past year, he has also had an increased weight gain of 30 pounds, and now weighs 150. Dylan will be starting high school in 2 months. He is currently in a manual wheelchair that he has had for 2 years. His current chair is too small, and he cannot propel it with the restrictions from the surgery. Right now his mom pushes him in the manual chair, and in school, a student peer is pushing him from one class to another.

● INTRODUCTION

Myelomeningocele is one of a group of disorders, referred to as neural tube disorders (NTDs). To understand NTDs, we will start with a discussion of the formation of the nervous system, during gestation, and how disruption of this formation results in a variety of defects of the CNS. NTDs are the second most frequent congenital anomaly with only heart defects occurring more frequently.[1] Since these occur during early gestation, they can result in complex sequelae, associated with the site and extent of the defect; some are so severe that they result in miscarriages, or even if birth occurs, life cannot be sustained.

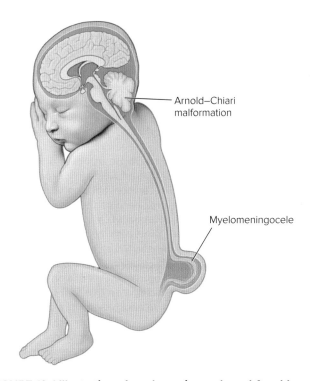

Arnold–Chiari malformation

Myelomeningocele

FIGURE 19-1 Illustration of myelomeningocele and Arnold–Chiari defects. The spinal defect (myelomeningocele) typically presents in the thoracolumbar spine as a bulging sac with neural and meningeal contents; the associated Arnold–Chiari malformation is illustrated at the craniocervical flexure with the cerebellum herniating down into the foramen magnum.

Neural Tube Defects

NTDs occur within the first 3 to 4 weeks of conception, during formation of the neural tube, a process called neurulation (see Box 19-1). The neural tube is the first structure of the developing brain and spinal cord.[2–4]

The initial closure of the neural tube first happens in the middle of the tube in the area of the rhombencephalon (see Figure 19-3); this occurs around day 21 of embryonic development. Closure then proceeds in both cephalic and caudal

Box 19-1	Development of the Nervous System (Neurulation)[3,4]

To understand NTDs, one must first understand a little about embryonic development. Within a few days of fertilization, the embryo is defined by three layers of tissue: the **endoderm** (inner layer) that will form into most of the internal organs; the **mesoderm** (middle layer) that will form into muscle and connective tissue as well as the cardiovascular system; and the **ectoderm** (outer layer) that forms the skin and nervous system. Within the ectoderm, the nervous system forms out of the centralized portion, known as the **neural plate**. The neural plate, over time, folds in on itself (invagination) to first create the **neural groove** that then comes together at the dorsal aspect to form the **neural tube** (Figure 19-2). Some of the neural crest cells remain outside of the neural tube and form the dorsal root and sympathetic ganglia of the nervous system. Once the tube is formed, cell proliferation occurs unequally along the tube such that a series of vesicles emerge along with bending of the tube to allow its expansion within the confines of the developing fetus. Early on, three vesicles emerge at the rostral aspect of the tube, referred to as the (1) **prosencephalon** – the most rostral portion that will become the cerebral hemispheres; (2) **mesencephalon** or middle portion that will become the midbrain; and (3) **rhombencephalon** – the most caudal vesicle that will become the pons, cerebellum, and medulla, see Figure 19-3A. Further cell proliferation results in a five-vesicle structure (Figure 19-3B) that will ultimately expand into the mature brain areas. The prosencephalon will expand into the telencephalon that will become the cerebral hemispheres as well as the **diencephalon**, which will ultimately form the neural portion of the eyes (retina, lens) and the hypothalamus, thalamus, epithalamus, and subthalamus; the **mesencephalon** remains a singular structure that will mature into the midbrain. The rhombencephalon diverges into two vesicles: the **metencephalon** that forms the pons and cerebellum and the **myelencephalon** that forms the medulla. The myelencephalon is contiguous with the remaining neural tube that will form the spinal cord. As the vesicle structures emerge, the tube begins to flex in on itself to afford space for further expansion with first two flexures: one between the mesencephalon and rhombencephalon (**cephalic flexure**) and the other between the rhombencephalon and the remaining neural tube (**cervical flexure**). The five-vesicle structure exhibits a third flexure between the metencephalon and myelencephalon known as the **pontine flexure** (Figure 19-3C). The central opening of the neural tube develops into the ventricles, cerebral aqueduct, and spinal canal, containing the cerebrospinal fluid.[4]

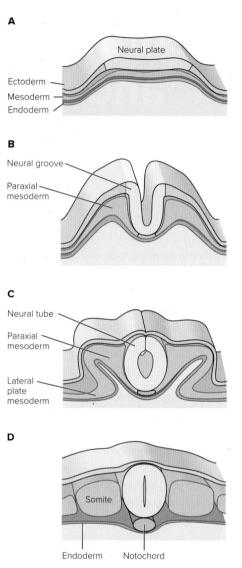

FIGURE 19-2 Neural tube development. A. 3 layers of tissue that will develop into the fetus with the central portion of the ectoderm, comprising the neural plate. **B.** Invagination creates the neural grove. **C.** The neural folds come together to form the neural tube. **D.** The neural tube sits above the notochord, which will develop into the spinal column, and is flanked on each side by somites, which will develop into cartilage and muscle. (Reproduced with permission from Kandel ER, Schwartz JH, et al., *Principles of Neural Science*, 5th Ed, New York, NY: McGraw-Hill; 2013.)

directions simultaneously with rostral closure complete by the 25th day and caudal closure by day 28[3] (Figure 19-4). Please remember that neurulation happens extremely early in embryotic development, so the expecting mother may not know she is pregnant or may have just missed a menstrual cycle.

NTDs can be characterized as open or closed. An open defect occurs when the neural contents protrude and are exposed to the environment. In closed defects, the epithelium covers the defect, so the neural contents are not exposed; thus, closed defects tend to be less severe than open defects.[2] In addition, to this distinction, NTDs are defined by their location and size. The location, size, and contents of the neural tube defect are important for not only life and viability but

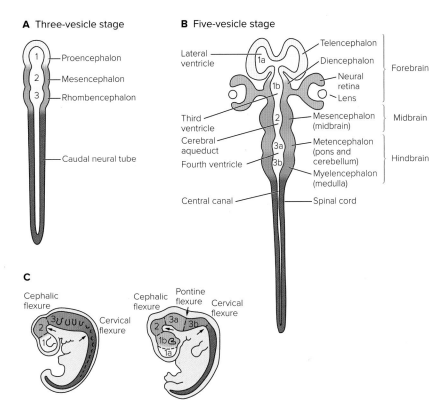

FIGURE 19-3 Neural vesicle development. A. 3 vesicle stage of neural tube development. **B.** 5 vesicle stage of neural tube development; C - flexing of the neural tube occurs first at 2 points (cephalic flexure and cervical flexure), with a third flexure (pontine) developing later. (Reproduced with permission from Kandel ER, Schwartz JH, et al., *Principles of Neural Science*, 5th Ed, New York, NY: McGraw-Hill; 2013.)

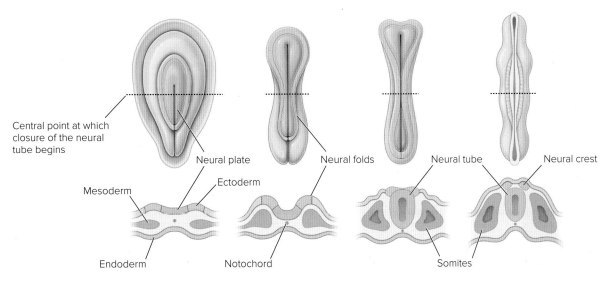

FIGURE 19-4 Neural tube closure. The closure of the neural tube begins in the center and proceeds both rostrally and caudally.

also for prediction of future disability. The location is the site where closure fails, occurring at some point along the cranial or caudal closure. The size is how big the lesion is or how much of the brain structures or vertebral column it spans, ranging from very small to very large. The length and position of the damaged segment (lack of closure of the neural tube) dictate its severity. The contents are what are inside the sac and can include components of the brain, skull, spinal cord, peripheral nerves, meninges, and cerebral spinal fluid or any combination of these.[2,3,5]

Lesions of the Cranial Neural Tube

There are three main types of cranial NTDs, associated with a failure of closure of the rostral neural tube. **Anencephaly** is an extremely rare open defect (3 per 10,000 pregnancies), occurring when the cranial neural tube fails to close; the exposed brain tissue is destroyed by exposure to the amniotic fluid with ultimate loss of the forebrain (cerebral hemispheres, thalamus, and midbrain) and skull; the lower brainstem and spinal cord are typically intact. These infants rarely survive gestation, but if they do, die within the first few hours of birth.[2] **Hydranencephaly** is a related disorder, where there's an absence of the cerebral hemispheres or cerebral cortex, which is replaced with cerebral spinal fluid. The skull and meninges are intact as are the basal ganglia, cerebellum, brainstem, and spinal cord. Hydranencephaly is not really a NTD but rather occurs during the second trimester of gestation after neurulation is complete; however, it is presented here because of its similarity to anencephaly. Causes are hypothesized to be severe bilateral stroke of the anterior cerebral circulation, infection, hypoxia, toxic exposure, or leukomalacia. The defect can be identified by ultrasound in later gestation, but if not detected in utero, may not be apparent at birth. Typically, the cerebellum and brainstem are formed, so reflexes, such as sucking and swallowing, and spontaneous arm and leg movements can be present; mothers report normal fetal movement, during pregnancy. Hydranencephaly is very rare at less than 1 in 10,000 pregnancies but only 1 to 3 per 100,000 live births, since often they end in miscarriage or death prior to birth. For those born alive, they typically start demonstrating symptoms within their first weeks of life, including irritability, feeding difficulties, and significant motor delay and often seizures and breathing problems. These infants rarely live beyond the first year, so treatment is supportive.[6] An **encephalocele** is a closed defect that involves partial protrusion of the meninges (meningocele) and/or brain (**encephalomeningocele**) through a small skull defect.[2] They are most often found in the frontal or occipital regions (Figure 19-5). Occipital encephaloceles are more common in North America, while frontal lesions (facial area) are more common in Asia. Surgical repair to close this lesion is required.

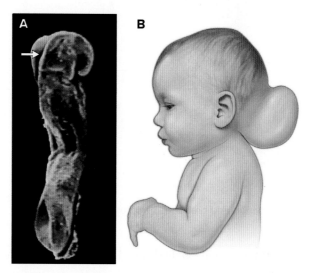

FIGURE 19-5 Illustration of encephalocele. A. Arrow marks the point of the neural tube where a failure of closure likely results in an encephalocele defect. **B.** As development continues, the encephalocele will present as a bulging sac at the site of the cranial defect with meningeal and neural contents within the sac.

Encephalocele is also rare at 1.4 per 10,000 live births.[7] If there is brain tissue in the sac, then the damage is more severe and can be life threatening. If there is no brain tissue in the sac, even large cysts can be removed; brain damage in this case is focal with resultant neurological impairment based on brain-injury location. If the contents of the sac do not include brain tissue, then the repair and prognosis are generally good but dependent on the location of the defect. Hydrocephalus is a frequent comorbidity of encephalocele.[7]

Lesions at the Spinal Levels

NTDs are much more common at the spinal level with the lower thoracic and lumbar levels most common. As a reminder, there are 7 cervical vertebra, 12 thoracic vertebra, 5 lumbar vertebra, and 5 fused sacral vertebra. Each vertebral body is different in shape and size based on the location. The boney spinal column offers a lot of protection to the spinal cord. The lamina forms and covers the spinal canal, where the spinal cord is located, with facet joints that articulate with the vertebra above and below. During development, each vertebra forms in a similar fashion to the neural tube, bending in on itself and coming together at the back into the spinous process. **Spinal dysraphism**, also historically referred to as spina bifida, is a defect of the closure of the spinous process or processes at some level of the spinal column. **Spinal dysraphism occulta** or **spina bifida occulta** is the mildest and most common form, present in 12-13% of healthy babies. In this case, there is no lamina or spinous process but the spinal cord, meninges, and cerebral spinal fluid are contained in the spinal canal. There is skin covering the defect and there may be a dimple, a small patch of hair, changes in pigment or a small fatty lump over the missing spinous process. Typically, this kind of defect does not cause any neurologic problem, and most people do not know they have it. However, there is a higher incidence of spinal cord tethering with spinal dysraphism occulta where the spinal cord is attached (tethered) to the surrounding tissue. Spinal cord tethering gets increasingly more serious as children get older because their growth can cause damage to the cord as the tethering pulls on the spinal cord as the spinal column grows. Notably, cord growth is slower and to a lesser degree than the spinal column; thus, growth induces stretching, and thereby damage, to the cord with neurologic symptoms presenting as the child grows.[8]

When the caudal neural tube fails to close, the vertebral body is unable to close as well, resulting in an absence or malformation of the vertebral body.[3] Similar to the variability of defects that occur with failure in closure of the cranial portion (encephaloceles), caudal failure can present with a continuum of defects, depending on what neural components are involved in the defect (see Figure 19-6). The mildest defect is referred to as a **meningocele**, which manifests as an absence of the lamina or spinous process, but the spinal cord remains contained within the spinal canal; however, there is a protrusion of the meninges (arachnoid and dura) and cerebral spinal fluid outside of the spinal canal. Meningocele is rare, but it is possible for the membrane or cyst to be surgically removed with little to no damage of any neural pathways.[2] When there is no lamina or spinous process and the protruding sac contains components of the spinal cord, meninges, and cerebral spinal fluid outside of the spinal canal, it is called a **myelomeningocele**. This is the most severe form of neural tube defect associated with spina bifida, and this means that during fetal development, the spinal cord is outside of the body in either a closed or open sac. If the sac is closed, meaning covered with skin, then the contents within have some protection. The sac can be long and thin, resembling a tail or finger, or round and wide. The sac can also be open where there are tissues and nerves exposed to amniotic fluid in utero and exposed to anything in the environment after birth. As such, infants with open lesions are at a greater risk for serious infections and subsequent neural damage. Myelomeningocele is the most common form of neural tube defect with spina bifida. Because of this prevalence, these two terms, myelomeningocele and spina bifida are often used interchangeably by clinicians; however, it is important to remember that they are actually variations of the spina bifida condition. With both meningoceles and myelomeningoceles, there is a visible defect on the baby and variable degrees of neural damage; while spina bifida refers actually to the spinal abnormality.[2]

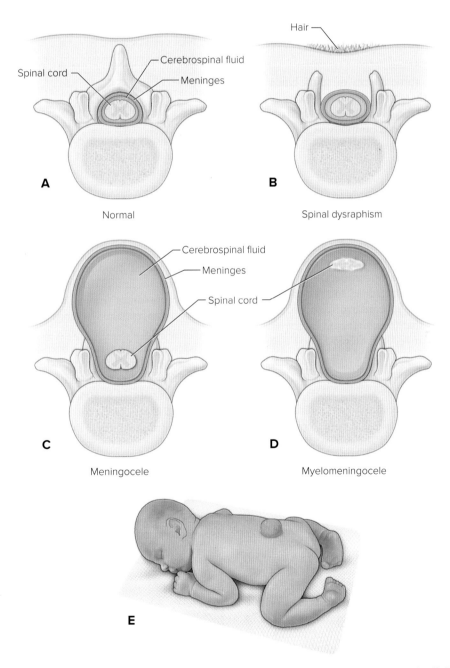

FIGURE 19-6 Spina bifida defects. A. Normal spinous process and vertebra. **B.** Spinal dysraphism occulta (failure of spinous process closure without protrusion of the spinal canal contents) with hair patch on skin above. **C.** Meningocele – fluid-filled sac of meninges protrudes through the spinal defect with spinal cord contained in the spinal canal. **D.** Myelomeningocele – spinal cord components within the meningeal sac protrude through the spinal defect. **E.** Appearance of myelomeningocele defect on infant at birth.

Myelomeningocele (MMC)

CASE A, PART II

In our case, Dylan presented in utero with an MMC at L1/L2, meaning the sac was between the first and second lumbar vertebra, which is a very common location for these lesions. He was diagnosed in utero via ultrasound and presented at birth or soon after with several common comorbidities (Arnold–Chiari malformation [A–CM], hydrocephalus, and hip dislocation). In the following discussion, we will examine how diagnosis of MMC occurs, the functional presentation of MMC, and the comorbidities associated with this defect.

Since MMC is the most common form of spina bifida and requires extensive physical therapy management, we will focus much of this chapter on this disorder. The term "spina bifida" is often used by the rehabilitation community as synonymous with MMC, but we will try to distinguish the two for clarity in the following discussion.

Location

The location of the lesion in patients with MMC is typically in the thoracic, lumbar, or sacral level of the spine and rarely in the cervical spine; this is also true of meningoceles and spina bifida occulta. Motor and sensory deficits include paralysis and loss of sensation, including touch, pain, temperature, and proprioception, below the lesion level. Bowel, bladder, and sexual dysfunction are similar to patients with spinal cord injury (see Chapter 13). While the damage parallels that for spinal cord injury, since it occurs during gestation it impedes musculoskeletal development in utero.[2]

Causes

The specific cause(s) of NTD is (are) unknown but is likely multifactorial. Risk factors include nutritional status, environmental toxins, and genetic contributions.[5] The evidence for a genetic cause or predisposition stems largely from the increased likelihood of a second NTD occurring, when a sibling or the mother has spina bifida or there has been a previous pregnancy with a neural tube defect.[5] However, for a relatively small group of infants, there is a defined chromosomal anomaly with trisomy 18 the most common.[9] Multiple genes have been implicated in NTDs; however, current research suggests that there is likely more than one causative gene and even more likely that there is a combination of genetic predisposition with other factors. Environmental factors that have been linked to NTDs include Valproic acid (an anticonvulsant); maternal fever, obesity, and diabetes; and excessive hot tub use. Yet, how these factors trigger NTD formation is unknown.[5] Additionally, early studies identified a deficit in folic acid in mothers, who had infants with NTDs, especially in those without access to prenatal care and subsequent studies found that providing a folic acid supplement reduced recurrence. Thus, women are encouraged to start taking 400 mcg of folic acid supplement every day when *planning* a pregnancy and not just after they become pregnant. One reason for starting supplementation early is that neural tube formation occurs very early after conception.[10] Overall, it is thought that a combination of nutritional, environmental, epigenetic, and genetic factors contribute to spina bifida and its associated NTD.

Incidence

CASE A, PART III

In our case, Dylan's defect was diagnosed by fetal ultrasound at 20 weeks; ultrasound at this time point is common and often identifies this defect, during the second trimester of fetal development.

MMC is reported in 1.8 per 10,000 live births.[2] It is a lifelong disability. Early diagnosis of MMC initially involved a blood test to measure the presence of alpha-fetoprotein in the blood, which had an accuracy of 70 to 80% in diagnosing an NTD.[11] However, ultrasound is now the most common method of identification and is routinely done in the 2nd trimester (18-24 weeks) with up to 98% accuracy.[9] Due to folic acid supplementation and improved nutrition during early pregnancy, the rates of MMC have been decreasing and are thought to be stabilizing.[10]

Surgical Management

Until 2011, most children with MMC received surgery after birth to close the lesion. However, the MOMS trial demonstrated improved outcomes (motor and cognitive) and lesser occurrence of hydrocephalus. Notably, there was a 20% improvement in the number of children able to ambulate by 30 months of age.[12] Since that time, there's been an increase in the tendency to repair the defect in utero to avoid the secondary damage that occurs via exposure to amniotic fluid and other environmental elements with 40 to 60% of cases eligible for in utero repair (see Box 19-2 for criteria for inclusion and exclusion).[9] Multiple factors contribute to these improved outcomes specifically prevention of damage from exposure to the amniotic environment and avoidance of secondary complications common in MMC, as described in the subsequent section (i.e., Arnold–Chiari malformation and hydrocephalus).[12]

Box 19-2 Criteria for and Complications of In Utero Repair of MMC (adapted from Meller 2021)[9]

Inclusion: (1) maternal age greater than 18; (2) gestational age 19-25 weeks; (3) thoracic-sacral location; (4) Chiari II malformation; (5) location near appropriate treatment center.

Exclusion: (1) Other fetal anomaly; (2) multiple fetuses; (3) high risk for preterm birth; (4) placental anomalies; (5) maternal obesity (BMI>35); (6) maternal infection (HIV, hepatitis); (7) previous hysterectomy; (8) psychosocial concerns.

Complications: (1) Potential uterine rupture in the current or subsequent pregnancies; (2) premature birth due to premature rupture of amniotic sac.

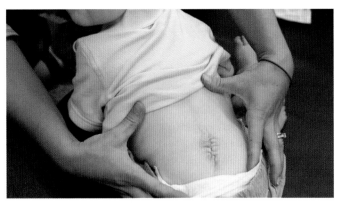

FIGURE 19-7 Postsurgical repair scarring. The need to pull skin over the space occupied by the myelomeningocele typically results in a large scar that further expands as the child grows. (Used with permission from Jill C. Heathcock, MPT, PhD, The Ohio State University.)

For children, who do not have an intrauterine repair, immediate surgical repair is necessary for protection and prevention of further injury to the spinal cord and peripheral nerves. This focuses on closure of the lesion (see Box 19-3 and Figure 19-7). Presently, once the spinal cord and peripheral nerves are damaged, there is no surgical fix. The goal of surgery is to put the neural tissue back in the spinal column, protect it from future damage, and guard against infection. Spina bifida is almost always identified in utero, unless there is an absence of prenatal care, and a C-section is scheduled to avoid any trauma to the skin and membranes around the sac and lesion that might occur with a vaginal delivery. Remarkably, fetuses with unknown spina bifida have been delivered vaginally without rupture of the sac or membrane. The surgery to close the lesion is typically done in the first 24 hours after birth. Surgery involves using skin and either fascia or muscle or both to close and protect the open area. After surgery, the primary goals are aimed at healing and protection of the surgical site. The role of the PT following surgery includes examination of the skin and position changes to avoid skin breakdown and pressure sores; initial positioning is prone with rotation to side-lying every 2 hours for at least 6 weeks to protect the repair.[13] Throughout childhood, the PT has a large role in stimulating age-appropriate activities and mobility.

Box 19-3	Surgical Closure of the Lesion[13]

Repair of the myelomeningocele lesion involves further extension of the skin opening to allow sufficient room to work and eventually sufficient skin to pull over the opening. Some neural elements that are caught in the sac itself may need to be sacrificed. Other neural contents that can be saved are enclosed in the dura mater, which may require augmentation with paravertebral muscles or fascia, and the dura closed. These elements (paravertebral muscles and fascia) are also used to provide some additional protection over the dural closure, and then, the skin is closed. An extensive scar will be left; notably, the spinal column defect is typically not repaired but rather soft tissue is used to cover the opening to protect the spinal cord.

Common Sensorimotor Characteristics in Myelomeningocele

The location and extent of damage are important for understanding common sensorimotor characteristics of MMC. Infants, children, and adults with MMC often show both upper and lower motor neuron signs, similar to what has been described in Chapter 13 for spinal cord injuries. Upper motor neuron (UMN) signs are observed when there is damage to the UMNs within the cortex or their projections (axons) within the brainstem, corticospinal tracts, or spinal cord. UMN signs are specific to the descending motor pathways in MMC. Cerebral palsy (Chapter 20) is a common pediatric UMN disorder, and stroke is a common UMN adult disorder. Typical ways to assess UMN and LMN signs are to examine muscle tone, reflexes, and involuntary movements. In children with UMN signs, you will see increased tone (hypertonia), spasticity, and often clonus as well as poor muscle control and synergistic movements (see Table 19-1 for descriptions). Patients with MMC often have bilateral but asymmetrical lesions due to the nature of the defect, similar to patients with traumatic spinal cord injuries. This means that one leg might have more or different function than the other leg. In terms of muscle development, there is always disuse atrophy and incomplete muscle development with UMN and LMN lesions in children. Patients with MMC will have a different developmental trajectory than infants with typical development, and they will not show the same types of antigravity movements, such as kicking, that effect their muscle growth and development over time. Disuse atrophy is typically widespread across all antigravity muscles below the lesion. Voluntary movements with UMN injuries are very difficult, ranging from impaired to absent.

Lower motor neuron signs result from damage to specific locations and structures including cranial nerves and nuclei, parts of the spinal cord including anterior horn cells (alpha motor neurons) and spinal roots, and any peripheral nerve damage, which innervates skeletal muscle. Peripheral nerve damage often comes in the form of pulling, stretching, or tearing of any part of the nerve(s) that connect(s) the spinal cord to a specific muscle. One of the most common pediatric injuries that cause LMN signs is brachial plexus palsy, an injury that occurs during birth (see Chapter 16). A hallmark of LMN injury is flaccid paralysis and areflexia, but with partial innervation, hypotonia, and hyporeflexia may be present (see Table 19-1 for definitions). Also, fasciculations are common; such small and occasional muscle twitches occur occasionally in a typical population (e.g., eyelid twitches), but those from LMN injury are more frequent and measurably different on EMG.[14] In MMC, weakness and paralysis are segmental and focal, based on the lesion site, and often asymmetrical with one side more affected than the other. Complications to the muscle and to muscle development include neurogenic atrophy, since the affected muscles may have never received appropriate nerve signals; this results in immediate and severe focal wasting, ultimately leading to current and future disuse and further atrophy. Voluntary movements with LMN injuries are either weak or absent. Notably, LMN signs are common in muscles innervated at the level of the spinal cord defect; UMN signs will be present at levels below the defect

TABLE 19-1	Signs of Upper and Lower Motor Neuron Damage	
UMN signs	Hypertonia	Increased muscle tone
	Spasticity	Velocity-dependent resistance to passive stretch such that a quick stretch elicits more resistance and a slow stretch less resistance.
	Hyperreflexia	Hyper-responsive monosynaptic stretch reflexes (brisk), elicited by a tendon tap.
	Clonus	Repetitive muscle contraction in response to a quick stretch. This is most common with a quick stretch of the gastrocnemius, elicited by quickly moving the foot into dorsiflexion. The number of beats of extension can be counted as an indication of severity
	Babinski sign	An upward movement of the hallux and splaying of the toes in response to a stroke (heel to toe) on the sole of the foot. This is a normal response in children under 4–6 months and abnormal after that. A negative sign in a mature child/adult is a downward movement of the hallux with minimal or absent toe movement.
	Autonomic reflexes	With the loss of UMN control of brainstem centers, an increase in blood pressure, heart rate, and sweating is often seen.
	Synergistic movement	Movement in flexor or extensor patterns that make voluntary control difficult (e.g., when flexing the elbow, the wrist and fingers also flex; when extending the elbow, the hand opens).
	Muscle weakness (paresis)/poor force generation	UMN's activate alpha motor neurons in the spinal cord, so damage to them results in difficulty in activating muscles and resultant diminished force generation
LMN signs	Flaccid paralysis	A loss of active muscle control and reflex activity due to damage of alpha motor neurons in the spinal cord or cranial nerve nuclei
	Hypotonia	Decreased muscle tone, often associated with increased joint laxity
	Areflexia	Absent reflex activity due to loss of alpha motor neurons or Ia afferents in the spinal cord
	Hyporeflexia	Diminished reflex activity due to partial damage to the alpha motor neurons, Ia afferents, or both
	Fasciculations	Small involuntary muscle twitches of skeletal muscle associated with denervation of the muscle

where the spinal reflexes remain intact in the absence of supraspinal control.[15]

Comorbidities Associated with Myelomeningocele/Spina Bifida

Associated Brain Abnormalities

Hydrocephalus and Arnold Chiari malformation (A-CM) are two complications associated with MMC that can affect the brain and cause additional CNS damage. Both can occur in the absence of spina bifida but are common comorbidities of this disorder.

Arnold Chiari Malformation (A–CM): A–CM is the displacement of the brainstem and cerebellar tonsils inferiorly through the foramen magnum and subsequent disruption of the flow of cerebral spinal fluid within the cerebral aqueduct or fourth ventricle, referred to as obstructive hydrocephalus (Figure 19-8). There are four levels of A–CM with Level I being the least severe and Level IV being the most severe. Level II is associated with MMC. For children that do not have an intrauterine repair, who have a thoracic or higher lesion, the occurrence of

AC–M II is above 95%; for those with lumbar or lower lesions, the occurrence is nearly 90%.[16] For children, who undergo an intrauterine repair, the incidence in the initial MOMS study (Management of Myelomeningocele Study) was much lower at roughly 64%.[12] It is thought that the MMC lesion allows cerebral spinal fluid to escape, thereby limiting the filling of the ventricular system, which in turn, allows the brainstem and cerebellum to move downward into the spinal column. This also creates tension on forebrain structures such as the corpus collosum, which can compromise executive function. A-CM II is associated with decreased cerebellar size and subsequent reorganization of cerebellar structures; thus, children with MMC may demonstrate changes in arm, trunk, and eye movements, associated with altered cerebellar function. Presentation of A-CM varies, depending on the magnitude of compression. For some infants, they demonstrate compromise of brainstem function at birth and require immediate management to survive. For others, brainstem and cerebellar compromise occur as they grow, including cerebellar signs such as ataxia. Symptoms of cranial nerve disruption can also emerge with further compression of the brainstem, where these nerves originate, which manifests as

A

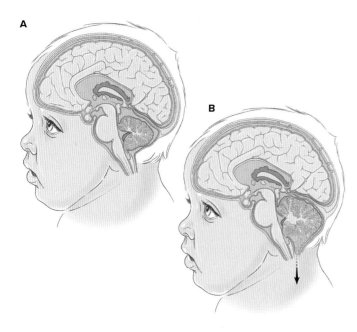

B

FIGURE 19-8 Arnold–Chiari malformation. A. Typical brain image with brainstem and cerebellum above the foramen magnum. **B.** Arnold–Chiari malformation with elongation of cerebellum into foramen magnum (type 1); in type II, which is common in MMC, there is further subluxation of the cerebellum and brainstem into the spinal canal, indicated by the arrow in the figure. (Reproduced with permission from Carney PR, & Geyer JD (Eds). *Pediatric Practice Neurology*. New York, NY: McGraw-Hill; 2010.)

disruption of eating (dysphagia), speech (dysphonia, dysarthria, vocal cord palsy) and respiration. In adolescents and adults, complaint of headache and/or dizziness is common.[17]

Medical management of A-CM II: Since the A-CM II defect occurs with hydrocephalus, the first treatment focuses on managing the hydrocephalus with external ventricular drainage and shunting (see hydrocephalus in subsequent section). Subsequent surgical intervention targets decompression of the brainstem and cerebellum through craniectomy and cervical laminoplasty. Respiratory compromise is an immediate indicator for surgery. Surgery consists of opening the upper cervical lamina and the dura to relieve pressure, and then some form of osteoplasty to support the opened vertebrae. Sometimes, especially in infants, a tracheotomy and insertion of a percutaneous endoscopic gastrostomy or jejunostomy (PEG/J) tube is required, so that food can be directly fed into the stomach or jejunum portion of the small intestine, respectively. These life-supporting methods are temporary for most children; occasionally, they become permanent, if the damage to the brainstem is

CASE A, PART IV

What brain malformation might we expect in Dylan?

- He has an A–CM and a history of hydrocephalus. He has had one shunt placement when he was an infant.

**Is this typical?*

Yes; here we discuss these two common comorbidities of MMC and their relationship to each other.

significant. Craniectomy is always supported by implantation of a shunt to manage hydrocephalus.[17]

Hydrocephalus is an accumulation of cerebral spinal fluid (CSF) in the ventricles, leading to increased intracranial pressure; hydrocephalus has multiple causes, including genetic anomalies and brain malformations such as A–CM. This increased intracranial pressure and accumulation of fluid expands the ventricles, compressing the brain against the skull and stretching white matter, which causes damage to brain structures and disrupts brain development. Untreated it can disrupt neural metabolism and induce neuroinflammation, gliosis, demyelination, and ultimately cell death.[18]

Hydrocephalus can be congenital (present at birth) or acquired. In some cases of congenital hydrocephalus, the cause is a genetic mutation, and in a subset of these it is inherited, most commonly as an x-linked inheritance. In other cases, it results from structural anomalies with unknown etiology, including A–CM. Acquired cases often follow an injury to the brain such as hemorrhage (stroke) or trauma; a complication from a tumor, cyst, or infection, a developmental malformation that eventually impedes CSF flow, or overproduction of CSF[19] (see Box 19-4). Overall hydrocephalus affects less than 1 out of 1000 live births in the United States but is much more frequent in developing countries, largely secondary to maternal infections. Signs and symptoms of hydrocephalus include a bulging fontanelle and scalp veins, behavioral changes, high-pitched

Box 19-4 The Ventricular System

The brain is supported structurally and chemically via the ventricular system and the cerebrospinal fluid (CSF) that circulates within it. The ventricular system is a series of ventricles and their connecting passages (Figure 19-9). The largest of the ventricles are the lateral ventricles within the cerebral hemispheres; these connect to the third ventricle, which is centered between the two thalamic nuclei, via the intraventricular foramina. The third ventricle connects to the fourth ventricle in the brainstem via the cerebral aqueduct. The fourth ventricle is contiguous with the central canal of the spinal cord; it also connects to the subarachnoid space through two foramina (Magendie and Luschka). This allows CSF to flow through the subarachnoid space that lies between the arachnoid and pia maters and provides some cushioning of the brain within the cranial cavity. Further, the subarachnoid space continues within the spinal canal between its arachnoid and pia mater linings, allowing fluid to move down the cord, pooling in the lumbar cistern, and moving back up the ventral side of the cord. From the cerebral subarachnoid space, CSF is absorbed through a specialized network of valves, called the arachnoid villi, into the venous sinuses, primarily the superior sagittal sinus, allowing it to enter the venous blood flow as it returns to the heart. CSF is produced in the choroid plexuses, located within the ventricles. CSF serves many functions, including providing a cushion for the brain and spinal cord from their bony enclosures as well as from external blows to the head, serving as a source of nutrients for the surrounding brain tissue, and absorbing metabolic waste from those brain tissues (Figure 19-10).

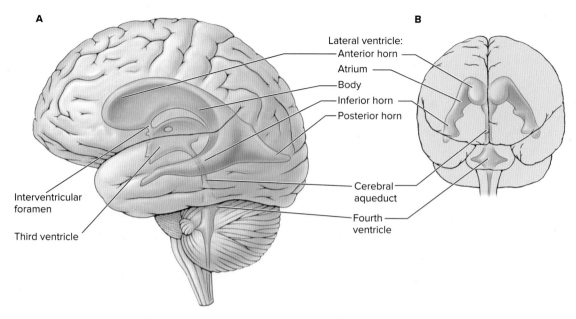

FIGURE 19-9 Ventricular system. A. Lateral (sagittal view) depicting ventricular system. **B.** Frontal section, depicting ventricular system. (Reproduced with permission from Martin JH (Ed). *Neuroanatomy Text and Atlas*, 4th Ed. New York, NY: McGraw-Hill; 2012.)

Box 19-5   Other Causes of Hydrocephalus in Children

Although MMC-associated hydrocephalus is the most common type of hydrocephalus, it can occur in the absence of MMC. Hydrocephalus without MMC occurs due to either (1) obstruction of the CSF pathway secondary to malformation (**noncommunicating hydrocephalus**) or blockage (**obstructive hydrocephalus**) or (2) overproduction or decreased absorption of CSF, known both as **communicating or nonobstructive** hydrocephalus. Overproduction is most commonly associated with a benign tumor (papilloma) within the choroid plexus, while diminished absorption is typically related to abnormal function within the subarachnoid villi, often associated with subarachnoid hemorrhage. Posthemorrhagic hydrocephalus is a common consequence of prematurity.[22]

Regardless of the cause of hydrocephalus, expansion of the ventricles due to excessive CSF, produces both stretching of white matter and compression of the adjacent brain tissue; further, disruption of CSF flow may interrupt the nutritional support to the brain or removal of metabolic waste typically provided by CSF, resulting in additional compromise to brain tissue. In infants, prior to fontanel closure, ventricular expansion is accompanied by expansion of the cranium. **Prior to the implementation of surgical shunting, children with congenital hydrocephalus experienced extreme enlargement of the cranium until eventually death ensued; this may still occur in 3rd world countries.** Now, surgical implantation of a shunt is done very early to minimize the ventricular expansion and secondary brain tissue damage, and thus, maximizes brain preservation and neurologic function. Many children with congenital hydrocephalus live normal lives without any or with very mild complications. However, hydrocephalus may be associated with diminished intelligence (lower IQ scores on testing) and greater incidence of nonverbal learning disabilities; the cause of these cognitive disabilities is likely multifaceted with disrupted early brain development as well as damage from surgical implantation of the shunt as contributing factors. Motor characteristics of hydrocephalus include poor fine motor skills such as handwriting with minimal effect on gross motor skills; however, early development may be delayed due to the enlarged head.[23]

---

cries, seizures, vomiting, and changes in appetite. **Fontanelles** (also spelled fontanels) are the "soft spot" on newborns' heads where the cranial sutures have not yet come together or fused. Patients with hydrocephalus typically have a large head due to fluid accumulation in the ventricles that causes the cranial bones to separate as the fontanelles stretch. Hydrocephalus may cause additional deficits in learning and memory, hearing loss, headaches, sensorimotor dysfunction, and impaired vision due to compression of brain tissue as the ventricles expand; deficits are related to the degree and location of tissue compression. These deficits can be severe, including intellectual disabilities, epilepsy, and cerebral palsy[18-20]

The treatment for hydrocephalus, with or without MMC, historically has been shunting. A shunt is a tube that is placed with one end typically in one of the lateral ventricles of the brain (can also be placed in the subarachnoid space), threaded down the neck just behind the ear, and terminates in the abdominal cavity (ventriculoperitoneal), atrium of the heart (ventriculo-atrial), or pleural cavity (ventriculopleural), allowing the excess fluid to drain. The fluid is then reabsorbed back into the body (see Figure 19-11). The shunt can be visible and palpable on the side of the infants' head behind the ear and typically includes a small valve or pump that can be externally massaged to prevent blockages; usually, two segments of tubing are used with one segment

(1) CSF is produced by the choroid plexus in the ventricles.

(2) CSF flows from the third ventricle through the cerebral aqueduct into the fourth ventricle.

(3) CSF in the fourth ventricle flows into the subarachnoid space by passing through the paired lateral apertures or the single median aperture, and into the central canal of the spinal cord.

(4) As the CSF flows through the subarachnoid space, it removes waste products and provides buoyancy to support the brain.

(5) Excess CSF flows into the arachnoid villi, then drains into the dural venous sinuses. Pressure allows the CSF to be released into the blood without permitting any venous blood to enter the subarachnoid space. The greater pressure on the CSF in the subarachnoid space ensures that CSF moves into the venous sinuses.

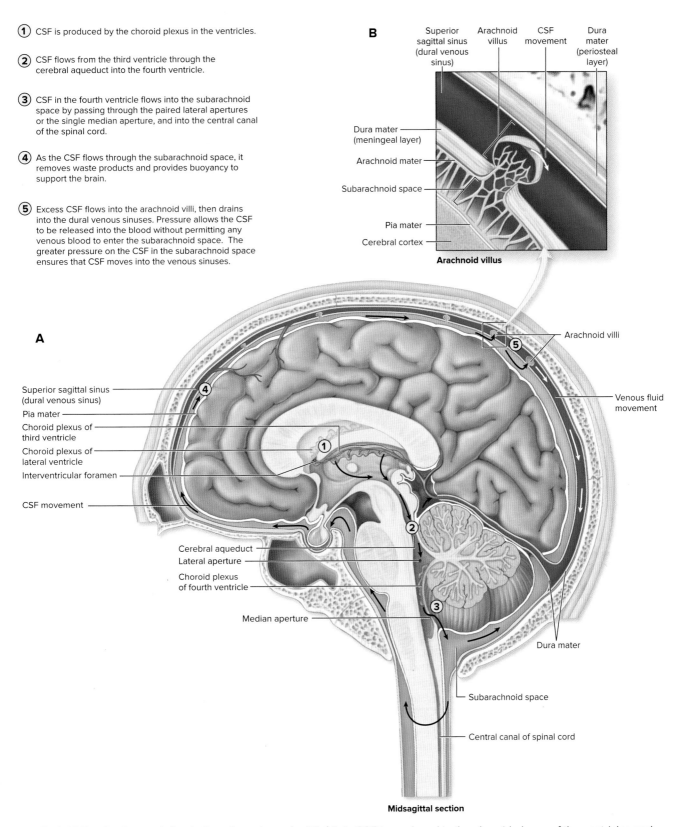

FIGURE 19-10 Production and circulation of cerebrospinal fluid. A. CSF is produced in the choroid plexus of the ventricles and circulates from the lateral ventricles (not pictured) to the third and fourth ventricles and within the central spinal canal; fluid then moves into the subarachnoid space of the brain and spinal canal, providing a compliant cushion for these structures. **B.** Small portals within the arachnoid mater (arachnoid villi) allow the CSF to move from the subarachnoid space to the superior sagittal sinus as well as other dural sinuses. (Reproduced with permission from McKinley M, O'Laughlin VD. *Human Anatomy*. 3rd Ed, New York, NY: McGraw-Hill; 2012.)

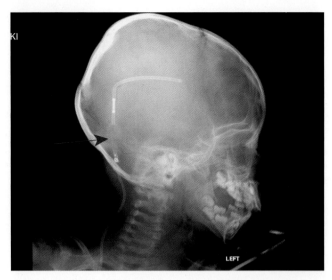

FIGURE 19-11 Illustration of shunting for hydrocephalus.
This is a radiograph illustration of a ventriculoperitoneal shunt, extending from the lateral ventricle to the peritoneum. The red arrow is pointing to the shunt valve, which is translucent. (Reproduced with permission from Shah BR, Lucchesi M, Amodio J, Silverberg M, eds. *Atlas of Pediatric Medicine*, 2nd ed. New York, NY: McGraw-Hill; 2013. Fig. 13.54: Photo contributor: John Amodio, MD).

running from the lateral ventricle to the junction behind the ear (proximal segment) and the second (distil segment) running from this junction to the point of fluid distribution (abdomen, heart). This allows replacement of the lower portion as the child grows without disruption of the proximal segment. There is a relatively high rate of shunt failure or malfunctioning with most children requiring some repair within 5 years of initial placement, so there must be ongoing neurosurgical follow-up to make sure the shunt stays in place, especially during growth and development, and to make sure there are no blockages. Monitoring of behavioral signs of shunt failure is necessary across all health care professions and caregivers. Hydrocephalus and shunt placements have several implications for PT, including knowledge of the signs of shunt failure, which mimic the signs of increased intracranial pressure discussed above, and its counterpart – over drainage that results in a depression of the fontanel with associated dizziness and headache. These are both treated as medical emergencies. Education of caregivers to recognize the signs of shunt failure is critical as is routine shunt follow-up with a physician. Severe neck flexion should be avoided in all patients with a shunt as it can cause a kink in the tubing or a separation of the shunt at the junction behind the ear. Common signs of shunt problems include (1) a change in motor status, tone (e.g., increased spasticity) or postural control; (2) nausea or vomiting; or (3) behavioral change, such as irritability, or more subtle poorer school performance.[18,19]

Since congenital hydrocephalus can often be detected with ultrasound in the second trimester, there have been multiple attempts to implant shunts in utero to prevent neural damage. However, these attempts have been fraught with problems, including fetal death, premature delivery, and displacement of the shunt, requiring replacement at birth. In addition, while

there has been no large clinical trial for comparisons, the outcomes for the children with intrauterine placement seem as variable as those with postnatal implantation.[20]

For children with MMC, a retrospective study of 1050 children found that for those, who underwent an intrauterine repair of the spinal defect, the occurrence of both AC–M and hydrocephalus was markedly reduced. In fact, none of the children developed AC–M, and only 7% required treatment for hydrocephalus.[21] However, in the MOMS outcomes, 40% of those with intrauterine repair required shunt placement.[12] Despite the discrepancy between these two reports, it appears that intrauterine repair holds promise in decreasing the occurrence of AC–M II and hydrocephalus.

Although motor deficits in children with hydrocephalus but not MMC are typically mild, **hydrocephalus with MMC can exaggerate already compromised gait, transfers, and postural abnormalities**. Balance and coordination are often poor in children with hydrocephalus, especially in infancy, as they have a larger head, elevating their center of gravity further. Early postural training may include necessary activities like strengthening of the neck muscles. After the shunt is placed, patients with hydrocephalus can participate in almost any activity (including sports) that is based on their level of function; gymnastics with its many somersaults and severe neck flexion positions and contact sports, such as football and soccer, should be avoided due to the likelihood of shunt damage. The PT should avoid positions and interventions that increase intracranial pressure, such as inversion (head lower than trunk).[19]

Latex Allergies

Infants with spina bifida are at high risk for developing latex allergies. This is something that everyone on the health care team, especially the physical therapist, needs to know. Repeated exposure to latex is the primary reason for an increased risk of the allergy. Infants with spina bifida are exposed to latex during the initial surgical procedure to close the spinal column, frequently have other surgeries (orthopedic, shunt implants for hydrocephalus), and have frequent bladder catheterizations. Notably, gloves, balloons, and balls all can have latex in them. The symptoms of latex allergies include skin rashes, common nasal signs like sneezing, itching, and a runny nose, and more serious signs like difficulty breathing, confusion, wheezing, and anaphylaxis, which can be life threatening. Therefore, it is important to limit the number of exposures to latex. In many pediatric physical therapy clinics, all the equipment, including the gloves, are latex free. To avoid repeated exposures, parents will be instructed by their physician to ask and require that all equipment used during rehabilitation be latex free.[24]

CASE A, PART V

In Dylan's case, as with many children, the hydrocephalus was not apparent at birth and manifested in the first weeks of life. This delayed presentation has led to much speculation that closure of the spinal defect plays a role in its development. Since hydrocephalus in MMC is almost always associated with the A–CM, additional speculation focused on compression of structures in the brainstem as a contributing factor in the development of hydrocephalus; a more recent hypothesis is that leakage of CSF through the spinal defect creates more room in the foramen magnum, allowing the A–CM, which in turn, creates the hydrocephalus. Notably, A–CM blocks the outlets for the 4th ventricle, impeding CSF flow into the subarachnoid space. It is likely that this combination of factors contributes to the development of hydrocephalus in most children with MMC.

In Dylan's case, immediate shunting upon identification of hydrocephalus was the common course of treatment until fairly recently. Dylan has normal intelligence but has been diagnosed with a visual learning disability, so he has his books on tape and takes his tests orally. Currently, with folic acid supplementation and the increasing use of prenatal MMC repair, the occurrence of A–CM and hydrocephalus in MMC is decreasing. Further, shunting is often delayed to determine the relative progressiveness of the hydrocephalus with only about 50% of infants having early shunt insertion currently; recent findings suggest that the hydrocephalus may spontaneously arrest, and thus, early shunting may not be necessary. Infection, post-shunting in children with MMC, is also much higher than in congenital hydrocephalus alone, so waiting to determine absolute need is becoming the preferred management method; these challenging medical decisions are based on infection and surgical risk, pressure on periventricular white matter, and severity of the hydrocephalus.[21,22] Also, there is an increasing use of endoscopic **ventriculostomy**, which creates a stoma in the front of the third ventricle to allow CSF to drain into the prepontine cistern of the subarachnoid space, thereby bypassing the obstructed cerebral aqueduct.[25] If successful, this avoids the complications of shunt revisions and subsequent infections that often occur with shunting.[26]

Since infancy and childhood are rapid periods of growth and development, changes associated with growth should be a consideration for the PT. With **Arnold–Chiari (A–C) malformations**, pressure on the brainstem, spinal cord, or cerebellum can be exaggerated with growth, causing increased pressure of CSF within the spinal cord. One of the signs of increased A–CM compression can be weakness in the upper extremities. Any changes in sensorimotor status should be taken seriously. Characteristics of cerebellar involvement may also increase with growth. Major growth-related changes to the A–CM may require cranioplasty as previously explained in this chapter. **Spinal cord tethering** occurs when the spinal cord adheres to the spinal column, thought to be due to scarring at the site of the lesion closure, and is a common condition in patients with MMC; when the children grow, there can be additional pulling that can produce serious damage to the spinal cord that may require a surgical release. This occurs in 10-30% of children with repaired MMC.[27,28] Symptoms include changes in strength, gait, and bowel/bladder function as well as worsening of scoliosis or other orthopedic deformity; the emergence of pain can also be an indicator.[27] While fetal repair diminishes many of the secondary consequences of MMC, the occurrence of tethered cord is slightly higher in those that undergo intrauterine repair with 33% experiencing this issue.[28] Surgical "untethering" is the only option for alleviating symptoms.[27]

Orthopedic Complications of Myelomeningocele

Orthopedic complications of MMC are common. Causes include (1) abnormal positioning in utero due to diminished muscle activity and movement; (2) asymmetrical muscle pull at the trunk and many lower extremity joints; and (3) poor or absent antigravity movement, specifically hip and knee extension, resulting in excessive flexor muscle activity that is exacerbated by time spent in flexed postures (e.g., sitting). It is critical to remember that the neurologic compromise to the spinal components, associated with MMC, is almost always asymmetric, and thus, results in normal or partial innervation of some muscles while others exhibit flaccid (at the level of lower motor neuron injury) or spastic (below the level of the lesion) paralysis. This asymmetry of muscle pull has an exaggerated effect in the young child, compared to his adult spinal cord injured counterpart, because it is occurring during development with no period of normal innervation. Notably, infants with MMC have limited extensor muscle activity that in combination with the baby's flexed posture in late-stage gestation contributes to positional changes in bone and joint alignment. Additionally, the baby may have limited mobility after birth, compounding these positional changes.[29]

Club foot, hip dysplasia, and **scoliosis** are three of the most common orthopedic complications commonly associated with MMC; others include leg length discrepancies, valgus or varus knee deformity, dislocated knees, and muscle contractures.[30] Both club foot and hip dysplasia are often apparent at delivery; scoliosis is more likely to develop over childhood as the child grows. Management of these orthopedic complications prioritizes optimizing spinal growth and stability, avoidance of pulmonary restriction, preventing skin breakdown, stabilization of lower extremity deformities, including achieving a plantigrade foot, and maximization of mobility.[31] With the exception of club feet, fetal repair decreases the occurrence of these orthopedic deformities.[30]

Club Foot

A patient can have club foot without MMC, and the overall incidence of club foot is 1 in 1000 live births.[32] Of those who have club foot, 50% are bilateral, and males are twice as likely as females to have club foot. A family history and maternal smoking increases the risk of club foot by twentyfold. Club foot is typically congenital and the cause may be multifactorial, including (1) teratologic – due to environmental toxin exposure such as cigarette smoke; (2) postural – secondary to a poor position in utero; (3) neurogenic – secondary to impaired innervation of foot musculature as in MMC; (4) syndromic – having a co-occurrence with other syndromes such as Down syndrome; or (5) genetic – although a specific gene hasn't been identified, there is a strong family occurrence and monozygotic twins have a 30% chance of both being afflicted.[32,33] In club foot, the patients' foot is severely deformed due to the misalignment of the bones, ligaments, and muscles. There are four general characteristics of club foot: forefoot Cavus and Adduction, heal Varus and

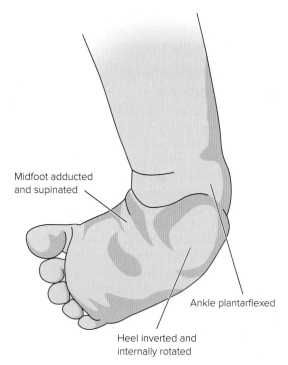

Midfoot adducted and supinated

Ankle plantarflexed

Heel inverted and internally rotated

FIGURE 19-12 Club foot deformity. (Reproduced with permission from Skinner HB & McMahon PJ (Eds): *Current Diagnosis & Treatment in Orthopedics*, 5th ed. New York, NY: McGraw-Hill; 2014.)

Equinus, making the mnemonic device CAVE (Figure 19-12). With unilateral clubfoot, the affected limb may be shorter with a thinner calf and shorter foot. There is a muscle imbalance with the lateral muscles more stretched and the medial muscles tight. Common motor characteristics are focused around gait abnormalities where PT can have a large role in evaluation and treatment. Club foot can be categorized by the Dimeglio system[34] (see Box 19-6).

Common gait abnormalities, associated with clubfoot, include decreased dorsiflexion, foot drop, in-toeing, decreased plantarflexion strength, and compensatory increases in knee hyperextension and hip external rotation. Range of motion at the foot and ankle is very important in patients with club foot with or without MMC. Contractures of the Achilles tendon can be the most common and most limiting. In addition, without any

correction of the clubfoot deformity, the lateral surface of the ankle becomes the weight-bearing surface, making walking difficult, if not impossible. Implications for PT include awareness of any precautions, early treatment, and promotion of motor development within the context of MMC. Infants with idiopathic club foot (and not MMC) scored worse on motor skill development on scales at 12 and 18 months of age. These ages represent a time period when motor skills include pulling-to-stand and walking that demand more of the foot and ankle. So, infants with club foot are at risk for motor delay even in the absence of MMC. The first goal of treatment for club foot is correction of the deformity. The most common method for treating clubfoot is the Ponsetti method, which consists of serial casting with casts changed every week; surgical lengthening of the Achilles tendon is performed prior to final casting, if the equinus deformity remains, which occurs in nearly 90% of cases. Three weeks of casting is required after tendonotomy. Once corrected, the foot is braced continuously (23 hours per day) for 3 weeks and then at nap and nighttime until the age of 4.[32,33] Clubfoot is present in 50 to 90% of children with MMC at birth, since they almost always have limited and/or asymmetric muscle activity at the foot/ankle, and thereby, are more at risk for abnormal posturing during gestation.[35]

Developmental Dysplasia of the Hip

Developmental dysplasia of the hip (DDH) is a condition that ranges in severity from mild ligamentous laxity in the hip, to mild changes in the development of the hip joint (acetabulum, femur, or both) with or without subluxation (partial dislocation), to complete dislocation that cannot be manually reduced (head of femur relocated into the acetabulum). It is diagnosed in 1 to 1.5 per 1000 live births in otherwise typically developing infants but is quite common in children with MMC. During typical development, as infants achieve weight-bearing postures, the acetabulum increases in depth and the femoral head develops a spherical shape; these two changes create a stable hip joint. Risk factors for DDH include female sex, as 80% of patients with hip dysplasia are girls, Native American descent, and a breach position in utero. When the acetabulum and/or femoral head demonstrate abnormal development, subluxation or dislocation is more likely. In some cases of DDH, the femoral head remains dislocated and a secondary, or artificial joint, develops as weight is born, pushing the femur into a higher point on the posterior

Box 19-6	Dimeglio Clubfoot Classification – Adapted from Canavese (2021)[34]		
The classification is determined, based on passive attempts to correct each aspect of the deformity (forefoot adduction, calcaneo-tarsal internal rotation; heel varus and equinus), scored 1-4 with 1 = 1= completely reducible through full range; 2 = reducible to neutral; 3 = reducible to less than neutral (e.g., −20°); 4 = rigid. Then, 1 point is given for the presence of each of these: (1) medial crease in forefoot, (2) posterior crease at the ankle joint, (3) foot cavus, and (4) hypertonia.			
Grade I – Benign	≤5	Can be passively reduced; little resistance	
Grade II – Moderate	6-10	Partially reducible (>50%) with some resistance	
Grade III – Severe	11-15	Increased stiffness; partially reducible (<50%)	
Grade IV – Very Severe	16-20	Rigid, not passively reducible	

pelvis. Neither hip dysplasia nor dislocation is thought to be painful in infancy, but both are associated with pain in older children and adults.[36]

Signs of DDH: If the hip is subluxed or dislocated, the infant may display uneven skin folds on the thigh, limited abduction, and a longer affected limb (Figure 19-13). Limited hip abduction in the affected limb with a discrepancy of greater than 10 degrees is the most reliable clinical measure in childhood, indicating the child needs to be referred. There are two additional clinical tests for young infants that can be performed easily. The **Ortolani sign** is performed by flexing the infants' hips to 90 degrees and abducting the hip looking for a palpable and audible click, indicating that the femoral head is moving back into the acetabulum; however, some children will demonstrate a click due to ligaments moving over the greater trochanter, so this may result in a false positive. The **Barlow sign** is more aggressive, flexing the hip to 90 degrees and then adducting the hip, which, in an unstable hip, will allow the femoral head to dislocate from the acetabulum; again, some children with DDH will not dislocate with this test and may be missed. Motor milestones may be delayed in children with DDH, especially upright activities. Early detection is the key for effective management of DDH. Infants who are identified after 9 months of age have a higher prevalence of surgical reduction of the hip than those identified earlier. Although hip abduction differences and the Ortolani and Barlow signs are the most common and effective clinical tests, they have questionable reliability, so imaging is the only definitive test for DDH. DDH is common in children with MMC, especially at mid-lumbar levels, due to muscle imbalance because the hip flexors and adductors are innervated but the extensors are not, yet with higher lesions, there may be spasticity in the hip flexors and adductors or contractures due to a common flexed sitting position, which can contribute to DDH.[31]

Treatment for DDH: The most common treatment for DDH is the **Pavlik harness** (Figure 19-14), which forces the hips into a flexed and abducted position to achieve acetabular and femoral head development. The Pavlik harness has success rates between 85 and 95%. Infants with DDH should not be positioned in extreme hip extension or adduction, and side-lying should be avoided during sleeping because of the adducted position of the top leg. Parent education will be important for avoiding these positions. If untreated, complications include arthritis, pain, and difficulty with ambulation.[36,37]

DDH is very common in children with MMC because either (1) there is an absence of any activity at the hip, and therefore,

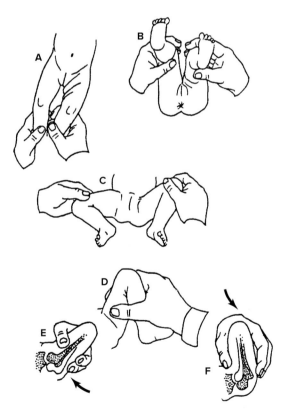

FIGURE 19-13 Early signs of developmental dysplasia of the hip. A. An adducted LE with uneven skin folds. **B.** Posterior uneven skin folds. **C.** Limited abduction. **D.** Pistoning of the hip with upward pull on the hip. **E.** Subluxation or dislocation with external rotation. **F.** Reseating of the hip with adduction. (Reproduced with permission from Skinner HB & McMahon PJ, eds. *Current Diagnosis & Treatment in Orthopedics*, 5th ed. New York, NY: McGraw-Hill; 2014. Fig. 10-4.)

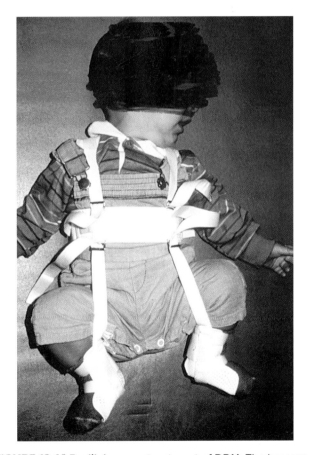

FIGURE 19-14 Pavlik harness treatment of DDH. The harness is optimal for infants prior to 6 months of age and is worn 24 hours/day for up to 12 weeks, and then, at night for another 4 to 6 weeks. (Reproduced with permission from Skinner HB & McMahon PJ, eds. *Current Diagnosis & Treatment in Orthopedics*, 5th ed. New York, NY: McGraw-Hill; 2014. Fig. 10-6.)

limited muscle pull to keep the head of the femur in the acetabulum or (2) there is an asymmetrical muscle pull such that the hip flexors and adductors remain innervated while hip extensors and abductors are not (L3/L4 level of activity), resulting in a pulling of the femoral head out of the shallow acetabulum. Both of these conditions are exacerbated by delayed weight-bearing; thus, early PT treatment should focus on weight-bearing postures (quadruped, standing). Surgery is not generally recommended to correct DDH in children with MMC, since DDH doesn't seem to be a limiting factor in ambulation status. Surgery is more often done in children with low lumbar or sacral lesions, for whom independent community ambulation is more likely.[31]

For infants with MMC and club foot or DDH, the timing of interventions can also create a very complicated picture, further limiting early weight-bearing. Surgical healing, after correction of each orthopedic condition, in combination with the need to develop motor skills requires careful consideration, when creating an appropriate treatment plan.

CASE A, PART VI

Dylan was treated with a Pavlik harness to correct his bilateral DDH; in children with MMC, that never achieve independent standing, it is more difficult to treat DDH, since weight-bearing is essential for normal acetabulum and femoral head development. In addition, it is likely that Dylan would have spastic paralysis of his hip flexors and adductors, since his lesion level is at L1/L2, and these muscles are innervated at L2–4. Spasticity of the hip flexors and adductors often can contribute to hip dislocation, especially when inadequate development of the acetabulum and femoral head are present. Yet, neural damage may be greater than the level of apparent spinal damage, so flaccid paralysis is also a possibility. Often, some degree of DDH persists in children with MMC despite early treatment, and if not painful, is left untreated in the older child. Even though children with this level of injury have limited potential for ambulation, standing is important to help combat hip flexion contractures, associated with prolonged sitting, and to assist development of the hip joint. An orthotic that supports the hips, knees, and ankles is essential for allowing standing. Ambulation may be achieved by a swing to or through gait (see description in Part IX), initially with a walker. However, few (<20%) children with an L1/L2 lesion will walk beyond early childhood due to the high energy cost of this type of ambulation.[38]

Scoliosis

Scoliosis is a curvature and possible rotation of the spine that can occur in typically developing children but is also quite common in neuromuscular disorders such as cerebral palsy, muscular dystrophy, and MMC due to asymmetrical muscle activity in the trunk or differences in leg length in ambulating children.

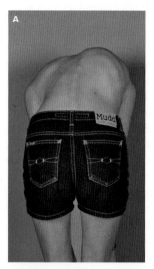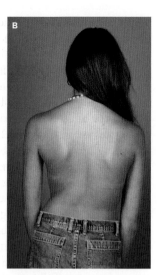

FIGURE 19-15 Presentation of S-curve scoliosis. A. Adam's forward bend test illuminates a prominent rib bump on the right consistent with a right thoracic concavity. **B.** Right lower shoulder and raised left hip are visually apparent in this right thoracic, left lumbar S-curve. (Reproduced with permission from Rudolph CD, Rudolph AM, Lister GE, First LR, Gershon AA, eds. *Rudolph's Pediatrics*, 22nd ed. New York, NY: McGraw-Hill; 2011. Fig. 216-5 and 216-4.)

The **Adam's forward bend test** is the most common screening measure for scoliosis, where the child bends forward from a standing position and a rib hump is prominent on one side but not the other (Figure 19-15).[39]

Scoliosis can be classified as (1) idiopathic; (2) congenital; (3) neuropathic; (4) myopathic; or (5) miscellaneous.[39] Idiopathic scoliosis has no known cause and can be diagnosed at any age, occurring in .5 to 5% of the general population. Curves of 10 degrees or less are considered minor and affect females and males almost equally (1.4 females:1 male). Curves of greater than 20 degrees affect females almost 7 times more frequently than males. Congenital scoliosis is caused by vertebral abnormalities (e.g., failure of vertebra to separate during development or only partial development of vertebra) that occur during spinal development but often do not induce a scoliosis until childhood or adolescence under periods of rapid bone growth.[39,40] Neuropathic causes include cerebral palsy, spinal muscular atrophy, and MMC, which impose altered muscle pull on the developing spine from spastic or asymmetric muscle activity. Similarly, myopathic scoliosis arises from conditions affecting the muscle itself, such as muscular dystrophy, but also results from an asymmetry of muscle activity. These two causes are often grouped together as neuromuscular scoliosis.[39] In children with MMC, the occurrence of scoliosis increases the higher the lesion in the spinal column with greater than 90% of children with thoracic lesions, 70% with high lumbar lesions, 43% with low lumbar lesions and 8% of those with sacral lesion presenting with scoliosis.[41]

Scoliosis can be further differentiated as (1) **structural**, meaning the curve is fixed and inflexible and is typically caused by abnormal vertebrae; or (2) **nonstructural**, meaning the curve corrects completely or partially with lateral bending and is commonly caused by positioning, muscle asymmetry, weakness, or neuropathy. In upright postures (standing or sitting), the height of the iliac crest and shoulders may be unequal with scoliosis of any etiology (Figure 19-15B). Frequently, scoliosis presents as an S-shaped deformity with a primary (largest) curve and secondary curve that compensates for the primary curve (see Table 19-2 for the Lenke classification of scoliosis). Terminology focuses on the convexity of the curves, structural versus nonstructural nature, and location (e.g., right primary thoracic structural curve and left secondary nonstructural lumbar curve). Associated issues include difficulty breathing due to the small intercostal space on the concave side of the curve and a large intercostal space on the convex side, weakness of the surrounding spinal musculature, and possible delays in motor milestone acquisition and other domains of development. The physical therapist has a role in the evaluation of scoliosis, and in patients with MMC, needs to be aware that it is a common co-occurrence. There is an overall poorer prognosis, if the vertebral growth plate is affected, which may occur in MMC. For children with curves greater than 40 degrees with vertebral rotation, spinal fusion is typically required for correction. Inpatient physical therapy

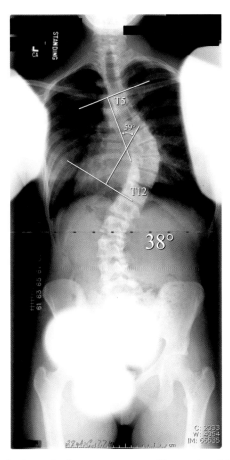

FIGURE 19-16 Scoliosis measurement. The angle of the curve is measured on an anterior-posterior radiographic image by identifying the top point of the curve (where it begins to realign) and the bottom point (where it begins to reverse itself); a line is drawn parallel to each of these points and then perpendicular lines are drawn into the curve till they intersect. This provides a measureable angle of 59 degrees for the primary curve in this image; the secondary curve measures 38 degrees (lines of measurement not shown). (Reproduced with permission from Rudolph CD, Rudolph AM, Lister GE, First LR, Gershon AA, eds. *Rudolph's Pediatrics*, 22nd ed. New York, NY: McGraw-Hill; 2011. Fig. 216-6.)

TABLE 19-2	Lenke Classification of Scoliosis[44]
LENKE CLASSIFICATION	**DESCRIPTION**
Lenke 1	Single structural thoracic curve with either a nonstructural compensation above (upper thoracic) or below (lumbar); correction of the thoracic curve results in spontaneous correction of the lumbar curve
Lenke 2 – Double thoracic curve	Two structural thoracic curves – the primary is typically midthoracic with a secondary upper thoracic curve; a nonstructural lumbar compensatory curve may also exist
Lenke 3 – Double major curves	A primary thoracic structural curve with a secondary lumbar structural curve; a nonstructural proximal thoracic compensatory curve is also present
Lenke 4 – Triple major curves	A midthoracic primary structural curve with both a proximal and lumbar secondary structural curves
Lenke 5 – Primary thoracolumbar or lumbar curve	A primary structural thoracolumbar or lumbar curve with a secondary thoracic nonstructural compensation
Lenke 6 – Thoracolumbar/ lumbar/thoracic curves	A primary structural lumbar curve with a structural thoracic secondary curve

after this surgery will include activities such as bed mobility (without rotation), lower extremity strengthening, orthoses, and parent and patient education on precautions and short- and long-term limitations. For children with curves between 20- and 40-degrees treatment involves bracing and spinal stabilization exercises; a brace is typically worn for up to 23 hours per day. The braces used are most often thoracolumbosacral orthoses (TLSO), since they enclose the trunk from just below the axilla to the sacrum; multiple types are available, providing slightly different methods of curve stabilization. Each allows some opening opposite points of pressure to afford room for the curve to correct to the opposite side.[39,42] Many of these children go on to have spinal fusion surgery, if their curve progresses to 40-45 degrees or is preventing them from maintaining a functional sitting position.[43] Figure 19-16 illustrates how scoliosis curves are measured.

CASE A, PART VII

Scoliosis correction is typically done in the teenage years, when growth is complete or almost complete. Surgery entails realigning the involved vertebrae and then fusing them together; this can partially correct the curve and then prevent further deformity. Small bone grafts are inserted between the vertebrae, which will then fuse with the vertebrae to create a solid bony structure; this procedure will change the mobility of the spine and stop all future growth in the area of the fusion, so that is why surgery is done when growth is nearly complete. Metal rods are also inserted and attached by either wires or screws to prevent movement during the healing process.[39] In Dylan's case, his fusion was accompanied by hip flexor tendon releases (cutting of the tendon, typically in a diagonal, and then reattaching the ends to allow increased length). His limitations in moving (avoidance of lifting, pushing his chair, twisting, etc.) will be in place for the first 3 months or so after surgery; then, he will gradually be able to return to his normal level of activity, although often with some diminished trunk mobility.

● PHYSICAL THERAPY MANAGEMENT

There are 2500 to 6000 babies born each year with MMC. Lesions are primarily in the lumbar and sacral regions, yet rarer cervical and thoracic lesions do occur. In terms of **general motor skill development**, the advent of fetal surgery has changed the functional outcome for many children. Historically, most children with MMC did not sit or crawl until 1 to 2 years of age and often did not walk or even pull-to-stand until they were 3 years of age or older. The ambulation outcomes for children with fetal repair demonstrate that 42% were able to ambulate independently by 30 months of age,[12] and 70% were able to be community ambulators, 68% without assistive device, at age 7[30]; thus, they are achieving higher levels of motor function and hitting them earlier than those repaired postnatally.[12] In fact, those undergoing intrauterine repair, often have motor function 1 to 2 spinal levels below the level of the spinal repair (e.g., repair at L3, function at L5). However, many children, adolescents, and adults with MMC, especially those repaired postnatally, use wheelchairs as their primary form of mobility even if, as young children, they took some steps.[12,30] Some of this is a shifting in goals by the child as they prefer to keep up with their peers in school and be more independent from their parents. Since MMC is a lifelong disability, there are implications for bone and muscle health at all ages. As a group, adolescent and adults with MMC have higher rates of obesity, poor fitness, and poor levels of independence.[45]

Movement Potential in MMC

Kicking behavior: Ultrasound observations indicate that fetuses with MMC move their legs and kick at the same rates as fetuses without MMC.[46] So, in utero, in a crowded and gravity-free environment, they move in equal amounts to typically developing infants. In addition, mothers of babies with and without MMC have done subjective kick counts and report similar amounts of movement and activity. Kicking behaviors in infancy are well studied, and there is a developmental progression of kicking that can be monitored and tracked. In terms of frequency, we know that older babies kick less than younger babies. In terms of pattern, babies start off by kicking in an alternating pattern; then as they get older, they start to show more single leg kicks, and as they get even older, they show more parallel kicks.[47] Since patients with MMC most commonly have thoracic, lumbar, and sacral lesions, PTs are most concerned about the sensorimotor function of the trunk and legs. There are a handful of studies that have quantified the leg movements of young infants with MMC. Infants who are 4 to 6 months of age with MMC show less movement and less variability in kicking patterns than typically developing infants[48]; yet, they can and do change their kicking frequency, based on their position, and they kick the most when in supine and in an open space. Physical therapists can use this information to modify the environment to improve the number of kicking repetitions as a strengthening exercise. Infants who are 1–6 months of age with MMC also show a shorter kicking duration, meaning their kicks do not last as long, with fewer movements and more asymmetry than infants with typical development.[49] Although there hasn't been a study to evaluate kicking behavior, following fetal MMC repair, these infants may show more typical kicking behavior than their postnatally repaired peers.

Ambulation: There are some predictors of ambulation ability based on lesion level with better prognosis for functional ambulation associated with lower lesion levels (Table 19-3). Bracing is a necessary component to facilitate ambulation for many children, and most children will also need crutches or a walker to achieve ambulation except for L5/sacral lesions that may ambulate with only minor bracing and no walking aid. Lesions above L1 result in absent lower extremity muscle function, and thereby, children with lesions at this level will require complete support of the hip, knee, and ankle to stand. Common abbreviations for orthotics use the first letter of each joint supported, such as a KAFO for the knee-ankle-foot orthosis. Lower lesions are associated with greater muscle control and less need for bracing.[50-53] Table 19-3 examines muscle activity and bracing needs for children with lumbar and sacral lesions.

This can be thought of as a guideline for prediction of ambulation status. Other published rates of ambulation include even more general characteristics. Twenty percent of patients with high lumbar lesions achieve some walking most often using a hip strategy. Eighty percent of patients with low lumbar lesions walk, likely because of the additional knee and ankle control. Ninety percent of patients with sacral lesions walk with sensorimotor function in the hip, knee, and ankle.[52,53] It is

TABLE 19-3	Ambulatory Potential Based on Lesion Level[50,51]		
LESION LEVEL	**EXPECTED MUSCLE FUNCTION**	**WALKING POTENTIAL**	**BRACING OPTIONS/ ASSISTIVE DEVICES**
L1 or above	No lower extremity muscle function; trunk function normal	Poor walking potential but may ambulate some within their household at young ages	Trunk-hip-knee-ankle-foot (THKAFO) orthosis or HKAFO with walker/crutches
L2	Possible hip flexion but no other lower extremity muscle function	Some household ambulation but will use a wheelchair for most settings and at older ages	Hip-knee-ankle-foot (HKAFO) or reciprocal gait orthosis (RGO) with walker/crutches
L3	Good to normal hip flexion and antigravity knee extension likely	Household ambulation likely but will use a wheelchair for community/school ambulation and often at older ages	Knee-ankle-foot (KAFO) or ankle-foot (AFO) orthosis with crutches
L4	Good to normal hip flexion and knee extension plus antigravity dorsiflexion	Household or community ambulation; may convert to wheelchair at older ages	Ankle-foot (AFO) orthosis with crutches
L5	Good to normal dorsiflexion plus good eversion/inversion and some plantarflexion, knee flexion, and hip extension (usually poor)	Community ambulation	AFO or supramalleolar orthosis, no crutches
S1	Antigravity hip extension and abduction and knee flexion plus some plantarflexion	Community ambulation	No orthotics
S2	Good to normal function at hip, knee, and ankle, missing some toe and foot muscle control		

also very common for younger children to ambulate to some degree but give it up as they get older despite motor function that would enable them to ambulate; this results from both the increased energy cost in moving a larger body mass and the need to move more quickly to keep up with peers. Each patient with MMC is unique and so is their functional status. Since the lesions are typically asymmetrical and incomplete, this results in unique functional features for each child. The exact level of lesion may be very important for a surgeon and much less important for the rehabilitation team. Some MMC clinics do not use lesion levels in the chart because it is not always accurate in describing the client's current level of performance. Functional abilities are charted directly instead of lesion level as that is more meaningful information to the rehabilitation team.

Orthotics

Orthotic prescription focuses on achieving joint alignment while not impeding function; it is important to not over brace, or in other words, to allow functional muscles to be active, even if they are only partially innervated. The joints of the orthotic should align with the anatomical joints, and orthotics should be comfortable, as easy to don and doff as possible, and as cosmetic as possible. Orthotics are typically made of

thermoplastics that can be molded to the child's extremity (Table 19-4).[54]

Role of the Physical Therapist

As a lifelong disability, patients with MMC will have multiple episodes of physical therapy throughout their lifespan. The role of the pediatric physical therapist is to provide training and skills necessary for functional independence to the best extent possible. This typically focuses on the achievement of early motor milestones, especially in infants and young children, as well as enhancing independent mobility (ambulation or wheelchair use) and maximizing stability to facilitate play, social development, learning, language, etc. Treatment will vary depending on the sensorimotor characteristics of the child and the treatment setting.

Episodes of physical therapy can happen in a variety of care settings (acute care, schools, rehabilitation, home, outpatient).

CASE A, PART VIII

In the NICU, Dylan was seen by the PT in the first days after his surgery. (If surgery is delayed, treatment may be initiated day 1 or 2 and then resume after surgery.) Initially, Dylan's treatment focused on positioning and handling techniques, promoting overall range of motion as well as protection of the spinal surgical site. Early education of the parents on how to handle Dylan facilitated early bonding. Once the shunt was placed in week 3, Dylan's parents were also educated on shunt protection (positions to be avoided) and signs of shunt dysfunction (this is typically done by the nursing or medical staff but should be emphasized by the PT). Dylan initially presented with excessive range of motion at the hips, so although early treatment focuses on promoting range of motion, excessive hip extension, and adduction were avoided to prevent hip subluxation or dislocation. Dylan's parents were also instructed to avoid tight swaddling of Dylan to avoid forcing his legs into an extended and adducted position; again, this can lead to further hip instability and subluxation/dislocation. In Dylan's case, his DDH was treated with a Pavlik harness that was fitted at about 1 month of age, after his initial surgeries to correct the lesion and implant the shunt were completed. In many children, the Pavlik harness may be fitted even earlier, if DDH is identified at birth. Pain management, providing an environment of developmental care to promote growth and development, and comprehensive parent education are key elements of NICU care for the infant with MMC.

From birth to 3 years of age, Dylan received early intervention services first in his home, and then, twice per week as part of his preschool program. Home-based services are common for EI before 3 years of age. Therapy, at this age, focused on maintaining/promoting normal range of motion and preventing contractures of the lower extremities; evaluating and teaching body awareness (e.g., exploring feet with hands); promoting positional and milestone development in supine, prone, sitting, and standing; promoting head and truck control and reaching, including object exploration; evaluating sensory dysfunction and developing sensory-precautions (e.g., bath water temperature, getting toes stuck in cribs or toys; see Box 19-7); enhancing sensory input for kicking and stepping development; promoting weight-bearing and independent mobility; learning of cause and effect relationships; avoiding learned disuse; and parent education on all of the above.

For children with MMC and associated hydrocephalus, early treatment must focus on developing head control, which is complicated by a slightly enlarged head and diminished lower extremity muscle activity that is needed to weight down the lower half of the body as the head is lifted. Trunk strengthening is also a focus of early treatment, since in the presence of lower extremity paresis, the trunk must work harder for the child to sit and achieve standing. Like other children with developmental disabilities, treatment also focuses on achieving developmental milestones. Table 19-5 presents ideas of early treatment activities for children with MMC.

| Box 19-7 | Sensory Loss in the Lower Extremities Requires Special Attention |

With MMC, there is a partial or complete loss of somatosensory function in the legs. This requires constant attention and vigilance to assure that the child does not injure themselves while moving or especially that the parents not injure the child unknowingly. For example, when putting on shoes, toes can become curled within the shoe; typically developing children will fuss if this happens, and the parents are alerted to the discomfort. Children with insensate feet will not fuss, and thus, can get pressure sores on their feet from getting a toe curled under the foot within a shoe. Similarly, ill-fitting shoes can create pressure sores that the child will not feel; even clothing can cause problems if too tight or it becomes wrinkled underneath the child. Frequent repositioning and parent attention can minimize the likelihood of pressure problems.

One of the more common problems that arise occurs as the child begins moving; creeping or crawling on rough surfaces can abrade the knees, shins, or toes without the child knowing it, so protection of these areas is critical as the child starts moving. Shoes or at least socks should be worn; long pants can protect the legs, or knee pads can be worn. Additionally, there needs to be constant vigilance with bath time. Parents must always check water temperature carefully so that the child is not placed in water that is too hot. Older children also need to be well educated in the dangers of getting into a tub without checking the water temperature with their hand. Much like the patient with a spinal cord injury, children with MMC need pressure relief so that they don't maintain a given position for too long. Typically developing children move constantly; however, children with MMC may demonstrate much less lower extremity movement, especially with high lumbar or thoracic lesions. Thus, parents must be instructed to vary the positioning of the infant so that pressure ulcers do not develop (every 4 hours at a minimum); using a pressure mattress cover (sheepskin or gel) can also be useful in preventing ulcer development in infants. As the child ages, they should be instructed in pressure relief at frequent intervals, at least every 15–20 minutes, if they are sitting in a wheelchair. The use of appropriate seating cushions will also help prevent ulcer development. Finally, a frequent cause of pressure sores for children with MMC are ill-fitting braces; it is critical that braces be frequently evaluated to assure a good fit in a growing child. It is quite common that the child enters a growth spurt and quickly the brace begins to rub in a given area. On removal of any brace, parents should be instructed to look for red spots; if these do not dissipate in 5 to 10 minutes, the brace needs to be adjusted.

Overlapping with early intervention and continuing throughout the lifespan, PTs will see patients of any age with MMC in an outpatient or school setting with similar objectives to those listed for the infant. PTs address milestone delay, develop functional training interventions, and provide adaptive equipment for mobility and transfers. For toddler and preschool ages, the PT may begin to have a large role in (1) identifying appropriate assistive devices (including canes, walkers,

TABLE 19-4	Orthotic Options for Children with MMC[54]
ORTHOTIC	**DESCRIPTION OF FIT AND USE**
Foot orthotic	Shoe insert that is fitted to support the arch of the foot and minimize pronation/supination
Supramalleolar	Fits around malleoli to stabilize forefoot (adduction/abduction), midfoot (pronation), and/or hindfoot (valgus/varus) while allowing dorsiflexion/plantarflexion.
Ankle-foot (AFO)	Typically fit to just below the knee to provide ankle stability with straps at the ankle and/or upper aspect
(1) Solid/Rigid	Blocks dorsiflexion and plantarflexion; controls foot (forefoot, midfoot, hindfoot) as needed
(2) Hinged/Articulating	Hinge at ankle between upper and foot segments; blocks plantarflexion with free or assisted dorsiflexion
(3) Floor reaction	An AFO with an anterior rigid, padded shell on the upper shin to control excessive dorsiflexion and assist knee extension at midstance
(4) Dynamic	Thinner material allows more flexibility; wraps around foot; resists plantarflexion and assists dorsiflexion; stabilizes foot
Knee-ankle-foot (KAFO)*	Typically constructed of a thermoplastic sleeve at the mid-thigh, with velcro strap(s) closure and a supporting metal frame both medial and lateral, connecting to an AFO. A drop lock at the knee joint allows the device to bend while sitting and then the lock to "drop" into place when the child assumes standing. In reality, the child typically locks the knee before pulling to stand and unlocks it after returning to sit.
Hip-knee-ankle-foot (HKAFO)*	Adds a pelvic band and hip joint to the KAFO. Locks at the hip joint will prevent hip flexion and extension, requiring both legs to move in unison (swing to or swing through gait).
Trunk-hip-knee-ankle-foot* (THKAFO)	An additional thoracic support, added to the HAFO, provides trunk support to the child with limited abdominal/spinal muscle activity.
Reciprocating gait (RGO)*	An HKAFO constructed with a cable connection between the two leg components to facilitate hip flexion on the unweighted leg and extension on the weight-bearing leg, creating an alternating or reciprocal gait pattern. Unweighting is typically achieved by lateral trunk bending, and hip extension is further enhanced by shoulder retraction and back extension on the side of the stance leg. For those with some hip flexion, an RGO will assist hip flexion while maintaining extension in the stance leg.
Parapodium*	A rigid THKAFO support (standing frame) that can allow some forward movement in a swing-to or swing-through manner. Typically have joints at the hip and knee to allow sitting when locks are disengaged.
Swivel walker*	A parapodium attached to a swivel base that achieves forward propulsion through alternating trunk rotation.

*All of these devices will require upper extremity assistance through the use of an assistive device, typically a walker initially and then crutches.

manual wheelchairs, power wheelchairs, standers, and orthotic devices); (2) enhancing independent mobility and transfers; (3) beginning a standing or walking program; and (4) providing the means for early social interactions with peers. Orthotic devices are very common for children with MMC; as listed in Table 19-6, orthotic device choice is predicated on lesion level with bracing providing support at joints with absent or minimal muscle function.

In **school-based settings**, PTs will see children with MMC to help with educational progress, including classroom mobility. This will include working closely with the teacher(s) and other support service providers (e.g., adaptive physical educators, occupational therapists) to adapt the classroom to meet the needs of the child, which may include assuring wider separation of desks to allow wheelchair access, encouraging longer

CASE A, PART IX

Given Dylan's lesion level, what type of orthotic would you likely recommend for Dylan as a toddler?

If you said a HKAFO or RGO, you're right; either of these would be appropriate for Dylan.

With an L1/L2 lesion, Dylan has only minimal hip flexion. When he was two, he was fitted with an HKAFO and was able to walk short distances within his home first with a standard walker and then with forearm crutches, using a swing-to-gait pattern, which refers to moving both crutches forward and then swinging both legs simultaneously toward the point of crutch placement; typically, the toes stay slightly behind the crutches. In older children, this may progress to a swing-through pattern, where the legs move past the crutches; this more advanced method requires considerable arm strength and balance; Dylan never achieved a swing-through pattern. Early therapy focused on strengthening his arms for not only ambulation but for wheelchair mobility, using lift-ups, wheelbarrow walking, and throwing activities with and without wrist cuff weights. By the age of three, he was able to get in and out of his wheelchair and keep up with his friends easily in the wheelchair. To get into his low wheelchair, he would pull up into a kneeling position and then pull to a supported standing position, pulling on the wheelchair arms, and then rotate to sit down. As he aged, he could push up into the chair from the floor by aligning himself with his back to the chair and placing both hands on the seat and performing a lift-up into the chair. As he grew, it became more and more energy intensive to walk even short distances; by the time he was 6, he primarily used a manual chair for both in-house and community mobility as this allowed him the speed and independence to keep up with his family and peers. Since his family had a two-story house, he managed the stairs by sitting and performing an arm lift up to pull himself backward up the stairs. Scooting down the stairs was fun but resulted in several instances of ischial sores until he learned to slowly go down the stairs, lifting up, and slowly dropping down to the next stair. His family was able to purchase a ranch-style home when he was five to eliminate the need to go up and down stairs. If this hadn't been possible, there are some seated stair lifts that might have been needed to facilitate stair ascent/descent as he aged.

transition times to afford the child sufficient time to move from one class to another, adaptation of bathroom facilities to allow catheterization (see Box 19-8 for information on bowel and bladder function), and education of the teacher on how to integrate a child with MMC into the classroom. For some children, a standing podium may be incorporated into some classroom activities to afford some time out of their wheelchair and weight bearing through the lower extremities each day. It is very important to be aware that patients with MMC are at an increased risk for obesity, sedentary behavior, and decreased physical fitness. Fitness should be addressed in all settings and at all ages.[45]

Notably, children with MMC have a higher incidence of learning disabilities and lower cognitive scores than the general population, likely related to hydrocephalus, yet many children with MMC have no learning disabilities and typical intelligence.

In **acute or inpatient rehabilitation settings**, the PT will see patients with MMC periodically throughout their lifespan for additional postsurgical (e.g., spinal fusion for scoliosis, other orthopedic surgery) or other rehabilitation needs. Evaluation and training for new orthotics, assistive devices, and wheelchairs

---

Box 19-8 Bowel and Bladder Management for Children with Myelomeningocele

Bowel and bladder management is a critical component of any program for patients with MMC, since they have disrupted bowel and bladder innervation. Often, there is a catheterization program for bladder voiding and a bowel program that may include dietary and pharmaceutical management as well as rectal stimulation. Bowel and bladder programs are taught to children so that they can be as independent as possible with toileting and not reliant on an adult for assistance as they age. Poor bladder management can cause back up into the kidneys, which can cause kidney damage. Fetal repair has also been associated with improved bowel and bladder function with one study reporting only 62% requiring intermittent catheterization compared to 87% in the postnatal repair group. For some children, surgical intervention is used to (1) enlarge the bladder (augmentation cystoplasty); (2) create a stoma to empty the bladder through the lower abdomen (vesicostomy); or (3) expansion of the urethra, which can narrow due to strictures (urethral dilation). The use of these procedures did not differ based on time of closure.[55] The physical therapist may be involved in training chair to commode transfers in the home and the school setting to facilitate bowel/bladder management.

CASE A, PART X

Dylan has been seen episodically over his school years to maximize function and assure maximum independence in the school setting, especially to help him transition from one school building to another as he progressed. In preschool and kindergarten, treatment focused on strengthening, ambulation, and wheelchair mobility in the classroom. However, by first grade, PT focused most on wheelchair mobility, including over ground propulsion (uneven surfaces such as ramps, gravel, and grass), wheelies to go over uneven surfaces, reaching for objects from his chair (laterally, overhead, and on the floor), and managing the cafeteria (carrying a tray and manipulating his chair). As he grew, continued UE strengthening was a focus along with transfers for toileting and moving to other surfaces (floor, bed, etc.) as well as wheelies for larger obstacles and righting the wheelchair if it tipped over (see Chapter 13 for wheelchair activities for the spinal cord patient). Following his scoliosis and tendon-lengthening surgery, his school-based therapist implemented a program to maximize the hip range of motion gained from the surgery; this involved getting Dylan out of his chair once per day to stretch his hip flexors for 5–10 minutes by lying prone and to evaluate his ability to propel his wheelchair with his limited mobility or to use powered mobility in the school setting (the school has been fortunate to have a number of chairs donated from other children as they were outgrown).

TABLE 19-5	Treatment Activities for Infants with MMC
TARGETED MOVEMENT	**ACTIVITY**
Upright head control	Babies first learn to hold their head upright, while being held, before any other position. Encouraging head control in sitting, while the trunk is well supported, can be done with the child sitting on the therapist's or parent's lap with the head and trunk against the trunk of the holder or with support at the shoulders and the child sitting away from the holder's trunk. Moving a toy in the visual field of the child will encourage head turning and lifting away from the support, especially if the toy is moved in a slow vertical motion (up-down). Also, tilting the child in each direction while encouraging him/her to look at a toy or another person, will encourage the head to be held upright. As some control is achieved, increasing the speed and range of toy movement or the degree of tilt will stimulate increased head control. These same activities will encourage trunk control with support at the lower trunk or hip. Also, working on prone and supine head control will facilitate upright head control.
Prone head lifting	Placing the child prone on a wedge or Thera-Ball so that head lifting can be done in a partial gravity-eliminated position will allow the child to develop neck extensor strength initially. Over time, the incline of the wedge or the position of the child on the ball can be adjusted to require more chin tucking while holding the head horizontal. An interesting toy should be used to stimulate head lifting.
	Parents can work on this by having their child lay on their belly across their lap. Placing one of their feet on a stool will help create an incline so that the child can work with gravity partially eliminated. Placing a toy for the child to look at on the floor, slightly in front of the child will encourage head lifting. As the child gains strength, decreasing the incline and moving the toy higher onto a chair or eventually a table will stimulate head lifting toward 90 degrees.
Supine head lifting	Similar to prone head lifting activities, a wedge or ball is a good way to work on supine head lifting by having the child move toward upright from an angled position; this will strengthen the neck flexors. Decreasing the incline as the child gains strength, will make this more challenging until the child is able to be pulled to sitting with the chin tucked.
	Parents can work on this by sitting on the floor in a partially reclined position with their back against the wall or a piece of furniture, their hips and knees flexed and their feet flat on the floor. The infant can then be placed on their lap with their head and trunk against their parent's thighs. Encouraging the child to look at a toy on the parent's stomach or just come to an upright position, without losing control of the head, will encourage neck flexor strength. Parents can support the child by holding the child's hands or as strength is gained, supporting the child's upper trunk and eventually the hips.
Rolling – prone to supine	For many children with MMC, rolling is done entirely with the head and upper body since leg movement may be minimal. Encouraging the child to look at a toy from a prone prop position and reaching with the hand in the direction of the roll will encourage rolling. Assistance from the therapist or parent can be done at the hip, first to assist, and then to resist the roll to further strengthen the trunk. Starting from a side-lying position will allow the child to strengthen the trunk initially, with the therapist resisting the roll at the hip and/or shoulder; also, using a wedge such that the child rolls "downhill" can make this easier early on.
Rolling – supine to prone	Similar to the prone to supine roll, children with MMC will roll supine to prone with minimal LE movement. Strong neck flexion will need to be achieved prior to successful rolling in this direction. Encouraging reaching for a toy across the body in the direction of the roll will facilitate this movement. Assisting lower extremity movement and trunk rotation is typically required early, but in children with hip flexor innervation, this motion should be encouraged as the child rolls. The side-lying and wedge methods, listed for prone–supine will also work for supine to prone.
Sitting	Sitting is a challenge for many children with MMC, since LE activity is typically needed to anchor the child while in sitting. However, most children will achieve some degree of independent sitting on the floor but may require some arm support, if their lesion is in the thoracic trunk. Lots of reaching with decreasing amounts of trunk and hip support are critical to develop sitting balance. Having the child straddle a roll or sit on a Thera-Ball with support at the lower trunk or hip can be good methods for working on sitting with reaching or weight shift activities. Tilting the roll or ball with encouragement to return to upright will strengthen the trunk and develop balance (provide verbal encouragement to return to upright; focus the child on the muscles that need to be working by touching or tapping them). Reaching to the side, the floor, and across midline will strengthen critical trunk muscles; support will need to be provided at the lower trunk and then the hip for most children to be successful in this activity.

(Continued)

TABLE 19-5	Treatment Activities for Infants with MMC (*Continued*)
TARGETED MOVEMENT	**ACTIVITY**
Abdominal strengthening	Assisted sit-ups, performed with the knees bent and holding the therapist's or parent's hands, can be an early way to begin abdominal strengthening, allowing the child to use some UE pull along with the abdominals. Slowly returning to supine (roll-down) will require eccentric abdominal activity, further strengthening the abdominals. Over time, decreasing and then eliminating the UE assistance should occur until none is provided. An incline can also be used to decrease the effect of gravity while performing a sit-up or roll-down to work on abdominal strengthening. Some support at the legs may need to be provided, since hip extension may be absent.
Upper extremity weight-bearing	Initial weight-bearing on the arms is critical for future functional movement. (1) For the infant, this can be done over a small roll or rolled towel to facilitate prone-propping. (2) For the older child, a larger roll may be used. Reaching for toys will facilitate weight shift and strengthen each arm while bearing weight on one and reaching with the other. (3) Once weight-bearing is achieved, having the child walk on their hands with support at their hip, a "wheelbarrow walk," will continue to strengthen the arms. (4) Performing "lift ups" (lifting the bottom off the support surface by pushing with the arms, while sitting) from a chair with arms or on the floor with the hands first on large block so that the elbows are flexed initially are also good ways to strengthen the arms, which will be critical in walking and wheelchair use.
Lower extremity weight-bearing/ strengthening	Lower extremity innervation and muscle strength will be determinants of the focus of physical therapy for children with MMC. Although most children with MMC will require some bracing for standing/walking, early therapy should include LE weight-bearing in a variety of positions with support from the therapist as appropriate. Strengthening of muscles will be critical to maximizing function in upright postures. (1) Weight-bearing in quadruped can be facilitated over a roll initially with the hands on the floor and therapist support at the hips; rocking forward and back or side to side will increase strength and stability over time; reaching for toys will also require weight-shifting to improve stability and trunk strength. (2) Kneeling or half-kneeling are great postures to strengthen the hips in those with some muscle function in the gluteal muscles; kneeling will also facilitate trunk muscle activity and upper extremity weight-bearing; reaching in these positions will strengthen trunk muscles and develop balance. For children with limited LE muscle activity, kneeling may still be appropriate to create some weight-bearing on the LE and especially the hips; however, this will require therapist control of the hips and considerable UE support by the child. (3) Weight-bearing in sitting astride a roll or in a low chair is also a good position for LE strengthening. Coming to standing and controlled return to sitting from standing will further strengthen the quadriceps as well as hip muscles, if innervated. For those with limited quad strength, pulling up with the arms will be required. (4) "Push-aways" are a simple way to strengthen the quads and potentially the gluts in young children. For this activity, the therapist holds the child's heels in their hands with the child supine and the therapist sitting and facing the child. Bend the knees to the chest and then have the child "push away" the therapist by straightening their legs. (5) Kicking a ball, with or without ankle weights, in sitting is another fun way to strengthen the quads for standing. (6) Squatting from standing and returning to standing is a great quad strengthening activity with or without UE support for the child with some quad strength; (7) Bridging in a supine position will increase gluteal strength in those with some innervation of these muscles; this can easily be a fun play activity with a car or ball to roll "under the bridge." (8) Early standing with appropriate bracing should be initiated when head and trunk control are sufficient; the use of appropriate assistive devices (e.g., wheeled walker, crutches) or other support (furniture, walls, therapist/parent hands) will likely be required. (9) Recent evidence suggests that body-weight supported treadmill training or weight-supported walkers may facilitate early weight-bearing activities with the potential to elicit walking at an earlier age.[56]

TABLE 19-6	Wheelchair Measurements
MEASUREMENT	**RATIONALE**
Seat to top of head Seat to occiput Seat to top of shoulder Seat to inferior angle of scapula	These measurements allow a determination of the height of the back of the chair and head rest, if needed. A head rest should hit at the occiput and support the head to its top. Most children with MMC will not need a head rest to maintain head control, but young children will have one to support their head for comfort or the back of the chair will go up to the top of the head to provide support when tired. For older children with limited trunk control but good head control, the chair back will typically end at the top of the shoulder; however, for teenagers and those with good trunk control, the back will end at the inferior angle of the scapula.
Seat to elbow	This measurement determines the height of the arm rest.
Seat to iliac crest	If a pelvic support is needed, this measurement will determine the height of the support. It can also identify pelvic obliquity (asymmetry) that may be addressed with the seat cushion to align the pelvis.
Chest width	If lateral trunk support is required, this will determine the width of the lateral supports. A measurement from the seat to the axilla will also be needed to determine the maximum height of the support, with 1–2 inches subtracted to prevent rubbing.
Chest depth	For children with limited trunk control, a chest harness may be needed, and this measurement will help determine the strap length. For transportation on a school bus, young children are required to have a chest harness.
Hip width – measure at widest point	Determines seat width; the seat should be at least 2 inches wider than this measurement to prevent pressure on the hips and allow a coat to be worn. Most pediatric chairs allow for the seat width to increase several inches over the life of the chair (the frame has the ability to expand) with or without replacement of the seat itself.
Thigh length (sacrum to popliteal fossa)	Determines seat depth; subtract 2 inches to prevent rubbing of the back of the leg by the seat. Similar to seat width, pediatric chair frames allow expansion of seat depth of several inches.
Knee to heel	Determines foot rest position; must allow 2 inches above the ground to allow clearance over uneven surfaces. Footrests are also typically adjustable to allow leg growth over the 5-year period.
Foot length	Determines foot rest depth

are also critical as the child ages to determine the best choice(s) and then train the child on appropriate use.

CASE A, PART XI

For Dylan, he was seen postoperatively to discuss movement limitations and to educate the family on transfer techniques, since he couldn't perform a push-up necessary for a chair to bed transfer. The parents were taught to perform a standing pivot transfer from the bed to the wheelchair and back.

Functional training, strengthening, electrical stimulation, exercise training, and motor skill training have been shown to be effective in improving impairments and function in children with MMC.[56] In addition, early step training that includes facilitated newborn stepping (leaning the baby forward over a stationary service), bouncing (stimulating weight-bearing by bouncing infant on lab in standing position) and supported stepping on a treadmill has been found to enhance motor development in children with lumbar lesions (L3 – S2), when initiated within one month of birth; in fact, they obtained motor milestones within the normal ranges of typical peers for sitting (6 months), crawling (12 months), standing alone (16.8 months) and independent walking (19.5 months). Infants also demonstrated a decrease in weight to length ratio.[57] Interestingly, there is very little research on the effectiveness of aquatic PT for these children with only one study that found a general improvement in cardiorespiratory endurance but not strength or motor skills after an aquatic program; however, only two of the children had MMC.[58] However, water can afford buoyancy that allows those with muscle weakness to move more easily than on land and, for those with spinal cord injury, has been reported to enhance ambulation ability.[59] Preventative techniques to avoid contractures, arthritis, skin breakdown (with pressure relief), and pain are all necessary components of a PT regimen. Pressure ulcers are reported by 15-25% of adults with MMC.[45] Therefore, pressure relief by tilting the wheelchair or doing an upper extremity sitting-pushup is prescribed every 15–20 minutes as are daily full body skin checks with a mirror. Exercise regimes or physical therapy to maintain function and prevent decline of current status is also important.

Adults with MMC also have decreased levels of fitness, decreased activity levels, and increased rates of obesity.[45] It is important to have comprehensive health programs that include nutrition and individual or group fitness for patients at all ages to maximize their health. Bone health should also be emphasized, since weight-bearing is necessary for bone development and maintenance; children, who are wheelchair dependent, are at a high risk for osteopenia and osteoporosis by adolescense.[60] It should be noted that these types of programs are not very common, but this is an area of potential growth in practice for PTs interested in maximizing function in adults with MMC.

Wheelchair Prescription

In many clinics and school settings, the PTs are responsible for deciding the type of wheelchair, including the seating and frame, for a child with MMC. Team evaluations and decision-making are common and typically include an equipment provider(s), a third-party payer representative, and the medical team. The PT is part of this team, evaluating the patient, problem-solving, and providing recommendations for design, purchase, and maintenance of wheelchairs as well as other adaptive equipment (Table 19-6). Toddlers and young children need to be able to navigate their environment on their own, so choosing the right mobility device involves a balance between safety and the importance of independent mobility for child development. Choosing the type of wheelchair and accessory components is very much a team activity with a lot of caregiver input. Most wheelchairs are customized to fit the size and unique sensorimotor, orthopedic, and functional abilities to meet the daily activities of each child. Yet, assuring appropriate positioning of the child by manipulating or adding features to a wheelchair due to changes in age, growth, development, functional status, orthotic conditions, etc. is commonplace.

The process from assessment of the patient to ordering a wheelchair and ultimately receipt of the wheelchair by the patient can take a lot of time. Demonstration chairs are often available from vendors or housed in clinics for patients to try out. Sometimes demonstration that patients are able to safely operate a wheelchair, especially with powered mobility, is required to justify the chair choice to third-party payers and sometimes the family. One critical aspect of wheelchair choice is the cognitive maturity of the child, including ability to understand the demands of a mobility device and impulse control, which is necessary to assure safety (e.g., slowing the chair in the presence of other children). Demonstration wheelchairs offer the opportunity to consult with the child and caregivers about what will work best for them with consideration of their ability to transport the chair and manage it in the home. Asking about the current equipment the family uses may give the PT an idea about what is working and what is needed. Ordering any kind of assistive equipment that the child or caregiver does not like will often result in that equipment being unused.

Part of the wheelchair evaluation will include a comprehensive medical history with emphasis on anything that might impact seating requirements or restrictions, including surgical history, orthopedic conditions, and respiratory or cardiac impairments. A new wheelchair is typically prescribed every 5 years, so the chair needs to have the ability to grow with the child and the potential for adapting to changes in the child's functioning over that time period; in some respects, this forces the PT to make "best guesses" of the future needs of the child. Despite our best efforts, children will sometimes change in unpredictable ways, including unexpected weight gain, surgery, or a change in function before the 5-year timeframe has passed, and the therapist and family will need to negotiate with the third-party payer for consideration of an early wheelchair replacement request.

A thorough evaluation of seating and postures, accounting for any deformities and ROM deficits, can be completed by the PT, including measurements as outlined in Table 19-6. Measurements are ideally taken in a seated position, typically a chair, if the patient has adequate postural and trunk control.

● WHEELCHAIR COMPONENTS

Considerations for wheelchairs for all children in need of one will include selection of appropriate components: (1) base (manual or powered); (2) frame; and (3) seating system as well as assessment of the environments, in which the child will function (home, school, other) and the activities, in which the child will participate, including for the older child, sporting activities.

Bases

The type of base, either powered or manual, should be determined first. Most children with MMC have adequate ROM and strength in their upper extremities to independently propel a manual wheelchair. After some training and daily use, young toddlers can be expert navigators of a manual wheelchair at home and in the community. Manual wheelchairs give children with MMC early functional mobility, the ability to keep up with age-matched peers, and a way to quickly explore their environment. The best choice for many young toddlers is an ultra-lightweight, rigid-frame chair that is low to the floor and can have a handle for parental control (Figure 19-17).[61] This will afford the child easier transfers into and out of the chair from the floor as well as put them at the eye-level of their peers. Many preschoolers can manipulate their wheelchairs through complex environments and, by early school age, to perform a wheelie to clear a low curb. If, and when, a power chair is needed, it is important to note that power bases are larger, heavier, and do not collapse as easily as manual bases, so consideration should also be given to maneuverability in the home and the ability of the family to transport the chair. Some children have declining function over their lifetime and might eventually need a power chair. Both manual and power bases are somewhat adaptable for different seating systems, accessories, and features. Accessories include arm rests, footrests, tilt or recline positioning, type of wheels and tires, hand rims, and brakes. Considerations for manual versus powered WCs include (1) whether the child or caregiver will be moving the chair; (2) the ability to self-propel, understand safety, and control impulsivity; (3) UE strength, overall endurance, and transfer abilities/potential; (4) cognition and vision; (5) any restrictions on mobility (e.g., orthopedic limitations like Dylan's); and (6) independence.

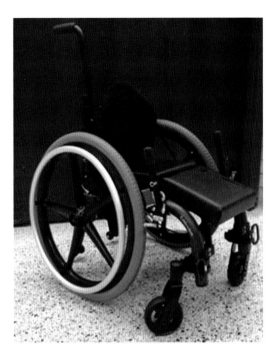

FIGURE 19-17 Manual wheelchair for toddler. This ultralight manual wheelchair is consistent with that described for Dylan, including a leg rest to support the whole lower extremity, a handle for the caregiver to control the chair. (Used with permission from Jill C. Heathcock, MPT, PhD, The Ohio State University).

CASE A, PART XII

By the time Dylan was two years old he had a custom-made manual wheelchair with a leg rest to support his entire lower extremities. The leg rest could bend to 90 degrees so as he got older and longer his legs could be in a flexed position at the knee and accessory foot rests added to the frame. The handle allowed his caregivers to maneuver the wheelchair in a similar manner as a stroller and provided safety support when needed, while allowing Dylan the ability to independently explore and participate in his environment at a speed equal to his peers. He used a reverse rolling walker with HKFOs for short distances at home and for lower extremity weight-bearing and upright ambulation training and exercise. Dylan continued to use standard light-frame manual wheelchairs as his primary form of independent mobility until the scoliosis surgery.

Frames

Frames can be rigid or folding. Folding frames allow for the WC to be collapsed and stored or transported in a small car trunk. Rigid frames cannot be folded but do allow for easy removal of the tires for storage and transport. Frames for WCs can be of many materials, including stainless steel, aluminum, and titanium. Traditional stainless steel frames are heavier than newer lightweight frames that are made of titanium or composite material.

Seating Systems

A seating system should create a functional sitting position that assures comfort, baseline pressure relief, adequate trunk support, and good postural alignment. The latter is especially important in children with thoracic lesions as they are likely to develop kyphosis, scoliosis, or both due to asymmetric trunk muscle activity. Scoliosis or pelvic obliquities can be observed in sitting posture and will result in asymmetrical seat to top of shoulder and seat to iliac crest measurements. Seat cushions vary greatly in firmness and pressure relief capacity, ranging from those made with air to those made of a hard foam. A balance is needed to minimize the sheer force (friction across the skin as the body moves on the seat), created by the seating material, with the need to find the best position for the child to maximize function while also protecting boney prominences and avoid pressure ulcers. For example, some positions, such as a reclined position, increase the potential for shear that needs to be offset by a higher friction seating material; however, this will make it more likely for movement to create excessive shear. The PT should obtain a history of skin integrity to determine cushion selection. If needed, pressure mapping systems are now available to accurately identify points of increased pressure where additional padding may be needed.

Notably, PTs should also provide patient and caregiver education on the type and timing of pressure relief for children with poor sensation in their buttocks/legs. Standard practices for pressure relief for older children include independent WC push-ups where the child uses the armrests to lift their lower body off the seat by pushing up with their arms; frequent weight shifts by leaning all the way forward and leaning side to side; having a caregiver tilt the chair back with proper body mechanics; and manually changing the position of the legs to unweight one side. With power chairs the reclining or tilt in space features can be used for pressure relief. Tilt-in-space frames retain the seat to back angle but the seat orientation to the ground changes. A tilt greater than 30 degrees has been shown to provide pressure relief in adults. Reclining chairs allow the back of the chair to change in relation to the seat, which affords pressure relief but increases the shear imposed on the skin.[62] Most seating systems are aligned in a 90-90-90 alignment, representing the hip, knee, and ankle angles.

Other options for seating systems include back height, headrest, lateral and pelvic supports, belt system, and footrest. Tall seat backs are common for children with low tone, poor sitting balance, and poor trunk control. A head rest can be included as an accessory if the patient child also has poor head control. A head rest is needed for head support during tilting or reclining in a power chair. A mid-seat back height, just below the scapula, allows freedom of the shoulders for propulsion as well as sports activities. Young toddlers with MMC, who have lower-level lesions and have adequate hip control, may use a standing WC that looks like Figure 19-17 but with a platform to stand with support at the knees and hips instead of a seat. Lap belts are necessary for young children, and chest harnesses are needed for those with poor trunk control or very young children, if they are transported in a school bus. Additional lateral supports may also be needed for the child with poor trunk control.

Environmental Factors

Final determination of the appropriate wheelchair system should include assessment of the home and school environments as well as the family's ability to manage the device. Assessment of the child's current home environment is critical to wheelchair selection, including the size and type of vehicle that is owned by the family and its capacity to transport a wheelchair, as well as the entry to the home to determine whether there are stairs to manage. Some third-party payers will require that a ramp is in place or currently being built before they will approve an order for a wheelchair. Home visits to evaluate individual needs are often conducted by a therapist and equipment provider. Smaller manual chairs for younger toddlers and children can be folded to fit in a small trunk and are lightweight, allowing for them to be carried up stairs, and thus eliminating the need for a ramp, since young children with or without impaired mobility are commonly carried into the home. Community needs including daycare, school, work, medical appointments, religious services, adaptive sports, and other unique considerations will also inform decision-making wheelchair specifications.

CASE A, PART XIII

***Is Dylan a candidate for power mobility?

There is not a simple answer to this question. First, his chair is only 2 years old, and his third-party payer typically only funds a new chair every 5 years; however, it may be possible to request consideration due to his change in status – recent weight gain and spinal fusion. As his PT, you would need to carefully document his change in status and evaluate his capacity to use a power chair, including whether he has any spatial perceptual deficits, associated with his visual learning disability. It is likely that he would be able to learn to control a power chair; however, if the limitations to his UE and trunk mobility are temporary, it will likely be better for him to continue to use a manual chair to maximize his physical activity and manage his health and weight. Independent mobility is also a major consideration. Dylan needs to be able to move around his environment by himself and a power chair might be the best solution at this time. His family may also need to obtain a lift to assist with transfers to avoid injuring themselves, if he continues to grow. Aging with MMC is often associated with weight gain, resulting in a decrease in functional status. Fitness programs should be developed to minimize this problem in older children and adults with MMC. Increased risk of cardiovascular problems may occur in adults with MMC due to decreased mobility, resulting in a sedentary lifestyle. It is important to have comprehensive health programs that include nutrition counseling and individual or group fitness for patients at all ages to maximize their health. Bone health should also be emphasized, since weight-bearing is necessary for normal bone development and maintenance; adults with MMC are at risk for osteoporosis and bone fractures, especially if they aren't walking.

COMPARISON TO SPINAL CORD INJURY

As mentioned earlier, there are some parallels between spinal cord injury and MMC. For example, in both, the spinal cord and neural tissue are damaged such that sensorimotor function is lost below the lesion level. The level gives necessary initial information about what kind of function a patient may have. Patients with SCI and MMC demonstrate a combination of UMN and LMS signs, and asymmetrical function is often present though the injury is typically bilateral. However, function and treatments are very different. For patients with a traumatic SCI, rehabilitation is *relearning* a skill that was already present, like walking. For infants with MMC, rehabilitation is the teaching of new skills such as the *emergence* of walking in a baby or child who has never walked before.

REFERENCES

1. Data & Statistics on Birth Defects. Centers for Disease Control and Prevention. Accessed on 1/10/22. https://www.cdc.gov/ncbddd/birthdefects/data.html.

2. Avagliano L, Massa V, George TM, Qureshy S. Bulfamante G, Finnell RH. Overview on neural tube defects: from development to physical characteristics. *Birth Defects Res.* 2019;111(19):1455-1467.

3. Greene NDE, Copp AJ. Development of the vertebrate central nervous system: formation of the neural tube. *Prenat Diagn.* 2009;29:303-311.

4. Borsani E, Vedova AMD, Rezzani R, Rodella LF, Cristini C. Correlation between human nervous system development and acquisition of fetal skills: an overview. *Brain Dev.* 2019;41:225-233.

5. Greene NDE, Copp AJ. Neural tube defects. *Annu Rev Neurosci.* 2014;37:221-242.

6. Sandoval JI, De Jesus O. Hydranencephaly. In: *StatPearls [Internet].* Treasure Island, FL: StatPearls Publishing; 2021. PMID: 32644417.

7. Rowland CA, Correa A, Cragan JD, Alverson CJ. Are encephaloceles neural tube defects? *Pediatrics.* 2006;118(3):916-923.

8. Graham P. Spina bifida occulta. *Orthopaedic Nurs.* 2021;40(4):259-261.

9. Meller C, Covini D, Aiello H, Isbisky G, Medina SP, Otano L. Update on prenatal diagnosis and fetal surgery for myelomeningocele. *Arch Argen Pediatr.* 2021;119(3):e215-e228.

10. Williams LJ, Rasmussen SA, Flores A, Kirby RS, Edmonds LD. Decline in the prevalence of spina bifida and anencephaly by race/ethnicity: 1995-2002. *Pediatrics.* 2005;116(3):580-586.

11. Trudell AS, Obido AO. Diagnosis of spina bifida on ultrasound: always termination? *Best Pract Res Clin Obstet Gynaecol.* 2014;28:367-377.

12. Saadai P, Farmer DL. Clinics in perinatology: fetal surgery for myelomeningocele. *Clin Perinatol.* 2012;39(2):279-288.

13. Brown OH, Makar KG, Ulma RM, et al. A simplified approach to myelomeningocele defect repair. *Annals Plastic Surg.* 2021;86(1):58-61.

14. Desai J, Swash M. Fasciculations: what do we know of their significance? *J Neurolog Sci.* 1991;152(S1):S43-S48.

15. Sival DA, van Weerden TW, Vles JSH, et al. Neonatal loss of motor function in human spina bifida aperta. *Pediatrics.* 2004;114(2):427-434.

16. Foss S, Flanders TM, Heuer GG, Schreiber JE. Neurobehavioral outcomes in patients with myelomeningocele. *Neurosurg Focus.* 2013;47(4):E6.

17. Talamonti G, Marcati E, Mastino L, Meccariello G, Picano M, D'Aliberti G. Surgical management of chiari malformation type II. *Child's Nerv System.* 2020;36:1621-1634.

18. McAllister JP II. Pathophysiology of congenital and neonatal hydrocephalus. *Semin Fetal Neonatal Med.* 2012;17:285-294.

19. Kahle KT, Kulkarni AV, Limbrick DD Jr, Watf BC. Hydrocephalus in children. *Lancet.* 2016;387:788-799.

20. Peiro JL, Fabbro MD. Fetal therapy for congenital hydrocephalus-where we came from and where we are going. *Childs Nerv Syst.* 2020;36:1697-1712.

21. Cavalheiro S, Silva de Costa MD, Barbosa MM, et al. Hydrocephalus in myelomeningocele. *Childs Nerv Syst.* 2021;37:3407-3415.

22. Oi S, Inagaki T, Shinoda M, et al. COE-Fetal and Congenital Hydrocephalus Top 10 Japan Study Group. Guideline for management and treatment of fetal and congenital hydrocephalus: center of excellence-fetal and congenital hydrocephalus top 10 Japan guideline 2011. *Childs Nerv Syst.* 2011;27:1563-1579.

23. Dalen K, Bruroy S, Wentzel-Larsen T, Laegreid LM. Intelligence in children with hydrocephalus, aged 4-15 years: a population-based, controlled study. *Neuropediatrics.* 2008;39:146-150.

24. Boettcher M, Goettler S, Exchenburg G, et al. Prenatal latex sensitization in patients with spina bifida: a pilot study. *J Neurosurg Pediatr.* 2014;13: 291-294.

25. Jallo GI, Kothbauer KF, Abbott IR. Endoscopi third vetriculostomy. *Neurosurg Focus.* 2005;19(6):E11.

26. Duru S, Peiro JL, Oria M, et al. Successful endoscopic third ventricuolostomy in children depends on age and etiology of hydrocephalus: outcome analysis in 51 pediatric patients. *Childs Nerv Syst.* 2018;34:1521-1528.

27. Hudgins RJ, Gilreath CL. Tethered spinal cord following repair of myeleomeningocele. *Neurosurg Focus.* 2004;16(2):E7.

28. Dewan MC, Wellons JC III. Fetal surgery for spina bifida. *J Neurosurg Pediatr.* 2019;24:105-114.

29. Swank M, Dias L. Myelomeningocele: a review of the orthopaedic aspects of 206 patients treated from birth with no selection criteria. *Dev Med Child Neurol.* 1992;34(12):1047-1052.

30. Houtrow AM, MacPherson C, Jackson-Coty J, et al. Prenatal repair and physical functioning among children with myelomeningocele: a secondary analysis of a randomized clinical trial. *JAMA Pediatr.* 2021;175(4):e205674.

31. Conklin MJ, Kishan S, Nanayakkara CB, Rosenfeld SR. Orthopedic guidelines for the care of people with spina bifida. *J Ped Rehabil Med.* 2020;13: 629-633.

32. Balasankar G, Luximon A, Al-Jumaily A. Current conservative management and classification of club foot: a review. *J Ped Rehabil Med.* 2016;9:257-264.

33. Gibbons PJ, Gray K. Update on clubfoot. *J Paediatr Child Health.* 2013;49:E434-E437.

34. Canavese F, Dimeglio A. Clinical examination and classification systems of congenital clubfoot: a narrative review. *Ann Transl Med.* 2021;9(13):1097.

35. Swaroop VT, Dias L. Orthopaedic management of spina bifida-part II: foot and ankle deformities. *J Child Orthop.* 2011;5:403-414.

36. Holroyd B, Wedge J. Developmental dysplasia of the hip. *Orthop Trauma.* 2009;32(3):162-168.

37. Dezateux C, Rosendahl K. Developmental dysplasia of the hip. *Lancet.* 2007;369:1541-1552.

38. Woodhouse CRJ. Myelomeningocele: neglected aspects. *Pediatr Nephrol.* 2008;23:1223-1231.

39. El-Hawary R, Chukwunyerenwa C. Update on evaluation and treatment of scoliosis. *Pediatr Clin N Am* 2014:61:1223-1241.

40. Konieczny MR, Senyurt H, Krauspe R. Epidemiology of adolescent idiopathic scoliosis. *J Child Orthop.* 2013;7:3-9.

41. Mummareddy N, Dewan MC, Mercier MR, Naftel RP, Wellons JC III, Bonfield CM. Scoliosis in myelomeningocele: epidemiology, management and functional outcome. *J Neurosurg Pediatr.* 2017;20:99-108.

42. Zaina F. De Mauroy JC, Hresko MT, et al. Bracing for scoliosis in 2014: state of the art. *Eur J Phys Rehabil Med.* 2014;50:93-110.

43. Negrini S, Donzelli S, Lusini M, Minnella S, Zaina F. The effectiveness of combined bracing and exercise in adolescent idiopathic scoliosis based on SRS and SOSORT criteria: a prospective study. *BMC Musculoskelet Disord.* 2014;15(1):263.

44. Hoashi JS, Cahill PJ, Bennett JT, Samdani AF. Adolescent scoliosis classification and treatment. *Neurosurg Clin N Am.* 2013;24:173-183.

45. Bendt M, Gabrielsson H, Riedel D, et al. Adults with spina bifida: a cross-sectional study of health issues and living conditions. *Brain Behav.* 2020; 10:e01736.

46. Korenromp MJ, van Gool JD, Bruinese HW, Kriek R. Early fetal leg movements in myelomeningocele. *Lancet.* 1986;1(8486):917-918.

47. Kamm K, Thelen E, Jensen JL. A dynamical systems approach to motor development. *Phys Ther.* 1990;70(12):763-775.

48. Chapman D. Context effects on the spontaneous leg movements of infants with spina bifida. *Pediatr Phys Ther.* 2002;14(2):62-73.

49. Rademacher N, Black DP, Ulrich BD. Early spontaneous leg movements in infants born with and without myelomeningocele. *Pediatr Phys Ther.* 2008;20(2):137-145.

50. Seitzberg A, Lind M, Biering-Sorensen F. Ambulation in adults with myelomeningocele: is it possible to predict the level of ambulation in early life? *Childs Nerv Syst.* 2008;24:231-237.

51. Bartonek A, Saraste H. Factors influencing ambulation in myelomeningocele: a cross-sectional study. *Dev Med Child Neurol.* 2001;43:253-260.

52. Findley TW, Agre JC, Habeck RV, Schmalz R, Birkebak RR, McNally MC. Ambulation in the adolescent with myelomeningocele. I: early childhood predictors. *Arch Phys Med Rehabil.* 1987;68(8):518-522.

53. Pauly M, Cremer R. Levels of mobility in children and adolescents with spina bifida: clinical parameters predicting mobility and maintenance of these skills. *Eur J Pediatr Surg.* 2013;23:110-114.

54. Knutson LM, Clark DE. Orthotic devices for ambulation in children with cerebral palsy and myelomeningocele. *Phys Ther.* 1991;71:947-960.

55. Brock JW III, Thomas JC, Baskin LS, et al. For the Eunice Kennedy Shriver NICHD MOMS Trial Group. Effect of prenatal repair of myelomeningocele on urological outcomes at school age. *J Urol.* 2019;202:812-818.

56. Dagenais LM, Lahay ER, Stueck KA, White E, Williams L, Harris SR. Effects of electrical stimulation, exercise training and motor skills training on strength of children with meningomyelocele: a systematic review. *Phys Occup Ther Pediatr.* 2009;29(4):445-463.

57. Lee DK, Sansom JK. Early treadmill practice in infants born with myelomeningocele: a pilot study *Pediatr Phys Ther.* 2019;31:68-75.

58. Fragala-Pinkham M, Haley SM, O'Neil ML. Group aquatic aerobic exercise for children with disabilities. *Dev Med Child Neurol.* 2008;50(11):822-827.

59. Wall T, Falvo L, Kesten A. Activity-specific aquatic therapy targeting gait for a patient with incomplete spinal cord injury. *Physiother Theory Pract.* 2017;33(4):331-344.

60. Apkon SD, Fenton L, Coll JR. Bone mineral density in children with myelomeningocele. *Dev Med Child Neurol.* 2008;51:63-67.

61. Meiser MJ, McEwen IR. Lightweight and ultralight wheelchairs: propulsion and preferences of two young children with spina bifida. *Pediatr Phys Ther.* 2007;19:245-253.

62. Groah SL, Schladen M, Pineda CG, Hsieh CHJ. Prevention of pressure ulcers among people with spinal cord injury: a systematic review. *Phys Med Rehabil.* 2015;7:613-636.

Review Questions

1. The form of spina bifida in which part of the spinal cord and nerves protrude through an incompletely closed spine is:
   A. Acute spinal defect
   B. Meningocele
   C. Myelomeningocele
   D. Spina bifida occulta

2. A baby is born with a small sac at the occiput of the cranium, filled with fluid and a small amount of neural tissue; this defect would correctly be called a/an:
   A. Anencephaly
   B. Encephalocele
   C. Hydrocele
   D. Meningocele

3. Which of the following regarding spina bifida is accurate:
   A. Myelomeningocele is the least severe form.
   B. The bony deformity involves malformation of the transverse process of the vertebral body.
   C. The most common location is within the cervical spine.
   D. Folic acid deficiency may contribute to spina bifida

4. The most appropriate orthosis for a child with myelomeningocele who has medial and lateral knee instability, has inadequate toe clearance during gait, has quad strength of 2, and is a household ambulator with limited community ambulation is:
   A. HKAFO
   B. KAFO
   C. SMA
   D. TKAFO

5. When a PT positions the infant in supine with hips flexed to 90 degrees and abducts one hip, causing the head of the femur to move posteriorly, the PT is using the
   A. Clunk test to determine hip symmetry
   B. Ober test to determine iliotibial band tightness
   C. Galeazzi sign to determine differences in thigh length
   D. Ortolani sign to identify hip dislocation

6. You're evaluating an infant with a myelomeningocele defect that has 4/5 ileopsoas and quad strength and 3/5 anterior tibialis strength. It is likely that this child's lesion is at level:
   A. L3
   B. L4
   C. L5
   D. S1

7. Children with myelomeningocele typically have
   A. A mixture of lower motor neuron and upper motor neuron dysfunction

B. A high likelihood of having mental retardation
   C. Normal bowel and bladder function
   D. A high probability of improvement in ambulation skills through the teenage years

8. Which of the following is most commonly associated with myelomeningocele?
   A. Intraventricular hemorrhage
   B. Congenital brain malformation involving the brainstem and foramen magnum
   C. Flaccidity below the level of the spinal lesion
   D. Intact sensation below the level of the lesion

9. The neural tube is created by what process
   A. Diaschisis
   B. Formulation
   C. Neurolation
   D. Tubalgation

10. Spina bifida is currently detected in utero by
    A. Amniocentesis
    B. Blood tests
    C. Decreased fetal kicking movements
    D. Ultrasound

11. Children with lesions above L1 are typically what type of ambulatory at school age?
    A. Household and limited community ambulators
    B. Household ambulators or non-walkers
    C. Unrestricted ambulators
    D. Community ambulators with assistive devices

12. A child presents with a 45-degree right thoracic and 25-degree left lumbar scoliosis. The best treatment for this child would be:
    A. Abdominal and back strengthening exercises
    B. Bracing
    C. Lateral wheelchair trunk supports
    D. Spinal fusion surgery

13. The following is a common complication of MMC?
    A. Brachial plexus palsy
    B. Club foot
    C. Peanut allergy
    D. Male gender

14. When ordering a wheelchair, the seat depth should be determined as:
    A. Greater trochanter to popliteal fossa plus 2 inches
    B. Greater trochanter to medial femoral condyle minus 2 inches
    C. Sacrum to popliteal fossa minus 2 inches
    D. Sacrum to medial femoral condyle plus 2 inches

15. **Which of the following activities, described in this chapter, can be used primarily to strengthen the arms in toddlers, preparing them to use their arms for ambulation and transfers?**
    A. Assisted sit-ups
    B. Bridging
    C. Push aways
    D. Wheelbarrow walking

16. **Neural tube disorders occur at which point in gestation?**
    A. At conception
    B. Within the first month
    C. By the end of the first trimester
    D. During the 2nd trimester

17. **Which of these neural tube disorders is associated with failure of closure of the caudal neural tube?**
    A. Anencephaly
    B. Encephalocele
    C. Hydranencephaly
    D. Myeomeningocele

18. **What is the most common side effect o intrauterine closure of a myelomeningocele defect?**
    A. Inceased occurrence of Arnold–Chiari malformation
    B. Increased occurrence of hydrocephalus
    C. Increased occurrence of premature delivery
    D. Increased occurrence of orthopedic conditions

19. **Arnold Chiari Malformation II includes which of the following?**
    A. Displacement of the cerebellum tonsils through the foramen magnum
    B. Enlargement of the cerebellum
    C. Shortening of the corpus callosum
    D. Enlargement of the 4th ventricle

20. **Which of the following symptoms of greater Arnold–Chiari impingement requires immediate surgical repair?**
    A. Ataxia
    B. Cranial nerve signs
    C. Dysphagia and dysphonia
    D. Headache

21. **When working with a child with hydrocephalus, what movement should be avoided?**
    A. Excessivee neck flexion
    B. Excessive trunk flexion
    C. Excessive neck extension
    D. Excessive trunk extension

22. **What type of assistive device would you expect a child with L5 sensory and motor function to use?**
    A. Crutches
    B. Manual wheelchair
    C. Power wheelchair
    D. None

Answers

1. C	2. B	3. D	4. B	5. D
6. B	7. A	8. B	9. C	10. D
11. B	12. D	13. B	14. C	15. D
16. B	17. D	18. C	19. A	20. C
21. A	22. D			

GLOSSARY

Adam's bend test. Forward bending of the trunk to look for rib hump (sign of scoliosis).

Anencephaly. Open neural tube defect with loss of cerebral hemispheres, thalamus, and midbrain.

Arnold Chiari malformation. Herniation of the brainstem and cerebellum through foramen magnum.

Barlow sign. Hip flexure to 90 degrees, followed by adduction while applying posterior pressure to see if hip dislocates (test for DDH).

Cephalic flexure. Bend in neural tube vesicle structure between mesencephalon and rhombencephalon.

Cervical flexure. Bend in neural tube vesicle structure between rhombencephalon and caudal tube.

Club foot. Forefoot cavus and adduction with heal varus and equinus.

Developmental dysplasia of the hip. Abnormal hip joint development.

Diencephalon. Vesicle that becomes the thalamus, hypothalamus epithalamus, subthalamus, retina, and lens.

Ectoderm. Outer layer of the neural tissue that forms the nervous system and skin.

Encephalocele. Closed defect with partial protrusion of meninges with or without neural tissue through skull defect.

Encephalomeningocele. Encephalocele with both meninges and neural tissue.

Endoderm. Inner layer of neural tissue that forms the internal organs.

Fontanelles (Fontanels). Soft spot between the cranial bones prior to fusion.

Hydranencephaly. Closed neural tube defect with loss of cerebral hemispheres.

Hydrocephalus. Buildup of cerebrospinal fluid (CSF) within the ventricles.

Communicating (non-obstructive). Abnormal production or absorption of CSF.

Noncommunicating. Malformation within the ventricular system that impedes CSF flow.

Obstructive. Blockage within the ventricular system that impedes CSF flow.

Lenke classification. System used to classify scoliosis.

Meningocele. Protrusion of meninges but not neural tissue.

Mesencephalon. Middle vesicle of neural tube; forms midbrain.

Mesoderm. Middle layer of neural tissue that forms muscle, connective tissue, and cardiovascular system.

Metencephalon. Vesicle that becomes the pons and cerebellum.

Myelencephalon. Vesicle that becomes the medulla.

Myelomeningocele. Neural tube disorder.

Neural groove. As the neural folds invaginate, they create this neural groove before they come together as the neural tube.

Neural plate. Central portion of ectoderm.

Neural tube defects. Disruption in the formation of the neural tube.

Ortolani sign. Hip flexion to 90 degrees, followed by abduction, to see if femoral head moves back into acetabulum (test for DDH).

Parapodium. Rigid THKAFO.

Pavlik harness. Treatment for DDH, forcing hip flexion and abduction.

Pontine flexure. Bend in five-vesicle neural tube structure between metencephalon and myelencephalon.

Prosencephalon. Rostral portion of neural tube, expands into telencephalon and diencephalon.

Rhombencephalon. Caudal vesicle of neural tube, expand into metencephalon and myelencephalon.

Scoliosis. Spinal curvature.

Nonstructural. Flexible curve that corrects with lateral bending.

Primary. Largest curve.

Secondary. Smaller compensatory curve.

Structural. Inflexible curve that doesn't correct with lateral bending.

Spina bifida occulta (spina dysraphism occulta). Absence of a lamina or spinous process of a vertebra.

Spinal cord tethering. Adherence of the spinal cord components or meninges to spinal column.

Spinal dysraphism (spina bifida). Failure of closure of the spinous process of spinal column.

Swivel walker. Parapodium that moves by alternating trunk rotation.

Ventriculostomy. Surgical creation of a stoma in the third ventricle to allow CSF to drain into the prepontine cistern.

ABBREVIATIONS

AFO	ankle foot orthosis
CAVE	Cavus and Adduction of forefoot; varus and Equinus of hindfoot
DDH	developmental hip dysplasia
HKAFO	hip-knee-ankle-foot orthosis
KAFO	knee-ankle-foot orthosis
MMC	myelomeningocele
RGO	reciprocating gait orthosis
THKAFO	trunk-hip-knee-ankle-foot orthosis

Cerebral Palsy 20

Jill C. Heathcock and Deborah S. Nichols-Larsen

OBJECTIVES

1) Understand the pathophysiology of cerebral palsy
2) Identify the common risk factors for cerebral palsy
3) Identify the typical characteristics of cerebral palsy
4) Identify common classification systems of cerebral palsy
5) Identify and choose optimal treatment interventions for children with cerebral palsy post-stroke

CASE A, PART I

Alejandro Lobo was born at 30 weeks gestation with a birth weight of 1.75 kg, length of 43 cm, and head circumference of 29 cm. He spent 7 weeks in the Neonatal Intensive Care Unit (NICU). On day of life 25, he had an ultrasound, which revealed a grade IV periventricular hemorrhage (PVL). He was born to Carmen and Paul Lobo and has an older sister Carla (2 years old, when he was born). Carmen is a physical education teacher at a local high school and Paul is a software developer.

PATHOPHYSIOLOGY

What Is Cerebral Palsy?

Cerebral palsy (CP) is a term that describes a collection of disorders of posture, movement, and balance that result from a defect or anomaly of the developing brain and is one of the top diagnoses of childhood disability, affecting 2 to 3 of every 1000 live births.[1] CP is nonprogressive, which means that there was an event (or discrete series of events) that caused damage to the brain by disrupting typical brain structure and function, but the brain damage does not worsen over time. Like brain injury in adults, CP presents with a disturbance of motor function but also may be accompanied by sensory dysfunction, cognitive impairments, language delay/dysfunction as well as medical disorders such as epilepsy and malnutrition. Although the lesion is nonprogressive, the presentation of CP may change as the child goes through developmental stages, and secondary musculoskeletal conditions are common as the child grows.[1] An estimated 760,000 people in the United States have CP with 65% under age 18.[2]

ETIOLOGY

CP may occur when there is an interruption of blood flow or damage to the developing brain, resulting in a permanent lesion with diverse consequences, depending on the location, severity, and time of insult. It should be noted that brain injury, during fetal development and early infancy, may not be immediately obvious, and therefore, the exact cause or timing of the insult may not be known. These events are typically single or a discrete series and not active at the time of diagnosis. Risk factors and the incidence of certain types of brain lesions are known, but the cause is often unknown.[1] Injury to the developing brain results in changes to otherwise predictable brain formation, growth, and maturation, as described in Chapters 8 and 19. However, it should be noted that CP can occur in those without known risk factors or obvious cause and is, then, referred to as idiopathic (without known cause). Notably, the causative brain injury for CP can occur during gestation, in the perinatal period (during labor, delivery, or shortly after delivery) or in the early developmental period.[1] The etiology of these injuries is heterogeneous, but the most common known causes will be discussed here. Notably, prematurity is one of the most common risk factors for CP; Box 20-1 describes the impact of prematurity on brain development and its association with CP.

Box 20-1 Sequelae of Prematurity

Babies born prior to the 37th week of gestation are considered premature, or preterm, but are further differentiated into **moderate to late preterm** (32–37 weeks), **very preterm** (28–32 weeks), and **extremely preterm** (<28 weeks).[3] Those born at 37-38[6/7] months are considered early term with those born at 39-41 weeks considered term and those born after 41 weeks considered late term.[4] They can be further differentiated into **low birth weight** (<2500 g), **very low birth weight** (<1500 g), and **extremely low birth weight** (<1000 g).[5] *It should be noted that babies with intrauterine growth restriction (see congenital anomalies in the next section) are also classified via these categories.* With improvements in the care for preterm infants, most are surviving; however, the incidence of neurologic impairment (CP, intellectual disability, learning disability) continues to be relatively high with up to 50% displaying some level of neurologic deficit. Not surprisingly, mortality and the incidence and severity of neurologic insult increase as the degree of prematurity increases (lower gestational age).[3,4,6] Notably, those classified as early term also have a greater incidence of mortality and neurologic morbidity than those born at 39-41 weeks, which has resulted in a decrease in the occurrence of early term elective deliveries.[6] The term used for neurologic injury secondary to prematurity is **encephalopathy of prematurity (EoP)**. However, there is not a singular cause of EoP.

A primary cause of EoP is **periventricular leukomalacia (PVL)**, characterized by large cysts within the white matter surrounding the ventricles. With improved neonatal care, there has been a decrease in the occurrence of PVL; however, diffuse white matter loss is now the most common cause of EoP. As described in Chapter 8, neurons are produced in the area surrounding the ventricles (subventricular zone – SVZ) and then migrate to their final destination within the brain; similarly the oligodendrocytes that produce central myelin begin as stem cells within the SVZ, yet myelination occurs much later in gestational development than neuronal migration. In fact, myelination is initiated in the last trimester of pregnancy and continues through the second year of life for projecting neurons and until early adulthood for intracortical neurons.[7] Thus, myelination is just beginning in babies born very preterm or extremely preterm. Inflammation secondary to hypoxia/ischemia or systemic infection brings microglia to the SVZ that apparently attack and kill the pre-oligodendrocyte cells, which are highly vulnerable at this stage. While there is an attempt by the system to replenish these lost cells, this may be insufficient, resulting in an arrest of myelination and reducing neuronal functional integrity. Further, this diffuse white matter disruption has downstream effects on the gray matter of the cortex and deep cerebral nuclei (hippocampus, basal ganglia, thalamus) with diminished dendritic arborization and fewer interneurons noted.[7] Notably, overall brain size and that of many brain regions are progressively smaller with increasing levels of prematurity, and these differences persist in many long term.[3]

Why is the premature brain at risk for hypoxia/ischemia? First, the blood vessels within the brain are still developing in the preterm infant, and thus, are at risk for hemorrhage or an ischemic incident. Second, the preterm infant lacks the capability to **autoregulate blood flow**, which is a necessary function to assure blood flow to the brain. For example, if the infant experiences an infection in another body system, blood may be diverted from the brain to meet the needs of the other system, resulting in brain hypoxia/ischemia, or if the infant is highly stressed, the blood pressure in these immature vessels may exceed the vessel capacity, resulting in hemorrhage. At particular risk for hemorrhage are the vessels in the endothelial lining of the ventricles; a hemorrhage in this area is referred to as an **intraventricular hemorrhage – IVH** – and is graded from level I (most mild) to IV (most severe); the most common place for IVH is in the frontal and parietal regions, making damage to the sensorimotor regions likely. Similar to PVL, hemorrhages in this area disrupt the development of oligodendrocytes and subsequent myelination of neurons, leading to neuronal death. However, the effect of IVH is typically more focal than that of PVL.[8]

IVH grades:

I: bleeding is confined to the germinal layer of the endothelium

II: bleeding into the ventricle(s) without enlargement of the ventricle

III: bleeding into the ventricle(s) with enlargement of the ventricle

IV: bleeding into the ventricle and adjacent brain tissue

Notably, both PVL and IVH can be detected by ultrasound.

Premature birth is caused by intrauterine infection in up to 40% of those born prematurely with increasing frequency at greater degrees of prematurity; in fact, it is a leading cause of neonatal mortality and spontaneous abortion. Intrauterine infection can lead to early onset sepsis, defined as a positive bacterial culture within 72 hours of birth. Prophylactic administration of antibiotics is a common practice in those born at VLBW. However, such administration is associated with other negative sequelae, including necrotizing enterocolitis.[9]

Necrotizing enterocolitis (NEC) is a condition of the bowel, characterized by death of the mucosal lining of the intestines and disruption of bowel function. While this can occur in full-term infants, it is much more common in preterm babies, with up to 12% of VLBW babies affected and a 20 to 30% mortality rate. This seems to be due to the immaturity of the bowel in preterm infants. When present, the intestine is susceptible to intestinal perforation, which can quickly generate into peritonitis and sepsis. It is a common cause of death in preterm infants and is linked to neurologic insults secondary to inflammation.[10]

CASE A, PART II

Alejandro was born at 33 weeks gestation and weighed 1.75 kg or 1750 g. Thus, he would be categorized as preterm with low birth weight. His IVH was a grade IV, indicating that there was blood in the ventricle and the adjacent tissue. Physical therapy for Alejandro began in the NICU, which is common practice for preterm infants. Within the NICU, physical therapy treatment focused on positioning to promote physiological flexion; facilitating autoregulation of autonomic functions, behavioral state, and sensorimotor responses; and assisting parents in the handling of their tiny son. Preterm infants do not experience the close confines of the latter part of gestation, so they typically present without the physiological flexion induced by that confinement; in fact, they may seem hypotonic at birth with limited antigravity movement. Thus, positioning of Alejandro focused on flexed postures to encourage increased flexor tone, especially side-lying, where he was able to begin bringing his hands together and toward his mouth to self-comfort. To facilitate autonomic autoregulation, he was swaddled after any medical procedure and when resting/sleeping, and his parents were encouraged to provide slow, gentle, calming massage or containment, when he was in his isolette, and to hold him against their skin (kangaroo care). These techniques lowered his respiration rate, heart rate, and blood pressure. As is true for many preterm infants, Alejandro demonstrated a stressful reaction to the many noises in the NICU and to all medical care (increased blood pressure, heart rate, and muted crying); therefore, he was protected from the environmental noise in a quieter area of the NICU. Handling was concentrated to allow longer periods between episodes, and then, gradually he was reintroduced to sounds and light, as his responses normalized, to prepare him to go home. Notably, changes in heart rate or respiration rate are often the primary signs of distress rather than crying in preterm infants, so these need to be carefully monitored by the physical therapist, while working in the NICU.[3,11–13]

Prenatal Causes of CP

CP most commonly results from an intrauterine event, accounting for nearly 80% of cases. Prior to 20 weeks, a disruption of development, during embryogenesis, may result in brain malformation, interfering with cell migration and maturation; such damage is associated with more severe impairment.[14] Potential causative factors can be maternal medical conditions (e.g., seizure disorder, heart disease, thyroid disorder, iodine insufficiency) or substance use (drugs, alcohol, or smoking), infections (see section below), placental insufficiency or thrombosis (clotting) of the placenta or umbilical cord.[15] **Placental insufficiency** disrupts gas, nutrient and waste exchange as well as immune and endocrine responses. **Placental insufficiency** can stem from structural abnormalities in the placenta, its attachment or blood flow to the baby.[16] This results in ongoing hypoxia and impaired nutrition of the developing fetus, which can result in a condition known as **intrauterine growth restriction** (IUGR) where overall growth of the fetus, including brain development, is impeded.[17] Babies with IUGR are at high risk of CP that has been reported as high as 30-fold; however, IUGR is also associated with other neurologic consequences such as epilepsy and intellectual disabilities.[18] Notably, multiple births are at greater risk for IUGR, and therefore, CP. There are also other reasons for the increased incidence of CP in pregnancies with multiple babies, including the likelihood of premature birth (Box 20-1).[19] Maternal metabolic disorders (e.g., diabetes), ingestion of toxins, and rare genetic syndromes are also known contributors to neurological disorders in childhood, including CP.[17] Events that occur in mid-gestation (24-32 weeks) are most likely to damage the perventricular white matter, since its blood supply is most vulnerable at that time; damage here is likely to affect white matter projections from the leg area of the motor cortex, resulting in diplegia. Near term events (peripartum) impact areas of highest metabolic need with damage dependent on magnitude (see perinatal asphyxia).[19]

Perinatal asphyxia refers to a disruption of oxygen, resulting in a period of anoxia to the developing brain, that takes place during fetal development, labor, delivery, or the neonatal period (after birth) that results in brain damage, referred to as **hypoxic-ischemic encephalopathy** (HIE).[20,21] Perinatal asphyxia accounts for about 10% of the cases of CP.[19] A short period of severe asphyxia in late term has its greatest effect on areas with high concentrations of neurons such as the thalamus and basal ganglia, producing an extrapyramidal pattern of rigidity.[15] In very severe cases, cysts develop subcortically, resulting in a severe form of quadriplegic CP with mental retardation.[14] Prolonged asphyxia that is less severe is more likely to produce diffuse damage in the subcortical white matter, which presents with upper motor neuron symptoms, including spasticity or a combination of spasticity and dystonia.[19] Notably, the vasculature of the fetal brain is very fragile, putting it at risk for an infarction or hemorrhage. The most common area of injury is the middle cerebral artery (MCA), which supplies blood to portions of the frontal, parietal, and temporal lobes. This means that a large proportion of brain tissue is at risk; if there is an infarction of the MCA (see Chapter 11 for information on the MCA), a hemiplegic pattern of injury will result.[19] Asphyxia can result from abnormalities of the placenta or thrombosis of the placenta or umbilical cord; however, there are many other causative events. During labor and delivery there is a possibility of the umbilical cord wrapping around the infant's neck and impeding respiration, during the initial moments of extrauterine life. Also, neonates may excrete their first bowel movement (**meconium** – a dark pasty stool) during labor, permitting aspiration of the substance by the baby that impedes breathing upon delivery.[19] **Placental previa** refers to an abnormal attachment of the placenta to the uterine wall such that it partially or completely covers the cervix; it may be associated with abnormal bleeding, during the pregnancy, especially in the last trimester, and thus, diminished oxygenation for the baby in the latter stages of gestation. Also, **placental abruption**, which refers to premature detachment of the placenta from the uterine wall, can also be a source of fetal hypoxia in utero and prematurity. Since partial abruption can occur fairly early (2nd to 3rd trimester), it can result in a period of prolonged hypoxia prior to delivery and, thereby, significant brain damage in the developing baby. Notably, abruption is also a cause for premature delivery.[16] Occasionally, the umbilical cord comes out of the vaginal canal before the head of the baby, referred to as **umbilical cord prolapse**; this is a medical emergency because of the immediate threat of cutting off the oxygen and blood supply to the fetus as well as the likelihood of abruption and subsequent maternal hemorrhage.[20,22] **Pre-eclampsia**, which is a maternal condition of pregnancy, is characterized by hypertension and proteinuria (protein in the urine) secondary to kidney dysfunction and can result in fetal growth restriction, premature birth, and placental abruption. Early onset pre-eclampsia (<34 weeks gestation) results from abnormal development of the placenta, and while less common, it is more likely to result in maternal or neonatal death or severe neonatal impairments, including CP. Late pre-eclampsia (after 34 weeks gestation) is less well understood but may be secondary to pathology of the placenta as well. Maternal consequences of pre-eclampsia are kidney or liver failure, pulmonary edema, and stroke, which is the most common cause of maternal fatality.[23] In early pre-eclampsia, mothers are carefully monitored to maintain the baby in utero for as long as possible without severely compromising the mother; in late pre-eclampsia, especially if after 37 weeks, delivery by C-section is typically conducted. The progression of pre-eclampsia to **eclampsia** is a life-threatening situation for both mother and baby; in eclampsia, the mother can experience convulsions, coma, and potentially death. The baby's life is also in jeopardy, since oxygenation can be disrupted, with the risk of CP or other developmental disorder likely, if the baby survives.[23]

Infection is a common cause of CP in both the natal and postnatal time frames. For the fetus, immune function is dependent on the maternal immune system. Some pathogens can cross the placenta and cause infection. Maternal illnesses can be unsafe for a fetus, causing spontaneous abortion or major developmental disorders (including CP), while others have no effect. Maternal infections such as chorioamnionitis (infection in the membranes surrounding the fetus), genitourinary tract or respiratory infections are associated with an increased occurrence of CP; in addition, the use of antibiotics, especially for multiple occurrences, seems tied to the incidence rate of CP.[24,25] Multiple viruses have been associated with congenital consequences with **rubella** (measles) the first to be identified; maternal infection with rubella is linked to deafness, eye abnormalities, congenital heart defects, developmental delay, learning disabilities, and CP; while rubella is uncommon in the United States due to vaccinations, it may still occur in developing countries or in those not vaccinated. **Cytomegalovirus (CMV)** is a variant of the herpes virus, which can lead to a chronic condition with mild symptoms in the mother but can cause IUGR and multiple neurologic consequences, including CP, other developmental problems with hearing loss most common, as well as multi-organ abnormalities. HIV has also been linked to both neurodevelopmental as well as neuropsychiatric disorders. The Zika virus outbreak of 2015 in south America highlighted the impact of RNA viruses on development; these are viruses encoded by ribonucleic acid; the Zika outbreak resulted in many infants born with microcephaly and other severe developmental consequences.[25,26]

Perinatal Birth Trauma can cause a lack of oxygen to the brain that can result in a brain injury and subsequent CP. **Obstructed labor** occurs when the fetus has difficulty fitting through the vaginal canal, typically from **cephalo-pelvic incompatibility** (the baby's head is too big for the mother's pelvis), resulting in too much and repeated force on the skull of the fetus as the mother attempts to push the baby out. This is uncommon in developed countries but continues to be a cause of brain damage and CP in undeveloped countries where cesarian births are inaccessible. Damage to the brachial plexus can also occur with obstructed labor, when the shoulders are too wide for the pelvis.[27] Historically, the use of forceps has been linked to the occurrence of CP; however, a recent report suggests that while non-surgical vaginal deliveries have the least occurrence of poor outcomes, forcep and cesarian deliveries have similar outcomes when prior fetal distress is taken into account, which explains the similar rate of CP as forcep use has decreased and cesarian deliveries have increased.[28]

Postnatal Causes of CP

A CP diagnosis is typically given to children that acquire brain injury in the first 3 years of life; approximately 8 to 10% of children with CP have a causative postnatal event.[1,14] Causes of such brain damage include (1) metabolic encephalopathy, (2) primary infections such as meningitis or malaria, (3) trauma such as shaken baby syndrome, or (4) infantile stroke.[14] Metabolic

encephalopathy can result from disrupted kidney or liver function, toxicity from an ingested or inhaled toxin (including alcohol or drug toxicity, which can be transmitted through breast milk), or subsequent to electrolyte disturbance, associated with an acute illness (e.g., diarrhea with a high fever). Shaken baby syndrome, as the name implies, results from shaking a baby, typically in the first year of life, causing stretching or shearing of white matter and capillaries. The resultant brain damage typically presents with quadriplegia.[14]

● RISK FACTORS

Although CP is not apparent at birth, there are many factors associated with an increased risk of CP. These factors are correlational, meaning there is an association, but they are not causal. Maternal risk factors have been extensively studied; paternal risk factors have been relatively ignored. In earlier sections, we have described maternal conditions that place one at risk for having a child with CP; these include substance abuse and medical conditions (seizure disorder, diabetes, thyroid disorders, cardiopulmonary disorders, including hypertension); in addition, women who have a history of delayed menstruation; prior miscarriage, preterm birth, or an existing child with a motor deficit; or are of advanced age are at greater risk for having a baby with CP and other developmental disorders (e.g., Down syndrome). Similarly, there is some suggestion that advanced paternal age can be a contributing factor. Low APGAR scores, which are an indication of fetal distress at birth (see Box 20-2) are also associated with greater occurrence of CP.

Box 20-2	Neonatal Assessment – APGAR

At delivery all newborns undergo a quick assessment, known as the APGAR to determine their overall well-being upon delivery; each is assessed at 1 and 5 minutes on each of the following:

A – appearance (skin color): pink all over = 2, pink body with blue extremities = 1, blue = 0

P – pulse: normal rate (>100 beats/min) = 2, slow (<100 beats/min) = 1, no pulse = 0

G – grimace (response to mild pinch): strong cry, extremity withdrawal or facial grimace = 2, milder response (weak cry, little movement) = 1, no response = 0

A – activity (muscle tone): actively moving = 2, some flexion of limbs = 1, no movement = 0

R – respiration (airway): strong cry = 2, weak cry or respiratory effort = 1, no breathing = 0

Obviously, a perfect score is 10, but since the birth process is fairly traumatic to a baby, many will score below that level, especially in terms of color as many babies have a blue hue in the first minutes after birth but will be fine. In fact, APGAR scores of 7 to 10 are considered normal; scores of 4 to 6 are of some concern, especially if they don't improve at the 5-minute assessment; scores of 0 to 3 indicate a need for immediate resuscitation and place the baby at risk for subsequent developmental problems. Infants with low APGAR scores are much more likely to have CP than those that score in the normal range.[29]

● DIAGNOSIS

Despite the precipitating injury typically occurring in the perinatal period, historically CP was commonly not diagnosed until 18 months to 2 years of age, when an obvious absence of major motor milestones (e.g., creeping and walking) and the presence of abnormal muscle tone became apparent. This is still true in many geographical areas and health systems. In 2017 an important paper was published on the diagnostic criteria for CP, which outlined magnetic resonance imaging, the Prechtl Qualitative Assessment of General Movements, and the Hammersmith Infant Neurological Examination to be used for early diagnosis.[30] With implementation of these criteria, many hospital systems and networks have reduced the average age of CP diagnosis.[31] Children with greater severity or often those with hemiplegia may be diagnosed earliest, but the early diagnostic criteria do not assess topography or severity. Those with greater severity often have associated eating problems, limited head control, and more severe muscle tone abnormalities such as hypotonia or spasticity that make diagnosis at an earlier age easier. Those with hemiplegia have an obvious disparity in limb movement, alerting observant parents and pediatricians to the limited use of one arm and leg. However, many physicians have historically taken a "wait and see" approach to the diagnosis in an attempt to avoid inappropriate labeling of the child, providing a "developmental delay" label initially and waiting to see if early intervention will resolve the delay. This approach has been shown to increase, rather than decrease parent well-being, so current recommendations are to use the tests listed above, which have strong sensitivity and specificity, to give a diagnosis when possible, or label at risk for CP, and then refer infants to CP-specific programs such as hip surveillance or constraint-induced movement therapy.[30] Often abnormalities of tone and delayed motor skill acquisition become more apparent in the 2nd year of life, making the diagnosis clear. From a medical perspective the diagnosis is based on the clinical presentation, requiring a combination of abnormal tone, altered deep tendon reflexes (e.g., Achilles tendon reflex), delayed motor development, and postural instability.[32] Neuroimaging can assist in a diagnosis to document a localized lesion, apparent brain malformation, or PVL (see Box 20-2) when present.[32] General movement analysis (GMA) involves categorizing infant movements, based on typical patterns. In brief, infants demonstrate what are called **writhing movements** (large slow extremity movement) from the third trimester of gestation to 9 weeks post-delivery and then transition to fidgety movements (small and irregular) at about 7 weeks, which continue until up to 20 weeks, when more purposeful movements become the majority of movements.[33] Altered writhing movements, called cramped synchronized, and atypical fidgety movements (either abnormal or absent), are predictive of CP. Cramped synchronized movements are characterized by a quick onset and offset (abrupt) and appear rigid.[34] **Fidgety movements** are considered abnormal when they are exaggerated in amplitude, speed, and smoothness (more jerky than normal); the absence of fidgety movements, during the expected timeframe, is also considered abnormal.[35]

CASE A, PART III

Alejandro was followed in a high-risk clinic for the first year of his life. One month after discharge from the NICU, he was diagnosed with myoclonic seizures that appeared like startle reactions without a precipitating stimulus and was given sodium valproate (see Table 20-4 later in this chapter when epilepsy is discussed). At his 3-month visit, the physical therapist noted that he had increased tone in his legs and always kicked with both legs simultaneously (no alternating kicks) with associated movements in the trunk and arms. The physical therapist used the GMA and categorized his spontaneous movements as "absent fidgety." Since Alejandro had objective signs of motor dysfunction using the GMA, abnormal neuroimaging on MRI with a lesion in the periventricular white matter *and* a perinatal birth history of prematurity and seizures, the physician and the therapist diagnosed "high risk of CP" and referred him to an early intervention program and the cerebral palsy clinic at their local hospital. In the EI program, he received PT 2–3 times per week within the class environment to facilitate the development of motor skills. He rolled in both directions by 8 months, pushed into quadruped by 11, and back into w-sitting by his first birthday. Therapy, at this time, was directed at increasing his ability to sit in different positions, reaching and weight-shift in quadruped to stimulate creeping, and standing activities (see later section on treatment).

Classification

Functional classification is descriptive of the way the child performs common functional motor activities. The most common, evidence-based, and helpful way to classify and predict future motor function of children with CP is the Gross Motor Function Classification System (GMFCS), which is a five-level system that categorizes children with CP, based on the motor function and limitation in daily motor abilities, based on the Gross Motor Function Measure (see Box 20-3). Classification levels are based on independent motor function and the use of assistive technology for mobility. They create meaningful comparisons for research studies, can guide treatment goal setting, and allow for accurate counseling, planning, and education for families and children with CP. Lower levels, starting with level I, indicate better motor function and fewer functional limitations. Broadly, children classified as GMFCS level I walk independently and have few motor impairments or limitations in daily life. Their impairments may not be noticeable until they perform high-level motor skills like advanced sports or skills that require precise coordination and timing (e.g., kicking a ball, climbing, riding a bike). Higher levels, ending with level V, indicate more severe limitations in motor function, limited independence, and higher use of assistive devices or powered mobility. Children with GMFCS level V have little to no antigravity movements or voluntary motor control and are dependent on a

---

Box 20-3   Gross Motor Function Measure

The Gross Motor Function Measure (GMFM) is an assessment tool for children ages 5 months to 16 years with CP that was used to develop the GMFCS levels. There are two versions of the GMFM, the GMFM-88 and GMFM-66, with the number corresponding to the number of items on the tool. All 66 items on the GMFM-66 are on the GMFM-88, so if the 88 is tested in the clinic, both 88 and 66 scores can be easily calculated. The GMFM is standardized and has five dimensions of gross motor function: (1) lying and rolling; (2) crawling and kneeling; (3) sitting; (4) standing; and (5) walking, running, and jumping. GMFCS levels have been plotted from GMFM-66 scores over time (age) to demonstrate when children show 90% of their maximal expected motor function. It is important to note that there is a plateau and/or decline in motor function for all levels after age 8, indicating the likelihood that children will not acquire new skills after this age and may lose skills, often secondary to increasing body size, greater influence of tone, and acquired orthopedic conditions that in insolation or combination make moving more difficult.[36]

---

caregiver for all aspects of care. They are transported by a caregiver or use a power chair with lots of postural support (see Box 20-4 for additional details).[37]

GMFCS levels are further clarified by age with separate descriptions for levels I-V in the following age ranges: less than 2, between 2 and 4, 4-6, 6–12, and 12-18. GMFSC levels are fairly stable overtime. For children classified after age 2, 82 to 87% stay at the same level; however, for those classified earlier than 2, there is more variability with up to 40% being reclassified by one or two levels.[38] Children in levels I and V are most likely to be reclassified.[36,37] While children in levels I and II tend to maintain their level of function, those at levels III-IV show a decline in function, during adolescence but remain in the same GMFCS level.[39] All information on the GMFCS levels and descriptions of each level can be found on the CanChild web page,[11] with free and meaningful assessment tools and descriptions of motor function for children with CP at different ages.[40]

Severity of Functional Impairment

The categories of mild, moderate, and severe are used to quickly and easily communicate general levels of impairment, when

---

Box 20-4   GMFCS Levels[37]

- Level I – Walks and runs independently in all settings but may be slower or less coordinated than peers
- Level II – Walks independently but has limitations in running, with uneven surfaces and stairs (may require handrail or two step/tread pattern)
- Level III – Walks with an assistive device in most settings and/or uses a manual wheelchair
- Level IV – Limited standing and walking ability, often with assistance; primarily uses power wheelchair
- Level V – Very limited mobility; reliant on caregiver support for movement and wheelchair propulsion; may use powered mobility

---

specific details are not needed. In general, **mild** means that the child can move and complete daily activities without assistance and may have limitations with higher-level motor skills such as sports or activities that require more advanced coordination. **Moderate** means that the child will need some assistance from a caregiver and/or adaptive equipment including braces, mobility aids, or technology in order to participate in daily activities. **Severe** means that the child cannot move very well independently, will need a wheelchair to move or be transported, and will need assistance from a caregiver for most or all daily activities. GMFCS levels are used when detail about functional status and prediction are necessary.

Typography (Body Area(s) Affected)

The categories of quadriplegia, diplegia, hemiplegia, and triplegia are used to describe the extremities affected by abnormal tone and movement impairment. **Quadriplegia** means all four limbs and the trunk/head are affected, often the arms more than the legs. Typically, those with quadriplegia are more disabled than those in the other typography groups and are more likely to have associated conditions. **Diplegia** means both lower extremities are affected, and the upper extremities are not affected or affected to a lesser degree than the lower extremities; the trunk and neck muscles are typically not impaired or only mildly impaired. **Hemiplegia** means that one side of the body, an ipsilateral upper and lower extremity are affected; in some, there is also an asymmetry of trunk involvement on the same side as the extremities. (*Much recent research suggests that the "non-affected" side in hemiplegia also has some changes in function though much more mild than the "affected" side, so terms like paretic and nonparetic are often used to distinguish the more involved side from the lesser involved side*).[14] These typography categories are illustrated in Figure 20-1. **Triplegia** is a term that is occasionally used when all four extremities are affected, but one extremity has much more function in comparison to the other three; the head and trunk are also affected. Movements of children with triplegia are initiated with the highest functioning extremity.[6]

Type (Predominate Motor/Muscle Tone Characteristic)

The categories of spastic, dyskinetic (athetosis, chorea), ataxic, and hypotonic are used to describe the primary motor characteristics of CP, including tone and accessory or involuntary movements, and the frequency of occurrence is consistent with the order in which they are listed. It should be noted that, since CP occurs in the developing brain, widespread brain damage may result rather than the focal damage discussed with stroke; thus, it is possible for CP to present with "mixed" types of muscle tone variations that may impact different body parts, be influenced by body position, or may present differently in infancy than at older ages. Up to 10% of children with CP will present with mixed muscle tone.[41] Some information on prevalence of motor characteristic and area of the brain implicated for the types of CP are discussed in Box 20-5.

Integration of topography, type, and severity classifications provides a comprehensive description of a child's presentation. However, the characteristics may change over time or children may present with mixed types, so this language can lead to confusion for families and medical professionals. GMFCS levels are the most widely used and reliable way to classify individual children with CP and group children with CP in research studies.

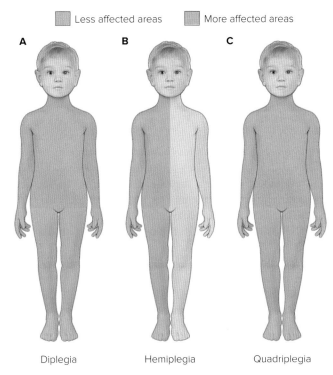

☐ Less affected areas   ☐ More affected areas

A   **B**   **C**

Diplegia   Hemiplegia   Quadriplegia

FIGURE 20-1 Representation of typography. A. Diplegia – greater involvement of the legs than arms and trunk.
B. Hemiplegia – greater involvement of the contralateral arm and leg with little trunk involvement and very mild ipsilateral involvement from the side of the lesion. **C.** Quadriplegia – all four extremities are involved (arms often more than legs and trunk).

CASE A, PART IV

At age 3, Alejandro presents with hypertonia and hyperreflexia in all four extremities (legs much greater than arms) and 5 degrees of hip and knee flexion contracture of both legs. He sits on the floor by "w-sitting," can creep on hands and knees without reciprocal leg movements, moving first both arms and then both legs, and takes steps in his preschool classroom using a reverse walker. No cognitive, learning, or language delays have been noted. He lives in a two-story house with one bathroom on the second floor; he is carried up and down the stairs.

Alejandro is presenting with moderate spastic diplegia with a GMFCS of III. Since he is 3, with spasticity and hyperreflexia of both arms and legs (mild in the arms and moderate in the legs), and limited walking at age 3, he has a moderate level of involvement. The combination of hypertonia and hyperreflexia is consistent with spasticity, and the presentation of greater involvement of the legs versus the arms meets the distribution (topography) of diplegia. He is beginning to ambulate with a reverse walker, so is not independent in his ambulation (GMFCS levels I and II), thus, placing him in GMFCS III. He is still using a stroller for community mobility but may be a candidate for a manual wheelchair soon.

Box 20-5   Motor Characteristics in CP[30,42,43]

Spastic – Spastic CP is characterized by hypertonia (spasticity) and hyperreflexia of deep tendon reflexes (DTRs). Remember, spasticity is a velocity-dependent resistance to passive stretch that can be measured with the modified Ashworth Scale (see Chapter 10 for details). Spastic CP is associated with damage to the cerebral cortex and pyramidal tracts. Damage to these areas also results in poor force generation in muscles and often an imbalance of muscle activity at joints. As is found with spasticity in adult conditions, the muscles typically affected in children are the UE flexors at all joints with the shoulder internal rotators and the hip flexors and adductors, the hamstrings at the knee, and the plantarflexors at the ankle. Children with spastic diplegia will have much less spasticity in their UE than LE but in these same muscle groups where present (some or all UE muscles may have normal tone). Children with spastic CP account for 85–90% of children with CP with decreasing occurrence from hemiplegia (38%), diplegia (37%), quadriplegia (24%), and triplegia (1%)[30]; therefore, the remaining types are sometimes grouped together as **non-spastic CP** and typically affect all four extremities

Dyskinetic (4-7%) – Disruption of the basal ganglia and its connections to the motor cortex produces abnormal involuntary movements and difficulty in movement coordination. This can present in multiple variations of movement that are distinguished by the speed and appearance of the involuntary movements. **Athetosis** is characterized by slow writhing (worm-like) movements that typically impact the distal portion of the limbs more than the proximal joints. **Chorea** is characterized by more rapid involuntary movements that can involve any part of the body (face, limbs, trunk). **Choreoathetosis** represents a combination of athetosis and chorea, in which both distal athetoid movements and proximal chorea movements occur. **Ballismus**, as the name suggests, involves quick jerky movements of the entire extremity as though the limb is "blasting" through the air, involving the proximal joints primarily. **Dystonia** is characterized by sustained co-contractions of muscles, leading to maintained postures often with twisting of the trunk or limbs and resulting from disrupted inhibition as a motion is initiated; these postures may be quite uncomfortable to the child, yet they will have difficulty moving out of the posture.

Ataxic (4-6%) – Ataxic CP is characterized by difficulty with coordination, balance, and initiating movement, resulting from damage of the cerebellum; like adults with cerebellar dysfunction, children with ataxic CP have trouble with co-contraction of muscles, so their movements are characterized by over and under-shooting of targets, swaying in a maintained posture, and a wide-based stance in weightbearing postures and when walking to provide stability. Notably, children with ataxic CP also display mild to moderate hypotonia as the cerebellum contributes to the generation of resting muscle tone. Thus, this is often referred to as hypotonic-ataxic CP, and some do not distinguish a separate hypotonic classification. In children with ataxic CP, DTRs are normal. Also, an **intention tremor** is common; with this type of tremor, the oscillation of the extremity increases during a directed movement (e.g., reaching).[42]

Hypotonic/Atonic (2%) – Hypotonic CP is characterized by low muscle tone and decreased DTRs and is thought to result of widespread brain damage most commonly in early fetal development. However, it should be noted that some children will present as hypotonic early in infancy but at later ages will present with dyskinetic, ataxic, or mixed CP. Also, some children with hypotonia will present with hyperreflexia rather than hyporeflexia. Some countries do not include this in their classification because it is so rare.

Mixed – Refers to a combination of the motor presentations of more than one of the above groups, often dyskinesia with spasticity.

MOTOR PATTERNS OF CHILDREN WITH CP

As should be evident from the preceding discussion, CP is a highly heterogeneous disorder, yet pediatric physical therapists can expect some common movement patterns in children with this disorder, depending on type of tone and its distribution and severity. General findings are that motor development will be delayed due to nervous system damage, abnormal tone and strength in major muscle groups, and potentially, the presence of other conditions such as orthopedic deformities and cognitive impairment (discussed later in this chapter). In addition, children with CP, especially those with spasticity, display impaired selective motor control, which refers to the ability to isolate flexion and extension movements at individual joints to create independent joint movement; thus, children with CP tend to move in patterns of total flexion or extension or experience unwanted co-contraction of flexors and extensors, when trying to move. Therefore, they are delayed in the development of motor skills as well as protective and equilibrium reactions (see Chapter 8 for description of each of these) and have decreased flexibility and variability in their movement patterns. For children with dystonic CP, this is coupled with involuntary movements that further impeded selective control.[44]

Head Control

Many children with CP will present with delayed development of head control. Surprisingly, children with hypertonia, dystonia, and hypotonia, including those that will develop ataxia, demonstrate poor antigravity neck strength and poor co-contraction of the neck muscles necessary for upright head control beyond the first few months of life, yet they often can momentarily lift their heads in prone, using their neck extensors but can't maintain it upright, since they lack co-contraction of the flexors and extensors necessary for this. When pulled to sit, they demonstrate poor neck flexion, similar to young infants, such that the head lags behind the shoulders (Figure 20-2), but those with spasticity will appear to have a strong arm pull that is not truly "strong," since it is generated by spasticity. Many children with tetraplegia, either with spasticity or dystonia, may never acquire adequate head control, and are likely to be classified as GMFCS IV or V. Not surprisingly, children with hemiplegia tend to develop head control much like their typical peers; those with diplegia may have a delay but will usually attain good head control.[42] Early PT should target head control, as it is a precursor for more advanced movements.

Rolling

Quadriplegia: Children with spastic or dystonic quadriplegia are not only delayed in their rolling, but if they are able to roll, will typically use a log roll, since they have difficulty dissociating the upper trunk from the lower trunk and the arms from the legs. In other words, they tend to move in patterns of total flexion or total extension. Also, they are often influenced by a persisting ATNR, which pulls their skull-side extremities into flexion, making it difficult for them to incorporate these limbs into the roll. So, when rolling prone to supine, they will extend their head and trunk, turn their head, and appear to "fall" into supine with little involvement of the extremities (they may push up with hands if able); this may be facilitated by the presence of the STNR, which triggers UE extension when the head is lifted and the ATNR, which will trigger some skull-side UE flexion as the head is turned. When rolling supine to prone, which is often quite delayed, if achieved at all, children with spastic quadriplegia or dystonia tend to assume a complete flexion pattern (head, trunk, legs), often leading with the legs, which may be less involved, and using the body-on-body reaction and much effort to move to prone. In those with limited neck flexor strength, the head doesn't contribute much to the roll. In addition, it is common for the arm, over which they are rolling, to be "caught" underneath them, and they may not have the ability to shift their weight to free it. For children with ataxia or hypotonia, rolling requires achieving sufficient antigravity strength to move out of supine or prone, and some will not be able to do so. However, those that do, lead with their strongest body part – head, arm, or leg, facilitated by the body-on-body reaction. Those at GMFCS level V often do not roll without assistance but those at level IV and above commonly achieve rolling.[45] When treating a child with quadriplegia to facilitate rolling, therapy targets head control, reaching across midline with both the arms and legs, increasing trunk rotation to move from a log to

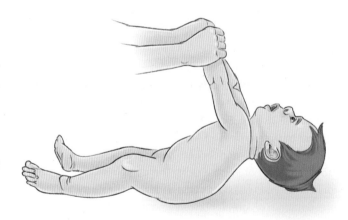

FIGURE 20-2 Head lag in cerebral palsy. Many children with cerebral palsy of all types will show early head lag when pulled to sit; as they age the LE and UE may show increased tone (spasticity) pulling the arms and legs into flexion but the head may still lag behind the shoulders. (Reproduced with permission from Carney PR, & Geyer JD, eds. *Pediatric Practice: Neurology.* New York, NY: McGraw-Hill; 2010. Fig. 11-1, Part A Only.)

a segmental roll, and weight-shift to facilitate freeing the arm, after rolling.

Diplegia: Since head control is typically good to normal in those with diplegia, children with this type of CP tend to roll close to the 6- to 8-month mark but may exhibit some of the total flexion/extension of their peers with quadriplegia, depending on the degree of tone expressed. Most will lead with their head and arms with little leg contribution; for many, the legs will be strongly extended, when rolling. They may also log roll longer than their typical peers but often will acquire a segmental roll, at least of the head and upper trunk, if not the legs.[46] Therapy targets trunk rotation, moving the leg past midline and achieving a segmental roll.

Hemiplegia: For children with hemiplegia, they may initially only roll in one direction toward or over their paretic side (supine to prone – will reach across their trunk with their non-paretic arm and leg and roll over their paretic side; prone to supine – will reach back with their non-paretic arm and leg and roll over their paretic side). Eventually, they will be able to roll in both directions, using a segmental roll. Therapy targets facilitating rolling in both directions.

Sitting

For children at GMFCS levels V, sitting is not achieved without external support or assistance. For those at GMFCS level IV, sitting will be delayed, but most will be able to sit, when placed into the position, but may not be able to assume the position; most will also require upper extremity support, of at least one arm, to maintain upright and will be delayed in developing protective and equilibrium reactions or may not develop them. Spasticity in their hamstrings may result in a posterior pelvic tilt that pulls them backward and makes sitting difficult; positions that diminish the effect of this spasticity (e.g., ring or tailor sitting) will be easier for them to maintain but harder to assume. Ring sitting is a position with the legs slightly bent in front of the child such that they form a "ring"; tailor sitting is a position where the knees and hips are flexed such that the heels are near the knee of the opposite leg (one or both may be under the knee). Children that can achieve sitting independently, especially those at GMFCS level III, often push back from prone or quadruped and assume a w-sitting position (bottom between heels) with an anterior pelvic tilt. Although this position strains the hips, which may already be at risk for hip dysplasia (see Table 20-1), it is easier to access than any other sitting posture and provides a wide base of support for those with poorer trunk control, so it is common for children with all types of CP except hemiplegia to prefer w-sitting. Overtime, many develop more flexibility in sitting with the ability to assume other sitting positions and acquire protective and equilibrium reactions to free their arms for play. Children at GMFCS I and II will easily assume sitting and will be able to move into and out of sitting easily, developing appropriate protective and equilibrium reactions. Those with hemiplegia tend to ring or side-sit initially with weight on the non-paretic arm; however, they typically are independent sitters with more flexibility than their peers with quadriplegic or diplegic presentations. To facilitate sitting, therapy should include sitting in a variety of positions, reaching in all directions, and disturbing the child's balance to stimulate equilibrium and protective responses while providing sufficient support so the child doesn't fall. Often balls or bolsters are used as sitting surfaces to allow mild disturbances of balance as the child reaches or plays at a table.

Crawling/Creeping

For clarification, crawling is used to describe movement on the belly that involves reciprocal and alternating movement of the arms and legs; in contrast, creeping is that same movement pattern in quadruped (all fours). Laymen usually call the latter crawling, so it may help the novice to think of this as belly crawling and quadruped creeping. Unhelpfully, some standardized tools and other countries use different definitions for crawling and creeping, so knowledge of the specific tool is paramount to scoring it correctly. Children at GMFCS levels V do not achieve either of these movement patterns. Those at level IV may achieve crawling but rarely creeping, and they tend to move with limited dissociation of limbs (total flexion, followed by total extension) Those at level III, especially those with spasticity, will also use a bilateral symmetrical UE/LE pattern and achieve both crawling and creeping (often called bunny hopping); the STNR may facilitate this pattern (*head extension leading to UE extension and LE flexion forward; head flexion with UE flexion and LE extension to propel them forward*). Some children mature into an alternating pattern; children with diplegia may alternate with their arms but not their legs, depending on severity. Children at levels I and II will achieve mature crawling and creeping, sometimes with mild asymmetry of movement.[53] *Note: children with hemiplegia may or may not crawl or creep due to their asymmetric presentation; it is not uncommon for these children to scoot in sitting, pulling, and pushing with their non-paretic arm and leg, respectively. Reaching activities in prone-prop (elbows or hands) or quadruped (with or without support of a bolster or wedge) can be used to increase UE strength and the ability to dissociate the movements of the arms. Wheelbarrow walking (walking on the hands with legs and/or trunk supported) is also a good way to increase UE strength and dissociation in those that are able to do so.*

Standing and Walking

Children at GMFCS level V do not stand or walk but may benefit from supported standing activities. Those at level IV will usually be able to achieve standing with assistance and may walk in a limited fashion with assistive devices and caregiver assistance, especially when turning; in contrast, those at level III can typically walk around their house or classroom with assistive devices but will use a wheelchair for community mobility, the playground, or longer distances within their school. By definition, those at levels I and II are independent community ambulators, differing most in the higher-level skills that they acquire (e.g., running, skipping, ball manipulation) with those in level I performing more activities with mild incoordination and those at level II typically not achieving jumping and running.[37] Children with hemiplegic CP can present with four different gait deviations: (1) foot drop during swing, associated with anterior tibialis weakness; (2) foot drop with plantarflexion during stance and knee hyperextension due to gastric and soleus spasticity; (3) characteristics of #2 plus limited knee flexion with excessive

TABLE 20-1	Orthopedic Conditions Associated with Cerebral Palsy	
JOINT	**CONDITION**	**DESCRIPTION**
Trunk[47]	Scoliosis	Asymmetry of muscle tone and strength in the trunk muscles can result in abnormal rotation and scoliosis of the trunk. Scoliosis is most common in those with spastic quadriplegia or dystonia.
	Kyphosis	Asymmetry between trunk flexors and extensors as well as posturing can result in a kyphotic deformity; this may also occur in combination with scoliosis.
Hip/thigh[48,49]	Hip dysplasia	Spasticity of the hip flexors, adductors, and internal rotators in association with elongated and weak hip extensors can allow the femoral head to be pulled in the direction of the spastic muscles. In addition, delayed standing can limit the deepening of the acetabulum that should occur. Together, these factors place the hip at risk for subluxation or dislocation. Sitting postures, especially w-sitting with the buttocks between the heels, further place the hip at risk. HD occurs in up to 30% of children with spasticity and 50% of those with quadriplegic spasticity. HD can also occur in the non-spastic forms of CP due to poor or asymmetrical muscle control at the hip, delayed or absent standing, and a reliance on abnormal postures (e.g., w-sitting).
	Femoral anteversion	Tight adductors and internal rotators can place an abnormal pull on the distal femur that over time increases the natural amount of femoral anteversion; this may contribute to other LE abnormalities.
Knee[50]	Flexion contracture	Spasticity of the hamstrings occurs in all forms of spastic CP; for those that spend most of their time in a wheelchair or seated position, significant shortening of the hamstrings with decreasing extensor strength at the knee can occur.
	Genu varum	With femoral anteversion, secondary to adductor and internal rotation spasticity/shortening, the knee is pulled medially and there is a lateral compensation of the lower leg. This contributes to a crouched gait along with hamstring spasticity/shortening, weak quadriceps and hip extensors, and equinovarus in the foot.
	Genu recurvatum	Knee recurvatum is most common in children with an equinus deformity at the ankle due to gastrocnemius spasticity or hamstrings that are too long (often after lengthening or dorsal rhizotomy) or too weak to oppose the gastroc spasticity; the pull of the gastrocnemius on the distal femur draws it posterior during stance as the proximal femur advances forward, resulting in hyperextension at the knee (recurvatum).
Ankle/foot[51]	Equinus	Spasticity of the gastrocnemius plus weak dorsiflexors can result in a plantar flexion deformity with secondary decrease in dorsiflexion and resultant gait abnormalities.
	Equinovalgus	Equinus of the ankle in association with eversion and pronation of the foot results from shortening of the gastroc and peroneal muscles; weight is born on the medial aspect of the foot.
	Equinovarus	Equinus of the ankle with inversion of the foot due to spasticity of the gastroc/soleus, flexor digitorum and hallucis, and posterior tibialis with weakness of the opposing muscles. This is the most common foot deformity in CP.
Shoulder[52]	Shoulder dysplasia	Spasticity of the internal rotators and adductors and secondary tightness of the joint capsule can pull the humeral head from the socket, resulting in subluxation or dislocation.
	Adductor contractures	Spasticity in the pectoralis major, teres major, and latissimus dorsi can occur, limiting abduction.
Elbow[52]	Flexor contractures	Spasticity of the biceps brachi and brachioradialis is common with the arm held in flexion at the elbow and loss of ROM over time.
Forearm[52]	Pronation contracture	Spasticity in the pronator teres and quadratus with weak supinators can lead to a contracture. Usually occurs with an elbow flexion contracture
Wrist[52]	Contracture	Spasticity in the flexor muscle(s) — flexor carpi ulnaris and radialis with weak wrist extensors can occur, especially in those with severe spasticity, limiting hand use.
Hand[52]	Swan-neck deformity	This is a deformity of hyperflexion of the distal IP joint with hyperextension of the proximal IP joint due to spasticity in the finger flexors and slippage of the extensor tendon laterally within its sheath
	Thumb in palm	Spasticity of the thumb adductors with weakness in thumb abduction can lead to an adducted thumb within the flexed fingers; this severely limits hand function.

hip flexion and lordosis during swing; and (4) characteristics of 1 and 3 with limited hip and knee excursion.[54] Children with spasticity, whether diplegic or quadriplegic, tend to have similar LE presentation of their spastic limbs when standing and walking, if these are achieved (see Figure 20-3). Four patterns are also noted: crouched, true equinus, jump (stiff knee), and apparent equinus. **Crouched gait** includes hip and knee flexion (crouching), internal rotation with adduction of the hip (genu valgum), and excessive dorsiflexion, usually with pes planus, during stance. **True equinus** presents with equinus throughout stance with hip and knee extension, often with knee recurvatum that masks the severity of the equinus. **Jump gait**, incorporates the former stiff knee gait, presenting with excessive ankle, hip, and knee flexion with an anterior pelvic tilt and excessive lordosis. The limb is rapidly progressed as though "jumped" from one stance phase to the next. During swing, children with a jump gait will have difficulty clearing their toes, due to limited limb flexion at all joints and may exhibit scissoring of the legs due to excessive adductor tone. In **apparent equinus**, as the name implies, there is an appearance of toe-walking due to excessive hip and knee flexion, but the ankle range of motion is normal.[54] All of these spastic gait patterns are characterized by a shortened stride length, shortened single limb stance phase, and increased energy expenditure during gait. Children with ataxia, if they achieve walking, will walk with a wide base, variable step length, greater lateral bending, and often stiff LE (limited flexion) to maximize stability.[55] For many children with all types of CP, the UE are commonly held in a high guard position for much longer than is typical in development, unless used for managing an assistive device, and may demonstrate increased tone, even in the level I or II child with spasticity, when speed or difficulty is increased (e.g., running, kicking).

Many children with spasticity will initially pull to stand without assuming a half-kneeling posture, as a typical child would, relying on the arms to do much of the work with little LE contribution until almost upright; this is especially true of the child with diplegia. Children at level III usually continue to require the UE to pull to stand and are unstable in attempts to squat to the floor to retrieve an object and return to stand without holding on to a support.

Children with hypotonia and/or ataxia perform functional movements by using a small (less than available) ROM, often hold stationary postures without adequate muscular activation (referred to as "hanging on ligaments"), move less, and seem to move from one static posture to another with poor stability during the movement. They often have kyphosis and lordosis, which puts them at risk for trunk deformities, including scoliosis, and contractures and dislocations of the limbs. Although children with hypotonia often begin with excessive ROM, they repeatedly use only a part of it and frequently have contractures secondary to this limited posturing.

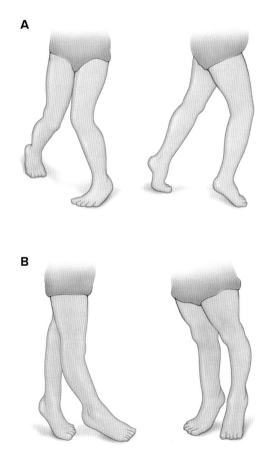

FIGURE 20-3 Crouched versus jump (stiff knee) gait.
A. Crouched gait — hip and knee flexion with femoral anteversion, tibial torsion, and equinus with pes planus. **B.** Jump (stiff knee) gait — knee extension with some scissoring of the legs during ambulation and equinovarus.

CASE A, PART V

Alejandro is demonstrating the stereotypical movement patterns of a child with spastic diplegia. He bunny-hops when he's creeping, walks with a crouched gait, w-sits, and lacks variation in his patterns of movement. For most typically developing children, they can sit in almost any position and walk slow, fast, on toes, backward, etc. For children with CP, they have a limited repertoire of movement and consistently move in one way (e.g., bunny hopping). Therapy is focused on increasing their repertoire of movements so that they have greater independence in their environments.

For Alejandro (AJ), a typical treatment session might look like this: First, the therapist might have Alejandro pick out a toy to play with and offer him some choices of motor activities. Physioballs can be fun for the child and promote antigravity movements and strengthening. When Alejandro is sitting on the ball and the therapist is stabilizing his pelvis, she encourages reaching in a variety of directions to elicit trunk rotation and strengthen the trunk muscles, as she stabilizes AJ at the hip on top of the ball. Bringing him down off the ball into a standing position with feet flat, the ball can now be pushed into the wall so that it bounces back, while AJ works on stance. Reaching with the arms and hands in this position is also done to further work on balance and trunk rotation. Squatting to the floor is a nice way to strengthen the quads and gluts, which are key muscles to oppose the spasticity of the hamstrings and hip flexors. For most children, reaching through their legs to a toy behind their heels (a 4-inch ball works nicely) will encourage a squat with the feet flat and knees apart; this avoids the child coming up on their toes with knees together, which is a common way that children with spasticity squat. It is critical that the therapist be able to identify tasks, such as this, that encourage more functional movement patterns, strengthen weak muscles, and allow the child to develop a greater repertoire of movements. Toward the end of the session, the therapist focuses on gait training, using an obstacle course with objects of various heights, an alternating ladder formation to step over, an incline to walk up, and many turns for Alejandro to negotiate. Stepping over obstacles stimulates a longer step with the "stepping foot" and induces increased single limb stance contralaterally. Obstacles and inclines can stimulate dorsiflexor activation to clear the obstacle and make it up the incline. Since dorsiflexors are typically weak and toe-walking common, these are good activities to encourage dorsiflexion and heel strike. Also, moving into and out of a variety of sitting postures should be addressed so that Alejandro has a greater repertoire for play and increased hip mobility; he may be able to move into side-sitting or tailor-sitting more easily by rotating as he pushes back from quadruped to assume these positions. However, in many children, their tight internal rotators and adductors make these positions quite difficult to assume and uncomfortable to maintain; it may be better for Alejandro to sit in a low chair some of the time to increase the number of options he has for functional play. As should be evident, therapists must be creative, making the tasks fun, yet finding ways to encourage child-directed movements that challenge the child's abilities.

Home tasks could include (1) long sitting or prone propping to provide passive stretch to his hamstrings and hip flexors, while watching TV or coloring; (2) stair climbing with assistance for quad strengthening; (3) half-kneeling for play to decrease reliance on bilateral symmetrical movement; (4) standing catch and throw with his sister, while a parent provides stability at the waist to increase standing balance and trunk rotation; and (5) kicking a ball, while standing with his walker, to increase single limb stance, dorsiflexion of the kicking leg, and balance. All of these can easily be built into the everyday activities of the family.

Upper Extremity Function

Characteristics of upper extremity impairment in children with CP include (1) posturing in shoulder adduction and internal rotation, elbow flexion, forearm pronation, and flexion of the wrist and fingers, including thumb adduction and flexion (thumb in the palm); (2) spasticity in the muscles contributing to this posture; (3) weakness of both spastic muscles and their antagonists;

(4) secondary loss of range of motion (contractures); (5) loss of sensation and proprioception; and (6) diminished dexterity and isolated finger motion.[56] The position of the elbow in flexion with forearm pronation puts the radial head in a position of risk for subluxation or dislocation. Contractures of the UE are common due to limited mobility and spasticity. For children with milder presentation, there is still diminished grip force, poor grip precision (inability to adjust to size and shape of the object), and reliance on more immature grasp methods.[52] While UE function may be primarily addressed by occupational therapists, the physical therapist should understand UE movement and reaching patterns and incorporate them into (1) reaching while addressing trunk control and balance, (2) weight-bearing on the UE while working on creeping, pulling to stand and standing, (3) strengthening of the UE through weight-bearing and play activities, and (4) more typical movement patterns (e.g., arm swing during gait).

● ASSOCIATED CONDITIONS OF CP

Orthopedic

Children with CP often either have insufficient muscle tone to support joint integrity or an imbalance of muscle tone and strength around joints that can result in soft tissue lengthening on one side and shortening on the other side. Such differences in muscle activity around joints can create instability and the potential for deformity over time. Further, delays in weight-bearing, especially standing, can affect bone health and joint maturation, especially at the hip where the acetabulum deepens with weight-bearing.[48,49] Table 20-1 outlines common orthopedic deformities associated with CP.

Intellectual Developmental Disability/Epilepsy

The term intellectual developmental disability (IDD) has replaced the use of mental retardation to describe individuals with deficits in cognitive function (reasoning, judgment, symbol use, memory, processing speed for acquiring new information) and adaptive behavior, which refers to the skills necessary to function in an age and culturally/environmentally appropriate manner, including social skills and behavioral management, that manifests during the developmental period (birth to age 18). This change in terminology reflects an increased emphasis on the limitations in adaptive behavior and a decreased reliance on IQ testing, in part, stemming from the problems inherent in IQ testing that may be biased against certain socioeconomic or racial/ethnic groups as well as those with motor or communication disorders where testing can be difficult.[57]

Children with IDD are further classified into levels of severity (mild, moderate, severe, and profound) based on IQ and adaptive functioning tests. The Wechsler Intelligence Scale in Children and its younger version for Preschool are the most used scales for determining IQ; they have a mean of 100 and an SD of 15, with a deficit of 2 SD below the mean defining IDD (<70). Similarly, tests of adaptive behavior allow corresponding categorization with a focus on conceptual skills (ability to learn concepts), practical skills (ability to learn daily living skills, including work-related skills), and social skills.[58] Table 20-2

TABLE 20-2	IDD Categories[57,58]	
LEVEL	**IQ RANGE**	**ADAPTIVE BEHAVIOR ABILITY/POTENTIAL**
Mild (85%)	69-56	Develop communication and social skills. Slow academic progress up to 6th grade level (unable to manage abstract concepts) by adulthood with mild limitations in coordination and higher-level motor skills; typically able to live independently, manage simple finances, and work in unskilled jobs.
Moderate (10%)	55-40	Slow acquisition of language, social, and motor skills with some difficulty in all areas at adulthood but acquire independent self-care abilities by adulthood with significant teaching; academic progress to 2nd grade level (simple reading and math); may live in the community with supervision and work a repetitive manual job.
Severe (3-4%)	39-25	Considerable limitations in acquisition of language, motor, and social skills; academic focus is on teaching practical and social skills; will require assistance/supervision with self-care; may work in supervised environment; will not live independently.
Profound (1-2%)	<25	Minimal practical skill acquisition, including mobility; will require assistance with most self-care skills.

provides descriptions of these categories of IDD with IQ level and adaptive behavior potential.

Approximately 50% of children with CP have IDD,[1] and when epilepsy is also present, the incidence increases to nearly 80%. This concomitant occurrence of IDD and epilepsy with CP should not be surprising given that each can individually be caused by damage to the developing brain, and therefore, can also be induced collectively by a single incident.[59]

Epilepsy (seizure disorder) is a condition of repetitive seizures in the absence of active disease; this is an important distinction, since seizures can occur in the presence of acute illness/disease, such as encephalitis, but will resolve once the disease has been treated unless brain damage occurs as a result of the disease. A **seizure** is an abnormal discharge of neurons in the brain, associated with motor, sensory, autonomic, emotional, or cognitive symptoms, dependent on the area of the brain affected. Damage to the brain can leave scar tissue that irritates surrounding intact tissue, thereby, inducing the abnormal activation that creates the seizure. Thus, seizures present in a variety of ways (see Table 20-3) that are differentiated, in part, as (1) **generalized**, referring to involvement of both hemispheres with a loss of consciousness, or (2) **partial**, indicating localization to one hemisphere and that some degree of consciousness remains intact. In the typically developing child population, epilepsy occurs in less than .4 to 1% of the population; in children with developmental disabilities, this incidence increases to 30–50%, and in children with CP it may be as high as 62%.[19,60] Children with more severe motor impairments (e.g., quadriplegia and very low birth weight) and those with IDD are more likely to develop seizures; additionally, epilepsy in children with CP is often more difficult to treat (refractory), requiring several medications to control the seizure activity. Up to 28% of children with CP, who have epilepsy, experience drug-resistant epilepsy.[61] Uncontrolled seizures can lead to additional

TABLE 20-3	Seizure Classifications[59]
SEIZURE TYPE	**DESCRIPTION**
Generalized	Loss of consciousness due to involvement of both cerebral hemispheres, includes tonic-clonic, absence, myoclonic, and atonic seizures
Tonic-clonic (grand mal)	A period of tonic (maintained) muscle co-contraction, followed by repetitive alternating muscle contractions of flexors and extensors (clonic phase).
Absence (petit mal)	Brief loss of consciousness (<10 seconds) associated with staring and loss of responsiveness that may go unnoticed by the child. Atypical absence seizures may have clonic, atonic, or stereotypic movements (e.g., swallowing, chewing, blinking) and last up to 20 seconds.
Myoclonic	Quick generalized muscle contraction similar in appearance to a startle response but without a precipitating stimulus.
Tonic	Generalized and maintained muscle contraction (identical to tonic phase of tonic-clonic) without a clonic phase.
Atonic	Generalized loss of muscle activity, resulting in complete collapse of the body (drops to floor)
Partial	Focal seizure without loss of consciousness, characterized by symptoms linked to the area of the brain in which the seizure occurs (e.g., sensory, motor, autonomic (changes in blood pressure, sweating, nausea), or emotion (fear, anxiety). Can progress to generalized seizure, commonly tonic-clonic.
Complex partial	Characterized by a variety of complex motor behaviors, such as chewing, picking at clothes, walking in circles with some disruption of awareness (not a complete loss of consciousness)

brain damage and in some instances, death secondary to a condition known as **status epilepticus**, where a prolonged seizure state persists (longer than 5 minutes) that places the child in a medically unstable condition, associated with diminished oxygen to the brain, neuroinflammation, and multiple system decline, including dysfunction in the cardiopulmonary system. The most common cause of status epilepticus in children without CP is infection or fever.[62] Despite the tendency for epilepsy to be difficult to treat in children with CP, up to 47% will achieve remission of their epilepsy by adolescence.[63]

Sensory Dysfunction

Concomitant disruption of vision is common in CP with up to 30%[64] to 70%[32] of children experiencing some change in their **visual system; 10% have a severe level of impairment**[32]; most commonly, this presents as poor visual acuity, but the causative pathology is different than diminished acuity in their peers. Visual deficits are most common in those born prematurely. Additionally, more severe changes can include blindness, retinopathy (especially in children with prematurity), and strabismus. **Strabismus** refers to poor coordination of the extraocular muscles, resulting in poor synchronization of eye movement and disruption of binocular vision. Other visual changes include refractive errors and visual field defects (see Chapter 11, "Stroke," for definitions).[64] **Hearing impairment** occurs in up to 18% of children with CP[1] with a moderate loss in 7% and a severe loss in 3 to 4%. These deficits stem from conductive, sensorineural, or central hearing impairments, secondary to neural damage.[65] **Vestibular dysfunction** has been reported in 48% of children with spasticity, associated with decreased saccular function. Taste and smell have not been routinely examined, but at least one study reported significant impairment of taste detection and identification in a group with quadriplegic CP.[66]

Deficits in **somatosensory function** are also common, presenting similarly to that described in Chapter 11 for stroke, including diminished touch perception, tactile discrimination abilities, and proprioception/kinesthesia.[60] Heightened pain sensitivity has also been reported in children with CP[67]; in addition, up to 75% of children with CP report pain, which can be secondary to orthopedic conditions, dystonia, or gastrointestinal issues.[64]

Language/Communication Disorders

Language disorders are common in children with CP, occurring in up to 74% of children and present similarly to the adult presentation, as described in Chapter 11 for stroke. The Speech Language Profile groups children into four categories of speech deficits: 1 = no disturbance; 2 = motor only (language is unaffected); 3 = motor and language impairment; 4 = no speech (anarthria) with language impairment.[68] In a population-based study, all children with anarthria demonstrated receptive language impairment; for those that were verbal, 93% had some receptive language impairment.[69] There seems to be a greater potential for plasticity in children, especially in those with hemiplegia, that allows for fairly normal speech development even with left hemisphere damage, likely resulting from the potential of the right hemisphere to control language when the left is damaged early. Notably, the most common language

disorder in CP is dysarthria, resulting from disrupted control of the oral muscles; three types of dysarthria have been described: spastic, ataxic, and hyperkinetic with similar presentations to the motor consequences of those conditions.[70] The severity of language impairment correlates with the severity of motor impairment, so those with severe spastic quadriplegia are most affected while those with diplegia are rarely affected. When IDD is also present, this will further impact the ability of the child to develop speech such that those with profound IDD rarely have functional speech.[69] Yet, there are children with severe CP presentation that have limited speech but without IDD; for these children, a communication device may unlock their world by allowing them to communicate through a synthesized voice or written word (see section on assistive technology).[71]

● MEDICAL MANAGEMENT OF THE CHILD WITH CP

The management of the child with CP is dependent on presentation and comorbidities; since each child will present uniquely, treatment needs to be directed at the specific needs of the child. For both medical and therapeutic management, the focus is on maximizing function and preventing secondary complications. From the discussion of this condition in previous sections, it should be apparent that medical management of the child with CP can include surgery for orthopedic conditions; pharmaceutical management of seizures, spasticity, or other conditions; prevention of secondary conditions, including orthopedic deformities; and maximizing growth and development through adequate nutritional management.

Management of Seizures

The primary treatment for seizures is pharmacological; unfortunately, antiseizure medications have a variety of side effects, including sedation/somnolence/lethargy, dyscoordination, poor attention, hyperactivity/agitation, irritability and aggression (see Table 20-4 for common medications, usage, and side effects). When combined with CP and IDD, these medications may significantly impact the child's ability to function, so treatment focuses on achieving the best seizure control while minimizing side effects to maximize function. In many instances, more than one drug is required to provide effective seizure control; obviously this may have an additive effect for the side effects as well.[19] For some children, epilepsy can be drug resistant and the likelihood of status epilepticus more common; for these children, families may be given rescue medications to administer. Common rescue medications are benzodiazapam derivatives (Conazepam, Diazepam, Midazolam, Lorazapam).[72] On rare occasions, surgery is indicated for the treatment of severe and refractory seizures. This may involve ablation of the seizure-generating neurons in focal epilepsy or severing of the corpus callosum in those with **generalized seizures** to stop the progression of the seizure activity from one hemisphere to the other. Of course, surgical intervention of this sort has its own set of consequences that will also impact the child's function.[74]

TABLE 20-4	Common Antiepileptic Medications[59,72,73]	
DRUG	**USES**	**COMMON SIDE EFFECTS**
Phenytoin (Dilantin)	Partial, generalized, absence	Unsteadiness, ataxia, sedation, attention deficits, disrupted problem-solving, slurred speech
Carbamazepine (Tegretol)	Focal, Partial, Generalized,	Disrupted sleep, irritability, attention deficit, ataxia, dyscoordination, dizziness, nausea
Phenobarbital	Partial or generalized	Hyperactivity, lethargy, sleep disruption, memory impairment, attention deficit
Valproic acid (Depakene/Depakote)	Absence, tonic-clonic, myoclonic	Sedation, minimal cognitive side effects
Lamotrigine (Lamictal)	Absence, Partial, complex partial, generalized	Tremor, changes in balance, fatigue, rash
Ethosuximide (Zarotin)	Absence	Decreased appetite, nausea, hyperactivity, rash, vomiting, disrupted sleep
Levetriacetam (Keppra)	Myoclonic (adults), focal/partial, absence (adults)	Irritability / agitation, ataxia, dizziness, fatigue/sleepiness, rash, mood changes
Oxcarbazepime (Trileptal)	Focal, partial, generalized	Dizziness/vertigo, ataxia, double vision, nausea, headache, rash, hyponatremia
Topiramate (Topamax)	Myoclonic	Weight loss, decreased sweating, word-finding problems
Zonisamide (Zonegran)	Focal, partial	Dizziness, insomnia, sleepiness, dyscoordination, loss of appetite, diarrhea
Gabapentin	Focal/partial, generalized (adults)	Ataxia, sleepiness, dizziness

Management of Spasticity

In children with spasticity, medical management is aimed at limiting the impact of spasticity on range of motion and movement, preventing orthopedic deformities, and minimizing pain, if present. Multiple **oral medications** can be used to decrease spasticity systemically, but they all have side effects that may compromise function, most commonly sedation. Further, many children with CP "rely" on their spasticity to achieve posture and movement; thus, they may experience a decrease in function when using an oral medication. Common oral medications are gamma aminobutyric acid (GABA) agonists (e.g., baclofen, diazepam, gabapentin, tiagabine), adrenergic agonists (tizanidine), and calcium channel blockers (sodium dantrolene). For children with severe spasticity or dystonia, **intrathecal baclofen** may be used to allow better positioning, hygiene, and mobility. This involves surgical placement of a catheter into the epidural lumbar space with a pump that is subcutaneous (just below the skin surface), which allows it to be refilled via injection. Although the effect of intrathecal baclofen can be widespread, including LE, UE, and trunk, it avoids the central effects, including sedation. Intrathecal baclofen has also been found to effectively diminish dystonia in some children.[75] For children with focal spasticity that is limiting mobility of single joints or a few joints, injections of **botulinum toxin** (Botox) may be effective in diminishing spasticity for up to 3 to 6 months so that therapy can focus on improving motor control and strength within the muscles to avoid surgery. Often Botox injections are accompanied by splinting (orthotics) to maintain improved range of motion, following the injection. The long-term effects of Botox injections is equivocal, since the spasticity will return as the effect of the injection wears off; however, with intensive physical therapy, long-term effects have been reported.[75,76] In some cases, surgery is required to increase range of motion and prevent further joint deformity (see surgical management in the next section). Of note, there is a surgical procedure that is focused on decreasing the spasticity itself, called a **selective dorsal rhizotomy**. In this procedure, the dorsal root afferents of the lumbar spine that are contributing to LE spasticity and hyperreflexia are lesioned; this is a tedious process that includes electrical stimulation to identify appropriate nerve roots to be sectioned and to preserve nerve roots that are least involved in the spasticity to maintain function. Following the surgery, intensive physical therapy is provided to work on strengthening, reeducation of muscles, and increasing mobility (6 weeks of daily therapy, 6 hours per day). This procedure is particularly effective for children with spastic diplegia at GMFCS levels II and III, reportedly, decreasing the need for orthopedic surgeries, enhancing the development of gross motor skills, and delaying the typical plateau of those skills.[1,75,77] Occasionally, dorsal rhizotomy is performed in children at GMFCS levels IV and V to improve hygiene care.[75]

Orthopedic Management

The first step in orthopedic management should be to prevent a deformity from developing through positioning, movement, orthotics, and stretching. In some cases, **serial casting** is used.

This technique casts the body part at an end of range position for a week or so; then, the cast is removed and reapplied at the new end of range position, gradually increasing the length of the soft tissue and increasing range of motion.[78] The goals of surgery are often different, depending on the functional level of the child: for those at higher GMFCS levels (II and III) the goal is improved function (ambulation or hand use); for those at lower GMFCS levels (IV and V), the goal is typically to minimize pain and/or improve hygiene care by the care providers. For the most part, surgery is not considered unless there is a fixed deformity, subluxation/dislocation, or significant impedance to mobility. Orthopedic surgeries can be categorized into four types: (1) lengthening of the tendon (tendonotomy) to improve range of motion; (2) transfer of a tendon to improve muscle balance at a joint (e.g., changing a spastic flexor carpi ulnaris to an extensor muscle by reattaching it to the dorsum of the wrist); (3) osteotomy (cutting the bone) to shorten, lengthen, or change the rotation of a bone to improve alignment (e.g., derotation osteotomy of the femur to correct excessive anteversion); and (4) fusion (arthrodesis) to fix the joint in an improved alignment (e.g., spinal arthrodesis for scoliosis).[79,80] Tendonotomies (lengthening) are typically done by cutting the tendon in a Z pattern (see Figure 20-4), which allows the two ends of the Z to be stitched together, thereby lengthening the tendon. Following surgery, splinting or casting is used in combination with therapy to maintain the new length, strengthen the lengthened and opposing muscles, and promote joint mobility. Serial casting done in connection with surgical lengthening of the muscle decreases the extent of the lengthening and maximizes the outcomes; this is commonly done with hamstring lengthening. When this is done, the initial cast is applied in the operating room. A wedge is cut into the cast just above the knee joint, allowing progressively larger plastic wedges to be inserted, thereby increasing the length of the elongated hamstring.[81] Notably, surgical procedures may be done in combination to achieve maximum results; for example, a femoral derotation osteotomy may be done in conjunction with an adductor lengthening to maximize outcome and prevent reoccurrence.[80] However, since growth can negate results, it is often recommended that the child be at least school age before such surgery is done to avoid reoccurrence and the need for subsequent surgeries.[82]

Nutritional Management

Inadequate nutritional intake is a common problem for children with CP; contributing factors include oromotor dysfunction, including poor lip closure and difficulty chewing and swallowing, postural instability, which impedes the ability to maintain the head and trunk in a suitable position for eating, and upper extremity dysfunction, which limits the ability to self-feed. Approximately 58% of children with CP at GMFCS levels III-V will have oropharyngeal dysphagia (disrupted motor control for eating) with 23% having a severe level of compromise; this can result in undernutrition in up to 46% of children with CP, especially those with greater severity and intellectual deficits. Dysphagia can make feeding a stressful time for parents and the child, requiring a longer feeding time; often the child has difficulty expressing hunger or fullness, so underfeeding can be common.[83] Additionally, these same children may suffer from **gastroesophageal reflux**, which refers to regurgitation of stomach contents to the esophagus, secondary to dysfunction of the lower esophageal sphincter, resulting in caloric loss.[84] Stomach acids can erode the esophagus, causing pain and further eating avoidance. Due to the many challenges in eating, many children with CP have very poor food consumption and are at risk for malnutrition that can further impede brain development and overall health, including bone health, which can limit bone density and place the child at risk for fractures.[85] In addition, aspiration of food is common in those with swallowing difficulties and can result in pneumonia or other respiratory consequence.[86] Initial treatment for feeding difficulty is to adjust the feeding process to make eating easier; this includes improved positioning, use of adaptive feeding methods (e.g., nipples with smaller holes, adaptive utensils for self-feeding), and alteration of foods to make eating easier (e.g., thickening of liquids to decrease aspiration). Increasing the caloric and nutrient content of food can help to maximize nutrition. Some children are also very picky eaters, which can further affect the nutrients ingested and further impede growth and development. **Nutritional supplements** may be prescribed to address imbalances, including increasing the caloric content of foods consumed. Children with spastic CP have been reported to require up to 70% more calories than their typically developing peers due to the energy costs of moving and/or wheelchair propulsion;[87] however, more recent reports suggest that caloric needs

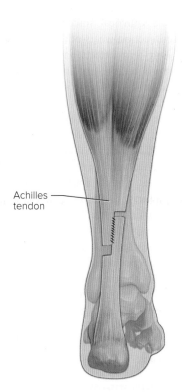

Achilles tendon

FIGURE 20-4 Z-plasty. To lengthen the Achilles tendon, a Z-incision is made in the tendon (above cut left to right) and then the two ends of the "Z" are sutured together to allow lengthening of the tendon.

have been over-estimated[83]; ambulatory children may have similar caloric requirements to their typical peers while those with limited movement may have lower requirements.[84] Yet, determining caloric intake and need can be quite challenging in children with severe disability; ongoing assessment of growth and weight gain is necessary along with analysis of food intake to ascertain diet adequacy. CP-specific growth charts have been developed to help guide nutrition assessment and planning.[83] Many children with CP also fail to consume sufficient quantities of fluids and fiber (e.g., fruits and vegetables), which can contribute to constipation; decreased intestinal motility and altered anal reflex activity can also contribute to constipation in children with CP.[88] For some children, oral feeding is insufficient to meet nutritional needs, and they require surgical intervention to assure nutritional intake. This determination is based on oral intake inadequacy, prolonged feeding time (>4-6 hr/day), growth failure, and triceps skinfold thickness below the 5th percentile.[83] The most common is surgical implantation of a tube into the stomach (**percutaneous endoscopic gastrostomy [PEG]**), which allows thick liquids to be pushed directly into the stomach, bypassing the mouth and esophagus.[83,86] For many children, this may also require an anti-reflux procedure that prevents further leakage of stomach contents into the esophagus.

CASE A, PART VI

Alejandro, like most children with diplegia, has no apparent language or intellectual delays; although he is still young to be certain that he won't display any learning disabilities. He has outgrown his seizures and is no longer taking medication. He is developing hip and knee flexion tightness that needs to be carefully managed. He may be a candidate for Botox injections in these muscles to temporarily block spasticity, while functional training program that includes movements that span range of motion and strengthening is implemented to improve knee and hip extension. At some point, he may also be a candidate for a selective dorsal rhizotomy, but typically, this is done after the child is 5 to 6 years of age and only if spasticity is severe enough to cause pain, worsening function, or limitation in self-care like toileting.

● PHYSICAL THERAPY MANAGEMENT

Treatment of the child with CP is aimed at maximizing function, increasing the variety of movements available to the child, and preventing secondary complications, especially orthopedic deformities. Similar to the treatment of adults with neurologic disorders, treatment of children is based on the growing body of evidence related to motor control and neuroplasticity, more specifically, what is needed to induce change in the nervous system (see Chapter 9). The basic tenets of inducing motor learning and plasticity are (1) plasticity requires intensity of practice that challenges the current level of function and thereby the nervous system, including numerous repetitions at the maximum ability of the individual; (2) practice needs to be task specific (e.g., to improve walking, the child should be walking); (3) practice of the whole activity is preferable to practicing part of the activity (e.g., although single limb stance is part of gait, practicing single limb stance may not improve stance during gait); (4) practice that requires problem-solving and variability is critical to learning and ultimately transferring the skill to new situations; (5) feedback should provide knowledge of performance (how the movement "looked") and results (success/failure) in limited amounts (more initially with less as the skill is acquired); and (6) feedback from the therapist should be weaned as the child becomes able to rely on his own sensory feedback (how the movement feels).[30,89] Handling the child to facilitate a movement should also be considered a form of feedback that limits the degrees of freedom available to the child and changes his own sensory experience of the movement; thus, like verbal feedback it should be used as little as necessary, greater initially with fading as each new skill is learned. Limiting feedback, including handling, allows the child to experience different solutions to solve a movement task, and this trial-and-error learning is thought to result in stronger learning and better generalization to new tasks.[90] In addition, therapy needs to be fun and interactive between therapist and the child but should also be focused on the family (family-centered), directed toward mutually developed goals, and in consideration of the family structure, culture, and daily activities. Therapists should be cognizant that they will spend, at best, a few hours per week with a child while the caregivers will spend up to 100 waking hours with their child per week. Thus, for therapy to be effective, the families must be able to implement components of the therapy in the home, yet this should not be overwhelming nor interfere with their function as a family.[32] Similarly, teachers should be part of the therapy program for the child, implementing components within the school day of the child to maximize effectiveness.

Managing the Effects of Abnormal Muscle Tone

Although abnormal tone should not be a primary focus of treatment, it often impacts treatment, and therefore, requires some attention. For example, in the child with spasticity, tone will increase when the child gets excited, so treatment in a quiet environment may be preferable initially, when focused on a new skill. Yet, as the skill is learned, the child must manage their enthusiasm and, thereby, tone, to function in the many environments that he might experience. There are techniques to increase tone in those with hypotonia and lower tone in spasticity/dystonia that may allow the child to move against gravity or move out of synergistic patterns temporarily. Techniques that may increase tone are bouncing on a ball/bolster, swinging, or joint compression (either manual or through weight-bearing); in contrast, slow rocking on a ball or bolster, passive rotation of the extremity or trunk, and active movements outside of synergistic patterns can diminish tone. However, it should be clear that these are transitory changes that can allow the child to move more easily momentarily but do not change the physiological causes of abnormal tone. So, it is important to strengthen antagonists and create movement opportunities that challenge the child's motor control system to generate new patterns of movement, breaking through synergistic patterns.

For children with significant spasticity or dystonia, the family should be instructed in range of motion exercises early to help prevent loss of motion and potential deformity; simple motions that can be done during diaper changes, bath time, and dressing (e.g., rocking into abduction, leg extension with dorsiflexion) will be easier for them to remember than a complex routine that takes a lot of time. Emphasis should be on LE extension, abduction, external rotation, and dorsiflexion as well as UE extension, abduction, external rotation, and supination. Making these a part of the caregivers' daily play time with the child will assure that they are completed. However, stretching is typically ineffective in maintaining ROM in the absence of a program of strengthening and task-specific motor training; active use of the muscle helps to increase the contractile elements of the muscle, which are altered in CP; stretching is insufficient in stimulating such changes.[91] Also, positioning of the child to minimize the effects of spasticity is also critical: (1) maintaining abduction during sitting (ring or tailor positions) or while being carried (e.g., straddling the parent's hip); (2) early standing to achieve hip and knee extension with feet flat; and (3) trunk and head support in sitting and when transporting for children with poor postural control to prevent scoliosis or kyphosis. These positioning suggestions are also important for children with dyskinetic, ataxic, or hypotonic CP. While children with ataxia and hypotonia have greater freedom of movement than the child with spasticity or dystonia, they also have diminished antigravity movement and stability so that they spend long periods of time in a single position (e.g., supported sitting), resulting in the potential for scoliosis or other orthopedic problems. Muscles will shorten if the legs are always flexed and abducted, whether spastic or hypotonic; thus, positioning is a critical component of preventative and therapeutic intervention for all children with CP. Notably, instructing the family in appropriate handling and carrying methods will also help them contend with a child that is difficult to handle.

Strengthening

Interestingly, weakness and poor force generation are common elements of CP regardless of type and varies with the GMFCS level with those at level I demonstrating the best strength, and those at level V the worst; thus, strengthening is an important part of treatment. However, the best method and expected results remain elusive with insufficient evidence to determine best practices. As is described for the child with myelomeningocele in Chapter 19, encouraging antigravity movement is the initial method for developing strength in neck and trunk muscles and hip extensors in infants and young children with CP via the same activities described in Table 19-5. Additionally, use of weight-bearing postures and functional activities (e.g., squatting and returning to stand; pushing away from the wall when rolled forward on a ball; maneuvering a scooter board with the hands) can further increase strength in children with CP. In many children, weight-training with free weights or resistive exercise equipment can improve strength (e.g., quadriceps

strength); however, it may not translate into improved function (e.g., knee extension during gait),[92] yet has been found to improve gait speed even in the absence of improved kinematics.[26] Performing 8 to 12 repetitions at a resistance of 50 to 80% of a single maximum repetition is recommended at a frequency of 3 times per week for at least 8 weeks to achieve measurable increases in strength.[93] This should be accompanied by task-specific training to improve function. Functional strength training can also be incorporated into treatment programs; for example, working on quad strengthening might include quad sets with weights, followed by squat to stand activities or stair climbing and eventually adding a weight belt to enhance strength.

Evidence-Based Treatment Approaches

Much research is now devoted to identifying best practices to maximize function in children with CP; approaches with sufficient evidence of effectiveness are all focused on increasing the intensity and variability of practice to achieve improved function and variability of movement.

Goals-Activity-Motor Enrichment (GAME) is a motor learning task-based approach that uses parent coaching and environmental enrichment to encourage early movement in infants at high risk for CP or diagnosed early (5-6 months). Therapists work with the parents to determine goals for each child and methods to encourage specific motor skills with complexity and variability increased as the child gains skills. Weight-bearing is encouraged early as is reaching and grasping. Parents are coached on appropriate toy selection and how to set up their home environment to encourage the identified goals.[30,94]

Treadmill training with/without partial body-weight support may facilitate earlier walking and allows the therapist to facilitate LE position and weight-shift, while not worrying about the child falling. A meta-analysis of treadmill training protocols found moderate to strong evidence that treadmill gait training improved gait endurance and speed as well as single limb stance (decreased double limb support) better than standard therapy; however, it didn't improve step length or cadence. It has also been reported to improve LE strength and bone density and decrease spasticity; however, it appears not to change the kinematics of the gait pattern with step length and cadence unchanged.[95] Similarly, partial body-weight support (BWS) can also be achieved with mobile systems that allow over ground walking; one randomized trial compared overground BWS to body-weight supported treadmill training (BWSTT) and found greater speed, greater stride length and speed, longer single leg stance, and longer swing phases when BWS was provided overground versus on the treadmill.[96] Thus, training overground with a BWS mobile system may result in greater improvements and facilitate better transfer of gait changes to the standard environment; however, additional research is needed.

Robotic-assisted therapy is being used for both gait training and arm training in children with CP. Robots can facilitate intense practice (many repetitions) with assistance or resistance that is task specific; this can be reaching or grasping with the arm/hand or step and dorsiflexion assistance for gait.[28,29] Concerns for robotic therapy have suggested that, like handling, it changes the sensory perception of a movement and diminishes the feedback and feed-forward mechanisms critical for voluntary movement, yet it has shown some promise. For example, **robotic resisted treadmill training**, where resistance was applied to the leg during swing phase, was found to improve fast walking speed, self-selected walking speed, and 6-minute walking distance while robotic-assisted treadmill training, where the swing phase was assisted, did not.[97] Further, a systematic review and meta-analysis reported robotic-assisted gait training was effective in increasing walking distance but the changes in gait speed and functionality, as measured by the GMFM, did not reach clinical significance.[98] It is likely that robotic training is best provided in conjunction with functional overground gait training to maximize its effectiveness. There are fewer studies that have examined robotic use for the UE in children, but there is some evidence that robot-assisted movement in combination with conventional task-specific training produced greater improvement in speed and movement smoothness than conventional training only.[99] **Biofeedback** in the forms of visual, auditory, or EMG to provide knowledge of performance or results has been used to improve motor performance as measured by standardized tests, kinematic (e.g., step length, speed), and kinetic (e.g., strength) measures. This can be as simple as demonstrating trajectory on a computer screen or providing an auditory cue each time heel strike occurs. A systematic review of biofeedback interventions found that using multiple modalities (visual and auditory) was common and had greater effectiveness than a single modality; similarly, targeting external variables such as accuracy was more effective than targeting internal movement variables such as joint angle. In addition, virtual reality immersive systems provide complex visual and auditory feedback that seems to have promise in achieving functional gains.[100] Determination of appropriate dosing and feedback parameters will be critical to guide clinical implementation. **Gaming** is being incorporated into therapy sessions and home programs with increasing frequency, using interactive systems, such as the Nintendo Wii™, PlayStation, and Kinect to improve weight-shift and balance , as well as gross motor and fine motor function. A systematic review found improvements in overall motor function, physical activity, dexterity, upper limb motor function, and balance, following gaming rehabilitation, which typically involves 3 to 4 sessions per week over 4 to 6 weeks. Gaming systems are a form of virtual reality. Parents and children report a positive experience with VR/gaming systems.[101] Another potential benefit of gaming is the easy ability of the systems to generate a high level of variability and are visually stimulating to engage the child, which may contribute to the enhanced outcomes reported.[102] **Constraint-induced Movement Therapy (CIMT)**, which has been used primarily for children with hemiplegia to increase use of the paretic UE, was initially designed as a treatment method for stroke but has been found to increase use of the paretic arm in children with hemiplegic CP. In this treatment paradigm, the non-paretic arm is typically splinted or casted, but gloves/mittens have been used, for several weeks (2-10, depending on the study) while intense therapy is focused on shaping of reaching, grasping, and manipulation activities with the paretic hand with feedback provided on results and performance. Shaping refers to the progressive changing of the complexity of the activity to work toward a desired targeted action. CIMT has been attempted with a broad age range of children (2-18) and some of the variability in outcomes may result from this variability in age. Yet, almost all studies have shown UE

improvement to some degree with this treatment.[30,103] More recently it has been applied to infants as young as 3 months with significant improvements in hand function, following 2- to 6-week periods of training with the hand "constrained" by a mitten; continued improvement was seen at 18 months.[104] For this reason, CIMT is amassing strong evidence of efficacy in children with hemiparetic CP.[30,105] Similarly, there is significant evidence to support intensive **bimanual hand-arm therapy** to improve UE function, initially designed for those with hemiplegic CP.[30,106] The original trial was called Hand-Arm Bimanual Intensive Therapy, so this is sometimes referred to as **HABIT**.[106] This treatment approach, like CIMT, focuses on intensive practice of functional tasks (both part and whole task practice), using both hands (e.g., flipping cards versus playing a game of cards). Traditionally, it is done in a 2-week paradigm for 6 hours/day.[105] It has also been trialed on children at higher functional levels (I-III) with bilateral CP and found to improve hand function in the less affected UE.[107] Building on the HABIT protocol, several groups have evaluated the inclusion of lower extremity and postural control activities in the HABIT protocol, referred to as **HABIT-ILE** (including lower extremity) for children with unilateral CP. In this paradigm, the UE functional activities are practiced while sitting on a ball or stool, standing (on the floor or a balance board), or moving (walking/running); Wii Fit and Kinect systems are also used to stimulate standing balance while using the UE to play. Like the other intensive programs, HABIT-ILE is provided over a 2-week period of daily practice. It has been found to improve both UE and LE function, including 6-meter walking time and GMFM-66 score, in school-aged children with unilateral[108] and bilateral CP at levels GMFCS II-IV.[109] Currently its being examined in younger children.[110] **Hippotherapy** is a form of treatment where a therapist uses a horse as a therapeutic tool to stimulate the visual, vestibular, and proprioceptive systems of the child; the therapist and aide(s) guide the horse's movements to challenge the child's posture and develop improved stability; this differs from therapeutic riding, where the focus is on teaching the child to ride a horse but the intent is also to improve balance and coordination. Hippotherapy has been studied much more than therapeutic riding and found to improve gross motor function, posture in standing and sitting, trunk strength, and reaching skills to a greater extent than standard treatment alone.[111] Another interesting treatment approach for children with CP is **aquatic therapy**, in which movement in water is used to improve mobility. Water is a supportive medium for children with CP as it provides buoyancy, decreasing the effect of gravity and allowing children with challenged balance and muscle weakness to move easier while in it. Most aquatic therapy is done in warm water that helps to relax the child, thereby, lowering spasticity; then, skills that might not be possible on land can be attempted, such as single limb stance, walking without an assistive device, squatting, jumping, or hopping. Additionally, water-specific skills are also introduced such as kicking with a kick board as an aerobic activity. As skills are developed in the water, they can, then, be attempted on land. The fun environment of the pool may keep the child engaged, while the buoyant setting allows a greater number of repetitions to be completed. Aquatic therapy has been found to improve gross motor skills but not to change overall spasticity measures.[112]

Assistive Technology

The function of children with CP can be enhanced with a large variety of assistive technology that includes mobility devices (e.g., crutches, walkers, wheelchairs, orthotics), adaptive equipment for activities of daily living (feeding, bathing, toileting), positioning equipment (standers, seating systems), communication devices, and environmental controls. With the expanding computer technology, the field of assistive technology is expanding exponentially so that it is quite challenging for the therapist to keep up with the changes.

Mobility Devices

In Chapter 19, we discussed orthotics, ambulation devices, and wheelchair fitting for the child with MMC; many of these same devices are also commonly used for children with CP. In the case of CP, the decision about what devices should be used is more complex in many ways than for the child with MMC, since tone is highly variable and the head, trunk, and arms are also commonly involved. While children with CP don't have the insensate issues that children with MMC have, they do require seating systems that provide appropriate support and protect from pressure ulcers, since often they are less mobile than their MMC peers.

Orthotics

The goals of orthotic prescription often differ for children at higher and lower GMFCS levels. Orthotics for those at GMFCS levels II and III aim primarily to increase function, especially gait, and prevent deformity while those for children at GMFCS levels IV and V aim principally at preventing deformity, especially scoliosis and hip dislocation. However, for many children at levels IV and V, orthotics can provide trunk support that allows greater arm and head function as well as managing scoliosis/kyphosis progression.[113]

The most common orthotic for ambulating children with CP is an AFO (Figure 20-5), to control the common equinovarus position of the foot that impedes the swing phase of gait as the toe drags and to assist with achieving heel strike. The child's ankle function (strength and ROM), presence of deformity, and tone along with the potential to improve or worsen gait will determine the kind of AFO that is preferable:

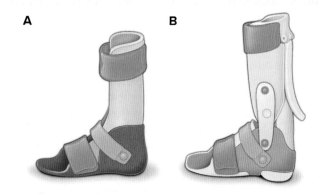

FIGURE 20-5 Solid versus articulating AFO. A. A single molded AFO with forefoot, ankle, and calf straps. **B.** An articulating AFO with plantarflexion stop.

articulating or non-articulating (solid or flexible).[109] A **non-articulating (solid-SAFO) AFO** is a single piece (no ankle joint) that is typically fit with the foot at a 90-degree angle with the calf. The thickness of the material allows for degrees of flexibility or rigidity. When the AFO is rigid, it will help the child achieve heel strike but limits push-off, since plantarflexion is blocked. Flexible AFOs allow some degree of plantarflexion for push-off and can assist dorsiflexion after toe off, since the elastic (spring) nature of the material pushes the foot into dorsiflexion to assist during swing and heel strike; for children, with mild spasticity this is appropriate, but for children with moderate to severe spasticity, it may elicit strong plantarflexion or clonus, which defeats the purpose of the AFO, and therefore, should be avoided. Also, it is important for the therapist to evaluate the effect of the AFO on knee position to assure that the AFO isn't making the crouch gait worse **Articulating AFOs** have a joint at the ankle and are constructed of two pieces. This allows active or active-assisted dorsiflexion via a spring mechanism but can block or limit plantarflexion. Either type of AFO can also assist with blocking knee hyperextension via a slightly forward positioning of the calf component; however, knee flexion often is not changed with either type of AFO.[114,115] It should be noted that up to 50% individuals, who are prescribed AFOs, fail to wear them due to discomfort, difficulty with doning/doffing them or getting into shoes, or damage to the AFO due to wear and the inability to replace them for financial reasons; this is especially true for children as they age. For some, they perceive the AFO to be ineffective.[116] Thus, it's important for the PT to monitor wear and assist with problem-solving to improve ease of use and determine appropriate fit or need for a new orthotic.

Adaptive Seating Systems/Wheelchairs

The goal for adaptive seating for children with CP is to maximize function by providing appropriate postural support that allows the best upper extremity use, controls abnormal tone, prevents deformity, and, in the case of wheelchairs, allows the most freedom of movement whether self-propelled or caregiver-propelled. Seating choices are dependent on the individual child's presentation (tone, deformities, and motor abilities), family situation, and growth potential. Thus, choosing a system for a child requires a comprehensive assessment and some trial and error with potential systems prior to purchase.

In Chapter 19, we discussed the general components of wheelchairs (bases, frames, seating systems) and measurements taken to determine the appropriate chair size and features. For children with CP, the combination of abnormal tone (e.g., spasticity or hypotonia), abnormal movements (e.g., dystonia, chorea, athetosis), and limited trunk control makes finding the right seating system and wheelchair challenging, especially for those at GMFCS levels IV and V, yet critical, not only to maximize function, minimize pain, and prevent deformities but also to maximize participation[117] Inadequate trunk support impedes head control and upper extremity function in those with a higher level of disability. Similarly, inadequate head control impedes communication, visual ability, and eating, so maximizing support and function are critical factors in choosing the right seating system.[118] While many studies have explored the various components of seating systems on the posture and function of children with CP, finding the right seat for an individual child is dependent on the child's presentation (tone, ROM, strength, function). For example, the orientation of the chair in space has received much consideration; this refers to the adjustment of the entire chair and not the back-hip angle, which may be maintained in a neutral position as the orientation is tipped. An **anterior-tilted chair** (see Figure 20-6), typically 5 to 15 degrees forward from upright, may facilitate an anterior pelvic tilt in those with a posterior pelvic tilt, decrease the effect of tight hamstrings, and encourage trunk extension, which may improve UE function in some children. Including an abduction orthosis when using an anteriorly tilted seat appears to contribute to the increased stability of children, who benefit from this position. However, in others, especially those with poor head control, a **posterior tilt** may be advantageous to facilitate improved head positioning and minimize LE extensor patterns; a posterior tilt is often used with a wedge seat to increase hip flexion to further diminish excessive extensor tone. Although this may improve head control and trunk posture, it may also put the child at increased risk for hip flexion contractures. While a wedged seat and posterior tilt are recommended for some children with excessive extensor tone, a seat to back angle of 110° has been reported to produce the best neutral head and trunk position for those without excessive extensor tone, while seated in a chair without a tilt.[118] A **head rest** may be essential to provide postural support for a child with poor head control, yet it may also stimulate an extensor thrust (full body extension triggered by pressure on the back of the head) unless positioned carefully; different positions may need to be evaluated to minimize the tendency to thrust into extension and to maximize the most upright head position possible. **Straps** or **harnessing** may be used to provide trunk support, maintain head position, and position the feet flat on the footrest. A **three-point lateral control system** can be used to support the trunk and minimize or prevent scoliosis; this system uses a pad at the hip and upper trunk just below the axilla on one side and a mid-thoracic pad on the other to align the trunk.[119] An **abduction device/orthosis** is often used to break up adductor tone and help position the legs in a position of abduction and mild external rotation; the use of an abduction orthosis is thought to assist in postural control and minimize extensor thrust but no specific research is available to substantiate this claim. Similarly,

saddle-style or **bolster seats** have been used in a number of commercially available systems to maintain hip abduction with some degree of external rotation and hip and knee flexion (usually ≥90 degrees) to break up tone, create an anterior pelvic tilt, and thereby, facilitate postural stability and afford better upper extremity function; again, there is little research on the effectiveness of these seats.[119] A **contour seat** or **seating system** (back, seat, lateral support) may be best for children and adults with CP that have complex postural control needs, including scoliosis, kyphosis, or hip dysplasia; a contour system is individually fit to the child through a molding process (there are several commercially available) that creates a seat that conforms to the body. Additional external hardware can also be attached to provide maximal support, as needed. A contour seat can often be removed from the chair for sitting on the floor or a standard chair at a table as well as within a wheelchair frame.[120] Figure 20-7 shows a wheelchair that has been adapted for a child with dystonia at GMFCS level V.

One of the first decisions to be made in choosing a wheelchair is whether it can be propelled by the child, either manually or via electric power, or will be pushed by the caregiver. Children, as young as 1 to 3 years of age, can propel a manual chair or learn to operate a power chair; however, few children with CP are successful in propelling a manual chair outdoors, so power mobility may afford early and robust mobility in more environments than a manual chair.[121] Especially for children at GMFCS levels IV and V, powered mobility provides the greatest likelihood of any independent mobility,[122] yet, it may also afford those at levels II and III greater mobility outdoors than walking or using a manual chair.[123,124] Providing a wheelchair early allows independent exploration of the child's environment and is expected to improve social interactions and ultimately cognitive development.[125] There are also many choices of control devices for power chairs that accommodate the limited motor abilities of some children with CP. However, the child must have sufficient cognitive and perceptual motor skills to comprehend cause and effect, problem solve their position relative to where they want to go, understand how the wheelchair functions, and be able to plan their movement within complex environments. This requires the ability to maintain attention and diligently scan the environment for obstacles.[120] Control systems for power chairs include joysticks, switches, touch pads, head systems, mouth controls (e.g., sip and puff), and voice controls.

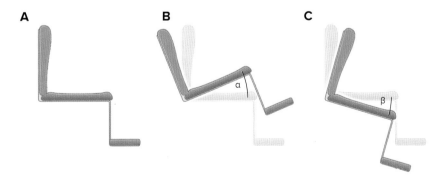

FIGURE 20-6 Seating orientation. A. A standard 90-90-90 seat representation that positions the hip, knee, and ankle at 90 degrees. **B.** A posterior tilt chair with additional hip flexion can be effective in controlling severe spasticity or dystonia yet limits active head motion. **C.** An anterior tilt chair can encourage an anterior pelvic tilt and an upright posture.

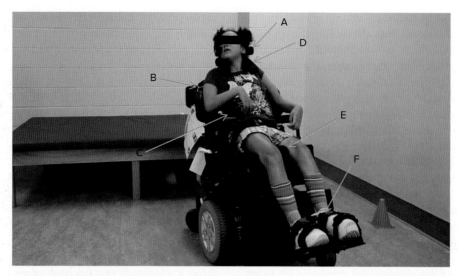

FIGURE 20-7 Power wheelchair for child with dyskinetic cerebral palsy. A. Head array allows control of the wheelchair by touch of cheek/head. **B.** Upper arm trough helps to control dystonic motions. **C.** Lateral trunk support to assist upright posture. **D.** Shoulder support pads to maintain shoulder contract with chair back. **E.** Abduction pommel maintains hip abduction. **F.** Footstraps on a rigid footplate maintain foot position. Note the seat is posteriorly tilted to assist with tone management.

Within each of these categories are numerous selections, allowing control of the wheelchair with a finger, fingers, or the hand; the chin, mouth, or head; or even the knee or foot. Thus, determining the best control device also requires trial and error with a variety of devices to find the best one. Fortunately, most wheelchair vendors will be able to outfit many devices to a given chair so that the right one can be determined.

Part of the decision of what type of wheelchair is appropriate for a given child includes an analysis of the home and school/work environments as well as the family's or for older adolescents/adults, the individual's ability to transport the chair. There needs to be a ramp into the home to allow entrance and exit; the household needs to have appropriate doorway clearance and minimal clutter to allow movement of the chair through the rooms. If the bedrooms are on an upper floor, there may need to be a home modification to allow the older child to have a bedroom on the main floor; young children may be easily carried upstairs, but this may be quite difficult for older children as they grow. A power chair requires a lift and van for transportation; yet even a manual chair that is fitted with many components may not be easily collapsible for transport in the trunk of a standard car, so a van or minivan may be required. Thus, physical therapists will play an important role in home assessment and the choice of the best wheelchair option for the child and family.

Ambulation Devices

For most children with CP needing ambulatory support, the first device will typically be a wheeled walker, most often a **posterior walker** (Figure 20-8); this type of walker places the walker frame behind the child with the grips at the side to encourage a more upright posture. Although anterior walkers are available for children, they can encourage a forward lean and flexed posture, so posterior walkers are more often the first device of choice.[126] Progression to **forearm crutches**

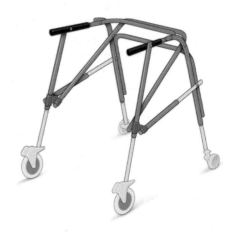

FIGURE 20-8 Posterior walker – the reverse walker encourages a more upright posture and is easier for the child to control than the standard anterior walker that can be pushed too far ahead of the child, resulting in forward falling.

is common as children gain upright stability, affording them the ability to maneuver on uneven terrains and stairs. No difference has been reported in the gait parameters (speed, kinematics) between using a posterior walker or forearm crutches; however, either device improves the child's gait (increased knee extension, less lateral trunk bend, and longer step length) over walking without a device.[127] Crutches will typically continue to be used through adulthood for those at GMFCS level III even when a wheelchair is used for community mobility.[122] For those at level IV, a wheeled walker may always be used if they are able to initiate steps with support, or they will walk only with assistance of a caregiver; wheelchair use (either self-propelled power wheelchair or pushed in a manual chair) will be their primary mobility. This will also be true of those at level V, but few will achieve independence with a power wheelchair (<20%).[122]

Positioning Devices

For children with a more severe level of disability, especially those at GMFCS level V, many devices are available to assist with positioning to increase weight-bearing and provide stability in a variety of postures for pressure release, deformity prevention, assistance with activities of daily living, and to enhance function.[128] There are a variety of **standers** that provide maximal support for the child, who is unable to stand on their own; standers often come with a tray or can be placed at a table or counter to allow the child to play (a necessity of childhood) while standing; this will also allow them to be eye-to-eye with peers as they play. Some power wheelchairs can also transform into a stander to afford the child time in standing to offset the hours spent in sitting. Early standing is thought to assist with LE bone development, prevent hip and knee flexion contractures, and enhance social interaction with peers, even in children at GMFCS level V, who do not have ambulation potential. Similarly, a standing program may improve ROM in adults at GMFCS levels IV and V.[129] **Sidelyers**, as the name suggests, assist in positioning a child in side-lying, which often allows the child more freedom of UE motion, including bringing the hands together for play, without excessive tone interference. There are also a variety of toileting and bathing devices to provide support for these activities, allowing greater independence for the child or adult with CP or assistance for their caregiver. As the child with severe disability ages, the family may need a **lifting device** to allow easier transitions from bed to wheelchair and for bathing and toileting. There are also a variety of lifts available (see Chapter 14 on multiple sclerosis).

Communication, Play, and Environmental Control Devices

For children with limited mobility, technology is making an incredible difference in their ability to communicate and interact with their environment. Computer technology is creating ever-expanding opportunities for the child and adult with severe mobility limitations. **Communication devices** can be a simple array of pictures, attached to a wheelchair tray, depicting common needs (e.g., foods, drink, family photos) to a complex computerized system that allows the child to indicate complex concepts or complete schoolwork through a synthesized voice or onscreen writing. Like wheelchairs, these devices can be activated by touch of an individual finger, the entire hand, the head, or even eye movement.[130] Note, many children with severe mobility impairment do not have intellectual deficits or have mild deficits, so these devices are opening up the world to them. For young children, many common toys can be modified with switches that enable the child with limited mobility to activate them; similarly, computer programs and video game systems can be modified so that small movements (e.g., eye movements) or voice activation are effective means for the child to control the program or game. Likewise, **environmental control systems** allow voice or switch activation of lights, computers, televisions, sounds systems, and almost any electric device. With the expansion of computer capabilities, it will be interesting to see what the next decade brings to the field of assistive technology and devices to assist those with disabilities to communicate and control their environments.

> ### CASE A, PART VII
>
> Alejandro was fitted with an articulating AFO with a plantarflexion block to help him achieve better heel strike and dorsiflexion during swing. Although he currently walks with a posterior walker, in the future, he may be a candidate for forearm crutches. Treadmill training might also be effective in improving his step length and speed of ambulation.[95–97]

● SUMMARY

As this chapter indicates, CP is a heterogeneous condition, presenting with a myriad of needs for the physical therapist and the rest of the school-based and rehabilitation-focused team members to address. As a lifelong condition, it requires treatment across the lifespan to assure the best outcome for the child and eventually the adult to function in their many environments (school, play, work, home, community). For children with severe disability, this also includes helping the family to manage the child and potentially the adult within the home. A growing area of need is to assist the adolescent's or young adult's transition to independence outside the family home. With such transitions, assessment of the new home and/or workplace with appropriate modifications may allow the adult with CP to function independently or with some care assistance in an independent living situation.

REFERENCES

1. Vitrikas K, Dalton H, Breish D. Cerebral palsy: an overview. *Am Fam Physician*. 2020;101(4):213-220.

2. Brain Injury Help Center. https://www.birthinjuryhelpcenter.org/cerebral-palsy-statistics.html. Accessed May 11, 2022.

3. Ream M, Lehwald L. Neurologic consequence of preterm birth. *Curr Neurol Neurosci Rep*. 2018;18:48.

4. Vohr BR, Msall ME, Wilson D, Wright LL, McDonald S, Poole WK. Spectrum of gross motor function in extremely low birth weight children with cerebral palsy at 18 months of age. *Pediatrics*. 2005;116(1):123-129.

5. Cutland CL, Lackritz EM, Mallett-Moore T, et al. The Brighton Collaboration Low Birth Weight Working Group. Low birth weight: case definition & guidelines for data collection, analysis, and presentation of maternal immunization safety data. *Vaccine*. 2017;35:6492-6500.

6. Vohr B. Long-term outcomes of moderately preterm, late preterm, and early term infants. *Clin Perinatol*. 2013;40:739-751.

7. Ophelders DRMG, Gussenhoven R, Klein L, et al. Preterm brain injury, antenatal triggers, and therapeutics: timing is key. *Cells*. 2020;9:1871.

8. Ortinau C, Neil J. The neuroanatomy of prematurity: normal brain development and the impact of preterm birth. *Clin Anat*. 2015;28(2):168-183.

9. Stinson LF, Payne MS. Infection-mediated preterm birth: bacterial origins and avenues for intervention. *Aust N Z J Obstet Gynaecol*. 2019;59:781-790.

10. Meister AL, Doheny KK, Travagli RA. Necrotizing enterocolitis: it's not all in the gut. *Exp Biol Med*. 2020;245:85-95.

11. McManus BM, Chambliss JH, Rapport MJ. Application of the NICU practice guidelines to treat an infant in a level III NICU. *Pediatr Phys Ther*. 2013;25:204-213.

12. Craig JW, Smith CR. Risk-adjusted/neuroprotective care in the NICU: the elemental role of the neonatal therapist (OT, PT, SLP). *J Perinatol*. 2020;40:549-559.

13. Khurana S, Kane AE, Brown SE, Tarver T, Dusing SC. Effect of neonatal therapy on the motor, cognitive, and behavioral development of infants born preterm: a systematic review. *Dev Med Child Neurol.* 2020;62(6):684-692.

14. Upadhyay J, Tiwari N, Ansari MN. Cerebral palsy: aetiology, pathophysiology and therapeutic interventions. *Clin Exp Pharmacol Physiol.* 2020;47:1891-1901.

15. Johnston MV, Hoon AH. Cerebral palsy. *Neuromolecular Med.* 2006;8:435-450.

16. Chin EM, Gorny N, Logan M, Hoon AH. Cerebral palsy and the placenta: a review of the maternal-placental-fetal origins of cerebral palsy. *Exp Neurol.* 2022;352:114021.

17. Halliday HL. Neonatal management of long-term sequelae. *Best Pract Res Clin Obstet Gynaecol.* 2009;23:871-880.

18. Wixey JA, Chand KK, Colditz PB, Bjorkman ST. Review: neuroinflammation in intrauterine growth restriction. *Placenta.* 2017;54:117-124.

19. Wimalasundera N, Stevenson VL. Cerebral palsy. *Pract Neurol.* 2016;16:184-194.

20. Rainaldi MA, Perlman JM. Pathophysiology of birth asphyxia. *Clin Perinatol.* 2016;43:409-422.

21. Herrera CA, Silver RM. Perinatal asphyxia from the obstetric standpoint: diagnosis and interventions. *Clin Perinatol.* 2016;43:423-438.

22. Wong L, Kwan AHW, Lau SL, Sin WTA, Leung TY. Umbilical cord prolapse: revisiting its definition and management. *Am J Obstet Gynecol.* 2021;225(4):357-366.

23. Bokslag A, van Weissenbruch M, Mol BW, de Groot CJM. Preeclampsia: short and long-term consequences for mother and neonate. *Early Hum Dev.* 2016;102:47-50.

24. Ahlin K, Himmelmann K, Hagberg G, et al. Cerebral palsy and perinatal infection in children born at term. *Obstet Gynecol.* 2013;122:41-49.

25. Bear JJ, Wu YW. Maternal infections during pregnancy and cerebral palsy in the child. *Pediatr Neurol.* 2016;57:74-79.

26. Ganguli S, Chavali PL. Intrauterine viral infections: impact of inflammation on fetal neurodevelopment. *Front Neurosci.* 2021;15:771557.

27. Leung TY, Chung TKH. Severe chronic morbidity following childbirth. *Best Pract Res Clin Obstet Gynaecol.* 2009;23:401-423.

28. Evans MI, Britt DW, Evans SM. Mid forceps did not cause "compromised babies" – "compromise" caused forceps: an approach toward safely lowering the cesarean delivery rate. *J Matern Fetal Neonatal Med.* 2022;35(25):5265-5273.

29. Phalen AG, Kirkby S, Dysart K. The 5 minute Apgar score: survival and short-term outcomes of extremely low-birth-weight infants. *J Perinat Neonatal Nurs.* 2012;26(6):166-171.

30. Novak I, Morgan C, Adde L, et al. Early, accurate diagnosis and early intervention in cerebral palsy: advances in diagnosis and treatment. *JAMA Pediatr.* 2017;171(9):897-907.

31. Byrne R, Noritz G, Maitre NL NCH Early Developmental Group. Implementation of early diagnosis and intervention guidelines for cerebral palsy in a high-risk infant follow-up clinic. *Pediatr Neurol.* 2017;76:66-71.

32. Morgan C, Fahey M, Roy B, Novak I. Diagnosing cerebral palsy in full-term infants. *J Paediatr Child Health.* 2018;54:1159-1164.

33. Hadders-Algra M. Early human motor development: from variation to the ability to vary and adapt. *Neurosci Biobehav Rev.* 2018;90:411-427.

34. Einspieler C, Marschik PB, Pansy J, et al. The general movement optimality score: a detailed assessment of general movements during preterm and term age. *Dev Med Child Neurol.* 2016;58:361-368.

35. Datta AN, Furrer MA, Bernhardt I, et al. The GM Group. Fidgety movements in infants born very preterm: predictive value for cerebral palsy in a clinical multicentre setting. *Dev Med Child Neurol.* 2017;59:618-624.

36. Hanna SE, Bartlett DJ, Rivard LM, Russell DJ. Reference curves for the gross motor function measure: percentiles for clinical description and tracking over time among children with cerebral palsy. *Phys Ther.* 2008;88:596-607.

37. Palisano R, Rosenbaum P, Walter S, Russell D, Wood E, Galuppi B. Development and reliability of a system to classify gross motor function in children with cerebral palsy. *Dev Med Child Neurol.* 1997;39(4):214-223.

38. Gorter JW, Ketelaar M, Rosenbaum P, Helders PJM, Palisano R. Use of the GMFCS in infants with CP: the need for reclassification at age 2 years or older. *Dev Med Child Neurol.* 2008;51:46-52.

39. Hanna S, Rosenbaum PL, Bartlett DJ, et al. Stability and decline in gross motor function among children and youth with cerebral palsy aged 2 to 21 years. *Dev Med Child Neurol.* 2009;51:295-302.

40. CanChild: https://www.canchild.ca/en/diagnoses/cerebral-palsy. Accessed on May 23, 2022.

41. Btandenburg JE, Fogarty MJ, Sieck GC. A critical evaluation of current concepts in cerebral palsy. *Physiology.* 2019;34:216-229.

42. Shevell M, Dagenais L, Hall N. The relationship of cerebral palsy subtype and functional motor impairment: a population-based study. *Dev med Child Neurol.* 2009;51:872-877.

43. Himmelmann K, Hagberg G, Wiklund LM, Eek MN, Uvebrant P. Sykinetic cerebral palsy: a population-based study of children born between 1991 and 1998. *Dev Med Child Neurol.* 2007;49:246-251.

44. Cahill-Rowley K, Rose J. Etiology of impaired selective motor control: emerging evidence and its implications for research and treatment in cerebral palsy. *Dev Med Child Neurol.* 2014;56:522-528.

45. Yokochi K, Hosoe A, Shimabukuro S, Kodama K. Motoscopic analysis of gross motor patterns in athetotic cerebral palsied children. *Brain Dev.* 1989;11:317-321.

46. Yokochi K, Hosoe A, Shimabukuro S, Kodama K. Gross motor patterns in children with cerebral palsy and spastic diplegia. *Pediatr Neurol.* 1990;6:245-250.

47. Brunner R. Development and conservative treatment of spinal deformities in cerebral palsy. *J Child Ortho.* 2020;14:2-8.

48. Modlesky CM, Zhang C. Complicated muscle-bone interactions in children with cerebral palsy. *Curr Osteoporos Rep.* 2020;18(1):47-56.

49. Valencia FG. Management of hip deformities in cerebral palsy. *Orthop Clin North Am.* 2013;41:549-550.

50. Young JL, Rodda J, Selber P, Rutz E, Graham HK. Management of the knee in spastic diplegia: what is the dose? *Orthop Clin North Am.* 2010;41:561-577.

51. Davids JR. The foot and ankle in cerebral palsy. *Orthop Clin North Am.* 2010;41:579-593.

52. Koman LA, Sarliakiotis T, Smith BP. Surgery of the upper extremity in cerebral palsy. *Orthop Clin North Am.* 2010;41:519-529.

53. Bottos M, Puato ML, Vianello A, Facchin P. Locomotion patterns in cerebral palsy syndromes. *Dev Med Child Neurol.* 1995;37:883-899.

54. Armand S, Decoulon G, Bonnefoy-Mazure A. Gait analysis in children with cerebral palsy. *EFORT Open Rev.* 2016;1:448-460.

55. Baker JM. Gait disorders. *Am J Med.* 2018;131:602-607.

56. Chin TYP, Duncan JA, Johnstone BR, Graham HK. Management of the upper limb in cerebral palsy. *J Pediat Ortho.* 2005;14(6):389-404.

57. Katz G, Lazeano-Ponce E. Intellectual disability: definition, etiological factors, classification, diagnosis, treatment and prognosis. *Salud Publica Mex.* 2008;50(S2):5132-5141.

58. Depositario-Cabacar DFT, Zelleke TG. Treatment of epilepsy in children with developmental disabilities. *Dev Disabil Res Rev.* 2010;16:239-247.

59. Odding E, Roebroeck ME, Stam HJ. The epidemiology of cerebral palsy: incidence, impairments and risk factors. *Disabil Rehabil.* 2006;28(4):183-191.

60. Purugganan O. Intellectual disabilities. *Pediatr Rev.* 2018;39(6):299-309.

61. Hanci F, Turay S, Dilek M, Kabakus N. Epilepsy and drug-resistant epilepsy in children with cerebral palsy: a retrospective observational study. *Epilepsy Behav.* 2020;112. doi.org/10.1016/j.yebeh.2020.107357.

62. Zimmern V, Korff C. Status epilepticus in children. *J Clin Neurophysiol.* 2020;37(5):429-433.

63. Tsbouchi Y, Tanabe A, Saito Y, Noma H, Maegaki Y. Long-term prognosis of epilepsy in patients with cerebral palsy. *Dev Med Child Neurol.* 2019;61:1067-1073.

64. Gulati S, Sondhi V. Cerebral palsy: an overview. *Indian J Pediatr.* 2018;85(11):1006-1016.

65. Richard C, Kjeldsen C, Findlen U, Gehred A, Maitre N. Hearing loss diagnosis and early hearing-related interventions in infants with or at high risk for cerebral palsy: a systematic review. *J Child Neurol.* 2021;36(10):919-929.

66. Naksahima T, Suzuki H, Sugiura S, Beppu R, Ishida K. Gustatory function in persons with cerebral palsy. *J Oral Rehabil.* 2020:47:523-527.

67. Riquelme I, Montoya P. Developmental changes in somatosensory processing in cerebral palsy and healthy individuals. *Clin Neurophysiol.* 2010;121:1314-1320.

68. Pennington L. Speech, language, communication, and cerebral palsy. *Dev Med Child Neurol.* 2016;58:530-540.

69. Mei C, Reilly S, Reddihough D, Mensah F, Pennington L, Morgan A. Language outcomes of children with cerebral palsy aged 5 years and 6 years: a population study. *Dev Med Child Neurol.* 2018;58:805-811.

70. Scholderle T, Haas E, Ziegler W. Dysarthria syndromes in children with cerebral palsy. *Dev Med Child Neurol.* 2021;63:444-449.

71. Tegler H, Pless M, Johansson MB, Sonnander K. Caregivers', teachers', and assistants' use and learning of partner strategies in communication using high-tech speech-generating devices with children with severe cerebral palsy. *Assist Technol.* 2021;33(1):17-25.

72. Fine A Wirrell EC. Seizures in children. *Pediatr Rev.* 2020;41(7):321-346.

73. Liu G, Slater N, Perkins A. Epilepsy: treatment options. *Am Fam Physician.* 2017;96(2):87-96.

74. Jayalakshmi S, Vooturi S, Gupta S, Panigrahi M. Epilepsy surgery in children. *Neurol India.* 2017;65(3):485-492.

75. Peck J, Urits I, Kassem H, et al. Interventional approaches to pain and spasticity related to cerebral palsy. *Psychopharmacol Bull.* 2020;50(4, suppl 1):108-120.

76. Papavasiliou AS. Management of motor problems in cerebral palsy: a critical update for the clinician. *Eur J Paediatr Neurol.* 2009;13:387-396.

77. Dudley RR, Parolin M, Gagnon B, et al. Long-term functional benefits of selective dorsal rhizotomy for spastic cerebral palsy. *J Neurosurg Pediatr.* 2013;12:142-150.

78. Milne N, Miao M, Beattie E. The effects of serial casting on lower limb function for children with cerebral palsy: a systematic review with meta-analysis. *BMS Pediatr.* 2020;20:324. https://doi.org/10.1186/s12887-020-02122-9.

79. Damiano DL, Alter KE, Chamber H. New clinical and research trends in lower extremity management for ambulatory children with cerebral palsy. *Phys Med Rehabil Clin N Am.* 2009;20(3):469-491.

80. Nahm NJ, Graham HK, Gormley ME, Georgiadis AG. Management of hypertonia in cerebral palsy. *Curr Opin Pediatr.* 2018;30:57-64.

81. Long JT, Cobb L, Garcia MC, McCarthy JJ. Improved clinical and functional outcomes in crouch gait following minimally invasive hamstring lengthening and serial casting in children with cerebral palsy. *Pediatr Orthop.* 2020;40(6):e510-e515.

82. Sharan D. Orthopedic surgery in cerebral palsy: instruction course lecture. *Indian J Orthop.* 2017;51:240-255.

83. Scarpato E, Stalano A, Molteni M, Terrone G, Mazzocchi A, Agostoni C. Nutritional assessment and intervention in children with cerebral palsy: a practical approach. *Int J Food Sci Nutr.* 2017;68(6):763-770.

84. Rempel G. The importance of good nutrition in children with cerebral palsy. *Phys Med Rehabil Clin N Am.* 2015;26:39-56.

85. Jesus AO, Stevenson RD. Optimizing nutrition and bone health in children with cerebral palsy. *Phys Med Rehabil Clin N Am.* 2020;31:25-37.

86. Benfer KA, Weir KA, Bell KL, Ware RS, Davies PSW, Boyd RN. Oropharyngeal dysphagia in preschool children with cerebral palsy: oral phase impairments. *Res Dev Disabil.* 2014;35:3469-3481.

87. Kuperminc MN, Gottrand F, Samson-Fang L, et al. Nutritional management of children with cerebral palsy: a practical guide. *Eur J Clin Nutr.* 2013;67:521-523.

88. Caramico-favero DCC, Guedes ZCF, de Morais MB. Food intake, nutritional status and gastrointestinal symptoms in children with cerebral palsy. *Arq Gastroenterol.* 2018;55(4):352-357.

89. Kleim JA, Jones TA. Principles of experience-dependent neural plasticity: implications for rehabilitation after brain damage. *J Speech Lang Hear Res.* 2008;51:S225-S239.

90. Robert MT, Sambasivan K, Levin MF. Extrinsic feedback and upper limb motor skill learning in typically-developing children and children with cerebral palsy: review. *Restor Neurol Neurosci.* 2017;35:171-184.

91. Kalkman BM, Baron L, O'Brian TD, Maganaris CN. Stretching interventions in children with cerebral palsy: why are they ineffective in improving muscle function and how can we better their outcome? *Front Physiol.* 2020;11:131.

92. Damiano DL, Arnold AS, Steele KM, Delp SL. Can strength training predictably improve gait kinematics? A pilot study on the effects of hip and knee extensor strengthening on lower-extremity alignment in cerebral palsy. *Phys Ther.* 2010;90:269-279.

93. Franki I, Bar-on L Molenaers G, et al. Tone reduction and physical therapy: strengthening partners in treatment of children with spastic cerebral palsy. *Neuropediatrics.* 2020;51(2):89-104.

94. Morgan C, Novak I, Dale RC, Guzzetta A, Badawi N. GAME (Goals-Activity-Motor Enrichment): protocol of a single blind randomized controlled trial of motor training, parent education and environmental enrichment for infants at high risk of cerebral palsy. *BMC Neurol.* 2014;14:203.

95. Han YG Yun CK. Effectiveness of treadmill training on gait function in children with cerebral palsy: meta-analysis. *J Ex Rehabil.* 2020;18(1):10-19.

96. Matsuno VM, Camargo MR, Palma GC. Alvero D, Berela AMF. Analysis of partial body weight support during treadmill and overground walking of children with cerebral palsy. *Rev Bras Fisioter.* 2010;14(5):404-410.

97. Wu M, Kim J, Gaebler-Spira DJ, Schmit BD, Arora P. Robotic resistance treadmill training improves locomotor function in children with cerebral palsy: a randomized controlled pilot study. *Arch Phys Med Rehabil.* 2017;98(11):2126-2133.

98. Volpani M, Aquino M, Holanda AC, Emygdio E, Polese J. Clinical effects of assisted robotic gait training in walking distance, speed and functionality are maintained over the long term in individuals with cerebral palsy: a systematic review and meta-analysis. *Disabil Rehabil.* 2022;44(19):5418-5428.

99. Gilliaux M, Renders A, Dispa D, et al. Upper limb robot-assisted therapy in cerebral palsy: a single-blind randomized controlled trial. *Neurorehabil Neural Repair.* 2015;29(2):183-192.

100. Macintosh A, Lam E, Vigneron V, Vignais N, Biddiss E. Biofeedback interventions for individuals with cerebral palsy: a systematic review. *Disabil Rehabil.* 2019;41(20):2369-2391.

101. Bonnechere B, Jansen B, Omelina L, Jan SVS. The use of commercial video games in rehabilitation: a systematic review. *Int J Rehabil Res.* 2016;39(4):277-279.

102. Chen Y, Fanchiang HD, Howard A. Effectiveness of virtual reality in children with cerebral palsy: a systematic review and meta-analysis of randomized controlled trials. *Phys Ther.* 2018;98:63-77.

103. Ramey SL, DeLuca SC, Stevenson RD, Conaway M, Darragh AR, Lo W. Constraint induced movement therapy for cerebral palsy: a randomized trial. *Pediatrics.* 2021;148(5):e2020033878.

104. Eliasson AC, Nordstrand L, Ek L, et al. The effectiveness of Baby-CIMT in infants younger than 12 months with clinical signs of unilateral-cerebral palsy: an explorative study with randomized design. *Res Dev Disabil.* 2018;72:191-201.

105. Chen YP, Pope S, Tyler D, Warren GL. Effectiveness of constraint-induced movement therapy on upper-extremity function in children with cerebral palsy: a systematic review and meta-analysis of randomized controlled trials. *Clin Rehabil.* 2014;28(10):939-953.

106. Gordon AM, Schneider JA, Chinnan A, Charles JR. Efficacy of a hand-arm bimanual intensive therapy (HABIT) in children with hemiplegic cerebral palsy: a randomized control trial. *Dev Med Child Neurol.* 2007;49:830-838.

107. Figueiredo PRP, Mancini MC, Feitosa AM, et al. Hand-arm bimanual intensive therapy and daily functioning of children with bilateral cerebral palsy: a randomized controlled trial. *Dev Med Child Neurol.* 2020;62:1274-1282.

108. Bleyenheuft Y, Arnould C, Brandao MB. Hand and arm bimanual intensive therapy including lower extremity (HABIT-ILE) in children with unilateral spastic cerebral palsy: a randomized trial. *Neurorehabil Neural Repair.* 2015;29(7):645-657.

109. Bleyenheuft Y, Ebner-Karestinos D, Surana B, et al. Intensive upper- and lower-extremity training for children with bilateral cerebral palsy: a quasi-randomized trial. *Dev Med Child Neurol.* 2017;59:615-633.

110. Araneda R, Sizonenko SV, Dinomais M, et al. and Early Habit-ILE group. Functional, neuroplastic and biomechanical changes induced by early hand-arm bimanual intensive therapy including lower extremities (e-HABIT-ILE) in preschool children with unilateral cerebral palsy: study protocol of a randomized control trial. *BMC Neurol.* 2020;20:133.

111. Silkwood-Sherer DJ, Killian CB, Long TM, Martin KS. Hippotherapy – an intervention to habilitate balance deficits in children with movement disorders: a clinical trial. *Phys Ther.* 2012;92:707-717.

112. Lai CJ, Liu WY, Yang TF, Chen CL, Wu CY, Chan RC. Pediatric aquatic therapy on motor function and enjoyment in children diagnosed with cerebral palsy of various motor severities. *J Child Neurol.* 2015;30(2):200-208.

113. Pettersson K, Rodby-Bousquet E. Prevalence and goal attainment with spinal orthoses for children with cerebral palsy. *J Pediatr Rehabil Med.* 2019;12:197-203.

114. Wright E, DiBello SA. Principles of ankle-foot orthosis prescription in ambulatory bilateral cerebral palsy. *Phys Med Rehabil Clin N Am.* 2020; 31:69-89.

115. Chisholm AE, Perry SD. Ankle-foot orthotic management in neuromuscular disorders: recommendations for future research. *Disabil Rehabil Assist Technol.* 2012;7(6):437-449.

116. Akaltun MS, Bicer OAS, Turan N, Gursoy S, Gur A. Use of lower extremity orthoses in patients with cerebral palsy and related factors. *Prosthet Orthot Int.* 2021;45(6):487-490.

117. Angsupaisal M, Maathuis CGB, Hadders-Algra M. Adaptive seating systems in children with severe cerebral palsy across international classification of functioning, disability and health for children and youth version domains: a systematic review. *Dev Med Child Neurol.* 2015;57:919-931.

118. Alkhateeb AM, Daher NS Forrester BJ, Martin BD, Jaber HM. Effects of adjustments to wheelchair seat to back support angle on head, neck, and shoulder postures in subjects with cerebral palsy. *Assist Technol.* 2020;33(6):326-332.

119. Chung J, Evans J, Lee C, et al. Effectiveness of adaptive seating on sitting posture and postural control in children with cerebral palsy. *Pediatr Phys Ther.* 2008;20:303-317.

120. Nace S, Tiernan J, Annaidh AN. Manufacturing custom-contoured wheelchair seating: a state-of-the-art review. *Prosthet Orthot Int.* 2019;43(4):382-395.

121. Kenyon LK, Jones M, Breaux B. Tsotsoros J, Gardner T, Livingstone R. American and Canadian therapists' perspectives of age and cognitive skills for paediatric power mobility: a qualitative study. *Disabil Rehabil: Assistive Technol.* 2020;15(6):692-700.

122. Palisano RJ, Hanna SE, Rosenbaum PL, Tieman B. Probability of walking, wheeled mobility, and assisted mobility in children and adolescents with cerebral palsy. *Dev Med Child Neurol.* 2010;52:66-71.

123. Rodby-Bousquet E, Paleg G, Casey J, wizert A, Livingstone R. Physical risk factors influencing wheeled mobility in children with cerebral palsy: a cross-sectional study. *BMC Pediatr.* 2016;16:165.

124. Rodby-Bousquet E, Hägglund G. Use of manual and powered wheelchair in children with cerebral palsy: a cross-sectional study. *BMC Pediatr.* 2010;10:59.

125. Livingstone R, Field D. Systematic review of power mobility outcomes for infants, children and adolescents with mobility limitations. *Clin Rehabil.* 2014;28(10):954-964.

126. Poole M, Simkiss D, Rose A, Li FX. Anterior or posterior walkers for children with cerebral palsy? A Systematic review. *Disabil Rehabil Assist Technol.* 2018;13(4):422-433.

127. Krautwurst BK, Dreher T, Wolf SI. The impact of walking devices on kinematics in patients with spastic bilateral cerebral palsy. *Gait Posture.* 2016;46:184-187.

128. Raul W, Sarmaci S, Khan I, Jawad M. Effect of position on gross motor function and spasticity in spastic cerebral palsy children. *J Pak Med Assoc.* 2021;71(3):801-805.

129. Rodby-Bousquet E, Agustsson A. Postural asymmetries and assistive devices used by adults with cerebral palsy in lying, sitting, and standing. *Front Neurol.* 2021;12:758706.

130. Reyes F, Niedzwecki C, Gaebler-Spira D. Technological advancements in cerebral palsy rehabilitation. *Phys Med Rehabil Clin N Am.* 2020;31: 117-129.

Review Questions

1. **Which of the following best describes the condition of cerebral palsy?**

   A. The initial lesion may progress as the child ages

   B. It always involves a motor impairment

   C. All children diagnosed with cerebral palsy have an apparent lesion on MRI

   D. The type of tone a child has will be constant over his/her lifetime

2. **A lesion in the germinal region of the developing brain that damages pre-oligodendrocytes is known as:**

   A. Intraventricular hemorrhage

   B. Necrotizing enterocolitis

   C. Neonatal stroke

   D. Periventricular leukomalacia

3. **A grade III intraventricular hemorrhage includes which area(s)?**

   A. Endothelial layer only

   B. Endothelial layer plus ventricle

   C. Endothelial layer, ventricle, and brain tissue

   D. Endothelial layer, ventricle, brain tissue, and cortex

4. **A child presents with spasticity in all four extremities, but her arms are more affected than her legs. This child is presenting with:**

   A. Spastic diplegia

   B. Spastic hemiplegia

   C. Spastic quadriplegia

   D. Spastic triplegia

5. **A swan-neck deformity involves which body part?**

   A. Ankle

   B. Finger

   C. Knee

   D. Trunk

6. A child you are working with stares off into space while chewing and picking at her clothes. This is most likely what type of seizure?
   A. Atonic
   B. Complex partial
   C. Myoclonic
   D. Tonic-clonic

7. An adolescent with IDD is learning to work at the grocery store, bagging groceries, is able to read street and bus signs to travel to and from the store, and has a few friends from high school with whom he likes to watch football games. This teenager is demonstrating what level of IDD?
   A. Mild
   B. Moderate
   C. Severe
   D. Profound

8. Your 7-year-old patient with diplegia walks with equinovarus, minimal knee flexion with recurvatum during stance, and frequently tripping when walking. She is demonstrating what gait pattern?
   A. Ataxic gait
   B. Crouched gait
   C. True equinus gait
   D. Scissor gait

9. Which of the following comorbidities occur in children with CP at the highest incidence rate?
   A. Epilepsy
   B. IDD
   C. Sensory dysfunction
   D. Malnutrition

10. A 4-year-old is walking with forearm crutches independently for all home and community activities except trips to the mall, zoo, or park. This child would likely be classified at which GMFCS level?
    A. Level I
    B. Level II
    C. Level III
    D. Level IV
    E. Level V

11. A child (GMFCS level V) has severe spasticity in both UE and LE that is impeding his parents' ability to bath and toilet him. The best spasticity management would most likely be?
    A. Botulinum toxin injections
    B. Intrathecal baclofen
    C. Surgical lengthening of all flexor tendons
    D. Oral gabapentin

12. A 3-year-old child at GMFCS level IV with no IDD but severe dystonia, right hip dislocation, and emerging scoliosis would be a candidate for what type of wheelchair?
    A. A manual chair for self-propulsion
    B. A manual chair for caregiver propulsion
    C. A power chair with an anterior-tilted seat
    D. A power chair with a contour seat

13. Therapy in the NICU is focused on which of the following?
    A. Facilitating acquisition of developmental milestones
    B. Facilitating self-regulation
    C. Inhibiting abnormal tone
    D. Maximizing stimulation

14. The "P" in APGAR stands for which of the following?
    A. Airway
    B. Heart rate
    C. Color
    D. Respiration
    E. Muscle activity

15. Which treatment method for children with CP is not focused on increasing postural control and gait?
    A. Aquatic therapy
    B. HABIT
    C. Hippotherapy
    D. Robotic therapy

16. A condition of pregnancy characterized by hypertension and proteinuria is?
    A. Prolapsed umbilical
    B. Placenta abruption
    C. Placental previa
    D. Pre-eclampsia

17. A baby is born at 34 weeks gestation, weighing 1300 g; this baby would appropriately be described as:
    A. Moderate preterm low birth weight
    B. Moderate preterm, very low birth weight
    C. Very preterm, low birth weight
    D. Very preterm, very low birth weight

18. The diagnostic criteria for early diagnosis of CP include which of the following?
    A. Abnormal MRI
    B. Abnormal MRI and Prechtl Qualitative Assessment of General Movements
    C. Abnormal MRI, Prechtl Qualitative Assessment of General Movements and the Hammersmith Infant Neurological Examination
    D. Abnormal MRI, abnormal tone, Prechtl Qualitative Assessment of General Movements and the Hammersmith Infant Neurological Examination

19. **Fidgety movements should be apparent at what age?**
    A. After 20 weeks of age
    B. Birth to 9 weeks of age
    C. During the first two trimesters
    D. From 7 to 20 weeks of age

20. **A child that you are working with displays sustained co-contraction of muscles that results in hyperextension of the neck and twisting of the trunk. This would be best categorized as:**
    A. Ataxia
    B. Ballismus
    C. Chorea
    D. Dystonia

21. **The characteristic upper extremity posture of a child with unilateral CP is:**
    A. Adduction and internal rotation of the shoulder with elbow, wrist, and finger flexion
    B. Adduction and internal rotation of the shoulder with elbow, wrist, and finger extension
    C. Adduction and external rotation of the shoulder with elbow, wrist, and finger flexion
    D. Adduction and external rotation of the shoulder with elbow, wrist, and finger extension

22. **Disrupted motor control for eating is referred to as:**
    A. Oropharyngeal dysarthria
    B. Oropharyngeal dysphagia
    C. Oromotor dysregulation
    D. Oromotor dysarthria

23. **Therapists should not encourage family members or caregivers to provide therapy in the home because they are likely to implement care incorrectly and make the child's condition worse.**
    A. True
    B. False

24. **Strengthening programs are inappropriate for children with spasticity because they will make the hypertonia worse and lead to greater likelihood of contractures.**
    A. True
    B. False

25. **The treatment approach that uses parent coaching, environmental enrichment and task-specific motor training is?**
    A. CIMT
    B. GAME
    C. HABIT
    D. HABIT-ILE

26. **A standing program for a child at GMFCS level V can be used for which of the following?**
    A. As a first step to independent standing
    B. To stimulate midline play
    C. To facilitate bone development in the LE
    D. A standing program is inappropriate for a child at level V.

Answers

1. B	2. D	3. B	4. C	5. B
6. B	7. B	8. C	9. C	10. C
11. B	12. D	13. B	14. B	15. B
16. D	17. B	18. C	19. D	20. A
21. B	22. B	23. B	24. B	25. C
26. C				

GLOSSARY

Aquatic therapy. Using water as a supportive treatment medium.

Apparent equinus gait. Excessive hip and knee flexion with apparent equinus but full range of motion at the ankle.

Articulating AFO. Ankle-foot orthotic with an ankle joint.

Ataxic CP. Associated with cerebellar damage, characterized by coordination, balance and movement dysfunction.

Athetosis. Slow writhing movements, greater in distal joints.

Atonic/hypotonic CP. Low muscle tone with altered deep tendon reflexes (hypo or hyperreflexia).

Ballismus. Quick, jerky movements of the entire limb.

Bimanual hand-arm therapy. Intensive treatment protocol that involves using both hands and arms in functional tasks.

Bimanual hand-arm therapy including lower extremities. Bimanual treatment that includes challenging sitting, standing and mobility activities.

Chorea. Rapid involuntary movements.

Choreoathetosis. Combination of athetosis and chorea.

Crouched gait. Hip and knee flexion, internal rotation and adduction of the hip, with excessive dorsiflexion.

Diplegia. Greater involvement of the legs than the arms; arms may not demonstrate involvement.

Dyskinetic CP. Basal ganglial damage associated with abnormal involuntary movements.

Dystonia. Sustained co-contraction of muscles.

Eclampsia. Progression of pre-eclampsia to a life-threatening condition for mother and baby.

Encephalopathy of prematurity. Neurologic injury secondary to prematurity.

Epilepsy. Repetitive seizures in the absence of active disease.

Fidgety movements. Small irregular movements made by neonates from 7 to 20 weeks.

Gastroesophageal reflex. Regurgitation of stomach contents into the esophagus.

Generalized seizure. Involves both hemispheres.

Hemiplegia. Unilateral involvement.

Hippotherapy. Use of a horse as a therapeutic tool to improve sensorimotor function.

Hypoxic-ischemic encephalopathy. Brain damage in the perinatal period secondary to anoxia.

Intrauterine growth restriction. A deficit in fetal growth during gestation.

Intraventricular hemorrhage. Hemorrhage in the endothelial lining of the ventricles.

Jump gait. Stiff knee with excessive ankle, knee and hip flexion, anterior pelvic tilt, and excessive lordosis.

Meconium. The dark pasty stool of the neonate.

Necrotizing enterocolitis. Death of the mucosal lining of the intestines.

Non-articulating AFO. Ankle-foot orthotic made of one piece.

Non-spastic CP. All other forms of CP (ataxic, dystonic, atonic).

Partial seizure. Involves one hemisphere with some degree of consciousness retained.

Percutaneous endoscopic gastrostomy. Surgical implantation of a tube into the stomach to provide direct feeding, bypassing the mouth.

Perinatal asphyxia. Disruption of oxygen that results in brain damage during gestation, delivery or the neonatal period.

Periventricular leukomalacia. Large cysts within the white matter near the ventricles.

Placental abruption. Premature detachment of the placenta.

Placental Insufficiency. Structural abnormality of the placenta that disrupts its normal function.

Placental previa. Attachment of the placenta too close to the cervix.

Pre-eclampsia. Kidney dysfunction resulting in hypertension and proteinuria.

Quadriplegia. Involvement of all four extremities with UE more involved or equally involved with LE.

Seizure. Abnormal discharge of neurons.

Selective dorsal rhizotomy. Surgical ablation of some dorsal root afferents to diminish spasticity.

Spastic CP. Characterized by hypertonia and hyperreflexia.

Strabismus. Poor coordination of extraocular muscles, resulting in blurred vision.

Triplegia. One extremity is less involved than the other three extremities.

True equinus gait. Equinus throughout stance with hip and knee (recurvatum) extension.

Umbilical cord prolapse. Delivery of the umbilical cord prior to the baby.

Writhing movements. Slow, whole extremity movement seen at late gestation and early infancy.

ABBREVIATIONS

AFO	ankle-foot orthosis
APGAR	appearance, pulse, grimace, activity, respiration
CIMT	constraint-induced movement therapy
ELBW	extremely low birth weight
EOP	encephalopathy of prematurity
GAME	goals, activity, motor enrichment
GMA	general movement assessment
GMFCS	gross motor classification system
HABIT	hand-arm bimanual intensive training
HABIT-ILE	hand-arm bimanual intensive training including lower extremity
HIE	hypoxic-ischemic encephalopathy
IDD	intellectual developmental disability
IUGR	intrauterine growth restriction
IVH	intraventricular hemorrhage
LBW	low birth weight
NEC	necrotizing enterocolitis
PEG	percutaneous endoscopic gastrostomy
PVL	periventricular leukomalacia
SAFO	solid ankle-foot orthosis
VLBW	very low birth weight

Developmental Disabilities

Deborah S. Nichols-Larsen and Jill C. Heathcock

21

OBJECTIVES

1) Differentiate the pathophysiology of common developmental disorders

2) Distinguish the diagnostic criteria of common developmental disorders

3) Compare the treatment needs of children with common developmental disorders from those discussed for children with cerebral palsy

● INTRODUCTION

The term "**developmental disorder**" or "**developmental disability**" refers to conditions that occur during the developmental period and disrupt the acquisition of typical developmental milestones, including motor, cognitive, language, and psychosocial skills.[1] Thus, this term includes a vast number of disorders; however, in this chapter, we are going to focus on those disorders commonly seen by physical therapists. We have separated out the two most common developmental disorders in respective chapters 19 (Neural tube) and 20 (Cerebral palsy) – cerebral palsy and myelomeningocele; however, it should be remembered that these are also developmental disorders.

As the time of onset (birth-22 years) indicates, developmental disabilities can manifest throughout childhood and adolescence. However, many are present at birth (**congenital**), occurring **prenatally** (prior to birth), or **perinatally** (during or close to the time of birth). Others occur **postnatally**, often the result of trauma or disease processes that impact the nervous system (e.g., meningitis). In this chapter, we will focus on those that are congenital; it should be noted that many congenital disorders are not diagnosed until much later in the developmental period. Causes of congenital disorders may be known (genetic – chromosomal anomaly or inherited, birth trauma, environmental exposure) or unknown (e.g., developmental coordination disorder), yet their presentations may be quite similar or highly unique. This chapter will focus on the common and unique elements of these disorders.

CASE A, PART I

Pauli Sabat is a 40-month-old little girl of Latino heritage, whose parents immigrated to the United States from Argentina a year before her birth, initially on student visas but now on work visas; both are college educated – Dr. Sabat is a PhD in physics and Mrs. Sabat is a computer scientist. They have scheduled an appointment at a diagnostic clinic for children with developmental disorders. They report that Pauli is not keeping up with the other kids at daycare; she doesn't run, doesn't catch or throw a ball like her peers, continues to walk up and down stairs with a two-step/stair pattern, while holding the railing, and tends to be easily distracted, rushing from one toy to another without spending more than 30 seconds with any one of them. She also has limited verbal language skills, mostly repeating syllables of words that she hears but not really initiating speech; she does say mama and papa appropriately but infrequently. Although she is being raised in a bilingual home, her parents report that her speech development is much slower than her two older siblings. However, she does seem to understand what is said to her, following directions like "come here" but inconsistently, both in English and Spanish. She feeds herself but prefers her fingers to utensils and is a very picky eater, eating pancakes, hot dogs, chicken nuggets, tater tots, and apples (peels removed) but no other foods. She can dress herself except for shoes and socks but is also very picky about the texture of the clothes that she wears, becoming very agitated in rough textures and requiring that all tags be removed from her clothing. She is not an affectionate child, rarely giving hugs as her siblings do, yet she is hardly ever fussy either. She tends to amuse herself with toys and still takes a 2-hour afternoon nap, while sleeping 10 hours at night, typically without waking. She is not toilet trained and has refused all attempts to do so. She also resists having her teeth brushed but will chew on the toothbrush; her hair is cut short because she hates to have it brushed or any type of barrette or band in it. Although she has received some medical care over the last 3 years, they have moved twice as a result of Mr. Sabat's change in work – first completing his doctorate, then a post-doc, and finally a faculty position. Thus, her developmental profile is incomplete, based on limited follow-up with medical providers.

MEDICAL DIAGNOSIS

The diagnosis of a given developmental disorder often begins with a diagnostic workup that will include a detailed family and pregnancy history, a comprehensive developmental assessment, and potentially laboratory, imaging, and genetic testing; although the physician will likely initiate the assessment with a comprehensive morphometric, neurologic, and physical examination, other professionals (physical therapist, occupational therapist, speech and language pathologist, and developmental psychologist) are typically involved in this comprehensive assessment. In the case of Pauli, she appears to have a global developmental delay (significant delay in two or more areas – motor, language, intellectual). Normally, this diagnosis is based on a delay of ≥2.0 standard deviations (SD) on a standardized test in each of these areas, so confirmation of this will occur via appropriate testing.[2]

CASE A, PART II

Pauli's parents report an uncomplicated pregnancy and full-term delivery. This was their third pregnancy and live birth. Mrs. Sabat received prenatal care at the University student clinic with one ultrasound at 15 weeks with no abnormalities noted; the delivery was vaginal after an 8-hour labor. The perinatal period was uncomplicated, and mother and baby were discharged home after 42 hours. Mrs. S reports that Pauli was a fussy baby, who didn't nurse like her other children (Lilliana, age 5, and Simon, age 7) and was primarily fed with a bottle, which worked much better. Pauli was slow to transition to soft foods; although she ate cereal fairly well, if quite thick, she did not progress to fruits and vegetables easily and has never eaten rice or pasta. Once her first eight teeth had erupted (approximately 13 months), she transitioned to solid foods, primarily those listed earlier. She will also eat snack foods, such as crackers and goldfish crackers as well as some plain hard cookies. Although Pauli began verbalizing as the other two children had, Mrs. S reports that she is more likely to grunt or point to make her needs known; her verbal speech consists of mama, papa, ball, up, down, and no. For the most part, she has been healthy except for two to three ear infections per year and has never required hospitalization. She rolled over at 6 months, sat and pulled to stand at 12 months, and began walking at 17 months. She uses both hands for play, not demonstrating any hand preference, scribbles when given a crayon, takes apart many of her toys, demonstrating good dexterity, but doesn't complete puzzles or put shapes in a shape-sorter.

The other two children in the household are in kindergarten and second grade, both achieving at or above age level in their schoolwork, despite moving to the United States just a few years ago, and participating in many extracurricular activities, including soccer, piano lessons, karate, and swimming. They are bilingual, speaking Spanish in the home and English at school and with friends. Neither has any health issue and their developmental history is unremarkable.

Physical Examination

The physical examination will typically begin with growth measurements: height, weight, and head circumferences. Growth tables are available to plot these measures across gender and age. Many children with developmental disabilities are small for age, which may relate to feeding or eating issues, such as displayed by Pauli, or growth differences may be part of a more complex pathology, such as **Down syndrome**. Similarly, extreme differences in head circumference (2 or more SD from the mean for age and gender) can be indicative of specific developmental syndromes or disorders. **Microcephaly** refers to a small head circumference; historically, 2 SD below the mean for age and gender was used, but more recently 3 SD has been used; there are genetic and non-genetic causes of microcephaly. The genetic causes are many; the non-genetic causes include congenital infections, exposure to teratogens, and vascular insufficiency. Similarly, **macrocephaly** refers to a head circumference that is 3 SD above age and gender norms, stemming from anatomic and metabolic causes and resulting in cellular overgrowth or proliferation. Thus, both microcephaly and macrocephaly are changes in brain and skull size.[3] The physical examination should also look for any other **dysmorphic feature**, which is an asymmetry or abnormality of a body structure that can be as simple as having one ear lower than the other or much more complex, such as the characteristic look of a child with Down syndrome; again, many developmental disabilities are associated with specific dysmorphic features, especially the many genetic syndromes that result in a specific array of features.[4] So, the physical examination looks for asymmetries in the face and body structure as well as general range of motion. Furthermore, a neurologic examination (as described in Chapter 9) should be conducted to assess reflexes, muscle tone, strength, and age-specific motor, language, and cognition skills. From a medical standpoint, this is typically a brief screening with subsequent referral to physical and/or occupational therapy, if delay is noted. In children with speech delay, a comprehensive hearing and speech evaluation should be conducted to assure adequate hearing to support speech perception and language development as well as to document any language delay; this should be conducted by an audiologist and speech/language pathologist, respectively.[2]

CASE A, PART III

Pauli measures at the 15th to 20th percentile for height, weight, and head circumference, so although generally small for age, she is at the 40th percentile of weight for height and is neither micro nor macrocephalic. She is mildly hypotonic with normal tendon reflexes and slight joint hypermobility (typically associated with hypotonia), including moderate pes planus (flat feet). At the physician's office, she did not respond to commands to walk forward or backward, stand on one foot, or jump, so she was referred to both physical and occupational therapy for further assessment. Due to her language delay, she was evaluated first by an audiologist, who found her responses to be inconsistent, although she startled to louder sounds, indicating some degree of hearing, but tended to ignore directions and softer sounds. The speech/language pathologist identified a significant language delay (see Chapter 8 for typical language milestones); her language skills are at the 9 to 12 month level.

Laboratory Testing

Genetic Testing

Genetic testing is not always done for children with developmental delay, especially when the cause is known (e.g., infantile stroke), but can help to rule out or diagnose potential causes of a global delay. Genetic disorders can be **inherited** from one or both parents (see Box 21-1) or the product of a genetic

---

Box 21-1	Methods of Genetic Inheritance

Our attributes (e.g., hair color, eye color, height, and body type) are the result of genetic inheritance. At conception, the chromosomes of the mother join with those of the father, resulting in gene pairing; it is this pairing that decides how the traits of our parents will be expressed (or not). Traits can be either dominant or recessive. For a dominant trait, only one allele (gene component that carries the trait) is necessary to express the trait (e.g., brown eyes); for a recessive trait, both genes must carry the trait in order for it to be expressed (e.g., blue eyes). In this example (eye color), if both parents have blue eyes, their children will all have blue eyes; however, as is depicted in Figure 21-1, when parents both have brown eyes or one has blue and the other brown, their children's eye color can be either brown or blue, depending on which genes are contained within the egg and sperm at conception. If two parents each have both alleles for brown eyes (BB), then all of their children will have brown eyes (the reverse of "A" in Figure 21-1). Traits carried on the X or Y gene are considered sex-linked; all others are considered autosomal.

Genetically inherited disorders can also be inherited through dominant or recessive transmission. With recessive inheritance, both parents must carry the genetic defect for the child to manifest the disorder; with dominant inheritance, the parent would also manifest the disease but often to a lesser degree than the child. Notably, there are many genetic disorders associated with the X chromosome. *Remember that girls have two X chromosomes, but boys have an X and a Y chromosome.* So, if a dominant defect is carried on one of the mother's X chromosomes and not the father's, 50% of the children (both boys and girls) will have the disorder (Figure 21-2A). However, if the defect is carried on the father's X chromosome and not the mother's, all of his daughters will have the disease, and none of his sons will

have the disease (Figure 21-2B). If the mother has a recessive mutation on the X chromosome, she will not manifest the disease but serves as a carrier, transmitting the defect to 50% of her daughters, who will also be carriers, and 50% of her sons, who will manifest the disorder (Figure 21-2C).

---

mutation, also referred to as an **acquired mutation**. Acquired genetic mutations that occur during gestation, typically occur at the point of conception or very soon afterward. If they occur at conception, every cell in the body will have the mutation; if they occur at a later point, only a portion of the body's cells will have the mutation and the presentation of the disorder will typically be milder than a defect that happens at conception. A genetic mutation is a disruption in the DNA sequence that occurs as cells are rapidly multiplying. *Remember that in typical cell mitosis, the two strands of DNA separate and then are duplicated, making two complete DNA strands that become part of the* **offspring cells**, *which in turn will duplicate the DNA strands and produce additional offspring cells.*

Mutations occur from four basic errors: (1) translocation – the gene or portion of the DNA chain replicates in a different location than normal; (2) duplication – when the DNA strands initially separate, one chromosome pair fails to separate and the resultant cells have three of a given chromosome; (3) deletion – loss of a part of the DNA strand; or (4) inversion – a gene or fragment of the strand breaks off and then reattaches in a reverse (upside down) orientation.[5]

For children with an obvious genetic defect (e.g., Down syndrome), for which there is a specific genetic test, a karyotyping analysis is done to confirm the presence of the abnormal or mutated gene and determine the percentage of cells with the mutation. Box 21-2 outlines the genetic manifestations of Down syndrome. When there is a global delay without an obvious

---

Box 21-2	Genetic Causes of Down Syndrome

A good example of the variability in acquired genetic mutations can be seen in Down syndrome (DS), which is caused by an additional 21st chromosome. In the most common presentation, **Trisomy 21**, which accounts for about 95% of children with this disorder, there is duplication at conception of the 21st chromosome in either the egg or sperm at fertilization, resulting in a third 21st chromosome in all cells of the body. However, in some children, this duplication happens at some time after conception, resulting in three 21st chromosomes in only a portion of the child's cells; this type of DS is referred to as **Mosaic Trisomy 21**, accounting for about 2% of children with DS. Finally, for some children (3-4%), the extra 21st chromosome (or a fragment of it) attaches at a different point in the DNA strand (**translocation**), commonly on the 14th chromosome. It should be noted that in a small percentage of children with translocation DS, the chromosomal mutation will be present in some cells of a parent, and thus, it is an **inherited mutation**. We will discuss the presentation of children with DS later in this chapter, but it should be noted that those with mosaicism or translocation will typically manifest the characteristics of the syndrome to a lesser degree than children with Trisomy 21.[6,7]

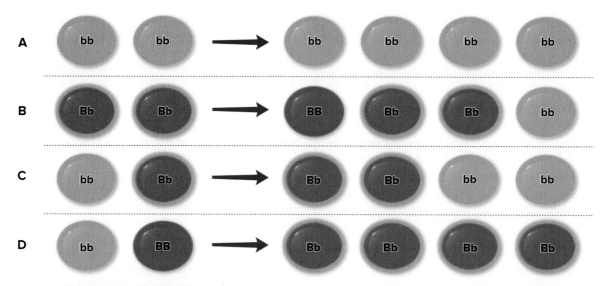

FIGURE 21-1 Genetic inheritance (potential trait expression with possible allele pairings). B, dominant gene for brown eyes; b, recessive gene for blue eyes. **A.** Two blue-eyed parents each have two genes for blue eyes (bb), so they will have all blue-eyed children (it is possible that both parents could have two genes for brown eyes [BB + BB], and then, similarly, all of their children will have brown eyes). **B.** Two brown-eyed parents with one gene for brown eyes (B) and one for blue eyes (b), depicted by the blue circle around the brown, have a 50/50 chance of contributing either the brown or blue-eyed gene to the embryo, and thus, there is a 75/25 chance that the child will have brown (BB or Bb) or blue eyes (bb). **C.** When there is one brown-eyed parent with both a blue and brown allele (Bb) and one blue-eyed parent (bb), the blue-eyed parent will always contribute a blue-eyed gene, but the brown-eyed parent has a 50/50 chance of contributing a brown or blue-eyed gene, resulting in only a 50% chance that the child will have brown eyes (Bb). **D.** A blue-eyed parent and a brown-eyed parent with both genes for brown eyes (BB), will always have brown-eyed children, but they will all carry a blue-eyed gene (Bb). (From Deborah S. Nichols Larsen, PT, PhD. The Ohio State University.)

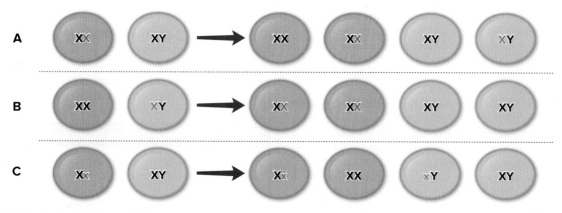

FIGURE 21-2 X-linked inheritance. A. Trait manifested in mother as a dominant gene; all children have a 50% chance of inheriting the trait; **B.** Dominant trait carried by father on the X chromosome will be manifested in all daughters. **C.** When a recessive trait is carried by mother, 50% of the daughters will be carriers and 50% of the sons will have the disorder. X = normal X chromosome; x = trait carrying; left side of diagram: pink oval, mother's genes; blue oval, father's genes; right side of diagram, genetic possibilities for offspring (pink, girls; blue, boys). (From Deborah S. Nichols Larsen, PT, PhD. The Ohio State University.)

genetic disorder, a chromosomal microarray (CMA) may be ordered. This type of analysis looks for duplications and deletions within the DNA strands, which can identify inherited conditions or acquired mutations.[5] For those with a normal CMA analysis, additional genetic testing may be done, including gene panels that examine specific genes, or X chromosome analysis because of the number of disorders associated with X chromosome abnormalities (e.g., Fragile X syndrome, Rett syndrome).[2,8] Table 21-1 describes common developmental disorders that are known to have a genetic mutation or inherited transmission that may be seen by a physical therapist.

Metabolic Testing

There are a group of disorders that result from what is known as inborn errors in metabolism, which stem from a disruption in enzymes or transport proteins that can be classified into two categories: (1) Category 1 involves a single system (e.g., immune system) or organ (kidney); (2) Category II involves a metabolic pathway that impacts multiple cells and organs (storage diseases) or a single organ that initiates a systemic effect (mitochondrial disorders). Category II disorders can further be divided into three subclassifications: (1) Group 1 – disorders of intermediary metabolism (phenylketonuria; Wilson's disease);

TABLE 21-1 Common Developmental Disorders with a Genetic Cause

GENETIC DISORDER	GENETIC ABNORMALITY	PRESENTATION	DIAGNOSIS	MEDICAL MANAGEMENT
Angelman syndrome[9-11]	Deletion of a gene (UBE3A) on the 15th chromosome, typically from the father, allowing overexpression of the maternal 15th chromosome[9]	Severe intellectual disability; global developmental delay with limited speech development; balance problems/ataxia; seizure disorder with abnormal EEG; hyperactivity, dysmorphic features (microcephaly, jaw protrusion, protruding tongue, teeth wide-spaced, deep-set eyes), hypopigmentation, sleep pattern disruption, happy disposition with arm/hand flapping[10]	Clinical presentation of global delay with limited speech, dysmorphic features, and unusually happy disposition. Genetic testing to identify the chromosomal anomaly.[10]	Pharmacological seizure management; treatment of associated disorders (gastrointestinal reflux, surgery to correct strabismus; surgical correction of associated orthopedic problems – scoliosis, plantarflexor shortening)[11]
Becker Muscular Dystrophy[12]	Mutation of the DMD gene on the X chromosome, which is critical for the development of dystrophin (a protein that anchors muscle fibers to the extracellular matrix), resulting in an abnormal form of dystrophin; occurs only in boys.	Progressive muscle weakness (proximal greater than distal), beginning in late childhood (age 10). Calf hypertrophy as in Duchenne but ambulate until late teens or early adulthood	Elevated creatine kinase; abnormal dystrophin in muscle biopsy; genetic analysis of the DMD gene	Similar to Duchenne MD but without corticosteroid treatment.
Charcot–Marie–Tooth disease[13]	Multiple genetic anomalies, some with autosomal dominant inheritance and others X-linked or autosomal recessive inheritance, with up to 40 genes involved	Most common progressive peripheral demyelinating neuropathy of both sensory and motor nerves (motor more impaired than sensory) with loss of reflexes, beginning distally, with variable onset (infancy–adulthood) and presentation. Pes cavus deformity is common, caused by loss of intrinsic foot muscle function.	Genetic testing	Surgical correction of orthopedic deformities; pharmacologic management of pain.
Cri-du-chat[14]	Deletion of the short-arm of chromosome 5	High-pitched "cat like" cry with facial dysmorphic features (broad nose, epicanthal folds, small jaw, microcephaly); small for age (weight more than height); severe mental retardation with global developmental delay and behavioral problems (hyperactivity, self-injurious or aggressive behavior, stereotypic behavior); hypotonia; potential organ malformations (heart, kidneys).	Initial diagnosis is often based on observation of the dysmorphic features and the cry with secondary karyotype genetic testing.	No specific medical management; only developmental support.

(Continued)

TABLE 21-1   Common Developmental Disorders with a Genetic Cause (Continued)

GENETIC DISORDER	GENETIC ABNORMALITY	PRESENTATION	DIAGNOSIS	MEDICAL MANAGEMENT
Cystic Fibrosis[15]	Autosomal inheritance of a mutation on chromosome 7, resulting in a deficiency of the transmembrane conductance regulator protein (CFTR) that functions to control permeability of the chloride ion channel.	Thickening of secretions in the lungs, intestines, pancreas, and gall bladder associated with chronic infections and nutritional issues.	Newborn screening for a pancreatic enzyme (immunoreactive trypsinogen); DNA testing; sweat test for elevated chloride (≥ 60 mmole/L).	Maintaining airways through postural drainage/percussion/chest compression; use of bronchodilators; frequent culturing for infections with early or prophylactic treatment; anti-inflammatory drug treatment; new CFTR modulating drugs to target chloride channel function.
Down syndrome	Mutation of chromosome 21 with duplication at conception (Trisomy 21) or later in cell proliferation (Mosaic Trisomy 21) or translocation (most frequently onto chromosome 14). Increased prevalence with maternal age.[7]	Abnormal brain development, mental retardation, hypotonia with joint laxity, dysmorphic features (epicanthal folds, small mouth that allows tongue to protrude, single palmar crease, short/curved little finger, low set ears), potential for cardiac, GI, or other organ malformations, with aging, Alzheimer's disease is common.[16]	Screening – Maternal blood test for elevated human chorionic gonadotropin and pregnancy-associated plasma protein-A with ultrasound to measure Nuchal Translucency (measures the amount of fluid at the upper cervical spine), which is greater with DS. Subsequent amniocentesis and karyotyping if DS is suspected. Diagnosis after birth includes observation of dysmorphic features and karyotyping.[7,17,18]	Well child care with attention to potential comorbidities and specific treatment for those present: (1) Auditory – otitis media, conductive hearing loss (2) Visual – congenital cataracts, strabismus, nystagmus, glaucoma (3) Oral – feeding issues, speech delay (4) Congenital heart defects (5) Endocrine – diabetes, hypo or hyperthyroidism (6) Hematologic – leukemia (7) Neurologic – seizures, mental retardation, autism, developmental delay (8) Orthopedic – joint laxity, atlanto-occipital instability (9) Dermatology – folliculitis, hyperkeratosis, seborrhea[7,17]
Duchenne Muscular Dystrophy	Mutation of the DMD gene on the X chromosome, resulting in a complete absence of functional dystrophin in affected boys[12,19]	Progressive muscle weakness (proximal more than distal) in early childhood (ages 2–5) with toe walking and muscle pseudohypertrophy (loss of muscle with fat replacement) early, followed by loss of ambulation ability (late childhood) and progressive respiratory and cardiac compromise, leading to death in late adolescence/early adulthood[12,19]	Elevated creatine kinase; absent dystrophin in muscle biopsy; genetic analysis of the DMD gene[12,19]	Corticosteroid treatment to support muscle function with management of the side effects of this treatment (weight gain, osteoporosis, cataracts, delayed sexual maturity); gene therapy; pharmacologic management of associated cardiomyopathy; respiratory exercises and support (ventilators); managing orthopedic changes (e.g., scoliosis) with potential surgery or bracing. Surgery needs to be carefully considered due to potential respiratory compromise.[12,19–21]

(Continued)

TABLE 21-1 Common Developmental Disorders with a Genetic Cause *(Continued)*

GENETIC DISORDER	GENETIC ABNORMALITY	PRESENTATION	DIAGNOSIS	MEDICAL MANAGEMENT
Fragile X syndrome	Disruption of a gene, named the Fragile X Mental Retardation gene 1 (FMR1), that is critical to the development of an RNA binding protein necessary for neuronal development, specifically dendrite formation. X chromosome linked with many adults (much more frequent in women) carrying an incomplete defect (permutation) without notable symptoms.[22]	Milder but more frequent presentation in girls than boys. Intellectual disability, global delay, hyperactivity and attention deficits with autistic symptoms, frequently seizures and sleep disturbances, facial dysmorphic features. Carriers may demonstrate hyperactivity, attention deficit, learning disabilities, and behavioral problems.[22]	Observation of developmental delay with subsequent X chromosomal analysis[22]	New focus on pharmacologic management, targeting GABA and glutamate receptors (antagonists), to control seizures, psychiatric, and behavioral symptoms.[23]
Niemann–Pick disease[24]	An autosomal inherited disorder of the NPC1 on chromosome 18 or NPC2 gene on chromosome 14 that disrupts lysosomal lipid storage (cholesterol, sphingomyelin, glycolipids) with secondary buildup in tissues.	Variable onset from infancy to adulthood with liver, spleen, and nervous system abnormalities, including vertical supranuclear palsy, and later respiratory failure. Early infantile onset (2 months–2 years) – enlarged liver/spleen, initial hypotonia that progresses to spasticity, motor delay and eventual loss of motor skills, intention tremor; typically die by age 5. Childhood onset (2–6 years) – ataxia, clumsiness, dysarthria, dysphagia, intention tremor, intellectual disability, vertical supranuclear palsy. Seizures and dystonia are also common. Survive to ages 7-12.	Delayed motor development and an enlarged liver/spleen are early signs in infants and children. Skin or liver biopsy plus serum analysis for abnormal cholesterol measures, followed by NPC1 and NPC2 sequencing.	Symptom specific (e.g., seizure medications to control seizures); recently, pharmacological administration of iminosaccaride inhibitors (e.g., miglustat) have had some success.
Prader–Willi syndrome	Deletion of multiple genes on the 15th chromosome, typically from the maternal contribution, allowing the paternal 15th chromosomal contribution to be overexpressed[9]	Initial failure to thrive, followed by excessive eating (hyperphagia) in childhood; global developmental delay; mental retardation or learning disabilities; behavioral problems, impaired psychosocial development; abnormal sleep patterns; hypogonadism with disrupted sexual maturation. Symptoms are related to hypothalamus malfunction.[25]	DNA methylation testing.[25]	Pharmacologic management with human growth hormone and sex steroid treatments. Behavioral treatment to control diet and provide a feeling of food security.[26]
Phenylketonuria (PKU)[27]	Autosomal recessive inheritance of a mutation of the phenylalanine hydroxylase (PAH) gene, resulting in an absence of PAH, which is a key enzyme necessary for neurotransmitter production	Without treatment, severe intellectual disability occurs; however, with neonatal diagnosis and implementation of standard treatment, children develop normally but poor bone density due to limited protein consumption is common. Diet lapses can result in deterioration of brain function.	Neonatal blood screening for elevated phenylalanine levels	Diet low in phenylalanine, which is found in many foods, especially proteins, and amino acid supplementation for brain development and neurotransmitter maintenance.

(Continued)

TABLE 21-1 Common Developmental Disorders with a Genetic Cause (Continued)

GENETIC DISORDER	GENETIC ABNORMALITY	PRESENTATION	DIAGNOSIS	MEDICAL MANAGEMENT
Rett syndrome[28]	X-linked chromosomal mutation of the gene that encodes methyl-CpG binding protein, resulting in disrupted synapse formation within neural networks, primarily in girls. Commonly lethal to boys in infancy; occasionally, males with XXY genotype survive with similar presentation to girls plus Klinefelter's syndrome.	Normal development up to 18 months with subsequent loss of neural function, resulting in intellectual disability, loss of motor skills, seizure onset and autistic behaviors (hand wringing, poor communication).	Observed loss of motor and communication skills with slowing head circumference growth and emergence of stereotypical movements (hand wringing). Genetic testing for the MECP2 gene mutation confirms the diagnosis in most girls.	Symptomatic (e.g., pharmacologic seizure management; orthopedic management of scoliosis that can develop)
Spinal Muscular Atrophy[29]	Deletion or mutation of the SMN1 gene, resulting in loss of the survival motor neuron (SMN) protein with ultimate loss of alpha motor neurons throughout the spinal cord and resultant loss of muscle fibers; inherited through autosomal recessive inheritance	Type I – present at birth, limited antigravity movement with no acquisition of motor milestones, life expectancy <2 years (leading genetic cause of infant death) Type II – diagnosis in first 18 months of life with progressive muscle weakness, will sit but not walk, life expectancy to teenage/early adulthood Type III – diagnosed after 18 months, walk independently with later progressive muscle weakness, life expectancy is near normal Type IV – diagnosed at adulthood, normal life expectancy	Genetic analysis to confirm the SMN1 mutation.	Symptomatic – respiratory support (oxygen, ventilator); nutrition support (feeding tubes); selection of adaptive equipment to maximize function and adapt the home for caregiving. Intrathecal Nusinersen to induce SMN2 (an homolgous SMN gene) to produce full length SMN protein is increasing life expectancy and function. Similarly, gene therapy with AVXS-101 (Zolgensma), applied through a viral vector is extending life and enhancing function.
Trisomy 18 (Edwards syndrome)	Genetic mutation at conception, resulting in three 18th chromosomes[30]	Multiple organ defects, especially congenital heart defects (many types) and dysmorphic features (e.g., skull malformations, finger anomalies); 75% mortality in first year of life with severe global developmental delay in survivors, some of whom have lived into their 20s.[30]	Physical appearance typically identifies the condition that is confirmed by karyotyping.[30]	Surgical correction of organ defects (CHD); respiratory support; assisted feeding (gastrointestinal tubes); in some cases, only palliative care is provided.[31]
Wilson's disease[32]	Mutations of the ATP7B gene, resulting in disruption of copper metabolism, with autosomal recessive inheritance.	Buildup of copper in tissues with brain and liver most vulnerable, resulting in progressive neural and liver damage.	Difficult diagnosis, often delayed until symptoms present, which can be as early as 4 but as late as 20+; no effective infant screening. Blood and urine tests for copper, confirmed by DNA testing are diagnostic.	Copper chelating agents plus zinc salts to decrease copper absorption from the gastrointestinal system, which can stabilize or result in improvements in symptoms.

(2) Group 2 – disorders of primary energy metabolism (mitochondrial disorders); and (3) Group 3 – disorders of complex molecules (lysosomal storage disorders). Common early presentation of these disorders includes (1) non-specific symptoms (lethargy, hyptonia); (2) seizures, most commonly myoclonic; and (3) severe motor dysfunction (hypertonia; dystonia). Blood testing or urinalysis will identify metabolite buildup in the blood or urine; other testing may include lumbar puncture or imaging.[33] The genetic defects for many of these disorders have been identified and are listed in Table 21-1. Some of these are treatable but others are not, resulting in progressive decline and eventually death. One example is Phenylketonuria (PKU), for which all newborns in the United States are screened prior to going home from the hospital; PKU is a genetic defect that disrupts a key enzyme for the production of epinephrine, norepinephrine, and dopamine. If untreated, it has severe neurologic consequences, including IDD; however, it is completely treatable by diet and nutritional supplementation.[27] Table 21-2 outlines Group 3 disorders that have neurologic presentations that may be seen by physical therapists.

Imaging

Imaging, specifically MRI, is being used more frequently in the diagnostic process. Success in conducting MRI imaging in sleeping infants without sedative medication has increased its use; infants are typically fed and swaddled, provided ear plugs to block the noise, and may be given a pacifier to help them sleep through the process.[38] However, a small percentage of

developmental disabilities require imaging for diagnosis, so it is only recommended for those with primarily a neurologic presentation, uncontrolled epilepsy, or developmental deterioration.[2]

CASE A, PART IV

Pauli's chromosomal array did not identify any genetic mutations nor did a secondary X chromosome analysis. Her metabolic tests were also normal. No imaging was ordered. Thus, Pauli's medical diagnosis for the time being will remain idiopathic global developmental delay, which means the cause is unknown. This is not an uncommon diagnosis, especially for children at a relatively young age (<4) with signs of mild to moderate global delay. Continued observation by the family physician and potentially a referral to a pediatric neurologist or physiatrist may occur. However, some diagnoses (e.g., autism spectrum disorders) become more evident as the child ages.

● PHYSICAL THERAPY ASSESSMENT

To evaluate Pauli, there are many standardized tests that can be used with the **Bayley Scales of Infant and Toddler Development** (BSITD)[39] and the **Peabody Developmental Motor Scales** (PDMS),[40] the most commonly used. Since the Bayley is aimed at children 0 to 3½ years of age and given Pauli's current

TABLE 21-2	Inborn Errors of Metabolism	
INBORN ERROR	**DESCRIPTION/PRESENTATION**	**DIAGNOSIS/TREATMENT**
Lysosomal storage disorders[34] • Autosomal recessive inheritance or X-linked inheritance • Examples: Hunter syndrome, Turner syndrome, Danon disease, Fabry disease, Niemann–Pick, Tay–Sachs	Variable, often neurologic with global developmental delay, ataxia, seizures, some variants have dysmorphic features; at older ages, strokes, neuropathies, and extrapyramidal symptoms may present. Liver and spleen enlargement due to accumulation of un-metabolized macromolecules. Tay–Sachs and other GM2 gangliosidosis disorders are neurodegenerative, characterized by loss of motor skills (head control, sitting), increasing hypotonia and exaggerated startle.[35]	Brain imaging, skeletal x-rays for abnormalities, and ultrasound for liver enlargement Symptomatic treatment (e.g., antiepileptics for seizures); enzyme replacement therapy or hematopoietic stem cell transplantation. No effective treatment for GM2 gangliosidosis disorders (Tay–Sachs), which are ultimately lethal before age 5.[34,35]
Sterol synthesis disorders[36] • Disruption in cholesterol storage/metabolism • Examples: Smith–Lemli–Opitz syndrome, Antley–Bixler syndrome, CK syndrome	Cholesterol is critical for neuronal cell membrane and myelin formation and derived from sterols (precursors). Presentation is highly variable but can include dysmorphic features (cleft palate, microcephaly, limb anomalies), GI symptoms, congenital heart defects, global developmental delay with motor and speech delays, sleep disturbances, self-injurious behaviors, tactile hypersensitivity, autistic behaviors.	Blood or urine analysis for specific markers; skin analysis for some disorders. No effective medical treatment.
Creatine deficiency disorders[37] • Autosomal recessive	Disruption in the metabolism of creatine, which is necessary to support cellular energy, especially in the brain and muscles. Mild to severe global delay, behavioral problems, and seizures.	Abnormal creatine in urine (high/low). Enzymatic assays, followed by genetic testing, is diagnostic. Treatment is focused on creatine supplementation or creatine precursor supplementation.

age (40 months), the therapist has chosen to use the Peabody, which will allow documentation of her motor skills through age 5 (or longer given a motor delay). For most developmental scales, the evaluator determines a basal level (the last level at which the child completes all items) and then a ceiling level (the first level at which the child doesn't pass any item). Then, there is a process for converting these raw scores into a standard score, typically a z-score, which indicates the difference from the mean (SD).

CASE A, PART V

Pauli's PDMS assessment indicated a basal level of 13 months and a ceiling level of 19 to 20 months for the gross motor subscales. This gave her a z-score of −3.53, which places her 3.5 SD from her age-matched peers and in the bottom percentile for children her age.[31] From this assessment, Pauli should be receiving physical therapy as part of an early intervention (EI) program. Goals for therapy should focus on (1) increasing strength to improve stability for single limb stance activities (stair climbing, kicking a ball); (2) improving locomotion skills such as stair climbing, negotiating obstacles and complex environments, walking backward or on a line, and running; and (3) object manipulation skills – throwing, catching, and kicking. A challenge for the therapist will be getting Pauli to follow directions and interact with the therapist for play skills such as throwing and kicking. Working with the educational team, the physical therapist should include behavioral management techniques to promote desired behaviors and minimize unwanted behaviors. Some group play activities will be beneficial to facilitate peer engagement and social skills such as turn taking.

COMMON DEVELOPMENTAL DISABILITIES

Down Syndrome

As mentioned earlier in the chapter, DS is one of the most common developmental disabilities; it results from a genetic mutation during conception or soon after, resulting in either three 21st chromosomes (Trisomy 21 or Mosaic Trisomy 21) or a translocation of the 21st chromosome, typically to the 14th chromosome. The occurrence of DS increases as maternal age increases with those 35 to 40 at greater risk; other risk factors include use of oral contraceptives, folic acid supplementation, and tobacco as well as exposure to solvents in the work environment.[6] Currently, most expectant mothers undergo a screening process to diagnose DS, other potential trisomies (e.g., Trisomy 18), and neural tube disorders (e.g., myelomeningocele), during the first trimester of pregnancy. Markers for DS include serum biomarkers (free β-hCG, pregnancy-associated plasma protein-A [PAPP-A]) and ultrasound examination of **Nuchal Translucency**, which measures an area of fluid buildup in the cervical spine between the cervical spine and the skin that is increased in children with DS as well as those with Trisomy 18.[7]

Intellectual Disability in DS

DS is the most common cause of **intellectual disability** (ID) in children, yet the degree of ID varies considerably in children with DS. Most children have a moderate level of ID (>70%) but some have a mild (7%) or severe (7%) level of ID. Interestingly, 7% of children with DS have normal intelligence. The ID in DS is characterized by poor short-term verbal and long-term explicit memory (facts, episodic), poor problem-solving and set-shifting but good visuospatial short-term and implicit (procedural) long-term memory. Further, the ID interacts with language development to result in a delay in language skills; receptive language typically exceeds expressive language. Children with DS also often demonstrate behavioral problems (attention deficit, hyperactivity, poor response inhibition, and autistic features, characterized by stereotypic behavior and withdrawal).[7,41]

Dysmorphic Features of DS

There are multiple features of DS that may be present in children with a DS diagnosis (Figure 21-3); not all children have all of these: (1) hypotonia – low muscle tone with joint hypermobility (often the first thing noted at birth); (2) epicanthal folds – an extra fold of skin on the upper eyelid between the nose and the eyebrow; (3) flat nasal bridge or facial profile; (4) brachycephaly (decreased anterioposterior cranial length) with wide fontanel; (5) short broad fingers and hands with curved 5th fingers; (6) single palmar crease; (7) low set ears with a folded meatus; (8) gap between the great toe and the 2nd toe; and (9) high palate and small oral cavity with hypotonia of the tongue, leading to a protruding tongue. Some of these, commonly hypotonia and epicanthal folds, are obvious at birth; others become more evident as the child ages.[7]

Organ Anomalies

In addition to the dysmorphic features listed above, there is an increased incidence of congenital organ anomalies in children with DS. Most common are **congenital heart defects** (atrioventricular septal defects, atrioventricular canal defects), which occur in approximately 50% of children with DS, so all children will undergo an electrocardiogram to screen for a defect in the first days of life. **Pulmonary hypertension (PH)** is also an issue for up to 34% of children born with DS; the likelihood of PH increases when a heart defect is also present. PH is thought to result from abnormalities in the vasculature of the lungs. Treatment involves respiratory support and nitric oxide therapy; PH often necessitates a longer NICU stay. **Gastrointestinal defects**, such as atresia of the esophagus or duodenum, tracheoesophageal fistulas, pyloric stenosis, Hirschsprung's disease or Meckel's diverticulum, and gastroesophageal reflux are also common.[42] Diagnosis of these disorders may require a GI series (barium enema with CT scan; barium swallow), and treatment requires immediate surgical correction. Eating problems are also common due to gastroesophageal reflux and oral musculature hypotonia, which may necessitate special feeding measures such as thickening of liquids and evaluation of different nipple types for best feeding. Reflux is worrisome as aspiration may occur; with repeated aspiration, lung infections, such as pneumonia, may occur, so it is critical to find feeding methods that prevent aspiration and maximize nutrition.[7,42,43]

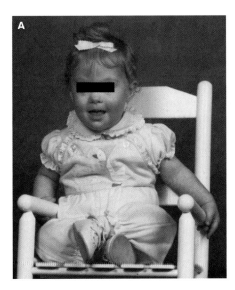

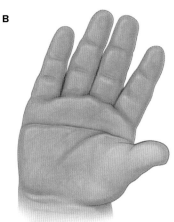

FIGURE 21-3 Dysmorphic features of Down syndrome.
A. This little girl demonstrates the common epicanthal folds (not visible with the eyes blacked out), flat nasal bridge, low-set ears, and lax oral musculature of Down syndrome. **B.** Single palmar crease associated with Down syndrome (note – this type of single crease is found in many children and adults without DS). (Part A: Reproduced with permission from Jorde LB, Carey JC, Bamshad MJ, White RL. *Medical Genetics.* St. Louis, MO: CV Mosby; 2000.)

Brain Differences in DS

There has been considerable research into the causative brain changes that are responsible for many of the cognitive, learning, motor, and behavioral deficits found in DS. The brain, itself, is small in DS as measured by total brain volume with deficient gray and white matter in all lobes but especially the frontal and temporal lobes, including the hippocampus and surrounding areas, as well as the cerebellum. Some of these changes aren't evident in early childhood but manifest later.[16] As discussed in Chapter 7, the temporal and frontal lobes are particularly critical to episodic memory and executive function, both of which are typically impaired with DS. The cerebellum has also been implicated in learning, especially motor learning, and muscle tone with damage typically resulting in hypotonia and postural control issues. Additionally, there are differences in neuronal function in those with DS, including decreased synaptic density

and fewer dendritic spines, which ultimately may disrupt the neural circuits that support learning and memory. Neurogenesis (new neuron formation) is also diminished within the hippocampus in DS and thought to contribute to the cognitive deficits in DS.[16,44]

Orthopedic Problems in DS

The hypotonia, associated with DS, is accompanied by ligamentous laxity that can contribute to joint instability. Common areas for this are at the atlanto-occipital joint or the atlantoaxial joint of the cervical spine. The occiput of the skull connects with the first cervical vertebra (C1), also called the atlas, resting on the superior articulating processes of C1, and is connected by thick ligaments between the occiput and C1, allowing for much of our cervical flexion and extension as well as lateral bending; however, in DS, the laxity of these ligaments may result in dangerous instability at this joint. Similarly, the joint between C1 and C2, also called the axis, is characterized by a protruding odontoid process from C2 that projects up into C1. This arrangement allows rotation of C1 on C2, accounting for much of our cervical rotation ability. Again, laxity of ligaments at this joint can result in dangerous laxity; both of these conditions pose potential risk for spinal cord injury. Neurologic symptoms, pain, abnormal head position, decreased head movements or deterioration of motor ability (gait, hand function) warrant further assessment with radiographs (x-rays); for many children, the condition is mild and asymptomatic; for asymptomatic individuals, physical activity is not limited except for contact sports (e.g., soccer or football). In some cases, the laxity is more severe and requires posterior fusion of C1 and C2.[45] Other common orthopedic issues include pes planus and hip and knee instability. Pes planus is found in almost all children and adults with DS; thus, it is important to fit the child with supportive shoes to enhance balance and minimize further deformity; rarely is surgical intervention required. Hypotonia at the hip and alterations in the acetabulum and femoral head angle allow excessive mobility of the hip joint, which can progress to hip subluxation or dislocation. Similarly, patellar instability can result in subluxation or dislocation. Orthotics or surgical intervention may be necessary to prevent or correct these hip and knee problems. Finally, an increase in inflammatory arthritis has been reported in children with DS, manifesting in early childhood and potentially resulting in joint damage; the most common sites are the wrists and hands.[45]

Other Health Complications in DS

Ear, **nose**, and **throat problems** are common in DS in association with malformation of these structures. Infections are often frequent, including otitis media, pneumonia, and rhinitis, and **hearing loss** may occur in association with repeated infection or malformation of the inner ear; estimates of hearing loss range from 38 to 78%.[42] A brainstem auditory evoked assessment can be used to evaluate the ability of the aural structures to transmit sound to the brain. This test involves measuring EEG (electroencephalography) responses to auditory stimulation and can be done in infants.[17] Similarly, children with DS may have **missing or misshaped teeth** or **late tooth eruption** that may impact eating, especially transitioning to solid foods, or require orthodontics.[17]

Other conditions that occur at a higher frequency in children with DS than typically developing children are **thyroid disease (hypothyroidism or hyperthyroidism)**, **eye problems** (amblyopia, congenital cataracts, glaucoma, nystagmus, strabismus, and refraction errors – myopia, astigmatism), diabetes, **epilepsy**, and **leukemia**.[17,42] Skin disorders such as seborrheic dermatitis and alopecia are also more common in children with DS.[42] Notably, children with DS are **smaller in stature (2 SD below average)** with shortened limbs than their typical peers; there are growth curves that have been developed specific to DS growth patterns for comparison. At older ages, **obesity** is often a problem, associated with decreased activity and thyroid issues, so weight management and a healthy diet should be initiated early and maintained.[42]

Motor Development in DS

Children with DS tend to be quiet, sleepy babies with diminished antigravity movement, especially in supine, and less engagement with their environment. In general, they develop motor skills at a slower rate to their typical peers that is even more delayed in upright postures. Rolling occurs close to that of typical peers, by 6 to 7 months, but most weight-bearing and mobility skills are more significantly delayed (see Table 21-3).[46] It is not uncommon for children with DS to delay walking until nearly 3 years of age, and many are unlikely to acquire higher level motor skills like climbing and ball skills (kicking, catching). There is likely an interaction between the ID and motor delay in children with DS; lack of interest in exploring the environment may delay motor behavior while delayed exploration may impede intellectual development. Also, independent walking requires attention to the environment and problem-solving for walking around and over obstacles, so it is likely to be more delayed in those with greater IDD. Further, walking may enhance cognitive and social development by enhancing the environmental experiences of the child and providing more social interactions.[47]

TABLE 21-3	Motor Skill Acquisition in Down Syndrome[46]	
SKILL	**MEAN AGE (MO)**	**RANGE (MO)**
Rolls supine to prone	6.5	4-9
Sits	10.3	7-15
Crawls on belly	14.2	9-23
Creeps hands and knees (quadruped)	17.9	1-29
Cruising	18.4	13-28
Walks 15 ft	26.0	1-40
Walks up and down stairs, mark time	40.5	29-60
Jumps once	48.0	33-68
Runs	49.5	34-68
Rides tricycle	57.6	41-78

Up to 87% of infants with DS are admitted to the NICU after birth, either due to an anomaly or the need for respiratory support; this is a critical time for assessment for any orthopedic issue and to prepare the parents for handling the child, who is floppy and hard to hold. Once at home, **early physical therapy treatment** focuses on developing antigravity movement and acquisition of motor milestones. Most children with DS will be enrolled in EI services, so physical therapy will be provided in an EI environment. Families should be encouraged to establish a bright and engaging environment and to create opportunities for the child to play in prone, supine, and supported sitting to minimize the time spent sleeping, sitting in an infant seat, or lying quietly. Instruction in handling and positioning techniques is important to facilitate the development of antigravity movement, head control, rolling, and sitting. These techniques mirror those used with children with MMC and CP, as described in Chapters 19 and 20, respectively. Starting therapy before 6 months of age has been found to reduce motor delay and lower the age of independent walking.[48,49] Similarly, early "tummy time" that was initiated prior to 3 months of age for 90 minutes daily, using play activities and positioning with a roll, on the caregiver's lap or chest, or a cushion, resulted in faster motor development that persisted to 12 months of age, compared to children, who began the intervention after 3 months of age.[50] Improved motor ability promotes cognitive, social, and emotional development as children are able to better explore their environment and engage with others.[49] Body-weight-supported treadmill training (BWSTT) has been found to be particularly effective in children with DS, facilitating earlier acquisition of independent walking and improving gait speed in older children.[51] Many children with DS have pes planus (flat feet) that may require some orthotic support – either a foot or supramalleolar orthotic; this has been reported to improve foot/ankle alignment and also to improve gait and balance; however, it may be beneficial to wait to provide orthotics until after the child starts walking as there is at least one study that documented faster gross motor acquisition of crawling, creeping, walking, running and jumping when treadmill training was done without orthoses compared to with orthoses.[52] Older children with DS benefit from therapy directed at improving upright postural control to assure safety, during play and school. Multiple intervention programs have been found to improve static and/or dynamic balance as well as gross motor skills, including WiiFit, backward walking training, whole body vibration, isokinetic training, and functional play skills like hopscotch in school-aged children and adolescents.[53]

Aging with DS

Although some children with DS succumb to congenital heart defects or other organ malformations; with improved surgical management, the majority of children are living to adulthood (>88%), and the average life expectancy is 50 years.[54] Thus, additional information relative to the aging of individuals with DS is pertinent to physical therapy practitioners. Notably, adults with DS demonstrate **accelerated aging** of many organ systems, including the brain; this abnormal aging is thought to be associated with disturbance of the immune system, allowing a condition of chronic inflammation, similar to that of aging, to exist.[55]

Adults with DS exhibit earlier aging of **the integumentary system** (wrinkles, graying, and hair loss), **earlier menopause** in women, advanced aging in the musculoskeletal system, resulting in early and widespread **osteoporosis**, increased occurrence of **cardiovascular problems** (atherosclerosis), and increased incidence of **Alzheimer's disease** (AD).[6,54,55] In those with DS, neurologic decline often appears as early as age 40; by age 60-69, 77% of those with DS are diagnosed with cognitive decline and this increases to 100% for those that live past 70;[6] there is some suggestion that those with mosaicism may be less likely to develop AD.[54] The anatomical changes, in those with DS and cogntivie decline, are consistent with AD on autopsy.[54] AD is associated with amyloid beta (Aβ) deposits in the extracellular areas of the brain; Aβ seems to be a catalyst for the development of the amyloid plaques and neurofibrillary tangles that are the characteristic anomalies of AD, ultimately resulting in neuronal death. Interestingly, the Aβ precursor gene has been localized to the 21st chromosome, which likely accounts for the exaggerated occurrence of AD in adults with DS.[54] Early symptoms of AD in adults with DS are often behavioral (aggression, change in sleep patterns, emotional outbursts), or in adults with seizures, increased seizure activity. Pharmacological treatments, typically used to treat AD have not been effective in the DS population.[56] For physical therapists, it is important to note that exercise programs (aerobic and strengthening) have been found to offset many of the aging problems of adults with DS, including osteoporosis, obesity, cardiovascular fitness, and decreased muscle mass.[57] Recent research has also linked increased sedentary behavior with the emergence of AD in those with DS, suggesting that moderate-to-vigorous activity may delay the onset of dementia in this population.[58]

Neuromuscular Degenerative Disorders (NMDs)

Within Table 21-1, there are a number of NMDs, including the muscular dystrophies, congenital myopathies, and spinal muscular atrophies that result from genetic mutations. While these groups of disorders have different pathologic etiologies, they all result in progressive loss of skeletal muscle, hypotonia, and weakness.[59] Exciting new medical treatment of children with some NMDs has progressed in the last decade through the development of disease-modifying therapies that target the genetic or muscle defect through preventing gene splicing, other genetic therapy, or replacement of the defective protein; some of these treatments require ongoing applications throughout the child's life while gene replacement is typically a one-time application.[29] While the science involved in these treatments is beyond the scope of this text, these new treatments are changing the role of physical therapy in the management of those disorders, for which disease-modifying treatments have been identified.

Muscular dystrophies are associated with changes in proteins that support the extracellular matrix of the muscle and the sarcolemmal membrane. **Duchenne Muscular Dystrophy** (DMD) is the most common and most severe of muscular dystrophies; as an x-linked recessive gene, it affects only males, with symptoms that begin between 2 and 5 years of age. Its pathology involves the deletion of part of the dystrophin gene necessary to produce the protein **dystrophin**, a critical component of skeletal and cardiac muscle membranes necessary for maintaining

muscle fiber strength.[19] The absence of dystrophin results in a cycle of muscle degeneration and regeneration, associated with chronic inflammation and replacement of muscle with fibrotic tissue. Boys with DMD typically present as toe walkers with calf hypertrophy and some motor delay, which is followed by a general decline in motor milestones, accompanied by respiratory and cardiac impairments and ultimately death. Since inflammation has been found to contribute to the degeneration of muscle fibers in DMD, multiple agents are being used to address this inflammation, including corticosteroids, which have been found to prolong function, including ambulation for as much as 3 years, and life by as much as a decade (from 14 to 25 years of age). Antioxidants and antifibrotics are also under investigation to delay muscle loss. However, the most promising work is targeting restoration of dystrophin through manipulation of the genetic defect (exon skipping or nonsense suppression) so that a form of dystrophin is produced. Exon skipping involves triggering the gene to "skip" the missing component and create a modified dystrophin protein; nonsense suppression similarly involves suppressing a "stop" mutation so that dystrophin is produced.[19] Eteplirsen is a compound that induces exon skipping, which has received FDA approval, resulting in increased dystrophin production by 23%, associated with improved walking distance; long-term effects are under investigation.[20] Gene therapy for DMD is focused on inserting small segments of the dystrophin gene via viral vectors to induce the production of dystrophin, referred to as microdystrophin gene transfer; multiple clinical trials are underway but findings are not yet available.[21] These treatments are likely to change the course of this disease as well as the less severe mucular dystrophies. For example, while DMD involves a complete loss of dystrophin, **Becker muscular dystrophy** involves a smaller genetic mutation with only partial loss of dystrophin; the disease progression is slower than DMD but presentation is similar. Those with BMD typically maintain walking ability into adulthood with only 40% becoming wheelchair dependent.[60]

Congenital myopathies involve protein deficits in the contractile elements of the muscle, resulting in generalized weakness, presenting in infancy or gestation (decreased fetal movement). Diagnosis involves muscle biopsy and genetic sequencing to distinguish the type of myopathy. Proximal muscle as well as facial, eye, and respiratory muscles are often most severely impacted, but this can vary by the type of myopathy. In contrast to muscular dystrophies, muscle weakness is slowly progressive or stable for many of the myopathies with some improvement possible.[59] The myopathies can be subdivided into five classes: (1) core – small myofibrillar areas of missing mitochondria; (2) nemaline – the presence of nemaline rods in the muscle sarcoplasma or nuclei; (3) centronuclear – with large irregular nuclei in the muscle fibers; (4) congenital fiber type disproportion – smaller and fewer type I muscle fibers; and (5) myosin storage – the presence of granular regions of hyaline bodies.[61] Currently, there are no approved pharmacological or medical treatments for congenital myopathies; however, similar to the muscular dystrophies, trials are underway that examine gene therapy for several specific types.[61]

Spinal muscular atrophies are autosomal recessive disorders, associated with loss of alpha motor neurons in the spinal cord and brainstem, resulting in denervation of skeletal muscle. They are associated with a mutation of the SMN1 gene on chromosome 5, which is necessary for the survival of motor neuron protein (SMN).[29] There are five types (0-IV) with SMA-0 the most severe and SMA-IV the least. SMA-0 is extremely rare but evident during gestation by an absence of fetal movement with a life expectancy of less than 6 months. SMA-I is diagnosed in infancy as these children won't sit and move very little with a life expectancy of 2 years unless ventilatory support is provided. SMA-II is diagnosed before 18 months, as these children sit but don't walk; most live into adulthood. SMA-III is diagnosed typically in childhood as children are able to walk but have proximal muscle weakness; walking may continue into adulthood but eventually require a wheelchair. Those with SMA-IV are diagnosed in adulthood and will continue to walk throughout their lives. Life expectancy for SMA-III and IV is normal.[62] The difference in severity is dependent on the presence of SMN2, which if present in the right amount can produce SMN; those with SMA I have 2 to 3 copies of SMN2 while those with SMA-III and IV have 3 to 5. Again, similar to what was described for DMD, a method of genetic manipulation to induce SMN2 to produce the SMN protein has been developed. Nusinersen, a synthetic compound that induces this SMN production, has been found to extend the life expectancy of those with infantile SMA and delay the need for ventilation but requires intrathecal application of 4 doses over 2 months and ongoing maintenance applications every 4 months. When applied to older children with other types of SMA, motor function was improved. The long-term effects of this treatment are still under investigation. Notably, a recombinant gene attached to the adeno-associated virus has been trialed in infants with SMA-I to induce SMN production (a method of gene therapy called AVXS-101). All 15 children in the trial were ventilator-free at 20 months of age; 12 patients acquired sitting and 2 walked independently, all but one could speak. This treatment has been approved in the United States for children under 2 and in Europe for those under 21 kg. Long-term follow-ups are underway.[29]

Physical Therapy Management of Children with NMDs

Physical therapy management focuses on optimizing motor function, preventing deformities, specifically muscle contractures that result from limited mobility and maintained postures, and selecting appropriate assistive technology to facilitate function and mobility. In addition, caregivers should be trained upon diagnosis in range of motion and static stretching activities (maintaining stretch at the end of the range) as well as proper positioning to minimize the risk for contractures and skeletal deformities (e.g., scoliosis); over the child's life, the therapist plays a critical role in the choice of seating and positioning devices that would adapt as the child grows and loses muscle control.[63,64]

There is some evidence to suggest that low resistive or isometric exercise can help to maintain strength or improve strength in those with some NMDs, yet there is concern that overwork can cause muscle injury, especially in those with muscular dystrophy with the use of eccentric contractions in strengthening programs especially detrimental.[60] It is recommended that eccentric training be avoided.[65] Strength training should target weak muscles as well as potential compensatory muscles, as muscle mass is lost in primary movers, to prolong function.[63] Aerobic exercise training, using a bicycle or upper extremity ergometer has been reported to increase aerobic capacity and strength without inducing muscle damage in those with BMD[60] and SMA-III.[65] Submaximal aerobic exercise is also recommended for DMD with swimming and cycling the activities of choice.[66] In addition, strengthening of respiratory muscles may improve ventilation and delay the need for a ventilator in those with mild or moderate weakness; however, it is not effective for those with severe weakness.[67] As the disease-modifying treatments continue to be developed, the role of PT in the management of treated children will need to be evaluated. One such study found that daily PT (5 times per week) provided in association with administration of Nusinersen in children with SMA (types I-III), resulted in greater achievement of motor milestones, compared to a group that received Nusinersen and PT no more than once per week. However, the details of the therapy provided were not included in the publication of this program, so research is needed to determine the best therapeutic activities.[62]

Therapists can also help the children adapt their movement patterns to progressively changing muscle strength to assist them to maintain function; this takes creativity to identify stronger muscles and potential movement patterns (e.g., side stepping up stairs to use both UE). The physical therapist also plays a critical role in determining when power mobility should be initiated, identifying other assistive technology needs (e.g., ambulation aids and lifting devices for transferring to and from the wheelchair, bed, toilet, or tub), and helping the family to adapt their home and the school to adapt the classroom to meet the needs of the child/adolescent.[66] Further, the physical therapist can contribute to the documentation of disease progression as well as treatment outcomes through careful recording of movement, strength, and range of motion (ROM). The CHOP-INTEND (**Test of Infant Motor Performance**) is a neurologic exam developed at the **Children's Hospital of Philadelphia** (CHOP); it was developed to evaluate infants with SMA Type I or other infants with progressive muscle weakness.[68,69] The **Hammersmith Functional Motor Scale Expanded** (HFMSE) was designed to document motor function in children and adults with SMA Types 2 and 3, especially for those enrolled in clinical trials.[70,71] While these two measures are designed for children with SMA, therapists can use them for other progressive congenital disorders.[68,70] For children with DMD, the **North Star Ambulatory Assessment** (NSAA) is typically used.[66,72] Alternatively, therapists can use timed measures of coming to standing from the floor and a chair, walking 10 m, ascending and descending stairs, or more standard measures such as the Timed Up and Go test to document functional mobility changes. Also, careful manual muscle testing to regularly document muscle strength is important as is observation of the child's ability to maintain a muscle contraction and recruit agonists for sustained muscle activity; using a handheld dynamometer will improve the therapist's ability to objectively quantify muscle strength. Finally, frequent ROM measurement should be completed to identify developing contractures to target positioning and stretching activities.[63]

It should be noted that in some cases contractures result from adaptation of movement that actually stabilizes the joint (e.g., the ankle), and overstretching can result in joint instability and loss of function. So, therapists must carefully evaluate the child's movements to determine how much stretching should be done. Again, static stretching that includes holding the stretch at the end of the ROM for 60 seconds or the use of night splints has been found to limit the progression of contractures.[64]

Developmental Coordination Disorder (DCD)

DCD is a disorder of fine and gross motor dyscoordination that affects new skill acquisition (motor learning and motor planning), activities of daily living, and participation in school and later work environments that affects up to 6% of school-aged children,[73] and boys much more commonly than girls[74]; the motor deficit includes poor balance and postural control as well as disrupted visual-spatial, executive function, attention and sensorimotor processing.[75] In addition, deficits in self-organization and time management skills are also common.[74] It is distinguished from other disorders, such as autism spectrum disorder and cerebral palsy, with its presentation of clumsiness, slow motor skill learning (both gross and fine motor) given the child's age and intellectual function, and absence of overt neurologic signs (spasticity, hyperreflexia, etc.).[74] Notably, soft neurologic signs may be present (wide-based gait, mild ataxia, ligamentous laxity). Although some children with DCD will present with intellectual deficits, this occurs in the same proportion as the general population and is not a diagnostic criterion; similarly, some children with DCD will also present with speech and language impairments, epilepsy, joint hypermobility, attention deficit/hyperactivity disorder (ADHD; see Box 21-3), or

dyslexia.[77] In fact, up to 60% of children with DCD present with ADHD, reading deficits, and/or language impairment. The impact of DCD spreads into the educational and social participation for children and adolescents with academic performance impeded by deficits in handwriting and organization; limitations in the acquisition of age-appropriate motor skills impede social participation, which may be further disrupted by speech intelligibility deficits that are often present.[78]

Etiology of DCD

A definitive cause for DCD has not been found; however, imaging studies have shown a general decrease in cortical thickness and decreased activation in the prefrontal, parietal, and cerebellar cortices as well as microstructural disorganization in the white matter of the corticospinal tracts and thalamic radiations. Thus, the neurologic changes are distributed across the sensorimotor system, including the connections with the prefrontal cortex necessary for predictive control.[79] Not surprisingly, DCD is more common in children born preterm, who have experienced neonatal encephalopathy.[73] Two theories have been proposed to explain the deficits of DCD: (1) a disruption in the ability to translate movements from a cognitive to an automatic phase and (2) a deficit in the internal representation of movement, which refers to the inability to compare the efference copy generated during motor planning to the execution of the movement in order to make a correction. Both of these theories emphasize the role of the cerebellum in this deficit; however, it is not felt that this is singularly a cerebellar problem. Interestingly, children with DCD show impaired anticipatory postural adjustments, requiring a reliance on feedback mechanisms for postural control that are ineffective for coordinated quick movements.[79]

Prognosis for Children with DCD

DCD is not just a pediatric disorder; rather, like so many developmental disabilities, it has a lifelong impact. Early diagnosis is associated with delayed motor skill acquisition and peer play. However, school-aged children demonstrate increasing difficulty with academic and social skills as well as emotional and behavioral concerns. Similar to their peers with DS, children with DCD are at risk for obesity and ultimately for cardiovascular conditions, resulting from decreased activity levels and community engagement. There are limited studies on adult outcomes for children with DCD, but it is expected that they will do best with employment opportunities that require limited motor skill.[80]

Treatment Approaches for DCD

Treatment recommendations for children with DCD include (1) process-focused approaches that address the impairments and functional limitations of DCD (e.g., balance, strength) and (2) task-focused paradigms that aim to improve motor planning and motor learning through task practice. In general, and not surprisingly, task-focused programs have been found to achieve greater improvements than process-focused programs.[81] One method that has been successful is the use of gaming, specifically the WiiFit™, which has been used to provide highly repetitive task practice that challenges postural control and interlimb coordination with improvements noted in those same areas as

Box 21-3	Attention Deficit Hyperactivity Disorder (ADHD)[76]

ADHD is another developmental disorder found in up to 5% of children and characterized by poor attention, impulsiveness, and exaggerated activity levels; although many children outgrow this disorder in adolescence/early adulthood, 50% or so will continue to demonstrate problems as adults with an impact on employment and social interactions. There is a strong familial hereditary component to ADHD, yet the actual genetic abnormality has not been identified. While attention deficit can occur in the absence of hyperactivity, and vice versa, these two disorders commonly occur together. ADHD is associated with decreased brain volume, involving many areas of the brain, including the basal ganglia, anterior cingulate, inferior parietal lobule, cerebellum, and hippocampus, as well as a general thinning of the cortex. In addition, diffusion tensor imaging has found white matter irregularities, especially in the superior longitudinal fasciculus that connects the inferior parietal lobe with the lateral prefrontal cortex, a critical pathway for attention. The most common treatment for ADHD is psychostimulants (e.g., methylphenidate, which blocks the reuptake of norepinephrine and dopamine) or selective norepinephrine reuptake inhibitors (e.g., atomoxetine) that have their primary influence on prefrontal, basal ganglial, and cerebellar brain regions, involved in attention.

well as running speed and agility, after a 6-week training program, using the "Balancing Games."[50] However, in a comparison of WiiFit Balance training and task training, focused on common playground games (e.g., tag, ball activities), greater improvement occurred in the task training group for strength, aerobic, and anaerobic measures.[82] Recently, motor imagery training, where the child is instructed to reflect on the feel and the visual image of a movement has also been found to enhance motor function. Further, group-based training in small groups has been recommended.[81] Thus, in planning treatment for children with DCD, therapists should keep in mind that a high level of repetition is likely required to improve motor performance but a variety of treatment options are available. For the evaluation of children with DCD, the **Movement Assessment Battery for Children** (MABC-2)[83] and the **Bruininks Oseretski Test of Motor Proficiency 2** (BOT-2) are recommended.[81,84]

Autism Spectrum Disorder

ASD is a common neurodevelopmental disorder with a myriad of symptomatology, most concentrated in impairments in language, social-emotional function, communication, and restrictive repetitive behaviors; many children also demonstrate impaired adaptive behavior and activities of daily living. As a spectrum disorder, the combinations of behavioral symptoms are varied such that no two children with ASD are the same. Current estimates of ASD are 1 in 59 children without racial or ethnic disproportions but with gender disproportions as there are four times more boys than girls diagnosed. Diagnosis is typically made by age five but early signs can be evident in infancy.[85] thus, it is recommended that all children be screened at 18 and 24 months of age, using the **Autism Diagnostic Interview-Revised** (ADI-R)[86] and the **Autism Diagnostic Observation Schedule-2** (ADOS-2).[87] The cause of ASD is unknown but both multiple genetic variations (over 800 identified), largely microdeletions or duplications, combined with environmental factors (in utero nutrition, toxin exposure, maternal infections) are implicated in its etiology.[88,89] A strong genetic component is suggested as up to 70 to 90% of monozygotic twins both express the disorder but 50% of dizygotic twins also both express the disorder, which also emphasizes the dual input of genetic and environmental factors. Further, there's a 25 to 30% manifestation in a third child, when two in a family have the diagnosis. Additionally, disruption in mitochondrial function has been implicated in some individuals with ASD.[88]

In some cases, regressive symptoms are identified with a decline in language and social skills in the second or third year of life. Even so, a high percentage of parents report that they were concerned about their baby's development at 1 and 2 years of age. The prevalence of ASD is higher in children with Fragile X or tuberous sclerosis and with older parents.[88] There is no cure or prenatal diagnostic tests for ASD. An ASD diagnosis is given by psychologists and psychiatrists using the DSM-V criteria, which include (1) lack of social-emotional or communication reciprocity; (2) verbal and/or nonverbal communication deficits; (3) inability or lack of interest in developing social relationships; (4) restricted or repetitive patterns of behavior or interests; and (5) sensory hyporeactivity or hyperreactivity.[90] Diagnosis requires at least three symptoms related to social behavior/communication and two symptoms of repetitive or restricted behavior.[91] Severity levels are distinguished by the level of support needed: (1) Level 1 requires some support for social communication and interactions, inflexible behavior, and organization skills; (2) Level 2 requires substantial support due to social impairments, verbal and non-verbal communication, and greater inflexibility of behavior, poor response to change, and greater level of restrictive/repetitive behaviors; (3) Level 3 requires very substantial support due to severe communication/social behavior impairments and severe inflexiblity, response to change, and restricted/repetitive behavior.[89] The DSM-V regrouped several pervasive developmental disorders into a single autism spectrum disorder. These included autism, **Asberger's syndrome**, pervasive developmental disorder not otherwise specified, Rett syndrome, and child disintegrative disorder. It also created a new diagnostic category of social communication disorder for children with the social/language characteristics of ASD but without the repetitive/restrictive behavior.[91] Children previously diagnosed with, Asperger's syndrome have been reclassified under the DSM-V as a high functioning level of ASD, but the term, Asberger's syndrome, is still used by many clinicians and lay persons. An AS diagnosis previously entailed two signs of social impairment and one of restrictive behavior without a deficit in cognition or other delay. Now, those diagnosed with ASD are classified into the three levels previously described, based on symptomology, as well as cognition into high functioning (IQ above 70) or low functioning (IQ ≤ 70); those previously diagnosed with AS are typically stratified into level one and described as high functioning.[92] Intellectual disabilities and other language impairments frequently co-occur with ASD and require additional testing and separate diagnostic categorization. See Box 21-4 for common features of ASD.

Brain Differences in ASD

There is considerable research examining the neurobiology of ASD. Overgrowth of the brain in the first two years of life has been well documented and the degree of overgrowth correlates to the severity of presentation; this is primarily an increase in the surface area and not the volume of the cortex within the frontal, parietal and temporal lobes as well as the visual cortex (see Chapter 9 for a description of brain development and pruning). Yet increased cortical thickness has been reported in older children and adults. Similarly, the amygdala and basal ganglial structures have been found to be enlarged in children and adults with ASD. Yet more recent findings suggest that gray matter volume is decreased in these same structures. White matter differences have also been reported in the corpus callosum, specifically the anterior portion connecting areas of the prefrontal cortex. Likewise, altered white matter projections in many areas of the brain have been reported, especially those related to social brain regions, including the superior longitudinal fasciculus that connects the superior temporal sulcus to the fusiform gyrus, which are involved in facial expression recognition.[93] fMRI studies have demonstrated decreased activity in the resting state network and social brain network as well as over activity in sensorimotor and visual networks.[94] Diffusion tensor imaging has identified decreased connectivity

Box 21-4	Common Features of ASD[85,88,89]

- Poor eye contact
- Lack of pointing or waving by 14 months
- Not responding to name by 12 months
- Few large smiles
- Language delay
- Self-stimulatory behaviors
- Delays or lack of pretend play and imagination
- Spinning body or objects repetitively
- Flapping hands and arms
- Rocking
- Echolalia – repeating what others have said
- Repeating phrases from television
- Narrow interests
- Perseverative movements and actions (repeating them over and over)
- Decreased social skills
- Inflexible routines
- Unusual sensory interests
- Difficulty initiating conversation
- Lack of understanding and use of gestures
- Wanting to be alone
- Decreased ability to describe feelings
- Poor emotional regulation
- Unusual reactions to new sensory information such as smell or taste
- Decreased ability to read facial expression
- Lack of understanding social cues
- Flat affect
- Using language in an unusual way
- Routine oriented
- Respond negatively to minor changes in routine
- Lack of the ability to direct another's attention to themselves or objects (joint attention)
- Difficulty with imitation
- Poor understanding of cause and effect

in three areas associated with emotions and social interactions: (1) the limbic system (cingulum bundle, uncinated fasciculus, mammillo-thalamic tract, and anterior thalamic projections); (2) the mirror neuron system that is involved in facial expression recognition with projections within the arcuate fasciculus, connecting the frontal, parietal, and temporal lobes; and (3) the face processing system that is responsible for face recognition as well as determination of the social implications of facial expression and involving areas of the occipital and temporal lobes with their interconnections. In young children, there seems to be an over-connectivity in many areas compared to their typical peers; while in older children, these same areas yield lower connectivity than their peers. Ultimately, neural changes may not be stable until late childhood or early adolescence.[95] Some of the same areas, associated with ASD symptomology, have also been identified as brain abnormalities in children with language

impairment, ADHD, sensory processing disorder, and other developmental disabilities.

Epilepsy in ASD

Epilepsy is a common occurrence in ASD with up to 46% of children with ASD also diagnosed with epilepsy; onset occurs at two time points – early childhood and adolescence. Epilepsy is more likely in females and those with a family history of epilepsy, more severe level of ASD (greater language deficits and IDD), or developmental regression.[96] Even those without an epilepsy diagnosis often demonstrate abnormal spontaneous brain activity on EEG (electroencephalogram), which has been hypothesized to indicate abnormal activity in the mirror brain network. The strong association between ASD and epilepsy and recent evidence of multiple genetic defects associated with both suggests a common mechanistic etiology that is influenced by environmental factors. Pharmacological management of seizures is necessary in most cases.[96] As discussed in Chapter 20, antiepileptic medications have many associated side effects, including drowsiness, dizziness, fatigue, weakness, irritability, anxiety, and confusion, that can exacerbate the symptomology of ASD. Physical therapists should be aware of these side effects and may need to time treatment sessions to avoid periods of fatigue and weakness.

Developmental Differences in ASD

The five domains of child development – cognitive, language, social, motor, and emotional – are all described as atypical in children with ASD.

Cognitive Function in ASD. There is a large range of intelligence in children with ASD. A 2018 report of a national network included analysis of 5058 children with ASD at age 8; of these, 35.2% were diagnosed with ID (IQ <70%), 23.1% had borderline IQ (71-85), and the remainder (41.7%) had an IQ above 85. Despite this range in IQ, only 12% of individuals with ASD have been reported to successfully live independently due to multiple factors – deficits in activities of daily living, incomplete educational preparation, under employment, and poor social skills.[89] Yet, some people with ASD can be successful when appropriate educational or vocational support is provided while others are able to complete college degrees and have successful careers. Still others with ASD exhibit savant behaviors, typically in one area, like math, memory, or music. Up to 37% of those with ASD are reported to have savant syndrome, which seems to be linked to greater sensory sensitivity, more obsessional behaviors, a greater tendency to systematize (organize information by systems), and have greater use of spatial imagery.[97]

Up to 63% of those with ASD are also diagnosed with ADHD; they also demonstrate difficulties with self-regulation, which refers to the ability to calm oneself or stop repetitive behaviors as well as the ability to block out distractions. Further, many children with ASD have difficulty with managing their emotions and may demonstrate irritability, depression, or emotion dysregulation. Children with greater language delay have been found to demonstrate greater self-regulation deficits; similarly, children with better self-regulation were found to have higher cognition. Thus, these deficits seem to combine to contribute to higher or lower functioning in children with ASD. While some adults with ASD live independently or with minimal assistance, supportive services are commonly needed as people with ASD and ID age.[98]

Language Development in ASD. A key feature of ASD is **delayed language**, both expressive and receptive, with children with ASD often not saying a first word until 2 or 3 years of age, and many children have no verbal skills. Notably, language acquisition plays a critical role in the development of self-regulation skills, which are usually taught through verbal instruction; therefore, the severity of the language dysfunction likely influences the degree of self-regulation dysfunction.[98] Sign language, picture exchange communication systems, or speech-generating devices are often introduced as a means of communication for children with limited speech. However, a recent systematic review found that augmentative and assistive communication (ACC), using any of these methods, was effective in increasing communication with the particular method employed and in some studies verbal communication also increased. Yet, this was not the case in all studies; importantly, speech did not decrease with the use of AAC.[99] Delays and differences in the language skills of children with ASD also include difficulty understanding simple sentences or words, speaking with unusual intonations, repetition of words with no intent to communicate (**echolalia**), understating or using humor inappropriately, and difficulty understanding abstract language and nonverbal cues – all contributing to difficulties in communication.[100] Another factor, contributing to the language delay of children with ASD seems to be auditory-visual misalignment; simply, this results from the child not attending visually to things that are verbally described or pointed out by caregivers so that they don't make the connection between words and the related objects or events.[101]

Socio-Emotional Development in ASD. Another feature of ASD is poor social skill development. Behaviors exhibited include a mismatch between facial expression, body language, gestures, and the environmental context as well as a lack of eye contact. Children with ASD often demonstrate a resistance to being touched, have difficulty understanding the perspective of others, and do not independently seek out social situations or express interest in what others are doing or experiencing. Children with ASD frequently have difficulty or cannot make friends with same-age peers. They avoid group situations and prefer spending time alone. Another feature of ASD is impairments in emotional development. Behaviors exhibited include (1) difficulty understanding facial expressions and the emotions of others – often described as a lack of empathy, (2) poor imitation of or use of facial expressions, (3) disrupted emotional control, and (4) inappropriate responsiveness to emotional situations.[95]

Motor Development in ASD. Impaired motor skill development is also a characteristic of ASD, although it is not part of the DSMV diagnostic criteria except for stereotypical repetitive movements. Interestingly, a high percentage of children with ASD qualify for supportive services such as physical therapy

with delays on standardized testing for fine and/or gross motor skills; in fact, they have many similarities to those with DCD,[99] including hypotonia; dysdiadochokinesis (inability to perform rapidly alternating movements), clumsiness, apraxia, and poor balance and postural control; delayed gross and fine motor skills; poor coordination in reaching and gait; difficulty with the learning of and execution of skilled movements (planning and refinement), performing movement sequences or rhythmic movements as well as poor ball skills; and impaired proprioception, strength, agility, and speed.[99,102] It is important to note that children with ASD often avoid new physical activities, placing them at higher risk for decreased endurance and resulting in less practice and exploration of new motor skills.

Since ASD is not typically diagnosed before 3 years of age, infants who go on to develop ASD may not be seen by physical therapists for ASD, but they could be referred to physical therapy for global developmental delay. Therapists should be aware of the early signs of ASD and the genetic predisposition in order to refer a family to appropriate healthcare professionals, if an ASD diagnosis is suspected in an infant or toddler. ASD screenings, using both parent surveys and clinical tools that are a combination of survey and clinical assessment, are routinely done at pediatrician's offices and can be incorporated into a physical therapy assessment, if needed. The **Modified Checklist for Autism in Toddlers** (M-CHAT)[103] is the most frequently used checklist for common features and behaviors that could be indicative of ASD, including social interaction, imaginative play, responses to sensory stimulation, and language and motor skills. This checklist is completed by a parent or caregiver and interpreted by a medical professional. EI (birth-3) should be available for children who are at risk for developmental disabilities, so some children with ASD may receive EI; however, since many children aren't diagnosed until 3, those with a late diagnosis may not receive EI services. Children with ASD commonly receive occupational therapy for sensory integration therapy (see description in Box 21-5), and **Applied Behavioral Analysis** (ABA) at home or school; ABA is an individualized program of one-on-one treatment to encourage positive behaviors (e.g., vocalizations, eye contact, modeling of facial expressions) while discouraging negative behaviors (e.g., hand flapping, aggression) in order to improve function and learning.[66] Treatment programs, for children with ASD who are receiving physical therapy, should incorporate behavioral modification techniques, including positive reinforcement for target behaviors (e.g., attention, eye gaze) and to minimize disruptive behaviors. Exercise interventions have been used to improve postural control as well as address autistic symptoms (communication and adaptive behavior, repetitive, injurious and aggressive behaviors) and to facilitate participation and social interactions; these include hippotherapy and therapeutic horseback riding, aquatic therapy, strength training, aerobic exercise (jogging, cycling), and exergames.[105,106] Further, exercise prior to academic work has been found to improve concentration and engagement, and exercise programs have been found to improve cardiovascular fitness and decrease obesity in older children, adolescents, and adults with ASD.[106] Yet, the majority of studies are with small cohorts, so there is still a need for high-quality studies on physical therapy interventions for children and adults with ASD. Using a

Box 21-5   Sensory Therapies for ASD

Sensory-focused treatments for ASD include both **sensory integration therapy** (SIT) and **sensory-based interventions** (SBI). SIT, developed by Ayres,[68] focuses on activities that require the child to process sensory information within a motor task; consistent with motor learning strategies, SIT challenges the child at the "peak" of their skill level, using vestibular (e.g., swings), proprioceptive (e.g., bouncing on therapy balls or trampolines), and tactile challenges (e.g., reaching for objects in sand). A critical component of SIT is the active engagement of the child to explore the sensory stimulation that is individualized to the child. A recent systematic review found strong evidence for the use of Ayre's based SIT for children 4 to 12 with ASD and an IQ above 65 to improve participation and sensorimotor function. SBIs apply either active or passive sensory stimulation to improve sensory processing, self-awareness, and self-regulation; techniques used include weight vests or therapeutic wrapping to increase proprioceptive awareness; sitting on a ball while playing at a table to improve postural control; massage to improve body awareness, responsiveness to touch or to calm the child; or auditory therapy to improve responsiveness to auditory stimuli. While there is fairly good evidence to support the use of SIT for children with ASD, there is limited evidence to support the use of SBI; however, this is likely due to the large variability in how it is applied and the methods for assessment.[104] Yet, the physical therapist, working with the child with ASD, may find some of these techniques helpful in their treatment strategies.

metronome for timing and sequencing of motor skills has been found to enhance the effectiveness of a physical therapy program, targeting gross motor skills, resulting in greater improvement in bilateral coordination, running, strength, and agility.[107]

Sensory Differences in ASD

From poor visual and auditory integration to sensorimotor impairments, sensory differences are commonplace in children with ASD with greater than 90% of children demonstrating atypical reactivity to sensory stimulation, referred to as **sensory integration disorder** (SID); this prevalence has made SID a component of the DSMV diagnostic criteria for ASD. SID refers to over- or under-responsiveness to sensory stimulation, thought to result for impaired sensory processing, and can impact leaning, motor function, and independence. As a result of SID, children with ASD either seek out sensory stimulation (e.g., spinning themselves or objects) or avoid sensory stimulation (e.g., smell aversions that affect eating, hypersensitivity to clothing textures that impact what the child will wear) with the child also demonstrating stereotypic behaviors to calm or stimulate themselves to meet this "sensory need." For many children, sensory symptoms are often the earliest sign of ASD and may contribute to the other manifestations of this disorder (e.g., social behavior). It is thought that sensory input is not integrated or organized appropriately in the brain, based on the disruption of connectivity described earlier. As a result of over- and under-responsiveness sensory stimuli can be disproportionally distressing or comforting to children with ASD.[108]

Other Treatments of ASD Symptoms

Pharmacology and dietary management of ASD symptoms are commonplace. Pharmacological management is difficult due to the vulnerability of individuals with ASD to the side effects of many medications. However, pharmacological management may be used to address ADHD, aggression, or self-injurious behavior, as well as insomnia and stereotypic behavior. Atypical antipsychotic medications are often used, with risperidone (commercially known as Risperdal) the most frequently prescribed, which has been found to decrease hyperactivity, irritability, aggression, and stereotypical behaviors (e.g., hand flapping) while improving social interactions. Unlike typical antipsychotics, like haloperidol, risperidone has fewer and less severe side effects, including weight gain, dizziness, tiredness, fatigue, fever, and nausea.[109] Other medications that have been tried include stimulant medications to address ADHD, but they have many side effects in this population, while non-stimulant medications such as alpha-2 agonists (e.g., guanfacine) are more effective with only minor side effects (sedation and lower blood pressure). For adults but not children with ASD, Fluoxetine has improved repetitive behaviors. In addition, melatonin has been found to improve sleep behavior in children with ASD.[88] Children with ASD often have food restrictions and secondary nutritional deficiencies as well as **gastrointestinal (GI) dysfunction**, including coeliac disease and inflammatory bowel disease, intestinal hyperpermeabiity, alterations of the microbiota, and frequent infections of the GI tract. Symptoms include diarrhea/constipation or esophageal reflux. Thus, dietary interventions have been investigated not only for the management of these GI conditions but also for attempting to address behavioral symptoms. Gluten-free (limiting wheat, barley, and rye products) and/or casein-free (limiting milk products) diets are the most commonly applied programs in ASD. The available evidence of their impact remains equivocal with some studies reporting improvements in ASD symptoms while others report no effect. The ketogenic diet (high fat, low carbohydrate) has also been used in individuals with ASD with some improvement in behavioral symptoms noted; however, a worsening of GI symptoms makes its use impractical.[110]

CASE A, PART VI

While Pauli does not have an ASD or ADHD diagnosis at this point, she does display many behaviors similar to those of these diagnoses. Therefore, physical therapy treatment should benefit from incorporating behavioral management techniques in her treatment program to improve her participation and diminish negative behaviors; working with the health care team, educational team and the family to develop strategies will be important to assure consistency across settings and maximize her outcomes. Further, her limited food choices and response to sensory stimuli (e.g., needing tags removed from clothes) suggest that she should be evaluated for sensory integration problems and potentially would benefit from a sensory integration treatment program as part of her occupational therapy treatment. Pauli is definitely a candidate for an educational program for children with developmental delays and a comprehensive treatment program; since she is almost 3, an IEP and preschool program should be identified. Like many young children with a global developmental delay, Pauli's condition does not fit into any definitive diagnostic category, and she will continue to be classified with a global developmental delay diagnosis. As she gets older, a more definitive diagnosis may be found, or she may continue with this diagnosis.

REFERENCES

1. Schalock RL, Luckasson R, Tasse MJ. The contemporary view of intellectual and developmental disabilities: implications for psychologists. *Psicothema.* 2019;31(3):223-228.

2. Belanger SA, Caron J. Evaluation of the child with global developmental delay and intellectual disability. *Paediatr Child Health.* 2018;23(6):403-410.

3. Pirozzi F, Nelson B, Mirzaa G. From microcephaly to megalencephaly: determinants of brain size. *Dialogues Clin Neurosci.* 2018;20(4):267-282.

4. Seggers J, Haadsma M, Bos AF, et al. Dysmorphic features and developmental outcome of 2-year-old children. *Dev Med Child Neurol.* 2014;56:1078-1084.

5. Weckselblatt B, Rudd MK. Human structural variation: mechanisms of chromosome rearrangements. *Trends Genet.* 2015;31(10):587-599.

6. Antonarakis SE, Skotko BG, Rafii MS, et al. Down syndrome. *Nat Rev Dis Primers.* 2021;6(1):9.

7. Gupta NA, Kabra M. Diagnosis and management of Down syndrome. *Indian J Pediatr.* 2014;81(6):560-567.

8. Flore LA, Milunsky JM. Updates in the genetic evaluation of the child with global developmental delay or intellectual disability. *Semin Pediatr Neurol.* 2012;19:173-180.

9. Nicholls RD. The impact of genomic imprinting for neurobehavioral and developmental disorders. *J Clin Invest.* 2000;105(4):413-418.

10. Duca DG, Craiu D, Boer M, et al. Diagnostic approach of Angelman syndrome. *J Clin Med.* 2013;8(4):321-327.

11. Buggenhout GV, Fryns JP. Angelman syndrome. *Eur J Hum Genet.* 2009; 17:1367-1373.

12. Flanigan KM. Duchenne and Becker muscular dystrophies. *Neurol Clin.* 2014;32:671-688.

13. Vallat JM, Mathis S, Funalot B. The various Charcot-Marie-Tooth diseases. *Curr Opin Neurol.* 2013;26(5):473-480.

14. Mainardi PC. Cri du Chat syndrome. *Orphanet J Rare Dis.* 2006;1(33):1-9.

15. Martiniano SL, Hoppe JE, Sagel SD, Zemanick ET. Advances in the diagnosis and treatment of cystic fibrosis. *Adv Pediatr.* 2014;61:225-243.

16. Hamner T, Udhnani MD, Osipowicz KZ, Lee NR. Pediatric brain development in Down syndrome: a field in its infancy. *J Int Neuropsychol Soc.* 2018;24(9):966-976.

17. Saenz RB. Primary care of infants and young children with Down syndrome. *Am Fam Physician.* 1999;59(2):381-390.

18. Spencer K. Screening for Down syndrome. *Scan J Clin Lab Invest.* 2014; 74(S244):41-47.

19. Leigh F, Ferlini A, Biggar D, et al. Neurology care, diagnostics, and emerging therapies of the patient with Duchene muscular dystrophy. *Pediatrics.* 2018;142(Suppl 2):S5-S16.

20. Datta N, Ghosh PS. Update on muscular dystrophies with focus on novel treatments and biomarkers. *Curr Neurol Neurosci Rep.* 2020;20:14.

21. Elangkovan N, Dickson G. Gene therapy for Duchenne muscular dystrophy. *J Neuromuscul Dis.* 2021;8:S303-S316.

22. Maurin T, Zongaro S, Bardoni B. Fragile X syndrome: from molecular pathology to therapy. *Neurosci Biobehav Rev.* 2014;46(Pt 2):242-255.

23. Gallagher A, Hallahan B. Fragile X-associated disorders: a clinical overview. *J Neurol.* 2012;259:401-413.

24. Vanier MT. Niemann-Pick disease type C. *Orphanet J Rare Dis.* 2010;5(16):1-18.

25. Jin DK. Systematic review of the clinical and genetic aspects of Prader-Willi syndrome. *Korean J Pediatr.* 2011;54(2):55-63.

26. Emerick JE, Vogt KS. Endocrine manifestations and management of Prader-Willi syndrome. *Int J Pediatr Endocrinol.* 2013;2013(1):14.

27. Ney DM, Blank RD, Hansen KE. Advances in the nutritional and pharmacological management of phenylketonuria. *Curr Opin Clin Nutr Metab Care.* 2014;17:61-68.

28. Briggs A. Primary care of a child with Rett syndrome. *J Am Assoc Nurse Pract.* 2014;26:471-480.

29. Nicolau S, Waldrop MA, Connolly AM, Mendell JR. Spinal muscular atrophy. *Semin Pediatr Neurol.* 2021;37:100878.

30. Rosa RFM, Rosa RCM, Zen PRG, Craziadio C, Paskulin GA. Trisomy 18: review of the clinical, etiologic, prognostic and ethical aspects. *Rev Paul Pediatr.* 2013;31(1):111-120.

31. Lorenz JM, Hardart GE. Evolving medical and surgical management of infants with trisomy 18. *Curr Opin Pediatr.* 2014;26:169-176.

32. Merle U, Schaefer M, Ferenci P, Stremmel W. Clinical presentation, diagnosis and long-term outcome of Wilson's disease: a cohort study. *Gut.* 2007: 56:115-120.

33. Saudubray JM, Garcia-Cazorla A. Inborn errors of metabolism overview: pathophysiology, manifestations, evaluation, and management. *Pediatr Clin North Am.* 2018;65:179-208.

34. Pastores GM. Neuropathic lysosomal storage disorders. *Neurol Clin.* 2013; 31(4):1051-1071.

35. Bley AE, Giannikopoulos OA, Hayden D, Kubilus K, Tifft CJ, Eichler FS. Natural history of infantile GM2 gangliosidosis. *Pediatrics.* 2011;128;e1233.

36. Kanungo S, Soares N, He M, Steiner RD. Sterol metabolism disorders and neurodevelopment: an update. *Dev Disabil Res Rev.* 2013;17:197-210.

37. Stockler-Ipsiroglu S, van Karnebeek CDM. Cerebral creatine deficiencies: a group of treatable intellectual developmental disorders. *Semin Neurol.* 2014;34:350-356.

38. Dong SZ, Zhu M, Bulas D. Techniques for minimizing sedation in pediatric MRI. *J Magn Reson Imaging.* 2019;50:1047-1054.

39. Bayley Scales of Infant and Toddler Development', 3rd ed. Pearson. 2005. http://www.pearsonclinical.com/psychology/products/100000123/bayley-scales-of-infant-and-toddler-development-third-edition-bayley-iii.html.

40. Folio MR, Fewell RR. Peabody Developmental Motor Scales. 3rd ed. Austin, TX: 2023. Available at: https://www.wpspublish.com/peabody-developmental-motor-scales-third-edition.html.

41. Grieco J, Pulsifer M, Seligsonn K, Skotko B, Schwartz A. Down syndrome: cognitive and behavioral functioning across the lifespan. *Am J Med Genetics. Part C.* 2015;169C:135-149.

42. Lagan N, Huggard D, McGrane F, et al. Multiorgan involvement and management in children with Down syndrome. *Acta Paediatr.* 2020;109:1096-1111.

43. Ravel A, Mircher C, Rebillat AS, Cieuta-Walti C, Megarbane A. Feeding problems and gastrointestinal diseases in Down syndrome. *Arch Pediatr.* 2020;27:53-60.

44. Lott IT, Dierssen M. Cognitive deficits and associated neurological complications in individuals with Down syndrome. *Lancet Neurol.* 2010;9:623-633.

45. Foley C, Killeen OG. Musculoskeletal anomalies in children with Down syndrome: an observational study. *Arch Dis Child.* 2019;104:428-487.

46. Winders P, Wolter-Warmerdam K, Hickey F. A schedule of gross motor development for children with Down syndrome. *J Intellect Disabil Res.* 2019;63(4):346-356.

47. Yamauchi Y, Aoki S, Koike J, Hanzawa N, Hashimoto K. Motor and cognitive development of children with Down syndrome: the effect of acquisition of walking skills on their cognitive and language abilities. *Brain Dev.* 2019;41:320-326.

48. Okada S, Uejo T, Hirano R, et al. Assessing the efficacy of very early motor rehabilitation in children with Down syndrome. *J Pediatr*. 2019;213:227-231.

49. Arslan FN, Dogan DG, Canaloglu SK, Baysal SG, Buyukavci R, Buyukavci MA. Effects of early physical therapy on motor development in children with Down syndrome. *North Clin Instanb*. 2022;9(2):156-161.

50. Wentz EE. Importance of initiating a "tummy time" intervention early in infants with Down syndrome. *Pediatr Phys Ther*. 2017;29:68-75.

51. Valentin-Gudiol M, Bagur-Calafat C, Girabent-Farres M, et al. Treadmill interventions with partial body weight support in children under six years of age at risk of neuromotor delay: a report of a Cochrane systematic review and meta-analysis. *Eur J Phys Rehabil Med*. 2013;49:67-91.

52. Looper J, Ulrich DA. Effect of treadmill training and supramalleolar orthosis use on motor skill development in infants with Down syndrome: a randomized clinical trial. *Phys Ther*. 2010;90:382-390.

53. Maiano C, Hue O, Lepage G, Morin AJS, Tracey D, Moullec G. Do exercise interventions improve balance for children and adolescents with Down syndrome? A systematic review. *Phys Ther*. 2019;99:507-518.

54. Rafil MS, Kleschevnikov AM, Sawa M, Mobley WC. Down syndrome. *Handb Clin Neurol*. 2019;167(3rd series):321-336.

55. Gensous N, Bacalini MG, Franceschi C, Garagnani P. Down syndrome, accelerated aging and immunosenescence. *Semin Immunopathol*. 2020;42:635-645.

56. Franceschi C, Garagnani P, Gensous N, Bacalini MG, Conte M, Salvioli S. Accelerated bio-cognitive aging in Down syndrome: state of the art and possible deceleration strategies. *Aging Cell*. 2019;18:e12903.

57. Barnhart RC, Connolly B. Aging and Down syndrome: implications for physical therapy. *Phys Ther*. 2007;87:1399-1406.

58. Fleming V, Pior-Gambetti B, Patrick A, Zammit M, Alexander A, et al. Physical activity and cognitive and imaging biomarkers of Alzheimers disease in Down syndrome. *Neurobiol Aging*. 2021.107;118-127.

59. Butterfield RJ. Congenital muscular dystrophy and congenital myopathy. *Curr Neurol Neurosci Rep*. 2020;20(6):14.

60. Lanza G, Pino M, Fisicaro F, et al. Motor activity and Becker's muscular dystrophy: lights and shadows. *Phys Sportsmed*. 2020;48(2):151-160.

61. Claeys KG. Congenital myopathies: an update. *Dev Med Child Neurol*. 2020;62:297-302.

62. Mirea A, Leanca MC, Onose G, et al. Physical therapy and Nusinersen impact on spinal muscular atrophy rehabilitative outcome. *Front Biosci*. 2022;27(6):179.

63. Johnson LB, Abresch JM. Physical therapy evaluation and management in neuromuscular diseases. *Phys Med Rehabil Clin N Am*. 2012;23:633-651.

64. Mercuri E, Finkel RS, Muntoni F, et al. Diagnosis and management of spinal muscular atrophy: Part 1: recommendations for diagnosis, rehabilitation, orthopedic and nutritional care. *Neuromuscul Disord*. 2018;28:103-113.

65. Bartels B, Montes J, van der Pol WL, de Groot JF. Physical exercise training for type 3 spinal muscular atrophy (review). *Cochrane Database Syst Rev*. 2019;3(3):CD012120.

66. Birnkrant DJ. Diagnosis and management of Duchenne muscular dystrophy, part 1: diagnosis, and neuromuscular rehabilitation, endocinem and gastrointestinal and nutritional management. *Lancet Neurol*. 2018;17(3):251-267.

67. Abresch RT, Carter GT, Han JJ, Mcdonald CM. Exercise in neuromuscular diseases. *Phys Med Rehabil Clin N Am*. 2012;23:653-673.

68. Glanzman AM, Mazzone E, Main M, et al. The children's hospital of Philadelphia infant test of neuromuscular disorders (CHOP INTEND): test development and reliability. *Neuromuscul Disord*. 2010;20(3):155-161.

69. CHOP-Intend. https://smauk.org.uk/files/files/Research/CHOP%20INTEND.pdf. Accessed on August 1, 2022.

70. Pera MC, Coratti G, Focina N, et al. Content validity and clinical meaningfulness of the HFMSE in spinal muscular atrophy. *BMC Neurol*. 2017;17(1):39.

71. HFMSE. https://www.biogenlinc.si/content/dam/intl/europe/slovenia/mta/hcp/biogenlinc-core/sl_SI/media/documents/spinal-muscular-atrophy/sign-and-symptoms/HFSM_scale_block_SLO.pdf. Accessed on 8/1/2022.

72. North Star Ambulatory Assessment. https://www.musculardystrophyuk.org/static/s3fs-public/2021-08/NSAA%20_Manual_%2015102020.pdf?VersionId=BaPGDWk5TxA3rtF2DDipAVYlOJ5Eoumo. Accessed on 8/3/2022.

73. Peters LHJ, Maathuis CGB, Hadders-Algra M. Neural correlates of developmental coordination disorder. *Dev Med Child Neurol*. 2013;55(suppl 4):59-64.

74. Kirby A, Sugden D, Purcell C. Diagnosing developmental coordination disorders. *Arch Dis Child*. 2014;99:292-296.

75. Vaivre-Douret L. Developmental coordination disorders: state of art. *Clin Neurophysiol*. 2014;44:13-23.

76. Friedman LA, Rapoport JL. Brain development in ADHD. *Curr Opin Neurobiol*. 2015;30:106-111.

77. Lingam R, Golding J, Jongmans MJ, Hunt LP, Ellis M, Emond A. The association between developmental coordination disorder and other developmental traits. *Pediatrics*. 2010;126:e1109-e1118.

78. Sylvestre A, Nadeau L, Charron L, Larose N, Lepage C. Social participation by children with developmental coordination disorder compared to their peers. *Disabil Rehabil*. 2013;35(21):1814 1820.

79. Jelsma D, Geuze RH, Mombarg R, Smits-Engelsman BCM. The impact of Wii Fit intervention on dynamic balance control in children with probable developmental coordination disorder and balance problems. *Hum Mov Sci*. 2014;33:404-418.

80. Zwicker JG, Missiuna C, Harris SR, Boyd LA. Developmental coordination disorder: a review and update. *Eur J Paediatr Neurol*. 2012;16:573-581.

81. Blank R, Barnett AL, Cairney J, et al. International clinical practice recommendations on the definition, diagnosis, assessment, intervention and psychosocial aspects of developmental coordination disorder. *Dev Med Child Neurol*. 2019;61:242-285.

82. Ferguson GD, Jelsma D, Jelsma J, Smits-Engelsman BCM. The efficacy of two task-orientated interventions for children with developmental coordination disorder: neuromotor task training and Nintendo Wii Fit training. *Res Dev Disabil*. 2013;34:2449-2461.

83. Movement Assessment Battery for Children. https://www.pearsonassessments.com/store/usassessments/en/Store/Professional-Assessments/Motor-Sensory/Movement-Assessment-Battery-for-Children-%7C-Second-Edition/p/100000433.html. Accessed on 8/3/2022.

84. Bruininks Ozeretski Test of Motor Proficiency 2. https://www.pearsonassessments.com/store/usassessments/en/Store/Professional-Assessments/Motor-Sensory/Bruininks-Oseretsky-Test-of-Motor-Proficiency-%7C-Second-Edition/p/100000648.html. Accessed on 8/3/2022.

85. Kodak T, Bergmann S. Autism spectrum disorder: characteristics, associated behaviors and early intervention. *Pediatr Clin North Am*. 2020;67:525-535.

86. Rutter M, LeCouteur A, Lord C. ADI-R: Autism Diagnostic Interview-Revised. Western Psychological Services. Los Angeles CA.2003. https://www.wpspublish.com/adi-r-autism-diagnostic-interviewrevised. Accessed on 8/3/2022.

87. Lord C.; Dilavore, PC, Gotham K, et al. *Autism Diagnostic Observation Schedule: ados-2*. Los Angeles, CA: Western Psychological Services; 2012.

88. Genovese A, Butler MG. Clinical assessment, genetics, and treatment approaches in autism spectrum disorder (ASD). *Int J Mol Sci*. 2020;21:4726.

89. Sanchack KE, Thomas CA. Autism spectrum disorder: primary care principles. *Am Fam Physician*. 2016;94(12):972-980.

90. Wright B, Spkins P, Pearson H. Should autism spectrum conditions be characterized in a more positive way in our modern world? *Medicina* 2020;56:233.

91. Sharma SR, Gonda X, tarazi FI. Autism spectrum disorder: classification, diagnosis and therapy. *Pharmacol Ther*. 2018;190:91-104.

92. De Giambattista C, Ventura P, Trerotoli P, Margari M, Palumbi R, Margari L. Subtyping the autism spectrum disorder: comparison of children with high functioning autism and asperger syndrome. *J Autism Dev Dis*. 2019;49:138-150.

93. Sato W, Uono S. The atypical social brain network in autism: advances in structural and functional MRI studies. *Curr Opin Neurol*. 2019.32:617-621.

94. Girault JB, Piven J. The neurodevelopment of autism from infancy through toddlerhood. *Neuroimaging Clin N Am.* 2020;30(1):97-114.

95. Ameis SH, Catani M. Altered white matter connectivity as a neural substrate for social impairment in autism spectrum disorder. *Cortex.* 2015;62:158-181.

96. Keller R, Basta R, Salerno L, Elia M. Autism, epilepsy, and synaptopathies: a not rare association. *Neurol Sci.* 2017;38:1353-1361.

97. Hughes JEA, Ward J, Gruffydd E, et al. Savant syndrome has a distinct psychological profile in autism. *Mol Autism.* 2018;9:53.

98. Nuske HJ, Pellecchia M, Kane C, et al. Self-regulation is bi-directionally associated with cognitive development in children with autism. *J Appl Dev Psychol.* 2020;68:101139.

99. White EN, Ayres KM, Snyder SK, Cagliani RR, Ledford JR. Augmentative and alternative communication and speech production for individuals with ASD: a systematic review. *J Autism Dev Dis.* 2021;51:4199-4212.

100. Mody M, Belliveau JW. Speech and language impairments in autism: insights from behavior and neuroimaging. *N Am J Med Sci.* 2013;5(3):157-161.

101. Venker CE, Bean A, Kover ST. Auditory-visual misalignment: a theoretical perspective on vocabulary delays in children with ASD. *Autism Res.* 2018;11(12):11621-1628.

102. Hilton CL, Zhang Y, Whilte MR, Klohr CL, Constantino J. Motor impairment in sibling pairs concordant and discordant for autism spectrum disorders. *Autism.* 2012;16(4):430-441.

103. Robins DL, Fein D, Barton ML, Green JA. The Modified Checklist for Autism in Toddlers: an initial study investigating the early detection of autism and pervasive developmental disorders. *J Autism Dev Disord.* 2001;31(2):131-144.

104. Schoen SA, Lane SJ, Mailloux Z, et al. A systematic review of Ayres sensory integration intervention for children with autism. *Autism Res.* 2019;12:6-19.

105. Ajzenman HF, Standeven JW, Shurtleff TL. Effect of hippotherapy on motor control, adaptive behaviors, and participation in children with autism spectrum disorder: a pilot study. *Am J Occup Ther.* 2013;67:653-663.

106. Srinivasan SM, Pescatello LS, Bhat AN. Current perspectives on physical activity and exercise recommendations for children and adolescents with autism spectrum disorders. *Phys Ther.* 2014;94:875-889.

107. El Shemy SA, El-Sayed MS. The impact of auditory rhythmic cueing on gross motor skills in children with autism. *J Phys Ther Sci.* 2018;30:1063-1068.

108. Robertson CE, Baron-Cohen S. Sensory perception in autism. *Nat Rev Neurosci.* 2017;18:671-684.

109. Whiteley P, Shattock P, Knivsberg AM, et al. Gluten- and casein-free dietary intervention for autism spectrum conditions. *Front Hum Neurosci.* 2013;6:344.

110. Ristori MV, Quagliariello A, Reddel S, et al. Autism, gastrointestinal symptoms and modulation of gut microbiota by nutritional interventions. *Nutrients.* 2019;11(11):2812.

Review Questions

1. **Global delay is defined as:**

   A. Delay in 1 SD in 3 or more developmental areas

   B. Delay of 1 SD in 2 or more developmental areas

   C. Delay of 2 SD in 3 or more developmental areas

   D. Delay of 2 SD in 2 or more developmental areas

2. **The current definitions of microcephaly and macrocephaly require a head circumference that is:**

   A. SD above/below the mean for age and gender

   B. SD above/below the mean for age and gender

   C. SD above/below the mean for age and gender

   D. SD above/below the mean for age and gender

3. **If both parents are carriers of a recessive genetic trait, they will have**

   A. A 25% chance of having a child with that trait

   B. A 50% chance of having a child with that trait

   C. A 75% chance of having a child with that trait

   D. A 100% chance of having a child with that trait

4. **The most common genetic cause of Down syndrome is?**

   A. Trisomy 21

   B. Mosaic Trisomy 21

   C. Translocation

5. **Which of the following is an X-linked disorder?**

   A. Cri-du-chat

   B. Duchenne Muscular Dystrophy

   C. Niemann–Pick disease

   D. Spinal Muscular Atrophy

6. **Which developmental disorder can be ameliorated through diet?**

   A. Fragile X

   B. Phenylketonuria

   C. Rett syndrome

   D. Trisomy 18

7. **Tay–Sachs is associated with what type of inborn error of metabolism?**

   A. Creatine deficiency

   B. Lysosomal storage

   C. Sterol synthesis

8. **Which of the following correctly describes the intellectual abilities of children with Down syndrome?**

   A. All children with Down syndrome have an intellectual deficit

   B. Most children with Down syndrome have severe intellectual deficits

C. Most children with Down syndrome have only a mild intellectual deficit

D. Most children with Down syndrome have a moderate intellectual deficit

9. **Down syndrome is associated with many dysmorphic features, which of the following correctly describes one of these features?**

A. Hypertonia

B. An eyelid that has an extra fold of skin

C. Longer 5th fingers

D. Multiple palmar creases

10. **Which of the following correctly describes the brain anomalies with Down syndrome?**

A. The brain is larger with deeper sulci

B. Neurogenesis is prolonged in those with Down syndrome

C. The cerebellum is smaller than expected with fewer synapses

D. The dendrites of those with DS have a greater number of dendritic spines

11. **Physical therapy for the child with Down syndrome will commonly include which of the following?**

A. Creation of a quiet environment to prevent overstimulation

B. The use of hip-knee-ankle (HKAFO) orthotics to provide support for gait training

C. Body-weight-supported treadmill training to stimulate independent ambulation

D. Avoidance of resistive exercises to prevent muscle fatigue

12. **For neuromuscular disorders, like Becker Muscular Dystrophy, which of the following treatment methods should be avoided?**

A. Concentric muscle strengthening

B. Eccentric muscle strengthening

C. Isometric muscle strengthening

13. **Developmental coordination disorder is thought to result from focal brain damage to the cerebellum.**

A. True

B. False

14. **Which of the following treatment methods is likely to have the best results for children with developmental coordination disorder?**

A. Balance training

B. Body-weight-supported treadmill training

C. Strength training

D. Task-specific training

15. **A motor delay is a diagnostic criterion for autism spectrum disorder.**

A. True

B. False

16. **Which of the following correctly describes the brain anomaly/anomalies associated with autism?**

A. Mild microcephaly

B. Thicker corpus callosum

C. More synapses

D. Hyperactive amygdala

17. **Which of the following statements about the motor behavior of children with ASD is correct?**

A. Many children with ASD have difficulty with rhythmic or sequential movements

B. Most children with ASD demonstrate typical motor development

C. Toe-walking in ASD is the result of hypertonia of the gastrocnemius

D. Despite many motor impairments, children with ASD excel at ball skills

18. **The sensory deficit(s) associated with ASD are correctly described by which of the following?**

A. Atypical sensory receptor function

B. Delayed sensory nerve conduction

C. Impaired sensory processing

19. **Which of the following correctly describes Sensory Integrative Therapy for ASD?**

A. Passive application of vibration or massage to hypersensitive body areas

B. Wearing a weighted vest to increase body awareness

C. Uses motor tasks with sensory challenges to improve sensory processing

D. Includes auditory stimulation to address communication deficits

20. **Which food products are often limited in the dietary management of children with ASD?**

A. Wheat, rye, barley, and milk products

B. Wheat, rye, barley, and red meat

C. Leafy vegetables and milk products

D. Milk products and red meat

21. **The most common reason for children with Down syndrome to be admitted to the NICU is:**

A. The need for respiratory support

B. The development of periventricular leukomalacia

C. To address orthopedic anomalies

D. To address feeding issues due to hypotonia

22. **Accelerated aging is associated with which developmental disorder?**
    A. Autism
    B. Developmental coordination disorder
    C. Down syndrome
    D. Phenylketonuria

23. **The NMD associated with an absence of dystrophin is:**
    A. Becker muscular dystrophy
    B. Congenital myopathy
    C. Duchenne muscular dystrophy
    D. Spinal muscular atrophy, type I

24. **Children with SMA Type II typically develop which motor milestone(s)?**
    A. Sitting
    B. Sitting and standing
    C. Sitting, standing, and walking
    D. None of these

25. **Which assessment is best used to document function in children with NMDs?**
    A. Bayley Scales of Motor Development
    B. Bruininks Oseretski Test of Motor Proficiency 2
    C. Hammersmith Functional Motor Scale Expanded
    D. Movement Assessment Battery for Children

26. **Screening for autism is recommended at what age?**
    A. 6-12 months of age
    B. 12-18 months of age
    C. 18-24 months of age
    D. 24-30 months of age

27. **Autism is most likely caused by:**
    A. Genetic mutation(s)
    B. Genetic mutation(s) in association with environmental influences
    C. Childhood vaccinations
    D. Environmental and dietary influences

28. **An adult with ASD is able to live on his own with assistance to pay his bills, maintain his daily schedule, and purchase groceries and other household needs. He would most likely be diagnosed at what level of ASD severity?**
    A. Level 1, high functioning
    B. Level 2, high functioning
    C. Level 3, high functioning

29. **A child presents with inattention, impulsivity, and heightened activity but typical language and motor skill development; this child is most likely diagnosed with:**
    A. Autims
    B. ADHD
    C. DCD
    D. SMA Type IV

30. **Which of the following conditions is associated with normal brain development?**
    A. Autism
    B. Developmental coordination disorder
    C. Down syndrome
    D. Muscular Dystrophies

Answers

1. D	**2.** C	**3.** A	**4.** A	**5.** B
6. B	**7.** B	**8.** D	**9.** B	**10.** C
11. C	**12.** B	**13.** B	**14.** D	**15.** B
16. C	**17.** A	**18.** C	**19.** C	**20.** A
21. A	**22.** C	**23.** C	**24.** A	**25.** C
26. C	**27.** B	**28.** A	**29.** B	**30.** D

GLOSSARY

Accelerated aging. Abnormal aging of body systems that occurs at a younger age than expected.

Acquired genetic mutation. Genetic defect that results from duplication, deletion, or translocation of part of a DNA strand.

Applied Behavioral Analysis. An individualized program of treatment to encourage positive behaviors and discourage negative behaviors in children with autism.

Asberger's syndrome. Formerly a mild form of autism now classified as level one high functioning.

Attention deficit hyperactivity disorder. DD associated with poor attention, impulsivity, and heightened activity.

Autism Diagnostic Interview Revised. Standardized parental interview to diagnose autism.

Autism Diagnostic Observation Schedule 2. Standardized observation assessment to diagnose autism.

Autism spectrum disorder. A neurodevelopmental disorder that manifests with impairments in language, social-emotional function, communication, and restrictive/repetitive behaviors.

Bayley Scales of Infant and Toddler Development. Fine and gross motor assessment for children under 42 months.

Becker muscular dystrophy. A milder form of muscular dystrophy that results from partial loss of dystrophin.

Bruininks Oseretski Test of Motor Proficiency 2. Assessment of motor skills, coordination, and balance, appropriate for children with DCD or other DD, ages 4 to 21.

Children's Hospital of Philadelphia Test of Infant Motor Performance. Assessment to document SMA I function.

Congenital. A condition present at birth.

Congenital myopathy. DDs associated with a protein deficit in the contractile elements of muscle.

Developmental coordination disorder. A disorder of fine and gross motor dyscoordination.

Developmental disability/disorder. A condition that occurs during the developmental period (birth to age 22) and disrupts the achievement of developmental milestones.

Down syndrome. A DD associated with an acquired genetic mutation of either three 21st chromosomes or translocation of the 21st chromosome to another site.

Dysmorphic features. Asymmetry or abnormality of a body structure.

Dystrophin. The protein missing in Duchenne and Becker muscular dystrophy.

Echolalia. Word repetition without the intent to communicate.

Hammersmith Functional Motor Scale Expanded. An assessment to document function in children with SMA Types 2 and 3 or other NMD.

Inherited mutation. A genetic defect that is inherited from one or both parents.

Macrocephaly. Head circumference larger than 3 SD above gender and age mean.

Microcephaly. Head circumference smaller than 3 SD below gender and age mean.

Modified Checklist for Autism in Toddlers. A checklist that documents behaviors and features of autism.

Movement Assessment Battery for Children. Evaluation for children with DCD.

Muscular dystrophies. A progressive degeneration of muscle due to a disturbance of proteins in the extracellular matrix or sarcolemmal membrane of muscle.

North Star Ambulatory Assessment. Assessment used with children with muscular dystrophy.

Nuchal translucency. Fluid buildup in the cervical spine between the spine and the skin that is increased in children with Down syndrome.

Peabody Scales of Motor Development. Fine and gross motor assessment for children from birth to 5 years.

Perinatal. At the time of birth.

Postnatal. After birth.

Prenatal. Before birth.

Sensory integration disorder. A sensory processing disorder and part of the diagnosis for autism.

Spinal muscular atrophy. Autosomal recessive disorder that results in loss of alpha motor neurons.

Trisomy 21. Three 21 chromosomes, associated with Down syndrome.

ABBREVIATIONS

AAC	augmentative and assistive communication
ABA	Applied Behavioral Analysis
ADHD	attention deficit hyperactivity disorder
ADI-R	Autism Diagnostic Interview Revised
ADOS-2	Autism Diagnostic Observation Schedule 2
BOT 2	Bruininks Oseretsky Test of Motor Proficiency 2
BSITD	Bayley Scales of Infant and Toddler Development
CHOP INTEND	Children's Hospital of Philadelphia Test of Infant Motor Performance
CMA	chromosomal microarray
DCD	developmental coordination disorder
DS	Down syndrome
EEG	electroencephalography
HFMSE	Hammersmith Functional Motor Scale Expanded
ID	intellectual disability
IDD	intellectual developmental disability
M-CHAT	Modified Checklist for Autism in Toddlers
NMDs	neuromuscular degenerative disorders
NSAA	North Star Ambulatory Assessment
PDMS	Peabody Developmental Motor Scales
SID	sensory integration disorder
SMA	spinal muscular atrophy
SMN	survival motor neuron protein
SMN1	gene on chromosome 5 that is necessry for the survival of SMN and is mutated in SMA

Appendix
Adult Outcome Measures by ICF Category and Diagnostic Group

	BODY STRUCTURE AND FUNCTION	ACTIVITY	PARTICIPATION
CVA	**Ashworth** Chedoke-McMaster Stroke Assessment Dynamometry Fugl-Meyer Assessment of Motor Performance NIH Stroke Scale Orpington Prognostic Scale Postural Assessment Scale for Stroke Patients Rivermead Motor Assessment Tardieu Spasticity Scale (Modified Tardieu)	**10 Meter Walk Test** (10MWT) **5 times sit to stand** **6 Minute Walk Test** (6MWT) 9 Hole Peg Test Action Research Arm Test (ARAT) **Activities-specific Balance Confidence Scale (ABC Scale)** Arm Motor Ability Test **Berg Balance Scale** (BBS) **Functional Gait Assessment** (FGA) (Dynamic Gait Index – Revised) Functional Ambulation Categories Functional Independence Measure (FIM) Functional Reach Motor Activity Log Timed Up and Go (TUG) Test Trunk Impairment Scale Wolf Motor Function Test	Assessment of Life Habits EuroQoL Falls Efficacy Scale (FES) Goal Attainment Scale Modified Rankin Scale Stroke Adapted SIP-30 Stroke Impact Scale Stroke Rehabilitation Assessment of Movement MS Impact Scale (MSIS-29)
MS	Box and Blocks Test Disease Steps Dizziness Handicap Inventory Fatigue Scale for Motor and Cognitive Functions Functional Assessment of MS FIM Guy's Neurological Disability Scale Maximal Inspiratory and Expiratory Pressure Rivermead Mobility Index MS Functional Composite	12-Item MS Walking Scale **6MWT** 9-Hole Peg Test **ABC Scale** **BBS** **FGA** (Dynamic Gait Index – Revised) Four Square Step Test Functional Assessment of MS FIM Functional Reach Hauser Ambulation Index Modified Fatigue Impact Scale MS Functional Composite Timed 25 Foot Walk TUG with Cognitive and Manual Trunk Impairment Scale Visual Analog Scale (fatigue) VO_2 max and VO_2 peak	FIM Goal Attainment Scale Guy's Neurological Disability Scale Medical Outcome Study (SF-36) Short Form Health Survey of Medical outcome study (SF-36) Functional Assessment of MS MS Functional Composite MS International Quality of Life Questionnaire MS Quality of Life (MS-QoL 54) MS Quality of Life Inventory

(Continued)

	BODY STRUCTURE AND FUNCTION	ACTIVITY	PARTICIPATION
TBI	Agitated Behavior Scale Apathy Evaluation Scale Ashworth Scale (Modified) Cog-Log and O(rientation)-Log Coma Recovery Scale-Revised Disorders of Consciousness Scale Dizziness Handicap Inventory Global Fatigue Index Moss Attention Rating Scale Patient Health Questionnaire Rancho Levels of Cognitive Function	12-Item MS Walking Scale **6MWT** Cognitive Functions Action Research Arm Test Balance Error Scoring Scale Barthel Index **BBS** Community Balance and Mobility Scale FIM Functional Assessment Measure High Level Mobility Assessment	Disability Rating Scale Sydney Psychosocial Reintegration Scale Quality of life after brain injury
SCI	Ashworth Scale (Modified) Bryce–Ragnarsson Pain Taxonomy Classification for Chronic Pain in SCI Donovan SCI Pain Classification Grasp and Release Test (GRT) Hand Held Myometry/ Myometry International Spinal Cord Injury Pain Classification (ISCIP) International Standards for Multidimensional Pain Inventory – SCI version Neurological Classification of Penn Spasm Frequency Scale, Spinal Cord Injury, ASIA Impairment Scale (AIS) Numeric Pain Rating Scale 6-Minute Arm Test (6-MAT) Spastic Reflexes (SCATS) Spinal Cord Assessment Tool for Spinal Cord Injury Spasticity Evaluation Tool (SCI-SET) Tardieu Scale, Modified Tardieu Scale Wheelchair Users Shoulder Pain Index (WUSPI)	**10MWT** **6MWT** ARAT **ABC Scale** Balance Evaluations Systems Test (BESTest) **BBS** Capabilities of UE Functioning Instrument (CUE) FES **FGA** (Dynamic Gait Index – Revised) FIM Functional Reach Test (FRT)/Modified Graded and Redefined Assessment of Sensibility Strength and Prehension (GRASSP) High Level Mobility and Assessment Tool (HiMAT) Jebsen–Taylor Hand Function Test TUG Test Toronto Rehabilitation Institute Hand Function Test Wheelchair Skills Test Functional Tests for Persons who Self Propel a Manual Wheelchair (4FTPSMW) Quadriplegia Index of Function (QIF) and short form	Craig Handicap Assessment and Reporting Technique (CHART) Craig Hospital Inventory of Environmental Factors (CHIEF) Impact on Participation and Autonomy Questionnaire (IPA) Life Satisfaction Questionnaire (LISAT-9) Needs Assessment Checklist (NAC) Quality of Well Being Short Form 36 (SF-36) Sickness Impact Profile 68 (SIP 68) Participation Assessment with Physical Activity Recall Assessment for People with Spinal Cord Injury (PARA-SCI) Quality of Life Index, Spinal Cord Version (QLI-SCI, Ferrans and Powers) Recombined Tools-Objective (PART-O) Reintegration to Normal Living Index (RNL) Satisfaction with Life Scale (SWLS, Deiner Scale) Spinal Cord Injury Lifestyle Scale (SCILS) World Health Organization Quality of Life-BREF (WHOQOL-BREF)
PD	Montreal Cognitive Assessment MDS UPDRS Parkinson's Fatigue Scale	**10MWT** **5 times sit to stand** **6MWT** 9-Hole Peg Test **ABC Scale** **FGA** (Dynamic Gait Index – Revised) Mini BESTest MDS UPDRS TUG Cognitive Freezing of Gait Questionnaire	Parkinson's Disease Quality of Life 39 or 8 item (PDQ-8 or PDQ-39)

(Continued)

	BODY STRUCTURE AND FUNCTION	ACTIVITY	PARTICIPATION
Vestibular	Dix–Hallpike Dynamic Visual Acuity (Instrumented) Dynamic Visual Acuity (Non-Instrumented) Head Impulse Test Modified Clinical Test of Sensory Interaction on Balance (mCTSIB) Romberg Sensory Organization Test (NeuroCom) Sharpened Romberg Vertigo Symptom Scale (VSS) Visual Analogue Scale (VAS) Visual Vertigo Analogue Scale (VVAS)	**ABC Scale** Balance Evaluation Systems Test (BEST) **BBS** Four Square Step Test **FGA** (Dynamic Gait Index – Revised) Mini Balance Evaluation Systems Test (Mini BEST) TUG Test	Dizziness Handicap Inventory
Motor Neuron Disease	ALS Depression Inventory 12 Ashworth Scale (Modified) Beck Depression Inventory Hospital Anxiety and Depression Scale Verbal fluency VASVAS Maximal Inspiratory and Expiratory Pressure Fatigue Severity Scale (FSS)	**10MWT** 9-Hole Peg Test **BBS** Functional Reach Test FIM Performance Oriented Mobility Assessment (POMA) TUG Test	Schedule for Evaluation of Individual Quality of Life-Direct Weighting Sickness Impact Profile Short Form-36
ALS		ALS Functional Rating Scale-Revised Appel ALS Scale ALS Severity Scale Norris Scale	ALS Assessment Questionnaire 40 (ALSAQ-40; ALSAQ-5) ALS-Specific QOL Instrument
GBS		Inflammatory Neuropathy Cause and Treatment group ODSS, modified GBS Disability Scale, modified Rankin Scale	
Developmental Disorders in Children	Bayley Scales of Infant and Toddler Development (1 month–42 months) Peabody Developmental Motor Scales (PDMS) (birth–6 years) Gross Motor Function Measure (GMFM) (5 months–16 years with CP)	Bayley Scales of Infant and Toddler Development (1 month–42 months) PDMS (birth–5 years) GMFM (5 months–16 years with CP) Pediatric Evaluation of Disability Inventory (PEDI) (birth–20 years)	Caregiver Priority and Child Health Index of Life with Disabilities (1–13 years old) Child Health and Illness Profile (11–17 years old) Child Health Questionnaire (5–18 years old) School Function Assessment (SFA) (K–6th grade)

Bolded measures are key measures to use in the neurologic population as they are the Core Measures recommended by Academy of Neurologic Physical Therapy (ANPT) and the EDGE task force groups.

Details on the ANPT's EDGE task force recommendations can be found at: http://www.neuropt.org/professional-resources/neurology-section-outcome-measures-recommendations

Detailed reviews of outcome measures cited here and others commonly used in therapy practice are available through RehabMeasures.org and include links to the actual instruments when available. Current website page address: http://www.rehabmeasures.org

Index

A

AAC (augmentative and assistive communication), 658
AALS (Appel ALS Scale), 462
ABA (Applied Behavioral Analysis), 658
Abarognosis, 187t
Abasia, 136b, 139f
Abducens nerve, 16, 186t
Abduction device/orthosis, 631
Abnormal neurogenesis, 293
ABR (auditory brainstem response), 105
Absence seizures, 623t
Absolute refractory period (ARP), 27, 27f
Abstract thought, 120
ACC (anterior cingulate cortex), 120f, 121
Accelerated aging, 652
Accessory cuneate nucleus (ACN), 54, 86
Accessory nerve, 186t
Accommodation, 94b
ACN (accessory cuneate nucleus), 54, 86
Acoustic neuroma, 514f, 514–515
Acquired dyslexia or alexia, 223
Action potential
  illustration of, 27f
  overview of, 26–28
  propagation of, 28, 29f
Action tremors, 541
Active forgetting, 124
Activities of daily living, 470
Activities-Specific Balance Confidence Scale (ABC Scale), 190, 522
Activity and participation, in neurologic exams, 190–191
Activity level assessments
  in amyotrophic lateral sclerosis, 460t, 461–462
  in Guillain–Barré syndrome, 478t
Acute anterior poliomyelitis, 481
Acute care facility
  bed exercises, 227t
  spinal cord injury, physical therapy for, 321–324
  stroke, physical therapy for, 226–235
Acute inflammatory demyelinating polyradiculoneuropathy (AIDP), 473
Acute respiratory distress syndrome (ARDS), 272
Adam's forward bend test, 594, 594f

Adaptive plasticity, 167–168, 168b
Adaptive seating systems, for cerebral palsy, 630–632
Adductor contractures, 620t
ADHD (attention deficit hyperactivity disorder), 655, 655b
ADI-12 (ALS Depression Inventory 12), 460
ADI-R (Autism Diagnostic Interview-Revised), 656
Adolescents, 153
ADOS-2 (Autism Diagnostic Observation Schedule-2), 656
Adult neurogenesis, 162
Adult outcome measures, 667–669
Advanced motor skill development, 204
Affect/mood, 182t
Afferent drive, 66
AFO (ankle-foot orthotics)
  articulating, 630
  for cerebral palsy, 630, 630f
  non-articulating, 630
  for stroke, 244–246, 245b–246b, 599t
Age-related neurologic changes
  brain changes, 557–559, 558t
  cognitive function, 561–562
  dementia, 562–573
  typical neuromuscular change with aging, 557–561
Aging
  accelerated, 652
  with Down syndrome, 652–653
  learning and, 561–562
  motor function and, 560
  negative plasticity as model of, 560t, 560–561
  teaching and, 561–562
Aging anorexia, 561b
Agitation, 278t, 283–285, 284t
Agraphia/dysgraphia, 223
AICA (anterior inferior cerebellar artery), 213, 219t
AIDP (acute inflammatory demyelinating polyradiculoneuropathy), 473
AIMS, 200
AIS (ASIA Impairment Scale), 305–306
Akathisia, 405
Akinesia, 402
AL (anterolateral system), 51–53

Alemtuzumab, 374t
Alexia, 223
Alexithymia, 121
Allocentric neglect, 221
Allodynia, 45, 187t, 339, 366
Allografts, 488
Alpha-synuclein, 528
ALS. See Amyotrophic Lateral Sclerosis (ALS)
ALS Depression Inventory 12 (ADI-12), 460
ALS Functional Rating Scale (ALSFRS), 455, 462
ALS Severity Scale (ALSSS), 462
ALSA (Amyotrophic Lateral Sclerosis Association), 457
ALS-Plus syndromes, 456
Alzheimer's disease (AD), 566–567, 653
Amacrine cellular networks, 95
Amantadine, 408t, 409
Ambulation
  in cerebral palsy patients, 632, 632f
  devices for, 632, 632f
  in myelomeningocele patients, 596–597, 597t
Amnesia, 268, 272b
Ampulla, 107, 107f
Amygdala, 6t, 11f, 12, 126
Amyloid plaques, 566
Amyotrophic lateral sclerosis (ALS)
  activity level assessments, 460t, 461–462
  adult outcome measures, 669
  clinical presentation of, 454–455
  cognitive dysfunction associated with, 459–460
  controlled exercise studies, 464t
  diagnosis of, 455–456
  El Escorial criteria for, 455t
  epidemiology of, 452–453
  fatigue associated with, 461
  general exercise guidelines, 467
  goal setting and exercise prescription, 462–464
  impairment, activity, and participation assessments, 460t
  intervention strategies for, 465t
  medical management, 457
  medical prognosis, 456–459
  muscle biopsies, 456f

Amyotrophic lateral sclerosis (ALS) (*cont.*)
  pathophysiology, 453f, 453–454
  physical therapy for, 459–462, 464, 467
  prognostic factors, 457t
  progression of, 454–455
  risk factors for, 452–453
  stages of, 465t
  symptomatic treatment of, 457–458t
  variants of, 455–456, 456t
Amyotrophic Lateral Sclerosis Association (ALSA), 457
Anal sphincter, 318f
Analgesia, 187t
Anencephaly, 581–582
Angelman syndrome, 645t
Angiogenesis, 163, 226, 573
Angular acceleration, 105, 106–108
Anisotropic diffusion, 168
Ankle strategy, 530
Ankle-foot orthotics (AFO)
  articulating, 630
  for cerebral palsy, 630, 630f
  non-articulating, 630
  for stroke, 244–246, 245b–246b, 599t
Annulospiral endings, 46
Anomalous trichromatic deficit, 99
Anosmia, 405
Anoxia, 268
Anteflexion, 133
Anterior cerebral arteries, 212, 217t
Anterior cingulate cortex (ACC), 120f, 121
Anterior commissure, 10f, 12
Anterior communicating artery, 213
Anterior inferior cerebellar artery (AICA), 213, 219t
Anterior limb of internal capsule, 12
Anterior lobe, 13
Anterior plane, 3, 4f
Anterior semicircular canal, 107f
Anterior spinal cord syndrome, 307, 307f
Anterior-tilted chair, 631, 631f
Anterograde amnesia, 123, 272b
Anterograde axonal transport, 28
Anterograde degeneration, 163, 267
Anterograde tracing, 31b
Anterograde transneuronal degeneration, 164
Anterolateral system (AL), 51–53
Anteropulsive, 402
Anthropometrics, 197
Anticipatory balance control, 538b
Anticipatory postural adjustments (APAs), 530
Antidromic volley, 449
Antiepileptic medications, 340, 625t
Anxiety, 290, 422
Anxious/ambivalent infants, 147b
APAs (anticipatory postural adjustments), 530
Apathy, 280t, 422
APGAR, 614b
Aphasia, 126–128, 222

Apogeotropic, 525
Apoptosis, 164–165
Apparent equinus, 621
Appel ALS Scale (AALS), 462
Applied Behavioral Analysis (ABA), 658
Apraxia, 216, 421
APTA (EDGE) Task Force, 322
Aquatic therapy, 629
Aqueous humor, 93
Arachnoid mater, 9, 9f
Arachnoid villi, 13
ARDS (acute respiratory distress syndrome), 272
Areflexia, 305
Arnold–Chiari malformation (A–CM), 579f, 586–587, 587f, 591
Arrhythmia, 309
Articulating ankle-foot orthotics, 630
Ascending sensory systems
  anterolateral system, 51–53
  dorsal-column-medial lemniscal pathway, 51
  spinocerebellar systems, 53–54
Ascending somatosensory pathways, 52f
ASD. See Autism spectrum disorder (ASD)
Ashworth Scale, 235
ASIA Impairment Scale (AIS), 305–306
ASIA Motor scores, 323t, 325t, 338t
Asperger's syndrome, 656
Assessment
  amyotrophic lateral sclerosis, 460t
  balance, 525–531, 529t
  basilar artery aneurysm, 251–252
  cognitive function, 277t
  coordination impairments, 189t
  movement impairments, 189t
  outpatient rehabilitation, 345
  peripheral neuropathies, 490–491
  sensory impairments, 187t
  spinal cord injury, 322–323
  stroke, 227–228
  vestibular disorders, 518–520
Assistance, levels of, 192t
Assisted gait, 417f
Assistive devices
  in cerebral palsy, 630–633
  in Parkinson's disease, 416–417, 417f
  in stroke, 240
Associative loop, 396b
Astasia, 136b, 139f
Astereognosis, 187t
Astrocytes, 34f, 34–35
Asymmetrical tonic neck reflex (ATNR), 135, 136t, 138f, 198t, 618
Ataxia, 376, 380–381, 540
Ataxic cerebral palsy, 617b
Ataxic dysarthria, 128, 543
Atelectasis, 315
Atherosclerosis (ATS), 568b
Athetosis, 617b
Atlas vertebra, 651
ATNR (asymmetrical tonic neck reflex), 135, 136t, 138f, 198t, 618

Atonic cerebral palsy, 617b–618b
Atonic seizures, 623t
Atopognosia, 187t
Attachment, 147b
Attention, 119b, 182t
Attention deficit hyperactivity disorder (ADHD), 655, 655b, 657
Auditory apparatus of the cochlea, 104f
Auditory brainstem response (ABR), 105
Auditory cueing, 416
Auditory evoked responses, 364
Auditory projections, 105f
Auditory system
  central processing of hearing, 103–104
  ear's organization and auditory apparatus, 103
  sound localization, 104
  testing of, 104–105
Auditory testing, 104–105
Augmentative and assistive communication (AAC), 658
Auricle, 103
Autism Diagnostic Interview-Revised (ADI-R), 656
Autism Diagnostic Observation Schedule-2 (ADOS-2), 656
Autism spectrum disorder (ASD)
  brain differences in, 656–657
  clinical features of, 657b
  cognitive function in, 657–658
  definition of, 656
  delayed language in, 658
  developmental differences in, 657–659
  epilepsy in, 657
  gastrointestinal dysfunction in, 659
  genetic factors, 656
  gluten-free diet for, 659
  intelligence in, 657
  language development in, 658
  motor development in, 658–659
  pharmacological treatment of, 659
  sensory differences in, 659, 659b
  sensory therapies for, 659b
  socio-emotional development in, 658
Autogenic inhibition reflex, 48
Autografts, 488
Autoimmune process of myelin damage, 363f
Autonomic dysfunction
  in Guillain–Barré syndrome, 477
  in multiple sclerosis, 371–372
  in Parkinson's disease, 403t, 403–404
  in spinal cord injury, 309
Autonomic dysreflexia, 309, 310f, 310t
Autonomic nervous system, 19
Autonomic neuropathy, 491, 493
Autophagy, 165
Avoidant infants, 147b
Awakenings (Sacks), 394
Axis vertebra, 651
Axon, 28
Axon hillock, 25, 26, 26f, 29f
Axon terminal, 26

Axonal transport, 267
Axonotmesis, 484

B
Babbling, 147
Babinski reflex/sign, 138f, 181b, 305, 586t
Backwards Release, 530
Baclofen, intrathecal, 625
Balance
    in amyotrophic lateral sclerosis, 461
    assessment of, 525–531, 529t
    in cerebellar disorders, 542, 544–545
    exercises, 380b
    in functional activities, 538b
    in multiple sclerosis, 370
    neurologic exam, 189
    in Parkinson's disease, 411, 415
Balance control, 112–113
Ballismus, 421, 617b
Bar-B-Que Roll maneuver, 534f
Barlow sign, 593
Basal ganglia
    disorders of. *See* Huntington's disease;
        Parkinson's disease
    emotion, 126
    function of, 5t, 85–86
    illustration of, 8f
    loops of, 85f, 396b
    overview of, 11–12
Basilar artery
    aneurysm of, 251–252
    description of, 213
    stroke-related symptoms of, 218t–219t
Bayley Scales of Infant and Toddler
        Development (BSITD), 200, 649
BBS (Berg Balance Scale), 189
BDNF (brain-derived neurotrophic factor),
        162, 572
Becker muscular dystrophy (BMD), 645t,
        653
Bed exercises, 227t
Bed mobility training, 231, 233t, 332t
Bed positioning, 230t
Beevor sign, 305
Behavioral audiometry, 104
Behavioral development, 154
Behavioral dyscontrol, 275
Behavioral dysfunction, 371, 376
Behavioral management techniques, 570b
Behavioral or self-regulation, 120
Behavioral self-management, 340
Bello-Haas, Dal, 464
Benign paroxysmal positional vertigo
        (BPPV), 515, 526t, 532–535
Berg Balance Scale (BBS), 189
BEST test, 189
Beta motor neurons, 47
Bilateral training, 236
Bilateral vestibular hypofunction (BVH),
        515, 539
Bi-level positive airway pressure (BiPAP),
        459
Bimanual hand-arm therapy, 629

Binocular visual field, 95f
Biofeedback, 629
Bipolar cells, 95, 100
Bladder dysfunction
    in multiple sclerosis, 372, 372t, 376–377
    in spinal cord injury, 311–313, 312f
Bladder management, in myelomeningocele,
        600b
Blind spot, 95
Blood vessels, of brain, 214f
Blood-oxygen-level-dependent (BOLD)
        signal, 169
BMD (Becker muscular dystrophy), 645t,
        653
Body mechanics, 462
Body-on-body reaction, 146f, 200f
Body structure and function
    balance, 189
    cerebellar disorders, 544
    communication, 183
    coordination and balance, 187–189
    cranial nerves, 185
    Huntington's disease, 429–430
    mental status examination, 181–183, 182t,
        183b
    motor examination, 183–185
    Parkinson's disease, 410–413
    sensory examination, 185–187
Body-weight support, 342
Body-weight supported treadmill training
        (BWSTT), 628, 652
BOLD (blood-oxygen-level-dependent)
        signal, 169
Bone conduction, 104
Bony labyrinth, 103, 105
Borg Exertion Scale, 229
BOT-2 (Bruininks Oseretsky Test of Motor
        Proficiency 2), 656
Botulinum toxin (Botox), 241, 313b, 625
Bowel dysfunction, 319t, 372, 372t, 376–377
Bowel management
    in myelomeningocele, 600b
    in spinal cord injury, 319t, 320–321
BPPV (benign paroxysmal positional
        vertigo), 515, 526t, 532–535
Brachial plexus injuries, 494–497, 495f, 614
Brachial plexus palsy, 495–497, 585
Bradycardia, 309
Bradykinesia, 86, 189t, 397, 399, 411
Bradyphrenia, 404
Brain
    acute neuroplasticity post-stroke, 226
    age-related changes in, 557–559, 558t
    blood vessels of, 214f
    cerebellum, 13–14
    cranial nerves, 15f, 16–17, 185, 186t
    in Down syndrome, 651
    gray and white matter, 4f
    lobes of, 9–11, 10f
    myelomeningocele-related abnormalities
        of, 586–590
    parts of, 4f, 8f, 8–9

spina bifida-related abnormalities of,
        586–590
    subcortical structures, 5t, 11–12
    ventricular system, 12–13, 587b, 588f
Brain-derived neurotrophic factor (BDNF),
        162, 572
Brain development
    description of, 135
    negative influences on, 153–154
    positive influences on, 154
Brain shifts, 273f
Brain tumor
    diagnosis, 293
    medical treatments of, 294
    pathogenesis of, 293–294
    physical therapy management of patient
        with, 294–295
    primary, 291–293
    symptoms, 293
Brainstem
    anatomy of, 4f, 8f, 14–17
    functions of, 6t
    herniation of, 273
Brainstem circulation, and stroke
        syndromes, 220f
Brainstem stroke, 250–251
Braintree Scale of Neurologic Stages of
        Recovery from Brain Injury, 269,
        270t–271t
Brandt–Daroff exercises, 532, 533f
Broca's area, 126f, 127, 223
Brown-Sequard injury, 306f, 306–307
Bruininks Oseretsky Test of Motor
        Proficiency 2 (BOT-2), 656
BSITD (Bayley Scales of Infant and Toddler
        Development), 200, 649
Bunge, Richard, 306
BVH (bilateral vestibular hypofunction),
        515, 539
BWSTT (body-weight supported treadmill
        training), 628, 652

C
C1, 651
C2, 651
CAA (cerebral amyloid angiopathy), 567,
        568b
Calcarine sulcus, 10f
Caloric test, 112
Camptocormia, 400
Canalithiasis, 515
Cannabinoids, for neuropathic pain, 340
Carbamazepine, 625t
Carbidopa, 408t
Cardiovascular deconditioning, 346
Cardiovascular disease (CVD), 346
Cardiovascular dysautonomia, 371–372
Cardiovascular function, 423
Cardiovascular/pulmonary system review,
        196
Carotid artery system, 212
Casani maneuver, 534f
Caspases, 164

Catabolism, 559b
Cataracts, 561b
Catechol-O-methyl transferase (COMT) inhibitors, 408t
Cauda equina syndrome, 308, 308f
Caudal direction, 3, 4f
Caudate nucleus, 6t, 11, 11f
Cawthorne habituation exercises, 536b–537b
CDP (computerized dynamic posturography), 519–520
Cell proliferation, 159f, 160
Cellular signaling, 25
Central cord syndrome, 304, 307, 307f
Central nervous system
    anatomy of, 159f
    injury to, 165–168
Central pattern generation circuits, 83
Central pattern generator (CPG), 69f, 69–71, 345
Central processing
    of hearing, 103–104
    of taste, 101
Central sulcus, 5t, 10, 10f
Central vestibular disorders, 516–517, 517, 531t, 539
Cephalic flexure, 580b, 581f
Cephalocaudal, 138
Cephalo-pelvic incompatibility, 614
Cerebellar ataxia, 545t
Cerebellar circuits, 87f
Cerebellar cortex, 5, 6t, 13
Cerebellar disorders
    anatomy and physiology of, 540
    balance, 542, 544–545
    body structure and function, 544
    cerebellar damage, 540t
    clinical presentation of, 540–543
    cognitive dysfunction in, 543
    medical management of, 543
    physical therapy examination, 543–544
    physical therapy treatment, 544–546
    signs and symptoms of, 541t
Cerebellar peduncles, 7t, 14, 14f
Cerebellar tentorium, 9
Cerebellopontine angle cistern, 13
Cerebellum
    function of, 6t, 85–88, 651
    images of, 14f
    lobes/regions of, 13–14
    overview of, 5
Cerebral amyloid angiopathy (CAA), 567, 568b
Cerebral aqueduct, 5t, 12
Cerebral artery, 212f, 215f
Cerebral circulation, 212–216
Cerebral cortex, 5, 8f, 11f
Cerebral hemispheres, 5, 8f, 223f
Cerebral palsy (CP)
    abduction device/orthosis for, 631
    adaptive seating systems for, 630–632
    ambulation devices for, 632, 632f
    anterior-tilted chair for, 631, 631f
    aquatic therapy for, 629

assistive technology for, 630–633
ataxic, 617b
atonic, 617b–618b
biofeedback for, 629
classification of, 615–616
communication devices for, 633
communication disorders in, 624
constraint-induced movement therapy for, 629
crawling/creeping movements in, 619
crouched gait in, 621, 621f
definition of, 611
diagnosis of, 615–616
dyskinetic, 617b
environmental control systems in, 633
epilepsy associated with, 622–624, 623t
etiology of, 611–614
evidence-based treatment approaches for, 628–629
fidgety movements associated with, 615
forearm crutches for, 632
functional classification of, 615–616
functional impairment in, 616
gait in, 621, 621f, 628
gaming for, 629
general movement analysis in, 615
goals-activity-motor enrichment for, 628
Gross Motor Function Classification System, 615, 616b
head control in, 618
head lag in, 618f
hearing impairment in, 624
hippotherapy for, 629
hypotonic, 617b–618b
intellectual developmental disability associated with, 622–624, 623t
language disorders in, 624
medical management of, 624–627
mobility devices for, 630
motor patterns in, 618–622
muscle tone abnormalities associated with, 627–628
nutritional management of, 625–627
oropharyngeal dysphagia in, 626
orthopedic conditions associated with, 620t, 622, 625–626
orthotics for, 630, 630f
pathophysiology of, 611
physical therapy management of, 627–633
positioning devices for, 633
posterior tilt chair for, 631, 631f
postnatal causes of, 614
prenatal causes of, 613–614
risk factors for, 614
robotic-assisted therapy for, 628–629
seizures associated with, 623t, 623–624, 625t
sensory dysfunction associated with, 624
sitting in, 619
spastic, 617b, 626
spasticity in, 621, 625
standers for, 633
standing in, 619, 621

strengthening techniques in, 628
three-point lateral control system for, 631
treadmill training for, 628
types of, 616, 617b–618b
typography of, 616, 617f
upper extremity function in, 622
vestibular disorders in, 624
visual impairment in, 624
walking in, 619, 621
wheelchairs for, 630–632, 632f
writhing movements associated with, 615
Cerebral peduncles, 7t, 15
Cerebrocerebellum, 13–14, 14f, 86
Cerebrospinal fluid (CSF)
    analysis of, 364
    circulation of, 589f
    functions of, 587b
    production of, 589f
Cerebrovascular accident. See Stroke
Cerebrum, 4f, 5t, 8f
Cervical flexure, 580b, 581f
Cervical spine, 63
Cervical VEMP (cVEMP), 519
Cervical weakness, 469
Cervicogenic dizziness, 518
Charcot–Marie–Tooth disease, 645t
Chemokines, 36
Child development. See also Infant development
    in 0 to 3 months, 135–142
    in 3 to 6 months, 143–144
    in 6 to 9 months, 145
    in 9 to 12 months, 146–148
    in 2nd year of life, 148–150
    adolescents, 153
    critical periods of, 135, 135b
    domains of, 133
    in fetal stage, 133–134
    language development, 142–143
    in middle childhood, 152–153
    oral motor development, 134, 142–143
    parachute response, 143, 146f, 200f
    preschoolers, 150–152
    sensitive periods of, 134, 135b
    sensory development, 134, 142–143
Children's Hospital of Philadelphia (CHOP), 654
CHOP-INTEND, 654
Chorea, 408, 421, 427, 617b
Choreoathetosis, 408, 617b
Choroid plexus, 5t, 12
Chromosomal microarray (CMA), 644
Chronic inflammatory demyelinating polyradiculopathy (CIDP), 490
Chronic traumatic encephalopathy, 291
CIMT (constraint-induced movement therapy), 243, 629
Cingulate cortex, 10–11
Cingulate gyrus, 10f
Cingulate sulcus, 5t, 10f
Circle of Willis, 213, 214f, 249
Circuit training, 242–243

Circumducted/circumduction gait pattern, 240b
Cisterna magna, 13
Clarke's column, 86
Clarke's nucleus, 53
Climbing fiber, 87
Clinical electromyography (EMG), 445, 449–451
Clonus, 305
Closed head injuries, 265
Closed-loop cueing, 416
Club foot, 591–592, 592b, 592f
CMA (chromosomal microarray), 644
CMAP (compound motor action potential), 449
CMV (cytomegalovirus), 614
Coccygeal segments, 4f
Cochlea, 103, 104f
Cochlear duct, 103
Cochlear nuclei, 16, 103
Cognition. *See also* Memory
    ability to learn by Ranchos LOC, 286b
    age-related changes in, 561–562, 563t–564t
    assessment, 277t
    declarative (explicit) memory, 122–123, 123f
    emotions, 124, 126
    executive function, 119–120, 120f
    forgetting, 124
    language, 126f, 126–128
    multiple sclerosis, 383
    neural networks supporting executive function, 120
    nondeclarative (implicit) memory, 121, 123f, 123–124
    physical therapy management, 276–277
Cognitive development
    in 3 to 6 months, 144
    in 6 to 9 months, 145
    in 9 to 12 months, 147–148
    in 2nd year of life, 148–150
    in adolescents, 153
    in infant, 144–145, 147–148
    in middle childhood, 152–153
    in newborn, 143
    Piagetian stages of, 144, 144b
    in preschoolers, 151–152
Cognitive dysfunction
    in amyotrophic lateral sclerosis, 459–460
    in cerebellar disorders, 543
    in Huntington's disease, 422
    in multiple sclerosis, 371, 376
    in Parkinson's disease, 403t, 404
    in stroke, 223–224
Cogwheel rigidity, 399
Coiling, 249
Colon sphincter, 318f
Color perception, 99
Color vision deficits, 99t
Coma, 269, 282–287
Communicating hydrocephalus, 588b
Communication, 183
Communication devices, 633

Communication disorders, 624
Compensation, bed mobility training and, 332t
Compensatory treatment techniques, 227
Complex partial seizures, 623t
Complex polyphasic potential, 450
Complex repetitive discharge, 451
Complex spike, 87
Compound motor action potential (CMAP), 449
Computer-controlled exoskeleton, 343
Computerized dynamic posturography (CDP), 519–520
COMT (catechol-O-methyl transferase) inhibitors, 408t
Concentration, 182t
Concrete operations period, 144b
Concrete thinking, 152
Concussion, 266t, 287t, 287–290
Condom catheter for males, 313b
Conduction aphasia, 128
Conduction velocity, 448–449
Conductive aphasia, 127, 223
Conductive hearing loss, 104
Cone cells, 93
Confabulation, 279t
Confusion, 278t, 283–285
Congenital, 641
Congenital heart defects, in Down syndrome, 650
Congenital hydrocephalus, 590
Congenital myopathies, 653
Congenital scoliosis, 594
Connectivity, 160–162
Constraint-induced movement therapy (CIMT), 243, 629
Constriction, pupillary, 94b
Contour seat, 631
Contracture prevention, 280–281
Contusions, 267
Conus medullaris, 307, 308f
Conventional compensatory gait training, 344
Cooksey habituation exercises, 536b–537b
Coordination, 187–189, 189t, 370, 381b. *See also* Balance
Cornea, 93
Corona radiata, 12
Corpus callosum, 7t, 11f, 12, 143
Cortex, 10–11
Cortical landmarks, 5t
Cortical motor areas, 77f
Cortical plate, 160
Cortical processing of olfaction, 100–101
Corticobasal ganglionic degeneration, 420
Corticomotoneuronal cells, 79
Cortico-ponto-cerebellar pathway, 14
Corticospinal tract
    destinations, 80
    functions, 80–81
    lateral system, 84
    origins and inputs, 79–80
CPG (central pattern generator), 69f, 69–71, 345

Cranial nerves (CN), 15f, 16–17, 185, 186t
Cranial nerve integrity, 461
Cranial neural tube disorders, 581–582
Crawling, 145
Creatine deficiency disorders, 649t
Crede method, 313b
Creeping, 143
Cri-du-chat syndrome, 645t
Crista, 107
Critical periods, 135, 135b
Crossed extensor reflex, 136t, 199t
Crouched gait, 621, 621f
Cruising, 139f, 147
Crystallized intelligence, 562b
CSF (cerebrospinal fluid) analysis, 364
CT scanning, 293, 293f
Cuneocerebellar tract, 54
Cupula, 107, 107f
Cupulolithiasis, 515
Cutaneous sensation, 43, 45, 187
CVD (cardiovascular disease), 346
CVEMP (cervical VEMP), 519
Cystic fibrosis, 646t
Cytokines, 36
Cytomegalovirus (CMV), 614

D
Dactylitis, 252
DAI (diffuse axonal injury), 267, 267f
Dawson's fingers, 364
DCD (developmental coordination disorder), 655–656
DCML (dorsal-column-medial lemniscal pathway), 51
DDH. *See* Developmental dysplasia of the hip (DDH)
Decerebrate posturing, 266b
Decision-making, 120
Declarative memory, 122–123
Decorticate posturing, 266b
Decreased dopamine levels in the striatum, 395
Deep brain stimulation (DBS), 409
Deep cerebellar nuclei (DCN), 6t, 13, 87
Deep nuclei, 5
Deep tendon reflex grades, 185t
Deep vein thrombosis (DVT), 309–310
Degrees of freedom, 85
Deletion, 643
Delirium, 565, 566t
Dementia
    behavioral management of, 570b
    causes of, 564b, 566t
    delirium vs., 565, 566t
    distinguishing features of, 569t
    medical management, 569–570
    motor learning, 571
    neurodegenerative causes of, 566–567
    normal pressure hydrocephalus, 568–569
    physical therapy for, 570–571
    screening for, 570–571
    vascular, 568
Demographics, 195

Dendritic tree, 25
Denervated muscle, 494
Dentate nucleus, 13, 14f
Denticulate ligaments, 17
Depolarization, 26
Depression
    in amyotrophic lateral sclerosis, 460
    dementia vs., 566t
    in Huntington's disease, 422
    after spinal cord injury, 342
    in traumatic brain injury, 280t, 290
Dermatomes, 49, 50f
Detrusor muscle, 311
Development. *See* Child development; Infant
    development
Developmental assessment, in pediatric
    neurologic evaluation, 200–201
Developmental coordination disorder
    (DCD), 655–656
Developmental disabilities/disorders
    adult outcome measures, 669
    age of onset, 641
    autism spectrum disorder. *See* Autism
        spectrum disorder (ASD)
    Becker muscular dystrophy, 645t, 653
    definition of, 641
    developmental coordination disorder,
        655–656
    diagnosis of, 642–644, 649
    Down syndrome. *See* Down syndrome
    Duchenne muscular dystrophy, 646t, 653
    genetic testing of, 643–644
    imaging of, 649
    laboratory testing of, 643–644, 649
    metabolic testing of, 644, 649
    muscular dystrophies, 645t, 653
    neuromuscular degenerative disorders. *See*
        Neuromuscular degenerative disorders
    physical examination of, 642
    physical therapy assessment of, 649–650
Developmental dysplasia of the hip (DDH)
    in cerebral palsy, 620t
    in myelomeningocele, 592–594, 593f
Developmental history, 195
Developmental neurogenesis, 159–162
Developmental neuroplasticity, 160–162
DGI (Dynamic Gait Index), 189, 416
DHI (Dizziness Handicap Inventory), 522
Diabetic autonomic neuropathy, 489
Diabetic distal symmetric polyneuropathy
    (DSP), 489
Diabetic neuropathies, 489–490, 490t
Diabetic radiculoplexus neuropathy
    (DRPN), 489
Diagnosis
    of amyotrophic lateral sclerosis, 455–456
    of brain tumor, 293
    of Guillain–Barré syndrome, 474–475,
        475t
    of Huntington's disease, 424
    of multiple sclerosis, 364–365
    in neurologic exam, 194
    of Parkinson's disease, 395t, 405–406

    of postpolio syndrome, 482
    of spinal cord injury, 304–305
Diaphragm, 314
Diaschisis, 322
Dichromatic vision, 99
Diencephalon, 8f, 580b
Differential diagnosis
    of Parkinson's disease, 395t
    of spinal cord injury, 304–305
Differentiation, 291
Diffuse axonal injury (DAI), 267, 267f
Diffusion, 28
Diffusion tensor imaging (DTI), 168–169,
    169f, 248, 656
Diffusion tensor tractography (DTT), 248
Dilation, of the pupil, 94b
"Diphasic dyskinesia," 409
Diplegia, 616, 617f, 619
Diplopia, 251, 367, 405
Direct pathway, 85
Disability Rating Scale, 269, 270t–271t
Disease-modifying therapy drugs (DMTs),
    373, 373t–374t
Disinhibition, 120, 279t, 423
Disorganized infants, 147b
Disuse atrophy, 585
Divergence, 66
Divided attention, 119b
Dix–Hallpike Test, 525, 526f, 526t
Dizziness, 518, 522t
Dizziness Handicap Inventory (DHI),
    522
DLPFC (dorsolateral prefrontal cortex), 120,
    120f
DMD (Duchenne muscular dystrophy),
    646t, 653
DMTs (disease-modifying therapy drugs),
    373, 373t–374t
Doll's eyes, 111
Dopamine, 86
Dopamine agonists, 408t, 409–410
Dorsal column, 51f
Dorsal horn, 63
Dorsal side, 3, 4f
Dorsal spinocerebellar tract, 53
Dorsal stream, 127
Dorsal-column-medial lemniscal pathway
    (DCML), 51
Dorsolateral prefrontal cortex (DLPFC), 120,
    120f
Dorsomedial default-mode network, 124
Down syndrome
    adults with, 653
    aging with, 652–653
    Alzheimer's disease and, 653
    body-weight-supported treadmill training
        in, 652
    brain differences in, 651
    cognitive decline associated with, 653
    congenital heart defects associated with,
        650
    description of, 642, 646t
    dysmorphic features of, 650, 651f

    ear, nose, and throat problems associated
        with, 651
    epicanthal folds associated with, 650, 651f
    gastrointestinal defects associated with,
        650
    genetic causes of, 643b
    hearing loss in, 651
    hypotonia associated with, 650–651
    intellectual disability in, 650
    ligamentous laxity associated with, 651
    motor development in, 652, 652t
    nuchal translucency measurements, 650
    obesity in, 652
    organ anomalies in, 650
    orthopedic problems in, 651
    patellar instability associated with, 651
    pes planus associated with, 651
    pregnancy screening for, 650
    pulmonary hypertension in, 650
    single palmar crease associated with, 650,
        651f
    skin disorders associated with, 652
    stature in, 652
    teeth issues in, 651
    thyroid disease in, 652
Drawing a circle test, 188b
DRPN (diabetic radiculoplexus neuropathy),
    489
DSP (diabetic distal symmetric
    polyneuropathy), 489
DTI (diffusion tensor imaging), 168–169,
    169f
DTI/DTT (diffusion tensor imaging/
    tractography), 248
Dual-tasking, 402
Duchenne muscular dystrophy (DMD),
    646t, 653
Duplication, 643
Dura mater, 9, 9f
DVA (dynamic visual acuity), 524
DVT (deep vein thrombosis), 309–310
Dynamic balance, 380b
Dynamic balance control, 537b–538b
Dynamic Gait Index (DGI), 189, 416
Dynamic postural control, 84–85
Dynamic splinting, 281
Dynamic visual acuity (DVA), 524
Dynamometers, 197
Dysarthria, 183, 223, 624
Dysautonomia/paroxysmal sympathetic
    hyperactivation (PSH), 275
Dysdiadochokinesia, 189t, 541
Dysesthesia, 187t, 336
Dysgraphia/agraphia, 223
Dyskinesia, 408, 411
Dyskinetic cerebral palsy, 617b
Dyslexia, 223
Dysmetria, 189t, 540–541
Dysmorphic feature, 642
Dysphagia, 626
Dyssynergia, 189t, 541
Dystonia, 402, 409, 421, 617b
Dystrophin, 653

E

EA (episodic ataxia), 540
EAE (experimental autoimmune encephalomyelitis), 362
Ear(s). *See also* Hearing
    anatomy of, 103, 103f
    development of, 134
Eardrum, 103
Echolalia, 658
Eclampsia, 613–614
Ectoderm, 580b
Edaravone, 457
EDGE (APTA) Task Force, 322
EDGE recommendations, 283t
Edinger–Westphal nucleus, 16, 94b
Edwards syndrome, 648t
Egocentric neglect, 221
El Escorial criteria, 455t
Electronystagmography (ENG), 518
Electrophysiologic testing
    clinical electromyography, 445, 449–451
    late waves (F-waves and H-reflexes), 449
    motor vs. sensory tests, 446–448
    nerve conduction studies (NCS), 445–446, 448–449
    neuropathies, 452t
    planning, 451
Electrophysiology, 77
Emboliform nucleus, 13, 14f
Embolism, 211
Emotion, 124, 126
Emotional competence, 147b
Emotional dyscontrol, 275
Emotional lability, 275
Emotional/behavioral dysfunction
    in Huntington's disease, 422–423
    in multiple sclerosis, 371
    in Parkinson's disease, 403t, 404
"En bloc" turning, 401
Encephalocele, 582, 582f
Encephalomeningocele, 582
Encephalopathy of prematurity (EoP), 612b
Encoding
    of information by neurons, 30–33
    in memory, 122
Endoderm, 580b
End of dose deterioration, 409
Endolymph, 103, 106
Endolymphatic hydrops, 515–516
Endpoint accuracy, 84
Energy conservation techniques, 383b
ENG (electronystagmography), 518
Entorhinal cortex, 11f
Environmental control systems, 633
Enzymatic degradation, 28
Enzymes, 28
EoP (encephalopathy of prematurity), 612b
Ependymal layer, 159
Epicanthal folds, 650, 651f
Epidemiology
    of amyotrophic lateral sclerosis, 452–453
    of Huntington's disease, 420
    of multiple sclerosis, 361–362

of Parkinson's disease, 393
Epidural stimulation, 342
Epilepsy
    antiepileptic medications for, 340, 625t
    in autism spectrum disorder, 657
    cerebral palsy and, 622–624, 623t
    traumatic brain injury and, 273–274
Episodic ataxia (EA), 540
Episodic memory, 122, 224
Epley maneuver, 532
EPSP (excitatory postsynaptic potential), 31, 31f, 32f
Equilibrium coordination tests, 188b–189b
Equilibrium reactions, 137t, 199t
Equinovalgus, 620t
Equinovarus, 620t
Equinus, 620t, 621
Ergonomics, 462
Errorless learning, 571
Eschar, 315
Ethosuximide, 625t
Eustachian tube, 103
Evaluation
    of amyotrophic lateral sclerosis, 459–462, 460t
    of balance, 525–531, 529t
    of basilar artery aneurysm, 251–252
    of cognitive function, 277t
    of movement and coordination impairments, 189t
    in neurologic exam, 180f, 194
    of outpatient rehabilitation, 345
    of peripheral neuropathies, 490–491
    of sensory impairments, 187t
    of spinal cord injury, 322–323
    of stroke, 227–228
    of vestibular disorders, 518–520
Evoked potential testing, 364
Examination
    of cerebellar disorders, 543–544
    of multiple sclerosis, 377–378
    of Parkinson's disease, 410–413
    in pediatric neurologic evaluation, 197–198
    of postpolio syndrome, 483
    of vestibular disorders, 520–531
Excitation, 30
Excitatory postsynaptic potential (EPSP), 31, 31f, 32f
Excitatory stripping, 166
Excitotoxicity, 164
Executive dysfunction, 269
Executive function (EF), 119–120, 120f
Exercise
    amyotrophic lateral sclerosis, 462–464, 464t, 467
    ataxia, 381b
    balance, 380b
    bed exercises, 227t
    dementia, 572–573
    designing of, general principles for, 484b
    gaze stability, 535–536, 536f
    habituation, 536–537, 537t

    motion sensitivity, 536–537
    multiple sclerosis, 383
    postural stability, 537
    progression principles in multiple sclerosis, 383b
    static balance, 380b, 537b
Experience-dependent plasticity, 167
Experimental autoimmune encephalomyelitis (EAE), 362
Explicit memory, 122–123, 123f
Expressive aphasia, 183, 223
Extensor thrust reflex, 136t, 199t
External acoustic meatus, 103
External ear, 103f
External urethral sphincter, 311
External ventricular drains, 273
Extrafusal fibers, 45
Extremely low birth weight, 611b
Extremely preterm, 611b
Extrinsic muscles, 81
Eye(s). *See also* Vision
    anatomy of, 93–95, 94f, 96f
    movement of, 96–98

F

Face, sensory projections from, 55
Facial nerve, 16, 186t
Falls, 401f, 417, 423
Falx cerebri, 9, 9f
FAM (Functional Assessment Measure), 285
Family adjustment to TBI, 286–287
Family history, 195
Fasciculation, 450
Fasciculus cuneatus, 16
Fasciculus gracilis, 16
Fast twitch muscle fibers, 64
Fastigial nucleus, 13, 14f
Fatigue
    in amyotrophic lateral sclerosis, 461
    in multiple sclerosis, 369–370, 370f, 376, 379
    in Parkinson's disease, 404–405, 411
Fatigue Severity Scale (FSS), 461
Feedforward control, 76
Femoral anteversion, 620t
FES (functional electrical stimulation), 236–237
Festination, 402
Fetus. *See also* Infant development; Newborn
    critical periods in, 135b
    generalized movements in, 133–134
    motor development in, 133–134
    movements by, 133–134
    nicotine exposure by, 153
    oral motor development in, 134
    rooting reflex in, 134
    sensitive periods in, 134
    sensory development in, 134
    thumb sucking by, 134
Fiber grouping, 559
Fiber tracts, 17, 17f
Fibrillation potential, 450
Fidgety movements, 137, 615

Filum terminale, 17
FIM (Functional Independent Measure), 345
Fine motor skills
  in 0 to 3 months, 139, 142
  in 3 to 6 months, 144
  in 6 to 9 months, 145
  in 9 to 12 months, 147
  in 2nd year of life, 148
  in adolescents, 153
  description of, 204
  in middle childhood, 152
  in preschoolers, 150
Finger to nose test, 188b
Finger to therapist's finger test, 188b
Fitness and wellness, 383, 419, 572–573
5 Times Sit to Stand, 190
Five Times Sit-to-Stand Test (FTSST), 529
Flaccid bladder, 312
Flaccid paralysis, 305
Flaccidity, 216, 326–328
Flexion contracture, 620t
Flexor contractures, 620t
Flexor withdrawal reflex, 136t, 199t
Flocculonodular lobe, 13
Flower spray endings, 46
Fluid intelligence, 562b
fMRI (functional magnetic resonance
    imaging)
  description of, 248
  neuroplasticity measurements using, 169,
    170f
  post-stroke, 170f
  resting state, 169–170
Focal peripheral mononeuropathies, 489
FOG (freezing of gait), 402, 411
FOGQ (Freezing of Gait Questionnaire),
    411, 416
Folstein Mini Mental Status Exam, 183b
Fontanelles, 135, 588
Foramen of Magendie, 5t, 12, 587b
Foramina of Luschka, 5t, 13, 587b
Force
  generation of, 66f
  production of, 65f, 183–184
Forearm crutches, 632
Forebrain, 8f
Forgetting, 124
Formal operations period, 144b
Fourth ventricle, 5t, 587b
Fragile X syndrome, 647t, 656
Freezing of gait (FOG), 402, 411
Freezing of Gait Questionnaire (FOGQ),
    411, 416
Frenzel lenses, 518
Friedreich's ataxia, 540
Frontal dysexecutive syndrome, 120
Frontal lobe, 5t, 8f, 10, 11f, 120f
Frontal operculum, 11f
Frontotemporal dementias (FTD), 568
FSS (Fatigue Severity Scale), 461
FST (Fukuda Stepping Test), 529
FTD (frontotemporal dementias), 568
FTSST (Five Times Sit-to-Stand Test), 529

Fukuda Stepping Test (FST), 529
Full interference pattern in EMG, 450
Functional Assessment Measure (FAM), 285
Functional deficits, 382–383
Functional electrical stimulation (FES),
    236–237
Functional goals, 194
Functional Independent Measure (FIM), 345
Functional losses, 412–413
Functional magnetic resonance imaging
    (fMRI)
  description of, 248
  neuroplasticity measurements using, 169,
    170f
  post-stroke, 170f
  resting state, 169–170
Functional mobility, 323t
Functional muscle testing, 184
Functional neuromuscular electrical
    stimulation (FNMES), 252
Functional Reach Test, 530
Functional status, 195–196, 462
Functional tasks, 84
Functional training, 494
Fused tetanus, 66
F-waves, 449

G
Gabapentin, 340, 625t
Gain, 518
Gait. *See also* Walking
  amyotrophic lateral sclerosis, 462,
    469–470
  assessment, 525–531
  cerebellar disorders, 542, 544–545
  in cerebral palsy, 621, 621f, 628
  clubfoot-related abnormalities of, 592
  control for, 85
  crouched, 621, 621f
  gait deviation, 240b
  Huntington's disease, 429
  intensive practice, 237–238
  jump, 621, 621f
  mobility, 201, 204
  multiple sclerosis, 370–371
  neurologic exam, 192–194
  Parkinson's disease, 401–402
  reciprocating, 599t
  systems review, 196
  task-oriented therapy, 238–239, 239t
Gait ataxia, 540, 542
Gait training, 232b, 342–344
Galant reflex, 136t, 198t
Galveston Orientation and Amnesia Test
    (GOAT), 269
GAME (goals-activity-motor enrichment),
    628
Gamma motor neurons, 47
Gap junctions, 29
Gastroesophageal reflux, 626
Gate theory of pain, 54b, 54f
Gaze stability exercises, 535–536, 536f
Gaze stabilization test (GST), 519

Gaze-holding nystagmus, 523
GBS. *See* Guillain–Barré syndrome (GBS)
GDNF (glial cell neurotrophic factor), 162
Gene-centered treatments, 294
General knowledge, 182
General motor skill development, 596
General movement analysis (GMA), 615
Generalized movements, in fetus, 133–134
Generalized seizures, 623t, 623–624
Genetic anticipation, 420
Genetic disorders, 643, 643b
Genetic inheritance, 643b, 644f
Genetic mutation, 643
Genu recurvatum, 620t
Genu varum, 620t
Giant potentials, 450
Glasgow Coma Scale, 266, 266b, 270t–271t
Glasgow Outcome Scale, 226
Glatiramer acetate, 373t
Glaucoma, 561b
Glial cell neurotrophic factor (GDNF),
    162
Glial cells, 34–37
Glioblastoma, 293f
Gliogenesis, 160
Glioma, 291, 292t
Global aphasia, 128, 223
Globose nucleus, 13, 14f
Globus pallidus, 6t, 11, 11f
Glossopharyngeal nerve, 16, 186t
Gluten-free diet, 659
GMFCS (Gross Motor Function
    Classification System), 615, 616b
GMFM (Gross Motor Function Measure),
    200, 616b
Goal setting, 462–464
Goals-activity-motor enrichment (GAME),
    628
GOAT (Galveston Orientation and Amnesia
    Test), 269
Golgi tendon organ (GTO), 46f, 47–48
Granule cells, 13, 87
Graphesthesia, 43
Grasp, 188b
Gray matter, 3–4, 4f, 7t, 63, 64f, 153
Gross limb movements, 83, 84
Gross Motor Function Classification System
    (GMFCS), 615, 616b
Gross Motor Function Measure (GMFM),
    200, 616b
Gross motor skills
  in 0 to 3 months, 135–139, 136t–137t,
    140t–141t
  in 3 to 6 months, 143–144
  in 6 to 9 months, 145
  in 9 to 12 months, 146–147
  in 2nd year of life, 148
  in adolescents, 153
  in middle childhood, 152
  in preschoolers, 150, 151t
Group Ib inhibitory interneurons, 66–67
GST (gaze stabilization test), 519
GTO (Golgi tendon organ), 46f, 47–48

Guidelines for the Use and Performance of Quantitative Outcome Measures in ALS Clinical Trials, 459
Guillain–Barré syndrome (GBS)
    activity level assessments in, 478t
    acute/progressive stage of, 479
    adult outcome measures, 669
    assessments of, 478t
    chronic/recovery stage of, 479–480
    clinical presentation of, 473–474
    diagnosis of, 474–475, 475t
    etiology of, 472–473
    functional scales, 477t
    incidence of, 472
    medical management of, 476
    pathologies of, 473f
    pathophysiology of, 472–473
    physical therapy evaluation, 476–477
    physical therapy interventions, 478–480
    prognosis, 475–476
    risk factors for, 472
    subtypes of, 474t
Gustation, 101–103, 102f

H
HABIT, 629
HABIT-ILE, 629
Habits, 124
Habituation
    description of, 124
    exercises for, 536–537, 537t
Hair cells, 106, 106f
Hammersmith Functional Motor Scale Expanded (HFMSE), 654
Hamstring stretching, 415f
Hand function, 419
Haptic perception, 43
Haptics, 56
Head control
    in cerebral palsy, 618
    in infant, 143
    in newborn, 135–137
Head impulse test (HIT), 524
Head lag, in cerebral palsy, 618f
Head position. *See* Vestibular system
Head-shaking induced nystagmus test (IISN), 524
Head-thrust test (HTT), 524
Hearing
    age-related changes in, 561b
    central processing of, 103–104
    in cerebral palsy, 624
    ear's organization and auditory apparatus, 103
    sound localization, 104
    testing, 104–105
Hearing tests, 520
Heel on shin test, 188b
Hematoma, 267, 269, 269b
Hemianesthesia, 221
Hemifield, 95
Hemiparesis, 216
Hemiplegia, 216, 616, 617f, 619

Hemorrhagic stroke, 215, 224–225
Heterotopic ossification (HO), 281, 309, 328
HFMSE (Hammersmith Functional Motor Scale Expanded), 654
HIE (hypoxic-ischemic encephalopathy), 614
High-contrast visual acuity, 98
High guard position, 145, 147
Higher cortical function, 182
Higher functioning, 182
Higher-level sensory processing, 55–57
Hindbrain, 8f
Hip dysplasia. *See* Developmental dysplasia of the hip (DDH)
Hip-knee-ankle-foot orthotic (HKAFO), 599t
Hip strategy, 530
Hippocampal formation, 11f, 12
Hippocampal-parahippocampal retrosplenial network, 124
Hippotherapy, 629
HIT (head impulse test), 524
HKAFO (hip-knee-ankle-foot orthotic), 599t
HO (heterotopic ossification), 281, 309, 328
Hoehn–Yahr Classification of Disability Scale, 406
Hoffman test/reflex, 181b
Home status assessment, 180b
Homonymous hemianopia, 222
Homonymous muscle, 47
Horizontal cellular networks, 95
Horizontal saccades, 96–97
H-reflexes, 449
HSN (head-shaking induced nystagmus test), 524
HTT (head-thrust test), 524
"Hung-up" reflexes, 421
Huntingtin gene, 420
Huntington's disease
    body structure and function, 429–430
    clinical course of, 424–425
    clinical presentation of, 421–424
    cognitive dysfunction in, 422
    diagnosis of, 424
    emotional/behavioral dysfunction in, 422–423
    epidemiology of, 420
    etiology of, 420
    late-stage, 430
    management of, 428–430
    medical management for, 425, 425t
    medications for, 425t
    pathophysiology of, 421
    physical therapy evaluation, 426–428
    progression of symptoms, 407t
    rating scale for impairments unique to, 426t
    risk factors for, 420
Hydranencephaly, 582
Hydrocephalus
    causes of, 588b

    communicating, 588b
    congenital, 590
    myelomeningocele as cause of, 586–590, 590f
    noncommunicating, 588b
    obstructive, 588b
    shunt for, 588, 588b, 590, 590f
    stroke and, 250
    ventriculostomy for, 591
Hyperalgesia, 45, 187t, 366
Hypercatabolism, 274–275
Hyperesthesia, 187t
Hyperhidrosis, 403
Hyperkinesia, 421
Hypermetabolism, 274–275
Hyperopia (farsightedness), 94b
Hyperreflexia, 234, 235f, 305
Hypersexuality, 403
Hypertonia, 234, 235f
Hypertonicity, 184, 230, 230t
Hyperventilation, 273
Hypoalgesia, 187t
Hypogastric nerve, 311
Hypoglossal nerve, 17, 186t
Hypokinesia, 86
Hypokinetic dysarthria, 128, 402
Hypokinetic state, 421
Hypomimia, 402
Hyponatremia, 250
Hypopituitarism, 290
Hypotension, 309
Hypothalamus, 6t, 8f, 12
Hypotonia, 189t, 621, 650
Hypotonic, 184
Hypotonic cerebral palsy, 617b–618b
Hypoxia, 268
Hypoxic ischemic brain injury, 268
Hypoxic-ischemic encephalopathy (HIE), 614

I
Ia inhibitory interneuron, 66–67, 67f
Ia inhibitory neuron, 67f
Ib inhibitory interneurons, 68f
ICARS (International Cooperative Ataxia Rating Scale), 544
ICH (intracranial hypertension), 272–273
IDD (intellectual developmental disability), 622–624, 623t
Idiopathic Parkinson's disease, 393–394
Idiopathic scoliosis, 594
Immediate recall, 181
Impairment level assessments, 459–461, 460t, 478t
Implantable FES systems, 343
Implicit learning, 123b
Implicit memory, 121, 123f, 123–124
Impulsivity, 278t, 423
Inability to self-reflect, 279t
Inborn errors of metabolism, 644, 649, 649t
Indirect pathway, 86
Indwelling catheter, 313b

Infant development
in 0 to 3 months, 135–142
in 3 to 6 months, 143–144
in 6 to 9 months, 145
in 9 to 12 months, 146–148
cognitive development, 143, 144–145
crawling, 145
critical periods, 135
equilibrium reactions, 137t
fine motor skills, 139, 142, 144
gross motor skills, 135–139, 136t–137t,
140t–141t, 145
head control, 135–137, 143
language development, 144–145, 149t
motor development, 138–139
movement, 137–139
neural maturation, 135, 143, 145–146
object permanence, 148
oral motor/language, 142–143, 145
oromotor development, 144–145, 147
parachute response, 143, 146f, 200f
physiologic flexion, 135, 139
posture, 135, 146f
primitive reflexes, 136b, 136t, 198t
prone popping, 136
protective reactions, 137t
pull to sit skill, 140f, 140t, 203b
righting reactions, 137t
rotational righting, 137t, 139
sensory development, 142–144
socioemotional development, 143,
144–145, 147–148
walking, 139f
Infantile stepping, 136b
Infection
cerebral palsy caused by, 614
urinary tract, 312–313
Inferior cerebellar peduncle, 14
Inferior olivary complex, 14, 16
Inferior olivary nucleus, 87
Inferior olive, 16
Inferior pincer grasp, 145
Inferior side, 3
Inferior (spinal) nucleus, 110t
Infiltrating tumors, 291
Inflammation, 164, 274, 362, 363f
Informal mental status exam, 181
Inherited mutation, 643b
Inhibition, 30, 119–120
Inhibitory interneurons, 69f
Inhibitory postsynaptic potential (IPSP), 30,
31f, 33
Initiation, 277t
Inner ear, 103f
INO (internuclear ophthalmoplegia), 367
In-patient rehabilitation setting
general approach to patient management,
325–328
physical therapy management, 328–338
spinal cord injury, 325–338
Insertional activity, 450
Insight, 182t
Insular cortex, 10, 11f, 126

Insular region, 5t
Integrative property of neurons, 30
Integumentary system review, 196, 461
Intellectual developmental disability (IDD),
622–624, 623t
Intellectual disability, in Down syndrome,
650
Intelligence, 182t, 562b
Intensive practice, 237–238
Intention tremors, 189t, 542, 617b
Interferon beta-1-a, 373t
Interhemispheric tracts, 169
Interleukin 1ß, 163
Intermediate zone, 63, 159–160
Intermittent catheter, 313b
Internal capsule, 6t, 11f, 12
Internal pathway, 164
International Association for the Study of
Pain, 338–339
International Cooperative Ataxia Rating
Scale (ICARS), 544
International Standards for Neurological
Classification of SCI (ISNCSCI), 305,
322
Interneuron(s), 25, 66–67
Interneuronal network, 68f
Internuclear ophthalmoplegia (INO), 367
Interventricular foramen, 12
Intracerebral hemorrhage, 211
Intracranial hypertension (ICH), 272–273
Intrafusal fibers, 45
Intrahemispheric tracts, 169
Intraparenchymal hematomas, 267
Intrastriatal transplantation, 4100
Intrathecal baclofen, 241, 625
Intrauterine growth restriction (IUGR), 614
Intraventricular hemorrhage (IVH), 612b
Inversion, 643
Ion(s), 27f
Ion channels, 28
Ionotropic receptors, 28, 30f
IPSP (inhibitory postsynaptic potential), 30,
31f, 33
Irritability, 423
Ischemic stroke, 212f, 224
Isolated muscle control, 216
IUGR (intrauterine growth restriction), 614

J
JFK Coma Recovery Scale – Revised, 269,
270t–271t
Joint motions by position, 227t
Joint range of motion, 411. See also Range of
motion (ROM)
Judgment, 182t, 277t
Jump gait, 621, 621f
"Just discernible" movements, 133
Juvenile Huntington's disease, 424

K
KAFO (knee-ankle-foot orthosis), 596, 599t
Kinesthesia, 45, 185–186

Kinetic tremors, 541
Kinocilium, 106
Knee-ankle-foot orthosis (KAFO), 596, 599t
Kyphosis, 620t

L
Labyrinthitis, 514
Lacerations, 267
Lack of initiation, 280t
Lacunar infarcts, 568
Lacunar stroke, 211
Lamotrigine, 625t
Landau reflex, 146f, 199t, 200f
Language
description of, 126f, 126–128
development of, 142–143, 145, 147–148
milestones of, 149t
Language development
in adolescents, 153
in autism spectrum disorder, 658
in middle childhood, 152
in preschoolers, 150
Language dysfunction
in cerebral palsy, 624
in stroke, 222–223, 223f
Last order interneuron, 66
Late waves (F-waves and H-reflexes), 449
Lateral corticospinal tract, 80
Lateral direction, 4f
Lateral geniculate nucleus, 95, 104
Lateral nucleus, 110t
Lateral reticulospinal tracts, 83
Lateral sensory cortex, 56–57
Lateral sulcus, 5t, 10f
Lateral systems, 83–84, 85
Lateral ventricle, 5t
Lateral vestibular nucleus, 82
Lateral vestibulospinal tract, 82, 109
Laterality index, 170
Latex allergies, 590–591
LBD (Lewy body dementia), 419, 567
Leadpipe rigidity, 399
Learned nonuse, 167, 227
Learning
aging and, 561–562
errorless, 571
experimental test of, 70f
implicit, 123b
motor. See Motor learning
negative, 560
procedural, 121, 123
Learning-associated neuroplasticity, 162–163
Lee Silverman Voice Treatment (LSVT), 418
Left hemisphere, 5
Left-beating nystagmus, 112
LEMS (lower extremity motor scores), 305
Lenke classification, of scoliosis, 595t
Lens, 93
Lens control, 94b
Letter sequence, 123b
Levels of cognitive functioning (LOC),
282–291
Levetiracetam, 625t

Levodopa (L-dopa), 407–408, 408t
"Lewy bodies," 395
Lewy body dementia (LBD), 419, 567
Lhermitte's sign, 366
Liberatory maneuver, 532, 533f
Limb ataxia, 540
Limb movement, 84, 540–541, 544
Limbic loop, 396b
Limbic region, 5t
Limbic system, 120f, 125f
Linear acceleration, 105, 108–109
LIS (locked-in syndrome), 251
Living environment, 195
LMN (lower motor neuron) signs
    brachial plexus palsy as cause of, 585
    in myelomeningocele, 585, 586t
    in spinal cord injury, 304
LOC (levels of cognitive functioning),
    282–291
Localized tumors, 291
Locked-in syndrome (LIS), 251
Locomotion
    central pattern generators for, 69f, 70b
    pediatric neurologic evaluation, 196
    task-dependent training for, 344–345
Locomotor training objectives, 344–345
Locus coeruleus, 15
Log rolling, 143
Lokomat system, 343
Long-term depression (LTD), 87, 123, 162
Long-term memory, 123f
Long-term potentiation (LTP), 87, 123,
    162–163
Low birth weight, 611b
Lower extremity motor scores (LEMS), 305
Lower motor neuron (LMN) signs
    brachial plexus palsy as cause of, 585
    in myelomeningocele, 585, 586t
    in spinal cord injury, 304
LSVT BIG, 418
LSVT (Lee Silverman Voice Treatment), 418
LTD (long-term depression), 87, 123, 162
LTP (long-term potentiation), 87, 123,
    162–163
Lumbar spine, 63, 70f
Lung-protective ventilation, 272
Lysosomal storage disorders, 649t

M

MABC-2 (Movement Assessment Battery for
    Children-2), 656
Macrocephaly, 642
Macrophages, 35
Macula, 93
Macular degeneration (MD), 561b
Magnetic resonance imaging (MRI), 168,
    168f, 364, 367f, 520
Magnocellular neurons, 81
Maladaptive plasticity, 167, 267
Mantel layer, 159
Manual muscle test (MMT), 183
Manual wheelchairs, 604, 605f, 631
Marcus Gunn pupil, 367

Marginal layer, 159
Marginal zone, 160
MCA. See Middle cerebral artery (MCA)
    infarction
M-CHAT (Modified Checklist for Autism in
    Toddlers), 658
MCI (mild cognitive impairment), 562
MCS (minimally conscious state), 290
MD (macular degeneration), 561b
MDA (Muscular Dystrophy Association),
    457
Measurable goals, 194
Mechanoreceptors, 43, 44f, 45
Meconium, 613
Medial direction, 4f
Medial lemniscus, 17, 17f
Medial longitudinal fasciculus (MLF), 17,
    17f, 109
Medial nucleus, 110t
Medial prefrontal cortex, 126
Medial reticulospinal tracts, 83
Medial temporal lobe, 122f
Medial vestibular nucleus, 82
Medial vestibulospinal tract, 82, 109
Medical history, 179–180, 195, 410, 520–523
Medical management
    of amyotrophic lateral sclerosis, 457
    of cerebellar disorders, 543
    of cerebral palsy, 624–627
    of dementia, 569–570
    of Guillain–Barré syndrome, 476
    of Huntington's disease, 425, 425t
    of multiple sclerosis, 373–377
    of Parkinson's disease, 406–409
    of pediatric stroke, 253
    of postpolio syndrome, 483
    of stroke, 224–226
    of vestibular disorders, 518–520
Medical management of spinal cord injury,
    308–321
    autonomic dysfunction, 309
    bladder dysfunction, 311–313
    neurogenic bowel, 317–321
    pressure ulcers and skin integrity,
        315–317
    pulmonary complication and respiratory
        dysfunction, 314–315
Medically stable client, 281–282
Medulla, 7t, 8f, 15–16
Medullary pyramids, 16
Membrane potential, 30–31
Membranous labyrinth, 103, 105–106
Memory
    consolidation of, 101
    explicit, 122–123, 123f
    implicit, 121, 123f, 123–124
    medial temporal lobe structures, 122f
    in neurologic exam, 181–182, 182t
    physical therapy management, 276–277
    retrieval of, 122
Ménière's disease, 515–516
Meninges, 5t, 8f, 9
Meningocele, 582, 583f

Mental status examination, 181–183, 182t,
    183b
MEP (motor evoked potential), 170
Mesencephalon, 580b
Mesoderm, 580b
Metabolic syndrome, 290
Metabotropic receptors, 28, 30f
Metencephalon, 580b
Meyer's loop, 95
Micro infarcts, 568
Microcephaly, 642
Microglia, 34f, 35–36
Microglial synaptic pruning, 163
Micrographia, 402, 419
Midbrain, 7t, 8f, 15
Middle cerebellar peduncle, 14
Middle cerebral arteries, 212–213, 217t, 613
Middle cerebral artery (MCA) infarction
    cognitive dysfunction secondary to,
        223–224
    language dysfunction secondary to,
        222–223, 223f
    motor dysfunction secondary to, 216, 221
    sensory dysfunction secondary to, 221
    visual field disruption secondary to, 222,
        222f
Middle childhood, 152–153
Middle ear, 103f
Migraine-associated dizziness, 517
Mild cognitive impairment (MCI), 562
Mild traumatic brain injury, 287t, 287–290
Mini-BESTest, 189
Minimally conscious state (MCS), 290
Mirror activities, 237
Mitoxantrone, 374t
Mitral cells, 100
MLF (medial longitudinal fasciculus), 17,
    17f, 109
MMC. See Myelomeningocele (MMC)
MND (motor neuron disease), 452
mNIHSS, 225t
Mobility
    in amyotrophic lateral sclerosis, 470
    bed, 231, 233t, 332, 332t
    in cerebral palsy, 630
    functional, 323t
    gait, 204
    in multiple sclerosis, 370–371
    in pediatric neurologic evaluation, 201,
        204
    prediction of, using level of spinal cord
        injury, 329t–330t
    primary form of, 204
    wheelchair, 333–334. See also Wheelchair
Mobility training, 415–418
MoCA (Montreal Cognitive Assessment),
    183b
Moderate to late preterm, 611b
Modified Ashworth Scale, 184b
Modified Checklist for Autism in Toddlers
    (M-CHAT), 658
Modified Rankin scale, 225–226
Monoamine oxidase inhibitors, 408t

Mononeuropathy, 484
Montreal Cognitive Assessment (MoCA), 183b
Mood/affect, 182t
Moro reflex, 136t, 138f, 198t
Morphogens, 160
Mosaic Trisomy 21, 643b
Mossy fibers, 86
Motion sensitivity exercises, 536–537
Motion sensitivity test, 524, 525t
Motion sickness, 517–518
Motor adaptation, 543
Motor control
    basal ganglia and cerebellum in, 85–88
    cortical motor areas, 77f
    descending systems for, 75–92, 78f
    example of a common movement task, 75–76
    functional scheme for understanding the tracts, 83–85
    overview of, 75
    pediatric neurologic evaluation, 196
Motor development
    in autism spectrum disorder, 658–659
    in Down syndrome infants, 652, 652t
    in fetus, 133–134
    in first 3 months, 138–139
    oral, 134
Motor dysfunction
    in Huntington's disease, 421–422
    in multiple sclerosis, 368–371
    in stroke, 216, 221
Motor evoked potential (MEP), 170
Motor examination, 183–185
Motor function, aging and, 560
Motor imagery, 231b
Motor impersistence, 421
Motor learning, 196
    cerebellar disorders, 543
    dementia, 571
    Huntington's disease, 421
    Parkinson's disease, 403
    physical therapy management, 277
Motor loop, 396b
Motor neuron disease and neuropathies
    adult outcome measures, 669
    amyotrophic lateral sclerosis, 451–471
    brachial plexus injuries, 494–497
    electrophysiologic testing, 445–451, 452t
    Guillain–Barré syndrome, 472–480
    introduction to, 445
    peripheral neuropathies, 484–494
    postpolio syndrome, 480–484
    radiculopathy, 451
Motor neuron disease (MND), 452
Motor neurons, 64–71, 455t
Motor skills, 204
Motor studies, 446, 447–448
Motor system function, 476–477
Motor unit, 64, 65t
Movement, 203b. *See also* Vestibular system
    examination of, 200–201
    in myelomeningocele, 596–597

Movement Assessment Battery for Children (MABC-2), 656
Movement decomposition, 541
Movement impairments, 189t
Movement scale, 411
Movement sense, 185–186
Movement task, common, 75–76
MRI (magnetic resonance imaging), 364, 367f, 520
MS EDGE Highly Recommended Outcome Measures and G-Codes, 378b
Multi-Directional Reach Test, 530
Multifocal mononeuropathy, 484
Multi-infarct dementia, 568
Multimodal sensory stimulation program, 282b
Multi-organ dysfunction syndrome (MODS), 274
Multiple mononeuropathy, 484
Multiple sclerosis
    adult outcome measures, 667
    autonomic dysfunction in, 372
    balance, 370–371
    clinical course of, 365f
    cognition in, 383
    cognitive dysfunction in, 371, 376
    course of, 364
    definition of, 361
    demographics of, 361–362
    diagnosis of, 364–365
    disease-modifying therapy drugs (DMTs), 373, 373t–374t
    disease-specific treatment strategies for, 383–384
    emotional/behavioral dysfunction in, 371
    epidemiology of, 361–362
    fatigue associated with, 369–370, 370f, 376, 379
    medical management of, 373–377
    motor dysfunction in, 368–371
    pain associated with, 366
    pathophysiology/pathogenesis, 362–363
    physical therapy management, 377–384
    prognosis of, 377
    risk factors, 361–362
    sensory dysfunction in, 365
    signs and symptoms, 364–373
    symptomatic medications, 375t–376t
    symptoms of, 368b
    treatment focus in, 378–379
    types of, 364b, 365f
    visual disturbances, 366–367
Multiple system atrophy, 420
Muscle(s), 64–71
Muscle activation, 65f
Muscle atrophy, 305
Muscle biopsies, 456f
Muscle force generation, 542
Muscle length, 411
Muscle performance, 401, 460–461
Muscle spindles, 45–47, 46f, 48
Muscle tone, 197
Muscle weakness, 469–470

Muscular dystrophies, 645t, 653
Muscular Dystrophy Association (MDA), 457
Musculoskeletal systems, 75, 196, 411–412
Music-based movement therapy, 418
Mutism, 402
MWF (myelin water fraction), 171
Myelencephalon, 580b
Myelin, 4, 28, 29f, 362, 363f
Myelin injury, 446, 449
Myelin water fraction (MWF), 171
Myelin Water Imaging, 170
Myelinated axon, 28
Myelination, 36, 134b
Myelomeningocele (MMC)
    acute rehabilitation settings and, 600, 603
    ambulation considerations, 596–597, 597t
    Arnold–Chiari malformation associated with, 586–587, 587f
    bladder management in, 600b
    bowel management in, 600b
    brain abnormalities associated with, 586–590
    causes of, 584
    club foot associated with, 591–592, 592b, 592f
    comorbidities associated with, 586–591
    definition of, 583
    description of, 579
    developmental dysplasia of the hip associated with, 592–594, 593f
    diagnosis of, 584
    general motor skill development affected by, 596
    hydrocephalus associated with, 586–590, 590f
    illustration of, 579f, 583f
    in utero repair of, 584b
    incidence of, 584
    inpatient rehabilitation settings and, 600, 603
    kicking behaviors in fetuses with, 596
    location of, 584
    lower motor neuron signs in, 585, 586t
    movement potential in, 596–597
    orthopedic complications of, 591–595
    orthotics for children with, 597, 599t
    physical therapist's role in, 597–604
    physical therapy management of, 596–604
    risk factors for, 584
    school-based settings and, 599–600
    scoliosis associated with, 594f–595f, 594–595, 595t
    sensorimotor characteristics of, 585–586, 586t
    sensory loss in lower extremities secondary to, 598
    spinal cord injury versus, 606
    spinal cord tethering associated with, 591
    surgical management of, 584–585, 585b, 585f
    treatment activities for infants with, 601t–602t

Myelomeningocele (MMC) (*cont.*)
upper motor neuron signs in, 585, 586t
wheelchair for, 603t, 604–606
Myoclonic seizures, 623t
Myoclonic twitches, 137
Myoclonus, 421
Myopathic potential, 451
Myopathic scoliosis, 594
Myopia (nearsightedness), 94b
Myotonic discharge, 451

N

Natalizumab, 374t
National Acute Spinal Cord Injury Studies
(NASCIS I, II, and III), 308
NAWM (normal-appearing white matter),
362
NCS (nerve conduction studies), 445–446
NEC (necrotizing enterocolitis), 612b
Necrosis, 226
Necrotizing enterocolitis (NEC), 612b
Negative learning, 560
Negative plasticity
as aging model, 560t, 560–561
description of, 267
Neglect syndrome, 221, 246f, 246–248
Nerve conduction studies (NCS), 445–446
Nerve conduit, 489
Nerve grafts, 488–489
Nerve recovery, grading system for, 488t
Nervous system
description of, 3, 4f
development of, 580b
Neural groove, 580b
Neural maturation
in 0 to 3 months, 135
in 3 to 6 months, 143
in 6 to 9 months, 145
in 9 to 12 months, 146
in 2nd year of life, 148
in adolescents, 153
in middle childhood, 152
in preschoolers, 150
Neural networks, 120
Neural plasticity, 33–34
Neural plate, 580b
Neural response to injury, 163–165
Neural stem cells (NSCs), 160
Neural tube
caudal, 582
closure of, 581f
development of, 580, 580f
Neural tube disorders (NTDs)
anencephaly, 581–582
closed, 580
cranial, 581–582
description of, 579f
embryology of, 580b, 580–581
encephalocele, 582, 582f
encephalomeningocele, 582
hydranencephaly, 582
meningocele, 582, 583f
myelomeningocele. *See* Myelomeningocele

open, 580
pathogenesis of, 580–583
spinal, 582–583, 583f
spinal dysraphism, 582, 583f
Neural vesicle, 581f
Neurapraxia, 484, 487
Neuroanatomy
autonomic nervous system, 19
brain, 8–11
brainstem, 14–17
cerebellum, 13–14
introduction to, 3–4
meninges, 9
peripheral nervous system, 19
spinal cord, 17–19
structures and functions in the nervous
system, 5t–7t
subcortical structures, 11–12
ventricular system, 12–13
Neurogenesis, 160
Neurogenic bowel, 317–321
Neurogenic shock, 309
Neuroimaging, 520
Neuroinflammation, 303–304
Neurologic exam
activity and participation, 190–191
body structure and function, 181–190
components of, 179–181
evaluation, 180f, 194
history, 179–180
overview of, 179
Parkinson's disease, 410–411
pediatric evaluation, 194–204
screening, 180–181
systems review, 180–181
treatment, 180f
Neuroma, 484
Neuromodulators, 29
Neuromuscular degenerative disorders
congenital myopathies, 653
muscular dystrophies, 645t, 653
physical therapy management of, 654–655
spinal muscular atrophies, 653–654
Neuromuscular electrical stimulation
(NMES), 343
Neuromuscular Recovery Scale (NRS), 306
Neuromuscular scoliosis, 594
Neuron(s)
description of, 25, 26f, 33
integrative functions of, 30
migration of, 160f
non-synaptic communication between, 29
transduction and encoding information
by, 30–33
typical, 25
Neuronal structure and function
glial cells, 34–37
introduction to, 25–34
neural plasticity, 33–34
overview of neural function, 26–29
Neuropathic pain, 338–341
Neuropathic scoliosis, 594
Neuroplasticity

acute, post-stroke, 226
adaptive, 167–168, 168b
adult neurogenesis, 162
after central nervous system injury,
165–167
developmental neurogenesis, 159–162
functional magnetic resonance imaging of,
169–170
in vivo measurements of, 168–171
learning-associated, 162–163
neural response to injury, 163–165
promoters of, 166
resting state functional magnetic
resonance imaging of, 169–170
structural imaging of, 168f–169f, 168–170
transcranial magnetic stimulation of, 170,
170f
treatment and, 248
Neuropsychiatric changes, 275–276
Neurotmesis, 484, 487, 496
Neurotransmitters, 558–559
Neurotrophins, 166
Neurulation, 580
Newborn. *See also* Infant development
APGAR assessment of, 614b
arm movements in, 139
cognitive development in, 143
encephalopathy in, 655
fine motor skills in, 139, 142
fontanelles of, 135, 588
gross motor skills in, 135–139, 136t–137t
head control in, 135–137
hyperkinetic movements in, 137–138
language development, 142–143, 149t
movement in, 137–139
oral motor development, 142–143
physiologic flexion of, 135, 139
posture in, 135
primitive reflexes in, 136b, 136t, 138f, 198t
prone popping, 136
pull to sit, 140f, 140t, 203b
rotational righting in, 137t, 139
sensory development in, 142–143
socioemotional development in, 143
Nicotine exposure, 153
Niemann–Pick disease, 647t
NIH Stroke Scale (NIHSS), 225, 225t
NIPPV (noninvasive positive-pressure
ventilation), 459
Nitrosative stress, 165
NMES (neuromuscular electrical
stimulation), 343
Node of Ranvier, 29f, 34
Noisy processing, 560
Non-articulating ankle-foot orthotics, 630
Noncommunicating hydrocephalus, 588b
Nondeclarative memory, 121, 123–124
Nonequilibrium coordination tests, 188b
Nonfluent aphasia, 126
Noninvasive positive-pressure ventilation
(NIPPV), 459
Nonparetic foot, 233b
Nonstructural scoliosis, 594–595

Non-synaptic communication between neurons, 29
Nordic walking, 418
Normal-appearing white matter (NAWM), 362
Normal pressure hydrocephalus (NPH), 568–569
Norris Scale, 462
North Star Ambulatory Assessment (NSAA), 654
NRS (Neuromuscular Recovery Scale), 306
NSAA (North Star Ambulatory Assessment), 654
NSCs (neural stem cells), 160
NTDs. *See* Neural tube disorders (NTDs)
Nuchal translucency, 650
Nucleus reticularis gigantocellularis, 82
Nucleus reticularis pontis caudalis, 82
Nutritional management
    of cerebral palsy, 625–627
    of Parkinson's disease, 410
Nutritional supplements, 626–627
Nystagmus, 112, 520, 526t, 529t

O

Object permanence, 148
Obstructed labor, 614
Obstructive hydrocephalus, 588b
Obstructive ventilator impairment, 314–315
Occipital lobe, 5t, 10
Ocrelizumab, 374t
Ocular alignment, 524
Ocular cranial nerve, 99t
Ocular tilt reaction (OTR), 524
Ocular VEMP (oVEMP), 519
Oculocephalic reflex, 111
Oculomotor dysfunction, 542
Oculomotor loop, 396b
Oculomotor nerve, 16, 186t
Odorants, 100
Ofalimumab, 373t
OFC (orbitofrontal cortex), 121
Offspring cells, 643
OFVMC (orbitofrontal ventromedial cortex), 121
OH (orthostatic hypotension), 371, 404
OKN (optokinetic nystagmus), 112
Olfaction, 100f, 100–101
Olfactory cortex, 101f
Olfactory nerve, 16, 100, 186t
Olfactory receptors, 100
Olfactory testing, 101
Oligoclonal immunoglobulin bands, 364
Oligodendrocyte precursor cells (OPCs), 37
Oligodendrocytes, 19, 34f, 36–37
On–off phenomenon, 409
OPCs (oligodendrocyte precursor cells), 37
Open head injuries, 265
Open-loop cueing, 416
Ophthalmoscope assessment, 99
Opioids, for neuropathic pain, 340
Opposition of fingers, 188b
Optic chiasm, 95

Optic muscle function, 99
Optic nerve, 16, 186t
Optic neuritis, 366–367
Optic projections, 95–96
Optic radiations, 95
Optic tract, 95
Optical righting reflex, 146f, 200f
Optokinetic nystagmus (OKN), 112
Optokinetic reflex, 112
Oral motor development
    in 0 to 3 months, 142–143
    in 3 to 6 months, 144–145
    in fetus, 134
Orbital-ventromedial prefrontal cortex, 120f
Orbitofrontal cortex (OFC), 121
Orbitofrontal ventromedial cortex (OFVMC), 121
Organ of Corti, 103
Oromotor development
    in infant, 144–145, 147
    in 2nd year of life, 148
    in preschoolers, 150
Oropharyngeal dysphagia, 626
Orthodromic volley, 449
Orthopedic conditions
    in cerebral palsy, 620t, 622, 625–626
    in Down syndrome, 651
Orthostatic hypotension (OH), 371, 404
Orthotics
    ankle-foot, 244–246, 245b–246b, 599t
    for cerebral palsy, 630, 630f
    hip-knee-ankle-foot, 599t
    knee-ankle-foot, 596, 599t
    for myelomeningocele, 597, 599t
    trunk-hip-knee-ankle-foot, 599t
Ortolani sign, 593
Oscillopsia, 111, 514
Osteoporosis, 328
Otoconia, 108
Otolith(s), 108
Otolithic membrane, 108–109, 109f
Otolithic organs, 105
OTR (ocular tilt reaction), 524
Outer hair cells, 103
Outpatient rehabilitation setting
    chronic complications of spinal cord injury, 338–339
    lifelong considerations, 346
    stroke, 241–248
Oval window, 103
OVEMP (ocular VEMP), 519
Oxcarbazepine, 625t
Oxidative stress, 165

P

Pain
    acute, 338–339
    in amyotrophic lateral sclerosis, 460
    antiepileptics for, 340
    behavioral self-management for, 340
    experience of, 53b
    gate theory of, 54b, 54f
    management of, 493

modulation of, 54b, 54f
    in multiple sclerosis, 366, 374
    neuropathic, 338–341
    opioids for, 340
    physical exercise/rehabilitation for, 340
    shoulder, 334, 469
    spinal cord injury-induced, 339–342
Pallidotomy, 409
Palmar grasp reflex, 136t, 138f, 198t
Parachute response, 143, 146f, 199t, 200f
Paradoxical breathing pattern, 314b
Parallel fibers, 87
Paramedian arteries, 215
Paraplegia, 304
Parapodium, 599t
Parasympathetic innervation
    of bladder and urethral sphincters, 312f
    of colon and anal sphincters, 318f
Parasympathetic nervous system, 16, 19
Paresthesias, 187t, 405
Parietal lobe, 5t, 10
Parietal ventral (PV) area, 56
Parietal–occipital sulcus, 5t, 10, 10f
Parkinson Disease Evidence Database to Guide Effectiveness (PDEDGE), 411, 412
Parkinsonism, 393
Parkinson-plus syndromes, 393, 419–420
Parkinson's disease (PD)
    adult outcome measures, 668
    balance, 411, 415
    body structure and function, 410–413
    clinical course of, 406
    clinical presentation, 397–403
    cognitive dysfunction, 403t, 404
    definition of, 393
    description of, 405
    diagnosis of, 405–406, 406t
    differential diagnosis, 395t
    drugs associated with, 395t
    emotional/behavioral dysfunction in, 403t, 404
    epidemiology of, 393
    etiology of, 393
    examination of, 410–413
    fatigue associated with, 404–405, 411
    Hoehn and Yahr staging of, 407t
    idiopathic, 393–394
    management of, 413–420
    medical management, 406–409
    medications for, 408t
    non-motor symptoms, 403t, 403–405
    Parkinson-plus syndromes, 394–395
    pathophysiology of, 395–397
    pharmacological management, 406–410
    primary motor symptoms, 397, 399–400
    progression of symptoms, 407t
    risk factors for, 393
    secondary motor symptoms, 401–403
    secondary Parkinsonism, 394
    surgical treatments for, 409–410
    symptoms of, 397, 399–403, 407t
    vascular Parkinsonism, 394

Partial seizures, 623, 623t

Participation level assessments, 460t, 462, 478t

Passive forgetting, 124

Pavlik harness, 593, 593f

PBTs (primary brain tumors), 291–293

PCEF (peak cough expiratory flow), 461

PDEDGE (Parkinson Disease Evidence Database to Guide Effectiveness), 411, 412

PDMS (Peabody Developmental Motor Scales), 200, 649

Peabody Developmental Motor Scales (PDMS), 200, 649

Peak cough expiratory flow (PCEF), 461

PED (pipeline embolization device), 250

PEDI, 196

Pediatric neurologic evaluation
  adaptive equipment, 204
  developmental assessment, 200–201
  examination, 197–198
  history, 195–196
  mobility, 201, 204
  movement examination, 200–201
  systems review, 196

Pediatric stroke, 252–253

PEDI-CAT, 196

Pedunculopontine nucleus, 15

PEG. *See* Percutaneous endoscopic gastrostomy (PEG)

Pencil test, 222f

Penumbra, 226

Perception, 182t

Percutaneous endoscopic gastrostomy (PEG), 627

Periaqueductal gray, 15

Perilymph, 103, 106

Perilymphatic fistula (PLF), 516

Perinatal, 641

Perinatal asphyxia, 614

Perinatal birth trauma, 614

Peripheral nervous system, 19, 559–560

Peripheral neuropathies
  autonomic neuropathy tests, 491, 493
  causes of, 485t–486t
  diabetic and related neuropathies, 489–490
  muscle denervation, 487
  nerve grafts, 488–489
  physical therapy assessment, 490–491
  physical therapy management, 493–494
  signs of recovery following neurotmesis, 487–488
  surgical repair, 487
  traumatic nerve injuries, 484, 487, 487t

Peripheral vestibular disorders, 513–515, 516t, 531, 531t

Peristalsis, 318

Periventricular leukomalacia, 612b

Perseveration, 119, 279t, 423

Personality, 277

Pervasive developmental disorders, 656

Pes planus, 651

PET (positron emission tomography), 248

PH (pulmonary hypertension), 650

Phasic neurons, 33

Phasic stretch reflex, 234

Phenobarbital, 625t

Phenylketonuria (PKU), 647t, 649

Phenytoin, 625t

Phonetics, 126

Phonology, 126

PHQ-2 Depression Screen, 564, 565b

Physical therapy management
  amyotrophic lateral sclerosis, 464, 467
  brachial plexus injuries, 494–497
  brain tumor, 294–295
  cerebellar disorders, 544–546
  cerebral palsy, 627–633
  cognition, 276–277
  dementia, 570–571
  Guillain–Barré syndrome, 478–480
  multiple sclerosis, 377–384
  myelomeningocele, 596–604
  neuromuscular degenerative disorders, 654–655
  peripheral neuropathies, 493–494
  postpolio syndrome, 483
  vestibular disorders, 532–539

Physical therapy management, for multiple sclerosis
  ataxia, 380–381
  disease stage-specific treatment, 383–384
  examination, 377–378
  exercise and cognition, 383
  fatigue, 369–370, 370f, 376, 379
  fitness, 383
  functional deficits, 382–383
  sensory changes, 379–380
  spasticity, 380
  treatment, 378–379, 383–384

Physical therapy management, for spinal cord injury
  acute, 323–324
  in-patient rehabilitation setting, 328–338
  outpatient rehabilitation setting, 342–346

Physical therapy management, for stroke
  acute care facility, 226–235
  assessment, 227–228
  assistance levels, 234
  assistive devices, 240
  circuit training, intensive task-oriented training, 242–243
  early interventions and prevention of complications, 229–230
  gait, 237b, 237–239
  general concepts, 226–227
  in home health and outpatient environments, 241–248
  neglect syndrome and pusher syndrome, 246–248
  in rehabilitation setting, 235–241
  rolling/bed mobility, 231
  sensory training post-stroke, 243–244
  spasticity, 234–235, 240–241
  task-oriented practice, 230
  task-oriented therapy, 238–239

transfers, task-oriented training, 242

uneven surfaces, task-oriented training, 242

upper extremity, 236–237

upright activities, 231–234

Physiologic flexion, 135, 139

Pia mater, 9, 9f

Piagetian stages of cognitive development, 144, 144b, 152

PICA (posterior inferior cerebellar artery), 215, 219t

Pincer grasp, 148

Pipeline embolization device (PED), 250

Pisa syndrome, 400

Pivot prone, 143

PKU (phenylketonuria), 647t, 649

Placental abruption, 613

Placental insufficiency, 614

Placental previa, 613

Plantar grasp reflex, 136t, 138f, 198t

Plantigrade walking, 147

Plasticity, 70f, 248–250, 332t

PLF (perilymphatic fistula), 516

PLS (primary lateral sclerosis), 455

PM (premotor cortex), 79

PNETs (primitive neuroectodermal tumors), 292

Polyneuropathy, 484

Pons, 7t, 8f, 11f, 15–16

Ponsetti method, 592

Pontine arteries, 213

Pontine flexure, 580b, 581f

Pontine nuclei, 7t, 15

Position, observation by, 202t–203t

Position sense, 186

Positional testing, 524–525

Positive Romberg sign, 188b

Positive sharp wave, 450

Positive support reflex, 136t, 198t

Positron emission tomography (PET), 248

Postcentral gyrus, 5t

Posterior cerebellum, 13

Posterior cerebral artery
  aneurysm of, 249f
  description of, 213
  stroke-related symptoms of, 218t

Posterior choroidal arteries, 215

Posterior communicating arteries, 213

Posterior inferior cerebellar artery (PICA), 215, 219t

Posterior limb of Internal capsule, 12

Posterior parietal association area, 5t

Posterior parietal cortex (PPC), 57

Posterior side, 3, 4f

Posterior spinal cord syndrome, 307, 308f

Posterior tilt chair, 631, 631f

Posterior walker, 632, 632f

Postnatal, 641

Postpolio syndrome (PPS)
  clinical presentation of, 481–482
  development and signs of, 481t
  diagnosis of, 482, 482b
  etiology of, 482–483

Postpolio syndrome (PPS) (*cont.*)
  factors associated with, 481t
  medical management, 483
  physical therapy for, 483
  polio virus, 481
  prognosis, 483
  psychosocial considerations, 483–484
Postrotatory nystagmus, 112
Postsynaptic neuron, 28
Post-traumatic amnesia (PTA), 197, 269
Post-traumatic epilepsy (PTE), 273–274
Post-traumatic Parkinsonism, 394
Posttraumatic stress disorder (PTSD), 480
Postural instability, 400
Postural orthostatic tachycardia syndrome
    (PoTS), 371–372
Postural reactions, 200f
Postural stability exercises, 537
Postural Stress Test, 530
Postural tremors, 189t, 541
Posture, 135, 462
Potassium, 27
PoTS (postural orthostatic tachycardia
    syndrome), 371–372
Power, 559b
Powered wheelchairs, 604, 631
PPC (posterior parietal cortex), 57
PPMS (primary progressive MS), 364b
Prader–Willi disease, 647t
PRAFO (pressure relief ankle foot orthosis),
    280
Precentral gyrus, 5t, 79
Pre-eclampsia, 613
Prefrontal cortex, 80
Pregabalin, 340
Premanifest stage of Parkinson's, 424
Prematurity
    adjustment for, 201b
    sequelae of, 611b–612b
Premotor cortex (PM), 79
Prenatal, 641
Preoperational period, 144b, 152
Presbycusis, 561b
Presbyopia, 94b, 561b
Preschoolers, 150–152, 151t
Pressure relief ankle foot orthosis (PRAFO),
    280
Pressure relief techniques, 316t
Pressure ulcers
    in myelomeningocele, 603
    in spinal cord injury, 315–317, 316t
Presynaptic neuron, 28
Presynaptic terminal, 28, 30f
Pretend play, 144b
Primary afferents (Ia), 46
Primary axonal damage, 474–475
Primary brain tumors (PBTs), 291–293
Primary fissure, 13
Primary form of mobility, 204
Primary injury, 303
Primary lateral sclerosis (PLS), 455
Primary progressive MS (PPMS), 364b
Primary respiratory muscles, 314f

Primary sensory cortex, 55–56
Priming, 124
Primitive neuroectodermal tumors (PNETs),
    292
Primitive reflexes, 136b, 136t, 138f,
    198t–199t
Primitive standing, 136t, 198t
Prioritization of attention, 119b
PRMS (progressive-relapsing MS), 364b
Procedural learning, 121, 123
Processing, speed of, 277t
Prognosis, 194
Programmed cell death, 160
Programs or related therapy services, 195
Progressive bulbar palsy, 456
Progressive muscular atrophy, 455
Progressive supranuclear palsy, 419–420
Progressive-relapsing MS (PRMS), 364b
Projection interneurons, 25
Projection neurons, 26f
Pronation, alternating, 188b
Pronation contracture, 620t
Prone popping, 136
Proprioception
    description of, 45–48, 196
    tests of, 185–187
Prosencephalon, 580b
Protective reactions, 137t, 199t
Protoplasmic astrocytes, 34
Pruning, 160, 161f
Pseudobulbar palsy, 456
PSH (dysautonomia/paroxysmal sympathetic
    hyperactivation), 275
Psychiatric impairments, 543
Psychosocial issues, 470–471
PTA (post-traumatic amnesia), 197, 269
PTE (post-traumatic epilepsy), 273–274
PTSD (posttraumatic stress disorder), 480
Pudendal nerve, 311
Pull Test, 530
Pull to sit, 140f, 140t, 203b
Pulmonary complication, 314–315
Pulmonary hypertension (PH), 650
Pupil
    control of, 94b
    definition of, 93
    responsiveness of, 99
Pupillary reflexes, 94b
Purkinje cells, 13, 87
Pusher syndrome, 221, 246–248
Putamen, 6t, 11, 11f
Pyramidal cell, 79

Q

Quadrantanopsia, 222
Quadriplegia, 616, 617f, 618–619
Quality of life (QOL), 462
Quick Mild Cognitive Impairment Screen
    (Qmci), 183b

R

Radial glial cell (RGC), 160, 160f
Radial palmar grasp, 145

Radiculopathy, 451
Radiologically isolated syndrome (RIS), 364
Ranchos Los Amigos Cognitive Recovery
    Scale, 269, 270t–271t, 282, 285
Ranchos Los Amigos levels of cognitive
    functioning (LOC), 282–291
    coma levels, 282
    level IV confused and agitated, 283–285
Range of motion (ROM), 197, 323, 411, 413,
    429
Raphe nuclei, 15
Rapid eye movement sleep behavior disorder
    (RBD), 405
Rapid postural reactions, 83
Rate coding, 31–32, 32f
Reaching, control for, 84–85
Reactive balance control, 538b
Reactive nitrogen species, 165
Reactive oxygen species, 165
Rebound, 541
Rebound test, 188b
Recent memory, 181
Receptive aphasia, 183, 223
Receptive fields, 45, 45f
Receptors, 44t
Reciprocating gait (RGO), 599t
Recombinant tissue-type plasminogen
    activator (rTPA), 224
Recurrent inhibition, 67
Recurrent vestibular disorders, 515–516
Red nucleus, 15, 81
Reflex integrity, 461
Reflexes. *See also specific reflex*
    description of, 185
    primitive, 136b, 136t, 138f, 198t–199t
Rehabilitation of function, keys to, 233b
Rehabilitation setting, 235–241
Relapsing-remitting MS (RRMS), 364b
Relative refractory period (RRP), 27, 27f
Release phenomenon, 234
Remote memory, 181–182
Renal calculi, 312
Renshaw cells, 67, 67f
Repetitive transcranial magnetic stimulation
    (rTMS), 341
Representational neglect, 221
Respiratory distress syndrome, 272
Respiratory dysfunction
    in amyotrophic lateral sclerosis, 457, 461
    in Huntington's disease, 423
    in Parkinson's disease, 404
    in spinal cord injury, 314–315
Respiratory muscles, 314f
Respiratory weakness, 469
Resting membrane potential (RMP), 26, 27f
Resting potential, 29f
Resting state functional magnetic resonance
    imaging (rs-fMRI), 169–170
Resting tremor, 189t
Restorative surgeries, 409
Restrictive ventilator impairment, 314
Retentive memory capability, 181
Reticular formation, 7t, 15

Reticulospinal tracts, 15, 82–83, 84
Retina
  anatomy of, 95, 96f
  definition of, 93
  detachment of, 561b
Retinal ganglion cell loss, 561b
Retinal slip, 535
Retroactive interference, 124
Retroflexion, 133
Retrograde amnesia, 197
Retrograde axonal transport, 28
Retrograde degeneration, 163, 267
Retrograde tracing, 31b
Retrograde transneuronal degeneration, 164
Rett syndrome, 648t
Reuptake, 31b
Reuptake inhibitors, 31b
Reverberating circuit, 68, 69f
Reverberating excitatory circuit, 69f
Reversal potential, 27f
RGC (radial glial cell), 160, 160f
RGO (reciprocating gait), 599t
Rhombencephalon, 580, 580b, 581f
Right hemisphere, 5
Righting reactions, 137t, 199t
Rigidity, 184, 399
Riluzole, 457
RIS (radiologically isolated syndrome), 364
Rivermead mobility test, 193
RMP (resting membrane potential), 26, 27f
Robotic resisted treadmill training, 629
Robotic-assisted therapy, 628–629
Robotics, 246
Rod and cone cells, 93
Roll test, 528f
Rolling/bed mobility, 231
ROM (range of motion), 197, 323, 411, 413, 429
Romberg Test, 189, 529
Rooting reflex, 134, 136t, 198t
Rostral direction, 3, 4f
Rostral spinocerebellar tract (RSCT), 54
Rotational chair testing, 518–519
Rotational righting, 137t, 139, 199t
Round window, 103
RRMS (relapsing-remitting MS), 364b
RRP (relative refractory period), 27, 27f
RSCT (rostral spinocerebellar tract), 54
rs-fMRI (resting state functional magnetic resonance imaging), 169–170
rTMS (repetitive transcranial magnetic stimulation), 341
rTPA (recombinant tissue-type plasminogen activator), 224
Rubella, 614
Rubrospinal tract, 81

S
Saccades, 523
Saccadic resetting movement, 112
Saccule, 82, 89f, 105, 108–109
Sacks, Oliver, 394
Salivatory nucleus, 16

Saltatory conduction, 36
SARA, 544
Sarcopenia, 559b
Satellite potentials, 450
SBI (sensory-based interventions), 659b
SCA (sickle cell anemia), 253b
Scarpa's ganglion, 109
SCCs (semicircular canals), 105, 105f, 106–108, 108f
Schwann cells, 19, 36
Sclera, 93
Scoliosis, 594f–595f, 594–595, 595t, 620t
Seated vertebral artery test, 523
Seating support, 337t
Seating systems, for cerebral palsy, 630–632
Seborrhea, 403
Seborrheic dermatitis, 404
Secondary afferents (II), 46–47
Secondary injury, 303–304
Secondary Parkinsonism, 393–394
Secondary-progressive multiple sclerosis (SPMS), 364b
Second-impact syndrome, 291
Secure infants, 147b
Seizures, in cerebral palsy
  management of, 624, 625t
  types of, 623t, 623–624
Selective dorsal rhizotomy, 625
Self-care, in preschoolers, 150
Self-perceived confidence, 147b
Self-regulation, 120
Semantic memory, 122
Semantics, 126
Semicircular canals (SCCs), 105, 105f, 106–108, 108f
Semont maneuver, 532
Senile plaques, 566
Sensation
  proprioception, 45–48
  receptive fields, 45
  touch, 43
Sense(s)
  auditory system, 103–105
  gustation, 101–103, 102f
  olfaction, 100f, 100–101
  taste and smell, relationship between, 101b, 561b
  vestibular system, 105–113
  vision, 93–100
Sensitive periods, 134, 135b
Sensitivity to antipsychotic medications, 567
Sensitization, 124
Sensorimotor period, 144b
Sensorimotor skills, 124
Sensorimotor systems, of spinal cord, 63–71
Sensorineural hearing loss, 104
Sensory changes, 365, 379–380
Sensory development
  in fetus, 134
  in infant, 144
  in newborn, 142–143
Sensory discrimination, 57f, 58t
Sensory dysfunction

  in autism spectrum disorder, 659, 659b
  in cerebral palsy, 624
  in Guillain–Barré syndrome, 477
  in Huntington's disease, 423
  in multiple sclerosis, 365
  in Parkinson's disease, 403t, 405
  in stroke, 221
Sensory examination, 185–187
Sensory impairment, 187t, 494
Sensory integration disorder (SID), 659
Sensory integration therapy (SIT), 659b
Sensory integrity, 198
Sensory neurons, 26f
Sensory organization, 538b
Sensory Organization Test (SOT), 189, 519f, 520t
Sensory projections from the face, 55
Sensory studies, 446–447, 447–448
Sensory testing, 57, 58t
Sensory therapies, for autism spectrum disorder, 659b
Sensory training post-stroke, 243–244
Sensory-based interventions (SBI), 659b
Sentinel hemorrhages, 249
Sequential resolution of spinal shock, 322t
Serial casting, 281, 625
Sexual dysfunction, 372, 377, 403
Sexual function, after spinal cord injury, 341t, 341–342
SHA (sinusoidal harmonic acceleration test), 518
Shadow plaques, 362
Sharpened Romberg, 188b, 529
Shifting attention, 119b
Shoulder dysplasia, 620t
Shoulder dystocia, 495
Shoulder pain, 334, 469
Shunt, for hydrocephalus, 588, 588b, 590, 590f
Sialorrhea, 402
Sickle cell anemia (SCA), 253b
Sickle-shaped erythrocyte, 252f
SID (sensory integration disorder), 659
Sidelyers, 633
Sidelying test, 527f
Silent synapse, 34
Sinemet, 407–408
Single-Leg Balance Stance Test (SLB), 529
Sinusoidal harmonic acceleration test (SHA), 518
SIRS (systemic inflammatory response syndrome), 274
SIT (sensory integration therapy), 659b
Sitting, 191
Sit-to-stand transfer, 238–239
6 Minute Walk Test, 190
Size principle, 65
Skeletomotor loop, 396b
Skill learning, 71
Skilled, voluntary movement, 81
Skin integrity, 229, 315–317
Skipping, 152
SLB (Single-Leg Balance Stance Test), 529
Sleep disorders, 403t, 405, 423

Slow twitch muscle fibers, 64
Slowly adapting cells, 33
Small vessel disease (SVD), 568b
Smell sense, 100f, 100–101, 134, 561b
Smooth pursuit, 523
SNpc (substantia nigra pars compacta), 395
Social competence, 147b
Socioemotional development
　in 6 to 9 months, 145
　in 9 to 12 months, 147–148
　in 2nd year of life, 148–150
　in adolescents, 153
　in autism spectrum disorder, 658
　in middle childhood, 152–153
　in newborn, 143
　in preschoolers, 151–152
Sodium potassium pump, 27
Solitary nucleus, 16
Soma, 25, 26f
Somatosensory functions
　in cerebral palsy, 624
　description of, 55t, 56f
Somatosensory pathways and perception, 52f
　central projection systems, 50–54
　dermatomes and spinal nerve
　　organization, 48–49
　higher-level sensory processing, 55–57
　introduction to, 43
　sensation, 43–48
　sensory projections from the face, 55
　testing methods, 58t
SOT (Sensory Organization Test), 189, 519f,
　520t
Sound localization, 104
Spared muscles, incorporating into
　rehabilitation, 324
Spastic bladder, 312
Spastic cerebral palsy, 617b, 626
Spasticity
　in cerebral palsy, 621, 625
　flaccidity vs., 326–328
　motor control, 81
　motor examination, 184
　in multiple sclerosis, 368, 374, 376, 380
　in spinal cord injury, 305
　in stroke, 234–235, 240–241
Spatial summation, 33
Specialty chairs, 419f
Speech, 13, 182t
　telegraphic, 148
Speech apraxia, 223
Speech audiometry, 104
Speech dysfunction, 371, 422, 543
Speech recognition, 104
Speed-dependent treadmill training,
　415–416
Sphincter dyssynergia, 312
Sphincter pupillae muscle, 93
Sphincterotomy, 313b
Spina bifida
　brain abnormalities associated with,
　　586–590
　comorbidities associated with, 586–591

description of, 582–583
　illustration of, 583f
　latex allergies associated with, 590–591
Spina bifida occulta, 582, 583f
Spinal accessory nerve, 16
Spinal cord
　anatomy of, 17
　external appearance of, 64f
　functions of, 7t
　gray and white matter, 4f, 64f
　illustration of, 8f, 18f
　internal appearance of, 64f
　overview of, 5
　segmental organization of, 17, 19
　sensorimotor systems of, 63–71
　structure and organization of, 63
　tethering of, 582, 591
　transection of, 69
Spinal Cord Independence Measure III, 345
Spinal cord injury
　acute physical therapy management,
　　323–324
　adult outcome measures, 668
　autonomic dysfunction in, 309
　bladder dysfunction in, 311–313
　cardiac changes associated with, 309
　chronic complications of, 338–339
　classification of, 305t, 305–308
　clinical presentation of, 306–308
　demographics of, 304
　differential diagnosis of, 304–305
　in-patient rehabilitation setting, 325–338
　lifelong considerations, 346
　limitations and seating support by level
　　of, 337t
　medical management. See Medical
　　management of spinal cord injury
　mobility and outcomes based on level of,
　　329t–330t
　myelomeningocele versus, 606
　neurogenic bowel, 317–321
　outpatient rehabilitation setting, 342–346
　pain caused by, 339–342
　pathophysiology, 303–305
　physical therapy assessment, 322–323
　physical therapy in acute setting, 321–324
　pressure ulcers associated with, 315–317
　pulmonary complications of, 314–315
　respiratory dysfunction in, 314–315
　sexual function after, 341t, 341–342
　skin integrity in, 315–317
　vasomotor changes secondary to, 309
Spinal dysraphism, 582
Spinal dysraphism occulta, 582, 583f
Spinal flexor withdrawal reflex, 68f
Spinal interneurons, 63, 66
Spinal muscular atrophies, 653–654, 648t
Spinal nerves, 48–49
Spinal shock, 322, 322t
Spinal stenosis, 304
Spinal trigeminal nucleus, 55
Spine
　cervical, 63

lumbar, 63, 70f
　neural tube disorders involving, 582–583,
　　583f
　scoliosis of, 594f–595f, 594–595, 595t
　thoracic, 63
Spinocerebellar ataxias, 540
Spinocerebellar systems, 53–54
Spinocerebellum, 13–14, 14f, 86
Spinomesencephalic tract, 53
Spinothalamic tract, 17f, 53, 134
Spiral ganglia, 103
Spiral organ, 103
SPMS (secondary-progressive MS), 364b
Spontaneous horizontal-rotatory nystagmus,
　514
Spontaneous nystagmus, 523
Spontaneous potentials, 450
Spontaneous recovery, 166
Spontaneous reorganization, 226
Sprouting, 33, 33f, 161f
Stairs, 429–430
Standard physical therapy, 415
Standardized clinical scales, 544
Standers, 633
Standing activities, 247
Stand-to-sit transfer, 238–239
Static balance exercises, 380b, 537b
Static head position, 108–109
Status epilepticus, 624
Stent, 249
Step Test Evaluation of Performance on
　Stairs (STEPS) Tool, 193
Stepping reflex, 136t, 198t
Stepping strategy, 530
STEPS (Step Test Evaluation of Performance
　on Stairs) Tool, 193
Stereocilia, 106, 109f
Stereognosis, 43, 57
Sternocleidomastoid, 314f
Sterol synthesis disorders, 649t
STNR (symmetric tonic neck reflex), 136t,
　138f, 198t, 618
Strabismus, 624
Stranger anxiety, 145
Strategic infarct dementia, 568
Strength, 183–184, 197, 411, 413–415, 559b
Strength training, 242–243
Stretching, 413, 415f, 429
Striatum, 6t, 11
Striola, 109
Stroke
　acute medical management, 224–226
　acute neuroplasticity after, 226
　adult outcome measures, 667
　basilar artery aneurysm and, 251–252
　brainstem, 220f, 250–251
　cerebral circulation in, 212–216
　cognitive dysfunction in, 223–224
　complication prevention in, 229–230
　consequences of, 213t, 215–216
　early intervention for, 229–230
　functional magnetic resonance imaging
　　of, 170f

Stroke (*cont.*)
  hemorrhagic, 215
  home health environment for, 241–248
  language dysfunction in, 222–223, 223f
  middle cerebral artery (MCA) infarction, 216–224
  motor dysfunction, 216, 221
  neuroplasticity, 226, 248
  outcomes of, 226
  pathophysiology of, 211
  pediatric, 252–253
  physical therapy management in acute care facility, 226–235
  physical therapy management in home health and out-patient environments, 241–248
  physical therapy management in rehabilitation setting, 235–241
  plasticity in, 248–250
  posterior cerebral artery aneurysm, 249f
  risk factors for, 212, 213t
  sensory dysfunction in, 221
  severity of, 225–226
  summary, 248–253
  syndromes and associated symptoms, 217t–219t
  upper extremity rehabilitation, 236–237
  variable symptoms and outcomes of, 212–215
  visual field disruption, 222, 222f
Structural imaging, 168f–169f, 168–170
Structural scoliosis, 594
Subarachnoid hemorrhage, 211
Subarachnoid space, 212f, 587b
Subcortical ischemic vascular dementia, 568
Subcortical structures, 5t
Subjective visual horizontal test, 520
Subjective visual vertical test, 520
Subplate, 160
Substantia nigra, 6t, 11f, 12, 15
Substantia nigra pars compacta (SNpc), 395
Subthalamic nucleus, 6t, 11
Subventricular zone, 159, 612b
Sucking, 142
Summation, 65–66
Superior cerebellar artery, 213, 215, 219t
Superior cerebellar peduncle, 14
Superior colliculus, 15, 95
Superior nucleus, 110t
Superior olivary nuclear complex, 104
Superior palmar grasp, 145
Superior plane, 3
Superior semicircular canal dehiscence, 516
Supination, alternating, 188b
Supplementary motor area, 79–80
Support system, 195
Supramalleolar orthosis, 245b, 599t
Suprapubic reflex, 136t
Suprapubic tapping, 313b
Surgical release, 281
Suspension strategy, 530
Sustained attention, 119
SVD (small vessel disease), 568b

Swallowing dysfunction, 371, 422
Swan-neck deformity, 620t
Swivel walker, 599t
Symmetric tonic neck reflex (STNR), 136t, 138f, 198t, 618
Sympathetic chain ganglia, 7t, 19
Sympathetic denervation, 404
Sympathetic innervation
    of bladder and urethral sphincters, 312f
    of colon and anal sphincters, 318f
Sympathetic nervous system, 19
Synapses, 26, 33, 33f
Synaptic cleft, 28
Synaptic function, 28–29, 30f
Synaptic modulation, 163
Synaptic scaling, 163
Synaptic terminals, 28
Synaptogenesis, 161f, 162
Synergistic motor control, 216
Synergistic movement patterns, 185
Synergy patterns, 230t
Syntax, 126
Syringomyelia, 346
Systemic inflammatory response syndrome (SIRS), 274
Systemic inflammatory syndrome, 274
Systems review, 180–181, 196

T

Tandem walking, 529
Tapping hand or foot, 188b
Task switching, 119
Task-based functional magnetic resonance imaging, 169
Task-dependent training for locomotion, 344–345
Task-oriented practice, 230, 238–239, 239t
Task-oriented training, 242–243
Tastants, 101
Taste buds, 134
Taste receptors, 101
Taste sense
    description of, 101–103, 102f, 561b
    development of, 134
    smell sense and, relationship between, 101b, 561b
    testing of, 103
tDCS (transcutaneous direct current stimulation), 340
Teaching, and aging, 561–562
Tectorial membrane, 103
Telegraphic speech, 148
Temper tantrums, 151
Temperament, 147b
Temporal-amygdala-orbitofrontal network, 124
Temporal coding, 32f, 32–33
Temporal dispersion, 446
Temporal lobe, 5t, 10, 11f
Temporal operculum, 11f
Temporal summation, 33
10 Meter Walk Test, 190
Tendonotomies, 626

TENS (transcutaneous electrical nerve stimulation), 341
Test of Infant Motor Performance, 654
Tetraplegia, 304
Texture discrimination, 43
Thalamotomy, 409
Thalamus, 6t, 11, 11f
Third ventricle, 5t, 587b
Thoracic spine, 63
Thoracolumbosacral orthoses (TLSO), 595
Thought processing, 182t
Three-point lateral control system, 631
Threshold, 26, 29f
Thrombotic stroke, 211
Thrombus, 211
Thumb sucking, 134
"Thunderclap" headache, 249
Thyroid disease, 652
TIA (transient ischemic attack), 211, 517
Time constant, 518
Timed Up and Go test (TUG), 189
Tinetti Mobility Test (TMT), 189, 416
Titubation, 542
TLSO (thoracolumbosacral orthoses), 595
TMS (transcranial magnetic stimulation), 170, 170f, 341
Toe to examiner's finger test, 188b
Tone, 184–185
Tonic-clonic seizures, 623t
Tonic labyrinthine reflex, 135, 136t
Tonic neurons, 33
Tonic seizures, 623t
Tonic stretch reflex, 234
Topiramate, 625t
Total functional capacity staging, 425t
Total parenteral nutrition (TPN), 275
Touch, 43
Touch perception, 58t
Touch receptors, 43
Toxic Parkinsonism, 394
Transcranial magnetic stimulation (TMS), 170, 170f, 341
Transcription factors, 294
Transcutaneous direct current stimulation (tDCS), 340
Transcutaneous electrical nerve stimulation (TENS), 341
Transcutaneous spinal cord stimulation, 326
Transduction, 30–33
Transfer training, 418
Transfers
    for amyotrophic lateral sclerosis, 470
    for Huntington's disease, 429
    in-patient rehabilitation setting, 333
    neurologic exam, 191–192
    sit-to-stand, 238–239
    stand-to-sit, 238–239
    task-oriented therapy, 239t, 242
    techniques for teaching, 231b
    training, 417f
Transient ischemic attack (TIA), 211, 517
Transitions, 196, 201
Translocation, 643

Transverse myelitis, 304
Traumatic brain injury
  adult outcome measures, 668
  behaviors associated with, 278t–279t, 285t
  chronic pain in, 290–291
  coma associated with, 269, 272
  concussion, 287–290
  consequences of, 269–282
  dysautonomia in, 275
  EDGE recommendations, 283t
  epilepsy and, 273–274
  executive dysfunction secondary to, 269, 272
  family adjustment, 286–287
  gastrointestinal dysfunction associated with, 274–275
  hypercatabolism associated with, 274–275
  hypermetabolism associated with, 274–275
  inflammation associated with, 274
  intracranial hypertension (ICH), 272–273
  introduction to, 265–266
  long-term outcomes, 290–291
  mild, 287–290
  neuropsychiatric changes secondary to, 275–276
  paroxysmal sympathetic hyperactivation (PSH) in, 275
  pathophysiology of, 267–269
  physical therapy management, 276–277
  post-traumatic amnesia associated with, 269, 272
  Ranchos Los Amigos levels of cognitive functioning, assessment and management based on, 282–291
  recovery measures in, 270t–271t
  respiratory distress syndrome, 272
  severity of, 266t
  signs of, 266b
Traumatic head injury, 517
Traumatic hematoma, 273f
Traumatic nerve injuries, 484, 487, 487t, 488f
Treadmill training
  for cerebral palsy, 628
  for Parkinson's disease, 415–416
  for stroke, 237, 237b
Tremor, 189t, 376, 397, 411, 421, 541–542, 544
Tricyclic antidepressants, for neuropathic pain, 340
Trigeminal ganglion, 55
Trigeminal nerve, 16, 186t
Trigeminal neuralgia, 366
Trigeminal nucleus, 15
Trigeminal pathways for somatosensory function, 56f
Triplegia, 616
Trisomy 18, 584, 648t
Trisomy 21, 643b, 650. *See also* Down syndrome
Trochlear nerve, 16, 186t
True equinus, 621
Truncal incurvation reflex, 136t, 198t

Trunk activities, 233t
Trunk control, 84
Trunk rotation, 412, 412f
Trunk stability, 84
Trunk-hip-knee-ankle-foot orthotic (THKAFO), 599t
Tuberothalamic arteries, 215
TUG (Timed Up and Go test), 189
Tullio's phenomenon, 516
Tumor(s)
  brain. *See* Brain tumors
  locations and characteristics of, 292t
  primitive neuroectodermal, 292
  symptoms of, 293
Tumor necrosis factor-α, 163
Two-point discrimination, 58t
2017 Revised McDonald Diagnostic Criteria for MS, 363, 366t
Tympanic duct, 103
Tympanic membrane, 103

U

Uhthoff's phenomenon, 372
Uhthoff's sign, 379
Ulnar nerve, 447f
Ulnar palmar grasp, 142
Umbilical cord prolapse, 613
Uneven surfaces, task-oriented training, 242
Unfused tetanus, 66
Unified Huntington's Disease Rating Scale (UHDRS), 424
Unified Parkinson's Disease Rating Scale (UPDRS), 406
Unilateral spatial neglect syndrome, 222f
Unilateral truncal (thoracic) radiculopathy, 489
Unilateral vestibular hypofunction (UVH), 513–514, 535–538, 537t
UNM (upper motor neuron) signs, 304
Unresponsive wakefulness syndrome (UWS), 269
Upper extremity
  in cerebral palsy, 622
  contractures of, 622
  in spinal cord injury, 334, 338
Upper extremity motor scores (UEMS), 305
Upper motor neuron (UNM) signs
  in myelomeningocele, 585
  in spinal cord injury, 304
Upright activities, 231–234, 233t
Urethral sphincter, 311, 312f
Urethral stents, 313b
Urinary tract infections (UTI), 312–313
Utilization time, 448
Utricle, 82, 105, 105f, 108–109
UWS (unresponsive wakefulness syndrome), 269

V

Vagus nerve, 16, 186t
Valproic acid, 625t
Valsalva maneuver, 313b
Vascular dementia (VaD), 568

Vascular Parkinsonism, 394, 419
Vasospasm, 250
Velocity step test, 518
Ventral corticospinal tract, 80
Ventral horn, 63
Ventral plane, 3, 4f
Ventral spinocerebellar tract (VSCT), 53
Ventral stream, 126
Ventral tegmental area, 15
Ventricle, 11f
Ventricular system, 12–13
Ventricular zone, 159
Ventriculostomy, 591
Ventromedial prefrontal cortex (VMPC), 121
Ventromedial systems, 84
Vertebral arteries, 213, 218t
Vertebrobasilar ischemic stroke/ insufficiency, 516–517
Vertical saccades, 97
Vertigo, 520, 521t
Very low birth weight, 611b
Very preterm, 611b
Vestibular Activities of Daily Living Scale (VD-ADL), 522
Vestibular disorders
  adult outcome measures, 669
  central, 516–517, 531, 531t, 539
  in cerebral palsy, 624
  cervicogenic dizziness, 518
  dizziness symptoms and possible causes, 522t
  medical and subjective histories, 520–523
  medical assessment and management, 518–520
  motion sickness, 517–518
  peripheral, 513–515, 531, 531t
  pharmacological treatment, 520
  physical therapy examination, 520–531
  physical therapy treatment, 532–539
  recurrent, 515–516
  tests and measures, 523–531
Vestibular duct, 103
Vestibular function tests, 518–520
Vestibular labyrinths, 105f, 105–106, 106f, 109
Vestibular migraine, 517
Vestibular neuritis, 514
Vestibular nuclei, 7t, 16, 110f, 110t
Vestibular pathways, 109–110
Vestibular Rehabilitation Benefit Questionnaire, 522
Vestibular schwannoma (VS), 514f, 514–515
Vestibular system
  anatomy and physiology of, 513
  angular acceleration, 106–108
  balance control, 112–113
  disorders of, 513–517
  linear acceleration and static head position, 108–109
  nystagmus, 112
  vestibular labyrinths, 105–106
  vestibular pathways, 109–110

Vestibular system (*cont.*)
  vestibulo-ocular reflex (VOR). *See*
    Vestibulo-ocular reflex (VOR)
  vestibulospinal reflex, 109, 111–112
Vestibular-evoked myogenic potential
  (VEMP), 519
Vestibule, 105, 105f
Vestibulocerebellum, 13, 14f, 86
Vestibulocochlear nerve, 16, 186t
Vestibulo-ocular reflex (VOR), 82, 109–111,
  110–111, 111f
Vestibulo-ocular reflex cancellation (VORc),
  523–524
Vestibulospinal reflex (VSR), 109, 111–112
Vestibulospinal tracts, 82, 84
Vibration testing, 186–187
Video games, 418–419
Videonystagmography (VNG), 518
Virtual reality, 246, 341, 629
Vision. *See also* Eye(s)
  age-related changes in, 561b
  optic projections and visual processing,
    95–96
  retina. *See* Retina
  testing of, 98–100
  visual fields. *See* Visual fields
  visual receptors, 93–95
Visual cortex, 96f
Visual cueing, 416
Visual disturbances
  in cerebral palsy, 624
  in multiple sclerosis, 366–367
  in Parkinson's disease, 405
Visual evoked potential (VEP), 96

Visual fields
  description of, 93, 95f, 99
  disruption in, 222, 222f
Visual hallucinations, 567
Visual image processing, 98f
Visual perception tests, 520
Visual processing, 95–96
Visual projections, 96f
Visual pursuit, 96–98
Visual receptors, 93–95
Visual testing, 98–100
Vitreous body, degeneration of, 561b
Vitreous humor, 93
Voltage-gated calcium channels, 28
Voltage-gated potassium channel, 26
Voltage-gated sodium channels, 26, 27f, 29f
VOR cancellation, 111
VOR gain, 518
VOR Phase, 518
VSCT (ventral spinocerebellar tract), 53

W
Walkers, 417f, 632, 632f
Walking. *See also* Gait
  description of, 192–194
  development of, 139f, 147, 204
  in multiple sclerosis, 376
  plantigrade, 147
Walking Index for Spinal Cord Injury II, 345
Wallerian degeneration, 163
Weakness, 368
Wearing-off, 409
Weight loss, 423–424
Wernicke's area, 126f, 127, 223

Wheelchair(s)
  base of, 604
  for cerebral palsy patients, 630–632,
    632f
  components of, 604–606, 630
  description of, 430
  environmental factors, 605
  frame of, 605
  illustration of, 419f
  manual, 604, 605f, 631
  measurements for, 603f
  mobility, 333–334
  for myelomeningocele patients, 603t,
    604–606
  powered, 604, 631
  prescription for, 604
  seating system for, 605
Wheelchair Skills Test, 334
White matter, 3–4, 4f, 5, 7t, 63, 64f, 153
Whole body vibration, 415
Wilson's disease, 648t
Withdrawal reflex, 68f
Word deafness, 126
Work simplification techniques, 383b
Working memory, 119–120, 224
Writhing, 134, 137, 615
Writing, 402, 419

X
X-linked inheritance, 644f

Z
Zonisamide, 625t
Z-plasty, 626f